Essentials of Psychiatric Nursing

Second Edition

Mary Ann Boyd, PhD, DNS, RN, PMHCNS-BC

Professor Emerita
Southern Illinois University Edwardsville
Edwardsville, Illinois

Rebecca Luebbert, PhD, RN, PMHCNS-BC

Associate Professor
Southern Illinois University Edwardsville
Edwardsville, Illinois

Philadelphia • Baltimore • New York • London
Buenos Aires • Hong Kong • Sydney • Tokyo

Not authorised for sale in United States, Canada, Australia, New Zealand, Puerto Rico, and U.S. Virgin Islands.

Vice President and Publisher: Julie K. Stegman
Director of Nursing Content Publishing: Renee Gagliardi
Acquisitions Editor: Michael Kerns
Director of Product Development: Jennifer K. Forestieri
Senior Development Editor: Meredith L. Brittain
Editorial Coordinator: Tim Rinehart
Editorial Assistant: Molly Kennedy
Marketing Manager: Brittany Clements
Design Coordinator: Joseph Clark
Art Director, Illustration: Jennifer Clements
Production Project Manager: Sadie Buckallew
Manufacturing Coordinator: Karin Duffield
Prepress Vendor: Aptara, Inc.

2nd Edition

Copyright © 2020 by Wolters Kluwer

Copyright © 2017 by Wolters Kluwer. All rights reserved. This book is protected by copyright. No part of this book may be reproduced or transmitted in any form or by any means, including as photocopies or scanned-in or other electronic copies, or utilized by any information storage and retrieval system without written permission from the copyright owner, except for brief quotations embodied in critical articles and reviews. Materials appearing in this book prepared by individuals as part of their official duties as U.S. government employees are not covered by the above-mentioned copyright. To request permission, please contact Wolters Kluwer at Two Commerce Square, 2001 Market Street, Philadelphia, PA 19103, via email at permissions@lww.com, or via our website at shop.lww.com (products and services).

9 8 7 6 5 4 3 2 1

Printed in China

Library of Congress Cataloging-in-Publication Data available upon request.
Library of Congress Control Number: 2019945806
978-1-9751-4864-5

This work is provided "as is," and the publisher disclaims any and all warranties, express or implied, including any warranties as to accuracy, comprehensiveness, or currency of the content of this work.

This work is no substitute for individual patient assessment based upon healthcare professionals' examination of each patient and consideration of, among other things, age, weight, gender, current or prior medical conditions, medication history, laboratory data and other factors unique to the patient. The publisher does not provide medical advice or guidance and this work is merely a reference tool. Healthcare professionals, and not the publisher, are solely responsible for the use of this work including all medical judgments and for any resulting diagnosis and treatments.

Given continuous, rapid advances in medical science and health information, independent professional verification of medical diagnoses, indications, appropriate pharmaceutical selections and dosages, and treatment options should be made and healthcare professionals should consult a variety of sources. When prescribing medication, healthcare professionals are advised to consult the product information sheet (the manufacturer's package insert) accompanying each drug to verify, among other things, conditions of use, warnings and side effects and identify any changes in dosage schedule or contraindications, particularly if the medication to be administered is new, infrequently used or has a narrow therapeutic range. To the maximum extent permitted under applicable law, no responsibility is assumed by the publisher for any injury and/or damage to persons or property, as a matter of products liability, negligence law or otherwise, or from any reference to or use by any person of this work.

shop.lww.com

To the Birnbaum's, Tsai's, and Lewis', with love and pride.
—Mary Ann Boyd

To Adam, with love and appreciation. Thank you for supporting my dreams.
—Rebecca Luebbert

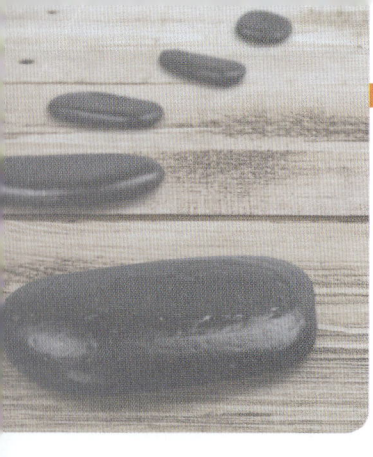

Contributors

CONTRIBUTORS TO *ESSENTIALS OF PSYCHIATRIC NURSING,* SECOND EDITION

Beverly Baliko, PhD, RN
Associate Professor
College of Nursing
University of South Carolina
Columbia, South Carolina
Chapter 17: Mental Health Care for Survivors of Violence

Andrea C. Bostrom, PhD, PMHCNS-BC
Professor
Kirkhof College of Nursing
Grand Valley State University
Grand Rapids, Michigan
Chapter 21: Schizophrenia and Related Disorders

Sheri Compton-McBride, DNP, RN
Director of RN/BS Nursing Program, Alternative Entry, and Contractual Management
Director of Acquisition of Clinical Sites and Instructor
School of Nursing
Southern Illinois University Edwardsville
Edwardsville, Illinois
Chapter 28: Sleep–Wake Disorders

Judith M. Erickson, PhD, PMHCNS-BC
Dean and Professor
School of Nursing
College of Mount Saint Vincent
Riverdale, New York
Chapter 18: Anxiety and Panic Disorders

Cheryl Forchuk, PhD, RN, OOnt, FCAHS
Beryl and Richard Ivey Research Chair in Aging, Mental Health, Rehabilitation and Recovery
Lawson Health Research Institute/Western University
London, Ontario
Chapter 9: The Nurse–Patient Relationship

Patricia E. Freed, EdD, MSN, RN, CNE
Associate Professor
Trudy Busch Valentine School of Nursing
Saint Louis University
St. Louis, Missouri
Chapter 20: Obsessive–Compulsive and Related Disorders

Kimberlee Hansen, MS, RN, NP
Nurse Practitioner
Jefferson Barracks Division
VA St. Louis Health Care System
St. Louis, Missouri
Chapter 24: Personality and Impulse-Control Disorders

Victoria Soltis-Jarrett, PhD, PMHCNS-BC, PMHNP-BC, FAANP
Carol Morde Ross Distinguished Professor of Psychiatric-Mental Health Nursing
University of North Carolina at Chapel Hill
Chapel Hill, North Carolina
Chapter 27: Somatic Symptom and Dissociative Disorders

Sandra P. Thomas, PhD, RN, FAAN
Editor, "Issues in Mental Health Nursing"
Sara and Ross Croley Endowed Professor in Nursing
College of Nursing
University of Tennessee, Knoxville
Knoxville, Tennessee
Chapter 14: Management of Anger, Aggression, and Violence

Barbara Jones Warren, PhD, RN, APRN, PMHCNS-BC, FNAP, FAAN
Professor, Clinical Nursing and Director
Psychiatric Mental Health Nurse Practitioner Specialty Track Director
ANA/NIMH Racial/Ethnic Minority Fellow
Martha S. Pitzer Center for Women, Children and Youth
College of Nursing
The Ohio State University
Columbus, Ohio
Chapter 21: Depression

For a list of the contributors for the ancillaries for the second edition, please visit http://thepoint.lww.com/BoydEssentials2e.

Jane H. White, PhD, PMHCNS-BC, FAAN
Vera E. Bender Professor of Nursing
College of Nursing and Public Health
Adelphi University
Garden City, New York
Chapter 26: Eating Disorders

CONTRIBUTORS TO *ESSENTIALS OF PSYCHIATRIC NURSING,* FIRST EDITION

Beverly Baliko, PhD, RN
Associate Professor
College of Nursing
University of South Carolina
Columbia, South Carolina
Chapter 30: Mental Health Care for Survivors of Violence

Andrea C. Bostrom, PhD, PMHCNS-BC
Professor
Kirkhof College of Nursing
Grand Valley State University
Grand Rapids, Michigan
Chapter 21: Schizophrenia and Related Disorders

Mary R. Boyd, PhD, RN
Associate Professor
College of Nursing
University of South Carolina
Columbia, South Carolina
Chapter 30: Mental Health Care for Survivors of Violence

Stephanie Burgess, PhD, APRN, FNP-BC
Associate Dean for Nursing Practice and Clinical Professor
College of Nursing
University of South Carolina
Columbia, South Carolina
Chapter 30: Mental Health Care for Survivors of Violence

Sheri Compton-McBride, DNP, RN
Director of RN/BS Program, Alternative Entry, and Contractual Management
Director of Clinical Acquisitions and Instructor
School of Nursing
Southern Illinois University Edwardsville
Edwardsville, Illinois
Chapter 26: Sleep–Wake Disorders

Judith M. Erickson, PhD, PMHCNS-BC
Dean
Harriet Rothkopf Heilbrunn School of Nursing
Long Island University
Long Island, New York
Chapter 16: Anxiety and Panic Disorders

Cheryl Forchuk, PhD, RN
Associate Director of Nursing Research
University of Western Ontario
Lawson Health Research Institute
Arthur Labatt Family School of Nursing and Department of Psychiatry
London, Ontario
Chapter 8: The Nurse-Patient Relationship

Kimberlee Hansen, MS, RN, NP
Nurse Practitioner
Jefferson Barracks Division
VA St. Louis Health Care System
St. Louis, Missouri
Chapter 22: Personality and Impulse-Control Disorders

Emily J. Hauenstein, PhD, LCP, MSN, RN
Unidel Katherine L. Esterly Chair in Health Sciences and Senior Associate Dean of Nursing and Healthcare
College of Health Sciences
University of Delaware
Newark, Delaware
Chapter 15: Suicide Prevention

Victoria Soltis-Jarrett, PhD, PMHCNS BC, PMHNP-BC
Associate Clinical Professor and Coordinator of the PMHNP Program
University of North Carolina at Chapel Hill
Chapel Hill, North Carolina
Chapter 23: Somatic Symptom and Dissociative Disorders

Sandra P. Thomas, PhD, RN, FAAN
Professor and Chair, PhD Program in Nursing
University of Tennessee, Knoxville
Knoxville, Tennessee
Chapter 13: Management of Anger, Aggression, and Violence

Barbara Jones Warren, PhD, RN, CNS-BC, PMH, FAAN
Professor, Clinical Nursing
Specialty Director, Psychiatric and Mental Health Nursing
National Institutes of Health/American Nurses Association Ethnic/Racial Minority Fellow
The Ohio State College of Nursing
Columbus, Ohio
Chapter 19: Depression

Jane H. White, PhD, PMHCNS-BC
Vera E. Bender Professor of Nursing and Associate Dean for Research and Graduate Programs
School of Nursing
Adelphi University
Garden City, New York
Chapter 24: Eating Disorders

CONTRIBUTORS TO *PSYCHIATRIC NURSING: CONTEMPORARY PRACTICE*, SIXTH EDITION

Beverly Baliko, PhD, RN, PMHNP-BC
Associate Professor
College of Nursing
University of South Carolina
Columbia, South Carolina
Chapter 41: Caring for Survivors of Violence and Abuse

Andrea C. Bostrom, PhD, PMHCNS-BC
Professor
Kirkhof College of Nursing
Grand Valley State University
Allendale, Michigan
Chapter 22: Schizophrenia and Related Disorders

Mary R. Boyd, PhD, RN
Professor Emerita
College of Nursing
University of South Carolina
Columbia, South Carolina
Chapter 41: Caring for Survivors of Violence and Abuse

Stephanie Burgess, PhD, APRN, FNP-BC, FAANP
Associate Dean for Nursing Practice/Health Policy and Clinical Professor
College of Nursing
University of South Carolina
Columbia, South Carolina
Chapter 41: Caring for Survivors of Violence and Abuse

Jeanne A. Clement, EdD, PMHCNS-BC, FAAN
Therapist
Central Ohio Behavioral Medicine, Inc.
Associate Professor Emeritus
College of Nursing
The Ohio State University
Columbus, Ohio
Chapter 12: Cognitive Interventions in Psychiatric Nursing

Sheri Compton-McBride, MS, RN
Director of Clinical Acquisitions and Instructor
School of Nursing
Southern Illinois University Edwardsville
Edwardsville, Illinois
Chapter 33: Sleep–Wake Disorders

Dorothy M. Corrigan, DMin, DNP(c), APRN, GNP-BC, CARN-AP
Nurse Practitioner
Tomah VA Medical Center
Tomah, Wisconsin
Chapter 43: Caring for Medically Compromised Persons

Catherine Gray Deering, PhD, APRN-BC
Professor
Clayton State University
Morrow, Georgia
Chapter 15: Mental Health Promotion for Children and Adolescents

Peggy El-Mallakh, PhD, RN, PMH APRN-BC
Associate Professor
College of Nursing
University of Kentucky
Lexington, Kentucky
Chapter 5: Mental Health Care in the Community

Judith M. Erickson, PhD, PMHCNS-BC
Dean
School of Nursing
College of Mount Saint Vincent
Riverdale, New York
Chapter 25: Anxiety Disorders

Cheryl Forchuk, PhD, RN, FCAHS, OOnt
Associate Director of Nursing Research
Distinguished University Professor
Nursing and Psychiatry
Western University
Assistant Director and Scientist
Lawson Health Research Institute
London Health Sciences Centre and St. Joseph's Health Care London
London, Ontario
Chapter 9: Communication and the Therapeutic Relationship

Patricia E. Freed, EdD, MSN, CNE
Associate Professor
School of Nursing
Saint Louis University
St. Louis, Missouri
Chapter 26: Obsessive Compulsive and Related Disorders

Vanya Hamrin, MSN, RN, APRN-BC
Associate Professor
School of Nursing
Vanderbilt University
Nashville, Tennessee
Chapter 35: Mental Health Assessment of Children and Adolescents

Kimberlee Hansen, MS, RN, CNS, NP
Nurse Practitioner
Jefferson Barracks Division
VA St. Louis Health Care System
St. Louis, Missouri
Chapter 29: Antisocial Personality and Disruptive, Impulse Control and Conduct Disorders

Peggy Healy, MSN, RN-BC, PMHN
Program Manager for Outpatient Mental Health Programs
VA St. Louis Health Care System
St. Louis, Missouri
Chapter 37: Mental Health Assessment of Older Adults

William Jacobowitz, MS, MPH, EdD, PMHCNS-BC
Assistant Professor
College of Nursing and Public Health
Adelphi University
Garden City, New York
Chapter 27: Trauma- and Stressor-Related Disorders

Victoria Soltis-Jarrett, PhD, PMHCNS-BC, PMHNP-BC, FAANP
Carol Morde Ross Distinguished Professor of Psychiatric-Mental Health Nursing
Family Psychiatric Nurse Practitioner
University of North Carolina at Chapel Hill
Chapel Hill, North Carolina
Chapter 32: Somatic Symptom and Related Disorders

Georgia L. Stevens, PhD, APRN, PMHCNS-BC
Director
P.A.L. Associates
Partners in Aging and Long-Term Caregiving
Washington, DC
Chapter 17: Mental Health Promotion for Older Adults

Sandra P. Thomas, PhD, RN, FAAN
Chair, PhD Program
Editor, "Issues in Mental Health Nursing"
Sara and Ross Croley Endowed Professor in Nursing
College of Nursing
University of Tennessee, Knoxville
Knoxville, Tennessee
Chapter 19: Management of Anger, Aggression, and Violence

Barbara Jones Warren, PhD, RN, PMHCNS-BC, FNAP, FAAN
Professor of Clinical Nursing
Director
Psychiatric Mental Health Nursing Across the Lifespan Specialty Track
NIH ANA Racial/Ethnic Minority Fellow
College of Nursing
The Ohio State University
Columbus, Ohio
Chapter 23: Depression

Sara Rich Wheeler, PhD, RN, PMHCNS-BC, LMHC
Principal, Grief, LTD, Covington, Indiana
Director of Education for the Society of Head and Neck Nurses
Chapter 20: Crisis, Loss, Grief, Response, Bereavement, and Disaster Management

Jane H. White, PhD, PMHCNS-BC, FAAN
Vera E. Bender Professor of Nursing and Associate Dean for Research
College of Nursing and Public Health
Adelphi University
Garden City, New York
Chapter 31: Eating Disorders

Deborah McNeil Whitehouse, PhD, RN-BC
Dean
College of Health Sciences
Eastern Kentucky University
Richmond, Kentucky
Chapter 28: Personality and Borderline Personality Disorder

Rhonda K. Wilson, MS, RN
Quality Coordinator for the Southern Region
Illinois Department of Mental Health
Chester Mental Health Center
Chester, Illinois
Chapter 42: Caring for Persons With Mental Illness and Criminal Behavior

Reviewers

Pamela Adamshick, PhD, RN, PMHCNS-BC
Associate Professor
Nursing and Public Health Department
Moravian College
Bethlehem, Pennsylvania

Abbey Devers, RN, BSN
Psychiatric/Mental Health Nursing Instructor
Nursing Program
Iowa Central Community College
Fort Dodge, Iowa

Nancy Elkins, EdD, MSN, RN
Associate Professor
School of Nursing
Marshall University
Huntington, West Virginia

Mary Beth Hutches, DNP, RN
Chair, BSN Programs
Assistant Professor
School of Nursing
Aurora University
Aurora, Illinois

Sheila G. Jacobs, RN, MSN
Professor, BSN Program
School of Nursing
George Mason University
Fairfax, Virginia

Deborah Johnson, MSN, RN
Assistant Professor
Department of Nursing
Ivy Tech Community College
Columbus, Indiana

Karen Lillie, RN, BS, MS, FNPC, PMHNP
Lecturer, Undergraduate Program Director
Department of Nursing
California State University, Bakersfield
Bakersfield, California

Kathy T. Morris, EdD, MSN, RN
Assistant Professor
School of Nursing
Georgia Southern University—Armstrong Campus
Savannah, Georgia

Colleen M. Quinn, EdD, MSN, RN
Professor
Department of Nursing
Broward College
Fort Lauderdale, Florida

Robi Thomas, PhD, RN, PMHNP-BC
Associate Professor
McAuley School of Nursing
University of Detroit Mercy
Grand Rapids, Michigan

Maureen Vidrine, DNP, APRN-PMH, BC
Associate Professor
Mary Inez Grindle School of Nursing
Brenau University
Gainesville, Georgia

Pamela Worrell-Carlisle, PhD, RN, MA, CHPN
Assistant Professor
School of Nursing
Georgia Southern University
Statesboro, Georgia

For a list of the reviewers for the ancillaries for the second edition, please visit http://thepoint.lww.com/BoydEssentials2e.

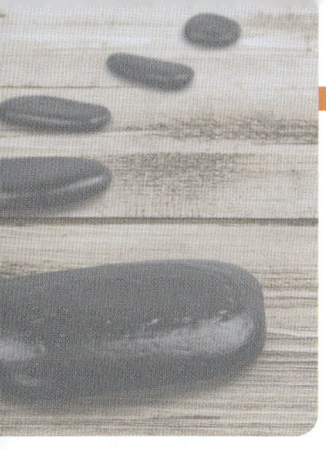

Preface

Mental health crises are increasingly affecting individuals, families, and communities. Opioid abuse is now of epidemic proportions. Suicide is touching families in small towns and large communities. Psychiatric–mental health nursing knowledge and skills are more important than ever to nursing practice. All nurses must be prepared to provide appropriate mental health care. Today the practicing nurse is required to have an extensive understanding of mental health disorders and the impact of the illness and treatment on the quality of life of the individual and family. Recovery from mental illness is a journey involving a partnership between health care professionals and the person with a mental health disorder. This individual not only needs support and treatment to recover from a serious disorder but also help in eradicating the stigma associated with a mental illness.

Essentials of Psychiatric Nursing, 2nd edition provides students with the evidence-based knowledge to develop recovery-oriented nursing interventions with the person with mental illness. This book incorporates updated content emphasizing communication skills, mental health promotion, and current, evidence-based, recovery-oriented nursing care of persons with common mental health disorders. A new chapter, Chapter 7: Recovery Framework for Mental Health Nursing, provides a framework to practice recovery-oriented nursing.

The book presents complex concepts in easy-to-understand language with multiple examples and explanations. The text is filled with meaningful information and is applicable to all areas of nursing practice.

Pedagogical features in the book plus dynamic online resources at http://thepoint.lww.com/BoydEssentials2e offer opportunities for students to challenge the stigma associated with mental disorders; please see discussions of these later in this preface. Case studies are central to the mental disorders discussions and provide students with the opportunity to link real-life experiences to theoretical concepts.

Our goal is to prepare nursing leaders who challenge the status quo, partner with their patients in the delivery of care, and use the latest evidence in their nursing practice.

Text Organization

Unit I, Essentials of Mental Health Care, discusses mental health and mental disorders as they relate to the concept of wellness. In Chapter 1, students will learn about the concepts of stigma and recovery. Chapter 2 discusses cultural and spiritual issues, and Chapter 3 covers patient rights and legal issues.

Unit II, Psychiatric–Mental Health Nursing Frameworks, provides a foundation for beginning practice with an explanation of ethics, standards, and nursing in Chapter 4; the theoretical foundation in Chapter 5; and the biologic foundations in Chapter 6. Chapter 7 further discusses recovery and presents a framework.

Unit III, Knowledge and Skills of Psychiatric–Mental Health Nursing, contains two communication chapters: Chapter 8, which focuses on therapeutic communication, and Chapter 9, which discusses the nurse–patient relationship. In addition, in this unit students will learn about psychiatric–mental health nursing assessment with a brief overview of typical nursing interventions in Chapter 10, pharmacology and other biologic interventions in Chapter 11, and group interventions in Chapter 12.

The chapters in Unit IV, Prevention of Mental Disorders, are not specific to persons with mental disorders. Content in this unit is applicable to all nursing practice settings. Chapter 13 presents a model of stress that is supported by strong evidence and that can be applied to all areas of nursing. Chapter 14 explains how to understand and manage angry and aggressive patients. Content in the other chapters in this unit, including crisis intervention (Chapter 15) and suicide prevention (Chapter 16), is also applicable to care of persons with or without mental disorders. This unit also includes an in-depth chapter (Chapter 17) on mental health care of survivors of violence.

The bulk of the content related to mental disorders is found in Unit V, Care and Recovery for Persons With Psychiatric Disorders, which consists of 12 chapters (Chapters 18 through 29). Each chapter discusses a mental disorder(s) and identifies priority nursing assessment and intervention strategies to promote recovery of persons with mental illness. Case studies are threaded throughout each chapter to demonstrate, in easy-to-understand language, the concepts being discussed. For some of these cases, videos and interactive cases at http://thepoint.lww.com/Boyd Essentials2e show nurses interacting with persons with the disorder(s) discussed in the chapter.

Unit VI, Care of Special Populations, consists of two chapters discussing mental health needs of special populations. Chapter 30 focuses on the mental disorders of children, and Chapter 31 describes the neurocognitive disorders of older adults.

Pedagogical Features

Essentials of Psychiatric Nursing incorporates a multitude of pedagogical features to focus and direct student learning.

Introductory and Chapter-Closing Features

- **Expanded Table of Contents** allows readers to find and refer to concepts from one location.
- **Learning Objectives, Key Terms,** and **Key Concepts** in the chapter openers cue readers to what will be encountered and what is important to understand in each chapter.
- **Summary of Key Points** lists at the end of each chapter provide quick access to important chapter content to facilitate study and review.
- **Critical Thinking Challenges** ask questions that require students to think critically about chapter content and apply psychiatric nursing concepts to nursing practice.
- **Movies** list current examples of movies that depict various mental health disorders and that are widely available on DVD for rent or purchase. Viewing points are provided to serve as a basis for discussion in class and among students.

Other Special Features

- **NCLEX Notes** help students focus on important application areas to prepare for the NCLEX.
- **Case Studies** are threaded throughout the Unit V disorder chapters. Each chapter begins with a case study that is highlighted throughout the chapter. This case study is used as the prototype for that chapter's Nursing Care Plan (at http://thepoint.lww.com/Boyd Essentials2e) and Therapeutic Dialogue. For some chapters, an accompanying video and interactive case study on thePoint are provided so students can view the symptoms and the nursing care for a patient with a specific disorder. For your convenience, a list of all the case studies, with their location in the book, appears in the "Case Studies in This Book" section later in this front matter.
- **Unfolding Patient Stories,** written by the National League for Nursing, are an engaging way to begin meaningful conversations in the classroom. These vignettes, which appear at the end of the first chapter in each unit, feature patients from Wolters Kluwer's vSim for Nursing | Mental Health (codeveloped by Laerdal Medical) and DocuCare products; however, each Unfolding Patient Story in the book stands alone, not requiring purchase of these products. For your convenience, a list of all these case studies, along with their location in the book, appears in the "Case Studies in This Book" section later in this front matter.
- **Emergency Care Alerts** highlight important situations in psychiatric nursing care that the nurse should recognize as emergencies.
- **Evidence-Based Nursing Care for Selected Disorders** sections provide an in-depth study of the more commonly occurring major psychiatric disorders.
- **Nursing Care Plans,** based on the case studies in the book and available at http://thepoint.lww.com/BoydEssentials2e, present clinical examples of patients with a particular diagnosis and demonstrate plans of care that follow patients through various diagnostic stages and care delivery settings.
- **Research for Best Practice** boxes highlight today's focus on evidence-based practice for *best practice*, presenting findings and implications of studies that are applicable to psychiatric nursing practice.
- **Therapeutic Dialogue** boxes compare and contrast therapeutic and nontherapeutic conversations to encourage students by example to develop effective communication skills.
- **Psychoeducation Checklists** identify content areas for patient and family education related to specific disorders and their treatment. These checklists support critical thinking by encouraging students to develop patient-specific teaching plans based on chapter content.
- **Clinical Vignette** boxes present reality-based clinical portraits of patients who exhibit the symptoms described in the text. Questions are posed to help students express their thoughts and identify solutions to issues presented in the vignettes.
- **Drug Profile** boxes present a thorough picture of commonly prescribed medications for patients with mental health problems. Examples include lorazepam (Ativan), an anxiolytic, and mirtazapine (Remeron), an antidepressant. The profiles complement the text discussions of biologic processes known to be associated with various mental health disorders.
- **Key Diagnostic Characteristics** summaries describe diagnostic criteria, target symptoms, and associated findings for select disorders, described in the *DSM-5* by the American Psychiatric Association.
- **Diagrams, illustrations, and photos** colorfully illustrate the interrelationship of the biologic, psychological, and social domains of mental health and illness.
- **Patient education, family,** and **emergency icons** highlight content related to these topics to help link concepts to practice.

A COMPREHENSIVE PACKAGE FOR TEACHING AND LEARNING

To further facilitate teaching and learning, a carefully designed ancillary package has been developed to assist faculty and students.

Instructor Resources

Tools to assist you with teaching your course are available upon adoption of this text at http://thepoint.lww.com/BoydEssentials2e.

- The **Test Generator** lets you put together exclusive new tests from a bank containing hundreds of questions to help you in assessing your students' understanding of the material. Test questions correspond to chapter learning objectives.
- A sample **Syllabus** provides guidance for structuring your course.
- An **e-book** allows access to the book's full text and images online.
- **Strategies for Effective Teaching** offer creative approaches.
- **Access to All Student Resources** is also provided.
- An extensive collection of materials is provided for each book chapter:
  - **Pre-Lecture Quizzes** (and answers) are quick, knowledge-based assessments that allow you to check students' reading.
  - **PowerPoint Presentations** provide an easy way for you to integrate the textbook with your students' classroom experience, either via slide shows or handouts. Multiple choice and true/false questions are integrated into the presentations to promote class participation and allow you to use i-clicker technology.
  - **Guided Lecture Notes** walk you through the chapters, objective by objective, and provide you with corresponding PowerPoint slide numbers.
  - **Discussion Topics** (and suggested answers) can be used as conversation starters or in online discussion boards.
  - **Assignments** (and suggested answers) include group, written, clinical, and Web assignments.
  - **Case Studies** with related questions (and suggested answers) give students an opportunity to apply their knowledge to a client case similar to one they might encounter in practice.
  - An **Image Bank** allows you to use the photographs and illustrations from this textbook in your PowerPoint slides or as you see fit in your course.

Student Resources

An exciting set of free resources is available to help students review and apply important concepts. Students can access these resources at http://thepoint.lww.com/BoydEssentials2e using the codes printed in the front of their textbooks.

- As indicated in the table of contents and in the appropriate places in the book, the following are found on the book's companion website at http://thepoint.lww.com/BoydEssentials2e: **Chapter 7** (Recovery Framework for Mental Health Nursing), **Chapter 28** (Sleep–Wake Disorders: Nursing Care of Persons with Insomnia and Sleep Problems), **Appendix A** (Brief Psychiatric Rating Scale), **Appendix B** (Abnormal Involuntary Movement Scale [AIMS]), and the **Glossary**.
- **NCLEX-Style Review Questions** for each chapter help students review important concepts and practice for the NCLEX.
- **Watch & Learn Videos:**
  - **Online video series,** *Lippincott Theory to Practice Video Series: Psychiatric–Mental Health Nursing*, includes videos of true-to-life patients displaying mental health disorders, allowing students to gain experience and a deeper understanding of mental health patients. The video series allows viewing of complete patient interviews and also gives the opportunity to view snippets of those interviews, for closer analysis or classroom discussion. The innovative videos feature patients found in the book and explore such topics as depression, eating disorders, and addiction.
  - A **Watch & Learn Video Clip** on cognitive functions is included from *Lippincott Video Guide to Psychiatric–Mental Health Nursing Assessment*.
- **Practice & Learn Interactive Case Studies:**
  - Most of these case studies relate to the *Lippincott Theory to Practice Video Series: Psychiatric–Mental Health Nursing videos* mentioned above (which in turn relate to the patients found in the book).
  - Other case studies, from *Lippincott Interactive Case Studies in Psychiatric–Mental Health Nursing*, relate to therapeutic communication, antidepressants, and dementia.
- **Journal Articles** provided for each chapter offer access to current research available in Wolters Kluwer journals.
- Plus, a **Spanish-English audio glossary, Lippincott Nursing Drug Handbook App, Nursing Professional Roles and Responsibilities, Heart and Breath Sounds,** and **Learning Objectives** from the textbook.

Adaptive Learning Powered by PrepU

Lippincott's Adaptive Learning Powered by PrepU helps every student learn more, while giving instructors the data they need to monitor each student's progress, strengths, and weaknesses. The adaptive learning system allows instructors to assign quizzes or students to take quizzes on their own that adapt to each student's individual mastery level. Visit http://thePoint.lww.com/prepU to learn more.

vSim for Nursing

vSim for Nursing, jointly developed by Laerdal Medical and Wolters Kluwer Health, offers innovative scenario-based learning modules consisting of Web-based virtual simulations, course learning materials, and curriculum tools designed to develop critical thinking skills and promote clinical confidence and competence. vSim for Nursing | Mental Health includes 10 mental health scenarios authored by the National League for Nursing. Students can progress through suggested readings, pre- and postsimulation assessments, documentation assignments, and guided reflection questions, and will receive an individualized feedback log immediately upon completion of the simulation. Throughout the student learning experience, the product offers remediation back to trusted Lippincott resources, including Lippincott Nursing Advisor and Lippincott Nursing Procedures—two online, evidence-based, clinical information solutions used in health care facilities throughout the United States. This innovative product provides a comprehensive patient-focused solution for learning and integrating simulation into the classroom.

Contact your Wolters Kluwer sales representative or visit http://thepoint.lww.com/vsim for options to enhance your mental health nursing course with vSim for Nursing.

Lippincott DocuCare

Lippincott DocuCare combines Web-based academic electronic health record (EHR) simulation software with clinical case scenarios, allowing students to learn how to use an EHR in a safe, true-to-life setting, while enabling instructors to measure their progress. Lippincott DocuCare's nonlinear solution works well in the classroom, simulation lab, and clinical practice.

Contact your Wolters Kluwer sales representative or visit http://thepoint.lww.com/DocuCare for options to enhance your mental health nursing course with DocuCare.

A COMPREHENSIVE, DIGITAL, INTEGRATED COURSE SOLUTION: LIPPINCOTT COURSEPOINT+

The same trusted solution, innovation, and unmatched support that you have come to expect from *Lippincott CoursePoint+* is now enhanced with more engaging learning tools and deeper analytics to help prepare students for practice. This powerfully integrated digital learning solution combines learning tools, case studies, virtual simulation, real-time data, and the most trusted nursing education content on the market to make curriculum-wide learning more efficient and to meet students where they are at in their learning. And now, it's easier than ever for instructors and students to use, giving them everything they need for course and curriculum success!

Lippincott Coursepoint+ includes:

- Engaging course content provides a variety of learning tools to engage students of all learning styles.
- A more personalized learning approach, including adaptive learning powered by PrepU, gives students the content and tools they need at the moment they need it, giving them data for more focused remediation and helping to boost their confidence.
- Varying levels of case studies, virtual simulation, and access to Lippincott Advisor help students learn the critical thinking and clinical judgment skills to help them become practice-ready nurses.
- Unparalleled reporting provides in-depth dashboards with several data points to track student progress and help identify strengths and weaknesses.
- Unmatched support includes training coaches, product trainers, and nursing education consultants to help educators and students implement CoursePoint+ with ease.

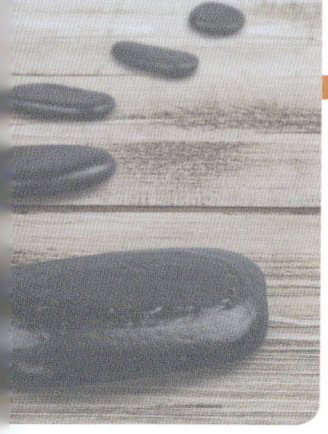

Acknowledgments

This text is a result of many long hours of diligent work by the contributors, editors, and assistants. Psychiatric nurses are constantly writing about and discussing new strategies for caring for persons with mental disorders. Consumers of mental health services provide directions for nursing care and validate the importance of nursing interventions. We wish to acknowledge and thank these individuals.

Michael Kerns, Meredith Brittain, Tim Rinehart, and Sadie Buckallew of Wolters Kluwer, as well as Karan Rana of Aptara, were extraordinary partners in this project during the development of this text. We want to especially acknowledge their attention to detail and commitment to the completion of this edition. They provided direction, support, and valuable input throughout this project.

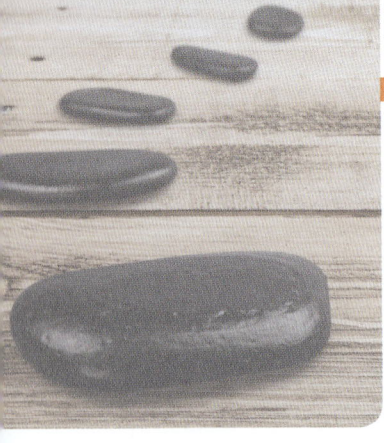

Contents

UNIT I ESSENTIALS OF MENTAL HEALTH CARE 1

1 Mental Health and Mental Disorders 1
Mental Health and Wellness 1
Overview of Mental Health Disorders 2
Recovery from Mental Illness 4

2 Cultural and Spiritual Issues Related to Mental Health Care 8
Cultural and Linguistic Competence 9
Cultural and Social Factors and Beliefs About Mental Illness 9
Spirituality, Religion, and Mental Illness 12

3 Patient Rights and Legal Issues 16
Self-Determinism: A Fundamental Right and Need 16
Protection of Patient Rights 17
Treatment and Patient Rights 19
Privacy and Confidentiality 22
Criminal Judicial Processes 23
Accountability for Nurses and Other Mental Health Care Professionals 25

UNIT II PSYCHIATRIC–MENTAL HEALTH NURSING FRAMEWORKS 29

4 Ethics, Standards, and Nursing Frameworks 29
Ethics of Psychiatric Nursing 29
Scope and Standards of Practice 30
The Biopsychosocial Framework 33
Tools of Psychiatric Nursing Practice 34
Challenges of Psychiatric Nursing 35

5 Theoretical Basis of Psychiatric Nursing 39
Psychodynamic Theories 39
Cognitive-Behavioral Theories 43
Developmental Theories 46
Social Theories 48
Nursing Theories 51

6 Biologic Foundations of Psychiatric Nursing 57
Neuroanatomy of the Central Nervous System 58
Neurophysiology of the Central Nervous System 63
Studies of the Biologic Basis of Mental Disorders 73
Diagnostic Approaches 76

7 Recovery Framework for Psychiatric–Mental Health Nursing 80
Chapter 7 is available at http://thepoint.lww.com/BoydEssentials2e and in the CoursePoint ebook.

UNIT III KNOWLEDGE AND SKILLS OF PSYCHIATRIC–MENTAL HEALTH NURSING 81

8 Therapeutic Communication 81
Self-Awareness 81
Effective Communication 82
Therapeutic Communication Strategies and Techniques 84
Boundaries and Body Space Zones 87
Defense Mechanisms 89
Communication Considerations for Patients with Mental Health Challenges 89

9 The Nurse–Patient Relationship 96
Effective Communication Needs in Relationships 96
The Nurse–Patient Relationship 97
Examples of Strategies Related to Therapeutic Relationships 101

10 The Psychiatric–Mental Health Nursing Process 104
Recovery-Oriented Psychiatric–Mental Health Nursing Assessment 104
Priority of Nursing Care 117
Developing Recovery Outcomes 117
Recovery-Oriented Nursing Interventions 117
Evaluating Outcomes 126

11 Psychopharmacology, Dietary Supplements, and Biologic Interventions 128
Psychiatric Medications 129
Psychopharmacology 129
Phases of Drug Treatment and the Nurse's Role 137
Major Psychopharmacologic Drug Classes 138
Integrative and Complementary Health Care 156
Other Biologic Treatments 157
The Issue of Adherence 159

12 Group Interventions 164
Preparing to Lead a Group 164
Leading a Group 166
Types of Groups 172
Common Nursing Intervention Groups 174

UNIT IV PREVENTION OF MENTAL DISORDERS 177

13 Stress and Mental Health 177
Biologic Perspectives of Stress 178
Psychosocial Perspectives of Stress 180
Responses to Stress 183
Coping 184
Adaptation 186
Nursing Care for the Person Experiencing Stress 186

14 Management of Anger, Aggression, and Violence 192
Anger 193
Aggression and Violence 197
Promoting Safety and Preventing Violence 199
Research and Policy Initiatives 205

15 Crisis, Loss, Grief Response, Bereavement, and Disaster Management 208
Crisis 208
Loss and Bereavement 210
Evidence-Based Nursing Care of Person in Crisis 213
Disaster and Terrorism 216
Evidence-Based Nursing Care of Persons Experiencing Disasters 218

16 Suicide Prevention 223
Suicide and Suicide Attempt 224
Treatment and Nursing Care for Suicide Prevention 230
Nurses' Reflection 235

17 Mental Health Care for Survivors of Violence 239
Types of Violence and Abuse 239
Theories of Violence 243
Establishing a Therapeutic Relationship 245
Evidence-Based Nursing Care for Persons Experiencing Violence 245
Treatment for the Abuser 254

UNIT V CARE AND RECOVERY FOR PERSONS WITH PSYCHIATRIC DISORDERS

18 Anxiety Disorders 257
Normal Versus Abnormal Anxiety Response 258
Phobias 260
Overview of Anxiety Disorders 260
Panic Disorder 261
Generalized Anxiety Disorder 276
Other Anxiety Disorders 277
Agoraphobia 277
Specific Phobia 277
Social Anxiety Disorder (Social Phobia) 278

19 Trauma- and Stressor-Related Disorders 282
Trauma and Resilience 282
Overview of Trauma- and Stressor-Related Disorders 283
Posttraumatic Stress Disorder 284
Dissociative Disorders 293
Other Trauma- and Stressor-Related Disorders 293

20 Obsessive–Compulsive and Related Disorders 296
Obsessions and Compulsions 296
Overview of Obsessive–Compulsive and Related Disorders 297
Obsessive–Compulsive Disorder 297
Trichotillomania 307
Excoriation (Skin-Picking) Disorder 307
Body Dysmorphic Disorder 307
Hoarding Disorder 308

21 Depression 311
Mood and Depression 311
Overview of Depressive Disorders 312
Major Depressive Disorder 313
Other Depressive Disorders 330

22 Bipolar Disorders 334
Mania 334
Bipolar Disorders 335
Bipolar I Disorder 335
Other Bipolar and Related Disorders 350

23 Schizophrenia and Related Disorders 354
Schizophrenia Spectrum Disorder 355
Schizophrenia 355
Schizoaffective Disorder 385
Delusional Disorder 386
Schizophreniform Disorder 386
Brief Psychotic Disorder 386
Psychotic Disorders Attributable to a Substance 386

24 Personality and Impulse-Control Disorders 391
Overview of Personality Disorders 392
Cluster A: Paranoid, Schizoid, and Schizotypal Personality Disorders 392
Paranoid Personality Disorder 392
Schizoid Personality Disorder 393
Schizotypal Personality Disorder 394
Cluster B Disorders: Borderline, Antisocial, Histrionic, and Narcissistic Personality Disorders 395
Borderline Personality Disorder 395
Antisocial Personality Disorder 408
Histrionic Personality Disorder 413
Narcissistic Personality Disorder 415
Cluster C Disorders: Avoidant, Dependent, and Obsessive-Compulsive Personality Disorders 416
Avoidant Personality Disorder 416
Dependent Personality Disorder 416
Obsessive-Compulsive Personality Disorder 417
Disruptive, Impulse-Control, and Conduct Disorders 418
Overview of Disruptive, Impulse-Control, and Conduct Disorders 418
Intermittent Explosive Disorder 421
Kleptomania 421
Pyromania 421
Continuum of Care for Disruptive, Impulse-Control Disorders 422

25 Addiction and Substance-Related Disorders 425
Overview of Substance Use and Abuse 425
Types of Substances and Related Disorders 427
Emerging Drugs and Trends 442
Gambling: A Non–Substance-Related Disorder 442
Evidence-Based Nursing Care for Persons With Substance-Related Disorders 443
Chemical Dependency and Professional Nurses 451

26 Eating Disorders 454
Anorexia Nervosa 455
Bulimia Nervosa 468
Binge-Eating Disorder 474
Other Eating Disorders 474
Purging Disorder 474
Night Eating Syndrome 474

27 Somatic Symptom and Related Disorders 477
Somatic Symptom Disorder 478
Illness Anxiety Disorder 489
Conversion Disorder (Functional Neurologic Symptom Disorder) 489
Factitious Disorders 489
Factitious Disorder 489
Factitious Disorder Imposed on Another 491

28 Sleep–Wake Disorders 494
Chapter 28 is available at http://thepoint.lww.com/BoydEssentials2e and in the CoursePoint ebook.

29 Sexual Disorders 495
Sexual Development 496
Sexual Responses 497
Sexual Health and Wellness 498
Sexual Dysfunctions and Problematic Behaviors 499
Female Orgasmic Disorder 499
Ejaculatory Dysfunction 502
Erectile Dysfunction 503
Female Sexual Interest/Arousal Disorder 505
Male Hypoactive Sexual Desire Disorder 506
Genitopelvic Pain/Penetration Disorder 506
Paraphilias 506
Gender Dysphoria 506

UNIT VI CARE OF SPECIAL POPULATIONS 511

30 Mental Health Disorders of Childhood and Adolescence 511
Neurodevelopmental Disorders of Childhood 512
Intellectual Disability 512
Autism Spectrum Disorder 513
Attention-Deficit Hyperactivity Disorder 517
Tic Disorders and Tourette Disorder 522
Separation Anxiety Disorder 524
Obsessive-Compulsive Disorder 526
Other Neurodevelopmental Disorders 527
Specific Learning Disorders 527
Communication Disorders 527
Other Mental Disorders 528
Mood Disorders 528
Childhood Schizophrenia 529
Elimination Disorders 529
Enuresis 529
Encopresis 529

31 Mental Health Disorders of Older Adults 534
Delirium 535
Alzheimer Disease 539
Other Dementias 555
Frontotemporal Neurocognitive Disorder 556
Neurocognitive Disorder With Lewy Bodies 556
Neurocognitive Disorder Due to Prion Disease 556
Neurocognitive Disorder Due to Traumatic Brain Injury 557
Substance/Medication-Induced Neurocognitive Disorder 557

Appendix A Brief Psychiatric Rating Scale 559

Appendix B Abnormal Involuntary Movement Scale (AIMS) 559

Glossary 559

Appendices A, B, and the Glossary are available at http://thepoint.lww.com/BoydEssentials2e and in the CoursePoint ebook.

Index 561

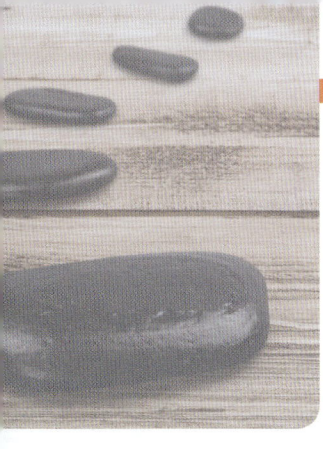

Case Studies in This Book

CASES THAT UNFOLD ACROSS UNITS

Unfolding Patient Stories: Andrew Davis
Unit V, Part 1   p. 280
Unit VI, Part 2   p. 531

Unfolding Patient Stories: David Carter
Unit III, Part 1   p. 95
Unit IV, Part 2   p. 190

Unfolding Patient Stories: George Palo
Unit IV, Part 1   p. 190
Unit VI, Part 2   p. 531

Unfolding Patient Stories: Li Na Chen
Unit I, Part 1   p. 7
Unit V, Part 2   p. 280

Unfolding Patient Stories: Linda Waterfall
Unit II, Part 1   p. 37
Unit V, Part 2   p. 280

Unfolding Patient Stories: Randy Adams
Unit II, Part 1   p. 37
Unit III, Part 2   p. 95

Unfolding Patient Stories: Sandra Littlefield
Unit I, Part 1   p. 7
Unit IV, Part 2   p. 190

Unfolding Patient Stories: Sharon Cole
Unit III, Part 1   p. 95
Unit V, Part 2   p. 280

CASES THAT UNFOLD WITHIN CHAPTERS

18 Anxiety Disorders
Doug, pp. 257, 262, 274

19 Trauma- and Stressor-Related Disorders
Susan, pp. 282, 284, 285, 288

20 Obsessive–Compulsive and Related Disorders
Tim, pp. 296, 298, 299, 301

21 Depression
Louise, pp. 311, 313, 316, 318

22 Bipolar Disorders
Christine, pp. 334, 335, 338, 339

23 Schizophrenia and Related Disorders
Arnold, pp. 354, 356, 367, 371

24 Personality and Impulse-Control Disorders
Rebecca, pp. 391, 396, 398, 401

25 Addiction and Substance-Related Disorders
Gladys, pp. 425, 427, 432, 444

26 Eating Disorders
Ellen, pp. 454, 468, 470, 471

27 Somatic Symptom and Related Disorders
Carol, pp. 477, 483, 484

28 Sleep–Wake Disorders 494
Michael, pp. e-9, e-14, e-17

Chapter 28 is available at http://thepoint.lww.com/BoydEssentials2e and in the CoursePoint ebook.

29 Sexual Disorders 495
Alice, pp. 495, 499, 500

UNIT I
ESSENTIALS OF MENTAL HEALTH CARE

1
Mental Health and Mental Disorders
Fighting Stigma and Promoting Recovery

Mary Ann Boyd

KEY CONCEPTS
- mental disorders
- mental health
- recovery
- stigma
- trauma
- wellness

LEARNING OBJECTIVES

After studying this chapter, you will be able to:

1. Relate the concept of mental health to wellness.
2. Identify the rationale for promoting wellness for people with mental health challenges.
3. Differentiate the concepts of mental health and mental illness.
4. Discuss the significance of epidemiologic evidence in studying the occurrence of mental disorders.
5. Describe the consequences of the stigma of mental illness on individuals and families.
6. Identify recovery components and their role in the treatment of mental illness.
7. Discuss the role of trauma-informed care in recovery-oriented nursing practice.

KEY TERMS

- cultural-bound syndrome • cultural explanation • cultural idiom of distress • cultural syndrome • *DSM-5* • epidemiology
- incidence • label avoidance • point prevalence • prevalence • public stigma • rate • recovery-oriented care • self-stigma
- syndrome • trauma-informed care

To understand health and illness in any practice area, nurses need a basic understanding of mental health and its relationship with wellness. This chapter discusses concepts of mental health and wellness, the diagnosis of mental disorders, how the stigma of mental illness can be a barrier to treatment, and the importance of focusing on recovery from mental illness.

MENTAL HEALTH AND WELLNESS

Mental health is defined as a state of well-being in which the individual realizes his or her own abilities, can cope with life's normal stresses, can work productively and fruitfully, and can make a contribution to society. A person cannot be healthy without being "mentally" healthy, but it is possible to be mentally healthy and have a mental or physical disorder (World Health Organization [WHO], 2013a). Mental health is essential to personal well-being, interpersonal relationships, and contributing to the community.

> **KEYCONCEPT** **Mental health** is the emotional and psychological well-being of an individual who has the capacity to interact with others, deal with ordinary stress, and perceive one's surroundings realistically. (Adapted from American Nurses Association, American Psychiatric Nurses Association, & International Society of Psychiatric–Mental Health Nurses, 2014).

Mental health is an important part of total wellness. The concept of wellness includes being in good physical and mental health. Problems in one area impact the other area. Wellness is not the absence of disease or stress; it involves having a purpose in life, being actively involved in satisfying work and play, having joyful relationships, having a healthy body and living environment, and being happy. It includes the mental, emotional, physical, occupational, intellectual, and spiritual aspects of a person's life (U.S. Department of Health and Human Services, Substance Abuse & Mental Health Services Administration [U.S. DHHS, SAMHSA], 2018a) (see Fig. 1.1).

> **KEYCONCEPT** **Wellness** is being in good physical and mental health. Improving physical health can benefit mental health, and vice versa. Wellness is not the absence of disease. There are eight dimensions of wellness: Emotional, financial, social, spiritual, occupational, physical, intellectual, and environmental (see Fig. 1.1).

Mental health problems significantly impact the process of wellness. Individuals with mental health problems are more likely to die decades earlier than the general public from preventable diseases (Heiberg et al., 2018). People with serious mental health problems often face social, economic, and/or environmental disadvantages that result in lack of access to health care, lack of information, and lack of culturally and linguistically competent care and programs (U.S. DHHS, SAMHSA, 2018b).

OVERVIEW OF MENTAL HEALTH DISORDERS

Mental disorders can disrupt mental health and result in one of the most common causes of disability. In this text, the terms "mental disorder" and "mental illness" will be used interchangeably.

> **KEYCONCEPT** **Mental disorders** are clinically significant disturbances in cognition, emotion regulation, or behavior that reflect a dysfunction in the psychological, biologic, or developmental processes underlying mental dysfunction. They are usually associated with distress or impaired functioning (American Psychiatric Association [APA], 2013).

A mental illness or mental disorder is a **syndrome**, a set of symptoms that cluster together that may have multiple causes and may represent several different disease states that have not yet been defined. Unlike many medical diseases, mental disorders are defined by clusters of behaviors, thoughts, and feelings, not underlying biologic pathology. Laboratory tests are not generally used in diagnosing mental disorders.

The landmark study *Global Burden of Disease 2010* found an alarming impact of mental and behavioral disorders on health and productivity in the world. Depression is one of the leading disease burdens in middle- and high-income countries such as the United States. By 2030, depression is projected to be the leading burden worldwide (WHO, 2013b). In 2017, in the United States, 1 in 5 adults, or 44.7 million people, had a mental illness (National Institute of Mental Health [NIMH], 2019).

Evidence for this very high occurrence of mental disorders is established through epidemiologic research. **Epidemiology**, the study of patterns of disease distribution and determinants of health within populations, contributes to the overall understanding of the mental health status of population groups, or aggregates, and associated factors. Epidemiologic studies examine associations among possible factors related to an area of investigation, but they do not determine causes of illnesses. The Centers for Disease Control and Prevention (CDC) tracks and reports mental health epidemiologic data. Throughout this book, epidemiologic data are included in discussions of mental health problems and

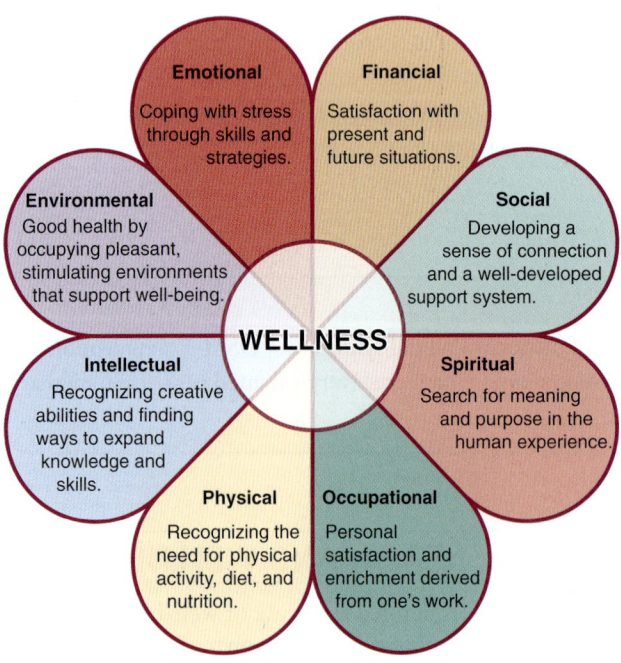

FIGURE 1.1 Eight dimensions of wellness. (Adapted from U.S. DHHS, SAMHSA. [2018a]. *The eight dimensions of wellness*. Retrieved from https://www.samhsa.gov/wellness-initiative/eight-dimensions-wellness)

> **BOX 1.1**
> **Epidemiologic Terms**
>
> In epidemiology, certain terms have specific meanings relative to what they measure. When expressing the number of cases of a disorder, population rates, rather than raw numbers, are used.
>
> **Rate** is the proportion of the cases in the population when compared with the total population. It is expressed as a fraction, in which the numerator is the number of cases and the denominator is the total number in the population, including the cases and noncases. The term *average rate* is used for measures that involve rates over specified time periods:
>
> $$\text{Rate} = \frac{\text{Cases in population}}{\text{Total population (cases and noncases)}}$$
>
> **Prevalence** refers to the total number of people who have the disorder within a given population at a specified time regardless of how long ago the disorder started.
>
> **Point prevalence** is the basic measure that refers to the proportion of individuals in the population who have the disorder at a specified point in time (t). This point can be a day on the calendar, such as April 1, 2015, or a point defined in relation to the study assessment, such as the day of the interview. This is also expressed as a fraction:
>
> $$\text{Point prevalence rate} = \frac{\text{Cases at } t}{\text{Population at } t}$$
>
> **Incidence** refers to a rate that includes only *new* cases that have occurred within a clearly defined time period. The most common time period evaluated is 1 year. The study of incidence cases is more difficult than a study of prevalent cases because a study of incidence cases requires at least two measurements to be taken: one at the start of the prescribed time period and another at the end of it.

mental disorders. See Box 1.1 for an explanation of terms.

Diagnosis of Mental Health Conditions

Mental disorders are organized and diagnosed according to the criteria published in the *Diagnostic and Statistical Manual of Mental Disorders–5* (*DSM-5*; APA, 2013). The current **DSM-5** system contains subtypes and other specifiers that further classify disorders. Although the *DSM-5* specifies criteria for diagnosing mental disorders, there are no absolute boundaries separating one disorder from another, and disorders often have different manifestations at different points in time.

In a mental disorder, alterations in behaviors, thoughts, and feelings are unexpected and are outside normal, culturally defined limits. If a behavior is considered normal within a specific culture, it is not viewed as a psychiatric symptom. For example, members of some religious groups "speak in tongues." To an observer, it appears that the individuals are hallucinating (see Chapter 23), but this behavior is normal for this group within a particular setting.

> **BOX 1.2**
> **Frequently Reported Cultural Syndromes and Idioms**
>
> ***Ataque de nervios:*** frequent episodes of loss of control, uncontrollable crying, tremors, and severe anxiety and sadness with somatization symptoms including muscle and headache, nausea, loss of appetite, insomnia, fatigue, and psychomotor agitation. Reported among women over 45 years old, with little education, and who have experienced a loss (such as a divorce) or acute distress.
>
> ***Susto:*** fright characterized by symptoms of psychomotor agitation, anorexia, insomnia, fever, diarrhea, confusion, apathy, depression, and introversion following an emotional trauma or witnessing a traumatic experience.
>
> (Adapted from Durá-Vilá & Hodes, 2012)

The amount of disability or impairment in functioning is an important consideration when assessing a person with a mental disorder. A person's ability to understand, communicate, and get along with others is important in the recovery process. If symptoms impair an individual's ability to independently perform self-care and daily activities, recovery will be more difficult. The WHO Disability Assessment Schedule 2.0 is an instrument that can be used for measuring the amount of impairment that the individual experiences.

Cultural-bound syndromes, which are illnesses that occur only within a specific culture, have been studied for years. The *DSM-5* replaced the term with three concepts: **Cultural syndrome** is a group of co-occurring symptoms that occur in one culture, for example, *ataque de nervios*. **Cultural idiom of distress** is a phrase or way of talking about distress within a culture; for example, *susto*. **Cultural explanation** or cause is an etiology that is culturally conceived (APA, 2013). There is little research that reliably describes cultural syndromes or idioms of distress, but there are two conditions, *ataque de nervios* and *susto*, that are frequently reported in a small number of persons (Durá-Vilá & Hodes, 2012) (Box 1.2).

Stigma

Stigma is one of the major barriers to treatment, recovery, and social integration. A major reason individuals with mental health problems do not seek or continue with treatment is the stigma they encounter. Stigma, myths, and misconceptions surrounding mental illness contribute to the discrimination and human rights violations experienced by people living with mental illness.

> **KEYCONCEPT Stigma** is a dynamic social/interactional process in which the stigmatized person is labeled as different and linked to negative stereotypes. Persons with stigmatizing beliefs socially distance themselves from the stigmatized person. Public stigma, self-stigma, and label avoidance are three types of stigma, people with mental illnesses experience.

Public Stigma

Public stigma occurs after individuals are publicly "marked" as having a mental illness. When they act or say things that are odd or unusual or tell others that they have a mental illness, these individuals are at risk of being subjected to prejudice and discrimination. Common stereotypes include being dangerous, unpredictable, and incapable of functioning independently. People with mental illness are sometimes treated as if they are responsible for their disabilities and are inaccurately accused of being weak or immoral (Corrigan & Al-Khouja, 2018). Stigmatization robs individuals of work, independent living, and meaningful relationships.

When people with mental illnesses or emotional problems are stigmatized by society, they are often ostracized by the society in which they live. The stigma associated with all forms of mental illness is strong but generally increases the more an individual's behavior differs from the cultural norm. Reducing stigma is identified as a public health priority (National Academy of Sciences, 2016).

Media perpetuates the stigma of mental disorders and treatment. TV and newspaper coverage often associate violence with mental illness (McGinty, Kennedy-Hendricks, Choksy, & Barry, 2016). Few describe successful treatment or recovery. Additionally, mental health treatment and providers are often stigmatized. In films, psychiatric hospitals are often portrayed as dangerous and unwelcoming places, such as in *The Snake Pit* (1948), *One Flew Over the Cuckoo's Nest* (1975), *Instinct* (1999), *Twelve Monkeys* (1995), *Sling Blade* (1996), *Girl, Interrupted* (1999), *Don Juan Demarco* (1994), *A Beautiful Mind* (2001), and *Analyze That* (2002). Nurses are dressed in white in contrast to the dark, gloomy surroundings, and patients have little to do other than to walk the halls of the institution, acting odd.

One of the best ways to counteract the negative effects of stigma is to have contact with the stigmatized group (Corrigan & Al-Khouja, 2018). Another way is to use nonstigmatizing language. Just as a person with diabetes mellitus should not be referred to as a "diabetic" but rather as a "person with diabetes," a person with a mental disorder should never be referred to as a "schizophrenic" or "bipolar" but rather as a "person with schizophrenia" or a "person with bipolar disorder." Using words such as "psycho," "nuts," "funny farm," and "maniac" reinforces negative images of mental illness. Jokes that depict people with mental illness as stupid, dangerous, or incompetent perpetuate negative myths.

Self-Stigma

Self-stigma occurs when negative stereotypes are internalized by people with mental illness. Patients are aware of the public's negative view of mental illness and agree with the public's perceptions. As they become aware of the negative stereotypes, they begin agreeing with the stereotype. Then they may begin applying the stigma to themselves: "I have a mental illness, so I must be incompetent." As a result of the application of the negative stereotype to self, they develop low self-esteem (Corrigan, 2016).

Label Avoidance

Label avoidance, avoiding treatment or care in order not to be labeled as being mentally ill, is another type of stigma, and one of the reasons, that so few people with mental health problems actually receive help. By avoiding treatment, they avoid the stigma of mental illness. For example, negative views of mental illness by several of the Asian cultures influence the willingness of its members to seek treatment. They may ignore their symptoms or refuse to seek treatment because of the stigma associated with being mentally ill (Corrigan, 2016).

RECOVERY FROM MENTAL ILLNESS

Recovery is the single most important goal for individuals with mental disorders. The following definition of recovery was released following a lengthy consensus process that began in 2010 and involved government agency officials, experts, consumers, family members, advocates, researchers, managed care representatives, and others.

> **KEYCONCEPT Recovery** from mental disorders and/or substance use disorders is a process of change through which individuals improve their health and wellness, live a self-directed life, and strive to reach their full potential (U.S. DHHS, SAMHSA, 2012).

Recovery-oriented treatment is based on the belief that mental illnesses and emotional disturbances are treatable, and that recovery is an expectation. There are four dimensions that support recovery, including *health* (managing disease and living in a physically and emotionally healthy way), *home* (a safe and stable place to live), *purpose* (meaningful daily activities and independence, resources, and income), and *community* (relationships and social networks). Consumers and families have real and meaningful choices about treatment options and providers. In **recovery-oriented care**, the person with a mental health problem develops a partnership with a clinician to manage the illness, strengthen coping abilities, and build resilience for life's challenges (Box 1.3). See Chapter 7 for further discussion.

Mental health recovery benefits not only the individual and family but also society by ultimately reducing the global burden of mental health problems. Recovery is guided by 10 fundamental principles (see Box 1.4).

BOX 1.3
Research for Best Practice: Cultural Change: Implementation of a Recovery Program

McDonagh, J. G., Haren, W. B., Valvano, M., et al. (2018). Cultural change: Implementation of a recovery program in a Veterans Health Administration Medical Center inpatient unit. *Journal of the American Psychiatric Nurses Association.* doi: 10.1177/1078390318786024.

THE QUESTION: How does an inpatient mental health unit implement recovery-oriented services?

METHODS: A recovery-oriented inpatient program on a 24-bed locked unit consisted of several critical components including the development of an interprofessional committee, creation of vision and mission statement, education of staff, integration of the peer support specialist role, development and delivery of recovery-oriented curriculum, development of the interprofessional program partnership, adoption of the Veterans Recovery Self-Help Resource book, and Veterans Recovery worksheet. An interprofessional Partnership for Wellness conducted 4 to 6 hours per day of evidence-based recovery and holistic health programs. The measurement indicators included veteran feedback, program requirements, and system measures.

FINDINGS: Preliminary indicators over a 2-year period suggest that when the veterans rated group content and relevance high, per-post psychiatric rehospitalization rates decreased by 46%, and fidelity to the recommended strategies was high.

IMPLICATIONS FOR NURSING: Recovery-oriented practice is realistic in an inpatient mental health unit if there is a committed interprofessional staff, effective training, and an organizational culture exemplifying recovery-oriented principles.

BOX 1.4
Guiding Principles of Recovery

Recovery emerges from hope: The belief that recovery is real provides the essential and motivating message of a better future—that people can and do overcome the internal and external challenges, barriers, and obstacles that confront them.

Recovery is person-driven: Self-determination and self-direction are the foundations for recovery, as individuals define their own life goals and design their unique path(s).

Recovery occurs via many pathways: Individuals are unique with distinct needs, strengths, preferences, goals, culture, and backgrounds including trauma experiences that affect and determine their pathway(s) to recovery. Abstinence is the safest approach for those with substance use disorders.

Recovery is holistic: Recovery encompasses an individual's whole life, including mind, body, spirit, and community. The array of services and supports available should be integrated and coordinated.

Recovery is supported by peers and allies: Mutual support and mutual aid groups, including the sharing of experiential knowledge and skills, as well as social learning, play an invaluable role in recovery.

Recovery is supported through relationship and social networks: An important factor in the recovery process is the presence and involvement of people who believe in the person's ability to recover; who offer hope, support, and encouragement; and who also suggest strategies and resources for change.

Recovery is culturally-based and influenced: Culture and cultural background in all of its diverse representations including values, traditions, and beliefs are key in determining a person's journey and unique pathway to recovery.

Recovery is supported by addressing trauma: Services and supports should be trauma-informed to foster safety (physical and emotional) and trust, as well as to promote choice, empowerment, and collaboration.

Recovery involves individual, family, and community strengths and responsibility: Individuals, families, and communities have strengths and resources that serve as a foundation for recovery.

Recovery is based on respect: Community, systems, and societal acceptance and appreciation for people affected by mental health and substance use problems—including protecting their rights and eliminating discrimination—are crucial in achieving recovery.

(From U.S. DHHS, SAMHSA, 2012)

Recovery-Oriented Care and Trauma-Informed Care

Mental health professionals increasingly focus on the harmful effects of trauma on health and mental health status. Individuals who experience trauma, particularly in childhood, have a higher incidence of chronic disease and behavior health issues. Trauma is a universal experience for people with mental and substance abuse disorders (U.S. DHHS, SAMHSA, 2014).

> **KEYCONCEPT** Individual **trauma** results from an event, series of events, or set of circumstances that is experienced by an individual as physically or emotionally harmful or life threatening and that has lasting adverse effects on the individual's functioning and mental, physical, social, emotional, or spiritual well-being (U.S. DHHS, SAMHSA, 2014).

An important aspect of recovery-oriented care is to prevent retraumatization by exposing individuals to triggers—such as confinement to a mental health unit or applying restraints—only when accompanied by the proper support and sensitivity (Davis & Maul, 2015).

Trauma-informed care is integral to recovery-oriented nursing care for people with emotional problems and mental disorders. Trauma-informed care incorporates a basic realization and understanding of the impact of trauma on individuals, families, groups, organizations, and communities. In trauma-informed care, nurses recognize the signs of trauma and respond by fully integrating knowledge about the trauma into policies, procedures, and practice.

Individuals with mental illnesses can regain mental health with the support of families, mental health providers, and society. The contributions of these individuals strengthen communities and support the overall health of a nation.

SUMMARY OF KEY POINTS

- Mental health is the emotional and psychological well-being of an individual. To be mentally healthy means that one can interact with others, deal with daily stress, and perceive the world realistically. Mental disorders are health conditions characterized by alterations in thinking, mood, or behavior and are associated with distress or impaired functioning.

- Good physical and mental health characterize wellness. Individuals can have a mental disorder and experience wellness.

- Epidemiology is important in understanding the distribution of mental illness and determinants of health within a given population. The rate of occurrence refers to the proportion of the population that has the disorder. Incidence is the rate of new cases within a specified time. Prevalence is the rate of occurrence of all cases at a particular point in time.

- Stigma toward mental illness can be viewed in three ways. Public stigma marks a person as having a mental illness. When a person with a mental illness shares the public's negative view of mental illness, self-stigma occurs. If a person with a mental illness does not seek treatment because of fear of being labeled "mentally ill," label avoidance occurs.

- The *DSM-5* organizes psychiatric diagnoses according to behaviors and symptom patterns.

- Cultural syndromes are specific disorders found within a particular locality or culture. There is little research on the syndromes, but *ataque de nervios* and *susto* are well documented.

- Mental health recovery is the single most important goal for the mental health delivery system. Recovery is viewed a process of changes through which individuals improve their health and wellness, live a self-directed life, and strive to reach their full potential.

- Trauma is experienced by many individuals as physically or emotionally harmful or life threatening and has lasting adverse effects on the individual. Trauma-informed care is integral to recovery-oriented care.

CRITICAL THINKING CHALLENGES

1. A person who is seeking help for a mental disorder asks why the individual's physical health is important to the nurse.
2. Compare the meaning of the epidemiologic terms *prevalence*, *incidence*, and *rate*. Access the CDC's website (www.cdc.gov) and identify major mental health problems in the United States.
3. Examine the description of people with mental illness in the media, including television programs, news, and newspapers. Are negative connotations evident?
4. Examine how family and friends describe people with mental illness. Do you think their description of mental illness is based on fact or myth? Explain.
5. Explain the three forms of stigma and give examples.
6. Discuss the negative impact of labeling someone with a psychiatric diagnosis.
7. Using the components of mental health recovery as a framework, compare the goals for a person with schizophrenia with those with a medical disease such as diabetes.
8. Discuss the application of trauma-informed care to a person who has experienced a trauma such as rape or a life-threatening event.

2015: *To Write Love on Her Arms*

This 2015 Substance Abuse and Mental Health Services Administration (SAMHSA) Voice Award winner is a true story that presents a vision of hope, healing, and redemption. Renee, played by Kat Dennings, is a Florida girl living with addiction and mental illness. She has also experienced abuse and is trying to come to grips with that trauma. Renee discovers the value of friendships and courageously embarks on a daunting journey toward recovery.

Viewing Points: Observe the stigma that is associated with having a mental illness. Identify the trauma Renee experienced and how it influences her ability to engage in treatment.

Chapter 1 • Mental Health and Mental Disorders

UNFOLDING PATIENT STORIES FOR UNIT I

Unfolding Patient Stories: Sandra Littlefield • Part 1

Sandra Littlefield is a 36-year-old female with borderline personality disorder. Her history includes several divorces, drug and alcohol abuse, poor impulse control, anxiety, cutting, suicide attempts, prostitution, and jail time. Why could Sandra be subject to stereotypes and bias? Describe the stigma of mental illness and how it can affect her as an inmate, in the community, and with recovery. What actions by Sandra may be influenced by internalizing the perceived stigma people have of her? (Sandra Littlefield's story continues in Unit IV.)

Care for Sandra and other patients in a realistic virtual environment: *vSim for Nursing* (thepoint.lww.com/vSimMental Health). Practice documenting these patients' care in DocuCare (thepoint.lww.com/DocuCareEHR).

Unfolding Patient Stories: Li Na Chen • Part 1

Li Na Chen is a 40-year-old Chinese female diagnosed with major depressive disorder who attempted suicide by drug overdose. She is married with two children, ages 12 and 14. Why is it important for the nurse to conduct a cultural assessment of the client and her family? Describe methods the nurse can use to demonstrate cultural competence and avoid inaccurate assumptions about the Chinese culture. What questions can the nurse ask to assess cultural beliefs, practices, and influences on Li Na's mental illness and family functioning? (Li Na Chen's story continues in Unit V.)

Care for Li Na and other patients in a realistic virtual environment: *vSim for Nursing* (thepoint.lww.com/vSimMental Health). Practice documenting these patients' care in DocuCare (thepoint.lww.com/DocuCareEHR).

REFERENCES

American Nurses Association, American Psychiatric Nurses Association, & International Society of Psychiatric–Mental Health Nurses. (2014). *Psychiatric–mental health nursing: Scope and standards of practice* (2nd ed.). Silver Spring, MD: American Nurses Association.

American Psychiatric Association. (2013). *Diagnostic and statistical manual of mental disorders* (5th ed.). Arlington, VA: Author.

Corrigan, P. W. (2016). Lessons learned from unintended consequences about erasing the stigma of mental illness. *World Psychiatry, 15*(1), 67–73.

Corrigan, P. W., & Al-Khouja, A. (2018). Three agendas for changing the public stigma of mental illness. *Psychiatric Rehabilitation Journal, 41*(1), 1–7.

Davis, R., & Maul, A. (2015). *Trauma-informed care: Opportunities for high-need, high-cost Medicaid population. Brief. Center for Health Care Strategies.* Retrieved August 28, 2018, from https://www.chcs.org/resource/trauma-informed-care-opportunities-high-need-high-cost-medicaid-populations

Durá-Vilá, G., & Hodes, M. (2012). Cross-cultural study of idioms of distress among Spanish nationals and Hispanic American migrants: Susto, nervios and ataque de nervios. *Social Psychiatry and Psychiatric Epidemiology, 47*(10), 1627–1637.

Heiberg, I. H., Jacobsen, B. K., Nesvåg, R., Bramness, J. G., Ted Reichborn-Kjennerud, T., Naess, Ø., et al. (2018). Total and cause-specific standardized mortality ratios in patients with schizophrenia and/or substance use disorder. *PLoS One, 3*(8), e0202028. doi: 10.1371/journal.pone.0202028.

McGinty, E. E., Kennedy-Hendricks, A., Choksy, S., & Barry, C. L. (2016). Trends in news media coverage of mental illness in the United States: 1995–2014. *Health Affairs, 35*(6), 1121–1129.

National Academy of Sciences. (2016). *Ending discrimination against people with mental substance use disorders; the evidence for stigma change.* Washington, DC: National Academies Press.

National Institute of Mental Health. (2019). Mental health information. *Transforming the understanding and treatment of mental illnesses.* Retrieved April 22, 2019, from https://www.nimh.nih.gov/health/statistics/mental-illness.shtml.

U.S. Department of Health and Human Services, Substance Abuse & Mental Health Services Administration (U.S. DHHS, SAMHSA). (2012). *SAMHSA's working definition of recovery updated.* Retrieved June 29, 2018, from https://www.store.samhsa.gov/product/SAMHSA-s-Working-Definition-of-Recovery/PEP12-RECDEF

U.S. Department of Health and Human Services, Substance Abuse & Mental Health Services Administration (U.S. DHHS, SAMHSA). (2014). *SAMHSA's concept of trauma and guidance for trauma-informed approach.* Retrieved from https://store.samhsa.gov/shin/content/SMA14-4884/SMA14-4884.pdf

U.S. Department of Health and Human Services, Substance Abuse & Mental Health Services Administration (U.S. DHHS, SAMHSA). (2018a). *The eight dimensions of wellness.* Retrieved August 25, 2018, from https://www.samhsa.gov/wellness-initiative/eight-dimensions-wellness

U.S. Department of Health and Human Services, Substance Abuse & Mental Health Services Administration (U.S. DHHS, SAMHSA). (2018b). *Health disparities. Wellness initiative.* Retrieved August 25, 2018, from https://www.samhsa.gov/health-disparities

World Health Organization (WHO). (2013a). *Comprehensive mental health action plan 2013–2020. Sixty-six World Health Assembly, Agenda Item 13.3.* Geneva, Switzerland: Author. Updated definition 2014. Retrieved August 25, 2018, from http://www.who.int/features/factfiles/mental_health/en

World Health Organization (WHO). (2013b). *Depression. A hidden burden.* Geneva, Switzerland: Author. Retrieved June 18, 2014, from http://www.who.int/mental_health/management/depression/flyer_depression_2012.pdf?ua=1

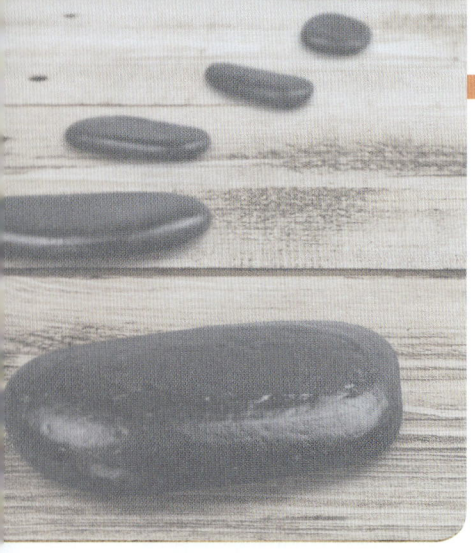

2
Cultural and Spiritual Issues Related to Mental Health Care

Mary Ann Boyd

KEY CONCEPTS
- culture
- cultural competence
- spirituality

LEARNING OBJECTIVES

After studying this chapter, you will be able to:

1. Discuss the ways that cultural competence is demonstrated in psychiatric–mental health nursing.
2. Describe the beliefs about mental health and illness in different cultural and social groups.
3. Differentiate concepts of religiousness and spirituality.
4. Discuss the role of spirituality and religiousness in persons with mental illness.
5. Discuss the beliefs of major religions and their role in shaping views on mental illnesses.

KEY TERMS
- acculturation
- cultural explanations
- cultural identity
- cultural idiom of distress
- linguistic competence
- religiousness

All cultural groups have sets of values, beliefs, and patterns of accepted behavior, and it is often difficult for those of one culture to understand those of another. This is especially true regarding mental illness—whereas some cultures view it as a condition for which the ill person must be punished and ostracized from society, other cultures are more tolerant and believe that family and community members are key to the care and treatment of mentally ill people. Nurses' and patients' religious backgrounds and cultural heritages may be different, so it is important for nurses to understand clearly the thinking and perspectives of other cultures and groups.

This chapter examines cultural and social mores of various cultural and religious groups. Understanding cultural and religious beliefs and the significance of spirituality is especially important when caring for people with mental health problems. These beliefs and practices can define and shape the experience of being mentally ill and influence the willingness to seek care. Treating mental disorders is intertwined with people's attitudes about themselves, their beliefs, values, and ways.

> **KEYCONCEPT Culture** is not only a way of life for people who identify or associate with one another on the basis of some common purpose, need, or similarity of background but also the totality of learned, socially transmitted beliefs, values, and behaviors that emerge from its members' interpersonal transactions. Culture is a term that goes beyond just race or ethnicity. It can also refer to such characteristics as age, gender, sexual orientation, disability, religion, income level, education, geographical location, or profession (U.S. Department of Health and Human Services [U.S. DHHS], 2018).

Cultures are dynamic and continually changing. When immigrants arrive in the United States with their own cultures, they begin to adapt to their new environment. **Acculturation** is the term used to describe the socialization process by which minority groups learn and adopt selective aspects of the dominant culture. Their culture changes because of the influences of the new environment. Eventually, a new minority culture evolves that is different than the native culture and also different from the dominant culture, which in turn is transformed by the new residents.

Everyone has a **cultural identity**, or a set of cultural beliefs with which one looks for standards of behavior. Because culture is broadly defined, many people consider themselves to have multiple cultural identities. Often, the nurse is challenged to provide culturally appropriate care for persons from cultures other than the nurse's culture. Uncertainty about cultural beliefs and practices can result in feelings of anxiety and vulnerability when interacting with patients from other cultures. Patients may interpret the nurse's anxiety as a lack of caring or competence (Markey, Tilki, & Taylor, 2018). It is important to learn and understand each patient's cultural background and identity to provide quality nursing care and avoid miscommunication and knowledge barriers.

CULTURAL AND LINGUISTIC COMPETENCE

Cultural and linguistic competence is especially important for psychiatric–mental health nurses because of the significance of therapeutic communication. There are several definitions of cultural and linguistic competence, but there is a consensus that cultural and linguistic competence involves an adjustment or recognition of one's own culture to understand the culture of another person.

Linguistic competence, the capacity to communicate effectively and convey information that is easily understood by diverse audiences, is an important part of cultural competence (Harris-Haywood et al., 2014). Linguistic competence not only refers to the appropriate use of words, grammar, and syntax, but also practical aspects such as choice of discussion topics, taking turns, use of metaphors, and the "hidden rules" of interactions. The following is an example of a hidden rule: For one patient, it is a cultural expectation for a nurse to sit down and "chit chat" before providing care; for another patient, limited eye contact is best. A nurse who is culturally competent understands and appreciates cultural differences in health care practices and similarities within, among, and between groups.

> **KEYCONCEPT Cultural competence,** the ability to interact effectively with people of different cultures, involves a set of academic and interpersonal skills that are respectful of and responsive to the health beliefs, health care practices, and cultural and linguistic needs of diverse patients to bring about positive health care outcomes (U.S. DHHS, 2018).

Cultural competence can reinforce a person's engagement in treatment, therapeutic relations, and treatment outcomes. It is essential in decreasing disparities in mental health services. There are linguistic variations within cultural groups as well as cultural variations within a language group. Speaking the same language does not guarantee shared meaning and understanding. Communication may be adversely affected when patients are unable to fully express themselves in English. Understanding the impact of literacy levels is integral to providing culturally competent care. Demonstrating an understanding that literacy levels contribute to the interpretation of personal, psychological experiences is critical (Substance Abuse and Mental Health Services Administration [SAMHSA], 2014).

CULTURAL AND SOCIAL FACTORS AND BELIEFS ABOUT MENTAL ILLNESS

Cultural beliefs and practices influence how patients communicate and manifest their symptoms, cope with their illnesses, and receive family and community support. The *DMS-5* differentiates **cultural idiom of distress**, a commonly used term or phrase that describes the suffering within a cultural group from **cultural explanations**, perceived causes for symptoms (American Psychiatric Association [APA], 2013). For example, the term *nervios* is an idiom used by Hispanics in the Western Hemisphere that explains a wide range of somatic and emotional symptoms such as headache, irritability, nervousness, insomnia, and difficulty concentrating. The term *susto* (extreme fright causing the soul to leave the body) is believed to be the cause of a group of varied symptoms including appetite disturbance, sleep problems, and low self-worth among people in Central and South America (see Chapter 1).

Social factors contribute to the development of mental disorders. Ethnic and racial minorities in the United States live in a social environment of inequality that increases their exposure to racism, discrimination, violence, and poverty, which contribute to the experience of their illnesses (SAMSHA, 2014). Racially and ethnically diverse groups are less likely to receive mental health services and more likely to receive poorer quality care. Poverty is found in all cultural groups and is present in other groups, such as older adults, people with physical disabilities, individuals with psychiatric impairments, and single-parent families. In the United States, 28% of people living below the poverty line are single mothers and their children; 37.4% of African Americans live below the poverty level, as do 34.3% of Hispanic Americans and 25.8% of white Americans (Fontenot, Jessica, & Kollar, 2018). Currently in the United States, the poverty guidelines for a family of four is a yearly income of $25,100 or less in the 48 mainland states; $31,380 or less in Alaska; and $28,870 or less in Hawaii (U.S. DHHS, 2018).

Families living in poverty are under tremendous financial and emotional stress, which may trigger or exacerbate mental problems. Along with the daily stressors of trying to provide food and shelter for themselves and their families, their lack of time, energy, and money prevents them from attending to their psychological needs. Often, these families become trapped in a downward economic spiral as tension and stress mount. The inability to gain employment and the lack of financial independence only add to the feelings of powerlessness and low self-esteem. Being self-supporting gives one a feeling of control over life and bolsters self-esteem. Dependence on others or the government causes frustration, anger, apathy, and feelings of depression and meaninglessness. Alcoholism, depression, and child and partner abuse may become a means of coping with such hopelessness and despair. The homeless population is the group most at risk for being unable to escape this spiral of poverty.

Hispanic Americans

The number of Hispanic Americans living in the United States has been gradually increasing, and this group is now the largest minority in the United States, constituting 58.8 million (18% of the total population). Countries of origin include Mexico (62%), Central and South America (15%), Puerto Rico (9%), and Cuba (4%). Hispanic populations are largest in urban areas, such as New York, Chicago, Los Angeles, San Francisco, and Miami–Fort Lauderdale (U.S. Census Bureau, 2017a).

Studies indicate that Hispanic Americans tend to use all other resources before seeking help from mental health professionals. Reasons for this are unclear, but barriers for treatment include beliefs that mental health facilities do not accommodate their cultural needs (e.g., language, beliefs, values), cost of care, availability of services, accessibility of services, and concerns regarding immigration status (Guzman, Woods-Giscombe, & Beeber, 2015; Lee, Laiewski, & Choi, 2014) (see Box 2.1).

BOX 2.1

Cultural Competence and Mental Health

- Learn about the patient's country of origin before assessment.
- Conduct a thorough social and cultural assessment.
- Demonstrate genuine interest in and respect for the individual.
- Educate patients about mental health issues, including available treatments, benefits of obtaining services, and contributions and abilities of individuals with a mental illness.
- Do not assume that all individuals of a racial or ethnic group are the same.
- Being quiet and lack of eye contact may be culturally appropriate and may indicate shyness, not depression or another mental illness.
- Tailor interventions to the individual; one intervention does not work for everyone.

Adapted from Acosta, H. (2009). *Hispanic mental health: Do's and don'ts when working with Hispanics in mental health.*

African Americans

In 2017, the estimated population of African Americans was 41 million, or 12.8% of the US population (U.S. Census Bureau, 2017a). Although African Americans share many beliefs, attitudes, values, and behaviors, there are also many subcultural and individual differences based on social class, country of origin, occupation, religion, educational level, and geographic location. Many African Americans have extensive family networks in which members can be relied on for moral support, help with child rearing, provide financial aid, and help in crises. In many African American families, older members are treated with great respect. But African Americans with mental illness suffer from the stresses of double stigma—not only from their own cultural group but also from longtime racial discrimination. To make matters worse, racial discrimination may come from within the health community itself (Box 2.2).

Several studies show that diagnoses and treatment for African Americans often are racially biased. African Americans are disproportionately diagnosed as having schizophrenia when compared to other groups. This disparity in diagnosis in schizophrenia has been stable over the past three decades. There is some indication

---

BOX 2.2

Research for Best Practice: Influence of Attitude and Stigma on African American and Latino Population

Ripp, A. A., & Carlson, R. G. (2017). Exploring the influence of attitude and stigma on participation of African American and Latino populations in mental health services. Journal of Multicultural Counseling and Development, 45(4), 80–94.

THE QUESTION: How do attitudes and stigma influence help-seeking behavior in African American and Latino community participants?

METHODS: African Americans ($n = 70\%$) and Latino adults ($n = 30\%$) who were receiving mental health services, had previously received treatment, had no experience with mental health, or were involved in the treatment of a loved one comprised the sample of 129 participants who completed surveys online. The average age of the participants was 25 years, with an average income ranging from $10,000 to $29,999 per year. Men represented 69% of the sample. Participants answered queries on three instruments: the Attitude Toward Seeking Professional Psychological Help, Intentions to Seek Counseling Inventory, and Self-Stigma of Seeking Health Scale.

FINDINGS: The findings suggested that positive attitudes about seeking professional help were associated with an intention to seek help and that as stigma increases, there is a decrease in the inclination to seek help.

IMPLICATIONS FOR NURSING: The nurse should consider the impact of stigma on the willingness to seek treatment for mental illness. There is a need for psychoeducation interventions designed to increase openness to psychological problems and reduce stigma.

that using a structured interview (rather than a subjective clinical interview) may reduce this disparity (Olbert, Nagendra, & Buick, 2018).

Asian Americans, Polynesians, and Pacific Islanders

In 2017, more than 18.9 million (5.7% of the US population) Asian Americans, Polynesians, and Pacific Islanders lived in the United States, and this group represents one of the fastest growing minority populations in the United States. This large multicultural group includes Chinese, Filipino, Japanese, Asian Indian, Korean, Vietnamese, Laotian, Cambodian, Hawaiian, Samoan, and Guamanian people. Most Chinese, Japanese, Korean, Asian Indian, and Filipino immigrants have migrated to urban areas; the Vietnamese have settled throughout the United States (U.S. Census Bureau, 2017a).

Generally, Asian cultures have a tradition of denying or disguising the existence of mental illnesses. In many of these cultures, it is an embarrassment to have a family member treated for mental illness, which may explain the extremely low utilization of mental health services. Only 17% of those experiencing problems seek care (Chu, Garcia, Koka, Wynn, & Kao, 2018).

Asian Americans may experience a culture-bound syndrome, such as neurasthenia, which is characterized by fatigue, weakness, poor concentration, memory loss, irritability, aches and pains, and sleep disturbances. Associated with the Korean culture, *hwa-byung*, "suppressed anger syndrome," is characterized by subjective and expressed anger, sensations of heat, and feelings of hate (Irn et al., 2018). Research regarding specific mental health problems in Asian cultures is sparse, but various data suggest that rates of suicide within Native Hawaiian adolescents are higher than those of other adolescents in the United States (American Foundation for Suicide Prevention, 2018).

Native Americans

In 2016, the estimated population of Native Americans was more than 6.7 million people, 2% of the US population (U.S. Census Bureau, 2017b). Native American cultures emphasize respect and reverence for the earth and nature, from which come survival and comprehension of life and one's relationships with a separate, higher spiritual being and with other human beings. Shamans, or medicine men, are central to most cultures. They are healers believed to possess psychic abilities. Healing treatments rely on herbal medicines and healing ceremonies and feasts. Self-understanding derives from an observing nature; relationships with others emphasize interdependence and sharing.

Traditional views about mental illnesses vary among the tribes. In some, mental illness is viewed as a supernatural possession, as being out of balance with nature. In certain Native American groups, people with mental illnesses are stigmatized. However, the degree of stigmatization is not the same for all disorders. In tribal groups that make little distinction between physical and mental illnesses, there is little stigma. In other groups, an event, such as suicide, is stigmatized. Different illnesses may be encountered in different Native American cultures and gene pools.

Arab Americans

The Arab American community includes immigrants and their descendants from several Arab world countries including Syria, Lebanon, Egypt, Palestine, Iraq, Jordan, and Yemen. There are an estimated 3.5 million Arab Americans in the United States with 94% living in metropolitan areas (Detroit, Los Angeles, New York, Chicago, Washington, DC). More than 80% are US citizens. Arab Americans have a strong commitment to family, economic and educational achievements, and making contributions to all aspects of American life. The first wave of Arab immigrants that came to the United States during the 19th and 20th centuries was primarily Christian. Since the 1960s, Muslim Arabs began immigrating in greater numbers to the United States. Most Arab Americans in the United States practice Christianity (Arab American Institute Foundation, 2014).

Mental illness and seeking mental health care are highly stigmatized in all Arab countries. Although there is little research about the views of Arab Americans, there is emerging evidence that stigma toward mental health treatment is preventing individuals from accessing treatment. They are more likely to visit a primary care provider with somatic problems that represent a mental health problem (Dallo et al., 2018; Dardas & Simmons, 2015; Jaber et al., 2015). An additional stressor is discrimination against the Muslim Arab American community, particularly for males (Assari & Lankarani, 2017).

Women of Minority Groups

Women within minority groups may experience more conflicting feelings and psychological stressors than do men in trying to adjust to both their defined role in the minority culture and a different role in the larger predominant society. Stress from acculturation, stigma toward mental illness, and lack of social support contribute to depression among immigrant women (Alhasanat-Khalil et al., 2018). Negative stereotypic attitudes of health care providers may also contribute to reluctance to access mental health care (Kapadia, Nazroo, & Tranmer, 2018).

Rural Cultures

Most mental health services are in urban areas because most people live near cities. Those living in rural areas have limited access to health care which leads to fewer people being diagnosed with a mental health problem. Even though rural residents are less likely than urban residents to have mental health diagnoses or receive mental health care, the suicide rate is higher in the rural areas with firearms most commonly used (Marino, Wolsko, Keys, & Pennavaria, 2016; Stein, Gennuso, Ugboaja, & Remington, 2017). Rural areas are also diverse in both geography and culture. For example, access to mental health for those in the Deep South is different from access for those with the same problems in the Northwest. Treatment approaches may be accepted in one part of the country but not in another. Suicide rates are higher in rural areas when compared to urban areas.

SPIRITUALITY, RELIGION, AND MENTAL ILLNESS

Both spirituality and religion are factors that may influence beliefs about mental illness and impact treatment and recovery.

KEYCONCEPT **Spirituality** develops over time and is a dynamic, conscious process. Although it is not easily defined, there is general agreement that five attributes best describe the essence of spirituality: meaning, belief, connecting, self-transcendence, and value (Stephenson & Berry, 2015).

Meaning involves making sense of life and having a purpose to exist. *Belief* provides a coping mechanism and facilitates hope by having something to have faith in. *Connecting* with a higher power and relationships with family and friends serve as important supports for persons in crisis. *Self-transcendence*, the experience and appreciation of a dimension beyond oneself, facilitates spiritual growth. *Value* identifies objects that have value to the person (Stephenson & Berry, 2015).

Related but different than spirituality, **religiousness** is the participation in a community of people who gather around common ways of worshiping. Spirituality can be expressed through adhering to a set of religious beliefs. Religious beliefs often define an individual's relationship within a family and community. Many different religions are practiced throughout the world. Judeo-Christian thinking tends to dominate Western societies. Other religions, such as Islam, Hinduism, and Buddhism, dominate Eastern and Middle Eastern cultures (Table 2.1). Because

TABLE 2.1 MAJOR WORLD RELIGIONS AND BELIEF FORMS

Source of Power or Force (Deity)	Historical Sacred Texts or Beliefs	Key Beliefs or Ethical Life Philosophy
Buddhism		
Buddha Individual responsibility and logical or intuitive thinking Buddhist subjects include: • *Lamaism* (Tibet), in which Buddhism is blended with spirit worship • *Mantrayana* (Himalayan area, Mongolia, Japan), in which intimate relationship with a guru and recitations of secret mantras are emphasized; belief in sexual symbolism and demons • *Ch'an* (China) *Zen* (Japan), in which self-reliance and awareness through intuitive understanding are stressed • *Satori* (enlightenment) may come from "sudden insight" or through self-discipline, meditation, and instruction	Tripitaka (scripture) Middle Path (way of life) The Four Noble Truths Eightfold Path (guides for life) The Texts of Taoism (include the Tao Te Ching of Lao Tzu and The Writings of Chuang Tzu) Sutras (Buddhist commentaries) Sangha (Buddhist community)	Buddhism attempts to deal with problems of human existence such as suffering and death. Life is misery, unhappiness, and suffering with no ultimate reality in the world or behind it. The cause of all human suffering and misery is desire. The "middle path" of life avoids the personal extremes of self-denial and self-indulgence. Visions can be gained through personal meditation and contemplation; good deeds and compassion also facilitate the process toward nirvana, the ultimate mode of existence. The end of suffering is the extinction of desire and emotion and ultimately the unreal self. Present behavior is a result of past deed.
Christianity		
God, a unity in tripersonality; Father, Son, and Holy Ghost	Bible Teachings of Jesus through the apostles and the church fathers	God's love for all creatures is a basic belief. Salvation is gained by those who have faith and show humility toward God. Brotherly love is emphasized in acts of charity, kindness, and forgiveness.
Confucianism		
No doctrine of a god or gods or life after death Individual responsibility and logical and intuitive thinking	Five Classics (confucian thought) Analects (conversations and sayings of Confucius)	A philosophy or a system of ethics for living rather than a religion that teaches how people should act toward one another. People are born "good." Moral character is stressed through sincerity in personal and public behavior. Respect is shown for parents and figures of authority. Improvement is gained through self-responsibility, introspection, and compassion for others.

TABLE 2.1	MAJOR WORLD RELIGIONS AND BELIEF FORMS *(Continued)*	
Source of Power or Force (Deity)	**Historical Sacred Texts or Beliefs**	**Key Beliefs or Ethical Life Philosophy**
Hinduism Brahma (the Infinite Being and Creator that pervades all reality) Other gods: Vishnu (preserver), Shiva (destroyer), Krishna (love)	Vedas (doctrine and commentaries)	All people are assigned to castes (permanent hereditary orders, each having different privileges in society; each was created from different parts of Brahma): 1. *Brahmans:* include priests and intellectuals 2. *Kshatriyas:* include rulers and soldiers 3. *Vaisyas:* include farmers, skilled workers, and merchants 4. *Sudras:* include those who serve the other three castes (servants, laborers, peasants) 5. *Untouchables:* the outcasts; those not included in the other castes
Islam Allah (the only God) Has two major sects: • *Sunni* (orthodox): traditional and simple practices are followed; human will is determined by outside forces • *Shiite*, practices are rapturous and trancelike; human beings have free will	Koran (the words of God delivered to Mohammed by the angel Gabriel) Hadith (commentaries by Mohammed) Five Pillars of Islam (religious conduct) Islam was built on Christianity and Judaism	God is just and merciful; humans are limited and sinful. God rewards the good and punishes the sinful. Mohammed, through the Koran, guides people and teaches them truth. Peace is gained through submission to Allah. The sinless go to Paradise, and the evil go to Hell. A "good" Muslim obeys the Five Pillars of Islam.
Judaism God	Hebrew Bible (Old Testament) Torah (first five books of the Hebrew Bible) Talmud (commentaries on the Torah)	Jews have a special relationship with God: obeying God's law through ethical behavior and ritual obedience earns the mercy and justice of God. God is worshiped through love, not out of fear.
Shintoism Gods of nature, ancestor worship, national heroes	Tradition and custom (the way of the gods) Beliefs were influenced by Confucianism and Buddhism	Reverence for ancestors and a traditional Japanese way of life are emphasized. Loyalty to places and locations where one lives or works and purity and balance in physical and mental life are major motivators of personal conduct.
Taoism All the forces in nature	Tao Te Ching ("The Way and the Power")	Quiet and happy harmony with nature is the key belief. Peace and contentment are found in the personal behaviors of optimism, passivity, humility, and internal calmness. Humility is an especially valued virtue. Conformity to the rhythm of nature and the universe leads to a simple, natural, and ideal life.
Tribal Beliefs *Animism:* Souls or spirits embodied in all beings and everything in nature (trees, rivers, mountains) *Polytheism:* Many gods, in the basic powers of nature (sun, moon, earth, water)	Passed on through ceremonies, rituals, myths, and legends Oral history, rather than written literature, is the common medium	All living things are related. Respect for powers of nature and pleasing the spirits are fundamental beliefs to meet the basic and practical needs for food, fertility, health, and interpersonal relationships and individual development. Harmonious living is comprehension and respect of natural forces.

Summary of Other Belief Forms
- *Agnosticism:* the belief that whether there is a God and a spiritual world or any ultimate reality is unknown and probably unknowable
- *Atheism:* the belief that no God exists because "God" is defined in any current existing culture of society
- *Maoism:* the faith that is centered in the leadership of the Communist Party and all the people; the major belief goal is to move away from individual personal desires and ambitions toward viewing and serving all people as a whole
- *Scientism:* the belief that values and guidance for living come from scientific knowledge, principles, and practices; systematic study and analysis of life, rather than superstition, lead to true understanding and practice of life.

Adapted from Axelson, J. A., & McGrath, P. (1998, 1993, 1985). *Counseling and development in a multicultural society.* Pacific Grove, CA: Brooks/Cole Publishing Company, a division of International Thomson Publishing, Inc.

BOX 2.3

Research for Best Practice: The Effects of Religiosity and Spirituality on Mental Health

Peres, M. F. P., Kamei, H. H., Tobo, P. R., & Lucchetti, G. (2018). Mechanisms behind religiosity and spirituality's effect on mental health, quality of life and well-being. *Journal of Religion & Health, 57*(5), 1842–1855.

THE QUESTION: What spirituality and religiosity aspects are related to quality of life, well-being, and mental health in a general population?

METHODS: A cross-sectional sample of 967 Brazilians were asked to complete questionnaires related to religiousness, faith–peace–meaning, optimism, life satisfaction, happiness, and quality of life.

FINDINGS: From the sample, 80% completed the survey. Participants had a mean age of 34 years, and 51% were female. All participants were married and had a university-level education. Participants identified as Catholics (43.5%), Protestants (7.4%), Spiritists (5.9%), and no religious affiliation or were atheists/agnostics (15.7%).

Meaning and peace were associated with less depressive symptoms and more physical, psychological, social, and environmental quality of life. Peace was also associated with less perceived stress. Faith was associated with more psychological and social quality of life. Meaning and peace were more strongly associated than religiousness with quality of life, mental health, and less stress. Religiousness participants found greater meaning and peace than nonreligious participants.

IMPLICATIONS FOR NURSING: Helping a person develop meaning and peace supports positive mental health and quality of life.

---

religious beliefs often influence approaches to mental health, it is important to understand the basis of various religions that appear to be growing in the United States. Both religion and spirituality can provide support and strength in dealing with mental illnesses and emotional problems.

People with mental illness benefit from spiritual assessment and interventions (see Chapter 10). Perception of well-being and health in persons with severe mental illness has been positively associated with spirituality and religiousness (Box 2.3). To carry out spiritual interventions, the nurse enters a therapeutic relationship with the patient and uses the self as a therapeutic tool. Examples of spiritual interventions include meditation; guided imagery; and, when appropriate, prayer to connect with inner sources of solace and hope.

SUMMARY OF KEY POINTS

- The term *culture* is defined as a way of life that manifests the learned beliefs, values, and accepted behaviors that are transmitted socially within a specific group. Culture also refers to age, gender, sexual orientation, disability, religion, income level, education, geographical location, or profession.

- Everyone has a cultural identity, which helps define expected behavior.

- Cultural and linguistic competence is based on a set of skills that allows individuals to increase their understanding and appreciation of cultural differences and similarities within, among, and between groups. Cultural competence is demonstrated by valuing the culture beliefs, bridging any language gap, and considering the patient's literacy level when planning and implementing care.

- Mental illnesses are stigmatized in many cultural groups. A variety of cultural and religious beliefs underlie the stigmatization.

- Access to mental health treatment is particularly limited for those living in rural areas or those who live in poverty.

- Spirituality can be a source of strength and support for both the patient with mental illness and the nurse providing the care.

- Religious beliefs are closely intertwined with beliefs about health and mental illness.

CRITICAL THINKING CHALLENGES

1. Assess your cultural competence with groups that have the following heritage: African, Asian, Hispanic, Arabic, and Native American.
2. Compare beliefs about mental illnesses within African and Asian American groups.
3. Compare the access to mental health services in your state or county in rural areas versus urban areas.
4. Discuss the differences between spirituality and religiousness. Is it possible that someone can be spiritual and not religious?
5. Identify the religious groups that are associated with the following sacred texts: Bible, Koran, Vedas, Texts of Taoism, Talmud.

2003: *House of Sand and Fog*

Colonel Massoud Amir Behrani, an Iranian immigrant played by Ben Kingsley, has spent most of his savings trying to enhance his daughter's chances of a good marriage. The rest of his funds were spent at an auction on a repossessed house owned by

Kathy Nicoli (Jennifer Connelly), an emotionally unstable, depressed young woman who failed to pay property taxes. The struggle for the house ensues with tragic results.

Viewing Points: Identify the cultural differences between the Behrani and Nicoli families. Are any cultural stereotypes depicted in the film? Discuss the role of prejudice and discrimination in the outcome of the movie. How did Kathy's mental illness and relationship with the police officer influence the negotiation for the house?

REFERENCES

Alhasanat-Khalil, D., Fry-McComish, J., Dayton, C., Benkert, R., Yarandi, H., & Giurgescu, C. (2018). Acculturative stress and lack of social support predict postpartum depression among U.S. immigrant women of Arabic descent. *Archives of Psychiatric Nursing, 32*(4), 530–535.

American Foundation for Suicide Prevention. (2018). *Suicide statistics*. New York: Author. Retrieved September 21, 2018, from http://www.spanusa.org

American Psychiatric Association. (2013). *Diagnostic and statistical manual of mental disorders, DSM-5* (5th ed.). Arlington, VA: American Psychiatric Association.

Arab American Institute Foundation. (2014). *Who are Arab Americans?* Retrieved September 19, 2018, from www.aaiusa.org/who-are-arab-americans

Assari, S., & Lankarani, M. M. (2017). Discrimination and psychological distress: Gender differences among Arab Americans. *Frontiers in Psychiatry, 8*(23), 1–10.

Chu, K. M., Garcia, S. M. S., Koka, H., Wynn, G. H., & Kao, T. C. (2018). Mental health care utilization and stigma in the military: Comparison of Asian Americans to other racial groups. *Ethnicity and Health*, 1–16. doi: 10.1080/13557858.2018.1494823.

Dallo, F. J., Prabhakar, D., Ruterbusch, J., Schwartz, K., Peterson, E. L., Liu, B., et al. (2018). Screening and follow-up for depression among Arab Americans. *Depression and Anxiety, 35*(12), 1198–1206.

Dardas, L. A., & Simmons, L. A. (2015). The stigma of mental illness in Arab families: A concept analysis. *Journal of Psychiatric and Mental Health Nursing, 22*(9), 668–679.

Fontenot, K., Jessica, S., & Kollar, M. (2018). *Income and poverty in the United States: 2017. U.S. census bureau, current population reports* (pp. 60–263). Washington, DC: U.S. Government Printing Office.

Guzman, E. D., Woods-Giscombe, C. L., & Beeber, L. S. (2015). Barriers and facilitators of Hispanic older adult mental health service utilization in the USA. *Issues in Mental Health Nursing, 36*(1), 11–20.

Harris-Haywood, S., Goode, T., Gao, Y., Smith, K., Bronheim, S., Flocke, S. A., et al. (2014). Psychometric evaluation of a cultural competency assessment instrument for health professionals. *Medical Care, 52*(2), e7–e15. Retrieved September 21, 2018, from www.lww-medicalcare.com

Irn, C. S., Baeg, S., Choi, J. H., Lee, M., Kim, H. J., Chee, I. S., et al. (2017). Comparative analysis of emotional symptoms in elderly Koreans with hwa-byung and depression. *Psychiatry Investigation, 14*(6), 864–870.

Jaber, R. M., Farroukh, M., Ismail, M., Najda, J., Sobh, H., Hammad, A., et al. (2015). Measuring depression and stigma towards depression and mental health treatment among adolescents in an Arab-American community. *International Journal of Culture and Mental Health, 8*(3), 247–254.

Kapadia, D., Nazroo, J., & Tranmer, T. (2018). Ethnic differences in women's use of mental health services: Do social networks plan a role? Findings from a national survey. *Ethnicity & Health, 23*(3), 293–306.

Lee, S., Laiewski, L., & Choi, S. (2014). Racial-ethnic variation in U.S. mental health service use among Latino and Asian non-U.S. citizens. *Psychiatric Services, 65*(1), 68–74.

Marino, E., Wolsko, C., Keys, S. G., & Pennavaria, L. (2016). A culture gap in the United States: Implications for policy on limiting access to firearms for suicidal persons. *Journal of Public Health Policy, 37* (Suppl 1), 110–121.

Markey, K., Tilki, M., & Taylor, G. (2018). Understanding nurses' concerns when caring for patients from diverse cultural and ethnic backgrounds. *Journal of Clinical Nursing, 27*(1-2):e259–e268.

Olbert, C. M., Nagendra, A., & Buick, F. (2018). Meta-analysis of Black vs. white racial disparity in schizophrenia diagnosis in the United States: Do structured assessments attenuate racial disparities? *Journal of Abnormal Psychology, 127*(1), 104–115.

Stein, E. M., Gennuso, K. P., Ugboaja, D. C., & Remington, P. L. (2017). The epidemic of despair among white Americans: Trends in the leading causes of premature death, 1999–2015. *AJPH Rural Health, 107*(10), 1541–1547.

Stephenson, P. S., & Berry, D. M. (2015). Describing spirituality at the end of life. *Western Journal of Nursing Research, 7*(9), 1229–1247.

Substance Abuse and Mental Health Services Administration. (2014). *Improving cultural competence. Treatment Improvement Protocol (TIP) Series No. 59*. HHS Publication No. (SMA) 14–4849. Rockville, MD: Substance Abuse and Mental Health Services Administration.

U.S. Census Bureau. (2017a). *Profile America Facts for Features*. Retrieved September 21, 2018, from https://www.census.gov/content/dam/Census/newsroom/facts-for-features/2017/cb17-ff17.pdf

U.S. Census Bureau. (2017b). *Facts for Features: American Indian and Alaska Native Heritage Month: November 2017*. Retrieved January 11, 2019, from https://www.census.gov/newsroom/facts-for-features/2017/aian-month.html

U.S. Department of Health and Human Services. (2018). The annual update of the HHS poverty guidelines. *Federal Register, 12*(83), 2642. Retrieved September 19, 2018, from https://www.gpo.gov/fdsys/pkg/FR-2018-01-18/pdf/2018-00814.pdf

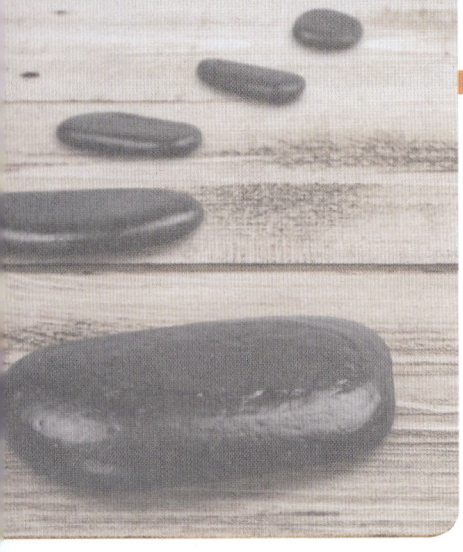

3
Patient Rights and Legal Issues

Rebecca Luebbert

KEY CONCEPT
- self-determinism

LEARNING OBJECTIVES

After studying this chapter, you will be able to:

1. Define self-determinism and its implications in mental health care.
2. Discuss the legal protection of the rights of people with mental illness.
3. Discuss the legal determination of competency.
4. Delineate the differences between voluntary and involuntary treatment.
5. Discuss the difference between privacy and confidentiality.
6. Discuss HIPAA and mandates to inform and their implications in psychiatric–mental health care.
7. Describe the populations with mental illnesses in forensic settings.
8. Discuss the stigma of mental illness and criminality.
9. Describe legal outcomes for persons with mental illness in forensic systems.
10. Identify the importance of accurate, quality documentation in electronic and nonelectronic patient records.

KEY TERMS

- accreditation • advance care directives • assault • breach of confidentiality • chemical restraint • competence • confidentiality • external advocacy system • forensic • incompetent • informed consent • internal rights protection system • involuntary commitment • least restrictive environment • living will • medical battery • negligence • power of attorney • privacy • restraint • seclusion • trauma-informed care • voluntary admission • voluntary commitment

Because individuals with mental disorders are often vulnerable to mistreatment and abuse, their legal rights and the ethical health care practices of mental health providers are ongoing concerns for psychiatric–mental health nurses. For example, can a person be forced into a hospital if his or her behavior is bizarre but harmless? What human rights can be denied to a person who has a mental disorder and under what circumstances? These questions are not easily answered. This chapter summarizes some of the key patient rights and legal issues that underlie psychiatric–mental health nursing practice across the continuum of care.

SELF-DETERMINISM: A FUNDAMENTAL RIGHT AND NEED

At the foundation of many questions related to the rights of mental health patients is the issue of self-determinism and preservation of this right.

KEYCONCEPT Self-determinism is based on a person's fundamental right to autonomy. Exercising this right, patients may choose to "accept, refuse, or terminate treatment without deceit, undue influence, duress, coercion, or prejudice" (American Nurses Association, 2015).

A self-determined individual is internally motivated to make choices based on personal goals, not to please others or to be rewarded. That is, a person engages in activities that are interesting, challenging, pleasing, exciting, or fun, requiring no rewards other than the positive feelings that accompany them because of inner goals, needs, drives, or preferences. Personal autonomy and avoidance of dependence on others are key values of self-determinism, which is integral to the recovery process (see Chapter 1).

In mental health care, self-determinism is the right to choose one's own health-related behaviors, which at times differ from those recommended by health professionals. A patient's right to refuse treatment, to choose an alternate treatment, and to seek a second opinion are all self-deterministic acts. In mental health care, adhering to treatment regimens may be at odds with the self-deterministic views of an individual. Patients may decline taking medication for many reasons, including denial or lack of insight into their illness, concerns about potential side effects or cost of medications, and perceived stigma associated with taking a psychotropic medication (Barloon & Hilliard, 2016). Supporting a person's ability to choose treatment becomes complex because of related issues of competency, **informed consent**, voluntary and **involuntary commitment**, and public safety; these issues are discussed later in this chapter.

PROTECTION OF PATIENT RIGHTS

Because people with psychiatric problems are vulnerable to mistreatment and abuse, laws exist that guarantee them legal protection. These laws offer protection of self-determinism, protection against discrimination in employment, and protection against mistreatment in health care settings.

Self-Determination Act

The *Patient Self-Determination Act* (PSDA) was implemented on December 1, 1991, as a part of the Omnibus Budget Reconciliation Act of 1990 and requires hospitals, health maintenance organizations, skilled nursing facilities, home health agencies, and hospices receiving Medicare and Medicaid reimbursement to inform patients at the time of admission of their right to be a central part of any and all health care decisions made about them or for them. Patients have the following rights:

- Be provided with information regarding advance care documents.
- Be asked at admission or enrollment whether they have an advance care document and that this fact be recorded in the medical record.
- Be provided with information on their rights to complete advance care documents and refuse medical care (Omnibus Budget Reconciliation Act, 1990).

The Act also requires health care institutions receiving Medicare and Medicaid reimbursement to educate health care personnel and the local community about advance care planning.

Advance Care Directives in Mental Health

At different times during the course of an illness, people with mental disorders may be unable to make sound decisions regarding their treatment and care. Fortunately, **advance care directives** legally protect them from their periodic poor decision-making abilities. A competent individual can make a decision about a treatment—a decision that can be honored even if the person is no longer able to make decisions. (See later discussion for how competency is determined.)

Advance care directives are written instructions for health care when individuals are incapacitated. **Living wills** and appointment directives, often referred to as **power of attorney** or health proxies, are recognized under state laws and their courts. A living will specifies what treatment should be omitted or refused in the event that a person is unable to make those decisions. A durable power of attorney for health care appoints a proxy, usually a relative or trusted friend, to make health care decisions on an individual's behalf if that person is incapacitated.

An advance directive does not need to be written, reviewed, or signed by an attorney. It must be witnessed by two people and notarized and applies only if the individual is unable to make his or her own decisions as a result of being incapacitated or if, in the opinion of two physicians, the person is otherwise unable to make decisions for him- or herself.

Psychiatric advance directives (PADs) are relatively new legal instruments and allow patients, while competent, to document their choices of treatment and care. This declaration must be made in advance and signed by the patient and two witnesses. Through the use of a PAD, individuals are empowered to direct their treatment such as choice of medication and hospitalization. Although a physician can override this declaration during times when the patient's decision-making capacity is clearly distorted because of mental illness, the patient must be informed first and the order made by the court. During periods of competency, the PAD can be revoked.

Bill of Rights for Mental Health Patients

Rights of people with mental disorders receive additional protection beyond that afforded to patients in other health care areas (Box 3.1). The *Mental Health Systems*

BOX 3.1

Bill of Rights for Persons Receiving Mental Health Services

- The right to treatment and services under conditions that support the person's personal liberty and restrict such liberty only as necessary to comply with treatment needs, laws, and judicial orders.
- The right to an individualized, written, treatment or service plan (to be developed promptly after admission), treatment based on the plan, periodic review and reassessment of needs, and appropriate revisions of the plan, including a description of services that may be needed after discharge.
- The right to ongoing participation in the planning of services to be provided and in the development and periodic revision of the treatment plan, and the right to be provided with a reasonable explanation of all aspects of one's own condition and treatment.
- The right to refuse treatment, except during an emergency situation, or as permitted under law in the case of a person committed by a court for treatment.
- The right not to participate in experimentation in the absence of the patient's informed, voluntary, written consent, the right to appropriate protections associated with such participation, the right to an opportunity to revoke such consent.
- The right to freedom from restraints or seclusion, other than during an emergency situation.
- The right to a humane treatment environment that affords reasonable protection from harm and appropriate privacy.
- The right to confidentiality of records.
- The right to access, upon request, one's own mental health care records.
- The right (in residential or inpatient care) to converse with others privately and to have access to the telephone and mails unless denial of access is documented as necessary for treatment.
- The right to be informed promptly, in appropriate language and terms, of the rights described in this section.
- The right to assert grievances with respect to infringement of the Bill of Rights, including the right to have such grievances considered in a fair, timely, and impartial procedure.
- The right of access to protection, service, and a qualified advocate in order to understand, exercise, and protect one's rights.
- The right to exercise the rights described in this section without reprisal, including reprisal in the form of denial of any appropriate, available treatment.
- The right to referral as appropriate to other providers of mental health services upon discharge.

From Title V of the Mental Health Systems Act [42 U.S.C. 9501 et seq.]. Retrieved from http://www4.law.cornell.edu/uscode/42/10841.html

---

Act [42 U.S.C. 9501 et seq.] of 1980 requires that each state review and revise, if necessary, its laws to ensure that mental health patients receive these human rights protections and services that they require.

Americans With Disabilities Act and Job Discrimination

The *Americans with Disabilities Act* of 1990 (ADA) ensures that people with disabilities, including those with mental illnesses and addictions, have legal protection against discrimination in the workplace, housing, public programs, transportation, and telecommunications. An employer is free to select the most qualified applicant available, but if the most qualified person has a mental disorder, this law mandates that reasonable accommodations need to be made for that individual. Accommodations are any adjustments to a job or work environment, such as restructuring a job, modifying work schedules, and acquiring or modifying equipment (U.S. Equal Employment Opportunity Commission, Office of the Americans with Disabilities Act, 2018).

Access to Mental Health Services

Mental health services are one of the ten designated Essential Health Benefits requiring coverage through plans established by the Patient Protection and Affordable Care Act. Services required include behavioral health treatment, counseling, and psychotherapy. The Mental Health Parity and Addiction Equity Act (MHPAEA) requires insurance plans to offer benefits and coverage for mental and substance disorders that are comparable to those offered for medical and surgical coverage. Treatment fees and limitations for mental health services cannot be any more restrictive than those designated for medical care (Substance Abuse and Mental Health Services Administration [SAMHSA], 2018).

Internal Rights Protection Systems

Mental health care systems have **internal rights protection systems**, or mechanisms to combat any violation of their patients' rights. *Public Law 99–319, the Protection and Advocacy for Mentally Ill Individuals Act of 1986*, requires each state mental health provider to establish and operate a system that protects and advocates for the rights of individuals with mental illnesses and investigates any incidents of abuse and neglect.

External Advocacy Systems

Health organizations such as the American Hospital Association, American Health Care Association, and the American Public Health Association serve as advocates for the rights and treatment of mental health patients and are a part of an **external advocacy system**. They are financially and administratively independent from the mental health agencies. These groups advocate through negotiation and recommendations but have no legal authority. They can resort to litigation that leads to lawsuits and consent decrees (legal mandates that are monitored by the U.S. Department of Justice) or, in some instances, a denial of **accreditation** to the health care institution by their certifying body.

Accreditation of Mental Health Care Delivery Systems

Patient rights are also assured of protection by an agency's accreditation, the recognition or approval of an institution according to the accrediting body's criteria. Accrediting bodies such as The Joint Commission require patient rights standards. The Centers for Medicare & Medicaid Services (CMS) sets patient rights standards for institutions seeking Medicare and Medicaid funding. Community mental health centers are not accredited by either the Joint Commission or CMS but by another agency, the Commission on Accreditation of Rehabilitation Facilities.

TREATMENT AND PATIENT RIGHTS

In caring for patients receiving mental health services or treatment, it is important for nurses to understand several issues related to the patient's rights to determine choices about his or her own treatment. These issues are related to competency, informed consent, **least restrictive environment**, and voluntary and involuntary treatment.

Competency

One of the most important concepts underlying the legal rights of individuals is competency to consent to or to refuse treatment. Although competency is a legal determination, it is not clearly defined across the states. It is generally agreed that competence, or the degree to which the patient can understand and appreciate the information given during the consent process, refers to a patient's cognitive ability to process information at a specific time. A patient may be competent to make a treatment decision at one time and not be competent at another time. Similarly, **competence** is also decision specific, so that a patient may be competent to decide on a simple treatment with a relatively clear consequence but may not be competent to decide about a treatment with a complex set of outcomes. A competent patient can refuse any aspect of the treatment plan.

Competency is different from rationality, which is a characteristic of a patient's decision, not of the patient's ability to make a decision. An irrational decision is one that involves hurting oneself pointlessly, such as stopping recommended treatment even though symptoms return. A person who is competent may make what appears to be an irrational decision, and it cannot be overruled by health care providers; however, if a person is judged **incompetent** (i.e., unable to understand and appreciate the information given during the consent process), it is possible to force treatment on the individual. Strong arguments are, however, made against forced treatment under these circumstances. Forced treatment denigrates individuals, and according to self-determinism theory and recovery concepts, individuals are not as likely to experience treatment success if it is externally imposed.

How is it determined that a patient is competent? Mental health legal experts generally agree that four areas should be directly assessed (Applebaum, 2007). Table 3.1 outlines these assessment areas. A patient who is competent to give informed consent should be able to achieve the following:

- Communicate choices.
- Understand relevant information.
- Appreciate the situation and its consequences.
- Use a logical thought process to compare the risks and benefits of treatment options.

TABLE 3.1 DETERMINATION OF COMPETENCY		
Assessment Area	**Definition**	**Patient Attributes**
Communicate choices	Ability to express choices	Patient should be able to clearly indicate treatment choice
Understand relevant information	Capacity to comprehend the meaning of the information given about treatment	Patient should be able to paraphrase understanding of treatment
Appreciate the situation and its consequence	Capacity to grasp what the information means specifically to the patient	Patient should be able to discuss the disorder, the need for treatment, the likely outcomes, and the reason the treatment is being suggested
Use a logical thought process to compare the risks and benefits of treatment options	Capacity to reach a logical conclusion consistent with the starting premise	Patient should be able to discuss logical reasons for the choice of treatment

Adapted from Applebaum, P. (2007). Assessment of patients' competence to consent to treatment. *New England Journal of Medicine*, 357(18), 1834–1840.

Informed Consent

Individuals seeking mental health care must provide **informed consent**, a legal procedure to ensure that the patient knows the benefits and costs of treatment. Merely signing a consent document does not imply an informed consent. To provide informed consent for care, the patient must be given adequate information upon which to base decisions and actively participate in the decision-making process. Informed consent is not an option but is mandated by state laws. In most states, the law mandates that a mental health provider must inform a patient in such a way that an average reasonable person would be able to make an educated decision about the interventions.

Informed consent is complicated in mental health treatment. A patient must be competent to give consent, but the individual's decision-making ability often is compromised by the mental illness. This dilemma might be illustrated by a situation in which a person who is informed of medication side effects refuses treatment, not because of the potential negative impact of the medication but because he or she denies the illness outright. The health care provider knows that when the person begins taking the medication, the symptoms of the illness may subside, and the decision-making ability will return.

Most institutions have policies that outline the nursing responsibilities within the informed consent process. The nurse has a key role in the process of informed consent, from structuring the written informed consent document to educating the patient about a particular procedure. The nurse makes sure that consent has been obtained before any treatment is given. Informed consent is especially important in research projects involving experimental drugs or therapies.

Least Restrictive Environment

The right to refuse treatment is related to a larger concept—the right to be treated in the **least restrictive environment**, which means that an individual cannot be restricted to an institution when he or she can be successfully treated in the community. In 1975, the courts ruled that a person committed to psychiatric treatment had a right to be treated in the least restrictive environment (Dixon v. Weinberger, 1975). Medication cannot be given unnecessarily. An individual cannot be restrained or locked in a room unless all other "less restrictive" interventions are tried first.

Seclusion and Restraint

Seclusion is the involuntary confinement of a person in a room or an area where the person is physically prevented from leaving (Centers for Medicare & Medicaid Services [CMS], 2015). A patient is placed in seclusion for purposes

---

BOX 3.2

Research for Best Practice: Evidence for Seclusion and Restraint Use

Sailas, E., & Fenton, M. (2012). Seclusion and restraint for people with serious mental illnesses. The Cochrane Database of Systematic Reviews, 2, CD001163.

THE QUESTION: How effective are seclusion, restraint, or alternative control measures for people with serious mental illness?

METHODS: A meta-analysis of the effectiveness of seclusion and restraint compared with the alternatives for persons with serious mental illnesses was conducted. Randomized controlled trials were included if they focused on the use of restraint or seclusion, or strategies designed to reduce the need for restraint or seclusion, in the treatment of serious mental illness. The search yielded 2,155 citations. Of these, 35 studies were obtained.

FINDINGS: No controlled studies exist that evaluate the effectiveness of seclusion or restraint in those with serious mental illness. There are reports of serious adverse effects for these techniques in qualitative reviews.

IMPLICATIONS FOR NURSING: Alternative ways of dealing with unwanted or harmful behaviors need to be developed. Because of the serious adverse effects reported, continuing use of seclusion or restraint must be questioned.

---

of safety or behavioral management. The seclusion room has no furniture except a mattress and a blanket. The walls are usually padded. The room is environmentally safe, with no hanging devices, electrical outlets, or windows from which the patient could jump. When a patient is placed in seclusion, he or she is observed at all times.

There are several types of seclusion arrangements. Some facilities place seclusion rooms next to the nurses' stations. These seclusion rooms have an observation window. Other facilities use a modified patient room and assign a staff member to view the patient at all times. Seclusion is an extremely negative patient experience; consequently, its use is seriously questioned, and many facilities have completely abandoned its practice (Box 3.2). Patient outcomes may actually be worse if seclusion is used.

The most restrictive safety intervention is the use of **restraint**, which is any manual method, physical or mechanical, that immobilizes or reduces the ability of the patient to move. The nurse must choose the least restrictive type of restraint to keep a patient safe. Wrist restraints restrict arm movement. Walking restraints or ankle restraints are used if a patient cannot risk the impulse to run from a facility but is safe to go outside and to activities. Four-point restraints (two wrists and two ankles) are applied. When five-point restraints are used, all extremities are secured, and another restraint is placed across the chest. **Chemical restraint** is the use of medications for restricting patients' behavior or their freedom of movement. Such restraints include medications that are not a part of their standard psychiatric treatment or that are a higher dosage of their standard medication.

Restraints should be applied only after all other interventions have been used and the patient continues to be a danger to self or others. Documentation must reflect a careful assessment of the patient that indicates the need for an intervention to protect the patient from harm (CMS, 2015). In addition, nurses should document all of the previously tried de-escalation interventions before the application of restraints (see Chapter 14). Restraints should be removed when the patient regains control over his or her behavior. The nurse should closely continuously observe the patient and protect him or her from self-injury while the patient is in seclusion and/or restraints.

There are definite risks associated with the use of seclusion and restraint; consequently, their use is seriously questioned (see Box 3.2). The use of seclusion and restraint can result in psychological harm and physical injury to both the patient and staff members involved in their use. Injury rates to staff in settings involving the use of seclusion and restraint are found to be higher than in other high-risk industries. Additionally, studies have shown that patients who have been secluded or restrained prolong their treatment time and are more likely to be readmitted for further treatment (SAMHSA, 2015).

In recovery-oriented practice, the nurse is particularly sensitive to recognizing the relationship between earlier trauma and retraumatizing a person by using restraint. **Trauma-informed care**–that is, being aware of, and sensitive to, doing no further harm to survivors of trauma–is important in recovery-oriented practice. A trauma-informed approach is characterized by the patient feeling connected, valued, informed, and hopeful of recovery, as well as the staff recognizing the connection between earlier trauma and adult mental health problems, and working in mindful and empowering ways with individuals and families (Muskett, 2014).

The use of both seclusion and restraints must follow the Medicare regulations contained in the Patients' Rights Condition of Participation (CMS, 2015). Agencies that do not follow the regulations may lose their Medicare and Medicaid certification and, consequently, their funding. The application of physical restraints should also follow hospital policies. Fundamental principles for the nurse to follow when considering the use of seclusion and restraints include:

- Seclusion or restraint must never be used out of convenience, as a punishment, or as a means of coercion.
- Seclusion or restraint must only be used as a last resort, when all other least restrictive means are shown to be ineffective.
- Seclusion or restraint must be used for the minimal amount of time necessary to ensure the safety of the patient or others.
- When mechanical restraint is necessary, the fewest number of restraint points must be used, and the individual must be under continuous observation.

(APNA Position Statement on the use of seclusion and restraint, 2018)

Voluntary and Involuntary Treatment

Accessing the mental health delivery system is similar to seeking any other type of health care. Whether in a public or private system, the treatment setting is usually outpatient. Treatment strategies (e.g., medication, psychotherapy) are recommended and agreed on by both the provider and the individual. Arrangements for treatment and follow-up are then made. The patient leaves the outpatient setting and is responsible for following the plan.

Inpatient treatment is generally reserved for patients who are acutely ill or have a **forensic** commitment. If hospitalization is required, the person enters the treatment facility, participates in the treatment planning process, and follows through with the treatment. The individual maintains all civil rights and is free to leave at any time even if it is against medical advice. In most settings, this type of admission is called a **voluntary admission**. If an individual is admitted to a public facility, the state statute may refer to the process as **voluntary commitment** rather than admission; however, in both instances, full legal rights are retained.

Involuntary commitment is the confined hospitalization of a person without the person's consent but with a court order. There are also legal provisions for people to be involuntarily committed to outpatient mental health facilities through state civil laws. Because involuntary commitment is a prerogative of the state agency, each state and the District of Columbia have separate commitment statutes; however, three common elements are found in most of these statutes. There must be evidence that the individual is (1) mentally disordered, (2) dangerous to self or others, or (3) unable to provide for basic needs (i.e., "gravely disabled").

Patients who are involuntarily committed have the right to receive treatment, but they also may have the right to refuse it. Arguments over the rights of civilly committed patients to refuse treatment first surfaced in 1975 when a federal district court judge issued a temporary restraining order prohibiting the use of psychotropic medication against the patient's will at a state hospital in Boston. Today, laws about commitment and refusal of medication vary from state to state. A separate judicial process may be necessary if an individual is determined to be incompetent to refuse medication. Forcing a patient to take medication against his or her will without a legal provision to do so may expose the nurse to liability (Barloon & Hilliard, 2017). Commitment procedures vary considerably among the states. Most have provisions for an emergency short-term hospitalization of 48 to 92 hours authorized by a certified mental health provider without court approval. These emergency hospitalizations are often initiated by a concerned family member or friend. At the end of this time-limited period, the individual either agrees to voluntary treatment or extended commitment procedures are begun. The judge must order the commitment, and the individual is afforded several legal rights, including notice of the proceedings, a full hearing (jury trial if requested) in which the government must prove the grounds for commitment, and the right to legal counsel at state expense.

> **NCLEXNOTE** Which patient is most likely a candidate for involuntary commitment? A patient who refuses to take medication or one who is singing in the street in the middle of the night disturbing the neighbors?
> Answer: The patient who is singing in the night disturbing the neighbors. Rationale: Patients have a right to refuse medication in many states and provinces. Refusing medication does not pose an immediate danger to self or others. The patient who is singing in the street is more likely to be judged as a danger to self or to others.

PRIVACY AND CONFIDENTIALITY

In addition to issues related to self-determinism, privacy and confidentiality are rights that need to be guaranteed and protected for mental health patients. **Privacy** refers to that part of an individual's personal life that is not governed by society's laws and government intrusion. Protecting an individual from intrusion is a responsibility of health care providers. **Confidentiality** pertains to an ethical duty of nondisclosure. Patients often share intimate details of their lives during the course of treatment, including personal thoughts, experiences, and behaviors. Providers who receive confidential information within the nurse–patient relationship must protect that information from being accessed by others and must not disclose it. Confidentiality involves two people: the individual who discloses and the person with whom the information is shared. If confidentiality is broken, a person's privacy is also violated; however, a person's privacy can be violated but confidentiality maintained. For example, if a nurse observes an adult patient reading pornography alone in his or her room, the patient's privacy has been violated. If the patient asks the nurse not to tell anyone and the request is honored, confidentiality is maintained.

A **breach of confidentiality** occurs when a nurse divulges a patient's personal information without the patient's consent. Examples of a breach in confidentiality include discussing a patient's problem with one of his or her relatives without the patient's consent and sharing patient information with another health professional who is not involved in the patient's care when the individual has not given permission for the information to be shared. Maintaining confidentiality is not as easy as it first appears. For example, family members are legally excluded from receiving any information about an adult member without consent even if that member is receiving care from the family. Ideally, a patient gives consent for information to be shared with the family or has psychiatric advance care directive. Ultimately, it is the nurse's duty to safeguard both personal and clinical information in the work setting as well as off duty in all venues, including social media (American Nurses Association, 2015).

HIPAA and Protection of Health Information

The Health Insurance Portability and Accountability Act (HIPAA) of 1996 provides legal protection in several areas of health care, including privacy and confidentiality. This act protects working Americans from losing existing health care coverage when changing jobs and increases opportunities for purchasing health care. It regulates the use and release of patient information, especially electronic transfer of health information. Effective April 2003, HIPAA regulations require patient authorization for the release of information with the exception of that required for treatment, payment, and health care administrative operations. The release of information related to psychotherapy requires patient permission. The underlying intent is to prevent the release of information to agencies not related to health care, such as employers, without the patient's consent. When information is released, the patient must agree to the exact information that is being disclosed, the purpose of disclosure, the recipient of the information, and an expiration date for the disclosure of information (U.S. Department of Health and Human Services, 2002).

The American Recovery and Reinvestment Act of 2009 includes several provisions affecting the management of health information. For the most part, this law focuses on maintaining privacy of electronic transfer and storage of health information and communication. In the clinical area, one way of maintaining privacy is by restricting access to records by staff members unless there is a specific reason such as caring for a patient.

Mandates to Inform

At certain times, health care professionals are legally obligated to breach confidentiality. When there is a judgment that the patient has harmed any person or is about to injure someone, professionals are mandated by law to report it to authorities. The legal "duty to warn" was a result of the 1976 decision of *Tarasoff v. Regents of the University of California*. In this case, a 26-year-old graduate student told university psychologists about his obsession with another student, Tatiana Tarasoff, whom he subsequently killed. Tatiana Tarasoff's parents initiated a separate civil action and brought a lawsuit against the therapist, the university, and the campus police, claiming that Tatiana's death was a result of **negligence** on the part of the defendants.

The plaintiffs claimed that the therapists should have warned Ms. Tarasoff that the graduate student presented a danger to her and that he should have been confined to a hospital. Both claims were originally dismissed in the lower courts, but in 1974, the California Supreme Court reversed the lower courts' decisions and said that Ms. Tarasoff should have been warned. The high court said that psychotherapists have a duty to warn the foreseeable victims of their patients' violent actions. Because of the outcry from professional mental health organizations, the court agreed to review the case, and in 1976, the original decision was revised by the ruling that psychotherapists have a duty to exercise reasonable care in protecting the foreseeable victims of their patients' violent actions. The results of this case have had far-reaching consequences and have influenced many decisions in the United States. Although many lawsuits have been based on the Tarasoff case, most have failed. Usually, if there are clear threats of violence toward others, the therapist is mandated to warn potential victims.

> **NCLEXNOTE** What guides the intervention for a patient who tells the nurse that he (she) wants to hurt a family member: mandate to inform or HIPAA?
> Answer: Mandate to inform. Rationale: Because others are at risk for injury, the Tarasoff decision will prevail.

CRIMINAL JUDICIAL PROCESSES

In mental health, the term **forensic** pertains to legal proceedings and mandated treatment of persons with a mental illness. Individuals with mental illnesses are at higher risk for arrest than the general population and are more likely to have encounters with the criminal justice system and be convicted of a crime than those without a mental illness (Gottfried & Christopher, 2017). Despite the large number of people with mental illnesses that commit crimes, the majority of the encounters with the justice system occur when individuals with mental illness are victims of crime (National Alliance on Mental Illness, 2018).

As the number of state hospitals was dramatically reduced beginning in the 1960s, the number of persons with mental illness incarcerated in jails and prisons increased. Individuals in crisis are more likely to encounter the police versus the mental health care system. Approximately 2 million individuals with mental illness are incarcerated in prisons and jails in the United States per year, including 15% of incarcerated men and 30% of incarcerated women (National Alliance on Mental Illness, 2018). High rates of substance use and substance use disorders are found in incarcerated adults and youth, and among both men and women. The prevalence of PTSD, mood, and anxiety disorders is also higher in incarcerated individuals than in the general population (Gottfried & Christopher, 2017). Individuals with schizophrenia or bipolar disorder are ten times more likely to be in a prison or jail than in a psychiatric treatment facility (Torrey, et al., 2014).

Individuals with mental illnesses are treated in a variety of forensic settings, including county jails, correctional facilities, psychiatric hospitals, and the community. The number of admissions to state psychiatric hospitals is increasing for the first time since the 1970s because of an increase of forensic patients (Torrey et al., 2014). Forensic patients often do not receive sufficient treatment for their illness while they are incarcerated, however, and as a result are at risk for further deterioration and revictimization (Gottfried & Christopher, 2017; National Alliance on Mental Illness, 2018).

Stigma of Criminality

Incarcerated patients suffer the combined effects of the stigma of mental illness and criminality. Although stigma is an issue for all persons with a mental illness, it is magnified for those who have committed a crime. There is often reluctance on the part of mental health professionals to treat these patients, especially if murder and childhood sexual abuse are involved. Even if the worry is unfounded, clinicians express safety concerns for themselves and other patients and may refuse to care for these patients.

When nonforensic patients receive the maximum benefit from hospitalization, they are normally discharged back into the community. For forensic patients, the community often wants a more stringent discharge threshold and unrealistically expects the hospital to guarantee compliance with community rules and structure. Treatment and the criminal justice systems are often in conflict with each other.

Fitness to Stand Trial

After a mental illness is diagnosed in a person who has committed a crime, the individual's **fitness to stand trial** is determined. Fitness means that a person is able to consult with a lawyer with a reasonable degree of rational understanding of the facts of the alleged crime and of the legal proceedings as spelled out in the court case of *Dusky v. United States* of 1960 (Beran & Tommey, 1979, p. 12).

A person is found **unfit to stand trial (UST)** if, because of mental or physical condition, he or she is unable to understand the nature and purpose of the proceedings or to assist in the defense (West, 2017).

In most states, when an individual with a mental illness is found UST, hospitalization in a forensic mental health facility follows. The goal of this hospitalization is to help the person become "fit" to stand trial, not to treat the mental illness. Sometimes the patient's mental illness has to be treated to attain fitness. Simply stated, to be fit to stand trial, the person must be able to communicate with counsel and assist in the defense; be able to appreciate his or her presence in relation to time, place, and things; be able to understand that he or she is in a court of justice charged with a criminal offense; show an understanding of the charges and their consequences, as well as court procedures and the roles of the judge, jury, prosecutor, and defense attorney; and have sufficient memory to relate the circumstances surrounding the alleged criminal offense.

An individual cannot be "unfit" forever. If fitness cannot be attained usually within 1 year, a hearing is held, during which the facts of the alleged crime are presented to a judge who rules on the case. If the charges are dismissed, the judge could order a civil commitment. If there is sufficient evidence to convict, the individual could be sent back to the hospital for further treatment to attain fitness. The maximum length of this additional treatment is based on the severity of the charge. For those accused of sexual-related offenses (because of mental disorder), states usually have special statutes for hospitalization and discharge (e.g., registration and community notification).

Not Guilty by Reason of Insanity

Once fitness to stand trial is established, the trial or hearing can proceed. One possible outcome is **not guilty by reason of insanity (NGRI)**. The accused is judged unable to distinguish right from wrong or to be unable to control his or her actions at the time of the crime. The rationale underlying this ruling is one of fairness. It is unfair to hold a person responsible if that individual does not know that the action is wrong or does not have control over his or her behavior.

Nearly all individuals found NGRI are also subject to involuntary commitment in a "secure" setting. The patient cannot leave hospital grounds without court approval. A person sentenced NGRI is given a date that is equal to the time or sentence to be served if he or she had been guilty of the crime.

Guilty but Mentally Ill

Different from NGRI, in which "not guilty" individuals are committed to the mental health system, **guilty but mentally ill (GBMI)** is a criminal conviction, and the person is sent to the correctional system. Mental illness is considered a factor in the crime but not to the extent that the individual is incapable of knowing right from wrong or controlling their actions. The sentence for the GBMI is the same type of determinate sentence any inmate receives. Before release, every effort is made to ensure that patients will receive proper follow-up care in the community and close monitoring by parole staff. Both NGRI and GBMI persons are treated for their mental disorders, but one is treated in jail and the other in a hospital. The conditions of release are different. Whereas individuals with a GBMI are subject to the correctional system's parole decisions, those with an NGRI are discharged from the hospital through the courts upon recommendations of the forensic mental health professionals.

Probation

Probation is a sentence of conditional or revocable release under the supervision of a probation officer for a specified time. For individuals with a mental illness who have committed minor offenses, probation is sometimes used instead of jail as long as care in a treatment facility can be arranged. If treatment and rehabilitation are successful, criminal charges may be dropped and a prison record avoided. Probation is also used when a criminal has served time and continued monitoring is needed after being released from the correctional facility.

Misconceptions Regarding Insanity Pleas

There are many misconceptions about the insanity plea. One is that the insanity defense provides a loophole through which criminals can escape punishment for illegal acts. In reality, the insanity defense is extremely difficult to use even in the cases of severely ill individuals. As a result, despite popular belief, the insanity defense is used in fewer than 1% of criminal cases (Box 3.3).

Countless newspaper articles, talk shows, and news commentaries concerning the insanity defense have bombarded the public. Some of the cases have been highly publicized. One such case was that of John Hinckley, who attempted to assassinate President Ronald Reagan in 1981 and who was found NGRI. On psychiatric examination, Hinckley was found to be living in a "fantasy world with magical and grandiose expectations of impressing and winning over" his love, actress Jodie Foster (Goldstein, 1995, p. 309). Hinckley attempted to commit a historic deed that would make him famous and unite him with the love object of his delusions. His acquittal stimulated public cries for reform of the insanity defense. Within 2.5 years of John Hinckley's acquittal, 34 states changed their insanity defense statutes to limit their use or to prevent the premature release of dangerous people.

> **BOX 3.3**
>
> **The Case of Andrea Yates**
>
> In March 2002, Andrea Yates, age 37 years, was convicted of murder for drowning her five children. She was sentenced to life in prison despite past treatment for postpartum depression and psychosis, four hospitalizations, and two suicide attempts. Andrea Yates was found guilty because in her testimony to the police, she stated that she knew the criminal justice system would punish her for her actions, implying that she knew the acts were wrong in the eyes of the law. Texas law does not recognize that for someone as ill as Andrea Yates, mental illnesses can create more powerful hierarchies of right and wrong than societal law. In July 2006, Andrea was granted a retrial because the previous verdict was overturned on appeal due to of erroneous testimony. At the second trial, Andrea was found not guilty by reason of insanity. She was committed to a state mental hospital with periodic hearings before a judge to determine whether she should be released (see https://www.biography.com/people/andrea-yates-235801 for more information).

Gun Laws and Mental Illness

The Brady Handgun Violence Prevention Act of 1993, commonly referred to as the Brady Act or Brady Bill, was originally proposed in response to Hinckley's assassination attempt on President Reagan. The Brady Act requires a background check on individuals seeking ownership of a firearm. Under this Act, individuals considered mentally incompetent, having severe mental illness, or those having been committed to a mental institution are prohibited from gun ownership.

There is much controversy surrounding gun control for persons with mental illness. Although the laws are intended to restrict firearms in those determined to be of significant danger to others, the reality is that only a very small percentage of all violent crimes are perpetrated by individuals diagnosed with mental illness. Therefore, insisting that gun violence is strictly a mental health problem unfairly stigmatizes those with mental illness (Philpott-Jones, 2018).

ACCOUNTABILITY FOR NURSES AND OTHER MENTAL HEALTH CARE PROFESSIONALS

Nurses and other health care professionals are accountable for the care they provide in mental health as well as any other practice area.

Legal Liability in Psychiatric Nursing Practice

Malpractice is based on a set of torts (a civil wrong not based on contract committed by one person that causes injury to another). An **assault** is the threat of unlawful force to inflict bodily injury upon another. An assault must be imminent and cause reasonable apprehension in the individual. Battery is the intentional and unpermitted contact with another. **Medical battery**, intentional and unauthorized harmful or offensive contact, occurs when a patient is treated without informed consent. For example, a clinician who fails to obtain consent before performing a procedure is subject to being accused of medical battery. Also, failure to respect a patient's advance directives is considered medical battery. False imprisonment is the detention or imprisonment contrary to provision of the law. Facilities that do not discharge voluntarily committed patients upon request can be subject to this type of litigation.

Negligence is a breach of duty of reasonable care for a patient for whom a nurse is responsible that results in personal injuries. A clinician who does get consent but does not disclose the nature of the procedure and the risks involved is subject to a negligence claim.

> **Concept Mastery Alert**
>
> Five elements are required to prove negligence:
> - Duty (accepting assignment to care for patient)
> - Breach of duty (failure to practice according to acceptable standards of care)
> - Cause in fact (the injury would not have happened if the standards had been followed)
> - Cause in proximity (harm actually occurred within the scope of foreseeable consequence)
> - Damages (physical or emotional injury caused by breach of standard of care)

Simple mistakes are not negligent acts.

Lawsuits in Psychiatric–Mental Health Care

Few lawsuits are filed against mental health clinicians and facilities compared with other health care areas. If psychiatric nurses are included in lawsuits, they are usually included in the lawsuit filed against agency. Common areas of litigation surround the nursing care of patients who are suicidal or violent. Maintaining and documenting an appropriate standard of care can protect nurses from complicated legal proceedings. The following can help prevent negative outcomes of malpractice litigations:

- Evaluate risks, especially when privileges broaden or care is transferred.
- Document decisional processes and reasons for choices among alternatives.
- Involve family in important decisions.
- Make decisions within team model and document this shared responsibility.
- Adhere to agency's policy and procedures.
- Seek consultation and record input.

Nursing Documentation

Careful documentation is important both to help ensure protection of patient rights and for nurse accountability. Documentation can be handwritten or electronic. It is very common in psychiatric facilities that all disciplines record one progress note. Nursing documentation is based on nursing standards (see Chapter 4) and the policies of the particular facility. Many documentation styles are problem focused. That is, documentation is structured to address specific problems that are identified on the nursing care plan or interdisciplinary treatment plan. No matter the setting or structure of the documentation, nurses are responsible for documenting the following:

- Observations of the patient's subjective and objective physical, psychological, and social responses to mental disorders and emotional problems
- Interventions implemented and the patient's response
- Observations of therapeutic and side effects of medications
- Evaluation of outcomes of interventions

Particular attention should be paid to the reason the patient is admitted for care. If the person's initial problem was suicide or homicidal ideation, the patient should routinely be assessed for suicidal and homicidal thoughts even if the treatment plan does not specifically identify suicide and homicide as potential problems. Careful documentation is always needed for patients who are suicidal, homicidal, aggressive, or restrained in any way. Medications prescribed on an as-needed (PRN) basis also require a separate entry, including reason for administration, dosage, route, and response to the medication.

A patient record is the primary documentation of a patient's problems, verifies the behavior of the patient at the point of care, and describes the care provided. The patient record is considered a legal document. Courts consider acts not recorded as acts not done. Patients also have legal access to their records. For handwritten documentation, the entries should always be written in pen with no erasures. If an entry is corrected, it should be initialed by the person making the correction. All entries should be clear, well written, and void of jargon. Judgmental statements, such as "patient is manipulating staff," have no place in patients' records. Only meaningful, accurate, objective descriptions of behavior should be used. General, stereotypic statements, such as "had a good night" or "no complaints" are meaningless and should be avoided.

With the universal use of electronic records, meaningful documentation is sometimes more difficult. Many institutions require health care workers to enter observations, assessment data, and interventions into a template that requires a "click" in a box on the monitor screen. Additional narrative entries are usually required to provide quality, individualized care. Nurses are held to the same standards of practice and documentation when entering electronic data as when entering data a nonelectronic record.

SUMMARY OF KEY POINTS

- The right of self-determination entitles all patients to refuse treatment, to obtain other opinions, and to choose other forms of treatment. It is one of the basic patients' rights established by Title II, Public Law 99–139, outlining the Universal Bill of Rights for Mental Health Patients.

- Laws and systems are established to protect the rights of people with mental health issues. Some of these include the Self-Determination Act, advance directives, a patient Bill of Rights, the ADA, internal rights protection systems, external advocacy systems, and accreditation of mental health care delivery systems.

- The internal rights protection system and the external advocates combat violations of human rights.

- Informed consent is another protective right that helps patients decide what can be done to their bodies and minds. It must be obtained from a competent individual before any treatment is begun to ensure that the information is not only received but understood.

- A competent person can refuse any treatment. Incompetence is determined by the court when the patient cannot understand the information.

- The right to the least restrictive environment entitles patients to be treated in the least restrictive setting and by the least restrictive interventions and protects patients from unnecessary confinement and medication.

- Seclusion or restraint should be used as a last resort and only when there is risk of harm to the patient or someone else. Patients secluded or restrained should be under continuous observation by staff.

- Involuntary commitment procedures are specified at the state level. Patients who are involuntarily committed have the right to refuse treatment and medication.

- Patient privacy is protected through HIPAA regulations related to the transfer and storage of information. A breach in confidentiality is legally mandated when there is a threat of violence toward others.

- There are special legal terms and considerations for individuals who have mental disorders and commit crimes. Those determined to be *UST* are mentally incompetent and unable to understand the proceedings against them or assist in their own defense. These patients are committed to a mental health facility for treatment until they achieve fitness. Those determined to be *NGRI* are those who demonstrate that they had no understanding of their actions and no control over them when they committed the crime. These patients are committed to a mental health facility for treatment and then discharged after treatment.

- *GBMI* applies to those who demonstrate that they knew the wrongfulness of their actions and had the ability to act otherwise. These patients enter the correctional system and receive treatment for their disorder but are returned after treatment to serve their sentences. For mentally disordered sex offenders, states usually have special statutes for hospitalization and discharge. Prisoners who develop mental illness while in prison are transferred to a mental hospital, treated, and returned to prison to complete their sentences.

- The goal for the person in a forensic setting is to coordinate mental health services and to provide a wide range of services that will help him or her successfully live within his or her community.

- Nursing documentation is guided by practice standards and policies of the agency. Nurses are responsible for individualized documentation in both electronic and nonelectronic health records.

CRITICAL THINKING CHALLENGES

1. Consider the relationship of self-determinism to competence by differentiating patients who are competent to give consent and those who are incompetent. Discuss the steps in determining whether a patient is competent to provide informed consent for a treatment.
2. Define competency to consent to or refuse treatment and relate the definition to the Self-Determination Act.
3. A patient is involuntarily admitted to a psychiatric unit and refuses all medication. After being unable to persuade the patient to take prescribed medication, the nurse documents the patient's refusal and notifies the prescriber. Should the nurse attempt to give the medication without patient consent? Support your answer.
4. A person who is homeless with a mental illness refuses any treatment. Although he is clearly psychotic and would benefit from treatment, he is not a danger to himself or others and seems to be able to provide for his basic needs. His family is desperate for him to be treated. What are the ethical issues underlying this situation?
5. Discuss the purposes of living wills and health proxies. Discuss their use in psychiatric–mental health care.
6. Identify the legal and ethical issues underlying the Tarasoff case and mandates to inform.
7. Compare the authority and responsibilities of the internal rights protection system with those of the external advocacy system.
8. Describe the differences between UST, NGRI, and GBMI. What are the criteria to be met by patients who are UST before they are determined to be fit to stand trial?

1987: *Nuts*
Starring Barbra Streisand, Richard Dreyfuss, Maureen Stapleton, Eli Wallach, and Robert Webber. A strong-willed, high-priced prostitute is accused of manslaughter. Her family and attorney want her to plead guilty by reason of insanity. The movie revolves around the family's attempt to have her declared incompetent to stand trial, which would commit her to a mental health center before she can go to trial. She insists on proving her sanity, and to discover the truth, her lawyer must battle his prejudice and her inexplicable belligerence.
Viewing Points: Watch how the family members attempt to use the competency hearings for maintaining family secrets.

REFERENCES

American Nurses Association. (2015). *Code of ethics for nurses with interpretive statements*. Silver Spring, MD: American Nurses Association.

American Psychiatric Nurses Association. (2018). *APNA Position Statement on the use of seclusion and restraint*. Retrieved from https://www.apna.org/i4a/pages/index.cfm?pageid=3728#PositionStatement

Applebaum, P. (2007). Assessment of patients' competence to consent to treatment. *New England Journal of Medicine*, 357(18), 1834–1840.

Barloon, L. F., & Hilliard, W. (2016). Legal considerations of psychiatric nursing practice. *Nursing Clinics of North America*, 51(2), 161–171.

Beran, N. J., & Tommey, B. G. (1979). *Mentally ill offenders and the criminal justice system. In Issues in forensic services* (p. 1–23). New York: Proeger Publishers, Proeger Special Studios.

Brady Handgun Violence Prevention Act of 1993. 18 U.S. Code § 921–922 (Public Law 103–159, 107 Stat. 1536, Nov. 30, 1993).

Centers for Medicare & Medicaid Services. (2015). Interpretive guidelines for hospital CoP for patient rights. *Quality of Care Information, Quality Standards 418.54*. Retrieved April 23, 2019 from https://www.cms.gov/Regulations-and-Guidance/Guidance/Manuals/

Dixon v. Weinberger, 405 F. Supp. 974 (D. D. C. 1975).

Goldstein, R. (1995). Paranoids in the legal system: The litigious paranoid and the paranoid criminal. *Psychiatric Clinics of North America*, 18(2), 303–315.

Gottfried, E. D., & Christopher, S. C. (2017). Mental disorders among criminal offenders: A review of the literature. *Journal of Correctional Health Care*, 23(3), 336–346.

Muskett, C. (2014). Trauma-informed care in inpatient mental health settings: A review of the literature. *International Journal of Mental Health Nursing, 23*(1), 51–59.

National Alliance on Mental Illness. (2018). "Jailing people with mental illness." Retrieved October 14, 2018, from https://www.nami.org/Learn-More/Mental-Health-Public-Policy/Jailing-People-with-Mental-Illness

Omnibus Budget Reconciliation Act of 1990. Public Law No. 101–158, Paragraph 4206, 4751.

Philpott-Jones, S. (2018). Mass shootings, mental illness, and gun control. *Hastings Center Report, 48*(2), 7–9.

Substance Abuse and Mental Health Services Administration (SAMSHA). (2015). *Alternatives to seclusion and restraint*. Retrieved from https://www.samhsa.gov/trauma-violence/seclusion

Substance Abuse and Mental Health Services Administration (SAMSHA). (2018). *Laws, regulations, and guidelines*. Retrieved from https://www.samhsa.gov/about-us/who-we-are/laws-regulations

Tarasoff v. *Regents of the University of California*, 551P. 2d 334 (Cal. 1976).

Torrey, E. F., Zdanowicz, M. T., Kennard, A. D., Lamb, H. R., Eslinger, D. F., Biasotti, M. C., et al. (2014). *The treatment of persons with mental illness in prisons and jails: A state survey*. Arlington, VA: Treatment Advocacy Center. Retrieved October 14, 2018, from http://www.treatmentadvocacycenter.org/storage/documents/treatment-behind-bars/treatment-behind-bars.pdf

U.S. Department of Health and Human Services. (2002). Standards for privacy of individually identifiable health information; final rule. *Federal Register, 65*, 53182–53273.

U.S. Equal Employment Opportunity Commission, Office of the Americans with Disabilities Act. (2018). *The ADA: Your employment rights as an individual with a disability*. Washington, DC: U.S. Government Printing Office. Retrieved from www.eeoc.gov/facts/ada18.html

West, T. (Ed.). (2017). *West's Illinois criminal law and procedure*. Chicago, IL: Thompson Reuters.

UNIT II
PSYCHIATRIC–MENTAL HEALTH NURSING FRAMEWORKS

4
Ethics, Standards, and Nursing Frameworks

Mary Ann Boyd

KEY CONCEPTS
- autonomy
- beneficence
- biopsychosocial framework
- standardized nursing language

LEARNING OBJECTIVES

After studying this chapter, you will be able to:

1. Identify ethical frameworks used in psychiatric nursing practice.
2. Delineate the scope and standards of psychiatric–mental health nursing practice.
3. Discuss the impact of psychiatric–mental health nursing professional organizations on practice.
4. Discuss the relationship of psychiatric–mental health nursing framework to the wellness and recovery models.
5. Discuss the basic tools of psychiatric–mental health nursing.
6. Discuss selected challenges of psychiatric–mental health nursing.

KEY TERMS

- advanced practice psychiatric–mental health registered nurses • clinical reasoning • fidelity • justice • nonmaleficence • nursing process • paternalism • psychiatric–mental health registered nurse • reflection • scope and standards of practice • veracity

This chapter opens with a discussion of the ethical concepts psychiatric nurses use daily. The scope and standards of practice are then highlighted. This chapter explains how a psychiatric–mental health nursing framework relates to the recovery and wellness models. The discussion of the challenges of psychiatric nursing sets the stage for the rest of the text through an overview of the dynamic nature of this specialty.

ETHICS OF PSYCHIATRIC NURSING

Psychiatric–mental health nursing actions are guided by the *Code of Ethics for Nurses with Interpretive Statements* (Box 4.1). The *Code* presents ethical values, obligations, duties and professional ideals, establishes an ethical standard, and confirms nursing's commitment to society. Psychiatric nurses face ethical problematic situations

> **BOX 4.1**
>
> **Code of Ethics for Nurses**
>
> 1. The nurse practices with compassion and respect for the inherent dignity, worth, and unique attributes of every person.
> 2. The nurse's primary commitment is to the patient, whether an individual, family, group, or community.
> 3. The nurse promotes, advocates for, and protects the rights, health, and safety of the patient.
> 4. The nurse has authority, accountability, and responsibility for nursing practice; makes decisions; and takes action consistent with the obligation to promote health and to provide optimal care.
> 5. The nurse owes the same duties to self as to others, including the responsibility to promote health and safety, preserve wholeness of character and integrity, maintain competence, and continue personal and professional growth.
> 6. The nurse, through individual and collective effort, establishes, maintains, and improves the ethical environment of the work setting and conditions of employment that are conducive to safe, quality health care.
> 7. The nurse, in all roles and settings, advances the profession through research and scholarly inquiry, professional standards development, and the generation of both nursing and health policy.
> 8. The nurse collaborates with other health professionals and the public to protect human rights, promote health diplomacy, and reduce health disparities.
> 9. The profession of nursing, collectively through its professional organizations, must articulate nursing values, maintain the integrity of the profession, and integrate principles of social justice into nursing and health policy.
>
> Reprinted with permission from American Nurses Association. (2015). *Code of ethics for nurses with interpretive statements.* Spring, MD: Nursesbooks.org. All rights reserved.

> **BOX 4.2**
>
> **Basic Questions for Ethical Decision Making**
>
> - What do I know about this patient situation?
> - What do I know about the patient's values and moral preferences?
> - What assumptions am I making that need more data to clarify?
> - What are my own feelings (and values) about the situation, and how might they be influencing how I view and respond to this situation?
> - Are my own values in conflict with those of the patient?
> - What else do I need to know about this case, and where can I obtain this information?
> - What can I never know about this case?
> - Given my primary obligation to the patient, what should I do to be ethical?
>
> Reprinted with permission from Davis, A. (2008). Provision two. In M. Fowler (Ed.). *Guide to the code of ethics for nursing: Interpretation and application* (p. 18). Washington, DC: Nursebooks.org.

daily (American Nurses Association [ANA], 2015). To determine the best ethical action, the nurse can reflect on a series of questions, outlined in Box 4.2.

Autonomy and beneficence are fundamental ethical concepts.

> **KEYCONCEPT** According to the principle of **autonomy**, each person has the fundamental right of self-determination. According to the principle of **beneficence**, the health care provider uses knowledge of science and incorporates the art of caring to develop an environment in which individuals achieve their maximal health care potential.

These principles can conflict when the patient is being guided by the principle of autonomy and the nurse by the principle of beneficence. For example, a patient wants to stop taking medication (autonomy), and the nurse urges the patient to continue (beneficence).

> **NCLEXNOTE** Be prepared to think in terms of patient scenarios that depict the principles of beneficence versus autonomy and identify differences between views of the patient and nurse.

Other ethical principles that guide mental health care include justice, nonmaleficence, paternalism, veracity, and fidelity. **Justice** is the duty to treat all fairly, distributing the risks and benefits equally. Justice becomes an issue in mental health when a segment of a population does not have access to health care. Basic goods should be distributed, so that the least advantaged members of society are benefited. **Nonmaleficence** is the duty to cause no harm, both individual and for all. **Paternalism** is the belief that knowledge and education authorize professionals to make decisions for the good of the patient. Mandatory use of seat belts and motorcycle helmets is an example of paternalism. This principle can be in direct conflict with the mental health recovery belief of self-determinism (see Chapters 1 and 7). **Veracity** is the duty to tell the truth. This is easier said than done. Patients may ask questions when the truth is unknown. For example, if I take my medication, will the voices go away? **Fidelity** is faithfulness to obligations and duties. It is keeping promises. Fidelity is important in establishing trusting relationships.

> **NCLEXNOTE** Tracking ethical decisions that the psychiatric nurse encounters in the inpatient versus outpatient setting may be a topic for examination.

SCOPE AND STANDARDS OF PRACTICE

The practice of psychiatric nursing is regulated by law but guided by scope and standards of practice. The legal authority to practice nursing is granted by the states and provinces, but **scope and standards of practice** are defined by the profession of nursing. The ANA and the psychiatric nursing organizations (discussed later in this chapter) collaborate in defining the boundaries of psychiatric–mental health nursing and informing society about the parameters of practice. The standards are authoritative statements that describe the responsibilities for which the practitioners are accountable.

Scope of Psychiatric–Mental Health Nursing Areas of Concern

The areas of concern for the psychiatric–mental health nurse include a wide range of actual and potential mental health problems or psychiatric disorders, such as emotional stress or crisis, self-concept changes, developmental issues, physical symptoms that occur with psychological changes, and symptom management of patients with mental disorders. To understand the problem and select an appropriate intervention, integration of knowledge from the biologic, psychological, and social domains is necessary.

Standards of Practice

Six standards of practice are organized according to the **nursing process** and include assessment, diagnosis, outcome identification, planning, implementation, and evaluation (Box 4.3). The nursing process serves as the foundation for clinical decision-making and provides a framework for nursing practice.

Each of these six standards includes competencies for which **Psychiatric–Mental Health Registered Nurse (PMH-RN)** and **Advanced Practice Psychiatric–Mental Health Registered Nurses** (PMH-APRN) are accountable. The fifth standard, implementation, has several subcategories that define standards for specific interventions. These standards of practice define the parameters of psychiatric–mental health nursing practice. It is important that nurses are prepared to practice according to these standards. Nurses ultimately are held accountable by society for practicing according to their standards.

Standards of Professional Performance

Ten standards of professional performance for psychiatric–mental health nurses follow the six standards of practice. These standards define and inform society about the professional role of psychiatric–mental health nurses and include ethics, education, evidence-based practice and research, quality of practice, communication, leadership, collaboration, professional practice evaluation,

---

BOX 4.3
Standards of Practice

STANDARD 1. ASSESSMENT
The PMH registered nurse collects and synthesizes comprehensive health data that are pertinent to the health care consumer's health and/or situation.

STANDARD 2. DIAGNOSIS
The PMH registered nurse analyzes the assessment data to determine diagnoses, problems, and areas of focus for care and treatment, including level of risk.

STANDARD 3. OUTCOMES IDENTIFICATION
The PMH registered nurse identifies expected outcomes and the health care consumer's goals for a plan individualized to the health care consumer or to the situation.

STANDARD 4. PLANNING
The PMH registered nurse develops a plan that prescribes strategies and alternatives to assist the health care consumer in attainment of expected outcomes.

STANDARD 5. IMPLEMENTATION
The PMH registered nurse implements the specified plan.

Standard 5A. Coordination of Care
The PMH registered nurse coordinates care delivery.

Standard 5B. Health Teaching and Health Promotion
The PMH registered nurse employs strategies to promote health and a safe environment.

Standard 5C. Consultation
The PMH advanced practice registered nurse provides consultation to influence the identified plan, enhance the abilities of other clinicians to provide services for health care consumers, and effect change.

Standard 5D. Prescriptive Authority and Treatment
The PMH advanced practice registered nurse uses prescriptive authority, procedures, referrals, treatments, and therapies in accordance with state and federal laws and regulations.

Standard 5E. Pharmacologic, Biologic, and Integrative Therapies
The PMH advanced practice registered nurse incorporates knowledge of pharmacologic, biologic, and complementary interventions with applied clinical skills to restore the health care consumer's health and prevent further disability.

Standard 5F. Milieu Therapy
The PMH advanced practice registered nurse provides, structures, and maintains a safe, therapeutic, recovery-oriented environment in collaboration with health care consumers, families, and other health care clinicians.

Standard 5G. Therapeutic Relationship and Counseling
The PMH registered nurse uses the therapeutic relationship and counseling interventions to assist health care consumers in their individual recovery journeys by improving and regaining their previous coping abilities, fostering mental health, and preventing mental disorder and disability.

Standard 5H. Psychotherapy
The PMH advanced practice registered nurse conducts individual, couples, group, and family psychotherapy using evidence-based psychotherapeutic frameworks and the nurse–client therapeutic relationship.

STANDARD 6. EVALUATION
The PMH registered nurse evaluates progress toward attainment of expected outcomes.

Reprinted with permission from American Nurses Association, American Psychiatric Nurses Association, & International Society of Psychiatric–Mental Health Nurses. (2014). *Psychiatric–mental health nursing: Scope and standards of practice* (2nd ed.). Silver Spring, MD: Nursesbooks.org.

TABLE 4.1 STANDARDS OF PROFESSIONAL PERFORMANCE

Standard	Area of Performance	Description
Standard 7	Ethics	Integrates ethical provisions in all areas of practice.
Standard 8	Education	Attains knowledge and competency that reflect current nursing practice.
Standard 9	Evidence-based practice and research	Integrates evidence and research findings into practice.
Standard 10	Quality of practice	Systematically enhances the quality and effectiveness of nursing practice.
Standard 11	Communication	Communicates effectively in a variety of formats in all areas of practice.
Standard 12	Leadership	Provides leadership in the professional practice setting and the profession.
Standard 13	Collaboration	Collaborates with the health care consumer, family, interprofessional health team, and others in the conduct of nursing practice.
Standard 14	Professional practice evaluation	Evaluates one's own practice in relation to the professional practice standards and guidelines, relevant statutes, rules, and regulations.
Standard 15	Resource utilization	Considers factors related to safety, effectiveness, cost, and impact on practice in the planning and delivery of nursing services.
Standard 16	Environmental health	Practices in an environmentally safe and healthy manner.

Reprinted with permission from American Nurses Association, American Psychiatric Nurses Association, & International Society of Psychiatric–Mental Health Nurses. (2014). *Psychiatric–mental health nursing: Scope and standards of practice* (2nd ed.). Silver Spring, MD: Nursesbooks.org.

resource utilization, and environmental health. Each standard of performance includes expected competencies (Table 4.1) (American Nurses Association, American Psychiatric Nurses Association, & International Society of Psychiatric–Mental Health Nurses, 2014).

Levels of Practice

There are two levels of psychiatric–mental health nursing practice. The first level is the PMH-RN with educational preparation within a bachelor's degree, associate's degree, or a diploma program. The next level is the PMH-APRN with educational preparation within a master's degree or doctoral degree program. At the PMH-APRN level, two subcategories exist including the mental health clinical nurse specialist (PMH-CNS) and psychiatric–mental health nurse practitioner (PMH-NP) (Box 4.4).

Psychiatric–Mental Health Nursing Practice

According to the *Psychiatric–Mental Health Nursing: Scope and Standards of Practice*, the **psychiatric–mental health nurse** is a registered nurse who demonstrates specialized competence and knowledge, skills, and abilities in caring for persons with mental health issues and problems and psychiatric disorders. Competency is obtained through both education and experience. The preferred educational preparation is at the baccalaureate level with credentialing by the American Nurses Credentialing Center (ANCC) or a recognized certification organization (ANA et al., 2014).

Nursing practice at this level is "characterized by the use of the nursing process to treat people with actual or potential mental health problems, psychiatric disorders and co-occurring psychiatric and substance use disorders" (ANA et al., 2014, p. 25). By using the nursing process, the PMH-RN promotes and fosters health and safety, assesses dysfunction and areas of strength, and assists individuals in achieving personal recovery goals. The nurse performs a wide range of interventions, including health promotion and health maintenance strategies, intake screening and evaluation and triage, case management, milieu therapy, promotion of self-care activities, psychobiologic interventions, complementary interventions, health teaching, counseling, crisis care, and psychiatric rehabilitation. An overview of psychiatric nursing interventions is presented in Unit 3.

BOX 4.4

Clinical Activities of Psychiatric–Mental Health Nurses

PSYCHIATRIC–MENTAL HEALTH REGISTERED NURSE
Health promotion and health maintenance
Intake screening, evaluation, and triage
Case management
Provision of therapeutic and safe environments
Milieu therapy
Promotion of self-care activities
Administration of psychobiologic treatment and monitoring responses
Complementary interventions
Crisis intervention and stabilization
Psychiatric rehabilitation

ADVANCED PRACTICE REGISTERED NURSE
Psychopharmacologic interventions
Psychotherapy
Community interventions
Case management
Program development and management
Clinical supervision
Consultation and liaison

Advanced Practice

The PMH-APRN is also a licensed registered nurse but is educationally prepared at the master's level and is nationally certified as a clinical nurse specialist or a psychiatric nurse practitioner by the ANCC. The doctorate in nursing practice (DNP) requires advanced education in systems function, analysis, and health policy; and advocacy may be at the PMH-RN level (RN administrators or educators) or at the APRN level (ANA et al., 2014). Researchers are prepared at the highest education level preparation with a doctorate in nursing science (DNS, DNSc) or a doctor of philosophy (PhD) degree.

Psychiatric–Mental Health Nursing Organizations

Whereas the establishment and reinforcement of standards go a long way toward legitimizing psychiatric–mental health nursing, professional organizations provide leadership in shaping mental health care. They do so by providing a strong voice for meaningful legislation that promotes quality patient care and advocates for maximal use of nursing skills.

The ANA is one such organization. Although its focus is on addressing the emergent needs of nursing in general, the ANA supports psychiatric–mental health nursing practice through liaison activities, such as advocating for psychiatric–mental health nursing at the national and state levels and working closely with psychiatric–mental health nursing organizations.

The American Psychiatric Nurses Association (APNA) and the International Society of Psychiatric Nursing (ISPN) are two organizations for psychiatric nurses that focus on mental health care. The APNA is the largest psychiatric–mental health nursing organization, with the primary mission of advancing psychiatric–mental health nursing practice; improving mental health care for culturally diverse individuals, families, groups, and communities; and shaping health policy for the delivery of mental health services. The ISPN consists of four specialist divisions: The Association of Child and Adolescent Psychiatric Nurses, International Society of Psychiatric Consultation Liaison Nurses, Society for Education and Research in Psychiatric–Mental Health Nursing, and Adult and Geropsychiatric–Mental Health Nurses. The purpose of ISPN is to unite and strengthen the presence and the voice of psychiatric–mental health nurses and to promote quality care for individuals and families with mental health problems. The International Nurses Society on Addictions (IntNSA) is committed to the prevention, intervention, treatment, and management of addictive disorders. These organizations have annual meetings at which new research is presented. Student memberships are available.

THE BIOPSYCHOSOCIAL FRAMEWORK

The biopsychosocial framework (Fig. 4.1) is a well-recognized, holistic model for organizing patient health care issues. The model delineates interactive domains of an individual's mental health and provides a framework for implementing the nursing process. For example, a nursing assessment can be conducted according to the physical, psychological, and social domains. This model is congruent with the recovery and wellness models and guides recovery-oriented care (see Chapter 1). Standardized nursing languages such as NANDA International/Nursing Interventions Classification (NIC), Nursing Outcomes Classification (NOC), Clinical Care Classification, and the Omaha System can be used with this framework (Butcher, Bulechek, Dochterman, & Wagner, 2018; Kerr et al., 2016; Martin, 2005; Moorhead, Swanson, Johnson, & Maas, 2018; NANDA-I, 2018; Saba, 2018).

> **KEYCONCEPT** The **biopsychosocial framework** consists of three separate but interdependent domains: biologic, psychological, and social. Each domain has an independent knowledge and treatment focus but interacts and is mutually interdependent with the other domains.

Biologic Domain

The *biologic* domain consists of the biologic theories related to mental disorders and problems as well as *all* the biologic activity related to other health problems. Biologic theories and concepts also relate to functional health patterns such as exercise, sleep, and adequate nutrition to mental health conditions. In addition, the

FIGURE 4.1 The biopsychosocial model.

neurobiologic theories also serve as a basis for understanding and administering pharmacologic agents (see Chapters 6 and 11).

Psychological Domain

The *psychological* domain contains the theoretical basis of the psychological processes—thoughts, feelings, and behavior (intrapersonal dynamics) that influence one's emotion, cognition, and behavior. The psychological and nursing sciences generate theories and research that are critical in understanding patients' symptoms and responses to mental disorders. Although there are neurobiologic changes in mental disorders, symptoms are psychological. For example, even though manic behavior is caused by dysfunction in the brain, there are no laboratory tests to confirm a diagnosis, only a pattern of behavior.

Many psychiatric nursing interventions are behavioral, such as cognitive approaches, behavior therapy, and patient education. Therapeutic communication techniques require nurses to develop awareness of their own, as well as their patients' internal feelings and behavior. For mental health nurses, understanding their own and their patients' intrapersonal dynamics and motivation is critical in developing a therapeutic relationship (see Chapter 8).

Social Domain

The *social* domain includes theories that account for the influence of social forces encompassing the patient, family, and community within cultural settings. Social and nursing sciences explain the connections within the family and communities that affect the mental health, treatment, and recovery of people with mental disorders. Psychiatric disorders are not caused by social factors, but their manifestations and treatment can be significantly affected by the society in which the patient lives. Family support can improve treatment outcomes. Moreover, family factors, including origin, extended family, and other significant relationships, contribute to the total understanding and treatment of patients. Community forces, including cultural and ethnic groups within larger communities, shape the patient's manifestation of disorders, response to treatment, and overall view of mental illness.

TOOLS OF PSYCHIATRIC NURSING PRACTICE

Self

The most important tool of psychiatric nursing is the self. Through relationship building, patients learn to trust the nurse who then guides, teaches, and advocates for quality care and treatment. Throughout this book, the patient–nurse relationship is emphasized.

Clinical Reasoning and Reflection

Sound **clinical reasoning** depends on the critical thinking skills and reflection. During critical thinking activities, such as problem solving and decision making, nurses analyze, evaluate, explain, infer, and interpret biopsychosocial data. Some critical thinking activities, such as nursing assessments, take time, but many decisions are moment to moment, such as deciding whether a patient can leave a unit or whether a patient should receive a medication. Clinical reasoning is important in sustaining care (Box 4.5).

Reflection involves continual self-evaluation through observing, monitoring, and judging nursing behaviors with the goal of providing ideal interventions. Reflective skills are used in all aspects of psychiatric nursing practice, from enhancing of self-awareness and examining nurse–patient interactions to evaluation of the system of care.

Interdisciplinary Care

The psychiatric–mental health nurse can expect to collaborate with other professionals and the patient in all settings. In the hospital, a patient may see a psychiatrist or psychiatric nurse practitioner who treats the symptoms

---

BOX 4.5

Research for Best Practices: Practice Development Strategies

Vella, N., Page, L., Edwards, C., & Wand, T. (2017). Sustaining a culture of practice development in an acute adolescent inpatient mental health unit. Journal of Child & Adolescent Psychiatric Nursing, 30(4), 195–200. Retrieved from https://doi.org/10.1111/jcap.12194

THE QUESTION: What processes, people, resources, and relationships enabled the successful implementation, and led to the sustainability, of a practice development program employed in an acute adolescent mental health unit.

METHODS: Following an external review of the unit, a meeting of key stakeholders was convened and subsequently an advisory panel formed to address specific issues facing nursing staff. This process resulted in the development of an educational package and adoption of the tidal model as the framework for mental health nursing practice in the unit. Clinical reasoning sessions and journal article presentations were incorporated to consolidate and maintain the change in nursing care.

FINDINGS: A planned, structured, and inclusive practice development program transformed the nursing culture and vastly improved the care provided to adolescents presenting in acute states of distress to this mental health unit.

IMPLICATIONS FOR NURSING: Nurses can spearhead a process that results in improved culture within a mental health unit by using clinical reasoning and evidence-based research.

and prescribes the medication; a case manager who coordinates care; a psychiatric social worker for individual psychotherapy; a psychiatric nurse for management of responses related to the mental disorder, administration of medication, and monitoring side effects; and an occupational therapist for transition into the workplace. In the community clinic, a patient may meet weekly with a therapist, monthly with a mental health provider who prescribes medication, and twice a week with a group leader in a day treatment program. These professionals bring a specialized skill to the patient's care.

Care Plan

Just like patients in medical–surgical settings, patients receiving psychiatric mental health services have written care plan. The patient and family (if appropriate) should be participants in the development of the plan. If only nursing care is being provided, such as in-home care, a nursing care plan may be used. If other disciplines are providing services to the same patient, which often occurs in a hospital, an interdisciplinary treatment plan may be used with or instead of a traditional nursing care plan. When an interdisciplinary plan is used, components of the nursing care plan should always be easily identified. The nurse provides the care that is judged to be within the scope of practice of the psychiatric–mental health nurse. Thus, the traditional nursing care plan may or may not be used, depending on institutional policies.

Whether a nursing care plan or an interdisciplinary treatment plan is used, these plans are important because they are individualized to a patient's needs. They are sometimes approved by third-party payers who reimburse the cost of the service. In this text, the emphasis is on developing nursing care plans because they serve as a basis of practice and can be included in a multidisciplinary or interdisciplinary individual treatment plan.

CHALLENGES OF PSYCHIATRIC NURSING

The challenges of psychiatric nursing are increasing. New knowledge is being generated, technology is shaping health care into new dimensions, and nursing practice is becoming more specialized and autonomous. This section discusses a few of the challenges.

Knowledge Development, Dissemination, and Application

Knowledge is rapidly expanding in the psychiatric–mental health field. Genetic research has opened a new area of investigation into the etiology of several disorders such as schizophrenia, bipolar disorders, dementia, and autism. Psychoneuroimmunology is investigating the role of the immune system in the development of mental disorders. The presence of comorbid medical disorders gains increasing importance in the treatment of mental disorders. For example, hypertension, hypothyroidism, hyperthyroidism, and diabetes mellitus all affect the treatment of psychiatric disorders. The challenge for psychiatric nurses today is to stay abreast of the advances in total health care to provide safe, competent care to individuals with mental disorders.

Additional challenges for psychiatric nurses include updating their knowledge, so that significant results of studies can be applied to the care of patients. Accessing new information through journals, electronic databases, and continuing education programs takes time and vigilance but provides a sound basis for application of new knowledge.

Overcoming Stigma

Nurses can play an important role in dispelling myths of mental illnesses. Stigma often prevents individuals from seeking help for mental health problems (see Chapter 1). Reducing stigma is every nurse's responsibility, whether or not the nurse practices psychiatric nursing. To reduce the burden of mental illness and improve access to care, nurses can educate all their patients about the etiology, symptoms, and treatment of mental illnesses.

Holistic Nursing Care

There was a time when psychiatric nursing care was viewed as being separate from medical nursing. This is no longer true. Even though the focus is on mental health issues, the psychiatric nurse practices from a holistic perspective and considers the medical and spiritual needs of the patient and their impact on the individual's mental health. The practice of psychiatric nursing is even more challenging as mental health promotion approaches include wellness concepts and approaches.

Health Care Delivery System Challenges

Additional continuing challenges for psychiatric nurses include providing nursing care within integrated community-based services where culturally competent, high-quality nursing care is needed to meet the emerging mental health care needs of patients. In caring for patients who require support from the social welfare system in the form of housing, job opportunities, welfare, and transportation, nurses need to be knowledgeable about these systems. Moreover, in some settings, the nurse may be the only one who has a background in medical disorders, such as human immunodeficiency virus, acquired immunodeficiency syndrome, and other somatic health problems. Assertive community treatment

TABLE 4.2 EXAMPLES OF THE RELATIONSHIP OF THE BIOPSYCHOSOCIAL MODEL TO STRUCTURED NURSING LANGUAGES

Nursing Language	Interventions		
	Biologic	*Psychological*	*Social*
NANDA International, NIC, and NOC *Diagnosis:* Insomnia	Encourage use of sleep medications that do not contain REM sleep suppressors.	Assist to eliminate bedtime stressors.	Regulate environmental stimuli.
Clinical Care Classification (CCC) *Diagnosis:* Sleep pattern disturbance	Care related to improving pattern of sleep.	Teach sleep pattern control.	Manage sleep pattern control.
Omaha System *Diagnosis:* Insomnia	Take medication therapy as prescribed.	Establish routine. Use guided imagery.	Use community resources.

Adapted from NANDA International. (2018). *Nursing diagnoses: Definitions and classification 2018–2020* (11th ed.). Stuttgart, Germany: Thieme; Saba, V. K. (2018). *Clinical Care Classification (CCC) system. A guide to nursing documentation.* New York: Springer Publishing Company; and Martin, K. S. (2005). *The Omaha System: A key to practice, documentation, and information management* (2nd ed.). St. Louis, MO: Elsevier Saunders.

reduces inpatient service use, promotes continuity of outpatient care, and increases the stability of people with serious mental illnesses (see Chapter 10). The nurse is involved in moving the currently fragmented health care system toward one focusing on consumer needs.

Impact of Technology and Electronic Health Records

Technologic advances have an unprecedented impact on the delivery of psychiatric nursing care and present new challenges. With the use of electronic health records, protection of patient confidentiality is more difficult in some ways. Patient records, once stored in remote areas and rarely viewed, are now readily available and easily accessed. Nurses need to be vigilant in maintaining privacy and confidentiality.

Electronic documentation enables nursing terminologies to be standardized and readily available to the nurse. The advantage of a standardized nursing language is improved patient care through better communication among nurses and other disciplines, increased visibility of nursing interventions, enhanced data collection, useful outcome evaluations, and greater adherence to standards of care.

There are several terminology sets being evaluated for use in electronic records (MLB Technologies, Clinovatons, 2017). Table 4.2 provides an example of how some of these standardized languages relate to the biopsychosocial framework. These terminologies vary in their scope of practice and their applicability to psychiatric nursing practice. For example, NANDA International/NIC/NOC is more inclusive of mental health phenomena than the Perioperative Nursing Data Set (PNDS). To be useful in psychiatric nursing, standardized languages must specifically address responses to mental disorders and emotional problems.

> **KEYCONCEPT** A **standardized nursing language** is readily understood by all nurses to describe care. It provides a common means of communication.

Telemedicine is a reality and takes many forms, from communicating with remote sites to completing educational programs. It is important for patients to be given the opportunity to use technology to learn about their disorders and treatment. Because many of the disorders can affect cognitive functioning, it is also important that software programs be developed that can be used by these individuals to facilitate cognitive functioning.

SUMMARY OF KEY POINTS

- Standards for ethical behaviors for professional nurses are set by national professional organizations such as the ANA.

- There are several ethical principles to consider when providing psychiatric nursing care, including autonomy, beneficence, justice, nonmaleficence, paternalism, veracity, and fidelity.

- *Psychiatric–Mental Health Nursing: Scope and Standards of Practice, published in 2014,* establishes the areas of concern, standards of practice according to the nursing process, and standards of professional performance and differentiates between the functions of the basic and advanced practice nurses.

- Several professional nursing organizations provide leadership in shaping mental health care, including the ANA, the APNA, ISPN, and IntNSA.

- The biopsychosocial framework focuses on the three separate but interdependent dimensions of biologic, psychological, and social factors in the assessment and treatment of mental disorders. This comprehensive and holistic approach to mental disorders is the foundation for effective psychiatric–mental health nursing practice and is integrated into recovery and wellness models.

- Nursing care plans and interdisciplinary treatment plans are written plans of care that are developed for each patient. Clinical reasoning skills are needed for developing and revising these tools.

- The psychiatric–mental health nurse interacts with other disciplines and many times acts as a coordinator in the delivery of care. There is always a plan of care for a patient, but it may be a nursing care plan or an individualized treatment plan that includes other disciplines.

- New challenges facing psychiatric nurses are emerging. Interpretation of research findings will assume new importance in the care of individuals with psychiatric disorders. The roles of nurses are expanding as nursing care becomes an established part of the community-based health care delivery system.

CRITICAL THINKING CHALLENGES

1. A 19-year-old patient with schizophrenia announces that he and a 47-year-old patient with bipolar disorder will be married the following week. They ask the nurse to witness the wedding. Discuss which ethical principles may be in conflict.
2. Compare the ethical concepts of *autonomy* and *beneficence*. Focus on the difference between legal consequences and ethical dilemmas.
3. Compare the variety of patients for whom psychiatric–mental health nurses care. Factors to be considered are age, health problems, and social aspects.
4. Visit the ANA's website for a description of the psychiatric–mental health nurse's certification credentials. Compare the basic level functions of a psychiatric nurse with those of the advanced practice psychiatric nurse.
5. Explain the biopsychosocial framework and apply it to the following three clinical examples:
   a. A first-time father is extremely depressed after the birth of his child, who is perfectly healthy.
   b. A child is unable to sleep at night because of terrifying nightmares.
   c. An older woman is resentful of moving into a senior citizen's residence even though the decision was hers.
6. Discuss the purposes of the following organizations in promoting quality mental health care and supporting nursing practice. Visit the organizations' websites for more information.
   a. ANA
   b. APNA
   c. International Society of Psychiatric–Mental Health Nurses
   d. IntNSA

UNFOLDING PATIENT STORIES FOR UNIT II

Unfolding Patient Stories: Linda Waterfall • Part 1

Linda Waterfall, a 48-year-old Native American with an aggressive form of breast cancer, is scheduled for a mastectomy. She is extremely nervous, refusing the preoperative medication, lorazepam, and reconsidering her family's request to meet with tribal healers. How can the code of ethics for nurses be applied to ethical issues identified in this situation? What values and beliefs of a nurse might conflict with Linda's? How does understanding the differences in values influence the nurse's response to Linda's beliefs and inform ethical decision making? (Linda Waterfall's story continues in Unit V.)

Care for Linda and other patients in a realistic virtual environment: **vSim** *for Nursing* (thepoint.lww.com/vSimMentalHealth). Practice documenting these patients' care in DocuCare (thepoint.lww.com/DocuCareEHR).

Unfolding Patient Stories: Randy Adams • Part 1

Randy Adams, a 28-year-old veteran exposed to bomb blasts during combat in the Middle East, has symptoms of posttraumatic stress disorder and neurocognitive problems. How can cognitive-behavioral and social theories be applied to his condition? How does an understanding of psychosocial theories assist the nurse in selecting suitable interventions to promote psychological and social functioning? (Randy Adams' story continues in Unit III.)

Care for Randy and other patients in a realistic virtual environment: **vSim** *for Nursing* (thepoint.lww.com/vSimMentalHealth). Practice documenting these patients' care in DocuCare (thepoint.lww.com/DocuCareEHR).

REFERENCES

American Nurses Association. (2015). *Code of ethics for nurses with interpretive statements*. Silver Spring, MD: Nursesbooks.org.

American Nurses Association, American Psychiatric Nurses Association, & International Society of Psychiatric–Mental Health Nurses. (2014). *Psychiatric–mental health nursing: Scope and standards of practice* (2nd ed.). Silver Spring, MD: Nursesbooks.org.

Butcher, H. K., Bulechek, G. M., Dochterman, J. M., & Wagner, C. M. (Eds.). (2018). *Nursing Interventions Classification (NIC)* (7th ed.). St. Louis: Elsevier.

Davis, A. (2008). Provision two. In M. Fowler (Ed.), *Guide to the code of ethics for nurses: Interpretation and application* (p. 18). Washington, DC: Nursebooks.org.

Kerr, M. J., Flaten, C., Honey, M. L., Gargantua-Aguila Sdel, R., Nahcivan, N. O., Martin, K. S., et al. (2016). Feasibility of using the Omaha System for community-level observations. *Public Health Nursing, 33*(3), 256–263.

Martin, K. S. (2005). *The Omaha System: A key to practice, documentation, and information management* (2nd ed.). St. Louis, MO: Elsevier Saunders.

MLB Technologies, Clinovatons. (2017). *Standard nursing terminologies: A landscape analysis*. The Office of the National Coordinator for Health Information Technology. Retrieved September 24, 2018, from https://www.healthit.gov/sites/default/files/snt_final_05302017.pdf

Moorhead, S., Swanson, E., Johnson, M., & Maas, M. L. (2018). *Nursing Outcomes Classification (NOC)* (6th ed.). St. Louis, MO: Elsevier.

NANDA International. (2018). *Nursing diagnoses: Definitions and classification 2018–2020* (11th ed.). Stuttgart, Germany: Thieme.

Saba, V. K. (2018). Clinical care classification system. Sabacare. Retrieved September 24, 2018, from https://www.sabacare.com/framework

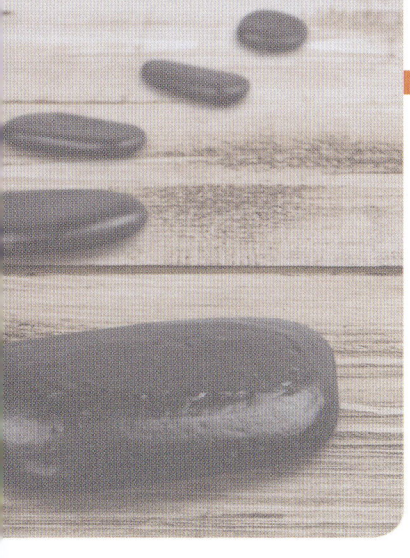

5
Theoretical Basis of Psychiatric Nursing

Mary Ann Boyd

KEY CONCEPTS
- anxiety
- empathic linkage

LEARNING OBJECTIVES

After studying this chapter, you will be able to:

1. Discuss psychosocial theories that support psychiatric nursing practice.
2. Identify the underlying theories that contribute to the understanding of human beings and behavior.
3. Compare the key elements of each theory that provides a basis for psychiatric–mental health nursing practice.
4. Identify common nursing theoretic models used in psychiatric–mental health nursing.

KEY TERMS

- behaviorism • classical conditioning • cognitions • cognitive theory • connections • countertransference • defense mechanisms • disconnections • empathy • family dynamics • formal support systems • informal support systems • interpersonal relations • libido • modeling • object relations • operant behavior • psychoanalysis • self-efficacy • self-system • social distance • transaction • transference • unconditional positive regard

This chapter presents an overview of selected psychodynamic, cognitive-behavioral, developmental, social, and nursing theories that serve as the knowledge base for psychiatric–mental health nursing practice. Many of these theories are covered in more depth in other chapters. Biologic theories are discussed in Chapters 6 and 11.

PSYCHODYNAMIC THEORIES

Psychodynamic theories explain the development of mental or emotional processes and their effects on behavior and relationships. Many of the psychodynamic concepts and models that are important in psychiatric nursing began with the Austrian physician Sigmund Freud (1856–1939). Since his time, Freud's theories have been enhanced by interpersonal and humanist models. These theories proved to be especially important in the development of therapeutic relationships, techniques, and interventions (Table 5.1).

Psychoanalytic Theory

In Freud's psychoanalytic model, the human mind is conceptualized in terms of conscious mental processes (an awareness of events, thoughts, and feelings with the ability to recall them) and unconscious mental processes (thoughts and feelings that are outside awareness and are not remembered).

Study of the Unconscious

Freud believed that the unconscious part of the human mind is only rarely recognized by the conscious, as in remembered dreams (see Movies at the end of this chapter). The term *preconscious* is used to describe unconscious material that is capable of entering consciousness.

TABLE 5.1	PSYCHODYNAMIC MODELS		
Theorist	**Overview**	**Major Concepts**	**Applicability**
Psychoanalytic Models			
Sigmund Freud (1856–1939)	Founder of psychoanalysis Believed that the unconscious could be accessed through dreams and free association Developed a personality theory and theory of infantile sexuality	Id, ego, superego Consciousness Unconscious mental processes Libido Object relations Anxiety and defense mechanisms Free associations, transference, and countertransference	Individual therapy approach used for enhancement of personal maturity and personal growth
Anna Freud (1895–1982)	Application of ego psychology to psychoanalytic treatment and child analysis with emphasis on the adaptive function of defense mechanisms	Refinement of concepts of anxiety, defense mechanisms	Individual therapy, childhood psychoanalysis
Neo-Freudian Models			
Alfred Adler (1870–1937)	First defected from Freud Founded the school of individual psychology	Inferiority	Added to the understanding of human motivation
Carl Gustav Jung (1875–1961)	After separating from Freud, founded the school of psychoanalytic psychology Developed new therapeutic approaches	Redefined libido Introversion Extroversion Persona	Personalities are often assessed on the introversion and extroversion dimensions
Otto Rank (1884–1939)	Introduced the idea of primary trauma of birth Active technique of therapy, including more nurturing than Freud Emphasized feeling aspect of analytic process	Birth trauma Will	Recognized the importance of feelings within psychoanalysis
Erich Fromm (1900–1980)	Emphasized the relationship of the individual to society	Society and individual are not separate	Individual desires are formed by society
Melanie Klein (1882–1960)	Devised play therapy techniques Believed that complex unconscious fantasies existed in children younger than 6 months of age Principal source of anxiety arose from the threat to existence posed by the death instinct	Pioneer in object relations Identification	Developed different ways of applying psychoanalysis to children; influenced present-day English and American schools of child psychiatry
Karen Horney (1885–1952)	Opposed Freud's theory of castration complex in women and his emphasis on the oedipal complex Argued that neurosis was influenced by the society in which one lived	Situational neurosis Character	Beginning of feminist analysis of psychoanalytic thought
Interpersonal Relations			
Harry Stack Sullivan (1892–1949)	Impulses and striving need to be understood in terms of interpersonal situations	Participant observer Parataxic distortion Consensual validation	Provided the framework for the introduction of the interpersonal theories in nursing
Humanist Theories			
Abraham Maslow (1908–1970)	Concerned himself with healthy rather than sick people Approached individuals from a holistic-dynamic viewpoint	Needs Motivation	Used as a model to understand how people are motivated and needs that should be met
Frederick S. Perls (1893–1970)	Awareness of emotion, physical state, and repressed needs would enhance the ability to deal with emotional problems	Reality Here-and-now	Used as a therapeutic approach to resolve current life problems that are influenced by old, unresolved emotional problems
Carl Rogers (1902–1987)	Based theory on the view of human potential for goodness Used the term *client* rather than *patient* Stressed the relationship between therapist and client	Empathy Positive regard	Individual therapy approach that involves never giving advice and always clarifying client's feelings

Personality and Its Development

Freud's personality structure consists of three parts: the id, ego, and superego (Freud, 1927). The *id* is formed by unconscious desires, primitive instincts, and unstructured drives, including sexual and aggressive tendencies that arise from the body. The *ego* consists of the sum of certain mental mechanisms, such as perception, memory, and motor control, as well as specific defense mechanisms (discussed below). The ego controls movement, perception, and contact with reality. The capacity to form mutually satisfying relationships is a fundamental function of the ego, which is not present at birth but is formed throughout the child's development. The *superego* is that part of the personality structure associated with ethics, standards, and self-criticism. A child's identification with important and esteemed people in early life, particularly parents, helps form the superego.

Object Relations and Identification

Freud introduced the concept of **object relations**, the psychological attachment to another person or object. He believed that the choice of a sexual partner in adulthood and the nature of that relationship depended on the quality of the child's object relationships during the early formative years.

The child's first love object is the mother, who is the source of nourishment and the provider of pleasure. Gradually, as the child separates from the mother, the nature of this initial attachment influences future relationships. The development of the child's capacity for relationships with others progresses from a state of narcissism to social relationships, first within the family and then within the larger community. Although the concept of object relations is fairly abstract, it can be understood in terms of a child who imitates her mother and then becomes like her mother in adulthood. This child incorporates her mother as a love object, identifies with her, and grows up to become like her. This process is especially important in understanding an abused child who, under certain circumstances, becomes an adult abuser.

Anxiety and Defense Mechanisms

For Freud, anxiety is the reaction to danger and is experienced as a specific state of physical unpleasantness. **Defense mechanisms** are coping styles that protect a person from unwanted anxiety. Although they are defined differently than in Freud's day, defense mechanisms still play an explanatory role in contemporary psychiatric–mental health practice. Defense mechanisms are discussed in the chapter on Communication and the Therapeutic Relationship (Chapters 8 and 9).

Sexuality

The energy or psychic drive associated with the sexual instinct, or **libido**, literally translated from Latin to mean "pleasure" or "lust," resides in the id. When sexual desire is controlled and not expressed, tension results and is transformed into anxiety (Freud, 1905). Freud believed that adult sexuality is an end product of a complex process of development that begins in early childhood and involves a variety of body functions or areas (oral, anal, and genital zones) that correspond to stages of relationships, especially with parents.

Psychoanalysis

Freud developed **psychoanalysis**, a therapeutic process of accessing the unconscious conflicts that originate in childhood and then resolving the issues with a mature adult mind. As a system of psychotherapy, psychoanalysis attempts to reconstruct the personality by examining free associations (spontaneous, uncensored verbalizations of whatever comes to mind) and the interpretation of dreams. Therapeutic relationships had their beginnings within the psychoanalytic framework.

Transference and Countertransference

Transference is the displacement of thoughts, feelings, and behaviors originally associated with significant others from childhood onto a person in a current therapeutic relationship (Moore & Fine, 1990). For example, a woman's feelings toward her parents as a child may be directed toward the therapist. If a woman were unconsciously angry with her parents, she may feel unexplainable anger and hostility toward her therapist. In psychoanalysis, the therapist uses transference as a therapeutic tool to help the patient understand emotional problems and their origin.

Countertransference, on the other hand, is defined as the direction of all of the therapist's feelings and attitudes toward the patient. Countertransference becomes a problem when these feelings and perceptions are based on other interpersonal experiences. For example, a patient may remind a nurse of a beloved grandmother. Instead of therapeutically interacting with the patient from an objective perspective, the nurse feels an unexplained attachment to her and treats the patient as if she were the nurse's grandmother. The nurse misses important assessment and intervention data.

Neo-Freudian Models

Many of Freud's followers ultimately broke away, establishing their own forms of psychoanalysis. Freud did not receive criticism well. The rejection of some of his basic tenets often cost his friendship as well. Various psychoanalytic schools have adopted other names because their doctrines deviated from freudian theory.

Adler's Foundation for Individual Psychology

Alfred Adler (1870–1937), a Viennese psychiatrist and founder of the school of individual psychology, was a student of Freud's who believed that the motivating force in human life is an intolerable sense of inferiority. Some people try to avoid these feelings by developing an unreasonable desire for power and dominance. This compensatory mechanism can get out of hand, and these individuals become self-centered and neurotic, overcompensate, and retreat from the real world and its problems.

Today, Adler's theories and principles are adapted and applied to both psychotherapy and education. Adlerian theory is based on principles of mutual respect, choice, responsibility, consequences, and belonging.

Jung's Analytical Psychology

One of Freud's earliest students, Carl Gustav Jung (1875–1961), a Swiss psychoanalyst, created a model called analytical psychology. Jung believed in the existence of two basically different types of personalities: extroverted and introverted. Whereas extroverted people tend to be generally interested in other people and objects of the external world, introverted people are more interested in themselves and their internal environment. According to Jung, both extroverted and introverted tendencies exist in everyone, but the libido usually channels itself mainly in one direction or the other. He also developed the concept of *persona*—what a person appears to be to others in contrast to who he or she really is (Jung, 1966).

Horney's Feminine Psychology

Karen Horney (1885–1952), a German American psychiatrist, challenged many of Freud's basic concepts and introduced principles of feminine psychology. Recognizing a male bias in psychoanalysis, Horney was the first to challenge the traditional psychoanalytic belief that women felt disadvantaged because of their genital organs. Freud believed that women felt inferior to men because their bodies were less completely equipped, a theory he described as "penis envy." Horney rejected this concept, as well as the oedipal complex, arguing that there are significant cultural reasons why women may strive to obtain qualities or privileges that are defined by a society as being masculine. For example, in Horney's time, most women did not have access to a university education, the right to vote, or economic independence. She argued that women truly were at a disadvantage because of the paternalistic culture in which they lived (Horney, 1939).

Other Neo-Freudian Theories

Otto Rank: Birth Trauma

Otto Rank (1884–1939), an Austrian psychologist and psychotherapist, was also one of Freud's students. He attributed all neurotic disturbances to the primary trauma of birth. For Rank, human development is a progression from complete dependence on the mother and family to physical independence coupled with intellectual dependence on society and finally to complete intellectual and psychological emancipation. A person's will guides and organizes the integration of self.

Erich Fromm: Societal Needs

Erich Fromm (1900–1980), an American psychoanalyst, focused on the relationship of society and the individual. He argued that individual and societal needs are not separate and opposing forces; their relationship is determined by the historic background of the culture. Fromm also believed that the needs and desires of individuals are largely formed by their society. For Fromm, the fundamental purpose of psychoanalysis and psychology is to bring harmony and understanding between the individual and society (Fromm-Rieichmann, 1950).

Melanie Klein: Play Therapy

Melanie Klein (1882–1960), an Austrian psychoanalyst, devised play therapy techniques to demonstrate how a child's interaction with toys reveals earlier infantile fantasies and anxieties. She believed that complex, unconscious fantasies exist in children younger than 6 months of age. She is generally acknowledged as a pioneer in presenting an object relations viewpoint to the psychodynamic field, introducing the idea of early identification, a defense mechanism by which one patterns oneself after another person, such as a parent (Klein, 1963).

Harry Stack Sullivan: Interpersonal Forces

Interpersonal theories stress the importance of human relationships; instincts and drives are less important. Harry Stack Sullivan (1892–1949), an American psychiatrist, viewed **interpersonal relations** as a basis of human development and behavior. He believed that the health or sickness of one's personality is determined by the characteristic patterns in which one deals with other people. For example, one man is passive aggressive to everyone who contradicts him. This maladaptive behavior began when he was unable to express his disagreement to his parents. Health depends managing the constantly changing physical, social, and interpersonal environment as well as past and current life experiences (Sullivan, 1953).

Humanistic Theories

Humanistic theories are based on the belief that all human beings have the potential for goodness. Humanist therapists focus on patients' ability to learn about and accept themselves. They do not investigate repressed memories. Through therapy, patients explore personal capabilities in order to develop self-worth. They learn to experience the world in a different way.

Rogers' Client-Centered Therapy

Carl Rogers (1902–1987), an American psychologist, introduced client-centered therapy. **Empathy**, the capacity to assume the internal reference of the client in order to perceive the world in the same way as the client, is used in the therapeutic process (Rogers, 1980). The counselor is genuine but nondirect and also uses **unconditional positive regard**, a nonjudgmental caring for the client. In this therapy, the counselor's attitude and nonverbal communication are crucial. The therapist's emotional investment (i.e., true caring) in the client is essential in the therapeutic process (Rogers, 1980).

Gestalt Therapy

Another humanistic approach is Gestalt therapy, developed by Frederick S. (Fritz) Perls (1893–1970), a German-born former psychoanalyst who immigrated to the United States. Perls believed the root of human anxiety is frustration with inability to express natural biologic and psychological desires in modern civilization. The repression of these basic desires causes anxiety. In Gestalt therapy, these unmet needs are brought into awareness through individual and group exercises (Perls, 1969).

Abraham Maslow's Hierarchy of Needs

Abraham Maslow's (1921–1970) hierarchy of needs is fixture in social science and nursing (Maslow, 1970) (Fig. 5.1). In nursing, Maslow's model is used to prioritize care. Basic needs (food, shelter) should be met before higher-level needs (self-esteem) can be met.

Applicability of Psychodynamic Theories to Psychiatric–Mental Health Nursing

Several psychodynamic concepts are important in the practice of psychiatric–mental health nursing, such as interpersonal relationships, defense mechanisms, transference, countertransference, and internal objects. In particular, a therapeutic interpersonal relationship is a core of psychiatric–mental health nursing intervention

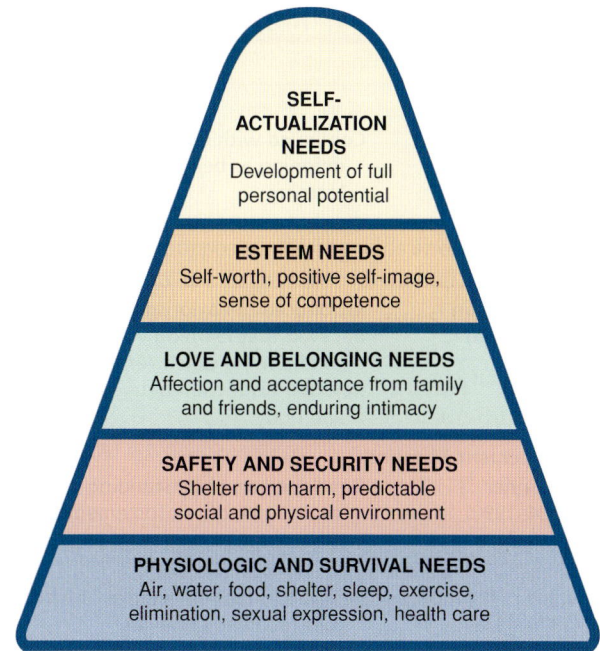

FIGURE 5.1 Maslow's hierarchy of needs.

(see Chapter 10 for nursing interventions). Even though there is general consensus that most of these theories are useful, the nurse should continue to critically analyze them for utility and relevance. For example, Maslow's theory may be useful when a person with mental illness is homeless and wants food and shelter. But, another person in a similar situation may reject food and shelter because self-esteem is associated with being free to reject the confines of an institution. In this case, self-esteem need is more important than food or shelter.

Recently, there is renewed interest in psychodynamic treatment for depression. Psychodynamic therapists have a strong emphasis on affect and emotional expression, examination of topics that the patient avoids, recurring patterns of behaviors, feelings, experiences and relationships, the past and its influence on the present, interpersonal relationships, and exploration of wishes, dreams, and fantasies (Soares et al., 2018).

COGNITIVE-BEHAVIORAL THEORIES

Behavioral Theories

Behavioral theories attempt to explain how people learn and act. Behavioral theories never attempt to explain the cause of mental disorders; instead, they focus on normal human behavior. Research results are then applied to the clinical situation. Two areas of behavioral theories relevant to psychiatric–nursing practice are stimulus–response theories and reinforcement theories (Table 5.2).

TABLE 5.2 BEHAVIORAL THEORISTS

Theorist	Overview	Major Concepts	Applicability
Stimulus–Response			
Edwin R. Guthrie (1886–1959)	Continued with understanding conditioning as being important in learning	Recurrence of responses tends to follow a specific stimulus	Important in analyzing habitual behavior
Ivan P. Pavlov (1849–1936)	Classical conditioning	Unconditioned stimuli Unconditioned response Conditioned stimuli	Important in understanding learning of automatic responses such as habitual behaviors
John B. Watson (1878–1958)	Introduced behaviorism Believed that learning was classical conditioning called *reflexes* Rejected distinction between mind and body	Principle of frequency Principle of recency	Focuses on the relationship between the mind and body
Reinforcement Theories			
B. F. Skinner (1904–1990)	Developed an understanding of the importance of reinforcement and differentiated types and schedules	Operant behavior Respondent behavior Continuous reinforcement Intermittent reinforcement	Important in behavior modification
Edward L. Thorndike (1874–1949)	Believed in the importance of effects that followed behavior	Reinforcement	Important in behavior modification programs

Early Stimulus–Response Theories

Pavlovian Theory

One of the earliest behavioral theorists was Ivan P. Pavlov (1849–1936), who noticed that stomach secretions of dogs were stimulated by triggers other than food reaching the stomach. He found that the sight and smell of food triggered stomach secretions, and he became interested in this anticipatory secretion. Through his experiments, he was able to stimulate secretions with a variety of other laboratory nonphysiologic stimuli. Thus, a clear connection was made between thought processes and physiologic responses.

In Pavlov's model, there is an unconditioned stimulus (not dependent on previous training) that elicits an unconditioned (i.e., specific) response. In his experiments, meat is the unconditioned stimulus, and salivation is the unconditioned response. Pavlov taught the dog to associate a bell (conditioned stimulus) with the meat (unconditioned stimulus) by repeatedly ringing the bell before presenting the meat. Eventually, the dog salivated when he heard the bell. This phenomenon is called **classical conditioning** (or pavlovian conditioning) (Pavlov, 1927/1960).

John B. Watson and the Behaviorist Revolution

At about the same time Pavlov was working in Russia, **behaviorism**, a learning theory that only focuses on objectively observable behaviors and discounts any independent activities of the mind, was introduced in the United States by John B. Watson (1878–1958). He rejected the distinction between body and mind and emphasized the study of objective behavior (Watson & Rayner, 1920). He developed two principles: frequency and recency. The *principle of frequency* states that the more often a response is made to a stimulus, the more likely the response to that stimulus will be repeated. The *principle of recency* states that the closer in time a response is to a particular stimulus, the more likely the response will be repeated.

Reinforcement Theories

Edward L. Thorndike

A pioneer in experimental animal psychology, Edwin L. Thorndike (1874–1949) studied the problem-solving behavior of cats to determine whether animals solved problems by reasoning or instinct. He found that neither choice was completely correct; animals gradually learn the correct response by "stamping in" the stimulus–response connection. The major difference between Thorndike and behaviorists such as Watson was that Thorndike believed that reinforcement of positive behavior was important in learning. He was the first reinforcement theorist, and his view of learning became the dominant view in American learning theory (Thorndike, 1906).

B. F. Skinner

One of the most influential behaviorists, B. F. Skinner (1904–1990), studied **operant behavior** or conditioning. In this type of learning, the focus is on the consequence of the behavioral response, not a specific stimulus.

If a behavior is reinforced or rewarded with success, praise, money, and so on, the behavior will probably be repeated. For example, if a child climbs on a chair, reaches the faucet, and is able to get a drink of water successfully, it is more likely that the child will repeat the behavior (Skinner, 1935). If a behavior does not have a positive outcome, it is less likely that the behavior will be repeated. Nurses use this knowledge to create behavior management plans to reinforce healthy, positive behaviors.

Cognitive Theories

The initial behavioral studies focused on human actions without much attention to the internal thinking process. When complex behaviors could not be accounted for by strictly behavioral explanations, thought processes became new subjects for study. **Cognitive theory**, an outgrowth of different theoretic perspectives, including the behavioral and the psychodynamic, attempted to link internal thought processes with human behavior (Table 5.3).

Albert Bandura's Social Cognitive Theory

Learning by watching others is the basis of Albert Bandura's (b. 1925) social cognitive theory. He developed his ideas after being concerned about television violence contributing to aggression in children. He showed learning occurs by internalizing behaviors of others through a process of **modeling** called pervasive imitation, or one person trying to be like another. The model does not have to be a real person but could be a character in history or generalized to an ideal person (Bandura, 1977, 1986).

An important concept of Bandura's is **self-efficacy**, a person's sense of his or her ability to deal effectively with the environment (Bandura, 1993). Efficacy beliefs influence how people feel, think, motivate themselves, and behave. The stronger the self-efficacy, the higher the goals people set for themselves and the firmer their commitment to them (McIntosh, 2003; Shin, Yun, Pender, & Jang, 2005).

One of Bandura's recent contributions is showing that intentions and self-motivation play roles in determining behavior, significantly expanding the reinforcement model. He believes that the human mind is not only reactive to a stimulus but is also creative, proactive, and reflective (Bandura, 2001).

Aaron Beck: Thinking and Feeling

American psychiatrist Aaron T. Beck (b. 1921) of the University of Pennsylvania devoted his career to understanding the relationship between cognition and mental health. For Beck, **cognitions** are verbal or pictorial events in the stream of consciousness. He realized the importance of cognitions when treating people with depression. He found that depression improved when patients began viewing themselves and situations in a positive light.

He believes that people with depression have faulty information-processing systems that lead to biased cognitions. These faulty beliefs cause errors in judgment that become habitual errors in thinking. These individuals incorrectly interpret life situations, judge themselves too harshly, and jump to inaccurate negative conclusions. A person may truly believe that he or she has no friends, and therefore no one cares. On examination, the evidence for the beliefs is based on the fact that there has been no contact with anyone because of moving from one city to another. Thus, a distorted belief is the basis of the cognition. Beliefs are important because they are related to a person's mood. For example, negative beliefs of caregivers of family members with Alzheimer disorder are related to depression (see Box 5.1). Beck continue to develop cognitive therapy, a successful approach for the treatment of depression (Beck, 2005).

Applicability of Cognitive-Behavioral Theories to Psychiatric–Mental Health Nursing

Basing interventions on behavioral theories is widespread in psychiatric nursing. For example, patient education interventions are usually derived from the behavioral

TABLE 5.3	COGNITIVE THEORISTS		
Theorist	Overview	Major Concepts	Applicability
Aaron Beck (b. 1921)	Conceptualized distorted cognitions as a basis for depression	Cognitions Beliefs	Important in cognitive therapy
Kurt Lewin (1890–1947)	Developed field theory, a system for understanding learning, motivation, personality, and social behavior	Life space Positive valences	Important in understanding motivation for changing behavior
Edward Chace Tolman (1886–1959)	Introduced the concept of cognitions: believed that human beings act on beliefs and attitudes and strive toward goals	Negative valences Cognition	Important in identifying person's beliefs

> **BOX 5.1**
>
> **Research for Best Practice: Caregiver Beliefs and Depression**
>
> Crano, C., Lucidi, F., & Violani, C. (2017). The relationship between caregiving self-efficacy and depressive symptoms in family caregivers of patients with Alzheimer disease: a longitudinal study. *International Psychogeriatrics, 29*(7), 1095–1103.
>
> **THE QUESTION:** Is there an association between caregiver's beliefs and depression?
>
> **METHODS:** A three-wave design was used with initial assessment and follow-ups 3 months later and 1 year later. One hundred and seventy caregivers of patients with AD responded to measures of caregiver burden, caregiving self-efficacy (including control over upsetting beliefs about caregiving), and depressive symptoms.
>
> **FINDINGS:** The caregiving burden at the time of the first assessment influenced the severity of depression 1 year later. The depressive symptoms were less severe when the caregivers believed that they had control over their upsetting thoughts about caregiving.
>
> **IMPLICATIONS FOR NURSING:** Interventions that target caregivers' negative thoughts about the caregiving role may help them in coping with their situation.

theories. Teaching patients new coping skills for their symptoms of mental illnesses is another example. Changing an entrenched habit involves helping patients identify what motivates them and how these new lifestyle habits can become permanent. In psychiatric units, behavioral interventions include the privilege systems and token economies. Behavioral approaches are discussed throughout this text.

DEVELOPMENTAL THEORIES

Developmental theories explain normal human growth and development over time. Many developmental theories are presented in terms of stages based on the assumption that normal development proceeds longitudinally from the beginning to the ending stage.

Erik Erikson: Psychosocial Development

Freud and Sullivan both published treatises on stages of human development, but Erik Erikson (1902–1994) outlined the psychosocial developmental model that is most often used in nursing. Erikson's model is an expansion of Freud's psychosexual development theory. Whereas Freud's model emphasizes intrapsychic experiences, Erikson's recognizes the role of the psychosocial environment. For example, parental divorce disrupts the family interaction pattern, and the financial and housing environment impact the development of the children.

Each of Erikson's eight stages are organized by age and developmental conflicts: basic trust versus mistrust, autonomy versus shame and doubt, initiative versus guilt, industry versus inferiority, identity versus role diffusion, intimacy versus isolation, generativity versus stagnation, and ego integrity versus despair. Successful resolution of a conflict or crisis leads to essential strength and virtues (Table 5.4). For example, a positive outcome of the trust versus mistrust crisis is the development of a basic sense of trust. If the crisis is unsuccessfully resolved, the infant moves into the next stage without a sense of trust. According to this model, a child who is mistrustful will have difficulty completing the next crisis successfully and, instead of developing a sense of autonomy, will more likely be full of shame and doubt (Erikson, 1963).

Identity and Adolescence

One of Erikson's major contributions is the recognition of the turbulence of adolescence and identity formation. When adolescence begins, childhood ways are given up, and bodily changes occur. An identity is formed. Trying to reconcile a personal view of self with society's perception can be overwhelming and lead to role confusion and alienation (Erikson, 1968).

Research Evidence for Erikson's Models

Evidence is mixed that every person follows the eight stages of development as outlined by Erikson. In an early

TABLE 5.4 ERIKSON'S EIGHT AGES OF MAN

Approximate Chronologic Age	Developmental Conflict[a]	Long-Term Outcome of Successful Resolution
Infant	Basic trust vs. mistrust	Drive and hope
Toddler	Autonomy vs. shame and doubt	Self-control and willpower
Preschool-aged child	Initiative vs. guilt	Direction and purpose
School-aged child	Industry vs. inferiority	Method and competence
Adolescence	Identity vs. role diffusion	Devotion and fidelity
Young adult	Intimacy vs. isolation	Affiliation and love
Adulthood	Generativity vs. stagnation	Production and care
Maturity	Ego integrity vs. despair	Renunciation and wisdom

[a]Successful outcome is evidenced by the development of the characteristic listed first.
Adapted from Erikson, E. (1963). *Childhood and society* (pp. 273–274). New York: Norton.

study, male college students who measured low on identity also scored low on intimacy ratings (Orlofsky, Marcia, & Lesser, 1973). These results lend support to the idea that identity precedes intimacy. In another study, intimacy was found to begin developing early in adolescence before the development of identity (Ochse & Plug, 1986). Studying fathers with young children, Christiansen and Palkovitz (1998) found that *generativity* (defined as the need or drive to produce, create, or effect a change) was associated with a paternal identity, psychosocial identity, and psychosocial intimacy. In addition, fathers who had a religious identification also had higher generativity scores than did others.

A longitudinal study of 86 men beginning at age 21 years with reassessment 32 years later at age 53 years supports Erikson's psychosocial eight-stage model (Westermeyer, 2004). In this study, 48 men (56%) achieved generativity at follow-up. Successful young adults as predicted by Erikson's model at midlife lived within a warm family environment; had an absence of troubled parental discipline; experienced a mentor relationship; and, most importantly, had favorable peer group relationships.

Erikson's model may apply differently to men and women. In one study, generativity is associated with well-being in both men and women, but in men, generativity is related to the urge for self-protection, self-assertion, self-expansion, and mastery. In women, the antecedents may be the desire for contact, connection, and union (Ackerman, Zuroff, & Moskowitz, 2000).

Studies show that generativity is significantly associated with successful marriage, work achievements, close friendships, altruistic behaviors, and overall mental health. Generativity is also associated with optimism and forgiveness in dealing with grandparenting problems within the family (Ehlman & Ligon, 2012; Pratt, Norris, Cressman, Lawford, & Hebblethwaite, 2008) and contemplating the meaning of life to older adults (Jonsén, Norberg, & Lundman, 2015).

Jean Piaget: Learning in Children

One of the most influential people in child psychology is Jean Piaget (1896–1980), who contributed more than 40 books and 100 articles on child psychology alone. Piaget's theory views intelligence as an adaptation to the environment. He proposes that cognitive growth is like embryologic growth: An organized structure becomes more and more differentiated over time. Piaget's system explains how knowledge develops and changes (Table 5.5).

Each stage of cognitive development represents a particular structure with major characteristics. Piaget's

TABLE 5.5 PIAGET'S PERIODS OF INTELLECTUAL DEVELOPMENT

Age (years)	Period	Cognitive-Developmental Characteristics	Description
Birth to 2	Sensorimotor	Divided into six stages, characterized by (1) inborn motor and sensory reflexes, (2) primary circular reaction and first habit, (3) secondary circular reaction, (4) use of familiar means to obtain ends, (5) tertiary circular reaction and discovery through active experimentation, and (6) insight and object permanence	The infant understands the world in terms of overt, physical action on that world. The infant moves from simple reflexes through several steps to an organized set of schemes. Significant concepts are developed, including space, time, and causality. Above all, during this period, the child develops the scheme of the permanent object.
2–7	Preoperational	Deferred imitation; symbolic play, graphic imagery (drawing); mental imagery; and language. Egocentrism, rigidity of thought, semilogical reasoning, and limited social cognition	Child no longer only makes perceptual and motor adjustment to objects and events. Child can now use symbols (mental images, words, gestures) to represent these objects and events; uses these symbols in an increasingly organized and logical fashion.
7–11	Concrete operations	Conservation of quantity, weight, volume, length, and time based on reversibility by inversion or reciprocity; operations: class inclusion and seriation	Conservation is the understanding of what values remain the same. For example, if liquid is poured from a short, wide glass into a tall, narrow one, the preoperational child thinks that the quantity has changed. For the concrete operation child, the amount stays the same.
11 through the end of adolescence	Formal operations	Combination system whereby variables are isolated and all possible combinations are examined; hypothetical–deductive thinking	Mental operations are applied to objects and events. The child classifies, orders, and reverses them. Hypotheses can be generated from these concrete operations.

theory was developed through observation of his own children and therefore never received formal testing.

The major strength of his model is its recognition of the central role of cognition in development and the discovery of surprising features of young children's thinking. For example, children in middle childhood become capable of considering more than one aspect of an object or situation at a time. Their thinking becomes more complex. They can understand that the area of a rectangle is determined by the length *and* width. For psychiatric–mental health nurses, Piaget's model provides a framework to recognize different levels of thinking in the assessment and intervention processes. For example, the assessment of concrete thinking is typical of some people with schizophrenia who are unable to perform abstract thinking.

Carol Gilligan: Gender Differentiation in Moral Development

Carol Gilligan (b. 1936) argues that most development models are male centered and therefore inappropriate for girls and women. She challenges Erik Erikson (psychosocial development) and Kohlberg's (moral) theories as being biased against women because they are based on primarily privileged, white men and boys. For Gilligan, attachment within relationships is the important factor for successful development. After comparing male and female personality development, she highlights differences (Gilligan, 2004). In developing identity, boys separate from their mothers, and girls attach. Girls probably learn to value relationships and become interdependent at an earlier age. They learn to value the ideal of care, begin to respond to human need, and want to take care of the world by sustaining attachments so no one is left alone. Her model of moral development, *Ethic of Care*, is divided into three stages beginning with *preconventional* or selfishness (what is best for me) to *conventional* or responsibility to others (self-sacrifice is goodness) to *postconventional* or do not hurt others or self (she is a person too) (Gilligan, 2011).

Gilligan's conclusion that female development depends on relationships has implications for everyone who provides care to women. Traditional models that advocate separation as the primary goal of human development immediately place women at a disadvantage. By negating the value and importance of attachments within relationships, the natural development of women is impaired. If Erikson's model is applied to women, their failure to separate then becomes defined as a developmental failure (Gilligan, 1982).

Jean Baker Miller: A Sense of Connection

Jean Baker Miller (1927–2006) conceptualized female development within the context of experiences and relationships. Her landmark book, *Toward a New Psychology of Women* (1976/1986), led to the development of the relational–cultural theory, which identified a sense of connection as the central organizing feature of women's development. The goal of development is to increase a woman's ability to build and enlarge mutually enhancing relationships (Miller, 1994). **Connections** (mutually responsive and enhancing relationships) lead to mutual engagement (attention), empathy, and empowerment. In relationships in which everyone interacts beneficially, mutual psychological development can occur. **Disconnections** (lack of mutually responsive and enhancing relationships) occur when a child or adult expresses a feeling or explains an experience and does not receive any response from others. The most serious types of disconnection arise from the lack of response that occurs after abuse or attacks. The theory is currently evolving and serves as a model for psychotherapy and nursing practice on psychiatric units (Kress, Haiyasoso, Zoldan, Headley, & Trepal, 2018; Walker & Rosen, 2004).

Applicability of Developmental Theories to Psychiatric–Mental Health Nursing

Developmental theories are used in understanding childhood and adolescent experiences and their manifestations as adult problems. When working with children, nurses can use developmental models to help gauge development and mood. However, because most of the models are based on the assumptions of the linear progression of stages and have not been adequately tested, applicability has limitations. Most do not account for gender differences and diversity in lifestyles and cultures.

SOCIAL THEORIES

Numerous social theories underlie psychiatric–mental health nursing practice. Chapter 2 presents some of the sociocultural issues and discusses various social groups. This section represents a sampling of important social theories that a nurse uses. This discussion is not exhaustive and should be viewed by the student as including a few of the important social theoretic perspectives.

Family Dynamics

Family dynamics are the patterned interpersonal and social interactions that occur within the family structure over the life of a family. Family dynamics models are based on systems theory in which the change of one part affects the total functioning of the system. The family is viewed organizationally as an open system in which one member's actions influence the functioning of the total system. Family theories are especially useful to nurses who are assessing family dynamics and planning interventions. Family systems models are used to help nurses form collaborative relationships with patients and families dealing with health problems. Generalist psychiatric–mental health nurses will not be engaged in family therapy. However, they will be caring for individuals and families. Understanding family dynamics is important in every nurse's practice.

Formal and Informal Social Support

Assisting patients in the recovery process means helping patients identify supportive family and community systems. **Formal support systems** are large organizations, such as hospitals and nursing homes that provide care to individuals. **Informal support systems** are family, friends, and neighbors. Individuals with strong informal support networks actually live longer than those without this type of support. Adolescents who are survivors of sexual assault are more likely to seek support from informal support systems than formal supports (Fehler-Cabral & Campbell, 2013). In addition, classic studies showed that those without informal support have significantly higher mortality rates when the causes of death are accidents (e.g., smoking in bed) or suicides (Litwak, 1985).

An important concept is **social distance**, the degree to which the values of the formal organization and primary group members differ. In the United States, the most closely located, accessible, and available family member is expected to provide the care to a family member. Spouses are the first choice, then children, other family members, friends, and finally formal support. On the other hand, care-related stress can result in the informal caregiver changing the balance by placing a family member in an institution (Friedemann, Newman, Buckwalter, & Montgomery, 2014).

Formal and informal support systems are balanced when they are at a midpoint of social distance, that is, close enough to communicate but not so close to destroy each other—neither enmeshment nor isolation (Litwak, Messeri, & Silverstein, 1990; Messeri, Silverstein, & Litwak, 1993). Conflicts arise when the relationship becomes unbalanced. For example, if the primary group and the formal care system begin performing similar caregiving services, there may be disagreements. Balance is reestablished when the formal system increases the social distance by developing relationships and providing support to the caregiver and reducing contact with the patient. Thus, a balance is maintained between the two systems. In another instance, when a patient relies only on the health care provider for care and support (e.g., calls the nurse every day, visits the physician weekly, refuses any help from family), balance can be reestablished by linking the patient to an informal support system for help with some of the caregiving tasks.

By applying frameworks of formal and informal support systems to their patients, psychiatric nurses can understand the complex social forces that patients with mental disorders and their caregivers experience (McPherson, Kayes, Moloczij, & Cummins, 2013) (Box 5.2). Nurses can help adjust the social distance between the formal and informal

> **BOX 5.2**
>
> **Research for Best Practice: Formal and Informal Support to Caregivers**
>
> Verbakel, E., Metzelthin, S. F., & Kempen, G. I. J. M. (2018). Caregiving to older adults: Determinants of informal caregivers' subjective well-being and formal and informal support as alleviating conditions. The Journals of Gerontology. Series B, Psychological Sciences and Social Sciences, 73(6), 1099–1111.
>
> **THE QUESTION:** Are there relationships among informal caregivers' subjective well-being and primary stressors, hours of informal caregiving, and burden? Does formal (professional home care) and informal support (from other caregivers, family, and friends) alleviate well-being losses due to providing informal care?
>
> **METHODS:** Data from 4,717 dyads of informal caregivers and their older care recipients were analyzed.
>
> **FINDINGS:** Caregivers' subjective well-being was directly related to the burden, hours of informal caregiving, and problem behavior of the care recipients. Formal and informal support reduced the impact of the primary stressors and caregiving hours. Reduction of formal/professional care may increase the negative well-being of caregivers.
>
> **IMPLICATIONS FOR NURSING:** Formal and informal support to caregivers can promote well-being for caregivers.

systems by identifying communication barriers and helping the two groups work together. For example, a patient misses an appointment because of a lack of transportation. The case manager helps the patient communicate the problem to the system to obtain another appointment. Informal caregivers are valued by the case manager, who recognizes the important services performed by family and friends. Thus, linkages between mental health providers (formal support) and the consumer network (informal support) are reinforced.

Role Theories

A role is a person's social position and function within an environment. Anthropologic theories explain members' roles that relate to a specific society. For example, the universal roles of healer may be assumed by a nurse in one culture and a spiritual leader in another. Societal expectations, social status, and rights are attached to these roles. Psychological theories, which are concerned about roles from a different perspective, focus on the relationship of an individual's role: the self. The responsibilities of a parent are often in conflict with the personal needs for time alone. All of the neo-freudian and humanist models that have been discussed focus on reciprocal social relationships or interactions that determine how the mind develops.

Role theories emphasize the importance of social interaction in either the individual's choice of a particular role or society's recognition of it. Psychiatric–mental health nursing uses role concepts in understanding group interaction and the role of the patient in the family and community. In addition, milieu therapy approaches discussed in later chapters are based on the patient's assumption of a role within the psychiatric environment.

Sociocultural Perspectives

Margaret Mead: Culture and Gender

American anthropologist Margaret Mead (1901–1978) is widely known for her studies of primitive societies and her contributions to social anthropology. She conducted studies in New Guinea, Samoa, and Bali and devoted much of her studies to the patterns of child rearing in various cultures. She was particularly interested in the cultural influences determining male and female behavior (Mead, 1970). Influenced by Carl Jung and Erik Erikson, she had a vision of unity and diversity of the psychosocial development of a single human species (Sullivan, 2004). Although her research is often criticized as not having scientific rigor and being filled with misinterpretations, it is accepted as a classic in the field of anthropology (Sullivan, 2004). She established the importance of culture in determining human behavior.

Madeleine Leininger: Transcultural Health Care

Concern about the impact of culture on the treatment of children with psychiatric and emotional problems led Madeleine Leininger (1924–2012) to develop a new field, transcultural nursing, directed toward holistic, congruent, and beneficent care. Leininger developed the *Theory of Culture Care Diversity and Universality*, which explains diverse and universal dimensions of human caring (Fig. 5.2). Nursing care in one culture is different from another because

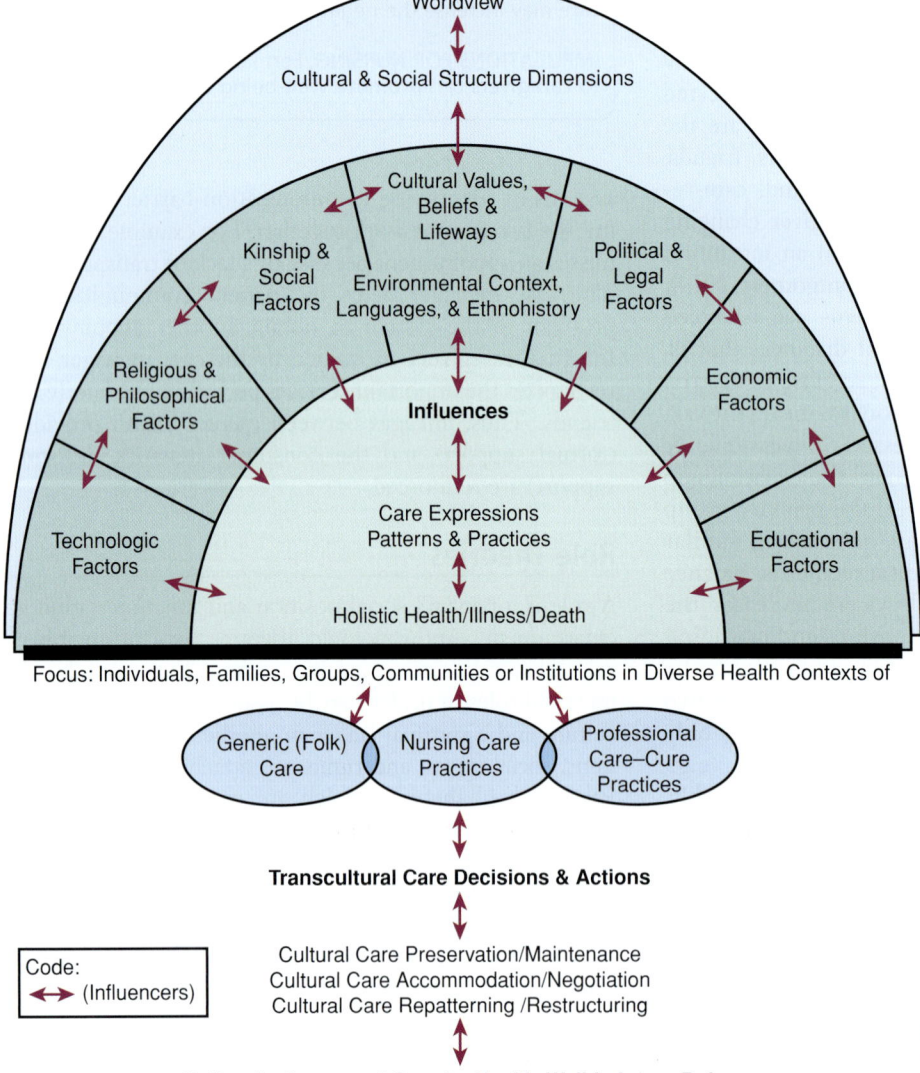

FIGURE 5.2 Leininger's Sunrise Model to depict theory of cultural care diversity and universality.

> **BOX 5.3**
>
> **Research for Best Practice: Cultural Knowledge of Mental Health Beliefs and Practices**
>
> Wolf, K. M., Zoucha, R., McFarland, M., Salman, K., Dagne, A., & Hashi, N. (2016). Somali immigrant perceptions of mental health and illness: An ethnonursing study. *Journal of Transcultural Nursing, 27*(4), 349–358.
>
> **QUESTION:** What are the mental health meanings, beliefs, and practices from the perspective of immigrant Somalis?
>
> **METHODS:** Qualitative ethnonursing research methods were used. Thirty informants (9 key and 21 general) were interviewed in community settings.
>
> **FINDINGS:** Analysis of the interviews revealed 21 categories and nine patterns. Two main themes emerged: Religion significantly influences their mental health, and religious beliefs and practices influence their health care choices.
>
> **IMPLICATIONS FOR NURSING:** Culturally congruent care will improve care for Somali immigrants.

definitions of health, illness, and care are culturally defined (Leininger & McFarland, 2006). The goal of Leininger's theory is to discover culturally based care (Leininger, 2007). Leininger's model continues to be used today as a framework for understanding mental health beliefs of various ethnic groups (Wolf et al., 2016) (see Box 5.3).

Applicability of Social Theories to Psychiatric–Mental Health Nursing

The use of social and sociocultural theories is especially important for psychiatric–mental health nurses. In any individual or family assessment, the sociocultural aspect is integral to mental health. It would be impossible to complete an adequate assessment without considering the role of the individual within the family and society. Interventions are based on the understanding and significance of family and cultural norms. It would be impossible to interact with the family in a meaningful way without an understanding of the family's cultural values. In the inpatient setting, the nurse is responsible for designing the social environment of the unit as well as ensuring that the patient is safe from harm. To accomplish this complex task, an understanding of the unit as a small social community helps the nurse use the environment in patient treatment (see Chapter 10). In addition, many group interventions are based on sociocultural theories (see Chapter 12).

NURSING THEORIES

Nursing theories are useful to psychiatric–mental health nursing in conceptualizing the individual, family, or community and in planning nursing interventions (see Chapter 10). The use of a specific theory depends on the patient situation. For example, in people with schizophrenia who have problems related to maintaining self-care, Dorothea Orem's theory of self-care is useful. By contrast, Hildegard Peplau's theories are appropriate when a nurse is developing a relationship with a patient. Because of the wide range of possible problems requiring different approaches, familiarity with several nursing theories is essential.

Interpersonal Relations Models

Hildegard Peplau: The Power of Empathy

Hildegard Peplau (1909–1999) introduced the first systematic theoretic framework for psychiatric nursing and focused on the nurse–patient relationship in her book *Interpersonal Relations in Nursing* in 1952 (Peplau, 1952). She led psychiatric–mental health nursing out of the confinement of custodial care into a theory-driven professional practice. One of her major contributions was the introduction of the nurse–patient relationship (see Chapter 9).

Peplau believed in the importance of the environment, defined as external factors considered essential to human development (Peplau, 1992): cultural forces, presence of adults, secure economic status of the family, and a healthy prenatal environment. Peplau emphasized the importance of empathic linkage.

> **KEYCONCEPT Empathic linkage** is the ability to feel in oneself the feelings experienced by another person.

The interpersonal transmission of anxiety or panic is the most common empathic linkage. According to Peplau, other feelings, such as anger, disgust, and envy, can also be communicated nonverbally by way of empathic transmission to others. Although the process is not yet understood, she explains that empathic communication occurs. She believes that if nurses pay attention to what they feel during a relationship with a patient, they can gain invaluable observations of feelings a patient is experiencing and has not yet noticed or talked about.

Anxiety is a key concept for Peplau, who contends that professional practice is unsafe if this concept is not understood.

> **KEYCONCEPT Anxiety**, according to Peplau, is an energy that arises when expectations that are present are not met.

If anxiety is not recognized, it continues to rise and escalates toward panic. There are various levels of anxiety, each having its observable behavioral cues (Box 5.4). These cues are sometimes called *defensive*, but Peplau argues that they are often "relief behaviors." For example, some people may relieve their anxiety by yelling

> **BOX 5.4**
> **Levels of Anxiety**
>
> **Mild:** awareness heightens
> **Moderate:** awareness narrows
> **Severe:** focused narrow awareness
> **Panic:** unable to function

and swearing; others seek relief by withdrawing. In both instances, anxiety was generated by an unmet security need.

> **NCLEXNOTE** Peplau's model of anxiety continues to be an important concept in psychiatric nursing. Severe anxiety interferes with learning. Mild anxiety is useful for learning.

The **self-system** is another important concept in Peplau's model. Drawing from Sullivan, Peplau defined the self as an "antianxiety system" and a product of socialization. The self proceeds through personal development that is always open to revision but tends toward stability. For example, in parent–child relationships, patterns of approval, disapproval, and indifference are used by children to define themselves. If the verbal and nonverbal messages have been derogatory, children incorporate these messages and also view themselves negatively.

The concept of need is important to Peplau's model. Needs are primarily of biologic origin but need to be met within a sociocultural environment. When a biologic need is present, it gives rise to tension that is reduced and relieved by behaviors meeting that need. According to Peplau, nurses should recognize and support the patients' patterns and style of meeting their health care needs.

Ida Jean Orlando

In 1954, Ida Jean Orlando (1926–2007) studied the factors that enhanced or impeded the integration of mental health principles in the basic nursing curriculum. From this study, she published *The Dynamic Nurse–Patient Relationship* to offer nursing students a theory of effective nursing practice. She studied nursing care of patients on medical–surgical units, not people with psychiatric problems in mental hospitals. Orlando identified three areas of nursing concern: the nurse–patient relationship, the nurse's professional role, and the identity and development of knowledge that is distinctly nursing (Orlando, 1961). A nursing situation involves the behavior of the patient, the reaction of the nurse, and anything that does not relieve the distress of the patient. Patient distress is related to the inability of the individual to meet or communicate his or her own needs (Orlando, 1961, 1972).

Orlando helped nurses focus on the whole patient rather than on the disease or institutional demands. Her ideas continue to be useful today, and current research supports her model (Olson & Hanchett, 1997). A small nursing study investigated whether Orlando's nursing theory–based practice had a measurable impact on patients' immediate distress when compared with nonspecified nursing interventions. Orlando's approach consisted of the nurse validating the patient's distress before taking any action to reduce it. Patients being cared for by the Orlando group experienced significantly less stress than those receiving traditional nursing care (Potter & Bockenhauer, 2000). Orlando's model has been used in many settings including fall prevention in a hospital (Abraham, 2011). Orlando's theory is also proposed as a model for teaching communication in nursing programs (Gaudet & Howett, 2018).

Existential and Humanistic Theoretical Perspectives

Rosemarie Rizzo Parse

The *Humanbecoming Theory* views humans as indivisible, unpredictable, ever-changing coauthors and experts about their lives (Parse, 1998, 2007). Three major themes underlie this theory: meaning (personal meaning to the situation), rhythmicity (the paradoxical patterning of the human–universe mutual processes—the ups and downs of life), and transcendence (power and originating of transforming) (Parse, 1996, 1998, 2008). The postulates involved in living a human life are *illuminating* (unbound knowing extended to infinity), *paradox* (intricate rhythm expressed as a pattern preference), *freedom* (liberation), and *mystery* (unexplainable) (Parse, 2007).

As one of the more abstract nursing theories, *humanbecoming* can used in understanding patients' life experiences and connecting psychologically with a patient. This theory has been widely studied in nursing and adds qualitative dimension to understanding the patient's human experience. For example, one of the studies addressed the positive effects of feeling strong within a community (Doucet, 2012). Parse's theory is recommended as an alternative to the medical approach for a grieving family who has experienced a pregnancy loss, still birth, or neonatal death. The theory of humanbecoming focuses on quality of life as experienced and the meaning of the experience as perceived by the parents (Wilson, 2016).

Jean Watson

The theory of transpersonal caring was initiated by Jean Watson (b. 1940). Watson believes that caring is the foundation of nursing and recommends that specific theories of caring be developed in relation to specific human conditions and health and illness experiences (Watson, 2005). Her conceptualizations transcend conventional views of illness and focus on the meaning of health and

> **BOX 5.5**
>
> **Nursing: Human Science and Human Care Assumptions, and Factors in Care**
>
> **ASSUMPTIONS**
> 1. Caring can be effectively demonstrated and practiced only interpersonally.
> 2. Caring consists of factors that result in the satisfaction of certain human needs.
> 3. Effective caring promotes health and individual or family growth.
> 4. Caring responses accept a person not only as he or she is now but also as what he or she may become.
> 5. A caring environment offers the development of potential while allowing the person to choose the best action for him- or herself at a given point in time.
> 6. Caring is more "healthogenic" than is curing. It integrates biophysical knowledge with knowledge of human behavior to generate or promote health and provide ministrations to those who are ill. A science of caring is complementary to the science of curing.
> 7. The practice of caring is central to nursing.
>
> **10 CARITAS PROCESSES™**
> 1. Embrace altruistic values and practice loving-kindness with self and others.
> 2. Instill faith, hope, and honor in others.
> 3. Be sensitive to self and others by nurturing individual beliefs and practices.
> 4. Develop helping–trusting–caring relationships.
> 5. Promote and accept positive and negative feelings as you authentically listen to another's story.
> 6. Use creative scientific problem-solving methods for caring decision making.
> 7. Share teaching and learning that addresses the individual needs and comprehension styles.
> 8. Create a healing environment for the physical and spiritual self that respects human dignity.
> 9. Assist with basic physical, emotional, and spiritual human needs.
> 10. Be open to mystery and allow miracles to enter.
>
> Watson Caring Science Institute, International Caritas Consortium. (2010). *Dr. Jean Watson's human caring theory: Ten Caritas Processes*. Retrieved from https://www.watsoncaringscience.org/

quality of life (Watson, 2007). There are three foundational concepts of her theory:

- Transpersonal Caring–Healing Relations: a relational process related to philosophic, moral, and spiritual foundation
- 10 Caritas Processes™: the original 10 Carative Factors have evolved into the 10 Caritas Processes™ (Box 5.5)
- Caritas Field: a field of consciousness created when the nurse focuses on love and caring as his or her way of being and consciously manifests a healing presence with others.

Watson's theory is especially applicable to the care of those who seek help for mental illness. This model emphasizes the importance of sensitivity to self and others; the development of helping and trusting relations; the promotion of interpersonal teaching and learning; and provision for a supportive, protective, and corrective mental, physical, sociocultural, and spiritual environment. A transpersonal caring intervention guide offers protocols to assist nurses in using caring intentionally and effectively in practice (Gallagher-Lepak & Kubsch, 2009). Watson's model is a model in the acute health care settings to guide the establishment of genuine therapeutic relationships (Hogan, 2013). Her approach is also used to determine cultural mental health care beliefs and practices.

Systems Models

Imogene M. King

The theory of goal attainment developed by Imogene King (1923–2007) is based on a systems model that includes three interacting systems: personal, interpersonal, and social. In this model, human beings interact with the environment, and the individual's perceptions influence reactions and interactions (Fig. 5.3). Nursing involves caring for the human being, with the goal of health defined as adjusting to the stressors in both internal and external environments (King, 2007). She defines nursing as a "process of human interactions between nurse and patient whereby each perceives the other and the situation; and through communication, they set goals, explore means, and agree on means to achieve goals" (King, 1981, p. 144). This model focuses on the process that occurs between a nurse and a patient. The process is initiated to help the patient cope with a health problem that compromises his or her ability to maintain social roles, functions, and activities of daily living (King, 1992).

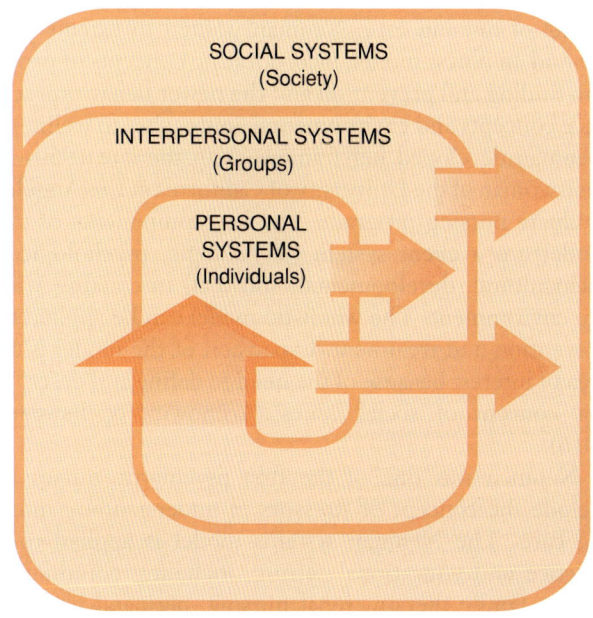

FIGURE 5.3 Imogene King's conceptual framework for nursing: dynamic interacting systems.

In this model, the person is goal oriented and purposeful, reacting to stressors, and is viewed as an open system interacting with the environment. The variables in nursing situations are as follows:

- Geographic place of the transacting system, such as the hospital
- Perceptions of the nurse and patient
- Communications of the nurse and patient
- Expectations of the nurse and patient
- Mutual goals of the nurse and patient
- The nurse and patient as a system of interdependent roles in a nursing situation (King, 1981, p. 88)

The quality of nurse–patient interactions may have positive or negative influences on the promotion of health in any nursing situation. It is within this interpersonal system of nurse and patient that the healing process is performed. Interaction is depicted in which the outcome is a **transaction**, defined as the transfer of value between two or more people. This behavior is unique, based on experience, and is goal directed.

King's work reflects her understanding of the systematic process of theory development. Her model continues to be developed and applied in national and international settings, including psychiatric–mental health care (Shanta & Connolly, 2013). The model also serves as a basis for a recent nursing theory related to work team/group empowerment. The theory is applied to improve nurses' empowerment within health care organizations (Friend & Sieloff, 2018).

Betty Neuman

Betty Neuman (b. 1924) uses a systems approach as a model of nursing care. Neuman wanted to extend care beyond an illness model, incorporating concepts of problem finding and prevention and the newer behavioral science concepts and environmental approaches to wellness. Neuman developed her framework in the late 1960s as chairwoman of the University of California at Los Angeles graduate nursing program. The key components of the model are a client system (physiologic, psychological, sociocultural, developmental, spiritual) interacting with the environment. The wholistic model can be applied to prevention and treatment. Expansion of the model is an area of interest because of the need to define and describe her concept of social issues (Aronowitz & Fawcett, 2016).

Neuman was one of the first psychiatric nurses to include the concept of stressors in understanding nursing care. The Neuman systems model is applied to a practice and educational setting, including community health, family therapy, renal nursing, perinatal nursing, and mental health nursing of older adults (Beckman, Boxley-Harges, & Kaskel, 2012; Neuman & Fawcett, 2011). This model has been applied to the practice and educational setting including international programs (Lee, 2014; Merks, Verberk, de Kuiper, & Lowry, 2012; Olowokere & Okanlawon, 2015).

Dorothea Orem

Self-care is the focus of the general theory of nursing initiated by Dorothea Orem (1914–2007) in the early 1960s. The Self-Care Deficit Nursing Theory consists of three separate parts: a theory of self-care, theory of self-care deficit, and theory of nursing systems (Biggs, 2008; Orem, 2001; Orem & Taylor, 2011). The theory of self-care defines the term as activities performed independently by an individual to promote and maintain personal well-being throughout life. The central focus of Orem's theory is the self-care deficit theory, which describes how people can be helped by nursing. Nurses can help meet self-care requisites through five approaches: acting or doing for, guiding, teaching, supporting, and providing an environment to promote the patient's ability to meet current or future demands. The nursing systems theory refers to a series of actions a nurse takes to meet the patient's self-care requisites. This system varies from the patient being totally dependent on the nurse for care to needing only some education and support.

Orem's model is used in psychiatric–mental health nursing because of its emphasis on promoting independence of the individual and on self-care activities (Burdette, 2012; Seed & Torkelson, 2012; Wazni & Gifford, 2017). Although many psychiatric disorders have an underlying problem, such as motivation, these problems are generally manifested as difficulties conducting ordinary self-care activities (e.g., personal hygiene) or developing independent thinking skills.

Other Nursing Theories

Other nursing models are applied in psychiatric settings. Martha Rogers' model of unitary human beings and Calista Roy's adaptation model have been the bases of many psychiatric nursing approaches.

SUMMARY OF KEY POINTS

- The traditional psychodynamic framework helped form the basis of early nursing interpersonal interventions, including the development of therapeutic relationships and the use of such concepts as transference, countertransference, empathy, and object relations.

- The behavioral theories are often used in strategies that help patients change behavior and thinking.

- Sociocultural theories remain important in understanding and interacting with patients as members of families and cultures.
- Nursing theories form the conceptual basis for nursing practice and are useful in a variety of psychiatric–mental health settings.

CRITICAL THINKING CHALLENGES

1. Discuss the similarities and differences among Freud's ideas and those of the neo-freudians, including Jung, Adler, Horney, and Sullivan.
2. Compare and contrast the basic ideas of psychodynamic and behavioral theories.
3. Compare and differentiate classic conditioning from operant conditioning.
4. Define the following terms and discuss their applicability to psychiatric–mental health nursing: classical conditioning, operant conditioning, positive reinforcement, and negative reinforcement.
5. List the major developmental theorists and their main ideas.
6. Discuss the cognitive therapy approaches to mental disorders and how they can be used in psychiatric–mental health nursing practice.
7. Define formal and informal support systems. How does the concept of social distance relate to these two systems?
8. Compare and contrast the basic ideas of the nursing theorists.

1962: *Freud*

MOVIES This film depicts Sigmund Freud as a young physician, focusing on his early psychiatric theories and treatments. His struggles for acceptance of his ideas among the Viennese medical community are depicted. This fascinating film is well done and gives an interesting overview of the impact of psychoanalysis.

Viewing Points: Watch for the impact on political thinking during the gradual acceptance of Freud's ideas. Discuss the "dream sequence" and its impact on the development of psychoanalysis as a therapeutic technique.

1990: *An Angel at My Table*

New Zealand. This three-part television miniseries tells the story of Janet Frame, New Zealand's premiere novelist and poet. Based on her autobiography, the film portrays Frame as a shy, awkward child who experiences a family tragedy that alienates her socially. She studies in England to be a teacher, but her shyness and social ineptness cause extreme anxiety. Seeking mental health care, she receives a misdiagnosis of schizophrenia and spends 8 years in a mental institution. She barely escapes a lobotomy when she is notified of a literary award. She then begins to develop friendships and a new life.

Viewing Points: Observe Janet Frame's childhood development. Does she "fit" any of the models that are discussed in this chapter? Consider her life in light of Gilligan and Miller's theories that it is important for women to have a sense of connection.

REFERENCES

Abraham, S. (2011). Fall prevention conceptual framework. *Health Care Manager (Frederick)*, 30(20), 179–184.
Ackerman, S., Zuroff, D. C., & Moskowitz, D. S. (2000). Generativity in midlife and young adults: Links to agency, communion, and subjective well-being. *International Journal of Aging and Human Development*, 5(1), 17–41.
Aronowitz, T., & Fawcett, J. (2016). Thoughts about social issues: A Neuman systems model perspective. *Nursing Science Quarterly*, 29(2), 173–176.
Bandura, A. (1977). *Social learning theory*. Englewood Cliffs, NJ: Prentice-Hall.
Bandura, A. (1986). *Social foundations of thought and action: A social-cognitive theory*. Englewood Cliffs, NJ: Prentice Hall.
Bandura, A. (1993). Perceived self-efficacy in cognitive development and function. American Educational Research Association Annual Meeting. *Educational Psychologist*, 28(2), 117–148.
Bandura, A. (2001). Social cognitive theory: An agentic perspective. *Annual Review of Psychology*, 52, 1–26.
Beck, A. T. (2005). The current state of cognitive therapy: A 40-year retrospective. *Archives of General Psychiatry*, 62(9), 953–959.
Beckman, S. J., Boxley-Harges, S. L., & Kaskel, B. L. (2012). Experience informs: Spanning three decades with the Neuman systems model. *Nursing Science Quarterly*, 25(4), 341–346.
Biggs, A. (2008). Orem's self-care deficit nursing theory: Update on the state of the art and science. *Nursing Science Quarterly*, 21(3), 200–206.
Burdette, L. (2012). Relationship between self-care agency, self-care practices and obesity among rural midlife women. *Self-Care, Dependent-Care & Nursing*, 19(1), 5–14.
Christiansen, S. L., & Palkovitz, R. (1998). Exploring Erikson's psychosocial theory and development: Generativity and its relationship to paternal identity, intimacy, and involvement in childcare. *The Journal of Men's Studies*, 7(1), 133–156.
Doucet, T. J. (2012). Feeling strong: A Parse research method study. *Nursing Science Quarterly*, 25(1), 62–71.
Ehlman, K., & Ligon, M. (2012). The application of a generativity model for the older adults. *International Journal of Aging and Human Development*, 74(4), 331–344.
Erikson, E. (1963). *Childhood and society* (2nd ed.). New York: Norton.
Erikson, E. (1968). *Identity: Youth and crisis*. New York: Norton.
Fehler-Cabral, F., & Campbell, R. (2013). Adolescent sexual assault disclosure: The impact of peers, families, and schools. *American Journal of Community Psychology*, 52(1–2), 73–83.
Freud, S. (1905). Three essays on the theory of sexuality. In J. Strachey, A. Freud, A. Strachey, & A. Tyson (Eds.). (1953). *The standard edition of the complete psychological works of Sigmund Freud* (pp. 135–248). London: Hogarth Press.
Freud, S. (1927). The ego and the id. In E. Jones (Ed.). (1957). *The international psychoanalytical library (No. 12)*. London: Hogarth Press.
Friedemann, M., Newman, F. L., Buckwalter, K. C., & Montgomery, R. J. (2014). Resource need and use of multiethnic caregivers of elders in their homes. *Journal of Advanced Nursing*, 70(3), 662–673.
Friend, M. L., & Sieloff, C. L. (2018). Empowerment in nursing literature: An update and look to the future. *Nursing Science Quarterly*, 31(4), 355–361.
Fromm-Reichmann, F. (1950). *Principles of intensive psychotherapy*. Chicago, IL: University of Chicago Press.
Gallagher-Lepak, S., & Kubsch, S. (2009). Transpersonal caring: A nursing practice guideline. *Holistic Nursing Practice*, 23(3), 171–182.
Gaudet, D., & Howett, M. (2018). Communication and technology: Ida Orland's theory applied. *Nursing Science Quarterly*, 31(4), 369–373.
Gilligan, C. (1982). *In a different voice*. Cambridge, MA: Harvard University Press.

Gilligan, C. (2004). Recovering psyche: Reflections on life-history and history. *Annual of Psychoanalysis, 32*, 131–147.

Gilligan, C. (2011). *Joining the resistance*. Malden, MA: Polity Press.

Hogan, B. K. (2013). Caring as a scripted discourse versus caring as an expression of an authentic relationship between self and other. *Issues in Mental Health Nursing, 34*(5), 375–379.

Horney, K. (1939). *New ways in psychoanalysis*. New York: Norton.

Jonsén, E., Norberg, A., & Lundman, B. (2015). Sense of meaning in life among the oldest old people living in a rural area in northern Sweden. *International Journal of Older People Nursing, 10*(3), 221–229.

Jung, C. (1966). On the psychology of the unconscious. The personal and the collective unconscious. In C. Jung (Ed.). *Collected works of C. G. Jung* (2nd ed., Vol. 7, pp. 64–79). Princeton, NJ: Princeton University Press.

King, I. (1981). *A theory for nursing: Systems, concepts, process*. New York: Wiley.

King, I. (1992). King's theory of goal attainment. *Nursing Science Quarterly, 5*(1), 19–26.

King, I. (2007). King's conceptual system, theory of goal attainment, and transaction process in the 21st century. *Nursing Science Quarterly, 20*(2), 109–116.

Klein, M. (1963). *Our adult world and other essays*. London: Heinemann Medical Books.

Kress, V. E., Haiyasoso, M., Zoldan, C. A., Headley, J. A., & Trepal, H. (2018). The use of relational-cultural theory in counseling clients who have traumatic stress disorders. *Journal of Counseling & Development, 96*(1), 106–114.

Lee, Q. (2014). Application of Neuman system model on the management of a patient with asthma. *Singapore Nursing Journal, 41*(1), 20–25.

Leininger, M. (2007). Theoretical questions and concerns: Response from the Theory of Culture Care Diversity and Universality perspective. *Nursing Science Quarterly, 20*, 9–13.

Leininger, M., & McFarland, M. (2006). *Cultural care diversity and universality theory. A theory of nursing* (2nd ed.). Seaburg, MA: Jones & Bartlett Publishers.

Litwak, E. (1985). Complementary roles for formal and informal support groups: A study of nursing homes and mortality rates. *Journal of Applied Behavioral Science, 21*(4), 407–425.

Litwak, E., Messeri, P., & Silverstein, M. (1990). The role of formal and informal groups in providing help to older people. *Marriage and Family Review, 15*(1–2), 171–193.

Maslow, A. (1970). *Motivation and personality* (rev. ed.). New York: Harper & Brothers.

McIntosh, D. (2003). *Testing an intervention to increase self-efficacy of staff in managing clients perceived as violent*. University of Cincinnati, PhD dissertation. Retrieved March 7, 2007, from http://etd.iohiolink.edu/view.cgi?acc_num=ucin1069786693

McPherson, K. M., Kayes, N. K., Moloczij, N., & Cummins C. (2013). Improving the interface between informal carers and formal health and social services: A qualitative study. *International Journal of Nursing Studies, 51*(3), 418–429.

Mead, M. (1970). *Culture and commitment: A study of the generation gap*. Garden City, NY: Natural History Press/Doubleday & Co.

Merks, A., Verberk, F., de Kuiper, M., Lowry, L. W. (2012). Neuman systems model in Holland: An update. *Nursing Science Quarterly, 25*(4), 364–368.

Messeri, P., Silverstein, M., & Litwak, E. (1993). Choosing optimal support groups: A review and reformulation. *Journal of Health and Social Behavior, 34*(6), 122–137.

Miller, J. B. (1976). *Toward a new psychology of women*. Beacon Press: Boston.

Miller, J. B. (1994). Women's psychological development. Connections, disconnections, and violations. In M. Berger (Ed.) *Women beyond Freud: New concepts of feminine psychology* (pp. 79–97). New York: Brunner Mazel.

Moore, B., & Fine, B. (Eds.). (1990). *Psychoanalytic terms and concepts*. New Haven, CT: The American Psychoanalytic Association and Yale University Press.

Neuman, B., & Fawcett, J. (Eds.). (2011). *The Neuman systems model* (5th ed.). Upper Saddle River, NJ: Prentice Hall.

Ochse, R., & Plug, C. (1986). Cross-cultural investigation of the validity of Erikson's theory of personality development. *Journal of Personality and Social Psychology, 50*(6), 1240–1252.

Olowokere, A. E., & Okanlawon, F. A. (2015). Application of Neuman system model to psychosocial support of vulnerable school children. *West African Journal of Nursing, 26*(1), 14–25.

Olson, J., & Hanchett, E. (1997). Nurse-expressed empathy, patient outcomes, and the development of a middle-range theory. *Image: The Journal of Nursing Scholarship, 29*(1), 71–76.

Orem, D. (2001). *Nursing concepts of practice* (6th ed.). St. Louis: Mosby.

Orem, D. E., & Taylor, S. G. (2011). Reflections on nursing practice science: The nature, the structure, and the foundation of nursing sciences. *Nursing Science Quarterly, 24*(1), 35–41.

Orlando, I. J. (1961). *The dynamic nurse–patient relationship*. New York: G. P. Putnam's Sons.

Orlando, I. J. (1972). *The discipline and teaching of nursing process*. New York: G. P. Putnam's Sons.

Orlofsky, J., Marcia, J., & Lesser, I. (1973). Ego identity status and the intimacy versus isolation crisis of young adulthood. *Journal of Personality and Social Psychology, 27*(2), 211–219.

Parse, R. R. (1996). Reality: A seamless symphony of becoming. *Nursing Science Quarterly, 9*, 181–184.

Parse, R. R. (1998). *The humanbecoming school of thoughts: A perspective for nurses and other health professionals*. London: Sage.

Parse, R. R. (2007). The humanbecoming school of thought in 2050. *Nursing Science Quarterly, 20*, 308–311.

Parse, R. R. (2008). The humanbecoming leading-following model. *Nursing Science Quarterly, 21*, 369–375.

Pavlov, I. P. (1927/1960). *Conditioned reflexes*. New York: Dover Publications.

Peplau, H. (1952). *Interpersonal relations in nursing*. New York: G. P. Putnam's Sons.

Peplau, H. (1992). Interpersonal relations: A theoretical framework for application in nursing practice. *Nursing Science Quarterly, 5*(1), 13–18.

Perls, F. (1969). *In and out of the garbage pail*. Lafayette, CA: Real People Press.

Potter, M. L., & Bockenhauer, B. J. (2000). Implementing Orlando's nursing theory. *Journal of Psychosocial Nursing and Mental Health Services, 38*(13), 14–21.

Pratt, M. W., Norris, J. E., Cressman, K., Lawford, H., & Hebblethwaite, S. (2008). Parents' stories of grandparenting concerns in the three-generational family: Generativity, optimism, and forgiveness. *Journal of Personality, 76*(3), 581–604.

Rogers, C. (1980). *A way of being*. Boston: Houghton Mifflin.

Seed, M. S., & Torkelson, D. J. (2012). Beginning the recovery journey in acute psychiatric care: Using concepts from Orem's self-care deficit nursing theory. *Issues in Mental Health Nursing, 33*(6), 394–398.

Shanta, L. L., & Connolly, M. (2013). Using King's interacting systems theory to link emotional intelligence and nursing practice. *Journal of Professional Nursing, 29*(3), 174–180.

Shin, Y., Yun, S., Pender, N. J., & Jang, H. (2005). Test of the health promotion model as a causal model of commitment to a plan for exercise among Korean adults with chronic disease. *Research in Nursing & Health, 28*(2), 117–125.

Skinner, B. F. (1935). The generic nature of the concepts of stimulus and response. *Journal of General Psychology, 12*, 40–65.

Soares, M. C., Mondin, T. C., Silva, G. D. G. D., Barbosa, L. P., Molina, M. L., Jansen, K., et al. (2018). Comparison of clinical significance of cognitive-behavioral therapy and psychodynamic therapy for major depressive disorder. *The Journal of Nervous and Mental Disease, 206*(9), 686–693.

Sullivan, G. (2004). A four-fold humanity: Margaret Mead and psychological types. *Journal of the History of the Behavioral Sciences, 40*(2), 183–206.

Sullivan, H. (1953). *The interpersonal theory of psychiatry*. New York: Norton.

Thorndike, E. L. (1906). *The principles of teaching, based on psychology*. New York: A. G. Seiler.

Walker, M., & Rosen, W. B. (2004). *How connections heal: Stories from relational-cultural therapy*. New York: Guilford Press.

Watson, J. (2005). *Caring science as sacred science*. Philadelphia, PA: F. A. Davis.

Watson, J. (2007). Theoretical questions and concerns: Response from a Caring Science Framework. *Nursing Science Quarterly, 20*, 13–15.

Watson, J. B., & Rayner, R. (1920). Conditioned emotional reactions. *Journal of Experimental Psychology, 3*, 1–14.

Wazni, L., & Gifford, W. (2017). Addressing physical health needs of individuals with schizophrenia using Orem's theory. *Journal of Holistic Nursing, 35*(3), 271–279.

Wolf, K. M., Zoucha, R., McFarland, M., Salman, K., Dagne, A., & Hashi, N. (2016). Somali immigrant perceptions of mental health and illness: An ethnonursing study. *Journal of Transcultural Nursing, 27*(4), 349–358.

Westermeyer, J. F. (2004). Predictors and characteristics of Erikson's life cycle model among men: A 32-year longitudinal study. *International Journal of Aging & Human Development, 58*(1), 29–48.

Wilson, D. R. (2016). Parse's nursing theory and its application to families experiencing empty arms. *International Journal of Childbirth Education, 31*(2), 29–33.

6
Biologic Foundations of Psychiatric Nursing

Mary Ann Boyd

KEY CONCEPTS
- neuroplasticity
- neurotransmitters

LEARNING OBJECTIVES

After studying this chapter, you will be able to:

1. Describe the association between biologic functioning and symptoms of psychiatric disorders.
2. Locate brain structures primarily involved in psychiatric disorders and describe the primary functions of these structures.
3. Describe basic mechanisms of neuronal transmission.
4. Identify the location and function of neurotransmitters significant to hypotheses regarding major mental disorders.
5. Discuss the role of genetics in the development of psychiatric disorders.
6. Discuss the basic utilization of new knowledge gained from fields of study, including psychoneuroimmunology and chronobiology.

KEY TERMS

- acetylcholine • amino acids • autonomic nervous system • basal ganglia • biogenic amines • biologic markers
- brain stem • cerebellum • chronobiology • circadian cycle • cortex • dopamine • extrapyramidal motor system
- frontal, parietal, temporal, and occipital lobes • functional imaging • GABA • genetic susceptibility • glutamate
- hippocampus • histamine • limbic system • locus caeruleus • neurocircuitry • neurohormones • neuromodulators
- neurons • neuropeptides • norepinephrine • phenotype • pineal body • population genetics • proband
- psychoneuroimmunology • receptor • serotonin • structural imaging • synaptic cleft • working memory • zeitgebers

All behavior recognized as human results from actions that originate in the brain and its amazing interconnection of neural networks. Modern research has increased understanding of how the complex circuitry of the brain interacts with the external environment, memories, and experiences. Through the spinal column and peripheral nerves, along with other systems, such as the endocrine and immune systems, the brain constantly receives and processes information. As the brain shifts and sorts through the amazing amount of information it processes every hour, it decides on actions and initiates behaviors, allowing each person to act in entirely unique and very human ways.

Mental disorders cannot be traced to specific physiologic problems but rather are complex syndromes consisting of symptoms that more or less cluster together. Therefore, it is important for the nurse to understand basic nervous system functioning, as well as some of the research that is exploring the biologic basis of mental disorders.

This chapter reviews the basic information necessary for understanding neuroscience as it relates to the role of the psychiatric–mental health nurse. It reviews basic central nervous system (CNS) structures and functions, the peripheral nervous system (PNS), general functions of the major neurotransmitters and **receptor**s, basic principles of neurotransmission, genetic models, circadian rhythms, and biologic tests. The chapter assumes that the reader has a basic knowledge of human biology, anatomy, and pathophysiology. It is not intended as a full presentation of neuroanatomy and physiology but rather as an overview of the structures and functions most critical to understanding the role of the psychiatric–mental health nurse. Psychiatric–mental health nurses must be able to make the connection between (1) patients' psychiatric symptoms, (2) the probable alterations in brain functioning linked to those symptoms, and (3) the rationale for treatment and care practices.

NEUROANATOMY OF THE CENTRAL NERVOUS SYSTEM

Although this section discusses functioning areas of the brain separately, each area is intricately connected with the others, and each functions interactively. The CNS contains the brain, **brain stem**, and spinal cord, and the PNS consists of the **neurons** that connect the CNS to the muscles, organs, and other systems in the periphery of the body. Whatever affects the CNS may also affect the PNS and vice versa.

Cerebrum

The largest region of the human brain, the cerebrum fills the entire upper portion of the cranium. The **cortex**, or outermost surface of the cerebrum, makes up about 80% of the human brain. The cortex is four to six cellular layers thick, and each layer is composed of cell bodies mixed with capillary blood vessels. This mixture makes the cortex gray brown (thus the term *gray matter*). The cortex consists of numerous bumps and grooves in a fully developed adult brain, as shown in Figure 6.1. This "wrinkling" allows for a large amount of surface area to be confined in the limited space of the skull. The increased surface area allows for more potential connections among cells within the cortex. The grooves are called *fissures* if they extend deep into the brain and *sulci* if they are shallower. The bumps or convolutions are called *gyri*. Together, they provide many of the landmarks for the subdivisions of the cortex. The longest and deepest groove, the longitudinal fissure, separates the cerebrum into left and right hemispheres. Although these two divisions are nearly symmetric, there is some variation in the location and size of the sulci and gyri in each hemisphere. Substantial variation in these convolutions is found in the cortex of different individuals.

Left and Right Hemispheres

The cerebrum can be roughly divided into two halves, or hemispheres. The left hemisphere is dominant in about 95% of people, but about 5% of individuals have mixed dominance. Each hemisphere controls functioning mainly on the opposite side of the body. Aside from controlling activities on the left side of the body, the right hemisphere also provides input into receptive nonverbal communication, spatial orientation and recognition, intonation of speech and aspects of music, facial recognition and facial

FIGURE 6.1 Lateral and medial surfaces of the brain. **Left:** The left lateral surface of the brain. **Right:** The medial surface of the right half of a sagittally hemisected brain. (From Bear, M. F., Conners, B. W., & Paradiso, M. A. [2016]. *Neuroscience: Exploring the brain* [3rd ed.]. Philadelphia, PA: Wolters Kluwer.)

expression of emotion, and nonverbal learning and memory. In general, the left hemisphere is more involved with verbal language function, including areas for both receptive and expressive speech control, and provides strong contributions to temporal order and sequencing, numeric symbols, and verbal learning and memory.

The two hemispheres are connected by the corpus callosum, a bundle of neuronal tissue that allows information to be exchanged quickly between the right and left hemispheres. An intact corpus callosum is required for the hemispheres to function in a smooth and coordinated manner.

Lobes of the Brain

The lateral surface of each hemisphere is further divided into four lobes: the **frontal, parietal, temporal, and occipital lobes** (see Fig. 6.1). The lobes work in coordinated ways, but each is responsible for specific functions. An understanding of these unique functions is helpful in understanding how damage to these areas produces the symptoms of mental illness and how medications that affect the functioning of these lobes can produce certain effects.

Frontal Lobes

The right and left frontal lobes make up about one fourth of the entire cerebral cortex and are proportionately larger in humans than in any other mammal. The precentral gyrus, the gyrus immediately anterior to the central sulcus, contains the primary motor area, or homunculi. Damage to this gyrus or to the anterior neighboring gyri causes spastic paralysis in the opposite side of the body. The frontal lobe also contains Broca area, which controls the motor function of speech. Damage to Broca area produces expressive aphasia, or difficulty with the motor movements required for speech. The frontal lobes are also thought to contain the highest or most complex aspects of cortical functioning, which collectively make up a large part of what we call personality. **Working memory** is an important aspect of frontal lobe function, including the ability to plan and initiate activity with future goals in mind. Insight, judgment, reasoning, concept formation, problem-solving skills, abstraction, and self-evaluation are all abilities that are modulated and affected by the actions of the frontal lobes. These skills are often referred to as *executive functions* because they modulate more primitive impulses through numerous connections to other areas of the cerebrum.

When normal frontal lobe functioning is altered, executive functioning is decreased, and modulation of impulses can be lost, leading to changes in mood and personality. The importance of the frontal lobe and its role in the development of symptoms common to psychiatric disorders are emphasized in later chapters that discuss disorders such

BOX 6.1
Frontal Lobe Syndrome

In the 1860s, Phineas Gage became a famous example of frontal lobe dysfunction. Mr. Gage was a New England railroad worker who had a thick iron-tamping rod propelled through his frontal lobes by an explosion. He survived, but suffered significant changes in his personality. Mr. Gage, who had previously been a capable and calm supervisor, began to show impatience, labile mood, disrespect for others, and frequent use of profanity after his injury (Harlow, 1868). Similar conditions are often called *frontal lobe syndrome*. Symptoms vary widely from individual to individual. In general, after damage to the dorsolateral (upper and outer) areas of the frontal lobes, the symptoms include a lack of drive and spontaneity. With damage to the most anterior aspects of the frontal lobes, the symptoms tend to involve more changes in mood and affect, such as impulsive and inappropriate behavior.

The skull of Phineas Gage, showing the route the tamping rod took through his skull. The angle of entry of the rod shot it behind the left eye and through the front part of the brain, sparing regions that were directly concerned with vital functions like breathing and heartbeat.

as schizophrenia, attention-deficit hyperactivity disorder (ADHD), and dementia. Box 6.1 describes how altered frontal lobe function can affect mood and personality.

Parietal Lobes

The postcentral gyrus, immediately behind the central sulcus, contains the primary somatosensory area. Damage to this area and neighboring gyri results in deficits in discriminative sensory function but not in the ability to perceive sensory input. The posterior areas of the parietal lobe appear to coordinate visual and somatosensory information. Damage to this area produces complex sensory deficits, including neglect of contralateral sensory stimuli and spatial relationships. The parietal lobes contribute to the ability to recognize objects by touch, calculate, write, recognize fingers of the opposite hands, draw, and organize spatial directions (e.g., how to travel to familiar places).

Temporal Lobes

The temporal lobes contain the primary auditory and olfactory areas. Wernicke area, located at the posterior aspect of the superior temporal gyrus, is primarily responsible for receptive speech. The temporal lobes also integrate sensory and visual information involved in control of written and verbal language skills as well as visual recognition. The hippocampus, an important structure discussed later, lies in the internal aspects of each temporal lobe and contributes to memory. Other internal structures of this lobe are involved in the modulation of mood and emotion.

Occipital Lobes

The primary visual area is in the most posterior aspect of the occipital lobes. Damage to this area results in a condition called *cortical blindness*. In other words, the retina and optic nerve remain intact, but the individual cannot see. The occipital lobes are involved in many aspects of visual integration of information, including color vision, object and facial recognition, and the ability to perceive objects in motion.

Association Cortex

Although not a lobe, the association cortex is an important area that allows the lobes to work in an integrated manner. Areas of one lobe of the cortex often share functions with an area of the adjacent lobe. When these neighboring nerve fibers are related to the same sensory modality, they are often referred to as *association areas*. For example, an area in the inferior parietal, posterior temporal, and anterior occipital lobes integrates visual, somatosensory, and auditory information to provide the abilities required for basic academic skills. These areas, along with numerous connections beneath the cortex, are part of the mechanisms that allow the human brain to work as an integrated whole.

Subcortical Structures

Beneath the cortex are layers of tissue composed of the axons of cell bodies. The axonal tissue forms pathways that are surrounded by glia, a fatty or lipid substance, which has a white appearance and gives these layers of neuron axons their name—white matter. Structures inside the hemispheres, beneath the cortex, are considered subcortical. Many of these structures, essential in the regulation of emotions and behaviors, play important roles in our understanding of mental disorders. Figure 6.2 provides a coronal section view of the gray matter, white matter, and important subcortical structures.

FIGURE 6.2 Coronal section of the brain, illustrating the corpus callosum, basal ganglia, and lateral ventricles. (From Bear, M. F., Conners, B. W., & Paradiso, M. A. [2016]. *Neuroscience: Exploring the brain* [3rd ed.]. Philadelphia, PA: Wolters Kluwer.)

The **basal ganglia** are subcortical gray matter areas in both the right and the left hemispheres that contain many cell bodies or nuclei. The primary subdivisions of the basal ganglia are the putamen, globus pallidus, and caudate. The basal ganglia are involved with motor functions and the learning and the programming of behavior or activities that are repetitive and, done over time, become automatic. The basal ganglia have many connections with the cerebral cortex, thalamus, midbrain structures, and spinal cord. Damage to portions of these nuclei may produce changes in posture or muscle tone. In addition, damage may produce abnormal movements, such as twitches or tremors. The basal ganglia can be adversely affected by some of the medications used to treat psychiatric disorders, leading to side effects and other motor-related problems.

Limbic System

The **limbic system** is essential to understanding the many hypotheses related to psychiatric disorders and emotional behavior in general. The limbic system is called a "system" because it comprises several small structures that work in a highly organized way. These structures include the hippocampus, thalamus, hypothalamus, amygdala, and limbic midbrain nuclei. See Figure 6.3 for identification and location of the structures within the limbic system and their relationships to other common CNS structures.

Basic emotions, needs, drives, and instinct begin and are modulated in the limbic system. Hate, love, anger, aggression, and caring are basic emotions that originate within the limbic system. Not only does the limbic system function as the seat of emotions, but because emotions are often generated based on our personal experiences, the limbic system also is involved with aspects of memory. Hypothesized changes in the limbic system play a significant role in many theories of major mental disorders, including schizophrenia, depression, and anxiety disorders (discussed in later chapters).

Hippocampus

The **hippocampus** is involved in storing information, especially the emotions attached to a memory. Our emotional responses to memories and our associations with other related memories are functions of how information is stored within the hippocampus. Although memory storage is not limited to one area of the brain, destruction of the left hippocampus impairs verbal memory, and damage to the right hippocampus results in difficulty with recognition and recall of complex visual and auditory patterns. Deterioration of the nerves of the hippocampus and other related temporal lobe structures found in Alzheimer disease produces the disorder's hallmark symptoms of memory dysfunction.

Thalamus

Sometimes called the "relay-switching center of the brain," the thalamus functions as a regulatory structure to relay all sensory information, except smell, sent to the CNS from the PNS. From the thalamus, the sensory information is relayed mostly to the cerebral cortex. The thalamus relays and regulates by filtering incoming information and determining what to pass on or not pass on to the cortex. In this fashion, the thalamus prevents the cortex from becoming overloaded with sensory stimulus. The thalamus is thought to play a part in controlling electrical activity in the cortex. Because of its primary relay function, damage to a very small area of the thalamus may produce deficits in many cortical functions, thus, causing behavioral abnormalities.

Hypothalamus

Basic human activities, such as sleep–rest patterns, body temperature, and physical drives such as hunger and sex, are regulated by another part of the limbic system that rests deep within the brain and is called the hypothalamus. Dysfunction of this structure, whether from disorders or because of an adverse effect of drugs used to treat mental illness, produces common psychiatric symptoms, such as appetite and sleep problems.

Nerve cells within the hypothalamus secrete hormones, for example, antidiuretic hormone, which when sent to the kidneys, accelerates the reabsorption of water; and oxytocin, which acts on smooth muscles to promote contractions, particularly within the walls of the uterus.

FIGURE 6.3 The structures of the limbic system are integrally involved in memory and emotional behavior. Theories link changes in the limbic system to many major mental disorders, including schizophrenia, depression, and anxiety disorders.

Because cells within the nervous system produce these hormones, they are often referred to as **neurohormones** (hormones that are produced by cells within the nervous system) and form a communication mechanism through the bloodstream to control organs that are not directly connected to nervous system structures.

The pituitary gland, often called the *master gland*, is directly connected by thousands of neurons that attach it to the ventral aspects of the hypothalamus. Together with the pituitary gland, the hypothalamus functions as one of the primary regulators of many aspects of the endocrine system. Its functions are involved in control of visceral activities, such as body temperature, arterial blood pressure, hunger, thirst, fluid balance, gastric motility, and gastric secretions. Deregulation of the hypothalamus can be manifested in symptoms of certain psychiatric disorders. For example, in schizophrenia, patients often wear heavy coats during the hot summer months and do not appear hot. Before the role of the hypothalamus in schizophrenia was understood, psychological reasons were used to explain such symptoms. Now it is increasingly clear that such a symptom relates to deregulation of the hypothalamus's normal role in temperature regulation and is a biologically based symptom (Lee, Jayathilake, Sim, & Meltzer, 2015).

Amygdala

The amygdala is directly connected to more primitive centers of the brain involving the sense of smell. It has numerous connections to the hypothalamus and lies adjacent to the hippocampus. The amygdala provides an emotional component to memory and is involved in modulating aggression and sexuality. Impulsive acts of aggression and violence have been linked to dysregulation of the amygdala, and erratic firing of the nerve cells in the amygdala is a focus of investigation in bipolar mood disorders (see Chapter 22).

Limbic Midbrain Nuclei

The limbic midbrain nuclei are a collection of neurons (including the ventral tegmental area and the **locus caeruleus**) that appear to play a role in the biologic basis of addiction. Sometimes referred to as the pleasure center or reward center of the brain, the limbic midbrain nuclei function to chemically reinforce certain behaviors, ensuring their repetition. Emotions such as feeling satisfied with good food, the pleasure of nurturing young, and the enjoyment of sexual activity originate in the limbic midbrain nuclei. The reinforcement of activities such as nutrition, procreation, and nurturing young are all primitive aspects of ensuring the survival of a species. When functioning in abnormal ways, the limbic midbrain nuclei can begin to reinforce unhealthy or risky behaviors, such as drug abuse. Exploration of this area of the brain is in its infancy but offers potential insight into addictions and their treatment.

Other Central Nervous System Structures

The **extrapyramidal motor system** is a bundle of nerve fibers connecting the thalamus to the basal ganglia and cerebral cortex. Muscle tone, common reflexes, and automatic voluntary motor functioning (e.g., walking) are controlled by this nerve track. Dysfunction of this motor track can produce hypertonicity in muscle groups. In Parkinson disease, the cells that compose the extrapyramidal motor system are severely affected, producing many involuntary motor movements. A number of medications, which are discussed in Chapter 11, also affect this system.

The **pineal body** is located above and medial to the thalamus. Because the pineal gland easily calcifies, it can be visualized by neuroimaging and often is a medial landmark. Its functions remain somewhat of a mystery despite long knowledge of its existence. It contains secretory cells that emit the neurohormone melatonin and other substances. These hormones are thought to have several regulatory functions within the endocrine system. Information received from light–dark sources controls release of melatonin, which has been associated with sleep and emotional disorders. In addition, a modulation of immune function has been postulated for melatonin from the pineal gland.

The locus caeruleus is a tiny cluster of neurons that fan out and innervate almost every part of the brain, including most of the cortex, the thalamus and hypothalamus, the cerebellum, and the spinal cord. Just one neuron from the caeruleus can connect to more than 250,000 other neurons. Despite its small size, the wide-ranging neuronal connections allow this tiny structure to influence the regulation of attention, time perception, sleep–rest cycles, arousal, learning, pain, and mood. It also plays a role in information processing of new, unexpected, and novel experiences. Some think its function or dysfunction may explain why individuals become addicted to substances and seek out risky behaviors despite awareness of negative consequences.

The brain stem, which is located beneath the thalamus and composed of the midbrain, pons, and medulla, has important life-sustaining functions. Nuclei of numerous neural pathways to the cerebrum are in the brain stem. They are significantly involved in mediating symptoms of emotional dysfunction. These nuclei are also the primary source of several neurochemicals, such as serotonin, that are commonly associated with psychiatric disorders.

The **cerebellum** is in the posterior aspect of the skull beneath the cerebral hemispheres. This large structure controls movements and postural adjustments. To

TABLE 6.1 PERIPHERAL ORGAN RESPONSE IN THE AUTONOMIC NERVOUS SYSTEM

Effector Organ	Sympathetic Response (Mostly Norepinephrine)	Parasympathetic Response (Acetylcholine)
Eye		
• Iris sphincter muscle	Dilation	Constriction
• Ciliary muscle	Relaxation	Accommodation for near vision
Heart		
• Sinoatrial node	Increased rate	Decrease is rare
• Atria	Increased contractility	Decrease in contractility
• Atrioventricular node	Increased contractility	Decrease in conduction velocity
Blood Vessels	Constriction	Dilation
Lungs		
• Bronchial muscles	Relaxation	Bronchoconstriction
• Bronchial glands		Secretion
Gastrointestinal Tract		
• Motility and tone	Relaxation	Increased
• Sphincters	Contraction	Relaxation
• Secretion		Stimulation
Urinary Bladder		
• Detrusor muscle	Relaxation	Contraction
• Trigone and sphincter	Contraction	Relaxation
Uterus	Contraction (pregnant) Relaxation (nonpregnant)	Variable
Skin		
• Pilomotor muscles	Contraction	No effect
• Sweat glands	Increased secretion	No effect
Glands		
• Salivary, lachrymal		Increased secretion
• Sweat		Increased secretion

regulate postural balance and positioning, the cerebellum receives information from all parts of the body, including the muscles, joints, skin, and visceral organs, as well as from many parts of the CNS.

Autonomic Nervous System

Closely associated with the spinal cord but not lying entirely within its column is the **autonomic nervous system**, a subdivision of the PNS. It was originally given this name for being independent of conscious thought, that is, automatic. However, it does not necessarily function as autonomously as the name indicates. This system contains efferent (nerves moving away from the CNS), or motor system neurons, which affect target tissues such as cardiac muscle, smooth muscle, and the glands. It also contains afferent nerves, which are sensory and conduct information from these organs back to the CNS.

The autonomic nervous system is further divided into the sympathetic and parasympathetic nervous systems. These systems, although peripheral, are included here because they are involved in the emergency, or "fight-or-flight," response as well as the peripheral actions of many medications (see Chapter 11). Figure 6.4 illustrates the innervations of various target organs by the autonomic nervous system. Table 6.1 identifies the actions of the sympathetic and parasympathetic nervous systems on various target organs.

NEUROPHYSIOLOGY OF THE CENTRAL NERVOUS SYSTEM

At their most basic level, the human brain and connecting nervous system are composed of billions of cells. Most are connective and supportive glial cells with ancillary functions in the nervous system.

> **KEYCONCEPT Neuroplasticity** is a continuous process of modulation of neuronal structure and function in response to the changing environment.

The changes in neural environment can come from internal sources, such as a change in electrolytes, or from external sources, such as a virus or toxin. Because of

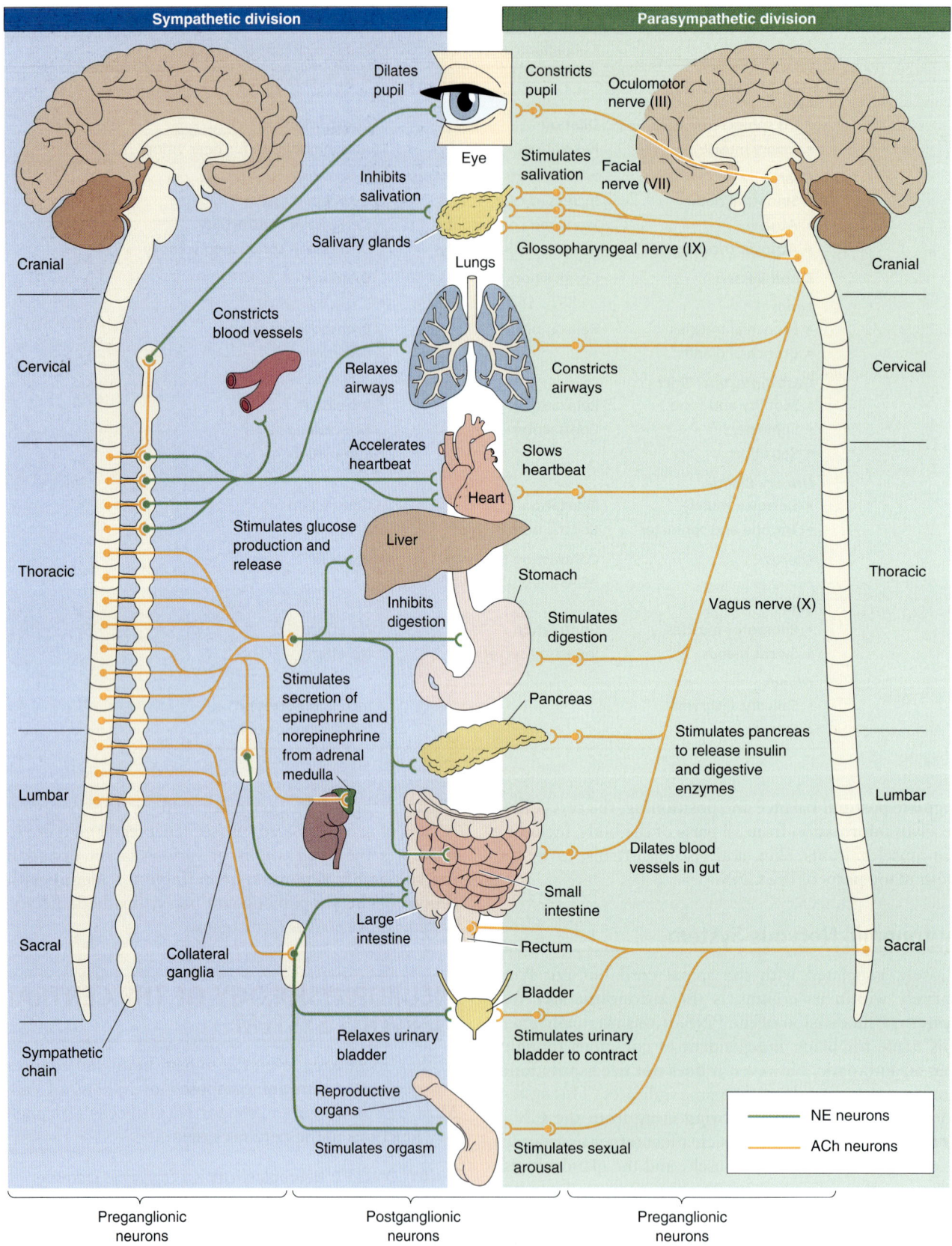

FIGURE 6.4 Diagram of the autonomic nervous system. Note that many organs are innervated by both sympathetic and parasympathetic nerves. (From Bear, M. F., Conners, B. W., & Paradiso, M. A. [2016]. *Neuroscience: Exploring the brain* [3rd ed.]. Philadelphia, PA: Wolters Kluwer.)

neuroplasticity, nerve signals may be rerouted, cells may learn new functions, the sensitivity or number of cells may increase or decrease, and some nerve tissue may undergo limited regeneration. Brains are mostly plastic during infancy and young childhood, when large adaptive learning tasks should normally occur. With age, brains become less plastic, which explains why it is easier to learn a second language at the age of 5 years than 55 years. Neuroplasticity contributes to understanding how function may be restored over time after brain damage occurs, or how an individual may react over time to continuous pharmacotherapy regimens.

Neurons and Nerve Impulses

In the human body, approximately 10 billion nerve cells, or neurons, function to receive, organize, and transmit information (Fig. 6.5). Each neuron has a cell body, or soma, which holds the nucleus containing most of the cell's genetic information. The soma also includes other organelles, such as ribosomes and endoplasmic reticulum, which carry out protein synthesis; the Golgi apparatus, which contains enzymes to modify the proteins for specific functions; vesicles, which transport and store proteins; and lysosomes, which are responsible for degradation of these proteins. Located throughout the neurons, mitochondria, containing enzymes and often called the "powerhouse" are the sites of many energy-producing chemical reactions. These cell structures provide the basis for secreting numerous chemicals by which neurons communicate.

It is not just the vast number of neurons that accounts for the complexities of the brain but also the enormous number of neurochemical interconnections and interactions among neurons. A single motor neuron in the spinal cord may receive signals from more than 10,000 sources of interconnections with other nerves. Although most neurons have only one axon, which varies in length and conducts impulses away from the soma, each has numerous dendrites, receiving signals from other neurons. Because axons may branch as they terminate, they also have multiple contacts with other neurons.

FIGURE 6.5 Cell body and organelles of neuron.

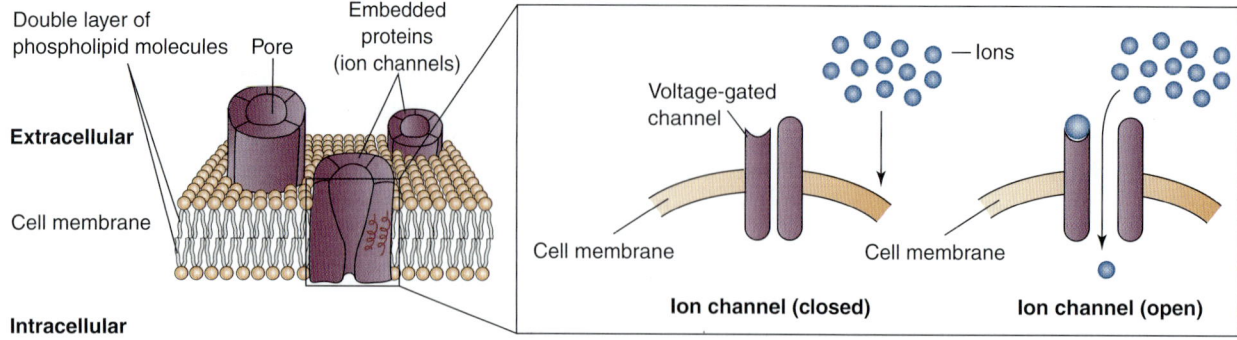

FIGURE 6.6 Initiation of a nerve impulse. The initiation of an action potential, or nerve impulse, involves the opening and closing of the voltage-gated channels on the cell membrane and the passage of ions into the cell. The resulting electrical activity sends communication impulses from the dendrites or axon into the body.

Nerve signals are prompted to fire by a variety of chemical or physical stimuli. This firing produces an electrical impulse. The cell's membrane is a double layer of phospholipid molecules with embedded proteins. Some of these proteins provide water-filled channels through which inorganic ions may pass (Fig. 6.6). Each of the common ions—sodium, potassium, calcium, and chloride—has its own specific molecular channel. Many of these channels are voltage gated and thus open or close in response to changes in the electrical potential across the membrane. At rest, the cell membrane is polarized with a positive charge on the outside and about a 270-mV charge on the inside, owing to the resting distribution of sodium and potassium ions. As potassium passively diffuses across the membrane, the sodium pump uses energy to move sodium from the inside of the cell against a concentration gradient to maintain this distribution. An action potential, or *nerve impulse*, is generated as the membrane is depolarized and a threshold value is reached, which triggers the opening of the voltage-gated sodium channels, allowing sodium to surge into the cell. The inside of the cell briefly becomes positively charged and the outside negatively charged. Once initiated, the action potential becomes self-propagating, opening nearby sodium channels. This electrical communication moves into the soma from the dendrites or down the axon by this mechanism.

Synaptic Transmission

For one neuron to communicate with another, the electrical process described must change to a chemical communication. The **synaptic cleft**, a junction between one nerve and another, is the space where the electrical intracellular signal becomes a chemical extracellular signal. Various substances are recognized as the chemical messengers among neurons.

As the electrical action potential reaches the ends of the axons, called *terminals*, calcium ion channels are opened, allowing an influx of Ca^{++} ions into the neuron. This increase in calcium stimulates the release of neurotransmitters into the synapse. Rapid signaling among neurons requires a ready supply of neurotransmitter. These neurotransmitters are stored in small vesicles grouped near the cell membrane at the end of the axon. When stimulated, the vesicles containing the neurotransmitter fuse with the cell membrane, and the neurotransmitter is released into the synapse (Fig. 6.7). The neurotransmitter then crosses the synaptic cleft to a receptor site on the postsynaptic neuron and stimulates adjacent neurons. This is the process of neuronal communication.

When the neurotransmitter has completed its interaction with the postsynaptic receptor and stimulated that cell, its work is done, and it needs to be removed. It can be removed by natural diffusion away from the area of high neurotransmitter concentration at the receptors by being broken down by enzymes in the synaptic cleft or through reuptake through highly specific mechanisms into the presynaptic terminal. The primary steps in synaptic transmission are summarized in Figure 6.7.

Neurotransmitters

As described in the overview above, neurotransmitters are key in the process of synaptic transmission. Neurotransmitters are small molecules that directly and indirectly control the opening or closing of ion channels. **Neuromodulators** are chemical messengers that make the target cell membrane or postsynaptic membrane susceptible to the effects of the primary neurotransmitter.

KEYCONCEPT Neurotransmitters are small molecules that directly and indirectly control the opening or closing of ion channels.

Excitatory neurotransmitters reduce the membrane potential and enhance the transmission of the signal between neurons. *Inhibitory neurotransmitters* have the commonly classified as the following: cholinergic, biogenic amine (monoamines or bioamines), amino acid, and neuropeptides. Table 6.2 summarizes some of the key neurotransmitters and their proposed functions.

Acetylcholine

Acetylcholine (ACh) is the primary cholinergic neurotransmitter. Found in the greatest concentration in the PNS, ACh provides the basic synaptic communication for the parasympathetic neurons and part of the sympathetic neurons, which send information to the CNS.

ACh is an excitatory neurotransmitter that is found throughout the cerebral cortex and limbic system. It arises primarily from cell bodies in the basal forebrain constellation, which provides innervations to the cerebral cortex, amygdala, hippocampus, and thalamus as well as from the dorsolateral tegmentum of the pons that projects to the basal ganglia, thalamus, hypothalamus, medullary reticular formation, and deep cerebellar nuclei (Fig. 6.8) (Siegel & Sapru, 2015). These connections suggest that ACh is involved in higher intellectual functioning and memory. Individuals who have Alzheimer disease or Down syndrome often exhibit patterns of cholinergic neuron loss in regions innervated by these pathways (e.g., the hippocampus), which may contribute to their memory difficulties and other cognitive deficits. Some cholinergic neurons are afferent to these areas bringing information from the limbic system, highlighting the role that ACh plays in communicating one's emotional state to the cerebral cortex.

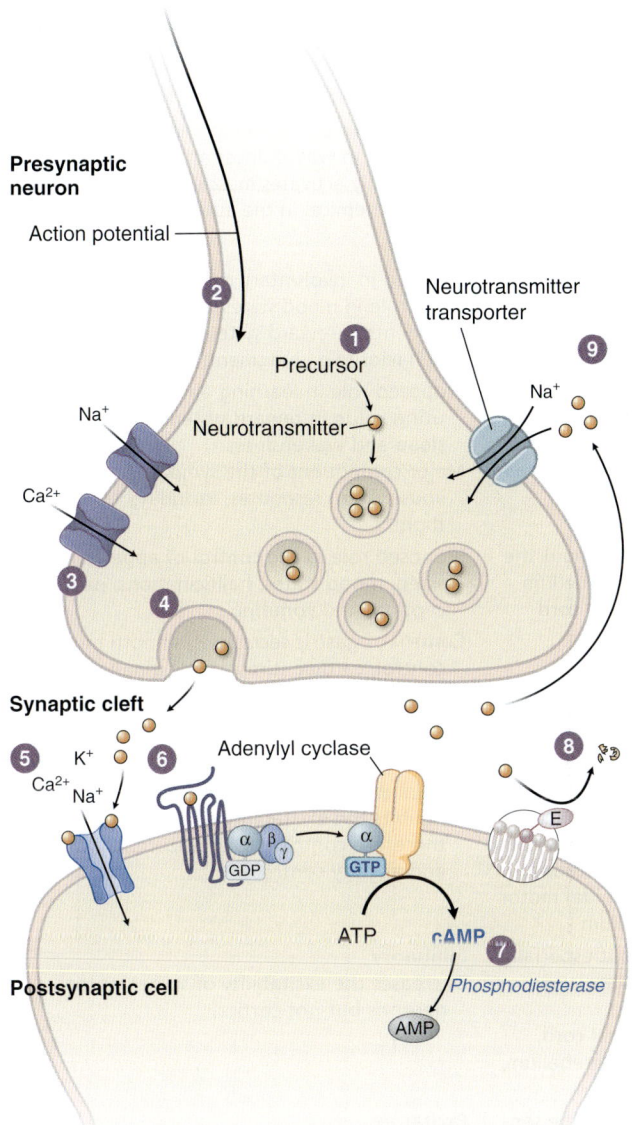

FIGURE 6.7 Synaptic transmission. The most significant events that occur during synaptic transmission: (*1*) the action potential reaches the presynaptic terminal; (*2*) membrane depolarization causes Ca++ terminals to open; (*3*) Ca++ mediates fusion of the vesicles with the presynaptic membrane; (*4*) transmitter molecules are released into the synaptic cleft by exocytosis; (*5*) transmitter molecules bind to postsynaptic receptors and activate ion channels; (*6*) conductance changes cause an excitatory or inhibitory postsynaptic potential, depending on the specific transmitter; (*7*) current flow spreads along the postsynaptic membrane; (*8*) transmitter remaining in the synaptic cleft returns to the presynaptic terminal by reuptake; and (*9*) diffuses into the extracellular fluid. (From Bear, M. F., Conners, B. W., & Paradiso, M. A. [2016]. *Neuroscience: Exploring the brain* [3rd ed.]. Philadelphia, PA: Wolters Kluwer.)

FIGURE 6.8 Cholinergic pathways. (From Bear, M. F., Conners, B. W., & Paradiso, M. A. [2016]. *Neuroscience: Exploring the brain* [3rd ed.]. Philadelphia, PA: Wolters Kluwer.)

opposite effect and slow down nerve impulses. Although some are synthesized from dietary precursors, such as tyrosine or tryptophan, most synthesis occurs in the terminals or the neuron itself. Neurotransmitters are

TABLE 6.2 CLASSIC AND PUTATIVE NEUROTRANSMITTERS: THEIR DISTRIBUTION AND PROPOSED FUNCTIONS			
Neurotransmitter	Cell Bodies	Projections	Proposed Function
Acetylcholine			
Dietary precursor: choline	Basal forebrain Pons Other areas	Diffuse throughout the cortex, hippocampus PNS	Important role in learning and memory Some role in wakefulness and basic attention Peripherally activates muscles and is the major neurochemical in the autonomic system
Monoamines			
Dopamine (dietary precursor: tyrosine)	Substantia nigra Ventral tegmental area Arcuate nucleus Retina olfactory bulb	Striatum (basal ganglia) Limbic system and cerebral cortex Pituitary	Involved in involuntary motor movements Some role in mood states, pleasure components in reward systems, and complex behavior (e.g., judgment, reasoning, insight)
Norepinephrine (dietary precursor: tyrosine)	Locus caeruleus Lateral tegmental area and others throughout the pons and medulla	Very widespread throughout the cortex, thalamus, cerebellum, brain stem, and spinal cord Basal forebrain, thalamus, hypothalamus, brain stem, and spinal cord	Proposed role in learning and memory, attributing value in reward systems, fluctuates in sleep and wakefulness Major component of the sympathetic nervous system responses, including "fight or flight"
Serotonin (dietary precursor: tryptophan)	Raphe nuclei Others in the pons and medulla	Very widespread throughout the cortex, thalamus, cerebellum, brain stem, and spinal cord	Proposed role in the control of appetite, sleep, mood states, hallucinations, pain perception, and vomiting
Histamine (precursor: histidine)	Hypothalamus	Cerebral cortex Limbic system Hypothalamus Found in all mast cells	Control of gastric secretions, smooth muscle control, cardiac stimulation, stimulation of sensory nerve endings, and alertness
Amino Acids			
GABA	Derived from glutamate without localized cell bodies	Found in cells and projections throughout the CNS, especially in intrinsic feedback loops and interneurons of the cerebrum Also in the extrapyramidal motor system and cerebellum	Fast inhibitory response postsynaptically inhibits the excitability of the neurons and therefore contributes to seizure, agitation, and anxiety control
Glycine	Primarily the spinal cord and brain stem	Limited projection, but especially in the auditory system and olfactory bulb Also found in the spinal cord, medulla, midbrain, cerebellum, and cortex	Inhibitory Decreases the excitability of spinal motor neurons but not cortical
Glutamate	Diffuse	Diffuse, but especially in the sensory organs	Excitatory Responsible for the bulk of information flow
Neuropeptides			
Endogenous opioids (i.e., endorphins, enkephalins)	A large family of neuropeptides that has three distinct subgroups, all of which are manufactured widely throughout the CNS	Widely distributed within and outside of the CNS	Suppress pain, modulate mood and stress Likely involvement in reward systems and addiction Also may regulate pituitary hormone release Implicated in the pathophysiology of diseases of the basal ganglia
Melatonin (one of its precursors: serotonin)	Pineal body	Widely distributed within and outside of the CNS	Secreted in dark and suppressed in light, helps regulate the sleep–wake cycle as well as other biologic rhythms
Substance P	Widespread, significant in the raphe system and spinal cord	Spinal cord, cortex, brain stem, and especially sensory neurons associated with pain perception	Involved in pain transmission, movement, and mood regulation
Cholecystokinin	Predominates in the ventral tegmental area of the midbrain	Frontal cortex, where it is often colocalized with dopamine Widely distributed within and outside of the CNS	Primary intestinal hormone involved in satiety; also has some involvement in the control of anxiety and panic

CNS, central nervous system; GABA, gamma-aminobutyric acid; PNS, peripheral nervous system.

Biogenic Amines

The **biogenic amines** (bioamines) consist of small molecules manufactured in the neuron that contain an amine group, thus the name. The catecholamines (amine attached to a catechol group) include dopamine, norepinephrine, and epinephrine, which are all synthesized from the amino acid tyrosine. Another monoamine, serotonin, is synthesized from tryptophan. Melatonin is derived from serotonin. All of these neurotransmitters are critical in many of the mental disorders.

Dopamine

Dopamine is an excitatory neurotransmitter found in distinct regions of the CNS and is involved in cognition, motor, and neuroendocrine functions. Dopamine is the neurotransmitter that stimulates the body's natural "feel-good" reward pathways, producing pleasant euphoric sensation under certain conditions. It is involved in the regulation of action, emotion, motivation, and attention. Dopamine levels are decreased in Parkinson disease, and abnormally high activity of dopamine has been associated with schizophrenia (discussed in more detail in Chapter 23). Abnormalities of dopamine activity within the reward system pathways are suspected to be a critical aspect of the development of drug and other addictions. The dopamine pathways are distinct neuronal areas within the CNS in which the neurotransmitter dopamine predominates. Three major dopaminergic pathways have been identified.

The *mesocortical* and *mesolimbic pathways* originate in the ventral tegmental area and project into the medial aspects of the cortex (mesocortical) and the limbic system inside the temporal lobes, including the hippocampus and amygdala (mesolimbic). Sometimes they are considered to be one pathway and at other times two separate pathways. The mesocortical pathway has major effects on cognition, including functions such as judgment, reasoning, insight, social conscience, motivation, the ability to generalize learning, and reward systems in the human brain. It contributes to some of the highest seats of cortical functioning. The mesolimbic pathway also strongly influences emotions and has projections that affect memory and auditory reception. Abnormalities in these pathways have been associated with schizophrenia.

Another major dopaminergic pathway begins in the substantia nigra and projects into the basal ganglia, parts of which are known as the *striatum*. Therefore, this pathway is called the *nigrostriatal pathway*. This influences the extrapyramidal motor system, which serves the voluntary motor system and allows involuntary motor movements. Destruction of dopaminergic neurons in this pathway has been associated with Parkinson disease.

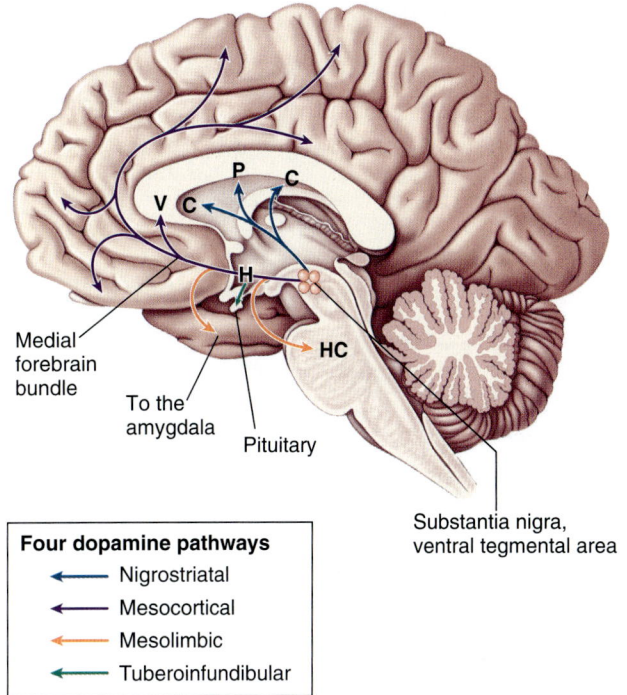

FIGURE 6.9 Dopaminergic pathways. *C*, caudate nucleus; *H*, hypothalamus; *HC*, hippocampal formation; *P*, putamen; *S*, striatum; *V*, ventral striatum. The dopaminergic diffuse modulatory systems arising from the substantia nigra and the ventral tegmental area. The substantia nigra and ventral tegmental area lie close together in the midbrain. They project to the striatum (caudate nucleus and putamen) and limbic and frontal cortical regions, respectively. (From Bear, M. F., Conners, B. W., & Paradiso, M. A. [2016]. *Neuroscience: Exploring the brain* [3rd ed.]. Philadelphia, PA: Wolters Kluwer.)

The final dopamine pathway originates from projections of the mesolimbic pathway and continues into the hypothalamus, which then projects into the pituitary gland. Therefore, this pathway, called the *tuberoinfundibular pathway*, has an impact on endocrine function and other functions, such as metabolism, hunger, thirst, sexual function, circadian rhythms, digestion, and temperature control. Figure 6.9 illustrates the dopaminergic pathways.

Norepinephrine

Norepinephrine is an excitatory neurochemical that plays a major role in generating and maintaining mood states. Because norepinephrine is so heavily concentrated in the terminal sites of sympathetic nerves, it can be released quickly to ready the individual for a fight-or-flight response to threats in the environment. For this reason, norepinephrine is thought to play a role in the physical symptoms of anxiety (Bastos et al., 2018).

Nerve tracts and pathways containing predominantly norepinephrine are called *noradrenergic* and are less clearly delineated than the dopamine pathways. In the

FIGURE 6.10 Noradrenergic pathways. (From Bear, M. F., Conners, B. W., & Paradiso, M. A. [2016]. *Neuroscience: Exploring the brain* [3rd ed.]. Philadelphia, PA: Wolters Kluwer.)

FIGURE 6.11 The serotonergic diffuse modulatory systems arising from the raphe nuclei. The raphe nuclei are clustered along the midline of the brain stem and project extensively to all levels of the CNS. (From Bear, M. F., Conners, B. W., & Paradiso, M. A. [2016]. *Neuroscience: Exploring the brain* [3rd ed.]. Philadelphia, PA: Wolters Kluwer.)

CNS, noradrenergic neurons originate in the locus caeruleus, where more than half of the noradrenergic cell bodies are located. Because the locus caeruleus is one of the major timekeepers of the human body, norepinephrine is involved in sleep and wakefulness. From the locus caeruleus, noradrenergic pathways ascend into the neocortex, spread diffusely (Fig. 6.10), and enhance the ability of neurons to respond to whatever input they may be receiving. In addition, norepinephrine appears to be involved in the process of reinforcement, which facilitates learning. Noradrenergic pathways innervate the hypothalamus and thus are involved to some degree in endocrine function. Anxiety disorders and depression are examples of psychiatric illnesses in which dysfunction of the noradrenergic neurons may be involved. (Refer to Table 6.1 for the effects of ACh on various organs in the parasympathetic system.)

Serotonin

Serotonin (also called 5-hydroxytryptamine or 5-HT) is primarily an excitatory neurotransmitter that is diffusely distributed within the cerebral cortex, limbic system, and basal ganglia of the CNS. Serotonergic neurons also project into the hypothalamus and cerebellum. Figure 6.11 illustrates serotonergic pathways. Serotonin plays a role in emotions, cognition, sensory perceptions, and essential biologic functions, such as sleep and appetite. During the rapid eye movement (REM) phase of sleep, or the dream state, serotonin concentrations decrease, and muscles subsequently relax. Serotonin is also involved in the control of food intake, hormone secretion, sexual behavior, thermoregulation, and cardiovascular regulation. Some serotonergic fibers reach the cranial blood vessels within the brain and the *pia mater* where they have a vasoconstrictive effect. The potency of some new medications for migraine headaches is related to their ability to block serotonin transmission in the cranial blood vessels. Descending serotonergic pathways are important in central pain control. Whereas depression and insomnia have been associated with decreased levels of 5-HT, mania has been associated with increased 5-HT. Some of the most well-known antidepressant medications, such as Prozac and Zoloft, which are discussed in more depth in Chapter 11, function by raising serotonin levels within certain areas of the CNS. Melatonin, which is derived from serotonin, is produced by the pineal gland and plays a role in sleep, aging, and mood changes.

Amino Acids

Amino acids, the building blocks of proteins, have many roles in intraneuronal metabolism. In addition, amino acids can function as neurotransmitters in as many as 60% to 70% of the synaptic sites in the brain. Amino acids are the most prevalent neurotransmitters. Virtually all of the neurons in the CNS are activated by excitatory amino acids, such as glutamate, and inhibited by inhibitory amino acids, such as gamma-aminobutyric acid (GABA) and glycine. Many of these amino acids coexist with other neurotransmitters.

Histamine

Histamine, derived from the amino acid histidine, has been identified as a neurotransmitter. Its cell bodies originate predominantly in the hypothalamus and project to all major structures in the cerebrum, brain stem, and spinal cord. Its functions are not well known, but it appears to have a role in autonomic and neuroendocrine regulation. Many psychiatric medications can block the effects of histamine postsynaptically and produce side effects such as sedation, weight gain, and hypotension.

Gamma-Aminobutyric Acid

GABA is the primary inhibitory neurotransmitter for the CNS. The pathways of GABA exist almost exclusively in the CNS, with the largest GABA concentrations in the hypothalamus, hippocampus, basal ganglia, spinal cord, and cerebellum. GABA functions in an inhibitory role in control of spinal reflexes and cerebellar reflexes. It has a major role in the control of neuronal excitability through the brain. In addition, GABA has an inhibitory influence on the activity of the dopaminergic nigrostriatal projections. GABA also has interconnections with other neurotransmitters. For example, dopamine inhibits cholinergic neurons, and GABA provides feedback and balance. Dysregulation of GABA and GABA receptors has been associated with anxiety disorders, and decreased GABA activity is involved in the development of seizure disorders.

Glutamate

Glutamate, the most widely distributed excitatory neurotransmitter, is the main transmitter in the associational areas of the cortex. Glutamate can be found in a number of pathways from the cortex to the thalamus, pons, striatum, and spinal cord. In addition, glutamate pathways have a number of connections with the hippocampus. Some glutamate receptors may play a role in the long-lasting enhancement of synaptic activity. In turn, in the hippocampus, this enhancement may have a role in learning and memory. Too much glutamate is harmful to neurons, and considerable interest has emerged regarding its neurotoxic effects.

Conditions that produce an excess of endogenous glutamate can cause neurotoxicity by overexcitation of neuronal tissue. This process, called excitotoxicity, increases the sensitivity of glutamate receptors, produces overactivation of the receptors, and is increasingly being understood as a critical piece of the cascade of events involved in physical symptoms of alcohol withdrawal in dependent individuals. Excitotoxicity is also believed to be part of the pathology of conditions such as ischemia, hypoxia, hypoglycemia, and hepatic failure. Damage to the CNS from chronic malfunctioning of the glutamate system may be involved in the psychiatric symptoms seen in neurodegenerative diseases such as Huntington, Parkinson, and Alzheimer diseases; vascular dementia; amyotrophic lateral sclerosis; and acquired immunodeficiency syndrome (AIDS)-related dementia. Degeneration of glutamate neurons is implicated in the development of schizophrenia.

Neuropeptides

Neuropeptides, short chains of amino acids, exist in the CNS and have a number of important roles as neurotransmitters, neuromodulators, or neurohormones. Neuropeptides were first thought to be pituitary hormones, such as adrenocorticotropin, oxytocin, and vasopressin, or hypothalamic-releasing hormones (e.g., corticotropin-releasing hormone and thyrotropin-releasing hormone [TRH]). However, when an endogenous morphine-like substance was discovered in the 1970s, the term *endorphin*, or endogenous morphine, was introduced. Although the amino acids and monoamine neurotransmitters can be produced directly from dietary precursors in any part of the neuron, neuropeptides are, almost without exception, synthesized from messenger RNA in the cell body. Currently, two types of neuropeptides have been identified. Opioid neuropeptides, such as endorphins, enkephalins, and dynorphins, function in endocrine functioning and pain suppression. The nonopioid neuropeptides, such as substance P and somatostatin, play roles in pain transmission and endocrine functioning, respectively.

There are considerable variations in the distribution of individual neuropeptides, but some areas are especially rich in cell bodies containing neuropeptides. These areas include the amygdala, striatum, hypothalamus, raphe nuclei, brain stem, and spinal cord. Many of the interneurons of the cerebral cortex contain neuropeptides, but there are considerably fewer in the thalamus and almost none in the cerebellum.

Receptors

Embedded in the postsynaptic membrane are a number of proteins that act as receptors for the released neurotransmitters. Each neurotransmitter has a specific receptor, or protein, for which it and only it will fit.

Lock and Key

The "lock-and-key" analogy has often been used to describe the fit of a given neurotransmitter to its receptor site. The target cell, when stimulated by the neurotransmitter, will then respond by evoking its own action potential and either producing some action common to that cell or acting as a relay to keep the messages moving throughout the CNS. This pattern of the electrical signal from one neuron, converted to chemical signal at the synaptic cleft, picked up by an adjacent neuron, again converted to an electrical action potential, and then to a chemical signal, occurs billions of times a day in billions of different neurons. This electrical–chemical communication process allows the structures of the brain to function together in a coordinated and organized manner.

Receptor Sensitivity

Both presynaptic and postsynaptic **receptors** have the capacity to change, developing either a greater-than-usual response to the neurotransmitter, known as supersensitivity, or a less-than-usual response, called subsensitivity. These changes represent the concept of neuroplasticity of brain tissue discussed earlier in the chapter. The change in sensitivity of the receptor is most commonly caused by the effect of a drug on a receptor site or by disease that affects the normal functioning of a receptor site. Drugs can affect the sensitivity of the receptor by altering the strength of attraction or affinity of a receptor for the neurotransmitter, by changing the efficiency with which the receptor activity translates the message inside the receiving cell, or by decreasing over time the number of receptors.

These mechanisms may account for the long-term, sometimes severely adverse, effects of psychopharmacologic drugs, the loss of effectiveness of a given medication, or the loss of effectiveness of a medication after repeated use in treating recurring episodes of a psychiatric disorder. Disease may cause a change in the normal number or function of receptors, thereby altering their sensitivity. For example, depression is associated with a reduction in the normal number of certain receptors, leading to an abnormality in their sensitivity to neurotransmitters such as serotonin and norepinephrine (Bewernick & Schlaepfer, 2015). A decreased response to continued stimulation of these receptors is usually referred to as *desensitization* or *refractoriness*. This suspected subsensitivity is referred to as *downregulation* of the receptors.

Receptor Subtypes

The nervous system uses many different neurochemicals for communication, and each specific chemical messenger requires a specific receptor on which the chemical can act. More than 100 different chemical messengers have been identified, with new ones being uncovered. In addition to the sheer number of receptors needed to accommodate these chemicals, the neurotransmitters may produce different effects at different synaptic sites.

Each major neurotransmitter has several different subtypes of receptors, allowing the neurotransmitter to have different effects in different areas of the brain. The receptors usually have the same name as the neurotransmitter, but the classification of the subtypes varies. For example, dopamine receptors are named D1,

TABLE 6.3	SELECTED NEUROTRANSMITTERS AND RECEPTORS
Neurotransmitter	**Receptor Subtypes**
Acetylcholine (ACH)	Muscarinic receptors (M_1, M_2, M_3, M_4, M_5) Nicotinic receptor
Glutamate (Glu)	AMPA, NMDA, kainate receptors
GABA	$GABA_A$, $GABA_B$
Serotonin (5-HT)	$5\text{-}HT_{1A}$, $5\text{-}HT_{1B}$, $5\text{-}HT_{1D}$, $5\text{-}HT_{1E}$, $5\text{-}HT_{2A}$, $5\text{-}HT_{2B}$, $5\text{-}HT_C$, $5\text{-}HT_4$, $5\text{-}HT_{5A}$
Dopamine (DA)	D1, D2, D3, D4, D5
Norepinephrine (NE)	α_1, α_2, β_1, β_2

Reprinted with permission from Bear, M. F., Connors, B. W., & Paradiso, M. A. (2016). *Neuroscience: Exploring the brain* (4th ed.). Philadelphia, PA: Wolters Kluwer.

D2, D3, and so on. Serotonin receptors are grouped in families such at $5\text{-}HT1_A$, $5\text{-}HT1_B$, and so on. The receptors for Ach have completely different names: muscarinic and nicotinic. Two specific subtype receptors have been identified for GABA: A and B (see Table 6.3).

Brain structures such as the prefrontal cortex, striatum, hippocampus, and amygdala are linked through complex neural functional networks (Plåschke et al., 2017). Recent research indicates that a dysfunctional **neurocircuitry** underlies most psychiatric disorders (Fig. 6.12).

FIGURE 6.12 Complex neural functional networks involved in psychiatric disorders. *Arrows* illustrate projections. *ACC,* anterior cingulate cortex; *Amy,* amygdala; *Cd,* caudate nucleus; *DPFC,* dorsal prefrontal cortex; *Ex Amy,* extended amygdala; *GP,* globus pallidus; *Hipp,* hippocampus; *MD,* medial dorsal nucleus of the thalamus; *MTL,* medial temporal lobe; *OFC,* orbital frontal cortex; *Pu,* putamen; *SN,* substantia nigra; *Thal,* thalamus; *vmPFC,* ventral medial prefrontal cortex; *VP,* ventral pallidum; *VS,* ventral striatum; *VTA,* ventral tegmental area. (Redrawn with permission from Haber, S. N., & Rauch, S. L. [2010]. Neurocircuitry: A window into the networks underlying neuropsychiatric disease. *Neuropsychopharmacology Reviews, 35*[1], 1–3.)

Various neurocircuits are the focus of study of different illness. For example, the cingulo-frontal-parietal network is associated with attention-deficit disorder, and the amygdalocortical circuitry is the focus in psychosis and schizophrenia.

STUDIES OF THE BIOLOGIC BASIS OF MENTAL DISORDERS

As described earlier, mental disorders are complex syndromes consisting of clusters of biopsychosocial symptoms. These syndromes are not specific physiologic disorders, and research efforts are focused on piecing the puzzle together. One important area of study is genetics; it is well established that genetic factors play an important role in the development of mental disorders. In addition, as the complexity of the nervous system and its interrelationship with other body systems and the environment have become more fully understood, new fields of study have emerged. One field worth noting is **psychoneuroimmunology** (PNI). Although it has long been observed that individuals under stress have compromised immune systems and are more likely to acquire common diseases, only recently have changes in the immune system been noted as widespread in some psychiatric illnesses. Another field, chronobiology, has provided new information suggesting that dysfunction of biologic rhythms may not only result from a psychiatric illness but also contribute to its development.

Genetics

The sequence of the human genome is the beginning of our understanding of complex genetic connections that leads to a **phenotype** or observable characteristics or expressions of a specific trait. The genome provides researchers with a road map of the exact sequence of the three billion nucleotide bases that make up human organisms. Many thought that after the human genome was mapped, it would be easy to determine the genes responsible for mental disorders. Unfortunately, it is not that simple. Knowing the location of the gene and its sequence are just pieces of the complex puzzle. The location of the genes does not tell us which genes are responsible for a mental illness or how mutations occur.

Population Genetics

Inheritance of mental disorders is studied by using epidemiologic methods that identify risks and patterns of illness or traits from generation to generation. Beginning with a **proband**, a person who has the disorder or trait, **population genetics** relies on the following principal epidemiologic methods:

- **Family studies** analyze the occurrence of a disorder in first-degree relatives (biologic parents, siblings, and children), second-degree relatives (grandparents, uncles, aunts, nieces, nephews, and grandchildren), and so on.
- **Twin studies** analyze the presence or absence of the disorder in pairs of twins. The *concordance rate* is the measure of similarity of occurrence in individuals with a similar genetic makeup.
- **Adoption studies** compare the risk for the illness developing in offspring raised in different environments. The strongest inferences may be drawn from studies that involve children separated from their parents at birth.

Mental disorders and their symptoms are not an expression of a single gene. The transmission pattern does not follow classic mendelian genetics in which the dominant allele (variant) on only one chromosome or recessive alleles on both chromosomes are responsible for manifestation of a disorder. Monozygotic (identical) twins do not manifest the same mental disorder with 100% concordance rate, but they have a higher rate of a disorder than dizygotic (fraternal) twins, who share roughly the same proportion of genes that ordinary siblings do (50%). Internal and external environmental events influence the development of a disorder with a genetic contribution. This interaction between the environment and a genetic predisposition underlies several mental disorders such as schizophrenia, autism, and ADHD.

Molecular Genetics

A gene comprises short segments of DNA and is packed with the instructions for making proteins that have a specific function. When genes are absent or malfunction, protein production is altered, and bodily functions are disrupted. In this fashion, genes play a role in cancer, heart disease, diabetes, and many psychiatric disorders. Although no conclusive evidence exists for a complete genetic cause of most psychiatric disorders, significant evidence suggests that strong genetic contributions exist for most (Corponi et al., 2018).

Intracellular genes direct protein production responsible for genetic expression. Individual nerve cells outside of the cell respond to these changes, modifying proteins to adapt to the new environment. This dynamic nature of gene function highlights the manner in which the body and the environment interact and in how environmental factors influence gene expression.

The study of molecular genetics in psychiatric disorders is in its infancy. It is likely that psychiatric disorders are polygenic. This means that psychiatric disorders develop when genes interact with each other and with environmental factors such as stress, infections, poor nutrition, catastrophic loss, complications during pregnancy, and exposure to toxins. Thus, genetic makeup conveys vulnerability, or a risk for the illness, but the right set of environmental factors must be present for the disorder to develop in an at-risk individual (Renzi et al., 2018).

Genetic Susceptibility

The concept of **genetic susceptibility** suggests that an individual may be at increased risk for a psychiatric disorder. Specific risk factors for psychiatric disorders are just beginning to be understood, and environmental influences are examples of risk factors. In the absence of one specific gene for the major psychiatric disorders, risk factor assessment is a logical alternative for predicting who is more likely to experience psychiatric disorders or certain conditions, such as aggression or suicidality (Lockhart, Sawa, & Niwa, 2018).

When considering information regarding risks for genetic transmission of psychiatric disorders, there are several key points to remember:

- Psychiatric disorders have been described and labeled quite differently across generations, and errors in diagnosis may occur.
- Similar psychiatric symptoms may have considerably different causes, just as symptoms such as chest pain may occur in relation to many different causes.
- Genes that are present may not always cause the appearance of the trait.
- Several genes work together in an individual to produce a given trait or disorder.
- A biologic cause is not necessarily solely genetic in origin. Environmental influences alter the body's functioning and often mediate or worsen genetic risk factors.

Psychoneuroimmunology

PNI examines the relationships among the immune system, nervous system, and endocrine system and our behaviors, thoughts, and feelings. The immune system is composed of the thymus, spleen, lymph nodes, lymphatic vessels, tonsils, adenoids, and bone marrow, which manufacture all the cells that eventually develop into T cells, B cells, phagocytes, macrophages, and natural killer (NK) cells (Fig. 6.13). Many contemporary stress research studies are examining the role of the NK cells in the early recognition of foreign bodies. Lower NK cell function is related to increased disease susceptibility. NK cell function is affected by stress-induced physiologic arousal in humans. NK cell activity has been shown to vary in response to many emotional, cognitive, and physiologic stressors, including anxiety, depression, perceived lack of personal control, bereavement, pain, and surgery (Furtado & Katzman, 2015; Kim, Na, Myint, & Leonard, 2015).

Overactivity of the immune system can occur in autoimmune diseases such as systemic lupus erythematosus (SLE), allergies, and anaphylaxis. Evidence suggests that the nervous system regulates many aspects of immune function. Specific immune system dysfunctions may result from damage to the hypothalamus, hippocampus, or pituitary and may produce symptoms of psychiatric disorders. Figure 6.14 illustrates the interaction between stress and the immune system. This figure also demonstrates the true biopsychosocial nature of the complex interrelationship of the nervous system, the endocrine system, the immune system, and environmental or emotional stress.

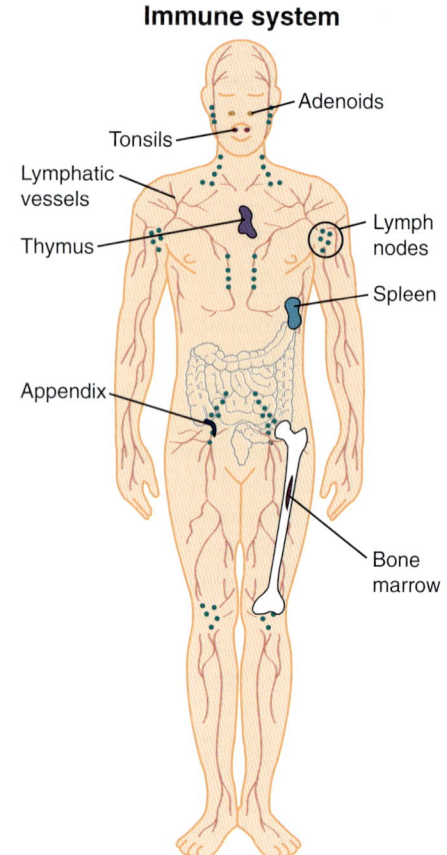

FIGURE 6.13 The immune system.

Immune dysregulation may also be involved in the development of psychiatric disorders. This can occur by allowing neurotoxins to affect the brain, damaging neuroendocrine tissue, or damaging tissues in the brain at locations such as the receptor sites. Some antidepressants have been thought to have antiviral effects. Symptoms of diseases such as depression may occur after an occurrence of serious infection, and prenatal exposure to infectious organisms has been associated with the development of schizophrenia. Stress and conditioning have specific effects on the suppression of immune function (Liu & Tang, 2018; Müller, Weidinger, Leitner, & Schwarz, 2015).

Normal functioning of the endocrine system is often disturbed in people with psychiatric disorders. For example, thyroid functioning is often low in those with bipolar disorder, and people with schizophrenia have a higher incidence of diabetes (see Unit V). The hypothalamus sends and receives information through

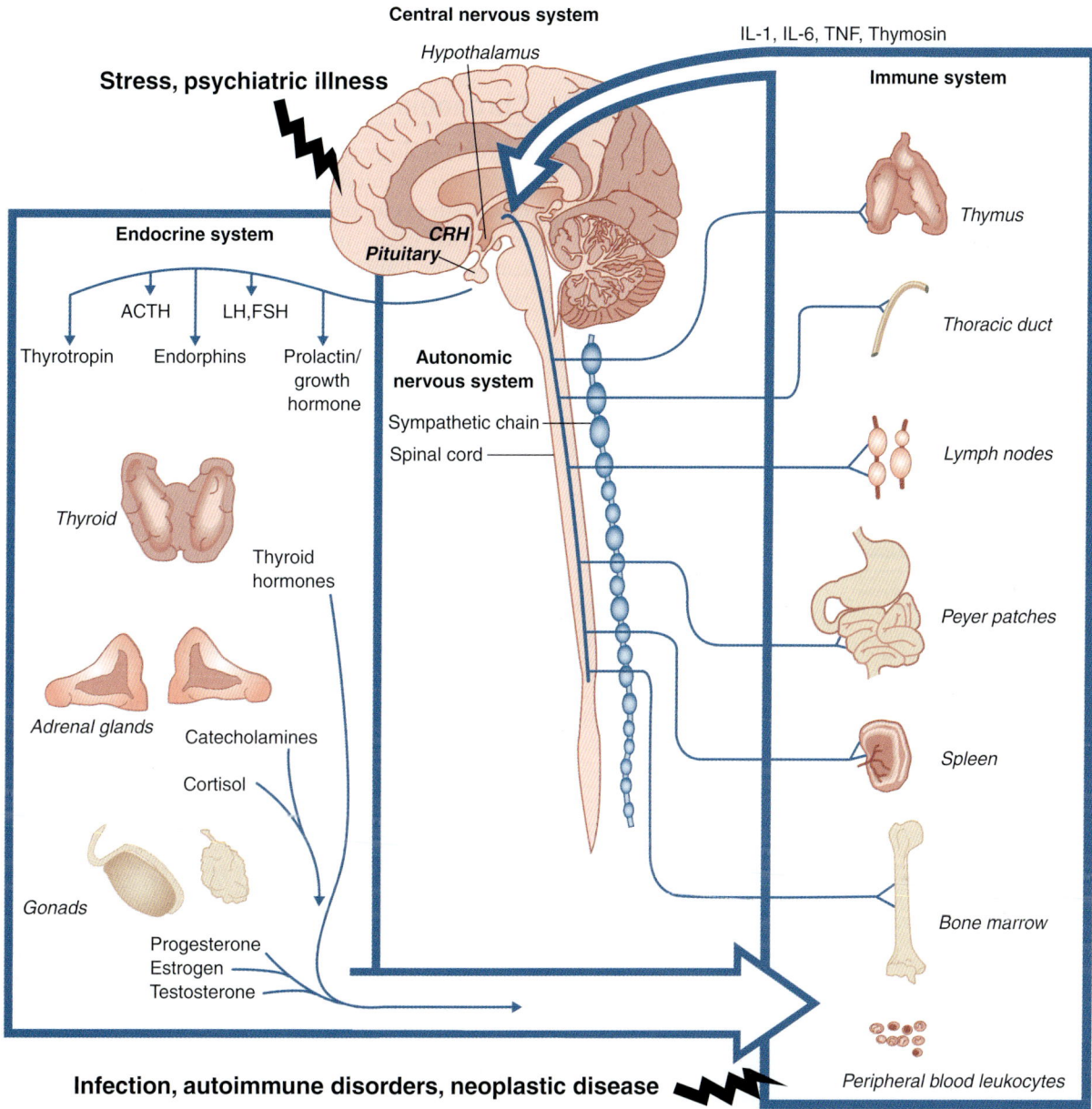

FIGURE 6.14 Examples of the interaction between stress or psychiatric illness and the immune system through the endocrine system. *ACTH*, adrenocorticotropic hormone; *CRH*, corticotropin-releasing hormone; *FSH*, follicle-stimulating hormone; *IL*, interleukin; *LH*, luteinizing hormone; *TNF*, tumor necrosis factor.

the pituitary, which then communicates with structures in the peripheral aspects of the body. Figure 6.15 presents an example of the communication of the anterior pituitary with a number of organs and structures.

Axes, the structures within which the neurohormones are providing messages, are the most often studied aspect of the neuroendocrine system. These axes always involve a feedback mechanism. For example, the hypothalamus–pituitary–thyroid axis regulates the release of thyroid hormone by the thyroid gland using TRH hormone from the hypothalamus to the pituitary and thyroid-stimulating hormone (TSH) from the pituitary to the thyroid. Figure 6.16 illustrates the hypothalamic–pituitary–thyroid axis. The hypothalamic–pituitary–gonadal axis regulates estrogen and testosterone secretion through luteinizing hormone and follicle-stimulating hormone. Interest in the endocrine system is heightened by various endocrine disorders that produce psychiatric symptoms. Addison disease (hypoadrenalism) produces depression, apathy, fatigue, and occasionally psychosis. Hypothyroidism produces depression and some anxiety. Administration of steroids can cause depression, hypomania, irritability, and in some cases, psychosis. Some psychiatric disorders have been associated with endocrine system dysfunction. For example, some individuals with mood disorders show

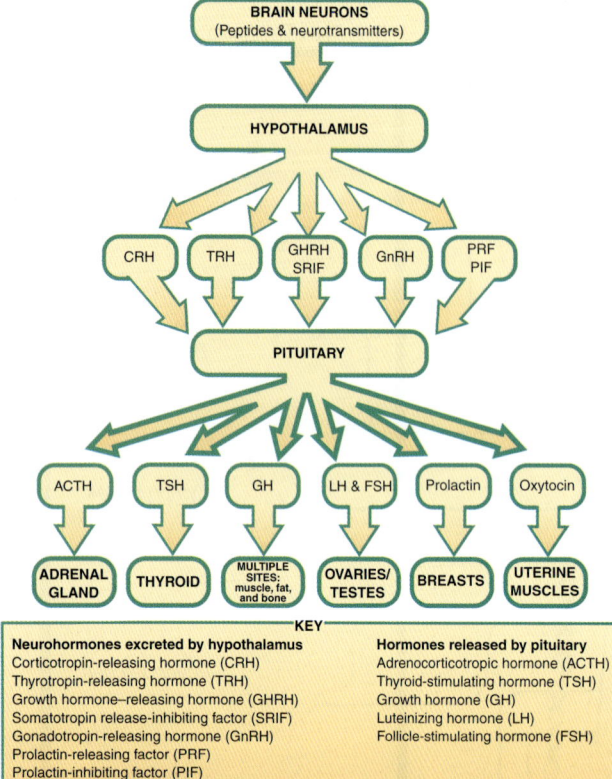

FIGURE 6.15 Hypothalamic and pituitary communication system. The neurohormonal communication system between the hypothalamus and the pituitary exerts effects on many organs and systems.

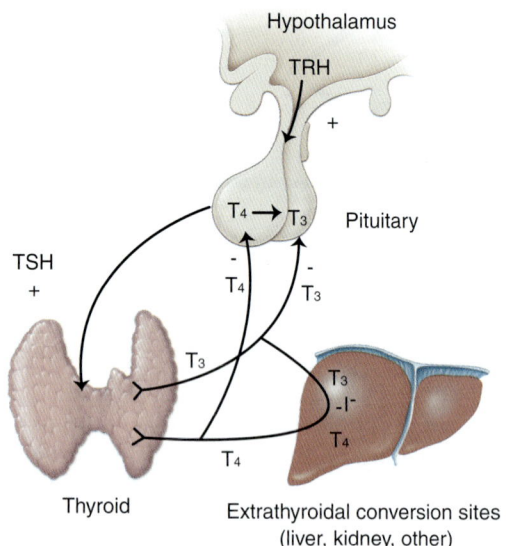

FIGURE 6.16 Hypothalamic–pituitary–thyroid axis. This figure shows the regulation of thyroid-stimulating hormone (TSH or thyrotropin) secretion by the anterior pituitary. Also depicted are the positive effects of thyrotropin-releasing hormone (TRH) from the hypothalamus and negative effects of circulating triiodothyronine (T_3) and T_3 from intrapituitary conversion of thyroxine (T_4).

evidence of dysregulation in adrenal, thyroid, and growth hormone axes (see Chapter 22).

Chronobiology

Chronobiology involves the study and measure of time structures or biologic rhythms. Some rhythms have a **circadian cycle**, or 24-hour cycle, but others, such as the menstrual cycle, operate in different periods. Rhythms exist in the human body to control endocrine secretions, sleep–wake, body temperature, neurotransmitter synthesis, and more. These cycles may become deregulated and may begin earlier than usual, known as a phase advance, or later than usual, known as a phase delay.

Zeitgebers are specific events that function as time givers or synchronizers and that set biologic rhythms. Light is the most common example of an external zeitgeber. The suprachiasmatic nucleus of the hypothalamus is an example of an internal zeitgeber. Some theorists think that psychiatric disorders may result from one or more biologic rhythm dysfunctions. For example, depression may be, in part, a phase advance disorder, including early morning awakening and decreased time of onset of REM sleep. Seasonal affective disorder may be the result of shortened exposure to light during the winter months. Exposure to specific artificial light often relieves symptoms of fatigue, overeating, hypersomnia, and depression (see Chapters 11, 22, and 28).

DIAGNOSTIC APPROACHES

Although no commonly used laboratory tests exist that directly confirm a mental disorder, they are still used as part of the diagnosis of these illnesses. **Biologic markers** are diagnostic test findings that occur only in the presence of the psychiatric disorder and include such findings as laboratory and other diagnostic test results and neuropathologic changes noticeable in assessment. These markers increase diagnostic certainty and reliability and may have predictive value, allowing for the possibility of preventive interventions to forestall or avoid the onset of illness. In addition, biologic markers could assist in developing evidence-based care practices. If markers are used reliably, it is much easier to identify the most effective treatments and to determine the expected prognoses for given conditions. The psychiatric–mental health nurse should be aware of the most current information on biologic markers so that information, limitations, and results can be discussed knowledgeably with the patient.

Laboratory Tests

For many years, laboratory tests have attempted to measure levels of neurotransmitters and other CNS substances in the bloodstream. Many of the metabolites of neurotransmitters can be found in the urine and cerebrospinal fluid (CSF) as well. However, these measures have had only limited utility in elucidating what is happening in the brain. Levels of neurotransmitters and metabolites in the bloodstream or urine do not necessarily equate with levels in the CNS. In addition, availability of the neurotransmitter or metabolite does not predict the availability of the neurotransmitter in the synapse, where it must act, or directly relate to the receptor sensitivity. Nonetheless, numerous research studies have focused on changes in neurotransmitters and metabolites in blood, urine, and CSF. These studies have provided clues but remain without conclusive predictive value and therefore are not routinely used.

Another laboratory approach to the study of some of the psychiatric disorders is the challenge test. A challenge test has been most often used in the study of panic disorders. These tests are usually conducted by intravenously administering a chemical known to produce a specific set of psychiatric symptoms. For example, lactate or caffeine may be used to induce the symptoms of panic in a person who has panic disorder. The biologic response of the individual is then monitored.

Beyond their role in helping to diagnose mental disorders, laboratory tests are also an active part of the normal care and assessment of patients with psychiatric disorders. Many physical conditions mimic the symptoms of mental illness, and many of the medications used to treat psychiatric illness can produce health problems. For these reasons, the routine care of patients with psychiatric disorders includes the use of laboratory tests such as complete blood counts, thyroid studies, electrolytes, hepatic enzymes, and other evaluative tests. Psychiatric–mental health nurses need to be familiar with these procedures and assist patients in understanding the use and implications of such tests.

Neurophysiologic Procedures

Several neurophysiologic procedures are used in mental health for diagnostic purposes.

Electroencephalography

Electroencephalography (EEG) is a tried and true method for investigating what is happening inside the living brain. Developed in the 1920s, EEG measures electrical activity in the uppermost nerve layers of the cortex. Usually, 16 electrodes are placed on the patient's scalp. The EEG machine, equipped with graph paper and recording pens, is turned on, and the pens then trace the electrical impulses generated over each electrode. Until the use of computed tomography (CT) in the 1970s, the EEG was the only method for identifying brain abnormalities. It remains the simplest and most noninvasive method for identifying some disorders. It is increasingly being used to identify individual neuronal differences.

An EEG may be used in psychiatry to differentiate possible causes of the patient's symptoms. For example, some types of seizure disorders, such as temporal lobe epilepsy, head injuries, or tumors, may present with predominantly psychiatric symptoms. In addition, metabolic dysfunction, delirium, dementia, altered levels of consciousness, hallucinations, and dissociative states may require EEG evaluation.

Spikes and wave-pattern changes are indications of brain abnormalities. Spikes may be the focal point from which a seizure occurs. However, abnormal activity often is not discovered on a routine EEG while the individual is awake. For this reason, additional methods are sometimes used. Nasopharyngeal leads may be used to get physically closer to the limbic regions. The patient may be exposed to a flashing strobe light while the examiner looks for activity that is not in phase with the flashing light or the patient may be asked to hyperventilate for 3 minutes to induce abnormal activity if it exists. Sleep deprivation may also be used. This involves keeping the patient awake throughout the night before the EEG evaluation. The patient may then be drowsy and fall asleep during the procedure. Abnormalities are more likely to occur when the patient is asleep. Sleep may also be induced using medication; however, many medications change the wave patterns on an EEG. For example, the benzodiazepine class of drugs increases the rapid and fast beta activity. Many other prescribed and illicit drugs, such as lithium, which increases theta activity, can cause EEG alterations.

In addition to reassuring, preparing, and educating the patient for the examination, the nurse should carefully assess the history of substance use and report this information to the examiner. If a sleep deprivation EEG is to be done, caffeine or other stimulants that might assist the patient in staying awake should be withheld because they may change the EEG patterns.

Polysomnography

Polysomnography is a special procedure that involves recording the EEG throughout a night of sleep. This test is usually conducted in a sleep laboratory. Other tests are usually performed at the same time, including electrocardiography and electromyography. Blood oxygenation, body movement, body temperature, and other data may be collected as well, especially in research settings. This procedure is usually conducted for evaluating sleep disorders, such as sleep apnea, enuresis, or somnambulism. However, sleep pattern changes are frequently researched in mental disorders as well.

Researchers have found that normal sleep divisions and stages are affected by many factors, including drugs, alcohol, general medical conditions, and psychiatric disorders. For example, REM latency, the length of time it takes an individual to enter the first REM episode, is shortened in depression. Reduced delta sleep is also observed. These findings have been replicated so frequently that some researchers consider them biologic markers for depression.

> **Concept Mastery Alert**
>
> Polysomnography involves recording an EEG throughout a night of sleep. A sleep deprivation EEG involves keeping a client awake the night before the EEG evaluation.

Structural and Functional Imaging

Neuroimaging of the brain involves **structural imaging**, which visualizes the structure of brain and allows diagnosis of gross intracranial disease and injury, and **functional imaging**, which visualizes processing of information. One of the most well-known examples of structural imaging is magnetic resonance imaging (MRI), which produces two- or three-dimensional images of brain structures without the use of x-rays or radioactive tracers. An MRI creates a magnetic field around the patient's head through which radio waves are sent. A functional MRI (fMRI) that creates functional images relies on the properties of oxygenated and deoxygenated hemoglobin to see images of changes in blood flow. The advantage of fMRI is that it is possible to see how the brain works when different stimuli are presented and problems that exist, such as a stroke. The fMRI has replaced most use of positron emission tomography (PET), which measures blood flow and oxygen and glucose metabolism. The emissions from the injected radioactive tracers are rapidly decayed and limit the monitoring of PET to short tasks.

Neuroimaging has limited clinical use in mental health, but its use is increasing in diagnosis and treatment of some disorders such as Alzheimer's and traumatic brain injury (Bayram, Caldwell, & Banks, 2018; Douglas, Muldermans, Wintermark, 2018). Neuroimaging has promising potential for unlocking the pathophysiology of several mental disorders. With the introduction of the fMRI, it is now possible to study the circuitry and pinpoint genetic-based predisposing factors. An MRI technique, diffusion tensor imaging, allows for viewing macroscopic changes that occur at the axon level (Tønnesen et al., 2018).

Other Neurophysiologic Methods

Evoked potentials (EPs), also called event-related potentials, use the same basic principles as an EEG. They measure changes in electrical activity of the brain in specific regions as a response to a given stimulus. Electrodes placed on the scalp measure a large waveform that stands out after the administration of repetitive stimuli, such as a click or flash of light. There are several different types of EPs to be measured, depending on the sensory area affected by the stimulus, the cognitive task required, or the region monitored, any of which can change the length of time until the wave occurrence. EPs are used extensively in psychiatric research. In clinical practice, EPs are used primarily in the assessment of demyelinating disorders, such as multiple sclerosis.

However, brain electrical activity mapping studies, which involve a 20-electrode EEG that generates computerized maps of the brain's electrical activity, have found a slowing of electrical activity in the frontal lobes of individuals who have schizophrenia.

SUMMARY OF KEY POINTS

- Neuroscientists now view behavior and cognitive function as a result of complex interactions within the CNS and its plasticity, or its ability to adapt and change in both structure and function.

- Each hemisphere of the brain is divided into four lobes: the frontal lobe, which controls motor speech function, personality, and working memory—often called the executive functions that govern one's ability to plan and initiate action; the parietal lobe, which controls the sensory functions; the temporal lobe, which contains the primary auditory and olfactory areas; and the occipital lobe, which controls visual integration of information.

- The structures of the limbic system are integrally involved in memory and emotional behavior. Dysfunction of the limbic system has been linked with major mental disorders, including schizophrenia, depression, and anxiety disorders.

- Neurons communicate with each other through synaptic transmission. Neurotransmitters excite or inhibit a response at the receptor sites and have been linked to certain mental disorders. These neurotransmitters include Ach, dopamine, norepinephrine, serotonin, GABA, and glutamate.

- Although no one gene has been found to produce any psychiatric disorder, significant evidence indicates that most psychiatric disorders have a genetic predisposition or susceptibility. For individuals who have such genetic susceptibility, the identification of risk factors is crucial in helping to plan interventions to prevent development of that disorder or to prevent certain behavior patterns, such as aggression or suicide.

- PNI examines the relationship among the immune system; the nervous system; the endocrine system; and thoughts, emotions, and behavior.

- Chronobiology focuses on the study and measure of time structures or biologic rhythms occurring in the body and associates dysregulation of these cycles as contributing factors to the development of psychiatric disorders.

- Biologic markers are physical indicators of disturbances within the CNS that differentiate one disease process from another, such as biochemical changes or neuropathologic changes. These biologic markers can be measured by several methods of testing, including challenge tests, EEG, polysomnography, EPs, CT scanning, MRI, PET, and single-photon emission CT; the psychiatric nurse must be familiar with all of these methods.

CRITICAL THINKING CHALLENGES

1. A woman who has experienced a "ministroke" continues to regain lost cognitive function months after the stroke. Her husband takes this as evidence that she never had a stroke. How would you approach patient teaching and counseling for this couple to help them understand this occurrence if the stroke did damage to her brain?

2. Your patient has "impaired executive functioning." Consider what would be a reasonable follow-up schedule for this patient for counseling sessions. Would it be reasonable to schedule visits at 1:00 PM weekly? Is the patient able to keep to this schedule? Why or why not? What would be the best schedule?

3. Mr. S is unable to sleep after watching an upsetting documentary. Identify the neurotransmitter activity that may be interfering with sleep. (Hint: fight or flight.)

4. Describe what behavioral symptoms or problems may be present in a patient with dysfunction of the following brain areas:
   a. Basal ganglia
   b. Hippocampus
   c. Limbic system
   d. Thalamus
   e. Hypothalamus
   f. Frontal lobe

5. Compare and contrast the functions of the sympathetic and parasympathetic nervous systems.

6. Discuss the steps in synaptic transmission, beginning with the action potential and ending with how the neurotransmitter no longer communicates its message to the receiving neuron.

7. Examine how a receptor's usual response to a neurotransmitter might change.

8. Compare the roles of dopamine and Ach in the CNS.

9. Explain how dopamine, norepinephrine, and serotonin all contribute to endocrine system regulation. Suggest some other transmitters that may affect endocrine function.

10. Discuss how the fields of PNI and chronobiology overlap.

11. Compare the methods used to find biologic markers of psychiatric disorders reviewed in this chapter. Consider the potential risks and benefits to the patient.

REFERENCES

Bastos, D. B., Sarafim-Silva, B. A. M., Sundefeld, M. L. M. M., Ribeiro, A. A., Brandão, J. D. P., Biasoli, É. R., et al. (2018). Circulating catecholamines are associated with biobehavioral factors and anxiety symptoms in head and neck cancer patients. *PLoS One*, *13*(8), e0202515.

Bayram, E., Caldwell, J. Z. K., Banks, S. J. (2018). Current understanding of magnetic resonance imaging biomarkers and memory in Alzheimer's disease. *Alzheimer's & Dementia (N. Y.)*, *4*, 395–413.

Bear, M. F., Conners, B. W., & Paradiso, M. A. (2016). *Neuroscience: Exploring the brain* (4th ed.). Philadelphia, PA: Wolters Kluwer.

Bewernick, B. H., & Schlaepfer, T. E. (2015). Update on neuromodulation for treatment-resistant depression. Review. *F1000 Faculty Rev*, *4*, 1389.

Corponi, F., Bonassi, S., Vieta, E., Albani, D., Frustaci, A., Ducci, G., et al. (2019). Genetic basis of psychopathological dimensions shared between schizophrenia and bipolar disorder. *Progress in Neuro-Psychopharmacology & Biological Psychiatry*, *89*, 23–29.

Douglas, D. B., Muldermans, J. L., & Wintermark, M. (2018). Neuroimaging of brain trauma. *Current Opinion in Neurology*, *31*(4), 362–370.

Furtado, M., & Katzman, M. A. (2015). Neuroinflammatory pathways in anxiety, posttraumatic stress, and obsessive compulsive disorders. *Psychiatric Research*, *229*(1–2), 37–38.

Haber, S. N., & Rauch, S. L. (2010). Neurocircuitry: A window into the networks underlying neuropsychiatric disease. *Neuropsychopharmacology Reviews*, *35*(1), 1–3.

Harlow, J. M. (1868). Recovery after severe injury to the head. *Publication of the Massachusetts Medical Society*, *2*, 327–346.

Kim, Y. K., Na, K. S., Myint, A. M., & Leonard, B. E. (2015). The role of pre-inflammatory cytokines in neuroinflammation, neurogenesis and the neuroendocrine system in major depression. *Progress in Neuro-psychopharmacology & Biological Psychiatry*, *64*, 277–284.

Lee, M. A., Jayathilake, K., Sim, M. Y., & Meltzer, H. Y. (2015). Decreased serotonin 2C receptor responses in male patients with schizophrenia. *Psychiatry Research*, *226*(1), 308–315.

Liu, Y., & Tang, X. (2018). Depressive syndromes in autoimmune disorders of the nervous system: Prevalence, etiology, and influence. *Frontiers in Psychiatry*, *9*, 451.

Lockhart, S., Sawa, A., & Niwa, M. (2018). Developmental trajectories of brain maturation and behavior: Relevance to major mental illnesses. *Journal of Pharmacological Sciences*, *137*(1), 1–4.

Müller, N., Weidinger, E., Leitner, B., & Schwarz, M. J. (2015). The role of inflammation in schizophrenia. *Frontiers in Neuroscience*, *9*, 372.

Pläschke, R. N., Cieslik, E. C., Müller, V. I., Hoffstaedter, F., Plachti, A., Varikuti, D. P., et al. (2017). On the integrity of functional brain networks in schizophrenia, Parkinson's disease, and advanced age: Evidence from connectivity-based single-subject classification. *Human Brain Mapping*, *38*(12), 5845–5858.

Renzi, C., Provencal, N., Bassil, K. C., Evers, K., Kihlbom, U., Radford, E. J., et al. (2018). From epigenetic associations to biological and psychosocial explanations in mental health. *Progress in Molecular Biology and Translational Science*, *158*, 299–323.

Siegel, A., & Sapru, H. N. (2015). *Essential neuroscience* (3rd ed.). Philadelphia, PA: Lippincott Williams & Wilkins.

Tónnesen, S., Kaufmann, T., Doan, N. T., Alnæs, D., Córdova-Palomera, A., Meer, D. V., et al. (2018). White matter aberrations and age-related trajectories in patients with schizophrenia and bipolar disorder revealed by diffusion tensor imaging. *Scientific Reports*, *8*(1), 14229.

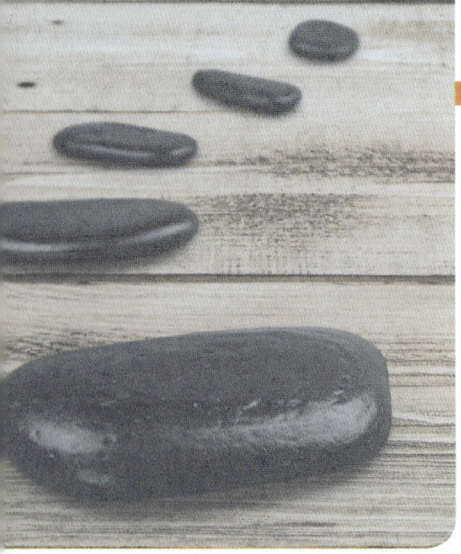

7
Recovery Framework for Psychiatric–Mental Health Nursing

Mary Ann Boyd

This chapter is available at http://thepoint.lww.com/BoydEssentials2e and in the CoursePoint ebook.

UNIT III
KNOWLEDGE AND SKILLS OF PSYCHIATRIC–MENTAL HEALTH NURSING

8
Therapeutic Communication

Rebecca Luebbert

KEY CONCEPTS
- self-awareness
- therapeutic communication

LEARNING OBJECTIVES

After studying this chapter, you will be able to:

1. Identify the importance of self-awareness in nursing practice.
2. Demonstrate the appropriate use of verbal and nonverbal communication skills.
3. Distinguish between active and passive listening.
4. Incorporate therapeutic communication strategies when working with patients.
5. Identify common barriers to therapeutic communication.
6. Understand the physical, emotional, and social boundaries of a therapeutic interaction.
7. Appreciate the significance of adaptive and maladaptive defense mechanisms.

KEY TERMS

- active listening • boundaries • communication blocks • content themes • defense mechanisms • introspective
- nonverbal communication • passive listening • process recording • self-disclosure • strength-based communication
- symbolism • verbal communication

Therapeutic communication is a necessary skill for all nurses. Effective communication between the nurse and patient is essential for patients to be active participants in their own care. This is especially true when working with patients with psychiatric disorders who may have difficulty communicating their needs. The purpose of this chapter is to help the nurse (1) develop self-awareness, (2) establish a pattern of therapeutic communication, and (3) recognize the significance and impact of a patient's use of defense mechanisms.

SELF-AWARENESS

Self-awareness is the process of understanding one's own beliefs, thoughts, motivations, biases, and limitations and recognizing how they affect others. Without self-awareness,

> **BOX 8.1**
>
> **"Know Thyself"**
>
> - What physical problems or illnesses have you experienced?
> - What significant traumatic life events (e.g., divorce, death of significant person, abuse, disaster) have you experienced?
> - What prejudiced or embarrassing beliefs and attitudes about groups different from yours can you identify from your family, significant others, and yourself?
> - Which sociocultural factors in your background could contribute to being rejected by members of other cultures?
> - How would the above experiences affect your ability to care for patients?

nurses will find it impossible to establish and maintain therapeutic relationships with patients. "Know thyself" is a basic tenet of psychiatric–mental health nursing (Box 8.1).

Nurses must carry out self-examination to create a well-developed sense of self-awareness. This introspection requires a willingness to examine their own personal beliefs, attitudes, and motivations. Although this process may be uncomfortable and time consuming, this objective contemplation is an essential exercise for a professional nurse that should be an ongoing process. Self-examination involves reflecting on the personal meaning of the current circumstances. This reflection can relate to the nurse's past situations and issues related to his or her own personal values. Self-examination is best performed with a trusted individual who can give objective but realistic feedback. Without the benefit of another's perspective, self-examination could lead to a biased view of self.

KEYCONCEPT **Self-awareness** is the process of understanding one's own beliefs, thoughts, motivations, biases, and limitations, and recognizing how they affect others.

Know Thyself

Each nurse brings a biopsychosocial self to nursing practice. The patient perceives the biologic dimension of the nurse in terms of physical characteristics: age, gender, body weight, height, ethnic or racial background, and any other observed physical characteristics. Additionally, the nurse's response to a patient can be influenced by unobservable personal physical characteristics, such as an existing chronic illness. The nurse's psychological state also influences how he or she analyzes patient information and selects treatment interventions. An emotional state or behavior can inadvertently influence the therapeutic relationship. For example, a nurse who has just learned that her child is using illegal drugs and who has a patient with a history of drug use may inadvertently project a judgmental attitude toward her patient, which would interfere with therapeutic communication. The nurse needs to examine underlying emotions, motivations, and beliefs and determine how these factors shape behavior.

The nurse's social biases can be particularly problematic for the nurse–patient interaction. Although the nurse may not verbalize these values to patients, some are readily evident in the nurse's behavior and appearance. A patient may perceive biases in the nurse as a result of how the nurse acts or appears at work. Other sociocultural values may not be immediately obvious to the patient, for example, the nurse's religious or spiritual beliefs or feelings about death, divorce, abortion, or homosexuality. These beliefs and thoughts can influence how the nurse interacts with a patient who is dealing with such issues.

Understanding Personal Feelings and Beliefs and Changing Behavior

Nurses must understand their own personal feelings and beliefs and try to avoid projecting them onto patients. The development of self-awareness will enhance the nurse's objectivity and foster a nonjudgmental attitude, which is so important for building and maintaining trust throughout the nurse–patient interaction. Soliciting feedback from colleagues and supervisors about how personal beliefs or thoughts are being projected onto others is a useful self-assessment technique. One of the reasons that ongoing clinical supervision is so important is that the supervisor really knows the nurse and can continually support positive interactions, observe for inappropriate communication, and question assumptions that the nurse may hold. Clinical supervision is different from administrative supervision in that the focus is on supporting the growth of the nurse and does not generally involve an administrative or reporting relationship.

After a nurse has identified and analyzed his or her personal beliefs and attitudes, behaviors that were driven by prejudicial ideas may change. The change process requires **introspective** analysis that may result in viewing the world differently. Through self-awareness and conscious effort, the nurse can change learned behaviors to engage effectively in therapeutic communication with patients. Nevertheless, sometimes a nurse realizes that some attitudes are too ingrained to support an effective interaction with a patient with different beliefs. In such cases, the nurse should refer the patient to someone with whom the patient is more likely to develop a successful therapeutic relationship.

EFFECTIVE COMMUNICATION

Effective communication, including verbal and nonverbal techniques, is a building block for all successful relationships (Box 8.2). Verbal communication, which is principally achieved by spoken words, includes the

> **BOX 8.2**
> **Principles of Therapeutic Communication**
>
> - The patient should be the primary focus of the interaction.
> - A professional attitude sets the tone of the therapeutic relationship.
> - Use self-disclosure cautiously and only when the disclosure has a therapeutic purpose.
> - Avoid social relationships with patients.
> - Maintain patient confidentiality.
> - Assess the patient's intellectual competence to determine the level of understanding.
> - Implement interventions from a theoretical base.
> - Maintain a nonjudgmental attitude. Avoid making judgments about the patient's behavior.
> - Avoid giving advice. By the time the patient sees the nurse, he or she has had plenty of advice.
> - Guide the patient to reinterpret his or her experiences rationally.
> - Track the patient's verbal interaction through the use of clarifying statements.
> - Avoid changing the subject unless the content change is in the patient's best interest.

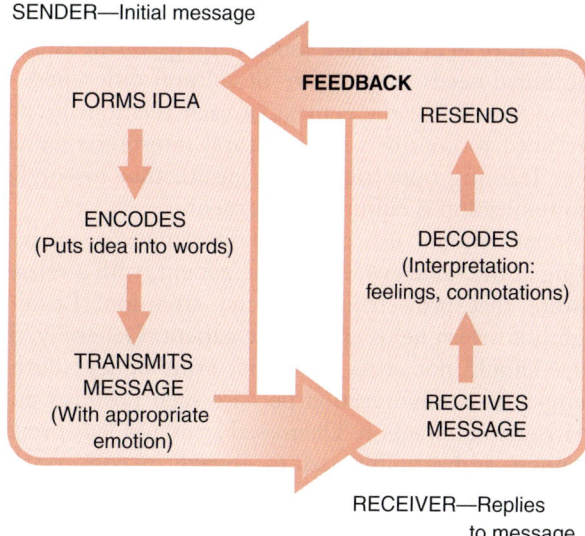

FIGURE 8.1 The communication process. (Adapted from Boyd, M. [1995]. Communication with patients, families, healthcare providers, and diverse cultures. In M. K. Strader, & P. J. Decker [Eds.]. *Role transition to patient care management* [p. 431]. Norwalk, CT: Appleton & Lange.)

underlying emotion, context, and connotation of what is actually said. Nonverbal communication includes gestures, expressions, and body language. Both the patient and the nurse use verbal and nonverbal communication. To respond therapeutically, the nurse assesses and interprets all forms of patient communication.

> **NCLEXNOTE** In analyzing patient–nurse communication, nonverbal behaviors and gestures are communicated first. If a patient's verbal and nonverbal communications are contradictory, priority should be given to the nonverbal behavior and gestures.

Verbal Communication

The process of **verbal communication** involves a sender, a message, and a receiver. The patient is often the sender, and the nurse is often the receiver, but communication is always two-way (Fig. 8.1). The patient formulates an idea, encodes that message (puts ideas into words), and then transmits the message with emotion. The patient's words and their underlying emotional tone and connotation communicate the individual's needs and emotional problems. The nurse receives the message, decodes it (interprets the message, including its feelings, connotation, and context), and then responds to the patient.

On the surface, this interaction is deceptively simple; unseen complexities lie beneath. Is the message the nurse receives consistent with the patient's original idea? Did the nurse interpret the message as the patient intended? Is the verbal message consistent with the nonverbal flourishes that accompany it? Validation is essential to ensure that the nurse has received the information accurately.

Nonverbal Communication

Gestures, facial expressions, and body language actually communicate more than verbal messages. Under the best circumstances, body language mirrors or enhances what is verbally communicated. However, if verbal and nonverbal messages conflict, the listener should rely on the nonverbal message. For example, if a patient says that he feels fine but has a sad facial expression and is slumped in a chair away from others, the message of sadness and depression, rather than the patient's words, will be accepted. The same is true of a nurse's behavior. For example, if a nurse tells a patient, "I am happy to see you," but the nurse's facial expression communicates indifference, the patient will receive the message that the nurse is bored.

People with psychiatric problems often have difficulty verbally expressing themselves and interpreting the emotions of others. Because of this, nurses need to continually assess the **nonverbal communication** needs of patients. Eye contact (or lack thereof), posture, movement (shifting in chair, pacing), facial expressions, and gestures are nonverbal behaviors that communicate thoughts and feelings. For example, a patient who is pacing and restless may be upset or having a reaction to medication. A clenched fist usually indicates that a person feels angry or hostile.

Nonverbal behavior varies from culture to culture. The nurse must, therefore, be careful to understand his or her own cultural context as well as that of the patient. For instance, in some cultures, it is considered disrespectful to look a person straight in the eye. Other examples of nonverbal communication that may vary considerably among cultures include whether one points with the finger, nose, or eyes, and how much hand gesturing is used. The nurse needs to be aware of cultural differences in communication in the context of each relationship and may need to consult with a cultural interpreter or use other learning opportunities to ensure that his or her communication is culturally congruent.

Nurses should use positive body language, such as sitting at the same eye level as the patient, with a relaxed posture that projects interest and attention. Leaning slightly forward helps engage the patient. Generally, the nurse should not cross his or her arms or legs during therapeutic communication because such postures pose a barrier to interaction. Uncrossed arms and legs project openness and a willingness to engage in conversation (Fig. 8.2). Any verbal response should be consistent with nonverbal messages.

THERAPEUTIC COMMUNICATION STRATEGIES AND TECHNIQUES

KEYCONCEPT **Therapeutic communication** is the ongoing process of interaction through which meaning emerges.

Therapeutic and social interactions are very different. In a therapeutic communication, the nurse focuses on the patient and patient-related issues. Activities should have a definite purpose, and conversation should focus only on the patient. The nurse must not attempt to meet his or her own social or other needs during the activity.

Limiting Self-Disclosure

One of the most important principles of therapeutic communication is to focus the interaction on the patient's concerns. **Self-disclosure**, telling the patient personal information, generally is not a good idea. The conversation should focus on the patient, not the nurse. If a patient asks the nurse personal questions, the nurse should elicit the underlying reason for the request. The nurse can then determine how much personal information to disclose, if any. In revealing personal information, the nurse should be purposeful and have identified therapeutic outcomes. For example, a male patient who was struggling with the implications of marriage and fidelity asked a male nurse if he had ever had an extramarital affair. The nurse interpreted the patient's statement as seeking role-modeling behavior for an adult man and judged self-disclosure in this instance to be therapeutic. He honestly responded that he did not engage in affairs and redirected the discussion back to the patient's concerns.

Nurses sometimes may feel uncomfortable avoiding patients' questions for fear of seeming rude. As a result, they might sometimes disclose too much personal information because they are trying to be "nice." However, being nice is not necessarily therapeutic. Redirecting the patient, giving a neutral or vague answer, or saying, "Let's talk about you," as appropriate, may be all that is necessary to limit self-disclosure. In some instances, nurses may need to tell the patient directly that the nurse will not share personal information (Table 8.1).

Active Listening

Listening is an ongoing activity in which the nurse attends to the patient's verbal and nonverbal communication. The art of listening is developed through careful attention to the content and meaning of the patient's speech. There are two types of listening: passive and active. **Passive listening** involves sitting quietly and letting the patient talk. A passive listener allows the patient

TABLE 8.1	SELF-DISCLOSURE IN THERAPEUTIC VERSUS SOCIAL RELATIONSHIPS	
Situation	Appropriate Therapeutic Response	Inappropriate Social Response With Rationale
A patient asks the nurse if she had fun over the weekend.	"The weekend was fine. How did you spend your weekend?"	"It was great. My boyfriend and I went to dinner and a movie." (This self-disclosure has no therapeutic purpose. The response focuses the conversation on the nurse, not the patient.)
A patient asks a student nurse if she has ever been to a particular bar.	"Many people go there. I'm wondering if you have ever been there?"	"Oh yes—all the time. It's a lot of fun." (Sharing information about outside activities is inappropriate.)
A patient asks a nurse if mental illness is in the nurse's family.	"Mental illnesses do run in families. I've had a lot of experience caring for people with mental illnesses."	"My sister is being treated for depression." (This self-disclosure has no purpose, and the nurse is missing the meaning of the question.)
While shopping with a patient, the nurse sees a friend, who approaches them.	To her friend: "I know it looks like I'm not working, but I really am. I'll see you later."	"Hi, Bob. This is Jane Doe, a patient." (Introducing the patient to the friend is very inappropriate and violates patient confidentiality.)

Through **active listening**, the nurse focuses on what the patient is saying, interprets the underlying meaning, and responds to the message objectively. The nurse's verbal and nonverbal behaviors indicate active listening. The nurse usually responds indirectly using techniques such as open-ended statements, reflection (see Table 8.2), and questions that elicit additional responses from the patient. In active listening, the nurse should avoid changing the subject and instead follow the patient's lead. At times, however, it is necessary to redirect a patient to focus on a specific topic or to clarify his or her thoughts or beliefs about that topic.

> **NCLEXNOTE** Self-disclosure can be used in very specific situations, but self-disclosure is not the first intervention to consider. In prioritizing interventions, active listening is one of the first to use.

Selection of Communication Techniques

Psychiatric nurses use many therapeutic techniques in establishing relationships and helping patients focus on their problems. Asking a question, restating, and reflecting are examples of such techniques. These techniques may at first seem artificial, but with practice, they can be useful. Table 8.2 lists some techniques along with examples. Choosing the best response begins with assessing and interpreting the meaning of the patient's communication—both verbal and nonverbal. For example, if a patient is angry and upset, the nurse might need to decide whether to invite the patient to sit down and discuss the problem, walk quietly with the patient, or simply observe the patient from a distance and not initiate conversation.

Nurses should not necessarily take verbal messages literally, especially when a patient is upset or angry. For example, one nurse walked into the room of a newly admitted patient who accused, "You locked me up and threw away the key." The nurse could have responded defensively that she had nothing to do with the patient being admitted; however, that response could have ended in an argument, and communication would have been blocked. Fortunately, the nurse recognized that the patient was communicating frustration at being in a locked psychiatric unit and did not take the accusation personally.

The next step is identifying the desired patient outcome. To do so, the nurse should engage the patient with eye contact and quietly try to interpret the patient's feelings. In this example, the desired outcome was for the patient to clarify the hospitalization experience. The nurse responded, "It must be frustrating to feel locked up." The nurse focused on the patient's feelings rather than the accusations, which reflected an understanding of the patient's feelings. The patient knew that the nurse accepted these feelings, which led to further discussion. It may seem impossible to plan reactions for each situation, but with practice, the nurse will begin to respond automatically in a therapeutic way.

FIGURE 8.2 Open and closed body language.

to ramble and does not focus or guide the thought process. This form of listening does not foster a therapeutic relationship. Body language during passive listening usually communicates boredom or indifference (Fig. 8.3).

FIGURE 8.3 Negative body language.

TABLE 8.2 VERBAL COMMUNICATION TECHNIQUES

Technique	Definition	Example	Use
Acceptance	Encouraging and receiving information in a nonjudgmental and interested manner	*Patient:* I have done something terrible. *Nurse:* I would like to hear about it. It's OK to discuss it with me.	Used in establishing trust and developing empathy
Confrontation	Presenting the patient with a different reality of the situation	*Patient:* My doctor won't talk to me. *Nurse:* I was in the room yesterday when you refused to speak with him.	Used cautiously to immediately redefine the patient's reality. However, it can alienate the patient if used inappropriately. A nonjudgmental attitude is critical for confrontation to be effective
Doubt	Expressing or voicing doubt when a patient relates a situation.	*Patient:* My best friend hates me. She never calls me. *Nurse:* From what you have told me, that does not sound like her. When did she call you last?	Used carefully and only when the nurse feels confident about the details. It is used when the nurse wants to guide the patient toward other explanations
Interpretation	Putting into words what the patient is implying or feeling	*Patient:* I could not sleep because someone would come in my room and rape me. *Nurse:* It sounds like you were scared last night.	Used in helping the patient identify underlying thoughts or feelings
Observation	Stating to the patient what the nurse is observing	*Nurse:* You are trembling and perspiring. When did this start?	Used when a patient's behaviors (verbal or nonverbal) are obvious and unusual for that patient
Open-ended statements	Introducing an idea and letting the patient respond	*Nurse:* Trust means… *Patient:* That someone will keep you safe.	Used when helping patient explore feelings or gain insight
Reflection	Redirecting the idea back to the patient for classification of important emotional overtones, feelings, and experiences; it gives patients permission to have feelings they may not realize they have	*Patient:* Should I go home for the weekend? *Nurse:* Should you go home for the weekend?	Used when patient is asking for the nurse's approval or judgment; use of reflection helps nurse maintain a nonjudgmental approach
Restatement	Repeating the main idea expressed; lets patient know what was heard	*Patient:* I hate this place. I don't belong here. *Nurse:* You don't want to be here.	Used when trying to clarify what the patient has said
Silence	Remaining quiet but nonverbally expressing interest during an interaction	*Patient:* I am angry! *Nurse:* (Silence) *Patient:* My wife had an affair.	Used when patient needs to express ideas but may not know quite how to do it; with silence, the patient can focus on putting thoughts together
Validation	Clarifying the nurse's understanding of the situation	*Nurse:* Let me see if I understand.	Used when nurse is trying to understand a situation the patient is trying to describe

Silence

Silence consists of deliberate pauses to encourage the patient to reflect and eventually respond. One of the most difficult but often most effective communication techniques is the use of silence during verbal interactions. By maintaining silence, the nurse allows the patient to gather thoughts and to proceed at his or her own pace. It is important that the nurse does not interrupt silences because of his or her own anxiety or concern of "not doing anything" if sitting quietly with a patient.

Validation

Another important technique is *validation*, which means explicitly checking one's own thoughts or feelings with another person. To do so, the nurse must own his or her own thoughts or feelings by using "I" statements (Orlando, 1961). The validation generally refers to observation, thoughts, or feelings and seeks explicit feedback. For example, a nurse who sees a patient pacing the hallway before a planned family visit may conclude that the patient is anxious. Validation may occur with a statement such as,

"I notice you pacing the hallway. I wonder if you are feeling anxious about the family visit?" The patient may agree ("Yes. I keep worrying about what is going to happen!") or disagree ("No. I have been trying to get into the bathroom for the last 30 minutes, but my roommate is still in there!").

Strength-Based Communication

Communication should be supportive, focusing on the patient's strengths instead of potential deficits. Language that promotes acceptance and respect should be favored over language that distracts from that goal. For example, instead of perceiving a patient to be manipulative, a more supportive view is that the person is resourceful or trying to get help. An entitled person might be seen alternatively as someone who is aware of his or her rights. Instead of noting that a patient is resistant to treatment, it may be that the person is instead choosing a different treatment. Nurses should incorporate language that promotes the strengths and unique characteristics of their patients (Ashcraft & Anthony, 2014).

Avoiding Blocks to Communication

Some verbal techniques block interactions and inhibit therapeutic communication (Table 8.3). One of the biggest blocks to communication is giving advice, particularly when others have already given the same advice. Giving advice is different from supporting a patient through decision making. The therapeutic dialogue presented in Box 8.3 differentiates between advice (telling the patient what to do or how to act) from therapeutic communication, through which the nurse and patient explore alternative ways of viewing the patient's world. The patient can then reach his or her own conclusions about the best approaches to use.

BOUNDARIES AND BODY SPACE ZONES

Boundaries are the defining limits of individuals, objects, or relationships. Boundaries mark territory, distinguishing what is "mine" from "not mine." Human beings have many different types of boundaries. Material boundaries, such as fences around property, artificially imposed state lines, and bodies of water, define territory as well as provide security and order. Personal boundaries include physical, psychological, and social dimensions. Physical boundaries are those established in terms of physical closeness to others—who we allow to touch us or how close we want others to stand near us.

Psychological boundaries are established in terms of emotional distance from others—how much of our innermost feelings and thoughts we want to share. Social boundaries, such as norms, customs, and roles, help us establish our closeness and place within the family, culture, and community. Boundaries are not fixed but dynamic. When boundaries are involuntarily infringed upon, the individual feels threatened and responds to the perceived threat. The nurse must elicit permission before implementing interventions that invade the patient's personal space.

TABLE 8.3	TECHNIQUES THAT INHIBIT COMMUNICATION		
Technique	Definition	Example	Problem
Advice	Telling a patient what to do	*Patient:* I am struggling at work. *Nurse:* You should probably find a new job.	The nurse solves the patient's problem, which implies that the nurse knows best, but the advice may not be the appropriate solution; it also encourages dependency on the nurse.
Agreement	Agreeing with a particular viewpoint of a patient	*Patient:* Abortions are sinful. *Nurse:* I agree.	The patient is denied the opportunity to change his or her view now that the nurse agrees.
Challenges	Disputing the patient's beliefs with arguments, logical thinking, or direct order	*Patient:* I'm a cowboy. *Nurse:* If you are a cowboy, what are you doing in the hospital?	The nurse belittles the patient and decreases the patient's self-esteem. The patient will avoid relating to the nurse who challenges.
Reassurance	Telling a patient that everything will be OK	*Patient:* I don't think I will ever get better. *Nurse:* Hang in there. Everything will turn out just fine.	The nurse makes a statement that may not be true. The patient is blocked from exploring his or her feelings.
Disapproval	Judging the patient's situation and behavior	*Patient:* I'm so sorry. I did not mean to kill my mother. *Nurse:* You should be. How could anyone kill their mother?	The nurse belittles the patient. The patient will avoid the nurse.

BOX 8.3 • THERAPEUTIC DIALOGUE • Giving Advice Versus Recommendations

Ms. J has just received a diagnosis of phobic disorder and has been given a prescription for fluoxetine (Prozac). She was referred to the home health agency because she does not want to take her medication. She is fearful of becoming suicidal. Two approaches are given below.

INEFFECTIVE COMMUNICATION (ADVICE)

Nurse: Ms. J, the doctor has ordered the medication because it will help with your anxiety.

Ms. J: Yes, but I don't want to take the medication. I'm afraid it will make me suicidal. Some psychiatric medication does that. I haven't had any attacks for 2 weeks, and it seems too risky since I'm doing better. I'm scared of the side effects.

Nurse: This medication has rarely had that side effect. You should try it and see if you have any suicidal thoughts.

Ms. J: (Remains silent for a while, crosses her legs, and looks away from the nurse and down at her feet) … okay.

(The nurse leaves, and Ms. J decides not take the medication. Within 1 week, Ms. J is taken to the emergency room with a panic attack.)

EFFECTIVE COMMUNICATION

Nurse: Ms. J, how have you been doing?

Ms. J: So far, so good. I haven't had any attacks for 2 weeks.

Nurse: I understand that the doctor gave you a prescription for medication that may help with the panic attacks.

Ms. J: Yes, but I don't want to take it. I'm afraid of becoming suicidal. Some of this psychiatric medication does that. I don't really want to take a needless risk since I've been feeling better.

Nurse: Those worries are understandable. Have you ever had feelings of hurting yourself?

Ms. J: Not yet.

Nurse: If you took the medication and had thoughts like that, what would you do?

Ms. J: I don't know, that's why I'm scared.

Nurse: I think I see your dilemma. This medication may help your panic attacks, but if the medication produces suicidal thoughts then it might compromise your progress and that's a pretty serious risk. Is that correct?

Ms. J: Yeah, that's it.

Nurse: What are the circumstances under which you would feel more comfortable trying the medication?

Ms. J: If I knew that I would not have suicidal thoughts. I would need to be assured of that.

Nurse: I can't guarantee that, but perhaps we could create an environment in which you would feel safe. I could call you every few days to see if you are having any of these thoughts and, if so, I could help you deal with them and make sure you see the doctor to review the medication.

Ms. J: Oh, that helps. If you do that, then I think that I will be alright.

(Ms. J successfully takes the medication.)

CRITICAL THINKING CHALLENGE

- Contrast the communication in the first scenario with that in the second.
- What therapeutic communication techniques did the second nurse use that may have contributed to a better outcome?
- Are there any cues in the first scenario that indicate that the patient will not follow the nurse's advice? Explain.

Personal Boundaries

Every individual is surrounded by four different body zones that provide varying degrees of protection against unwanted physical closeness during interactions. These were identified by Hall (1990) as the intimate zone (e.g., for whispering and embracing), the personal zone (e.g., for close friends), the social zone (e.g., for acquaintances), and the public zone (usually for interacting with strangers) (Fig. 8.4). The actual sizes of the different zones vary according to culture. Some cultures define the intimate zone narrowly and the personal zones widely. Thus, friends in these cultures stand and sit close while interacting. People of other cultures define the intimate zone widely and are uncomfortable when others stand close to them.

The variability of intimate and personal zones has implications for nursing. For a patient to be comfortable with a nurse, the nurse needs to protect the intimate zone of that individual. The patient usually will allow the nurse to enter the personal zone but will express discomfort if

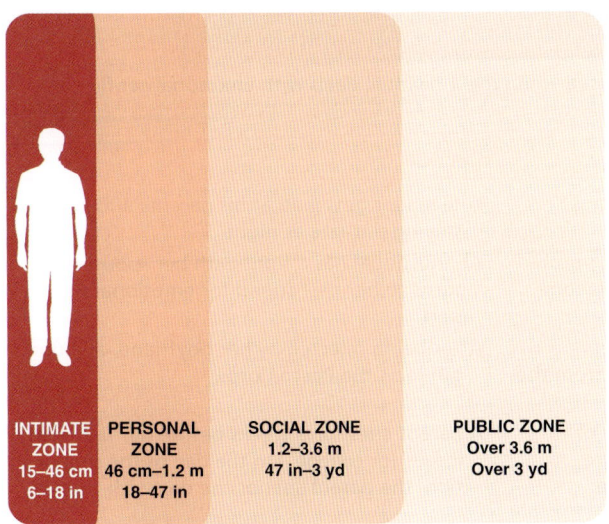

FIGURE 8.4 Body space zones.

the nurse breaches the intimate zone. For the nurse, the difficulty lies in differentiating the personal zone from the intimate zone for each patient.

The nurse's awareness of his or her own need for intimate and personal space is another prerequisite for therapeutic interaction with the patient. It is important that a nurse feels comfortable while interacting with patients. Establishing a comfort zone may well entail fine-tuning the size of body zones. Recognizing this will help the nurse understand occasional inexplicable reactions to the proximity of patients.

Professional Boundaries and Ethics

For nurses, professional boundaries are also essential to consider in the context of the nurse–patient interaction. Patients are often at a very vulnerable point in their life, and nurses need to be aware of professional boundaries to avoid exploitation of the patient. For example, in a friendship, there is a two-way sharing of personal information and feelings, but in nurse–patient relationship interactions, the focus is on the patient's needs, and the nurse generally does not share personal information or attempt to meet his or her own needs through the relationship.

DEFENSE MECHANISMS

When communicating with patients, it is also important for the nurse to be aware of the **defense mechanisms** patients may use. Defense mechanisms, (also known as coping styles), are psychological mechanisms that help an individual respond to and cope with difficult situations, emotional conflicts, and external stressors. Although defense mechanisms might seem to indicate the existence of problematic mental state, this is not true. Healthy individuals in many different contexts use defense mechanisms. The use of defense mechanisms may be conscious or unconscious. Some defense mechanisms (e.g., projection, splitting, acting out) are mostly maladaptive. Others (e.g., suppression, denial) may be either maladaptive or adaptive depending on the context in which they occur. The use of defense mechanisms becomes maladaptive when its persistent use interferes with the person's ability to function and quality of life (see Table 8.4).

For example, responding to a difficult life event altruistically is very often a healthy way to recover. On the other hand, defense mechanisms such as acting out, autistic fantasies, projection, and splitting are rarely adaptive. A defense mechanism such as repression can be a natural way to react to a traumatic experience, specifically when used in appropriate moderation. However, the unchecked repression of difficult thoughts or feelings can keep someone from coming to terms with their experiences. In developing a successful therapeutic relationship, and in establishing open communication, such knowledge of defense mechanisms will prove itself invaluable.

As nurses develop therapeutic communication skills, they will begin recognizing their patients' defense mechanisms. With experience, the nurse will evaluate the purpose of a defense mechanism and then determine whether or not it should be discussed with the patient. For example, if a patient is using humor to alleviate an emotionally intense situation, that may be very appropriate. On the other hand, if someone continually rationalizes antisocial behavior, the use of the defense mechanism should be discussed.

> **NCLEXNOTE** When studying defense mechanisms, differentiate similar defense mechanisms. For example, displacement, devaluation, and projection are similar, but not the same. Identify these mechanisms in your process recordings.

COMMUNICATION CONSIDERATIONS FOR PATIENTS WITH MENTAL HEALTH CHALLENGES

For patients with specific, known mental health problems or illnesses, the nurse must consider how these issues may impact the interactions.

Considering Specific Mental Health Issues

It is important to consider an individual's mental health challenges when selecting communication strategies. For example, patients with increased levels of anxiety may have poor concentration, requiring the nurse to use shorter and simpler statements or questions. Patients

TABLE 8.4 SPECIFIC DEFENSE MECHANISMS AND COPING STYLES

The following defense mechanisms and coping styles are commonly used when the individual deals with emotional conflict or stressors (either internal or external).

Defense Mechanism	Definition	Example
Acting out	Using actions rather than reflections or feelings during periods of emotional conflict	A teenager gets mad at his parents and begins staying out late at night.
Affiliation	Turning to others for help or support (sharing problems with others without implying that someone else is responsible for them)	An individual has a fight with her spouse and turns to her best friend for emotional support.
Altruism	Dedicating life to meeting the needs of others (receives gratification either vicariously or from the response of others)	After being rejected by her boyfriend, a young girl joins the Peace Corps.
Anticipation	Experiencing emotional reactions in advance or anticipating consequences of possible future events and considering realistic, alternative responses or solutions	A parent cries for 3 weeks before her last child leaves for college. On the day of the separation, the parent spends the day with friends.
Autistic fantasy	Excessive daydreaming as a substitute for human relationships, more effective action, or problem solving	A young man sits in his room all day and dreams about being a rock star instead of attending a baseball game with a friend.
Denial	Refusing to acknowledge some painful aspect of external reality or subjective experience that would be apparent to others (*psychotic denial* used when there is gross impairment in reality testing)	A teenager's best friend moves away, but the adolescent says he does not feel sad.
Devaluation	Attributing exaggerated negative qualities to self or others	A boy has been rejected by his long-time girlfriend. He tells his friends that he realizes that she is stupid and ugly.
Displacement	Transferring a feeling about, or a response to, one object onto another (usually less threatening), substitute object	A woman has an argument with her boss. She comes home from work and yells at her children.
Dissociation	Experiencing a breakdown in the usually integrated functions of consciousness, memory, perception of self or the environment, or sensory and motor behavior	An adult relates severe sexual abuse experienced as a child but does it without feeling. She says that the experience was as if she were outside her body watching the abuse.
Help-rejecting complaining	Complaining or making repetitious requests for help that disguise covert feelings of hostility or reproach toward others, which are then expressed by rejecting the suggestions, advice, or help that others offer (complaints or requests may involve physical or psychological symptoms or life problems)	A college student asks a teacher for help after receiving a bad grade on a test. Every suggestion the teacher has is rejected by the student.
Humor	Emphasizing the amusing or ironic aspects of the conflict or stressor	A person makes a joke right after experiencing an embarrassing situation.
Idealization	Attributing exaggerated positive qualities to others	An adult falls in love and fails to see the negative qualities in the other person.
Intellectualization	Excessive use of abstract thinking or the making of generalizations to control or minimize disturbing feelings	After rejection in a romantic relationship, the rejected explains the relationship dynamics to a friend.
Isolation of affect	Separation of ideas from the feelings originally associated with them	The individual loses touch with the feelings associated with a rape while remaining aware of the details.
Omnipotence	Feeling or acting as if one possesses special powers or abilities and is superior to others	An individual tells a friend about personal expertise in the stock market and the ability to predict the best stocks.
Passive aggression	Indirectly and unassertively expressing aggression toward others. There is a facade of overt compliance masking covert resistance, resentment, or hostility	One employee doesn't like another, so he secretly steals her milk from the office refrigerator. She is unaware of his hostile feelings.
Projection	Falsely attributing to another one's own unacceptable feelings, impulses, or thoughts	A child is very angry at a parent but accuses the parent of being angry.

TABLE 8.4 SPECIFIC DEFENSE MECHANISMS AND COPING STYLES (Continued)

Defense Mechanism	Definition	Example
Projective identification	Falsely attributing to another one's own unacceptable feelings, impulses, or thoughts. Unlike simple projection, the individual does not fully disavow what is projected. Instead, the individual remains aware of his or her own affect or impulses but misattributes them as justifiable reactions to the other person. Frequently, the individual induces the very feelings in others that were first mistakenly believed to be there, making it difficult to clarify who did what to whom first	A child is mad at a parent, who in turn becomes angry at the child but may be unsure of why. The child then feels justified at being angry with the parent.
Rationalization	Concealing the true motivations for one's own thoughts, actions, or feelings through the elaboration of reassuring or self-serving but incorrect explanations	A man is rejected by his girlfriend but explains to his friends that her leaving was best because she was beneath him socially and would not be liked by his family.
Reaction formation	Substituting behavior, thoughts, or feelings that are diametrically opposed to one's own unacceptable thoughts or feelings (this usually occurs in conjunction with their repression)	A wife finds out about her husband's extramarital affairs and tells her friends that she thinks his affairs are perfectly appropriate. She truly does not feel, on a conscious level, any anger or hurt.
Repression	Expelling disturbing wishes, thoughts, or experiences from conscious awareness (the feeling component may remain conscious, detached from its associated ideas)	A woman does not remember the experience of being raped in the basement but does feel anxious when going into that house.
Self-assertion	Expressing feelings and thoughts directly in a way that is not coercive or manipulative	An individual reaffirms that going to a ball game is not what she wants to do.
Self-observation	Reflecting feelings, thoughts, motivation, and behavior and responding to them appropriately	An individual notices an irritation at his friend's late arrival and decides to tell the friend of the irritation.
Splitting	Compartmentalizing opposite affect states and failing to integrate the positive and negative qualities of the self or others into cohesive images	Self and object images tend to alternate between polar opposites: exclusively loving, powerful, worthy, nurturing, and kind or exclusively bad, hateful, angry, destructive, rejecting, or worthless. One friend is wonderful and another former friend, who was at one time viewed as being perfect, is now believed to be an evil person.
Sublimation	Channeling potentially maladaptive feelings or impulses into socially acceptable behavior	An adolescent boy is very angry with his parents. On the football field, he tackles someone very forcefully.
Suppression	Intentionally avoiding thinking about disturbing problems, wishes, feelings, or experiences	A student is anxiously awaiting test results but goes to a movie to stop thinking about it.
Undoing	Words or behavior designed to negate or to make amends symbolically for unacceptable thoughts, feelings, or actions	A man has sexual fantasies about his wife's sister. He takes his wife away for a romantic weekend.

who are experiencing depression may have difficulty articulating their feelings or their thinking and responses may be slowed. The nurse will frequently use silence and empathic techniques throughout this interaction. The person who is depressed may also use communication styles such as overgeneralizing ("This always happens to me … everything always turns out for the worse…."). The nurse can assist the patient to be more specific (e.g., asking about a specific time or a specific exception).

Patients with schizophrenia may exhibit symptoms such as hallucinations or delusions. If a person is having auditory hallucinations (hearing sounds that no one else does), the nurse's voice may be one of several the patient is hearing. Clear, short sentences may assist in getting the patient's attention on the nurse's voice. A person experiencing delusions may use pronouns vaguely ("they" did it) or other forms of vague or unclear communication. Clarifying and assisting the patient to be more specific may assist the patient's thinking as well as communication.

As you read the chapters on various psychiatric disorders, consider how the signs and symptoms of each illness could have an impact on communication and the evolving therapeutic relationship.

Analyzing Interactions

Many patients with psychiatric disorders have difficulty communicating. They may have perceptual, cognitive, and information-processing deficits that interfere with their ability to express ideas, understand concepts, and accurately perceive the environment (Pounds, 2017). Because of the complexity of communication, mental health clinicians monitor their interactions with patients using various methods, including audio recording; video recording; and **process recording**, which entails writing a verbatim transcript of the interaction. A video or audio recording of an interaction provides the most accurate monitoring but is cumbersome to use. Process recording, one of the easiest methods to use, is adequate in most situations. Nurses should use it when first learning therapeutic communication and during times when communication becomes a problem. In a process recording, the nurse records, from memory, the verbatim interaction immediately after the communication (Table 8.5). Nonverbal communication, by both the patient and the nurse, should also be recorded.

The nurse then analyzes the content of the interaction in terms of the words and their meaning for both the patient and the nurse. The analysis is especially important because the ability to communicate is often compromised in people with mental disorders. Because words may not have the same meaning for the patient as they do for the nurse, clarification of meaning becomes especially important. The analysis can identify symbolic meanings, content themes, and blocks in communication.

Symbolism

Symbolism, the use of a word or phrase to represent an object, event, or feeling, is used universally. For example, automobiles are named for wild animals that represent speed, prowess, and beauty. In people with mental disorders, the use of words to symbolize events, objects, or feelings is often idiosyncratic, and they cannot explain their choices. For example, a person who is feeling scared and anxious may tell the nurse that bombs and guns are exploding. It is up to the nurse to make the connection between the bombs and guns and the patient's feelings and then validate this with the patient. Because of the patient's cognitive limitations, the individual may express feelings only symbolically. Another example is found in Table 8.6.

TABLE 8.5 PROCESS RECORDING

Setting: The living room of Mr. S's home. Mr. S is 23 years old and was hospitalized for 2 weeks. His diagnosis is bipolar mood disorder, and he is recovering from a depressive episode. His parents are in the room but cannot hear the conversation. Mr. S is sitting on the couch, and the nurse is sitting on a chair. This is the nurse's first visit after Mr. S's discharge from the hospital.

Patient	Nurse	Interpretation/Analysis
	How are you doing, Mr. S? (smiles and offers hand to shake)	*Plan:* Initially develop a sense of trust and initiate a therapeutic relationship.
I'm fine. It's good to be home (looking at floor, takes nurse's hand to briefly shake). I really don't like the hospital (shakes his head while still looking at floor).	You didn't like the hospital?	Interpretation: Validating assumption that Mr. S does not want to return to hospital. Nonverbal communication may indicate sadness or low self-esteem. This needs further exploration.
No. The nurses lock you up (maintains eye contact with nurse, frowning, arms crossed). Are you a nurse?		Patient validates assumption regarding hospital, but nonverbal behavior indicates there may be further concerns.
	I'm a nurse. I'm wondering if you think that I will lock you up (maintains eye contact and open posture)?	Interpretation: Mr. S may be wondering what my role is and whether I will put him back in the hospital. This assumption needs to be validated, and my role needs clarification.
You could tell my mom to put me back in the hospital (maintains eye contact with nurse).	Any treatment that I recommend will be thoroughly discussed with you first. I am here to help you stay out of the hospital. I will not discuss anything with your mother unless you give me permission to do so (nurse maintains eye contact and open posture).	Use interpretation to clarify Mr. S's thinking. Mr. S is wondering about my relationship with his mother. Explain my role and confidentiality.
(Patient maintains eye contact and uncrosses arms.)		Patient's nonverbal communication appears to indicate he is more comfortable with this clarification.

TABLE 8.6 USE OF SYMBOLISM

Setting: Mr. A has been diagnosed with schizophrenia and expresses himself through the use of television characters. A nurse observed another patient shoving him against the wall. As the nurse approached the two patients, the other patient ran, leaving Mr. A noticeably shaking. The nurse checked to see if Mr. A was all right.

Patient	Nurse	Interpretation/Analysis
	Mr. A, are you OK? (approaches patient)	
Robin Hood saved the day. (trembling, arms crossed)		Mr. A could not say, "Thank you for helping me." Instead, he could only describe a fictional character's response.
	You feel that you are saved?	The nurse focused on what Mr. A must be feeling if he felt that he had been rescued.
It's a glorious day in Sherwood Forest! (trembling decreases; smiles at nurse)		He seems to be happy now.
	Mr. A, are you hurting anywhere? (eyes scan over patient, using concerned tone of voice)	The nurse wanted to check whether the patient had been hurt when pushed against the wall.
The angel of mercy put out the fire. (continues to smile and extends hand to shake hands with nurse)		The patient is apparently not hurting now.

Some patients—for example, those with developmental disabilities or organic brain difficulties—may have difficulty with abstract thinking and symbolism. Conversations may be interpreted literally. For example, in response to the question: "What brings you to the hospital?" a patient might reply, "The ambulance." In these situations, the nurse must be cautious to avoid using symbols or metaphors. Concrete language, that is, language reflecting what can be observed through the senses, will be more easily understood.

Content Themes

Verbal behavior is also interpreted by analyzing **content themes**. Patients often express concerns or feelings repeatedly in several different ways. After a few sessions, a common theme emerges. Themes may emerge symbolically, as in the case with the patient who constantly talks about the "guns and bombs." Alternatively, a theme may simply be identified as a recurrent thread of a story that a patient retells at each session. For example, one patient often discussed his early abandonment by his family. This led the nurse to hypothesize that he had an underlying fear of rejection. The nurse was then able to test whether there was an underlying fear and to develop strategies to help the patient explore the fear (Box 8.4). It is important to involve patients in analyzing themes so they may learn this skill. Within the therapeutic relationship, the person who does the work is the one who develops the competencies, so the nurse must be careful to share this opportunity with the patient (Peplau, 1952; 1992).

Communication Blocks

Communication blocks are identified by topic changes that either the nurse or the patient makes. Topics are changed for various reasons. A patient may change the topic from one that does not interest him to one that he finds more meaningful. However, an individual usually changes the topic because he or she is uncomfortable with a particular subject. When a topic change is identified, the nurse or patient hypothesizes the reason for it. If the nurse changes the topic, he or she needs to determine why. The nurse may find that he or she is uncomfortable with the topic or may not be listening to the patient. Novice mental health nurses who are uncomfortable with silences or trying to elicit specific information from the patient often change topics. When communication blocks are recognized, the nurse should attempt to redirect the conversation back to the topic at hand unless the particular topic is too uncomfortable for the patient at that point in time. Is the patient

BOX 8.4
Themes and Interactions

Session 1: Patient discusses the death of his mother at a young age.
Session 2: Patient explains that his sister is now married and never visits him.
Session 3: Patient says that his best friend in the hospital was discharged and he really misses her.
Session 4: Patient cries about a lost kitten.
Interpretation: Theme of loss is pervasive in several sessions.

communicating one thing verbally and another non-verbally? The nurse must consider the patient's cultural background. Is the behavior consistent with cultural norms? For example, if a patient denies any problems but is affectionate and physically demonstrative (which is antithetical to her naturally stoic cultural beliefs and behaviors), the nonverbal behavior is inconsistent with what is normal behavior for that person. Further exploration is needed to determine the meaning of the culturally atypical behavior.

SUMMARY OF KEY POINTS

- To deal therapeutically with the emotions, feelings, and problems of patients, nurses must understand their own values and beliefs and interpersonal strengths and limitations.

- Verbal and nonverbal communications are both important, but body language, facial expressions, and gestures communicate more than verbal messages.

- Nonverbal behavior varies from culture to culture. The nurse must identify and understand the meaning of communication within the patient's culture.

- In therapeutic communication, the nurse limits self-disclosure, actively listens to the patient, and carefully selects communication techniques.

- **Strength-based communication** focuses on the patient's strengths rather than potential deficits.

- Nurses must maintain professional boundaries when caring for patients. The nurse should avoid establishing friendships with patients. In a friendship, both persons share personal information. In a professional relationship, the nurse focuses only on the patient.

- Reflection and analysis of interactions allow the nurse to identify significant content and themes, as well as evaluate therapeutic communication.

- Many persons with mental disorders have difficulty communicating. Nurses should understand the unique communication challenges of persons with these disorders.

CRITICAL THINKING CHALLENGES

1. Describe how you would do a suicide assessment on a distraught patient who comes to the physician's office expressing concerns about her ability to cope with her current situation. Describe how you would approach this patient if you determined she was suicidal. How might this assessment look different depending on the phase of the therapeutic relationship?

2. Describe how you would communicate with a patient who is concerned that the diagnosis of bipolar disorder will negatively affect his or her social and work relationships.

3. Your depressed patient does not seem inclined to talk about the depression. Describe the measures you would take to initiate a therapeutic relationship with him or her.

2002: *Analyze That*

In this comedy sequel to *Analyze This* (1999), Billy Crystal plays psychiatrist Dr. Ben Sobel. The patient is Paul Vitti (Robert De Niro), a mobster who has been sent to prison. Vitti is either having a psychotic break or is faking one, and his former psychiatrist is called back to assess the situation. Vitti is sent to Sobel's home for treatment. Both the psychiatrist and patient have unresolved feelings related to the deaths of their fathers.

Viewing Points: The issue of therapeutic boundaries is a source of comedy in this film. What normal therapeutic boundaries are being violated? Whose needs are being met throughout the film? What would be appropriate if a patient evoked personal unresolved issues for the therapist?

UNFOLDING PATIENT STORIES FOR UNIT III

Unfolding Patient Stories: Sharon Cole • Part 1

Sharon Cole, a 31-year-old female with bipolar disorder, had a surgical repair of an ankle fracture sustained in a fall during a manic episode. What verbal and nonverbal communication techniques can be used to establish a therapeutic relationship when she arrives on the orthopedic unit following surgery? Why is it important for the nurse to assess both verbal communication and nonverbal behavior? What methods can be used to facilitate a therapeutic interaction when Sharon is manic, talking constantly, expressing grandiose thoughts (that she is needed in Washington, DC, to solve political issues), and wanting to leave the hospital? What approaches can block effective communication? (Sharon Cole's story continues in Unit V.)

Care for Sharon and other patients in a realistic-virtual environment: *vSim for Nursing* (thepoint.lww.com/vSimMental Health). Practice documenting these patients' care in DocuCare (thepoint.lww.com/DocuCareEHR).

Unfolding Patient Stories: David Carter • Part 1

David Carter is a 28-year-old male with schizophrenia. He became violent and was brought to the emergency room with paranoid delusions and auditory hallucinations. During admission he was alternately agitated and withdrawn. Medications ordered include olanzapine 10 mg orally daily, venlafaxine 75 mg XR orally daily, lorazepam 2 mg orally every 8 hours as needed for agitation, and haloperidol 5 mg orally every 8 hours as needed for agitation. Describe the classification, action, dosing, and side effects for each medication. What monitoring should the nurse consider for each medication and when administering the as-needed medications? What client teaching should the nurse provide when administering the medications while considering his alternate states of agitation and withdrawal? (David Carter's story continues in Unit IV.)

Care for David and other patients in a realistic virtual environment: *vSim for Nursing* (thepoint.lww.com/vSimMental Health). Practice documenting these patients' care in DocuCare (thepoint.lww.com/DocuCareEHR).

Unfolding Patient Stories: Randy Adams • Part 2

Think back to **Randy Adams** in Unit II, a veteran with symptoms of posttraumatic stress disorder (PTSD) and neurocognitive problems that manifested after a recent car accident. He has resisted getting care from the Veterans Affairs hospital. How can Randy benefit from group therapy and be encouraged to attend? What group interventions would the nurse consider for a client with PTSD who is reexperiencing war events? How can the nurse foster communication and group interactions when Randy has decreased concentration and difficulty expressing his feelings?

Care for Randy and other patients in a realistic virtual environment: *vSim for Nursing* (thepoint.lww.com/vSimMental Health). Practice documenting these patients' care in DocuCare (thepoint.lww.com/DocuCareEHR).

REFERENCES

Ashcraft, L., & Anthony, W. (2014). *Tools for transforming language into therapeutic strength-based communication. (Person-centered alternatives to commonly used words and phrases)*. Presentation at Annual APNA Conference. Indianapolis, IN. Retrieved January 13, 2019, from https://www.apna.org/i4a/pages/index.cfm?pageid=6025

Boyd, M. (1995). Communication with patients, families, healthcare providers, and diverse cultures. In M. K. Strader, & P. J. Decker (Eds.). *Role transition to patient care management* (p. 431). Norwalk, CT: Appleton & Lange.

Hall, E. T. (1990). *The hidden dimension*. New York, NY: Anchor Books.

Orlando, I. J. (1961). *The dynamic nurse-patient relationship: Function, process and principles*. New York: G. P. Putnam's Sons.

Peplau, H. E. (1952; 1992). *Interpersonal relations in nursing*. New York: G. P. Putnam's Sons.

Pounds, K. G. (2017). A theoretical and clinical perspective on social relatedness and the patient with serious mental illness. *Journal of the American Psychiatric Nurses Association, 23*(3), 193–199.

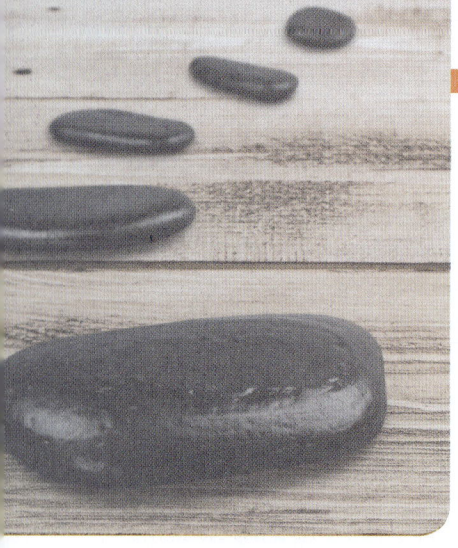

9
The Nurse–Patient Relationship

Cheryl Forchuk

KEY CONCEPT
- nurse–patient relationship

LEARNING OBJECTIVES

After studying this chapter, you will be able to:

1. Identify effective communication strategies that promote a therapeutic nurse–patient relationship.
2. Explain how the nurse can establish a therapeutic relationship with patients by using rapport and empathy.
3. Explain what occurs in each of the three phases of the nurse–patient relationship: orientation, working, and resolution.
4. Describe what characterizes a nontherapeutic relationship and a deteriorating nurse–patient relationship.
5. Recognize strategies and applications based on the principles of therapeutic nurse–patient relationships.

KEY TERMS

- countertransference • deteriorating relationship • empathic linkages • empathy • nontherapeutic relationship
- orientation phase • rapport • resolution phase • transference • working phase

The nurse–patient relationship is an important tool used to reach recovery goals. The purposes of this chapter are to (1) examine the specific stages or steps involved in establishing a therapeutic nurse–patient relationship, (2) explore the specific factors that make a nurse–patient relationship successful and therapeutic, and (3) differentiate therapeutic from nontherapeutic relationships.

EFFECTIVE COMMUNICATION NEEDS IN RELATIONSHIPS

When the nurse is establishing a nurse–patient relationship, the quality of communication is critical. This section describes the importance of rapport, empathy, recognition of empathic linkages, and the role of professional boundaries in nurse–patient interactions.

Rapport

Rapport is the development of interpersonal harmony characterized by understanding and respect, and is important in developing a trusting, therapeutic relationship. When rapport develops, a patient feels comfortable with the nurse and finds self-disclosure easier. People with psychiatric problems often feel alone and isolated. Establishing rapport helps lessen feelings of being alone. Nurses establish rapport by demonstrating interpersonal warmth, a nonjudgmental attitude, and their understanding. A skilled nurse will establish rapport that will alleviate the patient's anxiety in discussing personal problems.

Empathy

The use of **empathy** in a therapeutic relationship is central to psychiatric–mental health nursing. Empathy is sometimes confused with sympathy, which is the expression of compassion and kindness. Empathy is the ability to experience, in the present, a situation as another did at some time in the past. The nurse does not actually need to have had the experience for themselves, but must be able to imagine the feelings associated with it. For empathy to develop, there must be a "giving of self" to the other individual, as well as a reciprocal desire to know each other personally. The process involves the nurse receiving information from the patient with open, nonjudgmental acceptance, and communicating their understanding of the patient's experience and emotions so the patient feels understood.

Recognition of Empathic Linkages

While empathy is essential, it is important for the nurse to be aware of **empathic linkages**, or the *direct* communication of feelings (Peplau, 1952; 1992). This can commonly occur with anxiety. For example, a nurse may be speaking with a patient who is highly anxious, and the nurse may notice that his or her own speech is becoming more rapid in tandem with the patient's, or the nurse may have subjective feelings of anxiety. It may be difficult for the nurse to determine if the anxiety was communicated interpersonally, or if the nurse had a personal reaction to some content. However, being aware of one's own feelings, and having the ability to analyze them, is critical to determining the source of the feeling, and to address any associated problems.

Professional Boundaries in a Nurse–Patient Relationship

The importance of professional boundaries was discussed in Chapter 8. Maintaining professional boundaries may be more difficult in an ongoing therapeutic relationship. The patient may seek a friendship or sexual relationship with the nurse, but this would be inconsistent with the professional role, and is usually considered unethical.

Indicators that the relationship may be moving outside of professional boundaries are gift giving on either party's part, providing the patient with a personal phone number, spending more time than usual with a particular patient, strenuously defending or explaining the patient's behavior in team meetings, feelings by the nurse that only he or she truly understands the patient, keeping secrets, or frequently thinking about the patient outside of the work situation (Forchuk et al., 2006; Gardner, McCutcheon, & Fedoruk, 2017). State or provincial regulatory bodies provide guidelines and rules regarding professional or legal restrictions for sexual relationships. Guidelines are comparatively vague regarding the appropriateness of friendship, but such relationships are inappropriate when the nurse is actively providing care. Exceptions may be when a relationship preceded the nursing context, and another nurse is unavailable to provide care, such as in a rural area. Therapeutic relationships that meet the nurse's needs are also a breach of professional boundaries. When concerns arise related to therapeutic boundaries, the nurse must seek clinical supervision, or transfer the care of the patient immediately.

THE NURSE–PATIENT RELATIONSHIP

The **nurse–patient relationship** is a dynamic process that changes with time. It can be viewed in steps or phases with characteristic behaviors for both the patient and nurse. This text uses an adaptation of Hildegard Peplau's model, which she introduced in her seminal work, *Interpersonal Relations in Nursing* (Peplau, 1952; 1992). Emerging evidence suggests that a well-developed nurse–patient relationship positively affects patient care.

Phases

The nurse–patient relationship is conceptualized in three overlapping phases that evolve with time: orientation phase, working phase, and resolution phase. The **orientation phase** is the phase during which the nurse and patient get to know each other. During this phase, which can last from a few minutes to several months, the patient develops a sense of trust in the nurse. The second phase is the **working phase**, at which time the patient uses the relationship to examine specific problems and learn new ways of approaching them. The final stage, the **resolution phase**, is the termination stage of the relationship, and lasts from the time problems are actually resolved until the closing of the relationship. The relationship does not evolve in a simple linear pattern—it may be situated predominantly in one phase, with reflections of all phases seen in each interaction (Table 9.1).

KEYCONCEPT The nurse–patient relationship is a dynamic process that changes with time. It can be viewed in steps or phases with characteristic behaviors for both the patient and the nurse.

Orientation Phase

The orientation phase begins when the nurse and patient meet and ends when the patient begins to identify problems to be examined. During the orientation phase, the nurse discusses the patient's expectations, explains the purpose of the relationship and its boundaries, and facilitates the development of the relationship. The goal of the orientation phase is to develop trust and security within the nurse–patient relationship. During this initial phase,

TABLE 9.1 PHASES OF THE NURSE–PATIENT RELATIONSHIP

	Orientation	Working	Resolution
Patient	Seeks assistance Identifies needs Commits to a therapeutic relationship During the later part, begins to test relationship	Discusses problems and underlying needs Uses emotional safety of the relationship to examine personal issues Tests new ways of solving problems Feels comfortable with the nurse May use transference	May express ambivalence about the relationship and its termination Uses personal style to say "goodbye"
Nurse	Actively listens Establishes boundaries of the relationship Clarifies expectations Identifies countertransference issues Uses empathy Establishes rapport	Supports development of healthy problem solving Encourages patient to prepare for the future	Avoids returning to patient's initial problems Encourages independence Promotes positive family interactions

the nurse listens intently to the patient's history and perception of problems, begins to understand the patient, and identifies themes. The use of empathy facilitates the development of a positive therapeutic relationship.

During the first meeting, outlining the responsibilities of the nurse and patient is important. The nurse is responsible for providing guidance throughout the therapeutic relationship, protecting confidential information, and maintaining professional boundaries. The patient is responsible for attending agreed-upon sessions, interacting during the sessions, and participating in the nurse–patient relationship. The nurse should also explain clearly to the patient any expectations regarding meeting times, handling of missed sessions, and the estimated length of the relationship. Issues related to recording information, confidentiality, and how and what information will be shared within the interdisciplinary team, should also be made explicit. Restrictions regarding what can be shared, and with whom, are also covered by state or provincial mental health acts and health information acts.

Concept Mastery Alert
The nurse, not the patient, is responsible for active listening.

Usually, both the nurse and the patient feel anxious at the first meeting. The nurse should recognize these anxieties and attempt to alleviate them before the meeting. The patient's behavior during this first meeting may indicate to the nurse some of the patient's problems in interpersonal relationships. What the patient chooses to tell, or not tell, is also significant. In the beginning, patients may deny problems, employ various forms of defense mechanisms, or prevent the nurse from getting to know them. The patient is usually nervous and insecure during the first few sessions, and may exhibit behavior reflective of these emotions, such as rambling. Typically, by the third session, the patient can focus on a topic.

The first part of the orientation phase, also called the "honeymoon phase," is usually pleasant. However, the therapeutic team typically hits rough spots before completing this phase. The patient begins to test the relationship to be convinced that the nurse will really accept him or her. Typical "testing behaviors" include forgetting a scheduled session or being late for appointments. Patients may also express anger at something a nurse says, or may accuse the nurse of breaking confidentiality. Another common pattern is for the patient to first introduce a relatively superficial issue as if it were the major problem. The nurse must recognize that these behaviors are designed to test the relationship and establish its parameters, rather than an expression of rejection or dissatisfaction with the nurse. Student nurses often feel personally rejected during the patient's testing and may even become angry with the patient. If the nurse simply accepts the behavior and continues to be available and consistent with the patient, these behaviors usually subside. Testing needs to be understood as a normal way that human beings develop trust.

Working Phase

When the patient begins identifying problems to work on, the working phase of the relationship has started. By this phase, the patient has developed enough trust to identify problems so that strategies can be used to explore them. Problem identification can yield a wide range of issues, such as managing symptoms of a mental disorder, coping with chronic pain, examining issues related to sexual abuse, or dealing with problematic interpersonal relationships. In the working phase, the nurse can use various verbal and nonverbal techniques to help the patient examine problems and to support the patient through the healing process.

Transference (unconscious assignment to others the feelings and attitudes that *the patient* has originally associated with important figures) and **countertransference** (*the provider's* emotional reaction to the patient based on personal unconscious needs and conflicts) become important issues in the working phase. For example, a patient could be hostile to a nurse because of underlying resentment of authority figures, while the nurse, in turn, could respond defensively because of earlier, personal experiences with anger. The patient uses transference to examine problems. During this phase, the patient is psychologically vulnerable and emotionally dependent on the nurse. The nurse needs to recognize countertransference and prevent it from eroding professional boundaries.

Many times, nurses are eager to implement rehabilitation plans. However, this cannot be done until the patient trusts the nurse and identifies what issues he or she wishes to work on in the context of the relationship.

Resolution Phase

The final stage of the nurse–patient relationship is the resolution phase, which begins when actual problems are resolved and ends with the termination of the relationship. During this phase, the patient is redirected toward a life without this specific therapeutic relationship. The patient connects with community resources, solidifies a newly found understanding, and practices new behaviors. The patient takes responsibility for follow-up appointments and interacts with significant others in new ways. New problems are not addressed during this phase, except in terms of what was learned during the working stage. The nurse assists the client in strengthening relationships, making referrals, and recognizing and understanding signs of future relapse.

Termination begins on the first day of the relationship when the nurse explains that this relationship is time-limited and was established to resolve the patient's problems and help him or her handle them. Because a therapeutic relationship is dependent, the nurse must constantly evaluate the patient's level of dependence and continually support the patient's move toward independence. Termination is usually stressful for the patient, who must sever ties with the nurse—a person who has empathized with the patient's thoughts and feelings and who has given guidance and support over many sessions.

Depending on previous experiences with terminating relationships, some patients may not handle their emotions well during the termination phase. Some may not show up for the last session to avoid feelings of sadness and separation. Many patients display anger about the end of the relationship. Patients may express anger toward the nurse, or displace their anger onto others. For example, a patient may shout obscenities at another patient after being told that his therapeutic relationship with the nurse will end in a few weeks. One of the best ways to handle anger is to help the patient acknowledge it, explain that anger is a normal emotion when a relationship is ending, and reassure the patient that it is an acceptable feeling. The nurse should also reassure the patient that anger subsides after the relationship is over.

Another typical termination behavior is raising old problems that have already been resolved. The nurse may feel frustrated if during the termination phase, patients present resolved problems as if they were new. The nurse may feel that the sessions were unsuccessful, but in reality, patients are attempting to prolong the relationship to avoid its ending. Nurses should avoid addressing these problems. Instead, they should reassure patients that they have already covered those issues and learned methods to control them. They should explain that the patient may be feeling anxious about the relationship ending, and redirect the patient to newly found skills and abilities in forming new relationships, including opportunities through support groups and social groups. The final meeting should focus on the future (Box 9.1). The nurse can reassure the patient that the nurse will remember him or her, but the nurse should *not* agree to see the patient outside the relationship.

Nontherapeutic Relationships

Although it is hoped that all nurse–patient relationships will go through the phases of the relationship as described earlier, this is not always the case. In a **nontherapeutic relationship**, the nurse and patient both feel very frustrated and keep varying their approach with each other in an attempt to establish a meaningful relationship. This is different from a prolonged orientation phase in that the efforts are not sustained, but rather, vary constantly.

The nurse may try longer meetings, shorter meetings, being more or less directive, and varying the therapeutic stance from warm and friendly to aloof. Patients in this phase may try to talk about the past, but then change to discussions of the "here and now." They will talk about their family in one session, and in the next meeting, talk about their work goals. Both *grapple and struggle* to reach common ground, and both become increasingly frustrated with each other. Eventually, the frustration becomes so great that the pair gives up on each other and moves onto a phase of *mutual withdrawal*. The nurse may schedule seeing this patient at the end of the shift and "run out of time" so that the meeting never happens. The patient will leave the unit, or otherwise be unavailable during scheduled meeting times. If a meeting does occur, the nurse will try to keep it short, thinking, "What's the point—we just cover the same old ground anyway." The patient will attempt to keep it superficial and stay on safe topics ("You can always ask about your

> **BOX 9.1 • THERAPEUTIC DIALOGUE • The Last Meeting**

INEFFECTIVE APPROACH

Ms. J: Why did the other nurses bring you flowers and cards today?

Nurse: Well, that's because today is my last day, I'm transferring to the new hospital, across town.

Ms. J: Oh, um. I was just thinking, I need to talk to you about something important.

Nurse: What is it?

Ms. J: I have been worrying about my medication again.

Nurse: Oh, have you had any side effects?

Ms. J: No, but I might.

Nurse: I think you should tell the new nurse.

Ms. J: She is too new. She won't understand and you helped me last time. I feel so worried about your leaving. Is there any way you can stay? You said that you would check in, remember?

Nurse: Well, could I check on you tomorrow?

Ms. J: Oh, would you? I would really appreciate it if you would give me your new telephone number, that way I can tell you if anything happens.

Nurse: I don't know what the number will be, but you might be able to find it online.

EFFECTIVE APPROACH

Ms. J: Why did the other nurses bring you flowers and cards today?

Nurse: Oh, hello Ms. J. Do you remember? Today is my last day.

Ms. J: Oh, yes. Well, I need to talk to you about something important.

Nurse: We talked about that. Anything "important" needs to be shared with the new nurse.

Ms. J: But I want to tell you. You really made me feel better last time.

Nurse: Thank you, but remember that you improved a lot because you know what to do in order to continue progressing. Saying goodbye can be very hard.

Ms. J: I'll miss you.

Nurse: Your feelings are very normal when relationships are ending. I will remember you in a very special way.

Ms. J: Can I please have your telephone number in case I need to talk to you?

Nurse: No, I can't give that to you. It is important that we say goodbye today. And, remember, you can always talk to the new nurse about your concerns.

Ms. J: Okay, I know. Goodbye. Good luck.

Nurse: Goodbye.

CRITICAL THINKING CHALLENGE

- What were some of the mistakes the nurse in the first scenario made?
- In the second scenario, how does therapeutic communication in the termination phase differ from effective communication in the working phase?

---

medications—nurses love to health teach, you know") (Forchuk et al., 2000).

A **deteriorating relationship** is also nontherapeutic, and has been shown to have predictable phases (Coatsworth-Puspoky, Forchuk, & Ward-Griffin, 2006). This relationship starts in the *withholding* phase during which the nurse is perceived as "withholding" nursing support. The nurse fails to recognize that the patient is a person with an illness or health needs. The patient feels uncomfortable, anxious, frustrated, and guilty about being ill, and does not develop a sense of trust. A barrier exists between the patient and nurse.

The middle phase of a deteriorating relationship consists of two subphases: *avoiding* and *ignoring*. The patient begins to avoid the nurse, and perceives the nurse as avoiding him or her. The patient abides by the rules to avoid being perceived as causing problems. The nurse can be viewed as rude and condescending. The nurse ignores and avoids the patient's requests for help, and in turn, the patient becomes more anxious, frustrated, and fearful. Patients experiencing this phase report feelings of wanting to give up and of being rejected, not cared for, and not listened to.

The end phase of the deteriorating relationship is named *struggling with and making sense of*. In this final phase, the patient struggles with and tries to understand the unsatisfactory relationship. The patient feels hopeless and frustrated as a result of the lack of support received by the nurse. In a deteriorating relationship, the patient and nurse begin as strangers and end as enemies.

Obviously, no therapeutic progress can be made in a nontherapeutic or deteriorating relationship. The nurse may be hesitant to ask for a therapeutic transfer, assuming that a relationship would similarly fail with another nurse. However, each relationship is unique, and difficulties in one relationship do not predict difficulties in the next. Clinical supervision early on may assist the development of the relationship, but often a therapeutic transfer to another nurse is required.

EXAMPLES OF STRATEGIES RELATED TO THERAPEUTIC RELATIONSHIPS

This section presents two strategies related to therapeutic relationships: motivational interviewing and the transitional relationship model.

Motivational Interviewing

Motivational interviewing (MI) is a clinical method intended to engage a patient's own decision-making ability. By focusing and reinforcing the client's own arguments for change, MI can be used to achieve positive health outcomes. This is a collaborative process of directed counseling and focused discussions between the care provider and the patient. As a result, MI is inherently exploratory and adaptive.

There is a lot of evidence to suggest that MI contributes to positive health outcomes, and it can be particularly effective for patients who are not yet seeking mental health care (Lawrence, Fulbrook, Somerset, & Shulz, 2017); however, evidence also suggests that external factors can influence the success of MI for long-term outcomes. These external factors are often interpersonal and social in nature (Berg, Ross, & Tikkanen, 2011). Because much of the success of MI depends on the quality of interaction between the care provider and the patient, good communication practices are essential. The care provider needs to consider how the patient is receiving the communication, and whether the provider's comments are viewed as genuine and reflective of what the patient believes of themselves (Polcin et al., 2015). MI may not be appropriate for some patients (Vanderwaal, 2015). Therefore, careful attention to the effects of MI can make clear where MI may or may not be an ideal treatment option.

Because the success of MI is, in part, dependent on contingent factors, care providers require frequent instruction and feedback. Strong communication in the context of therapeutic relationships, as discussed in this chapter, especially self-awareness, empathetic linkages, active listening, and the avoidance of unhelpful varieties of defense mechanisms, requires ongoing training to affect therapeutic outcomes. While challenging to successfully implement, MI has produced positive health outcomes in many different settings (Colvara et al., 2018; Dillard, Zuniga, & Holstad, 2017; Schaefer & Kavookjian, 2017; Tylus-Earl & Jones, 2018). The use of MI is likely to vary according to patient needs. An example of provider-patient dialogue using MI techniques can be found in Crawley, Murphy, Regier, and McKee (2018). Miller and Moyers (2006) have identified eight features of MI that should appear in every application of this technique:

1. openness to collaboration with clients' own expertise,
2. proficiency in client-centered counseling, including accurate empathy,
3. recognition of key aspects of client speech that guides the practice of MI,
4. eliciting and strengthening client change talk,
5. rolling with resistance,
6. negotiating change plans,
7. consolidating client commitment, and
8. switching flexibly between MI and other intervention styles." (pg. 3)

Transitional Relationship Model/Transitional Discharge Model

The transitional relationship model (TRM; Forchuk et al., 2012; Forchuk et al., 2013) is theoretically grounded in the work of Hildegard Peplau, where healing occurs in relationships. Therapeutic relationships can be formed with the patient by either professionals or peer supporters. The TRM was first developed to ease the transition from long-term hospitalization to living within the community, but its use has now been expanded in a variety of transitional care processes. There are two essential components of the TRM:

1. The therapeutic relationship should be extended until a new relationship forms with another care provider (continuing the relationships formed in the hospital until new therapeutic relationships form in the community), and
2. Trained peer support (often through a consumer–survivor group) by a psychiatric survivor who has successfully transitioned into the community.

In addition to producing positive therapeutic outcomes, the TRM also reduces time spent in hospital and the number of readmissions (Reynolds et al., 2004) (see Box 9.2).

BOX 9.2

Research for Best Practice: Transitional Relationship Model

Forchuk, C., Martin, M. L., Jensen, E., Ouseley, S., Sealy, P., Beal, G., et al. (2013). Integrating an evidence-based intervention into clinical practice: 'Transitional relationship model'. Journal of Psychiatric and Mental Health Nursing, 20(7), 584–594.

THE QUESTION: The transitional relationship model (TRM) facilitates an effective discharge from the hospital to the community. Given this, what is the most effective way of implementing this model? What might facilitate the successful implementation of the TRM? What are the barriers to successful implementation?

METHODS: This study implemented the TRM in three waves across six wards using a delayed implementation control group design to study how the addition of new information changed the implementation of the TRM. Following the experiences of the wards in which the TRM was initially implemented, recommendations for successful implementation of the model were developed for the subsequent waves of wards. Recommendations were created using a combination of qualitative methods: monthly summaries, progress reports, meeting minutes, and focus groups.

FINDINGS: The results of this study can be divided into two categories: facilitators and barriers. The successful implementation of the TRM was aided by the use of educational modules (for both staff and peer training), on-site champions, and supportive documentation systems. Barriers included feeling swamped or overwhelmed, "death by process," pre-existing conflicts within teams, and changes in champions.

IMPLICATIONS FOR NURSING: The positive health outcomes associated with the TRM require careful preparation and constant attention to education, communication, and the effectiveness of the support given to caregivers.

SUMMARY OF KEY POINTS

- The nurse–patient relationship is built on therapeutic communication, including verbal and nonverbal interactions, between the nurse and the patient.

- Two of the most important communication concepts are empathy and rapport.

- In the nurse–patient relationship, as in all types of relationships, certain physical, emotional, and social boundaries and limitations need to be observed.

- The therapeutic nurse–patient relationship consists of three major and overlapping phases: the orientation phase, in which the patient and nurse meet and establish the parameters of the relationship; the working phase, in which the patient identifies and explores problems; and the resolution phase, in which the patient has learned to manage problems and the relationship can be terminated.

- The nontherapeutic relationship consists of three major and overlapping phases: the orientation phase, the grappling and struggling phase, and the phase of mutual withdrawal. A deteriorating relationship begins with a withholding phase, continues through the phases of avoiding and ignoring, and finally, ends unsatisfactorily with a phase named "struggling with and making sense of."

CRITICAL THINKING CHALLENGES

1. A patient who has followed all of the nurse's recommendations is very late for his appointment and announces that he is no longer going to take his medication. The nurse is quite surprised because she thought that he had been adhering to treatment recommendations. What phase of the therapeutic relationship are they entering? Explain. Discuss three different patient behaviors that could be expected during the resolution phase of the nurse–patient relationship. Discuss an ideal "working phase" of a nurse–patient relationship.

2. Think of a time when you worked with a patient who you did not like. What was behind the dislike? How did you handle the therapeutic relationship? What could you do differently?

1997: *Good Will Hunting*

Robin Williams plays therapist Dr. Sean Maguire. His patient, Will Hunting (Matt Damon), is a janitor at MIT who is also a troubled genius. Through a strong relationship, Will begins to realize his potential. This film deals with intense blocks to communication, as well as issues around justice system use and social status.

Viewing Points: Watch closely how the relationship develops between the characters played by Williams and Damon. How does the relationship change as the characters move through different stages of their relationship? Do you think that the level of self-disclosure depicted is therapeutic?

2008: *In Treatment*

This television show is about a Washington-based psychotherapist, Paul Weston (Gabriel Byrne). The series runs throughout the week. From Monday to Thursday, Dr. Weston meets with patients, and on Friday, he visits his own therapist (being analyzed yourself is an expectation for psychoanalysts).

Viewing Points: What aspects of therapeutic relationships can you identify in Dr. Weston's session? Look for ways in which transference and countertransference are portrayed. How is self-awareness developed for Dr. Weston?

2012: *Silver Linings Playbook*

This film portrays one man's struggle to return to society after he is released from a psychiatric inpatient hospital. Patrick (Bradley Cooper), who is trying to reconnect with his ex-wife and manage bipolar disorder, meets Tiffany (Jennifer Lawrence), who is struggling with depression following the death of her husband. Throughout the film, issues relating to stigma, establishing a therapeutic relationship, and providing mutual peer support are dealt with.

Viewing Points: As part of Patrick's release, he is mandated to continue meeting with a therapist. Think of this in relation to the TDM model discussed above. How is it similar and how is it different? Others often stigmatize Patrick and Tiffany. Can you identify where this happens and how such treatment might be avoided? Reflect on the fact that many other characters seem to have undiagnosed mental illnesses (such as OCD and anxiety). How do the characters help and hurt each other as they deal with the challenges of mental illness?

REFERENCES

Berg, R. C., Ross, M. W., & Tikkanen, R. (2011). The effectiveness of MI4MSM: How useful is motivational interviewing as an HIV risk prevention program for men who have sex with men? A systematic review. *AIDS Education and Prevention, 23*(6), 533–549.

Coatsworth-Puspoky, R., Forchuk, C., & Ward-Griffin, C. (2006). Nurse–client processes in mental health: Recipient's perspectives. *Journal of Psychiatric and Mental Health Nursing, 13*(3), 347–355.

Colvara, B. C., Faustino-Silva, D. D., Meyer, E., Hugo, F. N., Hilgert, J. B., & Celeste, R. K. (2018). Motivational interviewing in preventing early childhood caries in primary healthcare: A community-based randomized controlled cluster trial. *Journal of Pediatrics*, 201, 190–195.

Crawley, A., Murphy, L., Regier, L., & McKee, N. (2018). Tapering opioids using motivational interviewing. *Canadian Family Physician, 64*(8), 584–587.

Dillard, P. K., Zuniga, J. A., & Holstad, M. M. (2017). An integrative review of the efficacy of motivational interviewing in HIV management. *Patient Education and Counseling, 100*(4), 636–646.

Forchuk, C., Carmichael, C., Golea, G., Johnston, N., Martin, M. L., Patterson, P., et al. (2006). *Nursing best practice guideline: Establishing therapeutic relationships (revision)*. Toronto, Canada: Registered Nurses' Association of Ontario.

Forchuk, C., Martin, M. L., Jensen, E., Ouseley, S., Sealy, P., Beal, G., et al. (2012). Integrating the transitional relationship model into clinical practice. *Archives of Psychiatric Nursing, 26*(5), 374–381.

Forchuk, C., Martin, M. L., Jensen, E., Ouseley, S., Sealy, P., Beal, G., et al. (2013). Integrating an evidence-based intervention into clinical practice: 'Transitional relationship model'. *Journal of Psychiatric and Mental Health Nursing, 20*(7), 584–594.

Forchuk, C., Westwell, J., Martin, M. L., Bamber-Azzapardi, W., Kosterewa-Tolman, D., & Hux, M. (2000). The developing nurse-client relationship: Nurses' perspectives. *Journal of the American Psychiatric Nurses Association, 6*(1), 3–10.

Gardner, A., McCutcheon, H., & Fedoruk, M. (2017). The black and white and shades of grey of boundary violations. *Collegian, 24*(1), 45–51.

Lawrence, P., Fulbrook, P., Somerset, S., & Schulz, P. (2017). Motivational interviewing to enhance treatment attendance in mental health settings: A systematic review and meta-analysis. *Journal of Psychiatric Mental Health Nursing, 24*(9–10), 699–718.

Miller, W. R., & Moyers, T. B. (2006). Eight stages in learning motivational interviewing. *Journal of Teaching in the Addictions, 5*(1), 3–17.

Peplau, H. E. (1952; 1992). *Interpersonal relations in nursing*. New York: G. P. Putnam's Sons.

Polcin, D. L., Sterling, J., Brown, T., Brown, M., Buscemi, R., & Korcha, R. (2015). Client and therapist views about intensive and standard motivational interviewing. *Journal of Contemporary Psychotherapy, 45*(3), 167–176.

Reynolds, W., Lauder, W., Sharkey, S., Macivier, S., Veitch, T., & Cameron, D. (2004). The effects of transitional discharge model for psychiatric patients. *Journal of Psychiatric and Mental Health Nursing*, 11, 82–88.

Schaefer, M. R., & Kavookjian, J. (2017). The impact of motivational interviewing on adherence and symptom severity in adolescents and young adults with chronic illness: A systematic review. *Patient and Education Counseling, 100*(12), 2190–2199.

Tylus-Earl, N., & Jones, J. (2018). Motivational interviewing for patients with mood disorders. *Nursing, 48*(2), 18–20.

Vanderwaal, F. M. (2015). Impact of motivational interviewing on medication adherence in schizophrenia. *Issues in Mental Health Nursing, 36*(11), 900–904.

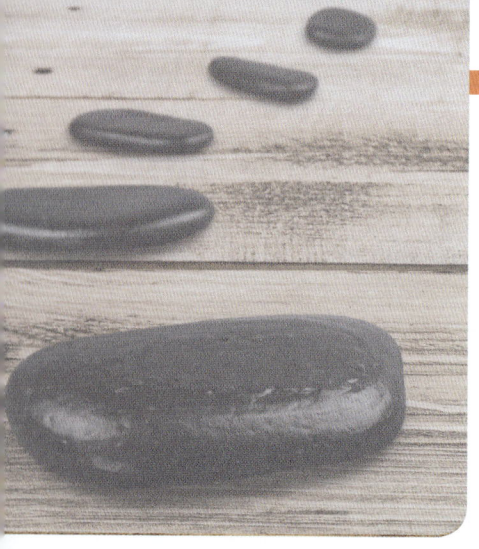

10

The Psychiatric–Mental Health Nursing Process

Mary Ann Boyd

KEY CONCEPTS
- assessment
- spirituality
- mental status examination
- outcomes
- recovery-oriented nursing interventions

LEARNING OBJECTIVES

After studying this chapter, you will be able to:

1. Define the recovery-oriented nursing process in psychiatric–mental health nursing.
2. Conduct a psychiatric–mental health nursing assessment.
3. Prioritize patient needs following a psychiatric nursing assessment.
4. Develop recovery-oriented outcomes in collaboration with the patient.
5. Apply recovery-oriented psychiatric–mental health nursing interventions by supporting patient strengths and addressing mental health problems and mental disorders.
6. Collaborate with the patient in evaluating outcomes.

KEY TERMS

- affect • behavior modification • behavior therapy • bibliotherapy • body image • conflict resolution • containment • counseling • cultural brokering • de-escalation • distraction • dysphoric • emotional well-being • environmental well-being • euphoric • euthymic • financial well-being • guided imagery • home visits • insight • intellectual well-being • judgment • labile • milieu therapy • mood • occupational well-being • open communication • patient observation • personal identity • physical well-being • psychoeducation • relaxation techniques • reminiscence • risk factors • seclusion • self-care • self-concept • self-esteem • social well-being • spiritual care assessment • spiritual support • structured interaction • token economy • validation

The psychiatric–mental health nursing process is approached from the perspectives of wellness and strength as well mental health problems. The process is guided by recovery principles (see Chapters 1 and 7). In this text, the nursing process is organized by the areas of assessment, priority of needs and outcome development, intervention, and evaluation. This chapter describes, but not all, of the commonly applied interventions. The nursing process targeting specific psychiatric disorders and emotional problems is discussed in later chapters.

RECOVERY-ORIENTED PSYCHIATRIC–MENTAL HEALTH NURSING ASSESSMENT

Assessment is the collection and interpretation of information related to health, wellness, strengths, functional status, and human responses to mental health problems. These data are collected within a collaborative relationship with the person seeking nursing care.

Assessment is not an isolated activity. Rather, it is a systematic and ongoing process that occurs throughout the nurse's care of the patient. The psychiatric–mental health nursing assessment (Box 10.1) is a basic guide to collecting assessment data. Assessment information is entered into the patient's written or computerized record, which may be presented in several different formats, including forms, checklists, narratives, and problem-oriented notes.

> **KEYCONCEPT Assessment** is the deliberate and systematic collection and interpretation of information or data to determine current and past health, wellness, strengths, functional status, and mental health problems, both actual and potential.

Assessment begins with the first contact with the patient when a collaborative relationship is initiated. Legal consent must be given by the patient, and the nurse must follow the Health Insurance Portability and Accountability Act of 1996 (HIPAA) guidelines (see Chapter 3). The patient must develop a sense of trust before he or she will be comfortable revealing intimate life details. It is of paramount importance that the nurse has a healthy knowledge of him- or herself as well (Box 10.2). The nurse's own biases and values, which may be different from those of the patient, can influence the nurse's interpretation of assessment data. A careful self-assessment helps the nurse interpret the data objectively.

Patient Interviews

An assessment interview usually involves direct questions to obtain facts, clarify perceptions, validate observations, interpret the meanings of facts, or compare information. The specific questions may take different forms. The nurse must clearly state the purpose of the interview and, if necessary, modify the interview process, so that both the patient and nurse agree on its purpose. The nurse may choose to use open- or closed-ended questions. Open-ended questions are most helpful when beginning the interview because they allow the nurse to observe how the patient responds verbally and nonverbally. They also convey caring and interest in the person's well-being, which helps to establish rapport. Nurses should use closed-ended questions when they need specific information. For example, "How old are you?" asks for specific information about the patient's age. These types of questions limit the individual's response but often serve as good follow-up questions for clarification of thoughts or feelings expressed.

Questions such as "How did you come to this clinic today?" allow patients to describe their experience in their own way. Some patients may answer this question concretely by saying, "I took a taxi" or "I came by car." Others may address this question by responding, "My family thought I should come, so they brought me" or "Well, I got up this morning ... I took a shower, got dressed ... and then, well you know, it's difficult sometimes to decide." Each of these answers helps the nurse assess the patient's thinking process as well as evaluate the content of the response.

Clarification is extremely important during the assessment process. Words do not have the same meaning to all people. Education, language, culture, history, and experience may influence the meaning of words. Sometimes simple and direct questioning provides clarification. In other situations, the nurse may clarify by providing a specific example for a more global thought the patient is trying to express. For example, a patient may say, "Things have been so strange since the children left." The nurse may respond with, "Sometimes, parents feel sad and empty when their children leave home. They don't know what to do with their time." Frequently summarizing what has been said allows the patient the opportunity to correct the nurse's interpretation. For example, verbalizing a sequence of events that the patient has reported may help to identify omissions or inconsistencies. Restating information or reflecting feelings that the patient has described also allows opportunity for clarification. It is essential that nurses understand exactly what patients are attempting to communicate before beginning to intervene. Box 10.3 provides a summary of other behaviors that enhance the effectiveness of an assessment interview.

Many psychiatric symptoms are beyond a patient's awareness. Family members, friends, and other health care professionals are important sources of information. Before seeking information from others, the nurse must obtain permission from the patient. The nurse needs to provide the patient with a clear explanation of why the information is needed and how it will be used. The nurse should explain that the strength-based assessment will include questions about wellness and strengths as well as mental health problems because these are all related to well-being.

Assessment of the Physical Domain

Many psychiatric disorders produce physical symptoms, such as the lack of appetite and weight loss associated with depression. A person's physical condition may also affect mental health, producing a recurrence or increase in symptoms. Many physical disorders may present first with symptoms considered to be psychiatric. For example, hypothyroidism often presents with feelings of lethargy, decreased concentration, and depressed mood. For these reasons, biologic information about the patient is always considered.

Current and Past Health Status

Beginning with a history of the patient's general medical condition, the nurse should consider the following:

- Availability of, frequency of, and most recent medical evaluation, including test results
- Past hospitalizations and surgical procedures
- Vision and hearing impairments

BOX 10.1

Biopsychosocial Psychiatric Nursing Assessment

I. Major reason for seeking help _____
II. **Initial information**
   Name _____
   Age _____ Marital status _____ Gender _____ Ethnic identification _____
III. **Present and past health status** _____ (Include Ht., Wt., BMI) _____
   Summary of strengths related to physical health

	Normal	Treated	Untreated
Physical functions: System review	☐	☐	☐
Elimination	☐	☐	☐
Activity/exercise	☐	☐	☐
Sleep	☐	☐	☐
Appetite and nutrition	☐	☐	☐
Hydration	☐	☐	☐
Sexuality	☐	☐	☐
Self-care	☐	☐	☐
Existing physical illnesses	☐	☐	☐
Medications (prescription and over the counter)	Dosage	Side effects	Frequency
Significant laboratory tests	Values	Normal range	

IV. **Mental health problems**
   Major concerns regarding mental health problem _____
   Major loss/change in past year: No _____ Yes _____
   Fear of violence: No _____ Yes _____
   Strategies for managing problems/disorder _____
V. **Mental status examination**
   General observations (appearance, psychomotor activity, attitude) _____
   Orientation (time, place, person) _____
   Mood, affect, emotions _____
   Speech (verbal ability, speed, use of words correctly) _____
   Thought processes (tangential, logic, repetition, rhyming of words, loose connections, disorganized) _____
   Cognition and intellectual performance _____
   Attention and concentration _____
   Abstract reasoning and comprehension _____
   Memory (recall, short-term, recent, and remote) _____
   Judgment and insight _____
VI. **Significant behaviors (psychomotor, agitation, aggression, withdrawn)** _____
VII. **Self-concept (body image, self-esteem, personal identity)** _____
VIII. **Stress and coping patterns** _____
IX. **Risk assessment**
   Suicide: High _____ Low _____ Assault/homicide: High _____ Low _____
   Suicide thoughts or ideation: No _____ Yes _____
   Current thoughts of harming self _____
   Plan _____
   Means _____
   Means available _____
   Assault/homicide thoughts: No _____ Yes _____
   What do you do when angry with a stranger? _____
   What do you do when angry with family or partner? _____
   Have you ever hit or pushed anyone? No _____ Yes _____
   Have you ever been arrested for assault? No _____ Yes _____
   Current thoughts of harming others _____
X. **Functional status**
   Changes in functioning (work, school, home) _____
XI. **Social systems**
   Cultural assessment
      Cultural group _____
      Cultural group's view of health and mental illness _____
      What cultural rules do you try to live by? _____
      Important cultural foods _____
   Family assessment
      Family members _____
      Members important to patient _____
      Decision makers, family roles, supportive members _____
   Community resources _____
XII. **Spiritual assessment**
XIII. **Economic status**
XIV. **Legal status**
XV. **Quality of life**
XVI. **SUMMARY OF PSYCHOSOCIAL STRENGTHS:**
Summary of significant data that can be used in prioritizing patient needs.
SIGNATURE/TITLE _____ Date _____

> **BOX 10.2**
> ### Self-Concept Awareness
>
> Self-awareness is important in any interaction. To understand a patient's self-concept, the nurse must be aware of his or her own self-concept. By answering these questions, nurses can evaluate self-concept components and increase their self-understanding. The more comfortable the nurse is with him- or herself, the more effective the nurse can be in each and every patient interaction.
>
> **BODY IMAGE**
> - How do I feel about my body?
> - How important is my physical appearance?
> - How does my body measure up to my ideal body? (How would I like to appear?)
> - What is positive about my body?
> - What would I like to change about my body?
> - How does my body image affect my self-esteem?
>
> **SELF-ESTEEM**
> - When do I feel confident and good about myself?
> - When do I feel unimportant?
> - What do I do when I feel good about myself? (Call friends, socialize?)
> - What do I do when I have negative feelings about myself? (Withdraw, dress poorly?)
> - When do I make negative statements?
> - Am I able to correct my negative self-statements?
>
> **PERSONAL IDENTITY**
> - How do I describe myself?
> - What three adjectives describe who I am?
> - Do I identify with a particular cultural group, family role, or place of residence?
> - What would I like to have on my tombstone?

> **BOX 10.3**
> ### Assessment Interview Behaviors
>
> The following behaviors carried out by the nurse will enhance the effectiveness of the assessment interview:
>
> - *Exhibiting empathy*—to show empathy to the patient, the nurse uses phrases such as, "That must have been upsetting for you" or "I can understand your hurt feelings."
> - *Giving recognition*—the nurse gives recognition by listening actively: verbally encouraging the patient to continue, and nonverbally presenting an open, interested demeanor.
> - *Demonstrating acceptance*—note that acceptance does not mean agreement or nonagreement with the patient but is a neutral stance that allows the patient to continue.
> - *Restating*—the nurse tries to clarify what the patient is trying to say by restating it.
> - *Reflecting*—the nurse presents the patient's last statement as a question. This gives the patient a chance to expand on the information.
> - *Focusing*—the nurse attempts to bring the conversation back to the questions at hand when the patient goes off on a tangent.
> - *Using open-ended questions*—general questions give the patient a chance to speak freely.
> - *Presenting reality*—the nurse presents reality when the patient makes unrealistic or exaggerated statements.
> - *Making observations*—the nurse says aloud what patient behaviors are observed to give the patient a chance to speak to those behaviors. For example, the nurse may say, "I notice you are twisting your fingers; are you nervous about something?"

- Cardiac problems, including cerebrovascular accidents (strokes), myocardial infarctions (heart attacks), and childhood illnesses
- Respiratory problems, particularly those that result in a lack of oxygen to the brain
- Neurologic problems, particularly head injuries, seizure disorders, or any losses of consciousness
- Endocrine disorders, particularly unstable diabetes or thyroid or adrenal dysfunction
- Immune disorders, particularly human immunodeficiency virus (HIV) and autoimmune disorders
- Use, exposure, abuse, or dependence on substances, including alcohol, tobacco, prescription drugs, illicit drugs, and herbal preparations

Physical Examination

Body Systems Review

After the nurse obtains historical information, he or she should examine physiologic systems to evaluate the patient's current physical condition. The psychiatric nurse should pay special attention to various systems that treatment may affect. For example, if a patient is being treated with antihypertensive medication, the dosage may need to be adjusted if an antipsychotic medication is prescribed. If a patient is overweight or has diabetes, some psychiatric medications can affect these conditions. Patients with compromised immune function (HIV, cancer) may experience mood alterations.

Neurologic Status

Particular attention is paid to recent head trauma; episodes of hypertension; and changes in personality, speech, or the ability to handle activities of daily living (ADLs). Cranial nerve dysfunction, reflexes, muscle strength, and balance are included in a thorough assessment. The nurse routinely assesses and documents movement disorders through the use of such tools as the Abnormal Involuntary Movement Scales (see Chapter 23 and Appendix B).

Laboratory Results

The nurse reviews and documents any available laboratory data, especially any abnormalities. Hepatic, renal, or urinary abnormalities are particularly important to document because these systems metabolize or excrete many psychiatric medications. In addition, the nurse notes abnormal white blood cell and electrolyte levels. Laboratory data are especially important, particularly if the nurse is the only person in the mental health team who has a "medical" background (Table 10.1).

TABLE 10.1 SELECTED HEMATOLOGIC MEASURES AND THEIR RELEVANCE TO PSYCHIATRIC DISORDERS

Test	Possible Results	Possible Cause or Meaning
Complete Blood Count (CBC)		
Leukocyte (white blood cell [WBC]) count	Leukopenia—decrease in leukocytes (white blood cells) Agranulocytosis—decrease in number of granulocytic leukocytes Leukocytosis—increase in leukocyte count above normal limits	May be produced by: phenothiazine, clozapine, carbamazepine Lithium causes a benign mild to moderate increase (11,000–17,000/mcL) Neuroleptic malignant syndrome (NMS) can be associated with increases of 15,000–30,000/mm^3 in about 40% of cases
WBC differential	"Shift to the left"—from segmented neutrophils to band forms	Shift often suggests a bacterial infection but has been reported in about 40% of cases of NMS
Red blood cell (RBC) count	Polycythemia—increased RBCs	Primary form—true polycythemia caused by several disease states Secondary form—compensation for decreased oxygenation, such as in chronic pulmonary disease Blood is more viscous, and the patient should not become dehydrated
	Decreased RBCs	Decrease may be related to some types of anemia, which requires further evaluation
Hematocrit (Hct)	Elevations	Elevation may be caused by dehydration
	Decreased Hct	Anemia may be associated with a wide range of mental status changes, including asthenia, depression, and psychosis 20% of women of childbearing age in the United States have iron-deficiency anemia
Hemoglobin (Hb)	Decreased	Another indicator of anemia; further evaluation of source requires review of erythrocyte indices
Erythrocyte indices, such as red cell distribution width (RDW)	Elevated RDW	Finding suggests a combined anemia as in that from chronic alcoholism, resulting from both vitamin B_{12} and folate acid deficiencies and iron deficiency Oral contraceptives also decrease vitamin B_{12}
Other Hematologic Measures		
Vitamin B_{12}	Deficiency	Neuropsychiatric symptoms, such as psychosis, paranoia, fatigue, agitation, marked personality change, dementia, and delirium may develop
Folate	Deficiency	The use of alcohol, phenytoin, oral contraceptives, and estrogens may be responsible
Platelet count	Thrombocytopenia—decreased platelet count	Some psychiatric medications, such as carbamazepine, phenothiazine, or clozapine, or other nonpsychiatric medications, may cause thrombocytopenia Several medical conditions are other causes
Serum Electrolytes		
Sodium	Hyponatremia—low serum sodium	Significant mental status changes may ensue. Condition is associated with Addison disease, the syndrome of inappropriate secretion of antidiuretic hormone (SIADH), and polydipsia (water intoxication) as well as carbamazepine use
Potassium	Hypokalemia—low serum potassium	Produces weakness, fatigue, electrocardiogram (ECG) changes; paralytic ileus and muscle paresis may develop Common in individuals with bulimic behavior or psychogenic vomiting and use or abuse of diuretics; laxative abuse may contribute; can be life-threatening
Chloride	Elevation	Chloride tends to increase to compensate for lower bicarbonate
	Decrease	Binging–purging behavior and repeated vomiting may be causes
Bicarbonate	Elevation	Causes may be binging and purging in eating disorders, excessive use of laxatives, or psychogenic vomiting
	Decrease	Decrease may develop in some patients with hyperventilation syndrome and panic disorder

TABLE 10.1	SELECTED HEMATOLOGIC MEASURES AND THEIR RELEVANCE TO PSYCHIATRIC DISORDERS (Continued)	
Test	Possible Results	Possible Cause or Meaning
Renal Function Tests		
Blood urea nitrogen (BUN)	Elevation	Increase is associated with mental status changes, lethargy, and delirium Cause may be dehydration Potential toxicity of medications cleared via the kidney, such as lithium and amantadine, may increase
Serum creatinine	Elevation	Level usually does not become elevated until about 50% of nephrons in the kidney are damaged
Serum Enzymes		
Amylase	Elevation	Level appears to increase after binging and purging behavior in eating disorders and declines when these behaviors stop
Alanine aminotransferase (ALT)—formerly serum glutamic pyruvic transaminase (SGPT)	ALT > AST Elevation	Disparity is common in acute forms of viral and drug-induced hepatic dysfunction Mild elevations are common with use of sodium valproate
Aspartate aminotransferase (AST)—formerly serum glutamic oxaloacetic transaminase (SGOT)	AST > ALT	Severe elevations in chronic forms of liver disease and postmyocardial infarction may develop
Creatine phosphokinase (CPK)	Elevations of the isoenzyme related to muscle tissue	Muscle tissue injury is the cause Level is elevated in neuroleptic malignant syndrome (NMS) Level is also elevated by repeated intramuscular injections (e.g., antipsychotics)
Thyroid Function		
Serum triiodothyronine (T_3)	Decrease	Hypothyroidism and nonthyroid illness cause decrease Individuals with depression may convert less T_4 to T_3 peripherally but not out of the normal range Medications such as lithium and sodium valproate may suppress thyroid function, but clinical significance is unknown
	Elevations	Hyperthyroidism, T_3, and toxicosis may produce mood changes, anxiety, and symptoms of mania
Serum thyroxine (T_4)	Elevations	Hyperthyroidism is a cause
Thyroid-stimulating hormone (TSH or thyrotropin)	Elevations	Hypothyroidism—symptoms may appear very much like depression except for additional physical signs of cold intolerance, dry skin, hair loss, bradycardia, and so on Lithium—may also cause elevations
	Decrease	Considered nondiagnostic—may be hyperthyroidism, pituitary hypothyroidism, or even euthyroid status

Physical Functions

Elimination

The nurse should inquire about and document the patient's daily urinary and bowel habits. Various medications can affect bladder and bowel functioning, so a baseline must be noted. For example, diarrhea and frequency of urination can occur with the use of lithium carbonate. Anticholinergic effects of antipsychotic medication can cause constipation and urinary hesitancy or retention.

Activity and Exercise

The patient's daily methods and levels of activity and exercise must be queried and documented. Activities are important interventions, and baseline information is needed to determine what the patient already enjoys or dislikes and whether he or she is getting sufficient exercise or adequate recreation. A patient may have altered activity or exercise in response to medication or therapies. In addition, many psychiatric medications cause weight gain, and nurses need to develop interventions that assist the patient to increase activities to counteract the weight gain.

Sleep

Changes in sleep patterns often reflect changes in a patient's emotions and are symptoms of disorders. If the patient responds positively to a question about changes in sleep patterns, it is important to clarify just what those changes are. For example, "difficulty falling asleep" means different things to different people. For a person who usually falls right to sleep, it could mean that it takes 10 extra minutes to fall asleep. For a person who normally takes 35 minutes to fall asleep, it could mean that it takes 90 minutes to do so.

Appetite and Nutrition

Changes in appetite and nutritional intake are assessed and documented because they can indicate changes in moods or relapse. For example, a patient who is depressed may not notice hunger or even that he or she does not have the energy to prepare food. Others may handle stressful emotions through eating more than usual. This information also provides valuable clues to possible eating disorders and problems with body image.

Obesity is one of the major health problems of many Americans, but it is particularly problematic for persons with psychiatric disorders. Many of the medications are associated with weight gain. A baseline body mass index (BMI) should be determined as treatment is initiated.

Hydration

Gaining perspective on how much fluid patients normally drink and how much they are drinking now provides important data. Some medications can cause retention of fluids, and others can cause diuresis; thus, the patient's current fluid status must be understood.

Sexuality

Questioning a patient on issues involving sexuality requires comfort with one's own sexuality. Changes in sexual activity as well as comfort with sexual orientation are important to assess. Issues involving sexual orientation that are unsettled in a patient or between a patient and family member may cause anxiety, shame, or discomfort. It is necessary to explore how comfortable the patient is with his or her sexuality and sexual functioning. These questions should be asked in a matter of fact but gentle and nonjudgmental manner. Initiating the topic of sexuality may begin with a question such as "Are you sexually active?" Birth control medications may also alter mood.

Self-Care

Self-care is the ability to perform ADLs successfully. Often, a patient's ability to care for him- or herself or carry out ADLs, such as washing and dressing, are indicative of his or her psychological state. For example, a depressed patient may not have the energy to change into clean clothes. This information may also help the nurse to determine actual or potential obstacles to a patient's compliance with a treatment plan.

Pharmacologic Assessment

The review of systems serves as a baseline from which the nurse may judge whether the initiation of a medication exacerbates symptoms or causes new ones to develop. It is important to determine which medications the patient takes now or has taken in the past. These include over-the-counter, herbal or nonprescription medications as well as prescribed medications. This assessment is important for reasons other than serving as a baseline. It helps target possible drug interactions, determines whether the patient has already used medications that are being considered, and identifies whether medications may be causing psychiatric symptoms.

Strengths and Wellness Assessment

During the assessment, the nurse should identify areas of strength and wellness including **physical well-being** or positive sleep patterns, healthy diet, or motivation to engage in healthy behaviors. Does the patient recognize the need for physical activity, diet, and nutrition? Recognition of this wellness dimension can help motivate the individual to improve these behaviors.

Psychological Assessment

The psychological domain is the traditional focus of the psychiatric nursing assessment. By definition, psychiatric disorders and emotional problems are manifested through psychological symptoms related to mental status, moods, thoughts, behaviors, and interpersonal relationships. This domain includes psychological strengths, psychological growth and development. The wellness domains, emotional and intellectual well-being should be included. Assessing this domain is important in developing a comprehensive picture of the patient.

Mental Health Problems

Individual concerns regarding a mental health problem or its consequences are included in the mental health assessment. A mental disorder, like any other illness, affects patients and families in many different ways. It is safe to say that a mental illness changes a person's life, and the nurse should identify what the changes are and their meaning to the patient and family members. Many patients experience specific fears, such as losing their job, family, or safety. Included in this part of the assessment is identifying current strategies or behaviors the patient uses in dealing with the consequences of disorder. A simple question such as "How do you deal with your voices when you are with other people?" may initiate a discussion about responses to the mental disorder or emotional problem.

> **BOX 10.4**
>
> **Narrative Mental Status Examination Note**
>
> M.J. is a 65-year-old widowed man who is slightly disheveled. He is cooperative with the interviewer and judged to be an adequate historian. His mood and affect are depressed and anxious. He becomes tearful throughout the interview when speaking about his wife. His flow of thought is hesitant but coherent when he is speaking about his wife. He is oriented to time, place, and person. He shows good recent and remote memory. He is able to recall several items given him by the interviewer. He shows poor insight and judgment regarding his sadness since the loss of his wife. He repeatedly says, "Mary wouldn't want me to be sad. She would want me to continue with my life."

Mental Status Examination

The mental status examination establishes a baseline, provides a snapshot of where the patient is at a particular moment, and creates a written record. Areas of assessment include general observations, orientation, mood and affect, speech, thought processes, and cognition. Box 10.4 provides a narrative note of the results from a patient's mental status examination.

> **KEYCONCEPT** The **mental status examination** is an organized systematic approach to assessment of an individual's current psychiatric condition.

General Observations

At the beginning of the interview, the nurse should record his or her initial impressions of the patient. These general observations include the patient's appearance, affect, psychomotor activity, and overall behavior. How is the patient dressed? Is the dress appropriate for weather and setting? What is the patient's affect (emotional expression)? What behaviors is the patient displaying? For example, the same nurse assessed two male patients with depression. At the beginning of the mental status examination, the differences between these two men were very clear. The nurse described the first patient as "a large, well-dressed man who is agitated and appears angry, shifts in his seat, and does not maintain eye contact. He interrupts often in the initial explanation of mental status." The nurse described the other patient as a "small, unshaven, disheveled man with a strong body odor who appears withdrawn. He shuffles as he walks, speaks very softly, appears sad, and avoids direct eye contact."

Orientation

The nurse can determine the patient's orientation by asking the date, time, and current location of the interview setting. If a patient knows the year but not the exact date, the interviewer can ask the season. A person's orientation tells the nurse the extent of confusion. If a patient does not know the year or the place of the interview, he or she is exhibiting considerable confusion.

Mood and Affect

Mood refers to the prominent, sustained, overall emotions that the person expresses and exhibits. Mood may be sustained for days or weeks, or it may fluctuate during the course of a day. For example, some patients with depression have a diurnal variation in their mood. They experience their lowest mood in the morning, but as the day progresses, their depressed mood lifts and they feel somewhat better in the evening. Terms used to describe mood include **euthymic** (normal), **euphoric** (elated), **labile** (changeable), and **dysphoric** (depressed, disquieted, and restless).

Affect refers to the person's capacity to vary outward emotional expression. Affect fluctuates with thought content and can be observed in facial expressions, vocal fluctuations, and gestures. During the assessment, the patient may exhibit anger, frustration, irritation, apathy, and helplessness while his or her overall mood remains unchanged.

Affect can be described in terms of range, intensity, appropriateness, and stability. Range can be full or restricted. An individual who expresses several different emotions consistent with the stated feelings and content being expressed is described as having a *full range* of affect that is congruent with the situation. An individual who expresses few emotions has a restricted affect. For example, a patient could be describing the recent tragic death of a loved one in a monotone with little expression. In determining whether this response is normal, the nurse compares the patient's emotional response with the cultural norm for that particular response. *Intensity* can be increased, flat, or blunted. The nurse determines whether the emotional response is *appropriate* for the situation. For example, an inappropriate response is shown by a patient who has an extreme reaction to the death of the victims of the September 11 tragedy as if the victims were personal friends. Another patient said that his life stopped when the World Trade Center towers came down. He could not eat or sleep for weeks afterward. *Stability* can be mobile (normal) or labile. If a patient reports feeling happy one minute and reduced to tears the next, the person probably has an unstable mood. During the interview, the nurse should look for rapid mood changes that indicate lability of mood. A patient who exhibits intense, frequently shifting emotional extremes has a labile affect.

Speech

Speech provides clues about thoughts, emotional patterns, and cognitive organization. Speech may be pressured, fast, slow, or fragmented. Speech patterns reflect the patient's thought patterns, which can be logical or illogical. To check the patient's comprehension, the nurse can show a patient an object (e.g., pen, watch) and ask the person to name them. During conversation, the nurse assesses the fluency and quality of the patient's speech. The nurse listens for repetition or rhyming of words.

Thought Processes

The nurse assesses the patient for rapid change of ideas; inability or taking a long time to get to the point; loose or no connections among ideas or words; rhyming or repetition of words, questions, or phrases; or use of unheard of words. Any of these observations indicates abnormal thought patterns. The content of what the patient says is also important. What thought is the patient expressing? The nurse listens for unusual and unlikely stories, fears, or behaviors; for example, "The FBI is tracking me" or "I am afraid to leave my house."

Cognition and Intellectual Performance

The nurse can assess for **intellectual well-being** by determining the extent that the patient recognizes his or her creative abilities and is able to learn new knowledge and skills. To assess the patient's cognition, that is, the ability to think and know, the nurse uses memory, calculation, and reasoning tests to identify specific areas of impairment. The cognitive areas include (1) attention and concentration, (2) abstract reasoning and comprehension, (3) memory, and (4) insight and judgment.

Attention and Concentration. To test attention and concentration, the nurse asks the patient, without pencil or paper, to start with 100 and subtract 7 until reaching 65 or to start with 20 and subtract 3. The nurse must decide which is most appropriate for the patient considering education and understanding. Subtracting 3 from 20 is the easier of the two tasks. Asking a patient to spell "world" backward is also useful in determining attention and concentration.

Abstract Reasoning and Comprehension. To test abstract reasoning and comprehension, the nurse gives the patient a proverb to interpret. Examples include "People in glass houses shouldn't throw stones," "A rolling stone gathers no moss," and "A penny saved is a penny earned."

Recall, Short-Term, Recent, and Remote Memory. There are four spheres of memory to check: recall, or immediate, memory; short-term memory; recent memory; and long-term, or remote, memory. To check immediate and short-term memory, the nurse gives the patient three unrelated words to remember and asks him or her to recite them right after telling them and at 5- and 15-minute intervals during the interview. To test recent memory, the nurse may question about a holiday or world event within the past few months. The nurse tests long-term or remote memory by asking about events years ago. If they are personal events and the answers seem incorrect, the nurse may check them with a family member.

Insight and Judgment. Insight and judgment are related concepts that involve the ability to examine thoughts, conceptualize facts, solve problems, think abstractly, and possess self-awareness. Insight is a person's awareness of his or her own thoughts and feelings and ability to compare them with the thoughts and feelings of others. It involves an awareness of how others view one's behavior and its meaning. For example, many patients do not believe that they have mental illness. They may have delusions and hallucinations or be hospitalized for bizarre and sometimes dangerous behavior, but they are completely unaware that their behavior is unusual or abnormal. During an interview, a patient may adamantly proclaim that nothing is wrong or that he or she does not have a mental illness. Even if a problem is recognized, the patient may lack insight regarding issues related to care.

Judgment is the ability to reach a logical decision about a situation and to choose a course of action after examining and analyzing various possibilities. Throughout the interview, the nurse evaluates the patient's ability to make logical decisions. For example, some patients may continually choose partners who are abusive. The nurse could logically conclude that these patients have poor judgment in selecting partners. Another way to examine a patient's judgment is to give a simple scenario and ask the person to identify the best response. An example of such a scenario is asking, "What would you do if you found a bag of money outside a bank on a busy street?" If the patient responds, "Run with it," his or her judgment is questionable.

Behavior

Throughout the assessment, the nurse observes any behavior that may have significance in understanding the patient's response or symptoms of the mental disorder or emotional problem. For example, a depressed patient may be tearful throughout the session, whereas an anxious patient may twist or pull his or her hair, shift in the chair, or be unable to maintain eye contact. The nurse may find that whenever a particular topic is addressed, the patient's behavior changes. The nurse needs to relate patterned behaviors to significant events by connecting behaviors with the assessment data. For example, a patient may change jobs frequently, causing family distress and financial problems. Exploration of the events leading up to job changes may elicit important information regarding the patient's ability to solve problems.

Self-Concept

Self-concept, which develops over a lifetime, represents the total beliefs about three interrelated dimensions of the self: body image, self-esteem, and personal identity. The importance of each of these dimensions varies among individuals. For some, beliefs about themselves are strongly tied to body image; for others, personal identity is most important. Still others develop personal identity from what others have told them over the years. The nurse carrying out an assessment must keep in mind that self-concept and its components are dynamic and variable. For example, a woman may have a consistent self-concept until her first pregnancy. At that time, the many physiologic changes of pregnancy may cause her body image to change. She may be comfortable and enjoy the "glow of pregnancy," or she may feel like a "bloated cow." Suddenly, her body image is the most important part of her self-concept, and how she handles it can increase or decrease her self-esteem or sense of personal identity. Thus, all of the components are tied together, and each one affects the others.

Self-concept is assessed through eliciting patients' thoughts about themselves, their ability to navigate in the world, and their nonverbal behaviors. A disheveled sloppy physical appearance outside cultural norms is an indication of poor self-concept. Negative self-statements, such as, "I could never do that," "I have no control over my life," and "I'm so stupid" reveal poor views of self. The nurse's own self-concept can shape the nurse's view of the patient. For example, a nurse who is self-confident and feels inwardly scornful of a patient who lacks such confidence may intimidate the patient through unconscious, judgmental behaviors, or inconsiderate comments.

A useful approach to measuring self-concept is asking the patient to draw a self-portrait. For many patients, drawing is much easier than writing and serves as an excellent technique for monitoring changes. Interpretation of self-concept from drawings focuses on size, color, level of detail, pressure, line quality, symmetry, and placement. Low self-esteem is expressed by small size, lack of color variation, and sparse details in the drawing. Powerlessness and feelings of inadequacy are expressed through a lack of a head, a mouth, arms, and feet in the drawing. A lack of symmetry (placement of figure parts or entire drawings off center) represents feelings of insecurity and inadequacy. As self-esteem builds, size increases, color tends to become more varied and brighter, and more details appear. Figure 10.1 shows a self-portrait of a

FIGURE 10.1 **Left:** Self-portrait of a 52-year-old woman at first group session following discharge from hospital for treatment of depression. **Right:** Self-portrait after 3 months of weekly group interventions.

patient at the beginning of treatment for depression and another drawn 3 months later.

Body Image

Body image represents a person's beliefs and attitudes about his or her body and includes such dimensions as size (large or small) and attractiveness (pretty or ugly). People who are satisfied with their body have a more positive body image than those who are not satisfied. Generally, women attach more importance to their body image than do men and may even define themselves in terms of their body.

Patients express body image beliefs through statements about their bodies. Statements such as "I feel so ugly," "I'm so fat," and "No one will want to have sex with me" express negative body images. Nonverbal behaviors indicating problems with body image include avoiding looking at or touching a body part; hiding the body in oversized clothing; or bandaging a particularly sensitive area, such as a mole on the face. Cultural differences must be considered when evaluating behavior related to body image. For example, the expectation of some cultures is that women and girls will keep their bodies completely covered and wear loose-fitting garments.

| **NCLEXNOTE** Be prepared to assess reactions to a body image change (e.g., loss of vision, paralysis, colostomy, amputation).

Self-Esteem

Self-esteem is the person's attitude about the self. Self-esteem differs from body image because it concerns satisfaction with one's overall self. People who feel good about themselves are more likely to have the confidence to try new health behaviors. They are also less likely to be depressed. Negative self-esteem statements include "I'm a worthless person" and "I never do anything right."

Personal Identity

Personal identity is knowing "who I am." Every life experience and interaction contributes to knowing oneself better. Personal identity allows people to establish boundaries and understand personal strengths and limitations. In some psychiatric disorders, individuals cannot separate themselves from others, which show that their personal identity is not strongly developed. A problem with personal identity is difficult to assess. Statements such as, "I'm just like my mother, and she was always in trouble," "I become whatever my current boyfriend wants me to be," and "I can't make a decision unless I check it out first" are all statements that require further exploration into the person's view of self.

Stress and Coping Patterns

Everyone has stress (see Chapter 18). One of the dimensions of wellness is **emotional well-being** or the ability to cope with stress through skills and strategies. Sometimes the experience of stress contributes to the development of mental disorders. Identification of major stresses in a patient's life helps the nurse understand the person and support the use of successful coping behaviors in the future. The nurse should explore how the patient deals with stress and identify successful coping mechanisms in order to encourage their use.

> **NCLEXNOTE** Every assessment should focus on stress and coping patterns. Identifying how a patient copes with stress can be used as a basis of care in all nursing situations. Include content from Chapter 19 when studying these concepts.

Risk Assessment

Risk factors are characteristics, conditions, situations, or events that increase the patient's vulnerability to threats to safety or well-being. Throughout this text, the sections concerning risk factors focus on the following:

- Risks to the patient's safety
- Risks for developing psychiatric disorders
- Risks for increasing, or exacerbating, symptoms and impairment in an individual who already has a psychiatric disorder

Consideration of risk factors involving patient safety should be included in each assessment. Examples of these risks include the risk for suicide and violence toward others or the risk for events, such as falling, seizures, allergic reactions, or elopement (unauthorized absence from health care facility). Nurses assess factors on a priority basis. For example, threats of violence or suicide take priority.

Suicidal Ideation

During the assessment, the nurse needs to listen closely to whether the patient describes or mentions thinking about self-harm. If the patient does not openly express ideas of self-harm, it is necessary to ask in a straightforward and gentle manner, "Have you ever thought about injuring or killing yourself?" If the patient answers, "Yes, I am thinking about it right now," the nurse knows not to leave the patient unobserved and to institute suicide precautions as indicated by the facility protocols. General questions to ask to ascertain suicidal ideation follow:

- Have you ever tried to harm or kill yourself? If yes, when?
- Do you have thoughts of suicide at this time? If yes, do you have a plan? If yes, can you tell me the details of the plan?
- Do you have the means to carry out this plan? (If the plan requires a weapon, does the patient have it available?)
- Have you made preparations for your death (e.g., writing a note to loved ones, putting finances in order, giving away possessions)?
- Has a significant episode in your life caused you to think this way (e.g., recent loss of spouse or job)?

If any of these responses are "yes," the nurse should explore the issue in detail, notify the supervisor, and clearly document the patient responses and nursing follow-up. The nurse is expected to follow the agency policies.

In order to assess patient strengths in coping with suicidal thoughts, the nurse can ask the patient to identify strategies that were used in resisting suicidal urges and actions. For example, one patient reported calling a family member to talk when the suicidal urges were really strong. The nurse can encourage patient to use these strategies in the future.

Assaultive or Homicidal Ideation

When assessing a patient, the nurse also needs to listen carefully to any delusions or hallucinations that the patient shares. If the patient gives any indication that he or she must or is being told to harm someone, the nurse must first think of self-safety and institute assaultive precautions as indicated by the facility protocols. General questions to ascertain assaultive or homicidal ideation follow:

- Do you intend to harm someone? If yes, who?
- Do you have a plan? If yes, what are the details of the plan?
- Do you have the means to carry out the plan? (If the plan requires a weapon, is it readily available?)

Assessment of the Social Domain

The assessment continues with examination of the patient's social domain. The nurse inquires about interactions with others in the family and community (work, church, or other organizations); the patient's parents and their marital relationship; the patient's place in birth order; names and ages of any siblings; and relationships with spouse, siblings, and children. The nurse also assesses work and education history and community activities. The nurse observes how the patient relates to any family or friends who may be in attendance. This component of the assessment helps the nurse anticipate how the patient may get along with other patients in an inpatient setting. It also allows the nurse to plan for any anticipated difficulties.

Functional Status

An important aspect of the assessment is determining the functioning of the patient (i.e., Is an adult working and living independently? Is a student attending classes?). How the patient copes with strangers and those with whom he or she does not get along is also important information.

Social Systems

A significant component of the patient's life involves the social systems in which he or she may be enmeshed. **Social well-being** involves developing a sense of connection and a well-developed support system. The social systems to examine include the family, the culture to which the patient belongs, and the community in which he or she lives.

Family Assessment

How the patient fits in with and relates to his or her family is important to know. General questions to ask include the following:

- Who do you consider family?
- How important to you is your family?
- How does your family make decisions?
- What are the roles in your family, and who fills them?
- Where do you fit in your family?
- With whom in your family do you get along best?
- With whom in your family do you have the most conflict?
- Who in your family is supportive of you?

Cultural Assessment

Culture can profoundly affect a person's world view (see Chapter 2). Culture helps a person frame beliefs about life, death, health and illness, and roles and relationships. During cultural assessment, the nurse must consider factors that influence the manifestations of the current mental disorder. For example, a patient mentions "speaking in tongues." The nurse may identify this experience as a hallucination when, in fact, the patient was having a religious experience common within some branches of Christianity. In this instance, knowing and understanding such religious practices will prevent a misinterpretation of the symptoms.

The nurse can elicit important cultural information by asking the following questions:

- To what cultural group do you belong?
- Were you raised in an ethnic community?
- How do you define health?
- How do you define illness?
- How do you define good and evil?
- What do you do to get better when you are physically ill? Mentally ill?
- Whom do you see for help when you are physically ill? Mentally ill?
- By what cultural rules or taboos do you try to live?
- Do you eat special foods?

Community Support and Resources

Many patients are connected to community resources, and the nurse needs to assess what they are and the patterns of usage. For example, a patient who is homeless may know of a church where he or she can sleep but may go there only on cold nights. Or a patient may go to the community center daily for lunch to be with other people. Examining the environment is a part of the individual's assessment. **Environmental well-being** involves living in pleasant, stimulating environments that support a healthy life style.

Occupational Status

Occupational well-being involves personal satisfaction and enrichment derived from one's work. The nurse should document the occupation the patient is now in as well as a history of jobs. If the patient has changed jobs frequently, the nurse should ask about the reasons. Perhaps the patient has faced such problems as an inability to focus on the job at hand or to get along with others. If so, such issues require further exploration.

Economic Status

Finances are very private for many people; thus, the nurse must ask questions about economic status carefully. However, **financial well-being** is satisfaction with present and future situations. What the nurse needs to ascertain is not specific dollar amounts but whether the patient feels stressed by finances and has enough for basic needs.

Legal Status

Because of laws governing people with mental illness, ascertaining the patient's correct age, marital status, and any legal guardianship is important. The nurse may need to check the patient's medical records for this information.

Quality of Life

The patient's perspective on quality of life means how the patient rates his or her life. Does a patient feel his life is poor because he cannot purchase everything he wants? Does another patient feel blessed because the sun is shining today? Listening carefully to the patient's discussion of his or her life and how he or she measures the quality of that life provides important information about self-concept, coping skills, desires, and dreams.

Psychosocial Strengths and Wellness Assessment

Throughout the assessment, the nurse should be able to identify areas of strength and wellness. A description of these areas should be validated with the patient and documented in the person's record.

Spiritual Assessment

> **KEY CONCEPT Spirituality** "is a way of being in the world in which a person feels a sense of connectedness to self, others, and/or a higher power or nature: a sense of meaning in life; and transcendence beyond self, everyday living, and suffering" (Weathers, McCarthy, & Coffey, 2015).

Several studies show that spirituality and religion are important in coping with mental disorders through providing hope, comfort, meaning of life, and serve as a resource for coping with symptoms, substance abuse, and protection against suicide (Das, Punnoose, Doval, & Nair, 2018; Paul, Corneau, Boozary, & Stergiopoulos, 2018). Nurses must be clear about their own spirituality to be sure it does not interfere with assessment of the patient's spirituality. Nurses also need to work within their area of competence and recognize the importance of referring patients to a health care chaplain or other spiritual care support.

The purpose of a **spiritual care assessment**, which is often the responsibility of the nurse, is to identify specific spiritual care needs and to formulate a care plan. A nursing spiritual assessment is usually included in the general nursing assessment, even when there are chaplains available (Timmins & Caldeira, 2017). The Joint Commission requires that spiritual care assessment and spiritual care delivery be directed to the patient or the patient's family but does not identify specific disciplines of the personnel who will conduct the assessment (The Joint Commission, 2018).

The spiritual assessment is based an individual's needs, which are discovered within an open, trusting dialogue. It is important that the nurse does not self-disclose personal values and beliefs during the assessment. The following questions can serve to initiate the assessment:

- How important is spirituality and/or religion in your life and coping with an illness?
- Are you involved in a religious or faith community?
- Would you like to address these issues in your mental health care?
- If yes, with whom would you like to address these issues?

Spiritual assessment questions need to correspond to the patient's readiness to discuss this topic. Patients and clinicians agree that it may take time for the patient to feel comfortable and ready to discuss spirituality. It is essential that questions are asked that focus on a patient's strengths. For example asking the question, "Was there a time in your life where you felt great peace and joy and maybe not so stressed out?" is less judgmental than the question "What were your sources of deep meaning, peace, joy, and strength … ?" The latter statement has an implied expectation that there should be sources (religious, spiritual) that exist.

Examples of questions that could help patients examine past or current spiritually related strengths and resources include the following (Gomi, Starnino, & Canda, 2014):

- Was there a time in your life when you really felt at peace?
- What do you do to get through the tough times (pray, meditate, visit nature, family)?
- When do you feel most positive about yourself?
- What brings inspiration to your life?

Questions that can help the individual connect to spiritual goals to recovery goals (if that is a goal of the person) include the following (Gomi et al., 2014):

- What helps you feel good or hopeful about your life?
- Is spirituality something you want to connect with in your recovery?
- Based on what you said, how would you say your spirituality could support your recovery?

PRIORITY OF NURSING CARE

After completing an assessment, the nurse and patient collaborate in identifying problem areas and planning for interventions within the scope of nursing practice. With experience, the nurse can cluster the assessment data to identify two or three immediate health or mental health problem issues related to promotion of health and well-being, prevention of illness, reduction of risks, or treat health care problems. The nurse may also use one of the nursing diagnostic taxonomies. See Chapter 4. The nurse and patient will then plan realistic goals that are consistent with and support recovery.

DEVELOPING RECOVERY OUTCOMES

Mutually agreed-upon goals flow from the prioritization of needs and provide guidance in determining appropriate interventions. Initial outcomes are determined and then are monitored and evaluated throughout the care process. Measuring outcomes not only demonstrates clinical effectiveness but also helps to promote rational clinical decision making and is reflective of the nursing interventions. Standardized tools are being developed through the National Institutes of Health and are being introduced to the clinical community. These tools measure patient-reported outcomes and use health attributes such as psychosocial illness impact, depression, pain, cognitive function, anxiety rather than specific disease measurements. These tools can be used in the clinical setting for measuring mental health outcomes (Broderick, DeWitt, Rothrock, Crane, & Forrest, 2013).

> **KEYCONCEPT Outcomes** are health experiences and evaluations reported by the patient or observed by the nurse related to symptoms, functioning, well-being, health perceptions, and satisfaction with care that can be attributed to nursing care at a given point in time (Broderick et al., 2013). An expected outcome is concise, stated in few words and in neutral terms (Table 10.2).

Expected outcomes are developed mutually with the patient and focus on the individual requesting mental health services. Nurses are accountable for documenting patient outcomes; nursing interventions; and any changes in health status or care plan, or both. Outcomes can be expressed in terms of the patient's actual responses (no longer reports hearing voices) or the health or mental health changes after implementation of nursing interventions.

The Nursing Outcomes Classification is a comprehensive, standardized classification of patient, family, and community outcomes. The purpose of this classification system is to evaluate the impact of interventions provided by nurses or other health care professionals (Moorhead, Swanson, Johnson, & Maas, 2018). There are 540 outcomes defined with a list of indicators that can be used.

RECOVERY-ORIENTED NURSING INTERVENTIONS

Recovery-oriented patient/nurse-initiated treatment is an autonomous action within the scope of nursing practice. It can also be physician-initiated treatment through an order written in the patient's record. In both instances, the nurse is held to a standard of nursing care.

> **KEYCONCEPT Recovery-oriented nursing interventions** are nursing actions or treatment, selected based on clinical judgment and mutual decision making with the patient, that are designed to achieve patient, family, or community outcomes. Interventions can be direct or indirect and can target specific symptoms, health needs, and strengths. See Box 10.5.

BOX 10.5

Research for Best Practice: Realities of Recovery-Oriented Rehabilitation

Parker, S., Dark, F., Newman, E., Korman, N., Rasmussen, Z., & Meurk, C. (2017). Reality of working in a community-based, recovery-oriented mental health rehabilitation unit: A pragmatic grounded theory analysis. *International Journal of Mental Health Nursing, 26*(4), 355–365.

THE QUESTION: What are the experiences of staff working at one recovery-oriented, community-based residential mental health rehabilitation unit?

METHODS: A pragmatic approach to grounded theory was used in the analysis of transcripts of staff across nursing, allied health, and nonclinical support roles. Semi-structured interviews were guided by four topics: (1) understanding of recovery-oriented, community-based care, (2) how working at the community care unit compares to other mental health settings, (3) expectations prior to beginning at the unit, and (4) reasons for continuing to work at the community care unit. Eight staff members participated.

FINDINGS: Four themes emerged: (1) rehabilitation is different than treatment requiring specialized skills and flexibility, (2) the community care unit is a positive transition space, (3) consumers have to be ready to change, and (4) recovery is central to rehabilitation.

IMPLICATIONS FOR NURSING: Recovery-oriented nursing practice focuses on collaborating with the patient (consumer) in helping the individual to be motivated to make the changes.

TABLE 10.2	EXAMPLE OF OUTCOMES	
Issue	**Outcome**	**Intervention**
Social isolation	Social involvement Indicators: a. Interact with other patients b. Attend group meetings	Using a contract format, explain role and responsibility of patients

There are several nursing interventions systems, including the Nursing Interventions Classification (NIC) (Butcher, Bulechek, Dochterman, & Wagner, 2018), the Clinical Care Classification system (Saba, 2017), and the Omaha nursing model (Martin, 2005; Martin & Kessler, 2017). All of these systems are recognized by the American Nurses Association (ANA). In this text, the *Psychiatric–Mental Health Nursing: Scope and Standards of Practice* guides the use of interventions (ANA, APNA, & ISPN, 2014). Some are adapted from classification systems and others from the psychiatric–mental health nursing literature.

Physical Interventions

Biologic interventions focus on physical functioning and are directed toward the patient's self-care, activities and exercise, sleep, nutrition, relaxation, hydration, and thermoregulation as well as pain management and medication management.

Promotion of Self-Care Activities

Many patients with psychiatric–mental health problems can manage ADLs or self-care activities such as bathing, dressing appropriately, selecting adequate nutrition, and sleeping regularly. Others cannot manage such self-care activities, either because of their symptoms or as a result of the side effects of medications.

In the inpatient setting, the psychiatric nurse structures the patient's activities, so that basic self-care activities are completed. During acute phases of psychiatric disorders, the inability to attend to basic self-care tasks, such as getting dressed, is very common. Thus, the ability to complete personal hygiene activities (e.g., dental care, grooming) is monitored, and patients are assisted in completing such activities. In a psychiatric facility, patients are encouraged and expected to develop independence in completing these basic self-care activities. In the community, monitoring these basic self-care activities is always a part of the nursing visit or clinic appointment.

Activity and Exercise Interventions

In some psychiatric disorders (e.g., schizophrenia), people become sedentary and appear to lack the motivation to complete ADLs. This lack of motivation is part of the disorder and requires nursing intervention. In addition, side effects of medication often include sedation and lethargy. Encouraging regular activity and exercise can improve general well-being and physical health. In some instances, exercise behavior becomes an abnormal focus of attention, as may be observed in some patients with anorexia nervosa.

When assuming the responsibility of direct care provider, the nurse can help patients identify realistic activities and exercise goals. As leader or manager of a psychiatric unit, the nurse can influence ward routine. Alternatively, the nurse can delegate activity and exercise interventions to nurses' aides. Some institutions have other professionals (e.g., recreational therapists) available for the implementation of exercise programs. As a case manager, the nurse should consider the activity needs of individuals when coordinating care.

Sleep Interventions

Many psychiatric disorders and medications are associated with sleep disturbances. Sleep is also disrupted in patients with dementia; such patients may have difficulty falling asleep or may frequently awaken during the night. In dementia of the Alzheimer type, individuals may reverse their sleeping patterns by napping during the day and staying awake at night.

Nonpharmacologic interventions are always used first because of the side-effect risks associated with the use of sedatives and hypnotics (see Chapter 11). Sleep interventions to communicate to patients include the following:

- Go to bed only when tired or sleepy.
- Establish a consistent bedtime routine.
- Avoid stimulating foods, beverages, or medications.
- Avoid naps in the late afternoon or evening.
- Eat lightly before retiring and limit fluid intake.
- Use your bed only for sleep or intimacy.
- Avoid emotional stimulation before bedtime.
- Use behavioral and relaxation techniques.
- Limit distractions.

Nutrition Interventions

Psychiatric disorders and medication side effects can affect eating behaviors. For varying reasons, some patients eat too little, but others eat too much. For instance, homeless patients with mental illnesses have difficulty maintaining adequate nutrition because of their deprived lifestyle. Substance abuse also interferes with maintaining adequate nutrition, either through stimulation or suppression of appetite or neglecting nutrition because of drug-seeking behavior. Thus, nutrition interventions should be specific and relevant to the individual's circumstances and mental health. In addition, recommended daily nutritional allowances are important in the promotion of physical and mental health, and nurses should consider them when planning care.

Some psychiatric symptoms involve changes in perceptions of food, appetite, and eating habits. If a patient believes that food is poisonous, he or she may eat sparingly or not at all. Interventions are then necessary to address the suspiciousness as well as to encourage adequate intake of recommended daily allowances. Allowing patients to examine foods, participate in preparations, and test the safety of the meal by eating slowly or after everyone else may be necessary. For patients who are paranoid, it is sometimes helpful to serve prepackaged foods.

Relaxation Interventions

Relaxation promotes comfort, reduces anxiety, alleviates stress, eases pain, and prevents aggression. It can diminish the effects of hallucinations and delusions. The many different **relaxation techniques** used as mental health interventions range from simple deep breathing to biofeedback to hypnosis. Although some techniques, such as biofeedback, require additional training and, in some instances, certification, nurses can easily apply simple relaxation, distraction, and imagery techniques.

Simple relaxation techniques encourage and elicit relaxation to decrease undesirable signs and symptoms. **Distraction** is the purposeful focusing of attention away from undesirable sensations, and **guided imagery** is the purposeful use of imagination to achieve relaxation or direct attention away from undesirable sensations (Box 10.6).

Relaxation techniques that involve physical touch (e.g., back rubs) usually are not used for people with mental disorders. Touching and massaging usually are not appropriate, especially for those who have a history of physical or sexual abuse. Such patients may find touching too stimulating or misinterpret it as being sexual or aggressive.

Hydration Interventions

Assessing fluid status and monitoring fluid intake and output are often important interventions. Overhydration or underhydration can be a symptom of a disorder. For example, some patients with psychotic disorders experience chronic fluid imbalance. Many psychiatric medications affect fluid and electrolyte balance (see Chapter 11). For example, when taking lithium carbonate, patients must have adequate fluid intake and pay special attention to testing serum sodium levels. Interventions that help patients understand the relationship of medications to fluid and electrolyte balance are important in their overall care.

Thermoregulation Interventions

Many psychiatric disorders can disturb the body's normal temperature regulation. Thus, patients cannot sense temperature increases or decreases and consequently cannot protect themselves from extremes of hot or cold. This problem is especially difficult for people who are homeless or live outside the protected environments of institutions and boarding homes. In addition, many psychiatric medications affect the ability to regulate body temperature.

Interventions include educating patients about the problem of thermoregulation, identifying potential extremes in temperatures, and developing strategies to

---

BOX 10.6
Relaxation Techniques: Descriptions and Implementation

RELAXED BREATHING
The goal of this exercise is to slow down your breathing, especially your exhaling.

STEPS
1. Choose a word that you associate with relaxation, such as CALM or RELAX or PEACEFUL.
2. Inhale through your nose and exhale slowly through your mouth. Take normal breaths, not deep ones.
3. While you exhale, say the relaxing word you have chosen. Say it very slowly, like this, "c-a-a-a-a-a-a-l-m" or "r-e-e-e-l-a-a-a-x."
4. Pause after exhaling before taking your next breath. If it's not too distracting, count to four before inhaling each new breath.
5. Repeat the entire sequence 10–15 times.

MUSCLE RELAXATION
The goal of this technique is to gently stretch your muscles to reduce stiffness and tension. The exercises start at your head and work down to your feet. You can do these exercises while sitting in a chair.

STEPS
1. Neck rolls. Drop your head to one side. Gently roll it around in a wide circle. Repeat 3–5 times. Then reverse directions, and gently roll your head in a wide circle the other way. Repeat 3–5 times.
2. Shoulder shrugs. Lift both shoulders in a shrugging motion. Try to touch your ears with your shoulders. Let your shoulders drop down after each shrug. Repeat 3–5 times.
3. Overhead arm stretches.[a] Raise both arms straight above your head. Interlace your fingers, like you're making a basket, with your palms facing down (toward the floor). Stretch your arms toward the ceiling. Then, keeping your fingers interlaced, rotate your palms to face upward (toward the ceiling). Stretch toward the ceiling. Repeat 3–5 times.
4. Knee raises. Reach down and grab your right knee with one or both hands. Pull your knee up toward your chest (as close to your chest as is comfortable). Hold your knee there for a few seconds, before returning your foot to the floor. Reach down and grab your left knee with one or both hands and bring it up toward your chest. Hold it there for a few seconds. Repeat the sequence 3–5 times.
5. Foot and ankle rolls. Lift your feet and stretch your legs out. Rotate your ankles and feet, 3–5 times in one direction, then 3–5 times in the other direction.

[a]If it is not comfortable to do step #3 with your arms overhead, try it with your arms reaching out in front of you.
Reprinted from Substance Abuse and Mental Health Services Administration. (2009). Illness management and recovery: Practitioner guides and handouts. HHS Pub. No. SMA-09-4462, Rockville, MD: Center for Mental Health Services, Substance Abuse and Mental Health Services Administration, U.S. Department of Health and Human Services.

protect the patient from the adverse effects of temperature changes. For example, reminding patients to wear coats and sweaters in the winter or to wear loose, lightweight garments in the summer may prevent frostbite or heat exhaustion, respectively.

Pain Management

Psychiatric nurses are more likely to provide care to patients experiencing chronic pain than acute pain. However, a single intervention is seldom successful for relieving chronic pain. In some instances, pain is managed by medication; in other instances, nonpharmacologic strategies, such as simple relaxation techniques, distraction, or imagery, are used. Indeed, relaxation is one of the most widely used cognitive and behavioral approaches to pain. Education, stress management techniques, hypnosis, and biofeedback are also used in pain management. Physical agents include heat and cold therapy, exercise, and transcutaneous nerve stimulation.

The key to managing pain is identifying how it disrupts the patient's personal, social, professional, and family life. Education focusing on the pain, use of medications for treatment, and development of cognitive skills are important pain management components. In some cases, redefining treatment success as improvement in functioning, rather than alleviation of pain, may be necessary. The interaction between stress and pain is important; that is, increased stress leads to increased pain. Patients can better manage their pain when stress is reduced.

Medication Management

The psychiatric–mental health nurse uses many medication management interventions to help patients maintain therapeutic regimens. Medication management involves more than the actual administration of medications. Nurses also assess medication effectiveness and side effects and consider drug–drug interactions. Monitoring the amount of lethal prescription medication is particularly important. For example, check if patients have old prescriptions of tricyclic antidepressants in their medicine cabinets. Treatment with psychopharmacologic agents can be lengthy because of the chronic nature of many disorders; many patients remain on medication regimens for years, never becoming free of medication. Thus, medication education is an ongoing intervention that requires careful documentation. Medication follow-up may include home visits as well as telephone calls.

Psychological Interventions

A major emphasis in psychiatric–mental health nursing is the psychological domain: emotion, behavior, and cognition. The basis of nursing care is establishing a therapeutic relationship with the patient. Because the therapeutic relationship was extensively discussed in Chapter 8, it is not covered in this chapter. This section does cover cognitive interventions, counseling, conflict resolution, bibliotherapy, reminiscence, behavior therapy, psychoeducation, health teaching, and spiritual interventions. Chapter 5 presents the theoretic basis for many of these interventions.

Cognitive Interventions

Evidence-based cognitive interventions are used in a variety of practice settings (inpatient and outpatient). The knowledge and skills inherent in cognitively based interventions have been extensively studied, and their effectiveness has been demonstrated for a variety of psychiatric disorders, especially depression (see Chapter 19) and anxiety and related disorders (see Chapters 16, 17, and 18).

Cognitive interventions are based on the concept of cognition. **Cognition** can be defined as an internal process of perception, memory, and judgment through which an understanding of self and the world is developed.

Cognitive interventions aim to change or reframe an individual's automatic thought patterns that have developed over time and that interfere with the individual's ability to function optimally. The skills and techniques developed on the basis of cognitive theory result in a new view of self and the environment.

Counseling Interventions

Counseling interventions are interactions between a nurse and a patient, family, or group experiencing immediate or ongoing difficulties related to their health or well-being. Counseling is usually short term and focuses on stabilizing symptoms, supporting personal recovery goals, improving coping abilities, reinforcing healthy behaviors, fostering positive interactions, or preventing illness and disability. Counseling strategies are discussed throughout the text. Psychotherapy, which differs from counseling, is generally a long-term approach aimed at improving or helping patients regain previous health status and functional abilities. Mental health specialists, such as advanced practice nurses, use psychotherapy.

Conflict Resolution and Cultural Brokering

Conflict resolution is a process of helping an individual or family identify a problem underlying a disagreement or dispute and developing alternative possibilities for solving the conflict (Weitzman & Weitzman, 2014). Conflict can be positive if individuals see the problem as solvable and providing an opportunity for growth and interpersonal understanding. The nurse may be in the position of actually teaching family members how to resolve their own conflicts positively. Key elements of any conflict resolution process are collaboration, motivation to seek a solution, and the ability to see the other person's point. Conflict resolution strategies are commonly taught to adolescents who are experiencing cyberbullying to adults in marital or romantic relationships (Garaigordobil & Martínez-Valderrey, 2015; Özgüç & Tanriverdi, 2018). Nurses are often in leadership positions and use conflict resolution skills to settle employee disputes.

At times, patients who are politically and economically powerless find themselves in conflict with the health care system. Differences in cultural values and languages among patients and health care organizations contribute to feelings of powerlessness. For example, immigrant families, migrant farm workers, people who are homeless, and people who need to make informed decisions under stressful conditions may be unable to navigate the health care system. The nurse can help to resolve such conflicts through **cultural brokering**, the act of bridging, linking, or mediating messages, instructions, and belief systems between groups of people of differing cultural systems to reduce conflict or produce change (Kam & Lazarevic, 2014).

For the "nurse as broker" to be effective, he or she establishes and maintains a sense of connectedness or relationship with the patient. In turn, the nurse also establishes and cultivates networks with other health care facilities and resources. Cultural sensitivity enables the nurse to be aware of and sensitive to the needs of patients from a variety of cultures. Cultural competence is necessary for the brokering process to be effective.

Bibliotherapy and Social Media

Bibliotherapy, sometimes referred to as bibliocounseling, is the reading of selected written materials to express feelings or gain insight under the guidance of a health care provider. The provider assigns and discusses with the patient a book, story, or article. The provider makes the assignment because he or she believes that the patient can receive therapeutic benefit from the reading. (It is assumed that the provider who assigned the reading has also read it.) The provider needs to consider the patient's reading level before making an assignment. If a patient has limited reading ability, the provider should not use bibliotherapy.

Literary works serve as a projective screen through which people see themselves in the story. Literature can help patients identify with characters and vicariously experience their reality. The use of bibliotherapy has been shown to improve depression when used with cognitive behavioral therapy (Müller, Rohde, Gau, & Stice, 2015). It can also expose patients to situations that they have not personally experienced—the vicarious experience allows growth in self-knowledge and compassion (Macdonald, Vallance, & McGrath, 2013). Bibliotherapy can also support recovery in inpatient units through reading books written in first person (Eisen, Lawlor, Wu, & Mason, 2018). Through reading, patients can enrich their lives in the following ways:

- *Catharsis:* expression of feelings stimulated by parallel experiences
- *Problem solving:* development of solutions to problems in the literature from practical ideas about problem solving
- *Insight:* increased self-awareness and understanding as the reader explores personal meaning from what is read
- *Anxiety reduction:* self-help written materials can reduce concerns about a diagnosed problem and treatment

Using the internet can be helpful to patients, but it also has drawbacks. Some websites can help patients gain insight into their problems through acquiring new knowledge and interacting with others in the privacy of their own surroundings. Web materials and chat groups are variable in quality and accuracy. Nurses should carefully evaluate the quality of the website.

Reminiscence

Reminiscence, the thinking about or relating of past experiences, is used as a nursing intervention to enhance life review in older patients. Reminiscence encourages patients, either in individual or group settings, to discuss their past and review their lives. Through reminiscence, individuals can identify past coping strategies that can support them in current stressful situations. Patients can also use reminiscence to maintain self-esteem, stimulate thinking, and support the natural healing process of life review. Activities that facilitate reminiscence include writing an account of past events, making a tape recording and playing it back, explaining pictures in old family albums, drawing a family tree, and writing to old friends.

Behavior Therapy

Behavior therapy interventions focus on reinforcing or promoting desirable behaviors or altering undesirable ones. The basic premise is that because most behaviors are learned, new functional behaviors can also be learned. Behaviors—not internal psychic processes—are the targets of the interventions. The models of behavioral theorists serve as a basis for these interventions (see Chapter 5).

Behavior Modification

Behavior modification is a specific, systematized behavior therapy technique that can be applied to individuals, groups, or systems. The aim of behavior modification is to reinforce desired behaviors and extinguish undesired ones. Desired behavior is rewarded to increase the likelihood that patients will repeat it, and over time, replace the problematic behavior with it. Behavior modification is used for various problematic behaviors, such as dysfunctional eating, addictions, anger management, and impulse control and often is used in the care of children and adolescents.

Token Economy

Used in inpatient settings and in group homes, a **token economy** applies behavior modification techniques to multiple behaviors. In a token economy, patients are rewarded with tokens for selected desired behaviors. They can use these tokens to purchase meals, leave the unit, watch television, or wear street clothes. In less restrictive environments, patients use tokens to purchase additional privileges, such as attending social events.

Token economy systems have been especially effective in reinforcing positive behaviors in people who are developmentally disabled or have severe and persistent mental illnesses. There is good evidence that the use of token economy for behavior and symptom management is effective in adults who are hospitalized, but there is little evidence to support transfer of the new behaviors outside the inpatient settings (Glowacki, Warner, & White, 2016). The strategy has been expanded to rehabilitation programs for children (Jones, Webb, Estes, & Dawson, 2013), and cocaine addiction (Farronato, Dursteler-Macfarland, Wiesbeck, & Petitjean, 2013).

Psychoeducation

Psychoeducation uses educational strategies to teach patients the skills they lack because of a psychiatric disorder. The goal of psychoeducation is a change in knowledge and behavior. Nurses use psychoeducation to meet the educational needs of patients by adapting teaching strategies to their disorder-related deficits (Box 10.7). As patients gain skills, functioning improves. Some patients may need to learn how to maintain their morning hygiene. Others may need to understand their illness and cope with hearing voices that others do not hear.

Specific psychoeducation techniques are based on adult learning principles, such as beginning at the point where the learner is currently and building on his or her current experiences. Thus, the nurse assesses the patient's current skills and readiness to learn. From there, the nurse individualizes a teaching plan for each patient. He or she can conduct such teaching in a one-to-one situation or a group format.

Psychoeducation is a continuous process of assessing, setting goals, developing learning activities, and evaluating for changes in knowledge and behavior. Nurses use it with individuals, groups, families, and communities. Psychoeducation serves as a basis for psychosocial rehabilitation, a service delivery approach for those with severe and persistent mental illness (see Chapter 23).

> **NCLEXNOTE** Apply knowledge from social sciences to help patients manage responses to psychiatric disorders and emotional problems.

Health Teaching

Health teaching is one of the standards of care for the psychiatric nurse. Teaching methods should be appropriate to the patient's development level, learning needs, readiness, ability to learn, language preference, and culture. Based on principles of learning, health teaching involves transmitting new information to the patient and providing constructive feedback and positive rewards, practice sessions, homework, and experimental learning. Health teaching is the integration of principles of teaching and learning with the knowledge of health and illness (Fig. 10.2).

BOX 10.7

Research for Best Practice: Psychoeducation Program for Family Members of Persons with First-Episode Psychosis

Petrakis, M., & Laxton, S. (2017). Intervening early with family members during first-episode psychosis: An evaluation of mental health nursing psychoeducation within an inpatient unit. Archives of Psychiatric Nursing, 31(1), 48–54.

THE QUESTION: Was the inpatient psychoeducation session helpful to family members of those with early psychosis?

METHODS: The psychoeducation session was conducted within the first week of the family members' admission. The data collection method of qualitative interviewing by telephone was used to facilitate the naturalness of the conversation and spontaneous feedback. There were 30 psychoeducation sessions delivered within a 5-month study period to 55 family members. Twenty-seven participated in a follow-up interview.

FINDINGS: The psychoeducation group showed significantly reduced levels of cognitive/inattention levels and improvement in social behavior. There were no differences in quality of life or family stress. Verbal information, psychosis fact sheets, and medication booklets were most helpful. This information was also distributed to family members who did not participate in the psychoeducation session.

IMPLICATIONS FOR NURSING: Early intervention for family members is helpful in developing an understanding of psychosis and necessary treatment.

FIGURE 10.2 Teaching evaluation model.

Thus, in health teaching, the psychiatric nurse attends to potential health care problems other than mental disorders and emotional problems. For example, if a person has diabetes mellitus and is taking insulin, the nurse provides health care teaching related to diabetes and the interaction of this problem with the mental disorder.

Spiritual Interventions

Spiritual care is based on an assessment of the patient's spiritual needs. Some interventions require actions such as listening, requesting a chaplain's presence, or providing readings; other interventions involve use of personal abilities and characteristics such as the use of the therapeutic relationship in supporting patient well-being. A nonjudgmental relationship and just "being with" (not doing for) the patient are key spiritual interventions. To assist people in spiritual distress, the nurse should know and understand the beliefs and practices of various spiritual groups. **Spiritual support**, assisting patients to feel balance and connection within their relationships, involves listening to expressions of loneliness, using empathy, and providing patients with desired spiritual articles (Caldeira & Timmons, 2017).

Interventions for the Social Domain

The social domain includes the individual's environment and its effect on his or her responses to mental disorders and distress. Interventions within the social domain are geared toward couples, families, friends, and large and small social groups, with special attention given to ethnicity and community interactions. In some instances, nurses design interventions that affect a patient's environment, such as helping a family member decide to admit a loved one to a long-term care facility. In other instances, the nurse actually modifies the environment to promote positive behaviors. Group interventions are discussed in Chapter 15.

Social Behavior and Privilege Systems in Inpatient Units

In psychiatric units, unrelated strangers who have problems interacting live together in close quarters, sometimes with two to four people sharing bedrooms and bathrooms. For this reason, most psychiatric units develop a list of behavioral expectations called unit rules that staff members post and explain to patients upon admittance. Their purpose is to facilitate a comfortable and safe environment; they have little to do with the patients' reasons for admission. Getting up at certain times, showering before breakfast, making the bed, and not visiting others' rooms are typical expectations. It is usually the nurse manager who oversees the operation of the unit and implementation of privilege systems.

Most psychiatric facilities use a privilege system to protect patients and to reinforce unit rules and other appropriate behavior (also see the previous section discussing token economies). The more appropriate the behavior, the more privileges of freedom the person has. Privileges are based on the assessment of a patient's risk to harm him- or herself or others and ability to follow treatment regimens. For example, a patient with few privileges may be required to stay on the unit and eat only with other patients. A patient with full privileges may have freedom to leave the unit and go outside the hospital and into the community for short periods.

Milieu Therapy

Milieu therapy provides a stable and coherent social organization to facilitate an individual's treatment. (The terms *milieu therapy* and *therapeutic environment* are often used interchangeably.) In milieu therapy, the design of the physical surroundings, structure of patient activities, and promotion of a stable social structure and cultural setting enhance the setting's therapeutic potential. A therapeutic milieu facilitates patient interactions and promotes personal growth. Milieu therapy is the responsibility of the nurse in collaboration with the patient and other health care providers. The key concepts of milieu therapy include containment, validation, structured interaction, and open communication.

Containment

Containment is the process of providing safety and security and involves the patient's access to food and shelter. In a well-contained milieu, patients feel safe from their illnesses and protected against social stigma. The physical surroundings are also important in this process and should be clean and comfortable, with special attention paid to promoting a noninstitutionalized environment. Pictures on walls, comfortable furniture, and soothing colors help patients relax. Most facilities encourage patients and nursing staff to wear street clothes, which help decrease the formalized nature of hospital settings and promote nurse–patient relationships.

Therapeutic milieus emphasize patient involvement in treatment decisions and operation of the unit; nurses should encourage freedom of movement within the contained environment. Patients participate in maintaining the quality of the physical surroundings, assuming responsibility for making their own beds, attending to their own belongings, and keeping an acceptable living area. Families are viewed as a part of the patient's life, and ties are maintained. In most inpatient settings, specific times are set for family interaction, education, and treatment. Family involvement is often a criterion for admission for treatment, and the involvement may include regular family attendance at therapy sessions.

Validation

In a therapeutic environment, **validation** is another process that affirms patient individuality. Staff–patient interactions should constantly reaffirm the patient's humanity and human rights. All interaction a staff member initiates with a patient should reflect his or her respect for that patient. Patients must believe that staff members truly like and respect them.

Structured Interaction

One of the most interesting milieu concepts is **structured interaction**, which is purposeful interaction that allows patients to interact with others in a useful way. For instance, the daily community meeting provides structure to explain unit rules and consequences of violations. Ideally, patients who are either elected or volunteer for the responsibility assume leadership for these meetings. In the meeting, the group discusses behavioral expectations, such as making beds daily, appropriate dress, and rules for leaving the unit. Usually, there are other rules, such as no fighting or name calling.

In some instances, the treatment team assigns structured interactions to specific patients as part of their treatment. Specific attitudes or approaches are directed toward individual patients who benefit from a particular type of interaction. Nurses consistently assume indulgence, flexibility, passive or active friendliness, matter-of-fact attitude, casualness, watchfulness, or kind firmness when interacting with specific patients. For example, if a patient is known to overreact and dramatize events, the staff may provide a matter-of-fact attitude when the patient engages in dramatic behavior.

Open Communication

In **open communication**, the staff and patient willingly share information. Staff members invite patient self-disclosure within the support of a nurse–patient relationship. In addition, they provide a model of effective communication when interacting with one another as well as with patients. They arrange an environment to facilitate optimal interaction and resocialization. Support, attention, praise, and reassurance given to patients improve self-esteem and increase confidence. Patient education is also a part of this support, as are directions to foster coping skills.

Milieu Therapy in Different Settings

Milieu therapy is applied in various settings. In long-term care settings, the therapeutic milieu becomes essential because patients may reside there for months or years. These patients typically have schizophrenia or developmental disabilities. Structure in daily living is important to the successful functioning of the individuals and the overall group but must be applied within the context of individual needs. For example, if a patient cannot get up one morning in time to complete assigned tasks (e.g., showering or making a bed) because of a personal crisis the night before, the nurse should consider the situation compassionately and flexibly, not applying the "consequences" rule or taking away the patient's privileges. In turn, the nurse must weigh individual needs against the collective needs of all the patients. For a patient who is consistently late for treatment activities, the nurse should apply the rules of the unit even if it means taking away privileges.

Recently, concepts of milieu therapy have been applied to short-term inpatient and community settings. In acute care inpatient settings, nursing actions provide limits to and controls on patient behavior and provide structure and safety for the patients. Milieu treatments are based on the individual needs of the patients and include relaxation groups, discussion groups, and medication groups. Spontaneous and planned activities are possible on a short-term unit as well as in a long-term setting. In the community, it is possible to apply milieu therapy approaches in day treatment centers, group homes, and single dwellings.

Promotion of Patient Safety

Although the use of social rules of conduct and privilege systems can enhance smooth operation of a unit, some potentially serious problems can be associated with these practices. A most critical aspect of psychiatric–mental health nursing is the promotion of patient safety, especially in inpatient units.

Observation

Patient observation is the ongoing assessment of the patient's mental status to identify and subvert any potential problem. An important process in all nursing practice, observation is particularly important in psychiatric nursing. In psychiatric settings, patients are ambulatory and thus more susceptible to environmental hazards. In addition, judgment and cognition impairment are symptoms of many psychiatric disorders. Often, patients are admitted because they pose a danger to themselves or others. In psychiatric nursing, observation is more than just "seeing" patients. It means continually monitoring them for any indication of harm to themselves or others.

All patients who are hospitalized for psychiatric reasons are continually monitored. The intensity of the observation depends on their risk to themselves and others. Some patients are merely asked to "check in" at different times of the day, but others have a staff member assigned to only them, such as in instances of potential suicide. Often "sharps," such as razors, are locked up and given to patients at specified times. Mental health facilities and units all have policies that specify levels of observation for patients of varying degrees of risk.

De-escalation

De-escalation is an interactive process of calming and redirecting a patient who has an immediate potential for violence directed toward self or others. This intervention involves assessing the situation and preventing it from escalating to one in which injury occurs to the patient, staff, or other patients. After the nurse has assessed the situation, he or she calmly calls to the patient and asks the individual to leave the situation. The nurse must avoid rushing toward the patient or giving orders (see Chapter 14). Nurses can use various interventions in this situation, including distraction, conflict resolution, and cognitive interventions.

Home Visits

Patients usually have been hospitalized or have received treatment for acute psychiatric symptoms before being referred to psychiatric home service. The goal of **home visits**, the delivery of nursing care in the patient's living environment, is to maximize the patient's functional ability within the nurse–patient relationship and with the family or partner as appropriate. The psychiatric nurse who makes home visits needs to be able to work independently, is skilled in teaching patients and families, can administer and monitor medications, and uses community resources for the patient's needs.

Home visits are especially useful in certain situations, including helping reluctant patients enter therapy, conducting a comprehensive assessment, strengthening a support network, and maintaining patients in the community when their condition deteriorates. Home visits are also useful in helping individuals comply with taking medication. The home visit process consists of three steps: the previsit phase, the home visit, and the postvisit phase. During previsit planning, the nurse sets goals for the home visit based on data received from other health care providers or the patient. In addition, the nurse and patient agree on the time of the visit. As the nurse travels to the home, he or she should assess the neighborhood for access to services, socioeconomic factors, and safety.

The actual visit can be divided into four parts. The first is the greeting phase, in which the nurse establishes rapport with family members. Greetings, which are usually brief, establish the communication process and the atmosphere for the visit. Greetings should be friendly but professional. In cultures that consider greetings important, this phase may involve more formal interactions, such as eating food or drinking tea with family members. The next phase establishes the focus of the visit. Sometimes the purpose of the visit is medication administration, health teaching, or counseling. The patient and family must be clear regarding the purpose. The implementation of the service is the next phase and should use most of the visit time. If the purpose of the visit is problem solving or decision making, the family's cultural values may determine the types of interaction and decision-making approaches. Closure is the last phase, the end of the home visit. It is a time to summarize and clarify important points. The nurse should also schedule any additional visits and reiterate patient expectations between visits. Usually, the nurse is the only provider to see the patient regularly. The nurse should acknowledge family members on leaving if they were not a part of the visit.

The postvisit phase includes documentation, reporting, and follow-up planning. This is also when the nurse meets with the supervisor and presents data from the home visit at the team meeting.

Community Action

Nurses have a unique opportunity to promote mental health awareness and support humane treatment for people with mental disorders. Activities range from being an advisor to support groups to participating in the political process through lobbying efforts and serving on community mental health boards. These unpaid activities are usually outside the realm of a particular job. However, an important role of professionals is to provide community service in addition to service through income-generating positions.

EVALUATING OUTCOMES

Evaluation of patient outcomes involves answering the following questions:

- What is the cost-effectiveness of the intervention?
- What benefits did the patient receive?
- What was the patient's level of satisfaction?
- Was the outcome specific or nonspecific to the patient's need?

Outcomes can be measured immediately after the nursing intervention or after time passes. For example, a patient may be able to resolve the acute depression and demonstrate confidence and improved self-esteem during a hospital stay. In various cases, it may be several months before the person can engage in positive interpersonal relationships.

SUMMARY OF KEY POINTS

- Assessment is the deliberate and systematic collection of information or data to determine current and past health, mental health, wellness, strengths, functional status, and present and past coping patterns.

- The assessment of the physical domain includes current and past health status, physical examination with review of body systems, review of physical functions, pharmacologic, strength, and wellness assessment.

- The psychological assessment includes the mental status examination, behavioral responses, and risk factor assessment.

- The mental status examination includes general observation of appearance, psychomotor activity, and attitude; orientations; mood; affect; emotions; speech; and thought processes.

- Behavioral responses are assessed as are self-concept and current and past coping patterns.

- Risk factor assessment includes ascertaining whether the patient has any suicidal, assaultive, or homicidal ideation.

- Psychological strengths and wellness attributes are summarized.

- The social assessment includes functional status; social systems; spirituality; occupational, economic, and legal status, quality of life, social strengths, and wellness attributes.

- The nursing assessment provides the data for nursing diagnoses and planning with the patient for mutually agreeable outcomes. Anticipated patient outcomes provide direction for psychiatric–mental health nursing interventions.

- Nursing interventions that are implemented for each domain include biologic (self-care, activity and exercise, sleep, nutrition, thermoregulation, and pain and medication management); psychological (counseling, conflict resolution, bibliotherapy, reminiscence, behavior therapy, psychoeducation, health teaching, and spiritual interventions); and social (behavior therapy and modification, milieu therapy, and various home and community interventions).

- Evaluation of patient outcomes involves assessing cost-effectiveness of the interventions, benefits to the patient, and the patient's level of satisfaction. Outcomes should be measurable, either immediately after intervention or after some time passes.

CRITICAL THINKING CHALLENGES

1. A 23-year-old white woman is admitted to an acute psychiatric setting for depression and suicidal gestures. This admission is her first, but she has experienced bouts of depression since early adolescence. She and her fiancé have just broken their engagement and moved into separate apartments. She has not yet told anyone that she is pregnant. She said that her mother had told her that she was "living in sin" and that she would "pay for it." The patient wants to "end

it all!" From this scenario, develop three assessment questions for each domain: biologic, psychological, and social.

2. Identify normal laboratory values for sodium, blood urea nitrogen, liver enzymes, leukocyte count, and differential and thyroid functioning. Why are these values important to know?

3. Write a paragraph on your self-concept, including all three components: body image, self-esteem, and personal identity. Explore the type of patient situations in which your self-concept can help your interactions with patients. Explore the types of patient situations in which your self-concept can hinder your interactions with patients.

4. Tom, a 25-year-old man with schizophrenia, lives with his parents, who want to retire to Florida. Tom goes to work each day but relies on his mother for meals, laundry, and reminders to take his medication. Tom believes that he can manage the home, but his mother is concerned. She asks the nurse for advice about leaving her son to manage on his own. What approach would you use?

5. Joan, a 35-year-old married woman, is admitted to an acute psychiatric unit for stabilization of her mood disorder. She is extremely depressed but refuses to consider a recommended medication change. She asks the nurse what to do. Using a nursing intervention, explain how you would approach Joan's problem.

6. A nurse reports to work for the evening shift. The unit is chaotic. The television in the day room is loud; two patients are arguing about the program. Visitors are mingling in patients' rooms. The temperature of the unit is hot. One patient is running up and down the hall yelling, "Help me, help me." Using a milieu therapy approach, what would you do to calm the unit?

REFERENCES

American Nurses Association, American Psychiatric Nurses Association, & and International Society of Psychiatric–Mental Health Nurses. (2014). *Psychiatric–mental health nursing: Scope and standards of practice* (2nd ed.). Silver Spring, MD: Nursebooks.org.

Broderick, J. E., DeWitt, E. M., Rothrock, N., Crane, P. K., & Forrest, C. B. (2013). Advances in patient-reported outcomes: The NIH PROMIS Measures. *EGEMS (Wash DC) (Generating Evidence & Methods to Improve Patient Outcomes)*, 1(1), 1015.

Butcher, H. K., Bulechek, G. M., Dochterman, J. M., & Wagner, C. M. (Eds.) (2018). *Nursing interventions classification (NIC)*, (7th ed) St. Louis: Elsevier.

Caldeira, S., & Timmins, F. (2017). Implementing spiritual care interventions. *Nursing Standard*, 31(34), 54–60.

Das, S., Punnoose, V. P., Doval, N., & Nair, V. Y. (2018). Spirituality, religiousness and coping in patients with schizophrenia: A cross sectional study in a tertiary care hospital. *Psychiatry Research*, 265, 238–243. doi: 10.1016/j.psychres.2018.04.030.

Eisen, K., Lawlor, C., Wu, C. D., & Mason, D. (2018). Reading and recovery expectations: Implementing a recovery-oriented bibliotherapy program in an acute inpatient psychiatric setting. *Psychiatric Rehabilitation Journal*, 41(1), 241–245.

Farronato, N. S., Dursteler-Macfarland, K. M., Wiesbeck, G. A., & Petitjean, S. A. (2013). A systematic review comparing cognitive-behavioral therapy and contingency management for cocaine dependence (Review). *Journal of Addictive Diseases*, 32(3), 274–287.

Garaigordobil, M., & Martínez-Valderrey, V. (2015). The effectiveness of cyberprogram 2.0 on conflict resolution strategies and self-esteem. *Journal of Adolescent Health*, 57(2), 229–234.

Glowacki, K, Warner, G., & White, C (2016). The use of a token economy for behavior and symptom management in adult psychiatric psychiatric inpatients: A critical review of the literature. *Journal of Psychiatric Intensive Care*, 12(2), 119–127.

Gomi, S., Starnino, V. R., & Canda, E. R. (2014). Spiritual assessment in mental health recovery, *Community Mental Health Journal*, 50(4), 447–453.

Jones, E. J., Webb, S. J., Estes, A., & Dawson, G. (2013). Rule learning in autism: The role of reward type and social context. *Developmental Neuropsychology*, 38(1), 58–77.

Kam, J. A., & Lazarevic, V. (2014). The stressful (and not so stressful) nature of language brokering: Identifying when brokering functions as a cultural stressor for Latino immigrant children in early adolescence. *Journal of Youth & Adolescence*, 43(12), 1994–2011.

Macdonald, J., Vallance, D., & McGrath, M. (2013). An evaluation of a collaborative bibliotherapy scheme delivered via a library service. *Journal of Psychiatric & Mental Health Nursing*, 20(10), 857–865.

Martin, K. S. (2005). *The Omaha system: A key to practice, documentation, and information, management* (2nd ed.). St. Louis, MO: Elsevier Saunders.

Martin, K. S., & Kessler, P. D. (2017). Omaha system: Improving the quality of practice and decision-support. In M. D. Harris (Ed.). *Handbook of home health care administration* (6th ed., pp. 235–248). Sudbury, MA: Jones and Bartlett.

Moorhead, S., Swanson, E., Johnson, M., & Maas, M., (Eds.). (2018). *Nursing outcomes classification (NOC): Measurement of health outcomes* (6th ed.). St. Louis, MO: Elsevier.

Müller, S., Rohde, P., Gau, J. M., & Stice, E. (2015). Moderators of the effects of indicated group and bibliotherapy cognitive behavioral depression prevention programs on adolescents' depressive symptoms and depressive disorder onset. *Behaviour Research and Therapy*, 75, 1–10.

Özgüc, S., & Tanriverdi, D. (2018). Relations between depression level and conflict resolution styles, marital adjustments of patients with major depression and their spouses. *Archives of Psychiatric Nursing*, 32(3), 337–342.

Paul, S., Corneau, S., Boozary, T., & Stergiopoulos, V. (2018). Coping and resilience among ethnoracial individuals experiencing homelessness and mental illness. *International Journal Social Psychiatry*, 64(2), 189–187.

Saba, V. K. (2017). *Clinical care classification (CCC) system (version 2.1) (User's Guide)* (2nd ed.). New York: Springer Publishing Company, LLC.

Substance Abuse and Mental Health Services Administration. (2009). *Illness management and recovery: Practitioner guides and handouts*. HHS Pub. No. SMA-09-4462. Rockville, MD: Center for Mental Health Services, Substance Abuse and Mental Health Services Administration, U.S. Department of Health and Human Services.

The Joint Commission Standards. (2018). Medical Record – Spiritual Assessment. Retrieved on November 5, 2018, from https://www.jointcommission.org/standards_information/jcfaqdetails.aspx?StandardsFaqId=1492&ProgramId=46.

Timmins, F., & Caldeira, S. (2017). Assessing the spiritual needs of patients. *Nursing Standard*, 31(29), 47–53.

Weathers, E., McCarthy, G., & Coffey, A. (2015). Concept analysis of spirituality: An evolutionary approach, *Nursing Forum*, 51(2), 79–96.

Weitzman, E. A., & Weitzman, P. F. (2014). In P. T. Coleman, M. Deutsch, & E. Marcus (Eds.). *The handbook of conflict resolution: Theory and practice* (3rd ed., pp. 203–229). San Francisco, CA: Jossey-Bass.

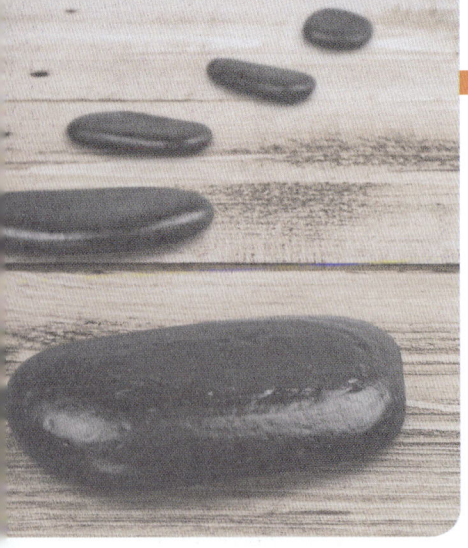

11

Psychopharmacology, Dietary Supplements, and Biologic Interventions

Mary Ann Boyd

KEY CONCEPTS
- agonists
- antagonists
- pharmacodynamics
- pharmacokinetics

LEARNING OBJECTIVES

After studying this chapter, you will be able to:

1. Differentiate target symptoms from side effects.
2. Identify nursing interventions for common side effects of psychiatric medications.
3. Explain the role of the governmental regulatory process in the approval of medication and the use of other biologic interventions.
4. Discuss the pharmacodynamics of psychiatric medications.
5. Discuss the pharmacokinetics of psychiatric medications.
6. Explain the major classifications of psychiatric medications.
7. Identify typical nursing interventions related to the administration of psychiatric medications.
8. Analyze the potential benefits of other forms of somatic treatments, including herbal supplements, nutrition therapies, electroconvulsive therapy, light therapy, transcranial magnetic stimulation, and vagus nerve stimulation.
9. Evaluate the significance of nonadherence and discuss strategies supportive of medication adherence.

KEY TERMS

- absorption • adherence • adverse reactions • affinity • akathisia • atypical antipsychotics • augmentation • bioavailability • biotransformation • boxed warning • carrier protein • chronic syndromes • clearance • compliance • conventional antipsychotics • cytochrome P450 (CYP450) system • desensitization • distribution • dosing • drug–drug interaction • dystonia • efficacy • enzymes • ethnopsychopharmacology • excretion • extrapyramidal symptoms (EPS) • first-pass effect • half-life • hypnotics • inhibitor • intrinsic activity • metabolism • metabolites • partial agonists • pharmacogenomics • phototherapy • polypharmacy • potency • prescribing information • protein binding • pseudoparkinsonism • relapse • repetitive transcranial magnetic stimulation • sedative–hypnotics • sedatives • selectivity • serotonin syndrome • side effects • solubility • steady state • tardive dyskinesia • target symptoms • therapeutic index • tolerance • toxicity • uptake receptors

Recent scientific and technologic developments have opened the door for the development of new medications that treat mental disorders. Nurses administer these medications, monitor their effectiveness, and manage side effects; they also have an important role in educating patients about their medications. Psychiatric medications are increasingly prescribed in primary care settings, and nurses practicing in nonpsychiatric settings now need an in-depth knowledge of them.

This chapter focuses on the pharmacodynamics and pharmacokinetics of psychiatric medications. Included in this chapter is an overview of the major classes of psychopharmacologic drugs used in treating patients with mental disorders and the role of herbal supplements and nutritional therapies. In addition, other biologic treatments are discussed, including electroconvulsive therapy (ECT), light therapy, **repetitive transcranial magnetic stimulation** (rTMS), and vagus nerve stimulation (VNS).

PSYCHIATRIC MEDICATIONS

As with any drug, psychiatric medications are designated for use in certain conditions for specific symptoms. The nurse quickly realizes that these symptoms are present in several conditions, leading to many medications being prescribed for different diagnoses. Because medications can have both desirable and undesirable effects, it is important for the nurse to understand these factors to help ensure patient safety.

Target Symptoms and Side Effects

Psychiatric medications and other biologic interventions are indicated for **target symptoms**, which are specific measurable symptoms expected to improve with treatment. Standards of care guide nurses in monitoring and documenting the effects of medications and other biologic treatments on target symptoms.

As yet, no drug has been developed that is so specific it affects only its target symptoms; instead, drugs typically act on a number of other organs and sites within the body. Even drugs with a high affinity and selectivity for a specific neurotransmitter will cause some responses in the body that are not related to the target symptoms. These unwanted effects of medications are called **side effects**. If unwanted effects have serious physiologic consequences, they are considered **adverse reactions**. The nurse monitors, documents, and reports the appearance of side effects and adverse reactions and implements nursing interventions for the relief of medication side effects (Table 11.1).

Drug Regulation and Use

The U.S. Food and Drug Administration (FDA) is responsible for ensuring the safety, efficacy, and security of human and veterinary drugs, biologic products, medical devices, nation's food supply, cosmetics, and products that emit radiation (www.FDA.gov). The FDA approves the labeling of medications and other biologic treatments after a thorough review of efficacy and safety data (Box 11.1). Nurses administering medications are responsible for knowing the labeling content, which is found in each medication's package insert or **prescribing information** (PI) and includes approved indications for the medication, side effects, adverse reactions,

---

BOX 11.1

Testing New Drugs for Safety and Efficacy

PHASES OF NEW DRUG TESTING
- Phase I: Testing defines the range of dosages tolerated in healthy individuals.
- Phase II: Effects of the drug are studied in a limited number of persons with the disorder. This phase defines the range of clinically effective dosage.
- Phase III: Extensive clinical trials are conducted at multiple sites throughout the country with larger numbers of patients. Efforts focus on corroborating the efficacy identified in phase II. Phase III concludes with a new drug application (NDA) being submitted to the U.S. Food and Drug Administration (FDA).
- Phase IV: Drug studies continue after FDA approval to detect new or rare adverse reactions and potentially new indications. During this period, adverse reactions from the new medication should be reported to the FDA.

IMPLICATIONS FOR MENTAL HEALTH NURSES
- Throughout the phases, side effects and adverse reactions are monitored closely. The studies are tightly controlled, and strict regulations are enforced at each step.
- To prove drug effectiveness, diagnoses must be accurate, strict guidelines are followed, and subjects usually are not taking other medications and do not have complicating illnesses.
- A newly approved drug is approved only for the indications for which it has been tested.

---

contraindications, and other important information. If the FDA identifies serious adverse reactions that can occur with the use of a specific medication, it may issue a warning found in a **boxed warning** in the PI. The nurse should be aware of these boxed warnings and monitor for the appearance of the adverse reactions. If a PI is not readily available, the labeling information is easily found on the FDA's website and in most pharmacy departments.

PSYCHOPHARMACOLOGY

A comparatively small amount of medication can have a significant and large impact on cell function and resulting behavior. When tiny molecules of medication are compared with the vast amount of cell surface in the human body, the fraction seems disproportionate. Yet the drugs used to treat mental disorders often have profound effects on behavior. To understand how this occurs, one needs to understand both where and how drugs work. The following discussion highlights important concepts relevant to psychiatric medications.

Pharmacodynamics: Where Drugs Act

Drug molecules act at specific sites, not on the entire cell surface. Psychiatric medications primarily target the central nervous system (CNS) at the cellular, synaptic

TABLE 11.1 MANAGING COMMON SIDE EFFECTS OF PSYCHIATRIC MEDICATIONS

Side Effect or Discomfort	Intervention
Blurred vision	Reassurance (generally subsides in 2 to 6 wks)
Dry eyes	Artificial tears may be required; increased use of wetting solutions for those wearing contact lens Alert ophthalmologist; no eye examination for new glasses for at least 3 wks after a stable dose
Dry mouth and lips	Frequent rinsing of mouth, good oral hygiene, sucking sugarless candies or lozenges, lip balm, lemon juice, and glycerin mouth swabs
Constipation	High-fiber diet; encourage bran, fresh fruits, and vegetables Metamucil (must consume at least 16 oz of fluid with dose) Increase hydration Exercise; increase fluids Mild laxative
Urinary hesitancy or retention	Monitor frequently for difficulty with urination, including changes in starting or stopping stream Notify prescriber if difficulty develops A cholinergic agonist, such as bethanechol, may be required
Nasal congestion	Nose drops, moisturizer, *not* nasal spray
Sinus tachycardia	Assess for infections Monitor pulse for rate and irregularities Withhold medication and notify prescriber if resting rate exceeds 120 bpm
Decreased libido, anorgasmia, ejaculatory inhibition	Reassurance (reversible); change to another medication
Postural hypotension	Frequent monitoring of lying-to-standing blood pressure during dosage adjustment period, immediate changes and accommodation, measure pulse in both positions; consider change to less antiadrenergic drug Advise patient to get up slowly, sit for at least 1 min before standing (dangling legs over side of bed), and stand for 1 min before walking or until lightheadedness subsides Increase hydration, avoid caffeine Elastic stockings if necessary Notify prescriber if symptoms persist or significant blood pressure changes are present; medication may have to be changed if patient does not have impulse control to get up slowly
Photosensitivity	Protective clothing Dark glasses Use of sun block; remember to cover all exposed areas
Dermatitis	Stop medication usage Consider medication change; may require a systemic antihistamine Initiate comfort measures to decrease itching
Impaired psychomotor functions	Advise patient to avoid dangerous tasks, such as driving Avoid alcohol, which increases this impairment
Drowsiness or sedation	Encourage activity during the day to increase accommodation Avoid tasks that require mental alertness, such as driving May need to adjust dosing schedule or, if possible, give a single daily dose at bedtime May need a cholinergic medication if sedation is the problem Avoid driving or operating potentially dangerous equipment May need change to less sedating medication Provide quiet and decreased stimulation when sedation is the desired effect
Weight gain and metabolic changes	Exercise and diet teaching Caloric control
Edema	Check fluid retention Reassurance May need a diuretic
Irregular menstruation or amenorrhea	Reassurance (reversible) May need to change class of drug Reassurance and counseling (does not indicate lack of ovulation) Instruct patient to continue birth control measures
Vaginal dryness	Instruct in use of lubricants

level at four sites: receptors, ion channels, enzymes, and carrier proteins.

> **KEYCONCEPT** **Pharmacodynamics** is the action or effects of drugs on living organisms.

Receptors

Receptors are specific proteins intended to respond to a chemical (i.e., neurotransmitter) normally present in blood or tissues (see Chapter 6). Receptors also respond to drugs with similar chemical structures. When drugs attach to a receptor, they can act as **agonists**—substances that initiate the same response as the chemical normally present in the body—or as **antagonists**—substances that block the response of a given receptor. Figure 11.1 illustrates the action of an agonist and an antagonist drug at a receptor site. A drug's ability to interact with a given receptor type may be judged by three properties: selectivity, affinity, and intrinsic activity.

> **KEYCONCEPT** **Agonists** (mimic the neurotransmitter) have all three properties: selectivity, affinity, and intrinsic activity. **Antagonists** (block the receptor) have only selectivity and affinity properties; they do not have intrinsic activity because they produce no biologic response by attaching to the receptor.

Some drugs are referred to as **partial agonists** because they have some intrinsic activity (although weak). Because there are no "pure" drugs affecting only one neurotransmitter, most drugs have multiple effects. A drug may act as an agonist for one neurotransmitter and an antagonist for another. Medications that have both agonist and antagonist effects are called mixed agonist–antagonists.

Selectivity

Selectivity is the ability of a drug to be specific for a particular receptor. If a drug is highly selective, it will interact only with its specific receptors in the areas of the body where these receptors occur and therefore not affect tissues and organs where its receptors do not occur. Using a "lock-and-key" analogy, only a specific, highly selective key will fit a given lock. The more selective or structurally specific a drug is, the more likely it will affect only the specific receptor for which it is meant. The less selective the drug, the more receptors are affected and the more likely there will be unintended effects or side effects.

Affinity

Affinity is the degree of attraction or strength of the bond between the drug and its biologic target. Affinity is strengthened when a drug has more than one type of chemical bond with its target. If a cell membrane contains several receptors to which a drug will adhere, the affinity is increased. The weaker the chemical bond, the more likely a drug's effects are reversible. Most drugs used in psychiatry adhere to receptors through weak chemical bonds, but some drugs, specifically the monoamine oxidase **inhibitors** (MAOIs; discussed later), have a different type of bond, called a covalent bond. A covalent bond is formed when two atoms share a pair of electrons. This type of bond is stronger and irreversible at normal temperatures. The effects of the drugs that form covalent bonds are often called "irreversible" because they are long-lasting, taking several weeks to resolve. Knowledge of a medication's affinity for receptors and subtypes of receptors may give some indication of the likelihood that specific target symptoms might improve and what side effects might be predicted.

Intrinsic Activity

A drug's ability to interact with a given receptor is its **intrinsic activity**, or the ability to produce a response after it becomes attached to the receptor. Some drugs have selectivity and affinity but produce no response. An important measure of a drug is whether or not it produces a change in the cell containing the receptor.

Ion Channels

Some drugs directly block the ion channels of the nerve cell membrane. For example, the antianxiety benzodiazepine

FIGURE 11.1 Agonist and antagonist drug actions at a receptor site. This schematic drawing represents drug–receptor interactions. At the **top**, drug D has the correct shape to fit receptor R, forming a drug–receptor complex, which results in a conformational change in the receptor and the opening of a pore in the adjacent membrane. Drug D is an agonist. At the **bottom**, drug A also has the correct shape to fit the receptor, forming a drug–receptor complex, but in this case, there is no conformational change and therefore no response. Drug A is, therefore, an antagonist.

drugs, such as diazepam (Valium), bind to a region of the gamma-aminobutyric acid (GABA)-receptor chloride channel complex, which helps to open the chloride ion channel. In turn, the activity of GABA is enhanced.

Enzymes

Enzymes are usually proteins that act as catalysts for physiologic reactions and can be targets for drugs. For example, monoamine oxidase (MAO) is an enzyme required to break down neurotransmitters associated with depression (norepinephrine, serotonin, and dopamine). The MAOI antidepressants inhibit this enzyme, resulting in more neurotransmitter activity.

Carrier Proteins: Uptake Receptors

A **carrier protein** is a membrane protein that transports a specific molecule across the cell membrane. Carrier proteins (also referred to as **uptake receptors**) recognize sites specific for the type of molecule to be transported. When a neurotransmitter is removed from the synapse, specific carrier molecules return it to the presynaptic nerve, where most of it is stored to be used again. Medications specific for this site block or inhibit this transport and therefore increase the activity of the neurotransmitter in the synapse. Figure 11.2 illustrates the reuptake blockade.

Clinical Concepts

Efficacy is the ability of a drug to produce a response and is considered when a drug is selected. The degree of receptor occupancy contributes to the drug's efficacy, but a drug may occupy a large number of receptors and not produce a response. Table 11.2 provides a brief summation of possible physiologic effects from drug actions on specific neurotransmitters. This information should serve only as a guide in predicting side effects because many physical outcomes or behaviors resulting from neural transmission are controlled by multiple receptors and neurotransmitters.

Potency refers to the dose of drug required to produce a specific effect. One drug may be able to achieve the same clinical effect as another drug but at a lower dose, making it more potent. Although the drug given at the lower dose is more potent because both drugs achieve similar effects, it may be considered to have equal efficacy.

In some instances, the effects of medications diminish with time, especially when they are given repeatedly, as in the treatment of chronic psychiatric disorders. This loss of effect is most often a form of physiologic adaptation that may develop as the cell attempts to regain homeostatic control to counteract the effects of the drug. There are many reasons for decreased drug effectiveness (Box 11.2).

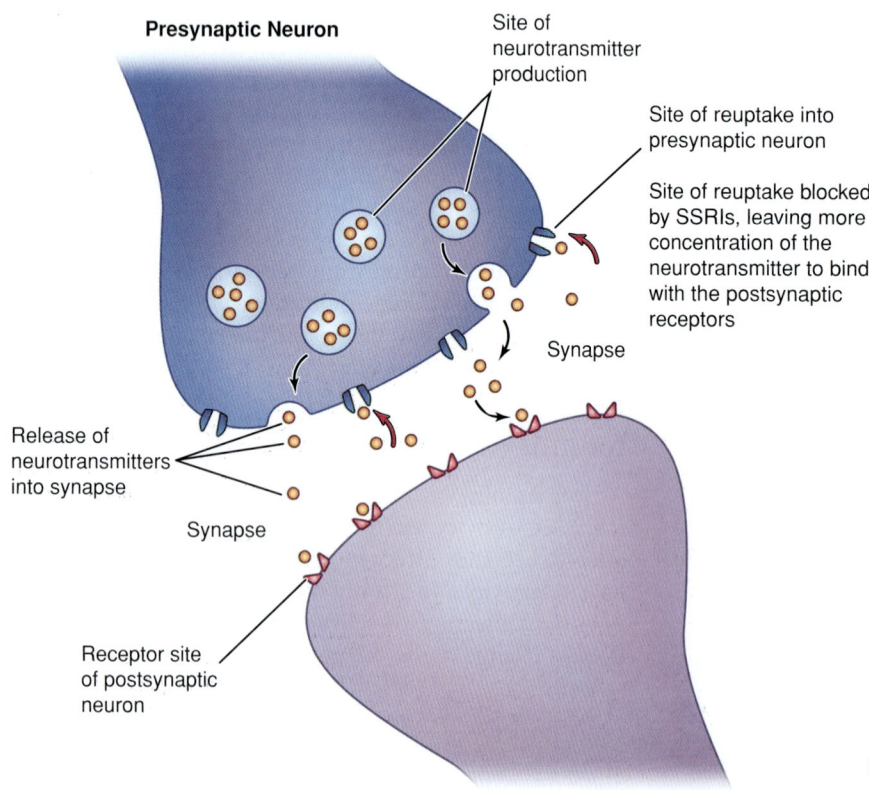

FIGURE 11.2 Reuptake blockade of a carrier molecule for serotonin by a selective serotonin reuptake inhibitor.

TABLE 11.2 DRUG ACTIONS ON NEUROTRANSMITTERS

Action by Drug on Neurotransmitter	Physiologic Effects	Example of Drugs
Reuptake Inhibition		
Norepinephrine reuptake inhibition	Antidepressant action Potentiation of pressor effects of norepinephrine Interaction with guanethidine Side effects: tachycardia, tremors, insomnia, erectile and ejaculation dysfunction	Desipramine Venlafaxine
Serotonin reuptake inhibition	Antidepressant action Antiobsessional effect Increase or decrease in anxiety (dose dependent) Side effects: gastrointestinal distress; nausea; headache; nervousness; motor restlessness; and sexual side effects, including anorgasmia	Fluoxetine Fluvoxamine
Dopamine reuptake inhibition	Antidepressant action Antiparkinsonian effect Side effects: increase in psychomotor activity, aggravation of psychosis	Bupropion
Receptor Blockade		
Histamine receptor blockade (H_1)	Side effects: sedation, drowsiness, hypotension, and weight gain	Quetiapine Imipramine Clozapine Olanzapine
Acetylcholine receptor blockade (muscarinic)	Side effects: anticholinergic (dry mouth, blurred vision, constipation, urinary hesitancy and retention, memory dysfunction) and sinus tachycardia	Imipramine Amitriptyline Olanzapine
Norepinephrine receptor blockade (α_1 receptor)	Potentiation of antihypertensive effect of prazosin and terazosin Side effects: postural hypotension, dizziness, reflex tachycardia, sedation	Amitriptyline Clomipramine Clozapine
Norepinephrine receptor blockade (α_2 receptor)	Increased sexual desire (yohimbine) Interactions with antihypertensive medications, blockade of the antihypertensive effects of clonidine Side effect: priapism	Amitriptyline Clomipramine Clozapine Trazodone Yohimbine
Norepinephrine receptor blockade (β_1 receptor)	Antihypertensive action (propranolol) Side effects: orthostatic hypotension, sedation, depression, sexual dysfunction (including impotence and decreased ejaculation)	Propranolol
Serotonin receptor blockade ($5\text{-}HT_{1A}$)	Antidepressant action Antianxiety effect Possible control of aggression	Trazodone Risperidone Ziprasidone
Serotonin receptor blockade ($5\text{-}HT_2$)	Antipsychotic action Some antimigraine effect Decreased rhinitis Side effects: hypotension, ejaculatory problems	Risperidone Clozapine Olanzapine Ziprasidone
Dopamine receptor blockade (D_2)	Antipsychotic action Side effects: extrapyramidal symptoms, such as tremor, rigidity (especially acute dystonia and parkinsonism); endocrine changes, including elevated prolactin levels	Haloperidol Ziprasidone

---

BOX 11.2
Mechanisms Causing Decreases in Medication Effects

- Change in receptors
- Loss of receptors
- Exhaustion of neurotransmitter supply
- Increased metabolism of the drug
- Physiologic adaptation

Desensitization is a rapid decrease in drug effects that may develop in a few minutes of exposure to a drug. This reaction is rare with most psychiatric medications but can occur with some medications used to treat serious side effects (e.g., physostigmine, sometimes used to relieve severe anticholinergic side effects). A rapid decrease can also occur with some drugs because of immediate transformation of the receptor when the drug molecule binds to the receptor. Other drugs cause a decrease in the number of receptors or exhaust the mediators of neurotransmission.

Tolerance is a gradual decrease in the action of a drug at a given dose or concentration in the blood. This decrease may take days or weeks to develop and results in loss of therapeutic effect of a drug. For therapeutic drugs, this loss of effect is often called *treatment refractoriness*. In the abuse of substances such as alcohol or cocaine, tolerance is a part of the addiction (see Chapter 25).

Toxicity generally refers to the point at which concentrations of the drug in the bloodstream are high enough to become harmful or poisonous to the body. Individuals vary widely in their responses to medications. Some patients experience adverse reactions more easily than others. The **therapeutic index** is the ratio of the maximum nontoxic dose to the minimum effective dose. A high therapeutic index means that there is a large range between the dose at which the drug begins to take effect and a dose that would be toxic to the body. Drugs with a low therapeutic index have a narrow range.

This concept of toxicity has some limitations. The range can be affected by drug tolerance. For example, when tolerance develops, the person increases the dosage, which makes him or her more susceptible to an accidental suicide. The therapeutic index of a medication also may be greatly changed by the coadministration of other medications or drugs. For example, alcohol consumed with most CNS-depressant drugs will have added depressant effects, greatly increasing the likelihood of toxicity or death.

Pharmacokinetics: How the Body Acts on the Drugs

The field of pharmacokinetics studies the process of how drugs are acted on by the body through absorption, distribution, metabolism (biotransformation), and excretion. Pharmacokinetics for specific medications is always explained in a drug's PI. Together with the principles of pharmacodynamics, this information is helpful in monitoring drug effects and predicting behavioral response.

> **KEYCONCEPT Pharmacokinetics** is the process by which a drug is absorbed, distributed, metabolized, and eliminated by the body.

Absorption and Routes of Administration

The first phase of **absorption** is the movement of the drug from the site of administration into the plasma. The typical routes of administration of psychiatric medications include oral (tablet, capsule, and liquid), deltoid and gluteal intramuscular (IM; short- and long-acting agents), and intravenous (IV; rarely used for treatment of the primary psychiatric disorder but instead for rapid treatment of adverse reactions). A transdermal patch antidepressant and oral inhalation are also available. The advantages and disadvantages of each route and the subsequent effects on absorption are listed in Table 11.3.

Drugs taken orally are usually the most convenient for the patient; however, this route is also the most variable because absorption can be slowed or enhanced by a number of factors. Taking certain drugs orally with food or antacids may slow the rate of absorption or change the amount of the drug absorbed. For example, antacids containing aluminum salts decrease the absorption of most antipsychotic drugs; thus, antacids must be given at least 1 hour before administration or 2 hours after.

Oral preparations are absorbed from the gastrointestinal tract into the bloodstream through the portal vein and then to the liver. They may be metabolized within the gastrointestinal wall or liver before reaching the rest of the body. This is called the **first-pass effect**. The consequence of first-pass effect is that only a fraction of the drug reaches systemic circulation. Oral dosages are adjusted for the first-pass effect. That is, the dose of the oral form is significantly higher than the IM or IV formulations.

Bioavailability describes the amount of the drug that actually reaches systemic circulation unchanged. The route by which a drug is administered significantly affects bioavailability. With some oral drugs, the amount of drug entering the bloodstream is decreased by first-pass metabolism, and bioavailability is lower. On the other hand, some rapidly dissolving oral medications have increased bioavailability.

> **Concept Mastery Alert**
>
> First-pass effect refers to the metabolism that a drug undergoes within the gastrointestinal wall or liver before reaching the rest of the body. Bioavailability describes the amount of a drug that actually reaches the systemic circulation unchanged.

Distribution

Distribution of a drug is the amount of the drug found in various tissues, particularly the target organ at the site of drug action. Factors that affect distribution include the size of the organ; amount of blood flow or perfusion within the organ; solubility of the drug; plasma **protein binding** (the degree to which the drug binds to plasma proteins); and anatomic barriers, such as the blood–brain barrier, that the drug must cross. A psychiatric drug may have rapid absorption and high bioavailability, but if it does not cross the blood–brain barrier to reach the CNS, it is of little use. Table 11.4 provides a summary of how some significant factors affect distribution. Two of these factors, solubility (ability of a drug to dissolve) and protein binding, warrant additional discussion with regard to how they relate to psychiatric medications.

TABLE 11.3 SELECTED FORMS AND ROUTES OF PSYCHIATRIC MEDICATIONS

Preparation and Route	Examples	Advantages	Disadvantages
Oral tablet	Basic preparation for most psychopharmacologic agents, including antidepressants, antipsychotics, mood stabilizers, anxiolytics, and so on	Usually most convenient	Variable rate and extent of absorption, depending on the drug May be affected by the contents of the intestines May show first-pass metabolism effects May not be easily swallowed by some individuals
Oral liquid	Also known as concentrates The antipsychotic risperidone The antidepressant fluoxetine Antihistamines, such as diphenhydramine Mood stabilizers, such as lithium citrate	Ease of incremental dosing Easily swallowed In some cases, more quickly absorbed	More difficult to measure accurately Depending on drug: • Possible interactions with other liquids such as juice, forming precipitants • Possible irritation to mucosal lining of mouth if not properly diluted
Rapidly dissolving tablet	Atypical antipsychotics, such as olanzapine, risperidone, asenapine	Dissolves almost instantaneously in mouth	Patient needs to remember to have completely dry hands and to place tablet in mouth immediately Tablet should not linger in the hand Handy for people who have trouble swallowing or for patients who let medication linger in the cheek for later expectoration Can be taken when water or other liquid is unavailable
Intramuscular	Some antipsychotics, such as ziprasidone, olanzapine, haloperidol, and chlorpromazine Anxiolytics, such as lorazepam Anticholinergics, such as benztropine mesylate No antidepressants No mood stabilizers	More rapid acting than oral preparations No first-pass metabolism	Injection site pain and irritation Some medications may have erratic absorption if heavy muscle tissue at the site of injection is not in use
Intramuscular depot (or long acting)	Risperidone (Risperdal Consta), paliperidone palmitate (Invega Sustenna), olanzapine (Olanzapine Pamoate), aripiprazole (Abilify Maintena), aripiprazole lauroxil (Aristada), haloperidol decanoate, fluphenazine decanoate	May be more convenient for some individuals who have difficulty following medication regimens	Pain at injection site
Intravenous	Anticholinergics, such as diphenhydramine, benztropine mesylate Anxiolytics, such as diazepam, lorazepam, and chlordiazepoxide	Rapid and complete availability to systemic circulation	Inflammation of tissue surrounding site Often inconvenient for patient and uncomfortable Continuous dosage requires use of a constant-rate IV infusion
Subcutaneous (abdominal)	Risperidone (Perseris)	More convenient than oral regime; injection in abdomen may be preferable to the gluteus.	Pain at injection site
Transdermal patch	Antidepressant, selegiline	Avoid daily oral ingestion of medication	Skin irritation
Oral inhalation	Conventional antipsychotic, loxapine	Rapidly absorbed to treat psychomotor agitation	Bronchospasm

IV, intravenous.

TABLE 11.4 FACTORS AFFECTING DISTRIBUTION OF A DRUG

Factor	Effect on Drug Distribution
Size of the organ	Larger organs require more drug to reach a concentration level equivalent to other organs and tissues.
Blood flow to the organ	The more blood flow to and within an organ (perfusion), the greater the drug concentration. The brain has high perfusion.
Solubility of the drug	The greater the solubility of a drug within a tissue, the greater its concentration.
Plasma protein binding	If a drug binds well to plasma proteins, particularly to albumin, it will stay in the body longer but have a slower distribution.
Anatomic barriers	Both the gastrointestinal tract and the brain are surrounded by layers of cells that control the passage or uptake of substances. Lipid-soluble substances are usually readily absorbed and pass the blood–brain barrier.

Solubility

Substances may cross a membrane in a number of ways, but passive diffusion is by far the simplest. To do this, the drug must dissolve in the structure of the cell membrane. Therefore, the **solubility** of a drug is an important characteristic. Being soluble in lipids allows a drug to cross most of the membranes in the body, and the tissues of the CNS are less permeable to water-soluble drugs than are other areas of the body. Most psychopharmacologic agents are lipid soluble and easily cross the blood–brain barrier. However, this characteristic means that psychopharmacologic agents also cross the placenta; consequently, most are contraindicated during pregnancy.

Protein Binding

Of considerable importance is the degree to which a drug binds to plasma proteins. Only unbound or "free" drugs act at the receptor sites. High protein binding reduces the concentration of the drug at the receptor sites. However, because the binding is reversible, as the unbound drug is metabolized, more drug is released from the protein bonds. Drugs are also released from storage in the fat depots. These processes can prolong the duration of action of the drug. When patients stop taking their medication, they often do not experience an immediate return of symptoms because they continue to receive the drug as it is released from storage sites in the body.

Metabolism

Metabolism, also called **biotransformation**, is the process by which a drug is altered and broken down into smaller substances, known as **metabolites**. Most metabolism occurs in the liver, but it can also occur in the kidneys, lungs, and intestines.

The **cytochrome P450 (CYP450) system**, a set of microsomal enzymes usually found in the liver, is important in the metabolism of a drug. There are more than 50 enzymes, but most of the metabolism occurs in only a few of them. The functioning of these enzymes is influenced by drugs and other chemical substances. Some drugs slow down, whereas other drugs speed up, an enzyme's ability to metabolize drugs. When the enzyme is inhibited from functioning, a drug may not be metabolized as expected, but instead it may be active longer. That leads to an increase in the plasma level, which may become toxic. On the other hand, some drugs speed up enzyme metabolism, resulting in the drug leaving the body faster than expected, with a concentration below the therapeutic level. A **drug–drug interaction** can occur if one drug inhibits an enzyme system, causing another drug to become toxic. The PI will inform the nurse which drugs should not be given together in order to prevent a drug–drug interaction.

Excretion

Excretion refers to the removal of drugs from the body either unchanged or as metabolites. **Clearance** refers to the total volume of blood, serum, or plasma from which a drug is completely removed per unit of time to account for the excretion. The **half-life** of a drug provides a measure of the expected rate of clearance. Half-life refers to the time required for plasma concentrations of the drug to be reduced by 50%. For most drugs, the rate of excretion slows, but the half-life remains unchanged. It usually takes four half-lives or more of a drug in total time for more than 90% of a drug to be eliminated.

Drugs bound to plasma proteins do not cross the glomerular filter freely. These lipid-soluble drugs are passively reabsorbed by diffusion across the renal tubule and thus are not rapidly excreted in the urine. Because many psychiatric medications are protein bound and lipid soluble, most of their excretion occurs through the liver, where they are excreted in the bile and delivered into the intestine. Lithium and gabapentin, mood stabilizers, are notable examples of renal excretion. Any impairment in renal function or renal disease may lead to toxic symptoms.

Dosing refers to the administration of medication over time so that therapeutic levels may be achieved or maintained without reaching toxic levels. In general, it is necessary to give a drug at intervals no greater than the half-life of the medication to avoid excessive fluctuation of concentration in the plasma between doses. With repeated dosing, a certain amount of the drug is accumulated in the body.

Steady-state plasma concentration, or simply **steady state**, occurs when absorption equals excretion and the therapeutic level plateaus. The rate of accumulation is determined by the half-life of the drug. Drugs generally reach steady state in four to five times the elimination half-life. However, because elimination or excretion rates may vary significantly in any individual, fluctuations may still occur, and dose schedules may need to be modified.

Individual Variations in Drug Effects

Many factors affect drug absorption, distribution, metabolism, and excretion. These factors may vary among individuals, depending on their age, genetics, and ethnicity.

Age

Pharmacokinetics is significantly altered at the extremes of the life cycle. Gastric absorption changes as individuals age. Gastric pH increases, and gastric emptying decreases. Gastric motility slows and splanchnic circulation is reduced. Normally, these changes do not significantly impair oral absorption of a medication, but addition of common conditions, such as diarrhea, may significantly alter and reduce absorption. Malnutrition, cancer, and liver disease decrease the production of the primary protein albumin. More free drug is acting in the system, producing higher blood levels of the medication and potentially toxic effects. The activity of hepatic enzymes also slows with age. As a result, the ability of the liver to metabolize medications may slow as much as a fourfold decrease between the ages of 20 and 70 years. Production of albumin by the liver generally declines with age. Changes in the parasympathetic nervous system produce a greater sensitivity in older adults to anticholinergic side effects, which are more severe with this age group.

Renal function also declines with age. Creatinine clearance in a young adult is normally 100 to 120 mL/min, but after age 40, this rate declines by about 10% per decade (Denic, Glassock, & Rule, 2016). Medical illnesses, such as diabetes and hypertension, may contribute to further decline of renal function. When creatinine clearance falls below 30 mL/min, the excretion of drugs by the kidneys is significantly impaired, and potentially toxic levels may accumulate.

Pharmacogenetics and Ethnopsychopharmacology

Pharmacogenomics is the study of how a person's genetic makeup affects his or her response to drugs. There are important genetic variations that influence the metabolism and action of psychotropic drugs in different ethnic groups. Various tests are used to predict genetic responses to drugs and the potential for adverse effects. For example, studies show that selecting antidepressants according to genetic profile can improve treatment outcomes for people with depression and anxiety (Bradley et al., 2018).

Overlapping pharmacogenetics is the field of **ethnopsychopharmacology,** the study of how culture and genetic differences in human groups determine and influence the response to medications. Ethnopsychopharmacology focuses on the impact of cultural practices, such as consuming foods or ingesting beverages, on genetic variations in metabolism, on complementary and alternate health care practices, and on herbal substances.

Although ethnic and racial groups are genetically heterogeneous, there are population differences in disease susceptibility (Dantra, Swart, Mpeta, Wonkam, & Masimirembwa, 2014). For example, some individuals of Asian descent produce higher concentrations of acetaldehyde with alcohol use than do those of European descent, resulting in a higher incidence of adverse reactions such as flushing and palpitations. Asians often require one half to one third the dose of antipsychotic medications and lower doses of antidepressants than whites require (Silva, 2013). In the African populations, there is a high degree of variability in the dosage of many medications (Alessandrini, Asfaha, Dodgen, Warnich, & Pepper, 2013).

PHASES OF DRUG TREATMENT AND THE NURSE'S ROLE

Phases of drug treatment include initiation, stabilization, maintenance, and discontinuation of the medication. The following discussion explains the role of the nurse in these phases.

Initiation Phase

Before the initiation of medications, patients must undergo several assessments.

- A psychiatric evaluation to determine the diagnosis and target symptoms
- A nursing assessment that includes cultural beliefs and practices (see Chapter 10)
- Physical examination and indicated laboratory tests, often including baseline determinations such as a complete blood count (CBC), liver and kidney function tests, electrolyte levels, urinalysis, and possibly thyroid function tests and electrocardiography (ECG), to determine whether a physical condition may be causing the symptoms and to establish that it is safe to initiate use of a particular medication.

During the initiation of medication, the nurse assesses, observes, and monitors the patient's response to the medication; teaches the patient about the action, dosage, frequency of administration, and side effects; and develops a plan for ongoing contact with clinicians. The first medication dose should be treated as if it were a "test" dose. Patients should be monitored for adverse reactions such as changes in blood pressure, pulse, or temperature; changes in mental status; allergic reactions; dizziness; ataxia; or gastric distress. If any of these symptoms develop, they should be reported to the prescriber.

Stabilization Phase

During stabilization, the prescriber adjusts or titrates the medication dosage to achieve the maximum amount of improvement with a minimum of side effects. Psychiatric–mental health nurses assess for improvements in the target symptoms and for the appearance of side effects. If medications are being increased rapidly, such as in a hospital setting, nurses must closely monitor temperature, blood pressure, pulse, mental status, common side effects, and unusual adverse reactions.

In the outpatient setting, nurses focus on patient education, emphasizing the importance of taking the medication, expected outcomes, and potential side effects. Patients need to know how and when to take their medications, how to minimize any side effects, and which side effects require immediate attention. A plan should be developed for patients and their families to clearly identify what to do if adverse reactions develop. The plan, which should include emergency telephone numbers or available emergency treatment, should be reviewed frequently.

Therapeutic drug monitoring is most important in this phase of treatment. Many medications used in psychiatry improve target symptoms only when a therapeutic level of medication has been obtained in the individual's blood. Some medications, such as lithium, have a narrow therapeutic range and must be monitored frequently and accurately. Nurses must be aware of when and how these levels are to be determined and assist patients in learning these procedures. Because of protein binding and lipid solubility, most medications do not have obtainable plasma levels that are clinically relevant. However, plasma levels of these medications may still be requested to evaluate further such issues as absorption and adverse reactions.

Sometimes the first medication chosen does not adequately improve the patient's target symptoms. In such cases, use of the medication will be discontinued, and treatment with a new medication will be started. Medications may also be changed when adverse reactions or seriously uncomfortable side effects occur or these effects substantially interfere with the individual's quality of life. Nurses should be familiar with the pharmacokinetics of both drugs to be able to monitor side effects and possible drug–drug interactions during this change.

At times, an individual may show only partial improvement from a medication, and the prescriber may try an **augmentation** strategy by adding another medication. For example, a prescriber may add a mood stabilizer, such as lithium, to an antidepressant to improve the effects of the antidepressant. **Polypharmacy**, using more than one group from a class of medications, is increasingly being used as an acceptable strategy with most psychopharmacologic agents to match the drug action to the neurochemical needs of the patient. Nurses must be familiar with the potential effects, side effects, drug interactions, and rationale for the treatment regimen.

Maintenance Phase

After the individual's target symptoms have improved, medications are usually continued to prevent **relapse** or return of the symptoms. In some cases, this may occur despite the patient's continued use of the medication. Patients must be educated about their target symptoms and have a plan of action if the symptoms return. In other cases, the patient may experience medication side effects. The psychiatric–mental health nurse has a central role in assisting individuals to monitor their own symptoms, identify emerging side effects, manage psychosocial stressors, and avoid other factors that may cause the medications to lose effect.

Discontinuation Phase

Some psychiatric medications will be discontinued; others will not. Some require a tapered discontinuation, which involves slowly reducing dosage while monitoring closely for reemergence of the symptoms. Some psychiatric disorders, such as mild depression, respond to treatment and do not recur. Other disorders, such as schizophrenia, usually require lifetime medication. Discontinuance of some medications, such as controlled substances, produces withdrawal symptoms; discontinuance of others does not.

MAJOR PSYCHOPHARMACOLOGIC DRUG CLASSES

Major classes of psychiatric drugs include antipsychotics, mood stabilizers, antidepressants, antianxiety and sedative–hypnotic medications, and stimulants.

Antipsychotic Medications

Antipsychotic medications can be thought of as "newer" and "older" medications. Newer or **atypical antipsychotics** appear to be equally or more effective but have fewer side effects than the traditional older agents. The term *typical or* **conventional antipsychotics** identifies the older

TABLE 11.5 ANTIPSYCHOTIC MEDICATIONS

Generic (Trade) Drug Name	Usual Dosage Range	Half-Life	Route of Administration
Atypical Antipsychotics			
Aripiprazole (Abilify)	10–30 mg/day	75–94 h	Oral tablets, injection, disintegrating tablet
Aripiprazole (Abilify MyCite)	10–30 mg/day	75–49 h	Oral tablet embedded with an ingestible event marker sensor intended to track drug ingestion
Aripiprazole (Maintena)	200–400 mg	29.9–46.6 days	Injection
Aripiprazole lauroxil (Aristada)	441–882 mg monthly	29.2–34.9 days	Injection
Asenapine (Saphris)	5–10 mg bid	24 h	Sublingual tablet
Brexpiprazole (Rexulti)	0.5–1.0 mg/day	86–91 h	Oral tablet
Cariprazine (Vraylar)	1.5–6.0 mg/day	2–4 days; 1–3 wks (metabolite)	Oral capsule
Clozapine (Clozaril, FazaClo, Versacloz)	300–900 mg/day	4–12 h	Oral tablet, disintegrating tablet, oral suspension
Iloperidone (Fanapt)	6–12 mg bid	18–33 h	Oral tablet
Lurasidone HCl (Latuda)	40 mg/day	18 h	Oral tablet
Olanzapine (Zyprexa)	5–15 mg/day; 2.5–10 mg/day IM	21–54 h	Oral tablet, disintegrating tablet; Injection
Olanzapine (Zyprexa Relprevv)	150–300 mg every 2–4 wks	30 days	Injection
Paliperidone (Invega extended release)	3–12 mg once daily in AM	23 h	Oral
Paliperidone palmitate (Invega Sustenna)	117 mg monthly	29–49 days	Injection
Pimavanserin (Nuplazid)	34 mg once daily	57 h for 17 mg	Oral tablet
Quetiapine fumarate (Seroquel)	150–750 mg/day	7 h	Oral tablet
Risperidone (Risperdal)	2–8 mg/day	20 h	Oral tablet, oral solution, disintegrating tablet
Risperidone (Risperdal Consta)	25–50 mg every 2 wks	3–6 days	Intramuscular Injection
Risperidone (Perseris)	90 or 120 mg once monthly	9–11 days	Abdominal subcutaneous injection
Ziprasidone HCl (Geodon)	40–160 mg/day; 10–20 mg/day IM	7 h	Oral capsule, oral suspension; Injection
Lurasidone HCl (Latuda)	40–80 mg	18 h	Oral tablet
Conventional (Typical) Antipsychotics			
Chlorpromazine	50–1,200 mg/day	2–30 h	Oral tablet
Fluphenazine	2–20 mg/day	4.5–15.3 h	Oral elixir, oral tablet, injection
Fluphenazine decanoate	12.5–25 mg every 3 wks		Injection
Perphenazine	12–64 mg/day	Unknown	Oral tablet
Trifluoperazine	5–40 mg/day	47–100 h	Oral tablet
Thiothixene (Navane)	5–60 mg/day	34 h	Oral capsule
Loxapine (Adasuve)	10 mg/day	7 h	Oral inhalation with inhaler
Haloperidol (Haldol)	2–20 mg/day	21–24 h	Oral tablet, oral concentration, injection
Haloperidol decanoate	50–100 mg every 3 wks	3 wks	Injection
Molindone	50–400 mg/day	1.5 h	Oral tablets
Pimozide (ORAP)	10 mg/day	55 h	Oral tablets

antipsychotic drugs. Table 11.5 provides a list of selected antipsychotics.

Indications and Mechanism of Action

Antipsychotic medications are indicated for schizophrenia, mania, and autism and to treat the symptoms of psychosis, such as hallucinations, delusions, bizarre behavior, disorganized thinking, and agitation (These symptoms are described more fully in later chapters). These medications also reduce aggressiveness, and inappropriate behavior associated with psychosis. Within the typical antipsychotics, haloperidol and pimozide are approved for treating patients with Tourette syndrome, reducing the frequency and severity of vocal tics. Some of the typical antipsychotics, particularly chlorpromazine, are used as antiemetics or for postoperative intractable hiccoughs.

The atypical antipsychotic medications differ from the typical antipsychotics in that they block serotonin receptors more potently than the dopamine receptors. The difference between the mechanism of action of the typical and atypical antipsychotics helps to explain their differences in terms of effect on target symptoms and in the degree of side effects they produce.

Pharmacokinetics

Antipsychotic medications administered orally have a variable rate of absorption complicated by the presence of food, antacids, smoking, and even the coadministration of anticholinergics, which slow gastric motility. Clinical effects begin to appear in about 30 to 60 minutes. Absorption after IM administration is less variable because this method avoids the first-pass effects. Therefore, IM administration produces greater bioavailability. It is important to remember that IM medications are absorbed more slowly when muscles are not used. Typically, the deltoid is used more than the gluteal muscles which may account for faster absorption of medication in the deltoid which has better blood perfusion.

Metabolism of these drugs occurs almost entirely in the liver with the exception of paliperidone palmitate (Invega Sustenna), which is not extensively metabolized by the liver but is excreted largely unchanged through the kidney and lurasidone HCl (Latuda) which is excreted through the urine and feces. Most antipsychotics are subject to the effects of other drugs that induce or inhibit the liver enzymes described earlier. Careful observance of concurrent medication use, including prescribed, over the counter, and substances of abuse, is required to avoid drug–drug interactions. For example, atypical antipsychotic concentrations may be affected by CYP450-inhibiting drugs such as paroxetine and fluoxetine.

Excretion of these substances tends to be slow. Most antipsychotics have a half-life of 24 hours or longer, but many also have active metabolites with longer half-lives. These two effects make it difficult to predict elimination time, and metabolites of some of these agents may be found in the urine months later. When a medication is discontinued, the adverse reactions may not immediately subside. The patient may continue to experience and sometimes need treatment for the adverse reactions for several days. Similarly, patients who discontinue their antipsychotic drugs may still derive therapeutic benefit for several days to weeks after drug discontinuation.

High lipid solubility, accumulation in the body, and other factors have also made it difficult to correlate blood levels with therapeutic effects. Table 11.5 shows the therapeutic ranges available for some of the antipsychotic medications. The potency of the antipsychotics also varies widely and is of specific concern when considering typical antipsychotic drugs.

Long-Acting Preparations

Currently, in the United States, atypical and conventional antipsychotics are available in long-acting forms. These antipsychotics are administered by injection once every 2 weeks to 3 months. Whereas the long-acting injectable atypical antipsychotics (risperidone, paliperidone, olanzapine, and aripiprazole) are water-based suspensions, the conventional antipsychotics are oil-based solutions. Long-acting injectable medications maintain a fairly constant blood level between injections. Because they bypass problems with gastrointestinal absorption and first-pass metabolism, this method may enhance therapeutic outcomes for the patient. The use of these medications is expected to increase the likelihood of adhering to a prescribed medication regimen.

Nurses should be aware that the injection site may become sore and inflamed if certain precautions are not taken. The oil-based injections (fluphenazine and haloperidol) are viscous liquids. For these injections, a large gauge needle (at least 21 gauge) should be used. Because the medication is meant to remain in the injection site, the needle should be dry, and a deep IM injection should be given by the Z-track method. (Note: Do not massage the injection site. Rotate sites and document in the patient's record.) Manufacturer recommendations should be followed.

Side Effects, Adverse Reactions, and Toxicity

Various side effects and interactions can occur with antipsychotics, with the conventional (typical) antipsychotics producing different side effects than the atypical antipsychotics. The side effects vary largely based on their degree of attraction to different neurotransmitter receptors and their subtypes.

Cardiovascular Side Effects

Cardiovascular side effects include orthostatic hypotension and prolongation of the QTc interval (a marker indicating an abnormal electrocardiogram that could cause serious irregular heart rhythms). Orthostatic hypotension is very common and depends on the degree of blockade of α-adrenergic receptors. Typical and atypical antipsychotics have been associated with prolonged QTc intervals and should be used cautiously in patients who have increased QTc intervals or are taking other medications that may prolong the QTc interval (Howland, 2015). Other cardiovascular side effects from typical antipsychotics have been rare, but occasionally they cause ECG changes that have a benign or undetermined clinical effect.

Anticholinergic Side Effects

Anticholinergic side effects resulting from blockade of acetylcholine are another common side effect associated with antipsychotic drugs. Dry mouth, slowed gastric motility, constipation, urinary hesitancy or retention, vaginal dryness, blurred vision, dry eyes, nasal congestion, and confusion or decreased memory are examples of these side effects. Interventions for decreasing the impact of these side effects are outlined in Table 11.1.

This group of side effects occurs with many of the medications used for psychiatric treatment. Using more than one medication with anticholinergic effects often increases the symptoms. Older patients are often most susceptible to a potential toxicity that results from high blockade of acetylcholine. This toxicity is called an *anticholinergic crisis* and is described more fully, along with its treatment, in Chapter 23.

Weight Gain

Weight gain is a common side effect of the atypical antipsychotics, particularly clozapine and olanzapine (Zyprexa), which can cause a weight gain of up to 20 lb within 1 year. Ziprasidone (Geodon), aripiprazole (Abilify), and lurasidone HCl (Latuda) are associated with little to no weight gain. If a patient becomes overweight or obese, switching to another antipsychotic should be considered and weight control interventions implemented.

Diabetes

One of the more serious side effects is the risk of type II diabetes. The FDA has determined that all atypical antipsychotics increase the risk for type II diabetes. Nurses should routinely assess for emerging symptoms of diabetes and alert the prescriber of these symptoms (see Box 11.3).

Sexual Side Effects

Sexual side effects result primarily from the blockade of dopamine in the tuberoinfundibular pathways of the hypothalamus. As a result, blood levels of prolactin may increase, particularly with risperidone and the typical antipsychotics. Increased prolactin causes breast enlargement and rare but potential galactorrhea (milk production and flow), decreased sexual drive, amenorrhea, menstrual irregularities, and increased risk for growth in pre-existing breast cancers. Other sexual side effects include retrograde ejaculation (backward flow of semen), erectile dysfunction, and anorgasmia.

Blood Disorders

Blood dyscrasias are rare but have received renewed attention since the introduction of clozapine (Clozaril).

BOX 11.3

Recommended Assessments Before and During Antipsychotic Therapy

- Weigh all patients and track BMI during treatment
  - Determine if overweight (BMI 25–29.9) or obese (BMI ≥30)
  - Monitor BMI monthly for the first 3 months; then quarterly
- Obtain baseline personal and family history of diabetes, obesity, dyslipidemia, hypertension, and cardiovascular disease
- Get waist circumference (at umbilicus)
  - Men: >40 in (102 cm)
  - Women: >35 in (88 cm)
- Monitor BP, fasting plasma glucose, and fasting lipid profile within 3 months and then annually (more frequently for patients with diabetes or have gained >5% of initial weight)
  - Prediabetes (fasting plasma glucose 100–125 mg/dL)
  - Diabetes (fasting plasma glucose >126 mg/dL)
  - Hypertension (BP >140/90 mm Hg)
  - Dyslipidemia (increased total cholesterol [>200 mg], decreased HDL, and increased LDL)

BMI, body mass index; BP, blood pressure; HDL, high-density lipoprotein; LDL, low-density lipoprotein.

Agranulocytosis is an acute reaction that causes the individual's white blood cell count to drop to very low levels often related to neutropenia, a drop in neutrophils. In the case of the antipsychotics, the medication suppresses the bone marrow precursors to blood factors. The exact mechanism by which the drugs produce this effect is unknown. The most notable symptoms of this disorder include high fever, sore throat, and mouth sores. Although benign elevations in temperature have been reported in individuals taking clozapine, no fever should go uninvestigated. Untreated neutropenia can be life threatening. Although severe neutropenia can occur with any of the antipsychotics, the risk with clozapine is greater than with the other antipsychotics. Therefore, prescription of clozapine requires weekly blood samples for the first 6 months of treatment and then every 2 weeks after that for as long as the drug is taken. Drawing of these samples must continue for 4 weeks after clozapine use has been discontinued. If sore throat or fever develops, medications should be withheld until a leukocyte count can be obtained. Hospitalization, including reverse isolation to prevent infections, is usually required. Severe neutropenia is more likely to develop during the first 18 weeks of treatment (Novartis, 2015).

Neuroleptic Malignant Syndrome

Neuroleptic malignant syndrome (NMS) is a serious complication that may result from antipsychotic medications. Characterized by rigidity and high fever, NMS is a rare condition that may occur abruptly with even one dose of medication. Temperature must always be monitored when administering antipsychotics, especially high-potency medications. This condition is discussed more fully in Chapter 23.

Other Side Effects

Photosensitivity reactions to antipsychotics, including severe sunburns or rash, most commonly develop with the use of low-potency typical medications. Sun block must be worn on all areas of exposed skin when taking these drugs. In addition, sun exposure may cause pigmentary deposits to develop, resulting in discoloration of exposed areas, especially the neck and face. This discoloration may progress from a deep orange color to a blue gray. Skin exposure should be limited and skin tone changes reported to the prescriber. Pigmentary deposits, retinitis pigmentosa, may also develop on the retina of the eye.

Antipsychotics may also lower the seizure threshold. Patients with an undetected seizure disorder may experience seizures early in treatment. Those who have a pre-existing condition should be monitored closely.

Medication-Related Movement Disorders

Medication-related movement disorders are side effects or adverse reactions that are commonly caused by typical antipsychotic medications but less commonly with atypical antipsychotic drugs. These disorders of abnormal motor movements can be divided into two groups: acute **extrapyramidal symptoms (EPS)**, which develop early in the course of treatment (sometimes after just one dose), and chronic syndromes, which develop from longer exposure to antipsychotic drugs.

Acute Extrapyramidal Symptoms. Acute EPS are acute abnormal movements that include dystonia, pseudoparkinsonism, and akathisia. They develop early in treatment, sometimes from as little as one dose. Although the abnormal movements are treatable, they are at times dramatic and frightening, causing physical and emotional impairments that often prompt patients to stop taking their medication. EPS occur when there is an imbalance of acetylcholine, dopamine, and GABA in the basal ganglia as a result of blocking dopamine.

Dystonia, sometimes referred to as an *acute dystonic reaction*, is impaired muscle tone that generally is the first EPS to occur, usually within a few days of initiating use of an antipsychotic. Acetylcholine is overactive because one of its modulators, dopamine, is blocked. Dystonia is characterized by involuntary muscle spasms that lead to abnormal postures, especially of the head and neck muscles. Acute dystonia occurs most often in young men, adolescents, and children. Patients usually first report a thick tongue, tight jaw, or stiff neck. Dystonia can progress to a protruding tongue, oculogyric crisis (eyes rolled up in the head), torticollis (muscle stiffness in the neck, which draws the head to one side with the chin pointing to the other), and laryngopharyngeal constriction. Abnormal postures of the upper limbs and torso may be held briefly or sustained. In severe cases, the spasms may progress to the intercostal muscles, producing more significant breathing difficulty for patients who already have respiratory impairment from asthma or emphysema. The treatment is the administration of a medication such as the anticholinergic agents that inhibit acetylcholine and thereby restore the balance of neurotransmitters (Table 11.6).

Drug-induced parkinsonism is sometimes referred to as **pseudoparkinsonism** because its presentation is identical to Parkinson disease. The difference is that the activity of dopamine is blocked in pseudoparkinsonism, and in Parkinson disease, the cells of the basal ganglia are destroyed. Older patients are at the greatest risk for experiencing pseudoparkinsonism (Marras, Austin, Bronskill, Diong, & Rochon, 2018). Symptoms include the classic triad of rigidity, slowed movements (akinesia), and tremor. The rigid muscle stiffness is usually seen in the arms. Akinesia can be observed by the loss of spontaneous movements, such as the absence of the usual relaxed swing of the arms while walking. In addition, masklike facies or loss of facial expression and a decrease in the ability to initiate movements also are present. Usually, tremor is more pronounced at rest, but it can also be observed with intentional movements, such as eating. If the tremor becomes severe, it may interfere with the patient's ability to eat or maintain adequate fluid intake. Hypersalivation is possible as well. Pseudoparkinsonism symptoms may occur on one or both sides of the body and develop abruptly or subtly but usually within the first 30 days of treatment. The treatment is the reduction in dosage or a change of antipsychotic that has less affinity for the dopamine receptor. Anticholinergic medication is sometimes given.

Akathisia is characterized by an inability to sit still or restlessness and is more common in middle-aged patients. The person will pace, rock while sitting or standing, march in place, or cross and uncross the legs. All of these repetitive motions have an intensity that is frequently beyond the explanation of the individual. In addition, akathisia may be present as a primarily subjective experience without obvious motor behavior. This subjective experience includes feelings of anxiety, jitteriness, or the inability to relax, which the individual may or may not be able to communicate. It is extremely uncomfortable for a person experiencing akathisia to be forced to sit still or be confined. These symptoms are sometimes misdiagnosed as agitation or an increase in psychotic symptoms. If an antipsychotic medication is given, the symptoms will not abate and will often worsen. Differentiating akathisia from agitation may be aided by knowing the person's symptoms before the introduction of medication. Whereas psychotic agitation does not

TABLE 11.6 DRUG THERAPIES FOR ACUTE MEDICATION-RELATED MOVEMENT DISORDERS

Agents	Typical Dosage Ranges	Routes Available	Common Side Effects
Anticholinergics			
Benztropine (Cogentin)	2–6 mg/day	PO, IM, IV	Dry mouth, blurred vision, slowed gastric motility causing constipation, urinary retention, increased intraocular pressure; overdose produces toxic psychosis
Trihexyphenidyl (Artane)	4–15 mg/day	PO	Same as benztropine, plus gastrointestinal distress. Older adults are most prone to mental confusion and delirium
Biperiden (Akineton)	2–8 mg/day	PO	Fewer peripheral anticholinergic effects. Euphoria and increased tremor may occur
Antihistamines			
Diphenhydramine (Benadryl)	25–50 mg qid to 400 mg daily	PO, IM, IV	Sedation and confusion, especially in older adults
Dopamine Agonists			
Amantadine (Symmetrel)	100–400 mg daily	PO	Indigestion, decreased concentration, dizziness, anxiety, ataxia, insomnia, lethargy, tremors, and slurred speech may occur with higher doses. Tolerance may develop on fixed dose
β-Blockers			
Propranolol (Inderal)	10 mg tid to 120 mg daily	PO	Hypotension and bradycardia. Must monitor pulse and blood pressure. Do not stop abruptly because doing so may cause rebound tachycardia
Benzodiazepines			
Lorazepam (Ativan)	1–2 mg IM; 0.5–2 mg PO	PO, IM	All may cause drowsiness, lethargy, and general sedation or paradoxical agitation. Confusion and disorientation in older adults
Diazepam (Valium)	2–5 mg tid	PO, IV	Most side effects are rare and will disappear if dose is decreased
Clonazepam (Klonopin)	1–4 mg/day	PO	Tolerance and withdrawal are potential problems

IM, intramuscular; IV, intravenous; PO, oral; qid, four times a day; tid, three times a day.

---

usually begin abruptly after antipsychotic medication use has been started, akathisia may occur after administration. In addition, the nurse may ask the patient if the experience is felt primarily in the muscles (akathisia) or in the mind or emotions (agitation).

Akathisia is the most difficult acute medication-related movement disorder to relieve. It does not usually respond well to anticholinergic medications. Rapid initiation of antipsychotics can increase the onset of akathisia (Yoshimura et al., 2018). The pathology of akathisia may involve more than just the extrapyramidal motor system. It may include serotonin changes that also affect the dopamine system. The usual approach to treatment is to change or reduce the antipsychotic. A number of medications are used to reduce symptoms, including β-adrenergic blockers, anticholinergics, antihistamines, and low-dose antianxiety agents with limited success. Frequently, combinations of these medications are used (Laoutidis & Luckhaus, 2013; Lohr, Eidt, Alfaraj, & Soliman, 2015).

A number of nursing interventions reduce the impact of these syndromes. Individuals with acute EPS need frequent reassurance that this is not a worsening of their psychiatric condition but instead is a treatable side effect of the medication. They also need validation that what they are experiencing is real and that the nurse is concerned and will be responsive to changes in these symptoms. Physical and psychological stress appears to increase the symptoms and further frighten the patient; therefore, decreasing stressful situations becomes important. These symptoms are often physically exhausting for the patient, and the nurse should ensure that the patient receives adequate rest and hydration. Because tremors, muscle rigidity, and motor restlessness may interfere with the individual's ability to eat, the nurse may need to assist the patient with eating and drinking fluids to maintain nutrition and hydration.

Risk factors for acute EPS include previous episodes of EPS. The nurse should listen closely when patients say they are "allergic" or have had "bad reactions" to antipsychotic medications. Often, they are describing one of the medication-related movement disorders, particularly dystonia, rather than a rash or other allergic symptom.

Chronic Syndromes: Tardive Dyskinesia. Chronic syndromes develop from long-term use of antipsychotics. They are serious and affect about 20% of the patients who receive typical antipsychotics for an extended period. These conditions are typically irreversible and cause significant impairment in self-image, social interactions, and occupational functioning. Early symptoms and mild forms may go unnoticed by the person experiencing them.

Tardive dyskinesia, the most well-known of the chronic syndromes, involves irregular, repetitive involuntary movements of the mouth, face, and tongue, including chewing, tongue protrusion, lip smacking, puckering of the lips, and rapid eye blinking. Abnormal finger movements are common as well. In some individuals, the trunk and extremities are also involved, and in rare cases, irregular breathing and swallowing lead to belching and grunting noises. These symptoms usually begin no earlier than after 6 months of treatment or when the medication is reduced or withdrawn. Once thought to be irreversible, considerable controversy now exists as to whether this is true.

The risk for experiencing tardive dyskinesia increases with age. Although the prevalence of tardive dyskinesia averages 15% to 20%, the rate rises to 50% to 70% in older patients receiving antipsychotic medications. The risk of probable tardive dyskinesia is three times lower in older adults receiving atypical antipsychotics compared to conventional antipsychotics (O'Brien, 2016). Women are at higher risk than men. Anyone receiving antipsychotic medication can develop tardive dyskinesia. Risk factors are summarized in Box 11.4. The causes of tardive dyskinesia remain unclear, but the most widely accepted theory is that dopamine antagonists block dopamine receptors, and evidence does suggest that imbalances of other neurotransmitters may be involved (Cornett, Novitch, Kaye, Kata, & Kaye, 2017).

Two medications recently approved by the FDA have shown promising results. Valbenazine (INGREZZA), a vesicular monoamine transporter 2 (VAMT2), was approved for the treatment of tardive dyskinesia. A related medication, deutetrabenazine (AUSTEDO), has a longer half-life than valbenazine, but twice-daily dosing with food is recommended (Citrome, 2017). Dietary precursors of acetylcholine, such as lecithin and vitamin E supplements, may prove to be beneficial.

The best approach to treatment remains avoiding the development of the chronic syndromes. Preventive measures include use of atypical antipsychotics, using the lowest possible dose of typical medication, minimizing use of as-needed (PRN) medication, and closely monitoring individuals in high-risk groups for development of the symptoms of tardive dyskinesia. All members of the mental health treatment team who have contact with individuals taking antipsychotics for longer than 3 months must be alert to the risk factors and earliest possible signs of chronic medication-related movement disorders.

Monitoring tools, such as the Abnormal Involuntary Movement Scale (AIMS) (see Appendix B), should be used routinely to standardize assessment and provide the earliest possible recognition of the symptoms. Standardized assessments should be performed at a minimum of 3- to 6-month intervals. The earlier the symptoms are recognized, the more likely they will resolve if the medication can be changed or its use discontinued. Newer, atypical antipsychotic medications have a much lower risk of causing tardive dyskinesia and are increasingly being considered first-line medications for treating patients with schizophrenia. Other medications are under development to provide alternatives that limit the risk for tardive dyskinesia.

Mood Stabilizers (Antimanic Medications)

Mood stabilizers, or antimanic medications, are psychopharmacologic agents used primarily for stabilizing mood swings, particularly those of mania in bipolar disorders. Lithium, the oldest, is the gold standard of treatment for acute mania and maintenance of bipolar disorders. Not all respond to lithium, and increasingly, other drugs are being used as first-line agents. Anticonvulsants, calcium channel blockers, adrenergic blocking agents, and atypical antipsychotics are used for mood stabilization.

Lithium

Lithium, a naturally occurring element, is effective in only about 40% of patients with bipolar disorder. Although lithium is not a perfect drug, a great deal is known regarding its use—it is inexpensive, it has restored stability to the lives of thousands of people, and it remains the gold standard of bipolar pharmacologic treatment.

Indications and Mechanisms of Action

Lithium is indicated for symptoms of mania characterized by rapid speech, flight of ideas (jumping from topic

---

BOX 11.4

Risk Factors for Tardive Dyskinesia

- Age older than 50 years
- Female
- Affective disorders, particularly depression
- Brain damage or dysfunction
- Increased duration of treatment
- Standard antipsychotic medication
- Possible higher doses of antipsychotic medication

to topic), irritability, grandiose thinking, impulsiveness, and agitation. Because it has mild antidepressant effects, lithium is used in treating depressive episodes of bipolar illness. It is also used as augmentation in patients experiencing major depression that has only partially responded to antidepressants alone. Lithium also has been shown to be helpful in reducing impulsivity and aggression in certain psychiatric patients.

The exact action by which lithium improves the symptoms of mania is unknown, but it is thought to exert multiple neurotransmitter effects, including enhancing serotonergic transmission, increasing synthesis of norepinephrine, and blocking postsynaptic dopamine. It has also been suggested that lithium's mood-stabilizing effects are related to the fact that it acts on cellular targets and exerting neuroprotective effects (Won & Kim, 2017). Lithium is actively transported across cell membranes, altering sodium transport in both nerve and muscle cells. It replaces sodium in the sodium–potassium pump and is retained more readily than sodium inside the cells. Conditions that alter sodium content in the body, such as vomiting, diuresis, and diaphoresis, also alter lithium retention. The results of lithium influx into the nerve cell lead to increased storage of catecholamines within the cell, reduced dopamine neurotransmission, increased norepinephrine reuptake, increased GABA activity, and increased serotonin receptor sensitivity. Lithium also alters the distribution of calcium and magnesium ions and inhibits second messenger systems within the neuron. The mechanisms by which lithium improves the symptoms of mania are complex and interrelated, involving the sum of all or part of these actions and more.

Pharmacokinetics

Lithium carbonate is available orally in capsule, tablet, and liquid forms. Slow-release preparations are also available. Lithium is readily absorbed in the gastric system and may be taken with food, which does not impair absorption. Peak blood levels are reached in 1 to 4 hours, and the medication is usually completely absorbed in 8 hours. Slow-release preparations are absorbed at a slower, more variable rate.

Lithium is not protein bound, and its distribution into the CNS across the blood–brain barrier is slow. The onset of action is usually 5 to 7 days and may take as long as 2 weeks. The elimination half-life is 8 to 12 hours and is 18 to 36 hours in individuals whose blood levels have reached steady state and whose symptoms are stable. Lithium is almost entirely excreted by the kidneys but is present in all body fluids. Conditions of renal impairment or decreased renal function in older patients decrease lithium clearance and may lead to toxicity. Several medications affect renal function and therefore change lithium clearance. See Chapter 22 for a list of these and other medication interactions with lithium. About 80% of lithium is reabsorbed in the proximal tubule of the kidney along with water and sodium. In conditions that cause sodium depletion, such as dehydration caused by fever, strenuous exercise, hot weather, increased perspiration, and vomiting, the kidneys attempt to conserve sodium. Because lithium is a salt, the kidneys retain lithium as well, leading to increased blood levels and potential toxicity. Significantly increasing sodium intake causes lithium levels to fall.

Lithium is usually administered in doses of 300 mg two to three times daily. Because it is a drug with a narrow therapeutic range or index, blood levels are monitored frequently during acute mania, and the dosage is increased every 3 to 5 days. These increases may be slower in older adult patients or patients who experience uncomfortable side effects. Blood levels should be monitored 12 hours after the last dose of medication. In the hospital setting, nurses should withhold the morning dose of lithium until the serum sample is drawn to avoid falsely elevated levels. Individuals who are at home should be instructed to have their blood drawn in the morning about 12 hours after their last dose and before they take their first dose of medication. During the acute phases of mania, blood levels of 0.8 to 1.4 mEq/L are usually attained and maintained until symptoms are under control. The therapeutic range for lithium is narrow, and patients in the higher end of that range usually experience more uncomfortable side effects. During maintenance, the dosage is reduced, and dosages are adjusted to maintain blood levels of 0.4 to 1 mEq/L.

Lithium clears the body relatively quickly after discontinuation of its use. Withdrawal symptoms are rare, but occasional anxiety and emotional lability have been reported. It is important to remember that almost half of the individuals who discontinue lithium treatment abruptly experience a relapse of symptoms within a few weeks. Some research suggests that if a person stops taking lithium, the drug will be less effective when the medication is restarted. Patients should be warned of the risks in abruptly discontinuing their medication and should be advised to consider the options carefully in consultation with their prescriber.

Side Effects, Adverse Reactions, and Toxicity

At lower therapeutic blood levels, side effects from lithium are relatively mild. These reactions correspond with peaks in plasma concentrations of the medication after administration, and most subside during the first few weeks of therapy. Frequently, individuals taking lithium complain of excessive thirst and an unpleasant metallic-like taste. Sugarless throat lozenges may be useful in minimizing this side effect. Other common side effects include increased frequency of urination, fine head tremor, drowsiness, and mild diarrhea. Weight gain occurs in about 20% of the individuals taking lithium. Nausea may be minimized by taking the medication with food or by use of a slow-release preparation. However, slow-release forms of lithium increase diarrhea. Muscle weakness, restlessness, headache, acne, rashes, and exacerbation of psoriasis have also been reported. See Chapter 23 for a summary of selected nursing interventions to minimize the impact of common side effects associated with lithium treatment. Patients most frequently discontinued their own medication use because of concerns with mental slowness, poor concentration, and memory problems.

As blood levels of lithium increase, the side effects of lithium become more numerous and severe. Early signs of lithium toxicity include severe diarrhea, vomiting, drowsiness, muscular weakness, and lack of coordination. Lithium should be withheld and the prescriber consulted if these symptoms develop. Lithium toxicity can easily be resolved in 24 to 48 hours by discontinuing the medication, but hemodialysis may be required in severe situations. See Chapter 23 for a summary of the side effects and symptoms of toxicity associated with various blood levels of lithium.

Monitoring of creatinine concentration, thyroid hormones, and CBC every 6 months during maintenance therapy helps to assess the occurrence of other potential adverse reactions. Kidney damage is considered an uncommon but potentially serious risk of long-term lithium treatment. This damage is usually reversible after discontinuation of the lithium use. A gradual rise in serum creatinine and decline in creatinine clearance indicate the development of renal dysfunction. Individuals with pre-existing kidney dysfunction are susceptible to lithium toxicity.

Lithium may alter thyroid function, usually after 6 to 18 months of treatment. About 30% of the individuals taking lithium exhibit elevations in thyroid-stimulating hormone (TSH), but most do not show suppression of circulating thyroid hormone. Thyroid dysfunction from lithium treatment is more common in women, and some individuals require the addition of thyroxine to their care. During maintenance, TSH levels may be monitored. Nurses should observe for dry skin, constipation, bradycardia, hair loss, cold intolerance, and other symptoms of hypothyroidism. Other endocrine system effects result from hypoparathyroidism, which increases parathyroid hormone levels and calcium. Clinically, this change is not significant, but elevated calcium levels may cause mood changes, anxiety, lethargy, and sleep disturbances. These symptoms may erroneously be attributed to depression if hypercalcemia is not investigated.

Lithium use must be avoided during pregnancy because it has been associated with birth defects, especially when administered during the first trimester. If lithium is given during the third trimester, toxicity may develop in a newborn, producing signs of hypotonia, cyanosis, bradykinesia, cardiac changes, gastrointestinal bleeding, and shock. Diabetes insipidus may persist for months. Lithium is also present in breast milk, and women should not breastfeed while taking lithium. Women expecting to become pregnant should be advised to consult with a physician before discontinuing use of birth control methods.

Anticonvulsants

In the psychiatric–mental health area, anticonvulsants are commonly used to treat patients with bipolar disorder and are considered mood stabilizers. The following discussion highlights the use of anticonvulsants as mood stabilizers in the treatment of bipolar disorder.

Indications and Mechanisms of Action

Valproate (valproic acid; Depakote), carbamazepine (Equetro), and lamotrigine (Lamictal) have FDA approval for the treatment of bipolar disorder and mania (see Chapter 23). In general, the anticonvulsant mood stabilizers have many actions, but their effects on ion channels, reducing repetitive firing of action potentials in the nerves, most directly decrease manic symptoms. No one action has successfully accounted for the anticonvulsants' ability to stabilize mood (Landgraf et al., 2016).

Pharmacokinetics

Valproic acid is rapidly absorbed, but the enteric coating of divalproex sodium adds a delay of as long as 1 hour. Peak serum levels occur in about 1 to 4 hours. The liquid form (sodium valproate) is absorbed more rapidly and peaks in 15 minutes to 2 hours. Food appears to slow absorption but does not lower bioavailability of the drug.

Carbamazepine is absorbed in a somewhat variable manner. The liquid suspension is absorbed more quickly than the tablet form, but food does not appear to interfere with absorption. Peak plasma levels occur in 2 to 6 hours. Because high doses influence peak plasma levels and increase the risk for side effects, carbamazepine should be given in divided doses two or three times a day. The suspension, which has higher peak plasma levels and lower trough levels, must be given more frequently than the tablet form.

These medications cross easily into the CNS, move into the placenta as well, and are associated with an increased risk for birth defects. Carbamazepine, valproic acid, and lamotrigine are metabolized by the CYP450 system. However, one of the metabolites of carbamazepine is potentially toxic. If other concurrent medications inhibit the enzymes that break down this toxic metabolite, severe adverse reactions are often the result. Medications that inhibit this breakdown include erythromycin, verapamil, and cimetidine (now available in nonprescription form).

Teaching Points

Nurses need to educate patients about potential drug interactions, especially with nonprescription medications. Nurses can also inform other health care practitioners who may be prescribing medication that these patients are taking carbamazepine. It is important to note that oral contraceptives may become ineffective, and female patients should be advised to use other methods of birth control.

Side Effects, Adverse Reactions, and Toxicity of Anticonvulsants

The most common side effects of carbamazepine are dizziness, drowsiness, tremor, visual disturbance, nausea, and vomiting. These side effects may be minimized by initiating treatment in low doses. Patients should be advised that these symptoms will diminish, but care should be taken when changing positions or performing tasks that require visual alertness. Giving the drug with food may diminish nausea. Adverse reactions include rare aplastic anemia, agranulocytosis, severe rash, rare cardiac problems, and syndrome of inappropriate secretion of the antidiuretic hormone (SIADH) caused by hyponatremia.

Valproic acid also causes gastrointestinal disturbances, tremor, and lethargy. In addition, it can produce weight gain and alopecia (hair loss). These symptoms are transient and should diminish with the course of treatment. Dietary supplements of zinc and selenium may be helpful to patients experiencing hair loss. Constipation and urinary retention occur in some individuals. Nurses should monitor urinary output and assist patients to increase fluid consumption to decrease constipation.

Benign skin rash, sedation, blurred or double vision, dizziness, nausea, vomiting, and other gastrointestinal symptoms are side effects of lamotrigine. In rare cases, lamotrigine (Lamictal) produces severe, life-threatening rashes that usually occur within 2 to 8 weeks of treatment. This risk is highest in children. Use of lamotrigine should be immediately discontinued if a rash is noted.

Transient elevations in liver enzymes occur with both carbamazepine and valproic acid but symptoms of hepatic injury rarely occur. If the patient reports abnormal pain or shows signs of jaundice, the prescriber should be notified immediately. Several blood dyscrasias are associated with carbamazepine, including aplastic anemia, agranulocytosis, and leukopenia. Patients should be advised to report fever, sore throat, rash, petechiae, or bruising immediately.

In addition, patients should be advised of the importance of completing routine blood tests throughout treatment. The risks for aplastic anemia and agranulocytosis with carbamazepine use still require close monitoring of CBCs during treatment. Valproate and its derivatives have had a similar course of development.

Antidepressant Medications

Medications classified as antidepressants are used not only for the treatment of depression but also in the treatment of anxiety disorders, eating disorders, and other mental health states (Table 11.7). They are used very cautiously in persons with bipolar disorder because of the possibility of precipitating a manic episode. The exact neuromechanism for the antidepressant effect is unknown in all of them. The onset of action also varies considerably and appears to depend on factors outside of steady-state plasma levels. Initial improvement with some antidepressants, such as the SSRIs, may appear within 7 days, but complete relief of symptoms may take several weeks. Antidepressants should not be discontinued abruptly because of uncomfortable symptoms that result. Discontinuance of use of these medications requires slow tapering. Individuals taking these medications should be cautioned not to abruptly stop using them without consulting their prescriber. Antidepressant medications are well absorbed from the gastrointestinal system; however, some individual variations exist. Most of the antidepressants are metabolized by liver enzymes so that other drugs metabolized by these enzymes may increase or decrease blood levels of the antidepressants. All of these medications have a "boxed warning" for increased risk of suicidal behavior in children, adolescents, and young adults.

Serotonin syndrome, or serotonin intoxication syndrome, can occur if there is an overactivity of serotonin or an impairment of the serotonin metabolism. Concomitant medications such as triptans used to treat migraines also can increase the serotonergic activity. With the advent of widely used antidepressants targeting the serotonergic systems, symptoms of this serious side effect should be assessed. Symptoms include mental status changes (hallucinations, agitation, coma), autonomic instability (tachycardia, hyperthermia, changes in blood pressure), neuromuscular problems (hyperreflexia, incoordination), and gastrointestinal disturbance (nausea, vomiting, diarrhea). Serotonin syndrome can be life threatening. The treatment for serotonin syndrome is discontinuation of the medication and symptom management.

Selective Serotonin Reuptake Inhibitors

The serotonergic system is associated with mood, emotion, sleep, and appetite and is implicated in the control of

TABLE 11.7	ANTIDEPRESSANT MEDICATIONS		
Generic (Trade) Drug Name	Usual Dosage Range (mg/day)	Half-Life (h)	Therapeutic Blood Level (ng/mL)
Selective Serotonin Reuptake Inhibitors			
Citalopram (Celexa)	20–50	35	Not available
Escitalopram (Lexapro)	10–20	27–32	Not available
Fluoxetine (Prozac)	20–80	2–9 days	72–300
Fluvoxamine (Luvox)	50–300	17–22	Not available
Paroxetine (Paxil)	10–50	10–24	Not available
Sertraline (Zoloft)	50–200	24	Not available
Serotonin Norepinephrine Reuptake Inhibitors			
Desvenlafaxine (Pristiq extended release)	50	11	Not available
Duloxetine (Cymbalta)	40–60	8–17	Not available
Levomilnacipran (Fetzima)	40–120	12	Not available
Nefazodone	100–600	2–4	Not available
Venlafaxine (Effexor)	75–375	5–11	100–500
Norepinephrine–Dopamine Reuptake Inhibitor			
Bupropion (Wellbutrin)	200–450	8–24	10–29
α$_2$-Antagonist			
Mirtazapine (Remeron)	15–45	20–40	Not available
Others			
Trazodone (Desyrel)	150–600	4–9	650–1,600
Vilazodone (Viibryd)	10–40	25	Not available
Vortioxetine (Brintellix)	5–20	66	Not available
Tricyclic Antidepressants			
Amitriptyline (Elavil)	50–300	31–46	110–250
Amoxapine	50–600	8	200–500
Clomipramine (Anafranil)	25–250	19–37	80–100
Imipramine (Tofranil)	30–300	11–25	200–350
Desipramine (Norpramin)	25–300	12–24	125–300
Doxepin	25–300	8–24	100–200
Nortriptyline (Aventyl, Pamelor)	30–100	18–44	50–150
Protriptyline (Vivactil)	15–60	67–89	100–200
Tetracyclic			
Maprotiline (Ludiomil)	50–225	21–25	200–300
Monoamine Oxidase Inhibitors			
Isocarboxazid (Marplan)	20–60	Not available	Not available
Phenelzine (Nardil)	15–90	24 (effect lasts 3–4 days)	Not available
Tranylcypromine (Parnate)	10–60	24 (effect lasts 3–10 days)	Not available
Selegiline (Emsam)	6–12 mg/24 h	25–50% delivered in 24 h	Not available

numerous emotional, physical, and behavioral functions (see Chapter 6). Decreased serotonergic neurotransmission has been proposed to play a key role in depression. In 1988, fluoxetine (Prozac) was the first of a class of drugs that acted "selectively" on serotonin, one group of neurotransmitters associated with depression. Other similarly selective medications, sertraline (Zoloft), paroxetine (Paxil), and fluvoxamine (Luvox), soon followed. The newest SSRI is escitalopram oxalate (Lexapro).

All of the SSRIs inhibit the reuptake of serotonin by blocking its transport into the presynaptic neuron, which in turn increases the concentration of synaptic serotonin. The concentration of synaptic serotonin is controlled directly by its reuptake; thus, drugs blocking serotonin transport have been successfully used for the treatment of depression and other conditions associated with serotonergic activity.

The SSRIs also have other properties that account for the common side effects, which include headache, anxiety, insomnia, transient nausea, vomiting, and diarrhea. Sedation may also occur, especially with paroxetine. Most often, these medications are given in the morning, but if daytime sedation occurs, they may be given in the evening. Higher doses, especially of fluoxetine, are more likely to produce sedation. Nausea and dizziness are common side effects which may subside within a few weeks. These side effects, along with sexual dysfunction, sedation, diastolic hypertension, and increased perspiration, tend to be dose dependent, occurring more frequently at higher doses. Other common side effects include insomnia, constipation, dry mouth, tremors, blurred vision, and asthenia or muscle weakness.

Sexual dysfunction is a relatively common side effect with most antidepressants. Erectile and ejaculation disturbances occur in men and anorgasmia in women. This side effect is often difficult to assess if the nurse has not obtained a sexual history before initiation of use of the medication. Anorgasmia is particularly common with the SSRIs and often goes unreported, frequently because nurses and other health care providers do not ask.

Serotonin Norepinephrine Reuptake Inhibitors

Decreased activity of the neurotransmitter norepinephrine is also associated with depression and anxiety disorders. Venlafaxine (Effexor), nefazodone (Serzone), duloxetine (Cymbalta), and desvenlafaxine (Pristiq) prevent the reuptake of both serotonin and norepinephrine at the presynaptic site and are classified as serotonin norepinephrine reuptake inhibitors (SNRIs). Desipramine (Norpramin) is technically a tricyclic antidepressant (TCA) and is usually categorized as such. It works, however, on both serotonin and norepinephrine, so it can also be considered an SNRI.

The side effects are similar to those of the SSRIs; there is also a risk for an associated increase in blood pressure. Elevations in blood pressure have been described, and nurses should monitor blood pressure, especially in patients who have a history of hypertension. Venlafaxine (Effexor) has little effect on acetylcholine and histamine; thus, it creates only mild sedation and anticholinergic symptoms. This medication is often used if a depressed patient is sleeping excessively and reports little energy. The most common side effects of nefazodone (Serzone) include dry mouth, nausea, dizziness, muscle weakness, constipation, and tremor. It is unlikely to cause sexual disturbance. Nefazodone also has a "boxed warning" for hepatic failure and should not be used in those with acute liver disease.

Norepinephrine–Dopamine Reuptake Inhibitors

Bupropion (Wellbutrin, Zyban) inhibits reuptake of norepinephrine, serotonin, and dopamine. Wellbutrin is indicated for depression and Zyban for nicotine addiction. The smoking cessation medication, Zyban, is given at a lower dose than Wellbutrin. Patients should not take Zyban if they are taking Wellbutrin. Bupropion has a chemical structure unlike any of the other antidepressants and somewhat resembles a few of the psychostimulants. Bupropion's activating effects may be experienced as agitation or anxiety by some patients. Others also experience insomnia and appetite suppression. For a few individuals, bupropion has produced psychosis, including hallucinations and delusions. Most likely, this is secondary to overstimulation of the dopamine system. Bupropion is contraindicated for people with seizure disorders and those at risk for seizures. The rate of seizures is similar to that with the SSRIs and mirtazapine but is lower than the rate associated with the older antidepressants. Most important, bupropion has a lower incidence of sexual dysfunction and often is used in individuals who are experiencing these side effects with other antidepressants (GlaxoSmithKline, 2014; Waldinger, 2015).

α_2-Antagonist

Mirtazapine (Remeron) boosts norepinephrine or noradrenaline and serotonin by blocking α_2-adrenergic presynaptic receptors on a serotonin receptor (5-HT_{2A}, 5-HT_{2C}, 5-HT_3). This is a different action than the other antidepressants. A histamine receptor is also blocked, which may explain its sedative side effect. Mirtazapine is indicated for depression. Side effects include sedation (at lower doses), dizziness, weight gain, dry mouth, constipation, and change in urinary functioning.

Other Antidepressants

Trazodone (Desyrel) blocks serotonin 2A receptor potently and blocks the serotonin reuptake pump less potently. It is indicated for depression but is often used off-label for insomnia and anxiety. Sedation is a very common side effect. Other side effects include weight gain, nausea, vomiting, constipation, dizziness, fatigue, incoordination, and tremor.

Other newly FDA-approved antidepressants target other receptor sites. For example, vilazodone (Viibryd) is a serotonin reuptake inhibitor and a partial agonist of 5-HT_{1A}; vortioxetine (Brintellix) inhibits reuptake of serotonin and norepinephrine, but is also a partial agonist to 5-HT_{1A}. These subtle differences translate into subtle clinical effects.

Tricyclic Antidepressants

The TCAs were once the primary medication used for treating depression. With the introduction of the SSRIs and other previously discussed antidepressants, the use of TCAs has significantly declined. In most cases, these medications are as effective as the other drugs, but

TABLE 11.8 — CYP450 METABOLISM OF COMMON ANTIDEPRESSANTS

Drug	How Metabolized	Induces	Inhibits
Bupropion	2B6	None	2D6
Citalopram	2C19, 2D6, 3A4	None	Mild 2D6
Desvenlafaxine	3A4	None	Mild 2D6
Duloxetine	1A2, 2D6	None	2D6
Escitalopram	2C19, 2D6, 3A4	None	Mild 2D6
Fluoxetine	2C9, 2C19, 2D6, 3A4	None	2C19, 2D6 3A4, norfluoxetine
Fluvoxamine	1A2, 2D6	None	1A2, 2C9, 2C19, 3A4
Mirtazapine	1A2, 2D6, 3A4	None	None
Nefazodone	2D6, 3A4	None	3A4
Paroxetine	2D6	None	2D6, 2B6
Selegiline	2A6, 2C9, 3A4/5	None	2D6, 3A4/5
Sertraline	2B6, 2C9, 2D6, 3A4	None	2B6, 2C9, 2C19, 2D6, 3A4 (dosage >200 mg)
St. John's Wort[a]	3A4	3A4	None
Trazodone	2D6, 3A4	None	None
Tricyclic antidepressants	2D6, others depending on drug	None	Mild 2D6
Venlafaxine	2D6	None	Mild 2D6
Vilazodone	3A4, 2C19, 2D6	None	2C8
Vortioxetine	2D6, 3A4/5, 2C9, 2A6, 2C8, 2B6	None	None

[a]Not a U.S. Food and Drug Administration–approved antidepressant.
Information from the Prescribing Information of each medication.

they have more serious side effects and a higher lethal potential (see Table 11.8). The TCAs act on a variety of neurotransmitter systems, including the norepinephrine and serotonin reuptake systems.

Pharmacokinetics

The TCAs are highly bound to plasma proteins, which make the association between blood levels and therapeutic clinical effects difficult. However, some plasma ranges have been established (see Table 11.7). Most of the TCAs have active metabolites that act in as much the same manner as the parent drug. Most of these antidepressants may be given in a once-daily single dose. If the medication causes sedation, this dose should be given at bedtime.

Side Effects, Adverse Reactions, and Toxicity

Because the TCAs act on several neurotransmitters in addition to serotonin and norepinephrine, these drugs have many unwanted effects. With the TCAs, sedation, orthostatic hypotension, and anticholinergic side effects are the most common sources of discomfort for patients receiving these medications. Other side effects of the TCAs include tremors, restlessness, insomnia, nausea and vomiting, confusion, pedal edema, headache, and seizures. Blood dyscrasias may also occur, and any fever, sore throat, malaise, or rash should be reported to the prescriber. Interventions to assist in minimizing these side effects are listed in Table 11.1.

The TCAs have the potential for cardiotoxicity. Symptoms include prolongation of cardiac conduction that may worsen pre-existing cardiac conduction problems. The TCAs are contraindicated with second-degree atrioventricular block and should be used cautiously in patients who have other cardiac problems. Occasionally, they may precipitate heart failure, myocardial infarction, arrhythmias, and stroke.

Antidepressants that block the dopamine (D_2) receptor, such as amoxapine, have produced symptoms of NMS. Mild forms of EPS and endocrine changes, including galactorrhea and amenorrhea, may develop.

Monoamine Oxidase Inhibitors

The MAOIs, as their name indicates, inhibit MAO, an enzyme that breaks down the biogenic amine neurotransmitters serotonin, norepinephrine, and others. By inhibiting this enzyme, serotonin and norepinephrine activity is increased in the synapse. In the United States, there are three oral formulations: phenelzine (Nardil), tranylcypromine (Parnate), and isocarboxazid (Marplan) and one available by a transdermal patch: selegiline (Emsam). These are considered MAOIs because they form strong covalent bonds to block the enzyme MAO. The inhibition of this enzyme increases with repeated administration of these medications and takes at least 2 weeks to resolve after discontinuation of use of the medication.

The major problem with the MAOIs is their interaction with tyramine-rich foods and certain medications that

TABLE 11.9 EXAMPLE OF A TYRAMINE-RESTRICTED DIET

Category of Food	Food With Tyramine	Food Allowed
Nonrefrigerated food	Spoiled foods or foods not refrigerated, handled, or stored properly	Food that is handled and stored properly
Cheese	All aged and mature cheeses, especially strong, aged, or processed cheeses such as American processed, cheddar, Colby, blue, brie, mozzarella, and parmesan; yogurt, sour cream	Fresh cottage cheese, cream cheese, ricotta cheese
Meat, fish, and poultry	Air-dried, aged, and fermented meats, sausages, and salamis Beef or chicken liver Dried and pickled herring Pepperoni Anchovies, meat extracts, meat tenderizers Meats prepared with tenderizers, improperly stored meat Spoiled or improperly stored animal liver	Fresh meat, poultry, and fish, including fresh processed meats (e.g., lunch meats, hot dogs, breakfast sausage, and cooked sliced ham)
Fruits and vegetables	Broad bean pods (Fava bean pods)	All other vegetables
Alcoholic beverages	All tap beers and other beers that have not been pasteurized; red wine, sherry, liqueurs; some alcohol-free and reduced alcohol beers	White wines may not contain tyramine
Miscellaneous foods	Marmite-concentrated yeast extract Sauerkraut Soy sauce and other soybean condiments	Soy milk Pizzas from commercial chain restaurants prepared with cheeses low in tyramine

U.S. Department of Health and Human Services Food & Drug Administration. (2010). *Avoid food-drug interactions. A guide from the National Consumers League and U.S. Food and Drug Administration. Publication no (FDA) CDER 10–1933.* Retrieved December 9, 2018, from www.fda.gov/drugs and Parke-Davis. (2007). Retrieved December 9, 2018, from http://www.accessdata.fda.gov/drugsatfda_docs/label/2007/011909s038lbl.pdf

can result in a hypertensive crisis. All of the MAOIs have dietary modification except the 6 mg/24 hours dose of selegiline. The enzyme monoamine is important in the breakdown of dietary amines (e.g., tyramine). When the enzyme is inhibited, tyramine, a precursor for dopamine, increases in the nerve cells. Tyramine has a vasopressor action that induces hypertension. If the individual ingests food that contains high levels of tyramine while taking MAOIs, severe headaches, palpitation, neck stiffness and soreness, nausea, vomiting, sweating, hypertension, stroke, and, in rare instances, death may result. Patients who are taking MAOIs are prescribed a low-tyramine diet (Table 11.9).

In addition to food restrictions, many prescription and nonprescription medications that stimulate the sympathetic nervous system (sympathomimetic) produce the same risk for hypertensive crisis as do foods containing tyramine. The nonprescription medication interactions involve primarily diet pills and cold remedies. Patients should be advised to check the labels of any nonprescription drugs carefully for a warning against use with antidepressants, especially the MAOIs, and then consult their prescriber before consuming these medications. In addition, symptoms of other serious drug–drug interactions may develop, such as coma, hypertension, and fever, which may occur when patients receive meperidine (Demerol) while taking an MAOI. Patients should notify other health care providers, including dentists, that they are taking an MAOI before being prescribed or given any other medication.

The MAOIs frequently produce dizziness, headache, insomnia, dry mouth, blurred vision, constipation, nausea, peripheral edema, urinary hesitancy, muscle weakness, forgetfulness, and weight gain. Older patients are especially sensitive to the side effect of orthostatic hypotension and require frequent assessment of lying and standing blood pressures. They may be at risk for falls and subsequent bone fractures and require assistance in changing position. Sexual dysfunction, including decreased libido, impotence, and anorgasmia, also is common with MAOIs.

Antianxiety and Sedative–Hypnotic Medications

Sometimes called *anxiolytics*, antianxiety medications, such as buspirone and sedative–hypnotic medications, such as lorazepam (Ativan), come from various pharmacologic classifications, including barbiturates, benzodiazepines, nonbenzodiazepines, and nonbarbiturate sedative–hypnotic medications, such as chloral hydrate. These drugs represent some of the most widely prescribed medications today for the short-term relief of anxiety or anxiety associated with depression.

Benzodiazepines

Commonly prescribed benzodiazepines include alprazolam (Xanax), lorazepam (Ativan), diazepam (Valium), chlordiazepoxide (Librium), flurazepam (Dalmane), and triazolam (Halcion). Although benzodiazepines are known to enhance the effects of the inhibitory neurotransmitter GABA, their exact mechanisms of action are not well understood. Of the various benzodiazepines in use to relieve anxiety (and treat insomnia), oxazepam (Serax) and lorazepam (Ativan) are often preferred for patients with liver disease and for older patients because of their short half-lives.

Pharmacokinetics

The variable rate of absorption of the benzodiazepines determines the speed of onset. Table 11.10 provides relative indications of the speed of onset, from very fast to slow, for some of the commonly prescribed benzodiazepines. Whereas chlordiazepoxide (Librium) and diazepam (Valium) are slow, erratic, and sometimes incompletely absorbed when given intramuscularly, lorazepam (Ativan) is rapidly and completely absorbed when given intramuscularly.

All of the benzodiazepines are highly lipid soluble and highly protein bound. They are distributed throughout the body and enter the CNS quickly. Other drugs that compete for protein-binding sites may produce drug–drug interactions. The degree to which each of these drugs is lipid soluble affects its duration of action. Most of these drugs have active metabolites, but the degree of activity of each metabolite affects duration of action and elimination half-life. Most of these drugs vary markedly in length of half-life. Oxazepam and lorazepam have no active metabolites and thus have shorter half-lives. Elimination half-lives may also be sustained for obese patients when using diazepam and chlordiazepoxide.

Side Effects, Adverse Reactions, and Toxicity

The most commonly reported side effects of benzodiazepines result from the sedative and CNS depression effects of these medications. Drowsiness, intellectual impairment, memory impairment, ataxia, and reduced motor coordination are common adverse reactions. If prescribed for sleep, many of these medications, especially the long-acting benzodiazepines, produce significant "hangover" effects experienced on awakening. Older patients receiving repeated doses of medications such as flurazepam at bedtime may experience paradoxical confusion, agitation, and delirium, sometimes after the first dose. In addition, daytime fatigue, drowsiness, and cognitive impairments may continue while the person is awake. For most patients, the effects subside as tolerance develops; however, alcohol increases all of these symptoms and potentiates the CNS depression. Individuals using these medications should be warned to be cautious when driving or performing other tasks that require mental alertness. If these tasks are part of the person's work requirements, another medication may be chosen. Administered intravenously, benzodiazepines often cause phlebitis and thrombosis at the IV sites, which should be monitored closely and changed if redness or swelling develops.

Because tolerance develops to most of the CNS depressant effects, individuals who wish to experience the feeling of "intoxication" from these medications may be tempted to increase their own dosage. Psychological dependence is more likely to occur when using these medications for a longer period. Abrupt discontinuation of the use of benzodiazepines may result in a recurrence of the target symptoms, such as rebound insomnia or anxiety. Other withdrawal symptoms appear rapidly, including tremors, increased perspiration, palpitations, increased sensitivity to light, abdominal discomfort or pain, and elevations in systolic blood pressure. These

TABLE 11.10 ANTIANXIETY AND SEDATIVE–HYPNOTIC MEDICATIONS

Generic (Trade) Drug Name	Usual Dosage Range (mg/day)	Half-Life (h)	Speed of Onset After Single Dose
Benzodiazepines			
Diazepam (Valium)	4–40	30–100	Very fast
Chlordiazepoxide (Librium)	15–100	50–100	Intermediate
Clorazepate (Tranxene)	15–60	30–200	Fast
Prazepam (Centrax)	20–60	30–200	Very slow
Lorazepam (Ativan)	2–8	10–20	Slow intermediate
Oxazepam (Serax)	30–120	3–21	Slow intermediate
Alprazolam (Xanax)	0.5–10	12–15	Intermediate
Halazepam (Paxipam)	80–160	30–200	Slow intermediate
Clonazepam (Klonopin)	1.5–20	18–50	Intermediate
Nonbenzodiazepine			
Buspirone (BuSpar)	15–30	3–11	Very slow

symptoms may be more pronounced with the short-acting benzodiazepines, such as lorazepam. Gradual tapering is recommended for discontinuing use of benzodiazepines after long-term treatment. When tapering short-acting medications, the prescriber may switch the patient to a long-acting benzodiazepine before discontinuing use of the short-acting drug.

Individual reactions to the benzodiazepines appear to be associated with sensitivity to their effects. Some patients feel apathy, fatigue, tearfulness, emotional lability, irritability, and nervousness. Symptoms of depression may worsen. The psychiatric–mental health nurse should closely monitor these symptoms when individuals are receiving benzodiazepines as adjunctive treatment for anxiety that coexists with depression. Gastrointestinal disturbances, including nausea, vomiting, anorexia, dry mouth, and constipation, may develop. These medications may be taken with food to ease the gastrointestinal distress.

Older patients are particularly susceptible to incontinence, memory disturbances, dizziness, and increased risk for falls when using benzodiazepines. Pregnant patients should be aware that these medications cross the placenta and are associated with increased risk for birth defects, such as cleft palate, intellectual disability, and pyloric stenosis. Infants born addicted to benzodiazepines often exhibit flaccid muscle tone, lethargy, and difficulties sucking. All of the benzodiazepines are excreted in breast milk, and breastfeeding women should avoid using these medications. Infants and children metabolize these medications more slowly; therefore, more drug accumulates in their bodies.

Toxicity develops in overdose or accumulation of the drug in the body from liver dysfunction or disease. Symptoms include worsening of the CNS depression, ataxia, confusion, delirium, agitation, hypotension, diminished reflexes, and lethargy. Rarely do the benzodiazepines cause respiratory depression or death. In overdose, these medications have a high therapeutic index and rarely result in death unless combined with another CNS depressant drug, such as alcohol.

Nonbenzodiazepines: Buspirone

Buspirone, a nonbenzodiazepine, is effective in controlling the symptoms of anxiety but has no effect on panic disorders and little effect on obsessive–compulsive disorder.

Indications and Mechanisms of Actions

Nonbenzodiazepines are effective for treating anxiety disorders without the CNS depressant effects or the potential for abuse and withdrawal syndromes. Buspirone is indicated for treating generalized anxiety disorder; therefore, its target symptoms include anxiety and related symptoms, such as difficulty concentrating, tension, insomnia, restlessness, irritability, and fatigue. Because buspirone does not add to depression symptoms, it has been tried for treating anxiety that coexists with depression. In some instances, it is thought to potentiate the antidepressant actions of other medications.

Buspirone has no effect on the benzodiazepine–GABA complex but instead appears to control anxiety by blocking the serotonin subtype of receptor, $5-HT_{1A}$, at both presynaptic reuptake and postsynaptic receptor sites. It has no sedative, muscle relaxant, or anticonvulsant effects. It also lacks the potential for abuse.

Pharmacokinetics

Buspirone is rapidly absorbed but undergoes extensive first-pass metabolism. Food slows absorption but appears to reduce first-pass effects, increasing the bioavailability of the medication. Buspirone is given on a continual dosing schedule of three times a day because of its short half-life of 2 to 3 hours. Clinical action depends on reaching steady-state concentrations; taking this medication with food may facilitate this process.

Buspirone is highly protein bound but does not displace most other medications. However, it does displace digoxin and may increase digoxin levels to the point of toxicity. It is metabolized in the liver and excreted predominantly by the kidneys but also via the gastrointestinal tract. Patients with liver or kidney impairment should be given this medication with caution.

Buspirone cannot be used on a PRN basis; rather, it takes 2 to 4 weeks of continual use for symptom relief to occur. It is more effective in reducing anxiety in patients who have never taken a benzodiazepine.

Buspirone does not block the withdrawal of other benzodiazepines. Therefore, a switch to buspirone must be initiated gradually to avoid withdrawal symptoms. Nurses should closely monitor patients who are undergoing this change of medication for emergence of withdrawal symptoms from the benzodiazepines and report such symptoms to the prescriber.

Side Effects, Adverse Reactions, and Toxicity

Common side effects from buspirone include dizziness, drowsiness, nausea, excitement, and headache. Most other side effects occur at an incidence of less than 1%. There have been no reports of death from an overdose of buspirone alone. Older patients, pregnant women, and children have not been adequately studied. For now, buspirone can be assumed to cross the placenta and is present in breast milk; therefore, its use should be avoided in pregnant women, and women who are taking this medication should not breastfeed.

Sedative–Hypnotics

Sedatives reduce activity, nervousness, irritability, and excitability without causing sleep, but if given in large enough doses, they have a hypnotic effect. **Hypnotics** cause drowsiness and facilitate the onset and maintenance of sleep. These two classifications are usually referred to as **sedative–hypnotics**—drugs that have a calming effect or depress the CNS. These medications include (1) benzodiazepines, (2) GABA enhancers, (3) melatonergic hypnotics, (4) antihistamines, and (5) the orexin receptor antagonist (Table 11.11). The benzodiazepines have been previously discussed. The GABA enhancers modulate GABA-A receptors. They do not cause a high degree of tolerance or dependence and are easier to discontinue than the benzodiazepines. Melatonergic hypnotics are melatonin agonists, and antihistamines block histamines, causing sedation (Stahl, 2014). The orexin receptor antagonists block the activity of orexins, neurotransmitters involved in wakefulness and arousal. These medications are discussed thoroughly in Chapter 28.

Stimulants and Wakefulness-Promoting Agents

Amphetamines were first synthesized in the late 1800s but were not used for psychiatric disorders until the 1930s. Initially, amphetamines were prescribed for a variety of symptoms and disorders, but their high abuse potential soon became obvious.

Currently among the medications known as stimulants are methylphenidate (Ritalin, Methylin, Metadate), amphetamine sulfate, amphetamine/dextroamphetamine (Adderall), dexmethylphenidate (Focalin), lisdexamfetamine (Vyvanse), and CNS stimulants. Modafinil (Provigil) and armodafinil (Nuvigil) are wakefulness-promoting agents used for narcolepsy and other sleep disorders.

Indications and Mechanisms of Action

Medical use of these stimulants is now restricted to a few disorders, including narcolepsy, attention-deficit hyperactivity disorder (ADHD), particularly in children, and obesity unresponsive to other treatments. However, stimulants are increasingly being used as an adjunctive treatment in depression and other mood disorders to address the fatigue and low energy common to these conditions.

Amphetamines indirectly stimulate the sympathetic nervous system, producing alertness, wakefulness, vasoconstriction, suppressed appetite, and hypothermia. Tolerance develops to some of these effects, such as suppression of appetite, but the CNS stimulation continues. Although the exact mechanism of action is not completely understood, stimulants cause a release of catecholamines, particularly norepinephrine and dopamine, into the synapse from the presynaptic nerve cell. They also block reuptake of these catecholamines. Methylphenidate is

TABLE 11.11 HYPNOTICS FOR INSOMNIA

Generic (Trade) Drug Name	Usual Dosage Range (mg/day)	Elimination Half-Life (h)	Speed of Onset After Single Dose
Benzodiazepine Hypnotics			
Flurazepam	15–30	47–100	Fast
Temazepam (Restoril)	15–30	9.5–20	Moderately fast
Triazolam (Halcion)	0.25–0.5	1.5–5	Fast
Quazepam (Doral)	0.75–15	39	Fast
Estazolam (ProSom)	1	10–24	Fast
Nonbenzodiazepine Hypnotics			
Eszopiclone (Lunesta)	2–3	6	Fast
Zaleplon (Sonata)	10	1	Fast
Zolpidem (Ambien)	5–10	2.6	Fast
Zolpidem tartrate (Ambien CR)	12.5	2.6	Fast
Melatonergic Hypnotics			
Melatonin	0.1–10	0.5–0.75	Fast
Ramelteon (Rozerem)	8	1–2.6	Fast
Antihistamines			
Hydroxyzine (Vistaril)	50–100	20	Fast
Doxylamine (Unisom)	25	10	Fast
Orexin Receptor Antagonist			
Suvorexant (Belsomra)	10–20 mg	12	Fast

structurally similar to the amphetamines but produces a milder CNS stimulation. Psychostimulants should be used very cautiously in individuals who have a history of substance abuse.

Although the stimulant effects of these medications may seem logically indicated for narcolepsy, a disorder in which the individual frequently and abruptly falls asleep, the indications for childhood ADHD seem less obvious. The etiology and neurobiology of ADHD remain unclear, but psychostimulants produce a paradoxical calming of the increased motor activity characteristic of ADHD. Studies show that medication decreases disruptive activity during school hours, reduces noise and verbal activity, improves attention span and short-term memory, improves ability to follow directions, and decreases distractibility and impulsivity. Although these improvements have been well documented in the literature, the diagnosis of ADHD and subsequent use of psychostimulants with children remain matters of controversy (see Chapter 30).

Modafinil (Provigil) and armodafinil (Nuvigil), wake-promoting agents, are used for treating excessive sleepiness associated with narcolepsy, sleep apnea, and residual sleepiness for shift work sleep disorder. Armodafinil is longer acting than modafinil. The mechanism of action is unclear, but it is hypothesized that they increase glutamate and suppress GABA in the hypothalamus, hippocampus, and thalamus. There is no evidence of direct effects on dopamine, but there may be action on a dopamine transport. These drugs may increase the risk of Stevens–Johnson syndrome (Dell'Osso, Dobrea, Cremaschi, Arici, & Altamura, 2014).

Pharmacokinetics

Psychostimulants are rapidly absorbed from the gastrointestinal tract and reach peak plasma levels in 1 to 3 hours. Considerable individual variations occur between the drugs in terms of their bioavailability, plasma levels, and half-lives. Table 11.12 compares the primary psychostimulants used in psychiatry. Some of these differences are age dependent because children metabolize these medications more rapidly, producing shorter elimination half-lives.

The psychostimulants appear to be unaffected by food in the stomach and should be given after meals to reduce the appetite suppressant effects when indicated. However, changes in urine pH may affect the rate of excretion. Excessive sodium bicarbonate alkalizes the urine and reduces amphetamine secretion. Increased vitamin C or citric acid intake may acidify the urine and increase its excretion. Starvation from appetite suppression may have a similar effect. All of these drugs are highly lipid soluble, crossing easily into the CNS and the placenta. Psychostimulants undergo metabolic changes in the liver, where they may affect, or be affected by, other drugs. They are primarily excreted through the kidneys; therefore, renal dysfunction may interfere with excretion.

Psychostimulants are usually begun at a low dose and increased weekly, depending on the improvement of symptoms and occurrence of side effects. Initially, children with ADHD are given a morning dose so their school performance may be compared from morning to afternoon. Rebound symptoms of excitability and overtalkativeness may occur when use of the medication is withdrawn or after dose reduction. These symptoms also begin about 5 hours after the last dose of medication, which may affect the dosing regimen for some individuals. The return of symptoms in the afternoon for children with ADHD may require that a second dose be given at school. Prescribers should work with parents to implement other interventions after school and on weekends when the psychostimulants are not used. The severity of symptoms may require that the medications be continued during these times, but this dosing schedule should be determined after careful evaluation on an individual basis. Use of these medications should not be stopped abruptly, especially with higher doses, because the rebound effects may last for several days.

Modafinil (Provigil) is absorbed rapidly and reaches peak plasma concentration in 2 to 4 hours. Armodafinil reaches peak plasma concentration later and is maintained for 6 to 14 hours. Absorption of both may be delayed by 1 to 2 hours if taken with food. Modafinil is eliminated via liver metabolism with subsequent excretion of metabolites through renal excretion. They may interact with drugs that are metabolized by liver

TABLE 11.12	PSYCHOSTIMULANT MEDICATIONS	
Generic (Trade) Drug Name	Usual Dosage Range (mg/day)	Elimination Half-Life
Dextroamphetamine (Dexedrine)	5–40	Highly variable depending on urine pH
Methylphenidate (Ritalin)	10–60	2.4 h (children); 2.1 h (adults)
Amphetamine/dextroamphetamine (Adderall)	2.5 mg (3–5 yrs) 5 mg (6 yrs) 5–60 mg for narcolepsy	9–11 h
Dexmethylphenidate extended release (Focalin XR)	5–40 mg	3 h
Lisdexamfetamine (Vyvanse)	30 mg	<1 h

enzymes including phenytoin, diazepam, and propranolol. Concurrent use of modafinil or armodafinil and other drugs metabolized by the liver enzyme system may lead to increased circulating blood levels of the other drugs.

Side Effects, Adverse Reactions, and Toxicity

Side effects associated with psychostimulants typically arise within 2 to 3 weeks after use of the medication begins. From most to least common, these side effects include appetite suppression, insomnia, irritability, weight loss, nausea, headache, palpitations, blurred vision, dry mouth, constipation, and dizziness. Because of the effects on the sympathetic nervous system, some individuals experience blood pressure changes (both hypertension and hypotension), tachycardia, tremors, and irregular heart rates. Blood pressure and pulse should be monitored initially and after each dosage change.

Rarely, psychostimulants suppress growth and development in children. These effects are a matter of controversy, and research has produced conflicting results. Although suppression of height seems unlikely to some researchers, others have indicated that psychostimulants may have an effect on cartilage. Height and weight should be monitored several times annually for children taking these medications and compared with prior history of growth. Weight should be monitored, especially closely during the initial phases of treatment. These effects also may be minimized by drug "holidays," such as during school vacations.

Rarely, individuals may experience mild dysphoria, social withdrawal, or mild to moderate depression. These symptoms are more common at higher doses and may require discontinuation of use of medication. Abnormal movements and motor tics may also increase in individuals who have a history of Tourette syndrome. Psychostimulants should be avoided by patients with Tourette symptoms or with a positive family history of the disorder. In addition, dextroamphetamine has been associated with an increased risk for congenital abnormalities. Because there is no compelling reason for a pregnant woman to continue to take these medications, patients should be informed and should advise their prescriber immediately if they plan to become pregnant or if pregnancy is a possibility.

Death is rare from overdose or toxicity of the psychostimulants, but a 10-day supply may be lethal, especially in children. Symptoms of overdose include agitation, chest pain, hallucinations, paranoia, confusion, and dysphoria. Seizures may develop, along with fever, tremor, hypertension or hypotension, aggression, headache, palpitations, rashes, difficulty breathing, leg pain, and abdominal pain. Toxic doses of dextroamphetamine are above 20 mg, with potential death resulting from a 400-mg dose. Parents should be warned regarding the potential lethality of these medications and take preventive measures by keeping the medication in a safe place.

Side effects associated with modafinil and armodafinil include nausea, nervousness, headache, dizziness, and trouble sleeping. If the effects continue or are bothersome, patients should consult the prescriber. Modafinil and armodafinil are generally well tolerated with few clinically significant side effects. It is potentially habit forming and must be used with great caution in individuals with a history of substance abuse or dependence (Cephalon, 2017).

INTEGRATIVE AND COMPLEMENTARY HEALTH CARE

Several integrative and complementary health care options are discussed in this section.

Herbal Therapies

Integrative health care expands and incorporates treatment modalities outside the norm of Western medicine. Herbal therapies are often used in addition to or in place of antidepressants and antianxiety medication (Shah, Becicka, Talen, Edberg, & Namboodiri, 2017). An in-depth discussion of herbal therapies is outside the scope of this text, and readers are encouraged to seek additional resources from the National Center for Complementary and Integrative Health (NCCIH) within the National Institutes of Health.

This chapter discusses dietary supplements and herbal therapies commonly used by persons receiving mental health care. These are exempt from the FDA's efficacy and safety standards because they are considered food. Lack of regulation does not mean that these supplements are ineffective or unsafe. These substances can be effective but can also have adverse reactions and interact with prescribed medications. Nurses need to understand these potential interactions and assess their patients for the impact of these substances.

St. John's Wort (SJW), derived from *Hypericum perforatum L.*, is used for depression, pain, anxiety, insomnia, and premenstrual syndrome. SJW is believed to modulate serotonin, dopamine, and norepinephrine. The risk of developing serotonin syndrome is increased when taken with other serotonergic drugs. It has the potential to interact with other medications (i.e., birth control pills, digoxin) and should not be taken with prescribed antidepressants (NCCIH, 2018; Warren, Cowen, & Harmer, 2018).

Kava, derived from the *Piper methysticum* plant, is used for anxiety reduction. Kava interacts with dopaminergic transmission, inhibits the MAO-B enzyme system, and modulates the GABA receptor. It may also inhibit uptake of noradrenaline. Kava is widely used by Pacific Islanders as a social and ceremonial tranquilizing drink. In 2002, the FDA issued warnings about the risk of severe liver injury associated with kava. Several countries have restricted its use. Thrombocytopenia, leukopenia, and hearing impairment have been reported with the use of kava (NCCIH, 2018; Savage, Firth, Stough, & Sarris, 2018).

Valerian (*Valeriana officinalis*), a member of the Valerianaceae family, is a perennial plant native to Europe and Asia and naturalized to North America. Valerian is a common ingredient in products promoted for insomnia and nervousness. The evidence of its effectiveness is inconclusive. The mechanism of action is unclear, but appears to be relatively safe. There are some reports that suggest hepatotoxicity in humans (NCCIH, 2018; Savage et al., 2018).

Vitamin, Mineral, and Other Dietary Supplements

The neurotransmitters necessary for normal healthy functioning are produced from chemical building blocks taken in with the foods we eat. Many nutritional deficiencies may produce symptoms of psychiatric disorders. Fatigue, apathy, and depression are caused by deficiencies in iron, folic acid, pantothenic acid, magnesium, vitamin C, or biotin. Logically, treating these deficiencies with dietary supplements should improve the psychiatric symptoms. The question becomes: Can nutritional supplements improve psychiatric symptoms that are not the result of such deficiencies?

Tryptophan, the dietary precursor for serotonin, has been most extensively investigated as it relates to low serotonin levels and increased aggression. Individuals who have low tryptophan levels are prone to have lower levels of serotonin in the brain, resulting in depressed mood and aggressive behavior (Badawy, 2018).

Dietary supplements such as melatonin and lecithin target CNS functioning. Melatonin, a naturally occurring hormone secreted from the pineal gland, is used for treatment of insomnia and prevention of "jet lag" in air travelers. Lecithin, a precursor to acetylcholine, is used to improve memory and treat dementia. The extent to which the level of acetylcholine is raised by ingestion of lecithin is unknown (Tayebati, 2018).

Medications may also influence the development of nutritional deficiencies that may worsen psychiatric symptoms. For example, drugs with strong anticholinergic activity often produce impaired or enhanced gastric motility, which may lead to generalized malabsorption of vitamins and minerals. In addition, many vitamin and mineral supplements have toxicities of their own when given in excess. For example, daily ingestion of more than 100 mg of pyridoxine (vitamin B_6) can produce neurotoxic symptoms, photosensitivity, and ataxia. More research is needed to identify the underlying mechanisms and relationships of dietary supplements and dietary precursors of the bioamines to mood and behavior and psychopharmacologic medications. For now, it is important for the psychiatric–mental health nurse to recognize that these issues may be potential factors in improvement of the patient's mental status and target symptoms.

OTHER BIOLOGIC TREATMENTS

Although the primary biologic interventions remain pharmacologic, other somatic treatments have gained acceptance, remain under investigation, or show promise for the future. These include neurosurgery, ECT, phototherapy, and (most recently) rTMS and VNS. The use of neurosurgery is very limited and outside the scope of this text.

Electroconvulsive Therapy

For hundreds of years, seizures have been known to produce improvement in some psychiatric symptoms. Camphor-induced seizures were used in the 16th century to reduce psychosis and mania. With time, other substances, such as inhalants, were tried, but most were difficult to control or produced adverse reactions, sometimes even fatalities. ECT was formally introduced in Italy in 1938. It is one of the oldest medical treatments available and remains safely in use today. It is one of the most effective treatments for severe depression but has been used for other disorders, including mania and schizophrenia, when other treatments have failed.

With ECT, a brief electrical current is passed through the brain to produce generalized seizures lasting 25 to 150 seconds. The patient does not feel the stimulus or recall the procedure. A short-acting anesthetic and a muscle relaxant are given before induction of the current. A brief pulse stimulus, administered unilaterally on the nondominant side of the head, is associated with less confusion after ECT. However, some individuals require bilateral treatment for effective resolution of depressive symptoms. Induction of a seizure is necessary to produce positive treatment outcomes. Because individual seizure thresholds vary, the electrical impulse and treatment method also may vary. In general, the lowest possible electrical stimulus necessary to produce seizure activity is used. Blood pressure and the ECG are monitored during the procedure. This procedure is repeated two or three times a week, usually for a total of 6 to 12 treatments. Because there is no particular difference in treatment efficacy and a twice-weekly regimen produces less accumulative memory loss, this treatment course is often chosen. After symptoms have improved, antidepressant medication may be used to prevent relapse. Some patients who cannot take or do not experience response to antidepressant treatment may continue to have ECT treatment. Usually, once-weekly treatments are gradually decreased in frequency to once monthly.

The number and frequency vary depending on the individual's response.

Although ECT produces rapid improvement in depressive symptoms, its exact mechanism of antidepressant action remains unclear. It is known to downregulate β-adrenergic receptors in much the same way as antidepressant medications. However, unlike antidepressant therapy, ECT produces an upregulation in serotonin, especially 5-HT$_2$. ECT also has several other actions on neurochemistry, including increased influx of calcium and effects on second messenger systems.

Brief episodes of hypotension or hypertension, bradycardia or tachycardia, and minor arrhythmias are among the adverse reactions that may occur during and immediately after the procedure but usually resolve quickly. Common aftereffects from ECT include headache, nausea, and muscle pain. Memory loss is the most troublesome long-term effect of ECT. Many patients do not experience amnesia, but others report some memory loss for months or even years. Evidence is conflicting on the effects of ECT on the formation of memories after the treatments and on learning, but most patients experience no noticeable change. Memory loss occurring as part of the symptoms of untreated depression presents a confounding factor in determining the exact nature of the memory deficits from ECT. It is important to remember that patient surveys are positive, with most individuals reporting that they were helped by ECT and would have it again (Brown, Nowlin, Sartorelli, Smith, & Johnson, 2018).

ECT is contraindicated in patients with increased intracranial pressure. Risk also increases in patients with recent myocardial infarction, recent cerebrovascular accident, retinal detachment, or pheochromocytoma (a tumor on the adrenal cortex) and in patients at high risk for complications from anesthesia. Although ECT should be considered cautiously because of its specific side effects, added risks of general anesthesia, possible contraindications, and substantial social stigma, it is a safe and effective treatment.

Psychiatric–mental health nurses are involved in many aspects of care for individuals undergoing ECT. Informed consent is required, and all treating professionals have a responsibility to ensure that the patient's and family's questions are answered completely. Available treatment options, risks, and consequences must be fully discussed. Sometimes memory difficulties associated with severe depression make it difficult for patients to retain information or ask questions. Nurses should be prepared to restate or explain the procedure as often as necessary. Whenever possible, the individual's family or other support systems should be educated and involved in the consent process. Educational videos are available, but they should not replace direct discussions. Language should be in terms the patient and family members can understand. Other nursing interventions involve preparation of the patient before treatment, monitoring immediately after treatment, and follow-up. Many of these considerations are listed in Box 11.5.

BOX 11.5

Interventions for the Patient Receiving Electroconvulsive Therapy

- Discuss treatment alternatives, procedures, risks, and benefits with patient and family. Make sure that informed consent for ECT has been given in writing.
- Provide initial and ongoing patient and family education.
- Assist and monitor the patient who must take NPO after midnight the evening before the procedure.
- Make sure that the patient wears loose, comfortable, nonrestrictive clothing to the procedure.
- If the procedure is performed on an outpatient basis, ensure that the patient has someone to accompany him or her home and stay with him or her after the procedure.
- Ensure that pretreatment laboratory tests are complete, including a CBC, serum electrolytes, urinalysis, ECG, chest radiography, and physical examination.
- Teach the patient to create memory helps, such as lists and notepads, before the ECT.
- Explain that no foreign or loose objects can be in the patient's mouth during the procedure. Dentures will be removed, and a bite block may be inserted.
- Insert an IV line and provide oxygen by nasal cannula (usually 100% oxygen at 5 L/min).
- Obtain emergency equipment and be sure it is available and ready if needed.
- Monitor vital signs frequently immediately after the procedure, as in every postanesthesia recovery period.
- When the patient is fully conscious and vital signs are stable, assist him or her to get up slowly, sitting for some time before standing.
- Monitor confusion closely; the patient may need reorientation to the bathroom and other areas.
- Maintain close supervision for at least 12 hours and continue observation for 48 hours after treatment. Advise family members to observe how the patient manages at home, provide assistance as needed, and report any problems.
- Assist the patient to keep or schedule follow-up appointments.

CBC, complete blood count; ECG, electrocardiogram; ECT, electroconvulsive therapy; IV, intravenous; NPO, nothing by mouth.

Light Therapy (Phototherapy)

Human circadian rhythms are set by time clues (*Zeitgebers*) inside and outside the body. One of the most powerful regulators of these body patterns is the cycle of daylight and darkness.

Research findings indicate that some individuals with certain types of depression may experience disturbance in these normal body patterns or of circadian rhythms, particularly those who experience a seasonal variation in their depression. These individuals are more depressed during the winter months, when there is less light; they improve spontaneously in the spring (see Chapter 23). These individuals usually have symptoms that are somewhat different from classic depression, including fatigue, increased need to sleep, increased appetite and weight gain, irritability, and carbohydrate craving. Sometimes, the symptoms appear in the summer, and some individuals have only subtle changes without developing the full pattern. Administering artificial light to these patients during winter months has reduced these depressive symptoms.

Light therapy, sometimes called **phototherapy**, involves exposing the patient to an artificial light source during winter months to relieve seasonal depression. Artificial light is believed to trigger a shift in the patient's circadian rhythm to an earlier time. Research remains ongoing (Penders et al., 2016). The light source must be very bright, full-spectrum light, usually 2,500 lux, which is about 200 times brighter than normal indoor lighting. Harmful ultraviolet light is filtered out. Exposure to this light source has produced improvement and relief of depressive symptoms for significant numbers of seasonally depressed individuals. It produces no change for individuals who are not seasonally depressed (Mårtensson, Pettersson, Berglund, & Ekselius, 2015).

Studies have shown that morning phototherapy produces a better response than either evening or morning and evening timing of the phototherapy session. Light banks with full-spectrum light may be put together by the individual or obtained from various companies now producing these light sources. Light visors (visors containing small, full-spectrum light bulbs that shine on the eyelids) have also been developed. The patient is instructed to sit in front of the lights at a distance of about 3 ft, engaging in a variety of other activities, but glancing directly into the light every few minutes. This should be done immediately on arising and is most effective before 8 am. The duration of administration may begin with as little as 30 minutes and increase to 2 to 5 hours. One to 2 hours is usually sufficient, and the antidepressant response begins in 1 to 4 days, with the full effect usually complete after 2 weeks. Full antidepressant effect is usually maintained with daily sessions of 30 minutes (Fisher et al., 2014).

Side effects of phototherapy are rare, but eye strain, headache, and insomnia are possible. An ophthalmologist should be consulted if the patient has a pre-existing eye disorder. In rare instances, phototherapy has been reported to produce an episode of mania. Irritability is a more common complaint. Follow-up visits with the prescriber or therapist are needed to help manage side effects and assess positive results. Phototherapy should be implemented only by a provider knowledgeable in its use.

Transcranial Magnetic Stimulation

Transcranial magnetic stimulation was introduced in 1985 as a noninvasive, painless method to stimulate the cerebral cortex. Undergirding this procedure is the hypothesis that a time-varying magnetic field will induce an electrical field, which, in brain tissue, activates inhibitory and excitatory neurons, thereby modulating neuroplasticity in the brain. The low-frequency electrical stimulation from rTMS triggers lasting anticonvulsant effects in rats, and the therapeutic benefits of rTMS in humans are thought to be related to an action similar to that produced by anticonvulsant medication. The rTMS has been used for both clinical and research purposes. The rTMS stimulation of the brain's prefrontal cortex may help some depressed patients in much the same way as ECT but without its side effects (Philip et al., 2018). Thus, it has been proposed as an alternative to ECT in managing symptoms of depression. The rTMS treatment is administered daily for at least 1 week, much like ECT, except that subjects remain awake. Although proven effective for depression, rTMS does have some side effects, including mild headaches.

Vagus Nerve Stimulation

VNS sends electrical impulses to the brain to improve depression. The vagus nerve has traditionally been considered a parasympathetic efferent nerve that was responsible only for regulating autonomic functions, such as heart rate and gastric tone. However, the vagus nerve (cranial X) also carries sensory information to the brain from the head, neck, thorax, and abdomen, and research has identified that the vagus nerve has extensive projections of its sensory afferent connections to many brain areas. Although the basic mechanism of action of VNS is unknown, incoming sensory, or afferent, connections of the left vagus nerve directly project into many of the very same brain regions implicated in neuropsychiatric disorders. These help us to understand how VNS is helpful in treating psychiatric disorders. VNS connections change levels of several neurotransmitters implicated in the development of major depression, including serotonin, norepinephrine, GABA, and glutamate, in the same way that antidepressant medications produce their therapeutic effect (Redgrave et al., 2018).

Approved by the FDA for the adjunctive treatment of severe depression for adults who are unresponsive to four or more adequate antidepressant treatments, VNS is a permanent implant. VNS is not a cure for depression, and patients must be seen regularly for assessment of mood states and suicidality.

THE ISSUE OF ADHERENCE

Medications and other biologic treatments work only if they are used. On the surface, **adherence**, or **compliance** to a therapeutic routine, seems amazingly simple. However, following therapeutic regimens, self-administering medications as prescribed, and keeping appointments are amazingly complex activities that often prevent successful

> **BOX 11.6**
>
> **Common Reasons for Not Taking Medications as Prescribed**
>
> - Uncomfortable side effects and those that interfere with quality of life, such as work performance or intimate relationships
> - Lack of awareness or denial of illness
> - Stigma
> - Feeling better
> - Confusion about dosage or timing
> - Difficulties in access to treatment
> - Substance abuse

treatment. In recovery-oriented practice, the patient makes the decision to take medications. It is important that the patient does not feel coerced into taking the medication. The nurse's role is to support the patient's decision-making process and provide honest, evidence-based advice.

Adherence exists on a continuum and can be conceived of as full, partial, or nil. Partial adherence, whereby a patient either attempts to take medications but misses doses or takes more than prescribed, is by far the most common. Recent estimates indicate that on the average, 50% or more of the individuals with schizophrenia taking antipsychotic medications stop taking the medications or do not take them as prescribed. It should be remembered that problems with adherence are an issue with many chronic health states, including diabetes and arthritis, not just psychiatric disorders. Box 11.6 lists some of the common reasons for nonadherence. Psychiatric–mental health nurses should be aware that a number of factors contribute to the decision to discontinue medications.

The most often cited reasons for not taking medications as prescribed are the side effects. Medication side effects may interfere with work performance or other important aspects of the individual's life. For example, a construction worker cannot afford to be drowsy and sedated while operating a crane at a construction site, and a woman in an intimate relationship may find anorgasmia intolerable. Even though symptom improvement may be observed by health care professionals, it may not be noticed by the patient. Nurses need to be sensitive to the patient's ability to tolerate side effects and to the impact that side effects have on the patient's life. Medication choice, dosing schedules, and prompt treatment of side effects may be crucial factors in helping patients continue with their treatment.

Cognitive deficits associated with some psychiatric disorders may make it difficult for the individual to self-monitor, develop insight, make choices, remember to fill prescriptions, or keep appointments. Forgetfulness, cost, and confusion regarding dosage or timing may also contribute to noncompliance. New advances in medication formulation are designed to address some of these issues. For example, long-acting injections are designed to reduce or eliminate the need to remember an oral medication regime. Recently, the FDA approved a tablet formulation of an antipsychotic aripiprazole embedded with a digital adherence-assessment device. The system consists of an ingestible sensor, a wearable sensor, and software applications that confirm adherence. More research is needed to confirm the practicality of using the device and its effectiveness in improving treatment adherence (Papola, Gastaldon, Ostuzzi, 2018).

Family members may have similar difficulties that influence the individual not to take the medication. They may misunderstand or deny the illness, thinking, for example, "My wife's better, so she doesn't need that medicine anymore." Family members may be distressed when observable side effects occur. Adherence concerns must not be dismissed as the patient's or family's problem. Psychiatric nurses should actively address this issue. A positive therapeutic relationship between the nurse and patient and family must provide a strong sense of trust that side effects and other difficulties in treatment will be addressed and minimized. When individuals report experiencing distressing side effects, the nurse should immediately respond with assessment and interventions to reduce these effects. It is important to assess compliance often, asking questions in a nonthreatening, nonjudgmental manner. It also may be helpful to seek information from others who are involved with the patient.

Adherence can be improved by psychoeducation. This approach is most helpful if it addresses the individual's specific symptoms and concerns. For example, if the patient is having difficulty with understanding the purpose of the medication, it may be helpful to link taking it to reduction of specific unwanted symptoms or improved functioning, such as continuing to work. Family members should also be included in these discussions.

Other factors that interfere with adherence should also be assessed and plans developed to minimize their effect. For example, an individual who is being considered for clozapine therapy may have missed a number of appointments in the past. On assessment, the nurse may discover that it takes the individual 2 hours on three different buses each way to reach the clinic. The nurse can then assist with arranging for a home health nurse to visit the patient's apartment, draw blood samples for analysis, and assess side effects, thus decreasing the number of trips the patient must make to the clinic.

SUMMARY OF KEY POINTS

- Target symptoms and side effects of medications should be clearly identified. The FDA approves the use of medications for specific disorders and symptoms.

- Psychiatric medications primarily act on CNS receptors, ion channels, enzymes, and carrier proteins. Agonists mimic the action of a specific neurotransmitter; antagonists block the response.

- A drug's ability to interact with a given receptor type depends on three qualities: selectivity—the ability to interact with specific receptors while not affecting other tissues and organs; affinity—the degree of strength of the bond between drug and receptor; and intrinsic activity—the ability to produce a certain biologic response.

- Pharmacokinetics refers to how the human body processes the drug, including absorption, distribution, metabolism, and excretion. Bioavailability describes the amount of the drug that actually reaches circulation throughout the body. The wide variations in the way each individual processes any medication often are related to physiologic differences caused by age, genetic makeup, other disease processes, and chemical interactions.

- Antipsychotic medications are drugs used in treating patients with psychotic disorders, such as schizophrenia. They act primarily by blocking dopamine or serotonin postsynaptically. In addition, they have a number of actions on other neurotransmitters. Older typical antipsychotic drugs work on positive symptoms and are inexpensive but produce more side effects than the newer atypical antipsychotic drugs which work on positive and negative symptoms.

- Medication-related movement disorders are a particularly serious group of side effects that principally occur with the typical antipsychotic medications and that may be acute syndromes, such as dystonia, pseudoparkinsonism, and akathisia, or chronic syndromes, such as tardive dyskinesia.

- The mood stabilizers, or antimanic medications, are drugs used to control wide variations in mood related to mania, but these agents may also be used to treat patients with other disorders. Lithium and the anticonvulsants are chemically unrelated and act in different ways to stabilize mood.

- Antidepressant medications are drugs used primarily for treating symptoms of depression. They act by blocking reuptake of one or more of the bioamines, especially serotonin and norepinephrine. These medications vary considerably in their structure and action. Newer antidepressants, such as the SSRIs, have fewer side effects and are less lethal in overdose than the older TCAs.

- Antianxiety medications also include several subgroups of medications, but the benzodiazepines and nonbenzodiazepines are those principally used in psychiatry. The benzodiazepines act by enhancing the effects of GABA, and the nonbenzodiazepine buspirone acts on serotonin. Benzodiazepines can be used on a PRN basis, but buspirone, the one available nonbenzodiazepine, must be taken regularly.

- Psychostimulants enhance neurotransmitter activity, acting at a number of sites in the nerves. These medications are most often used for treating symptoms related to ADHD and narcolepsy.

- ECT uses the application of an electrical pulsation to induce seizures in the brain. These seizures produce a number of effects on neurotransmission that result in the rapid relief of depressive symptoms.

- rTMS and VNS are two emerging somatic treatments for psychiatric disorders. They are both means to directly affect brain function through stimulation of the nerves that are direct extensions of the brain.

- Phototherapy involves the application of full-spectrum light in the morning hours, which appears to reset circadian rhythm delays related to seasonal affective disorder and other forms of depression. Nutritional therapies are in various stages of investigation.

- Adherence refers to the ability of an individual to self-administer medications as prescribed and to follow other instructions related to medication treatment. It can be full, partial, or nil. Nonadherence is related to factors such as medication side effects, stigma, and family influences. Nurses play a key role in educating patients and helping them to improve adherence.

CRITICAL THINKING CHALLENGES

1. Discuss how you would go about identifying the target symptoms for a specific patient for the following medications: antipsychotic, antidepressant, and antianxiety drugs.
2. Track the approval process from identification of a potential substance to marketing a medication. Compare at least three psychiatric medications that are in phase III trials (hint: www.FDA.gov).
3. Obtain the PIs for the three atypical antipsychotics, two SSRIs, and one SNRI. Compare their boxed

warnings, pharmacodynamics, pharmacokinetics, indications, side effects, and dosages.

4. Compare the oral and IM doses of lorazepam. Why are these doses similar?
5. Mr. J. has schizophrenia and was just prescribed an antipsychotic. His family wants to know the risks–benefits of the medication. How would you answer?
6. Identify the CYP450 enzyme that metabolizes the following medications: risperidone, olanzapine, quetiapine, clozapine, fluoxetine, venlafaxine, trazodone, nefazodone, and bupropion.
7. Find the four medications or substances that induce or inhibit the following CYP450 enzymes: 2D6, 2C19, 3A4, and 1A2.
8. Obtain the PI for clozapine, risperidone, quetiapine, and Risperdal Consta. Compare the half-lives of each drug. Discuss the relationship of the drug's half-life to the dosing schedule. When is steady state reached in each of these medications?
9. Explain the health problems associated with anticholinergic side effects of the antipsychotic medications.
10. Compare the type of movements that characterize tardive dyskinesia with those that characterize akathisia and dystonia and explore which one is easier for a patient to experience.
11. One patient is prescribed the MAOI Emsam, 6 mg/day, and another is taking another MAOI, Nardil, 15 mg/day. Are the dietary restrictions different?
12. A patient who is taking an MAOI asks you to explain what will happen if she eats pizza. Prepare a short teaching intervention beginning with the action of the medication and its consequences.
13. Explain how your nursing care would be different for a male patient taking lithium carbonate than for a female patient.
14. Patient A is taking valproic acid (Depakote) for mood stabilization, and patient B is taking lamotrigine (Lamictal). After comparing notes with each other, they ask you why patient A has to have drug blood levels and patient B does not. How are these two drugs alike? How are they different?
15. Two patients are getting their blood drawn. One patient is getting lithium and the other clozapine. What laboratory tests are being ordered?
16. A patient who is depressed has been started on sertraline. During the assessment, she tells you that she is also taking SJW, lecithin, and a multiple vitamin. What is your next step?
17. Compare different approaches that you might use with a patient with schizophrenia who has decided to stop taking his or her medication because of intolerance to side effects.

REFERENCES

Alessandrini, M., Asfaha, S., Dodgen, T., Warnich, L., & Pepper, M. S. (2013). Cytochrome P450 pharmacogenetics in African populations. *Drug Metabolism Reviews, 45*(2), 253–275.

Badawy, A. A. (2018). Modulation of tryptophan and serotonin metabolism as a biochemical basis of the behavioral effects of use and withdrawal of androgenic-anabolic steroids and other image- and performance-enhancing agents. *International Journal of Tryptophan Research, 11*, 1–16.

Bradley, P., Shiekh, M., Mehra, V., Vrbicky, K., Layle, S., Olson, M. C., et al. (2018). Improved efficacy with targeted pharmacogenetic-guided treatment of patients with depression and anxiety: A randomized clinical trial demonstrating clinical utility. *Journal of Psychiatric Research, 96*, 100–107.

Brown, S. K., Nowlin, R. B., Sartorelli, R., Smith, J., & Johnson, K. (2018). Patient experience of electroconvulsive therapy: A retrospective review of clinical outcomes and satisfaction. *Journal of ECT, 34*(4), 240–246.

Citrome, L. (2017). Clinical management of tardive dyskinesia: five steps to success. *Journal of the Neurological sciences, 383*, 199–204.

Cephalon. (2017). *Nuvigil (armodafinil) tablets*. Retrieved December 7, 2018, from http://www.accessdata.fda.gov/drugsatfda_docs/label/2015/021875s021lbledt.pdf

Cornett, E. M., Novitch, M., Kaye, A. D., Kata, V., & Kaye, A. M. (2017). Medication-induced tardive dyskinesia: A review and update. *Ochsner Journal, 17*(2), 162–174.

Dantra, C., Swart, M., Mpeta, B., Wonkam, A., & Masimirembwa, C. (2014). Cytochrome P450 pharmacogenetics in African populations: Implications for public health. *Expert Opinion on Drug Metabolism & Toxicology, 10*(6), 769–785.

Dell'Osso, B., Dobrea, C., Cremaschi, L., Arici, C., & Altamura, A. C. (2014). Wake-promoting pharmacotherapy for psychiatric disorders. *Current Psychiatry Reports, 16*(12), 524.

Denic, A., Glassock, R. J., & Rule, A. D. (2016). Structural and functional changes with the aging kidney. *Advances in Chronic Kidney Disease, 23*(1), 19–28.

Fisher, P. M., Madsen, M. K., McMahon, B., Holst, K. K., Andersen, S. B., Laursen, H. R., et al. (2014). Three-week bright-light intervention has dose-related effects on threat-related corticolimbic reactivity and functional coupling. *Biological Psychiatry, 76*(4), 332–339.

GlaxoSmithKline. (2014). *Wellbutrin prescribing information*. Retrieved December 9, 2018, from http://www.accessdata.fda.gov/drugsatfda_docs/label/2014/018644s048,020358s055lbl.pdf

Howland, R. H. (2015). Psychiatric medications and sudden cardiac death: Putting the risk in perspective. *Journal of Psychosocial Nursing and Mental Health Services, 53*(2), 23–25.

Landgraf, D., Joiner, W. J., McCarthy, M. J., Kiessling, S., Barandas, R., Young, J. W., et al. (2016). The mood stabilizer valproic acid opposes the effects of dopamine on circadian rhythms. *Neuropharmacology, 107*, 262–270.

Laoutidis, Z. G., & Luckhaus, C. (2013). 5-HT2A receptor antagonists for the treatment of neuroleptic-induced akathisia: A systematic review and meta-analysis. *International Journal of Neuropsychopharmacology, 17*(5), 823–832.

Lohr, J. B., Eidt, C. A., Alfaraj, A. A., & Soliman, M. A. (2015). The clinical challenges of akathisia. *CNS Spectrums, 20*(Suppl 1), 1–14.

Marras, C., Austin, P. C., Bronskill, S. E., Diong, C., & Rochon, P. A. (2018). Antipsychotic drug dispensing in older adults with Parkinsonism. *American Journal of Geriatric Psychiatry, 26*(12), 1244–1257.

Mårtensson, B., Pettersson, A., Berglund, L., & Ekselius, L. (2015). Bright white light therapy in depression: A critical review of the evidence. *Journal of Affective Disorders, 182*, 1–7.

National Center for Complementary and Integrative Health (NCCIH). (2018). *Herbs at a glance*. Retrieved December 7, 2018, from https://nccih.nih.gov/health/herbsataglance.htm

Novartis. (2015). *Clozaril (prescribing information)*. Retrieved December 9, 2018, from http://www.accessdata.fda.gov/drugsatfda_docs/label/2015/019758s074lbl.pdf

O'Brien, A. (2016). Comparing the risk of tardive dyskinesia in older adults with first-generation and second-generation antipsychotics: A systematic review and meta-analysis. *International Journal of Geriatric Psychiatry, 31*(7), 683–693.

Papola, D., Gastaldon, C., & Ostuzzi, G. (2018). Can a digital medicine system improve adherence to antipsychotic treatment? *Epidemiology and Psychiatric Sciences, 27*(3), 227–229.

Penders, T. M., Stanciu, C. N., Schoemann, A. M., Ninan, P. T., Bloch, R., & Saeed, S. A. (2016). Bright light therapy as augmentation of pharmacotherapy for treatment of depression: A systematic review and meta-analysis. *Primary Care Companion for CNS Disorders, 18*(5). doi: 10.4088/PCC.15r01906.

Philip, N. S., Leuchter, A. F., Cook, I. A., Massaro, J., Goethe, J. W., & Carpenter, L. L. (2018). Predictors of response to synchronized transcranial magnetic stimulation for major depressive disorder. *Depression & Anxiety, 36*(3), 1–8.

Redgrave, J., Day, D., Leung, H., Laud, P. J., Ali, A., Lindert, R., et al. (2018). Safety and tolerability of transcutaneous vagus nerve stimulation in humans; a systematic review. *Brain Stimulation, 11*(6), 1225–1238.

Savage, K. M., Firth, J., Stough, C., & Sarris, J. (2018). GABA-modulating phytomedicines for anxiety: A systematic review of preclinical and clinical evidence. *Phytotherapy Research, 32*(1), 3–18.

Shah, A. K., Becicka, R., Talen, M. R., Edberg, D., & Namboodiri, S. (2017). Integrative medicine and mood, emotions and mental health. *Primary Care, 44*(2), 281–304.

Silva, H. (2013). Ethnopsychopharmacology and pharmacogenomics. A review. *Advances in Psychosomatic Medicine, 33*, 88–96.

Stahl, S. M. (2014). *Stahl's essential psychopharmacology: Prescriber's Guide* (5th ed.). New York, Cambridge University Press.

Tayebati, S. K. (2018). Phospholipid and lipid derivatives as potential neuroprotective compounds. *Molecules, 23*(9). pii: E2257.

Waldinger, M. D. (2015). Psychiatric disorders and sexual dysfunction. *Handbook of Clinical Neurology, 130*, 469–489.

Warren, M. B., Cowen, P. J., & Harmer, C. J. (2018). Subchronic treatment with St John's wort produces a positive shift in emotional processing in health volunteers. *Journal of Psychopharmacology, 33*(2):194–201.

Won, E., & Yong-Ku, K. (2017). An oldie but goodie: Lithium in the treatment of bipolar disorder through neuroprotective and neurotrophic mechanisms. *International Journal of Molecular Sciences, 18*(12), pii: 2679.

Yoshimura, B., Sato, K., Sakamoto, S., Tsukahara, M., Yoshimura, Y., & So, R. (2018). Incidence and predictors of acute akathisia in severely ill patients with first-episode schizophrenia treated with aripiprazole or risperidone: Secondary analysis of an observational study. *Psychopharmacology, 236*(2),723–730.

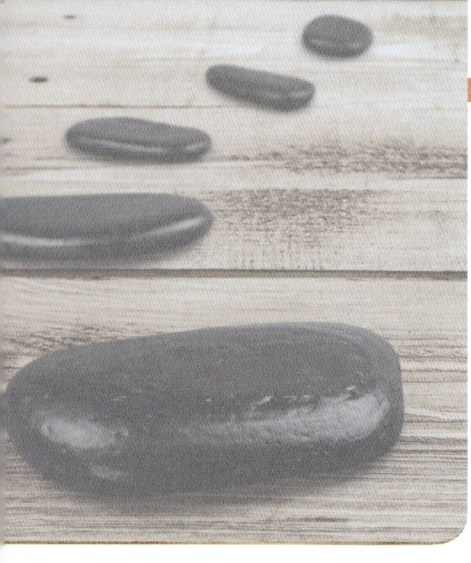

12

Group Interventions

Mary Ann Boyd

KEY CONCEPTS
- group
- group dynamics
- group process

LEARNING OBJECTIVES

After studying this chapter, you will be able to:

1. Discuss concepts used in leading groups.
2. Compare the roles that group members can assume.
3. Identify important aspects of leading a group, such as member selection, leadership skills, seating arrangements, and ways of dealing with challenging behaviors of group members.
4. Identify types of groups: psychoeducation, support, psychotherapy, and self-help.
5. Describe common nursing intervention groups.

KEY TERMS

- closed group • cohesion • coleadership • communication pathways • direct leadership • dyad • formal group roles
- group themes • groupthink • indirect leadership • individual roles • informal group roles • maintenance roles
- open group • task roles • triad

Group interventions are a key nursing strategy in mental health promotion and recovery. A group experience can help an individual enhance self-understanding, conquer unwanted thoughts and feelings, and learn new behaviors. In a group, members learn from each other as well as the leader. Group interventions are efficient because several patients can participate at one time, and they can be used in most settings. Groups can vary in purpose from being a social group attending a local ball game to an intensive psychotherapy group.

> **KEYCONCEPT** A **group** is two or more people who develop interactive relationships and share at least one common goal or issue. *A group is more than the sum of its parts.* A group develops its own personality, patterns of interaction, and rules of behavior.

Nurses in various roles and settings may use group interventions, such as when conducting patient education or leading support groups. This chapter discusses group concepts, considerations in group leadership, and types of groups that nurses commonly lead.

PREPARING TO LEAD A GROUP

Psychiatric nurses lead a wide range of groups (see later discussion of Types of Groups). Some are structured, such as a psychoeducation group, and others are unstructured (e.g., a social group). The purpose of the group will dictate the amount of structure and types of activities. In all groups, nurses maintain professional boundaries. Because some group activities are social in nature (unit parties, community trips), it is easy to forget that socialization is a treatment intervention. Nurses should avoid meeting personal social needs within this context.

Thoughtful planning and preparation make for a successful group. The following sections discuss important considerations when planning for a group.

Selecting Members

Individuals can self-refer or be referred to a group by treatment teams or clinicians, but the leader is responsible for assessing each individual's suitability for the group. In instances when a new group is forming, the leader assesses the individual's suitability for the group based on the following criteria:

- Does the purpose of the group match the needs of the potential member?
- Does the potential member have the social skills to function comfortably in the group?
- Will the other group members accept the new group member?
- Can the potential member make a commitment to attending group meetings?

Forming an Open or Closed Group

In planning for a group, one of the early decisions is whether the group will be open or closed. In an **open group**, new members may join, and old members may leave the group at different sessions. Because length of patient hospitalization is relatively short, open groups are typical on inpatient units. For example, a newly admitted patient may join an anger management group that is part of an ongoing program in an inpatient unit.

In a **closed group**, members begin the group at one time, and no new members are admitted. If a member leaves, no replacement member joins. In a closed group, participants get to know one another very well and can develop close relationships. Closed groups are more typical of outpatient groups that have a sequential curriculum or psychotherapy groups. These groups usually meet weekly for a specified period. Outpatient smoking cessation, psychotherapy, and psychoeducation groups are examples.

Determining Composition

Another decision is the group size. The size of a group will depend on the overall group goals and patients' abilities. Patients with challenging behaviors should be carefully screened and may be able to function in smaller rather than larger groups.

Small groups (usually no more than seven to eight members) become more cohesive, are less likely to form subgroups, and can provide a richer interpersonal experience than large groups (Yalom & Leszcz, 2005). A very small group is two people (**dyad**) or three (**triad**). Small groups function nicely with one group leader although many small groups are led by two people. Even though small groups cannot easily withstand the loss of members, they are ideal for patients who are highly motivated to deal with complex emotional problems, such as sexual abuse, eating disorders, or trauma or for those who have cognitive dysfunction and require a more focused group environment with minimal distractions.

In leading a small group, the leader gets to know the members very well but maintains objectivity. The nurse observes for transference of participants toward the leader or other member. If a member becomes a "favorite patient," the leader should reflect upon any underlying personal countertransference issues (see Chapter 9).

KEYCONCEPT Be prepared to select members and plan for a patient or family support group to help deal with the impact of mental illnesses on the family lifestyle.

Large groups (more than 8 to 10 members) are effective for specific problems or issues, such as smoking cessation or medication information. Large groups are often used in the workplace (Cahill & Lancaster, 2014). A large group can be ongoing and open ended. Usually, transference and countertransference issues do not develop.

However, leading a large group is challenging because of the number of potential interactions and relationships that can form and the difficulty in determining the feelings and thoughts of the participants. As the size of the group increases, the level of engagement decreases and conflict increases (LoCoco, Gullo, Lo Verso, & Kivlighan, 2013). It may be difficult to get everyone's attention to begin a group session. Subgroups can form, making it difficult to develop a cohesive group. If subgroups form that are detrimental to the group, the nurse can change the structure and function of communication within the subgroups by rearranging seating and encouraging the subgroup to interact with the rest of the group. Gender mix is also a consideration and can make a difference in the success of the group. For example, research shows that all-female and mixed gender groups rate their groups as more valuable and useful than did members of all-male groups. All-male groups and mixed groups are more task oriented than all-female groups. A high proportion of women in a mixed gender group might facilitate an early development of positive group climate (LoCoco et al., 2013).

Selecting a Leadership Style

A group is led within the context of the group leader's theoretic background and the group's purpose. For example, a leader with training in cognitive-behavioral therapy may focus on treating depression by asking members to think differently about situations, which in turn lead to feeling better. A leader with a psychodynamic orientation may focus on the feelings of depression by examining situations that generate the same feelings. Whatever the leader's theoretic background, his or her leadership behavior can be viewed on a continuum of direct to indirect.

Direct leadership behavior enables the leader to control the interaction by giving directions and information and allowing little discussion. The leader literally tells the members what to do. On the other end of the continuum is **indirect leadership**, in which the leader primarily reflects the group members' discussion and offers little guidance or information to the group. Sometimes the group needs a more direct approach, such as in a psychoeducation class; other times it needs a leader who is indirect. The challenge of providing leadership is to give sufficient direction to help the group meet its goals and develop its own group process but enough freedom to allow members to make mistakes and recover from their thinking errors in a supportive, caring, and learning environment.

Coleadership, when two people share responsibility for leading the group, is useful in most groups as long as the coleaders attend all sessions and maintain open communication. Coleadership works well when the coleaders plan together and meet before and after each session to discuss the group process.

Setting the Stage: Arranging Seating

Group sessions should be held in a quiet, pleasant room with adequate space and privacy. Holding a session in too large or too small a room inhibits communication. The sessions should be held in private rooms that nonmembers cannot access. Interruptions are distracting and can potentially compromise confidentiality. Arrangement of chairs should foster interaction and reduce communication barriers. Communication flows better when no physical barriers, such as tables, are between members. Group members should be able to see and hear each other. Arranging a group in a circle with chairs comfortably close to one another without a table enhances group work. No one should sit outside the group. If a table is necessary, a round table is better than a rectangular one, which implicitly increases the power of those who sit at the ends.

Group members tend to sit in the same places. Those who sit close to the group leader are more likely to have more power in the group than those who sit far away.

Planning the First Meeting

The leader sets the tone of the group at the first meeting. The leader and members introduce themselves. The leader may ask participants to share some introductory information such as why they joined the group and what do they hope to gain from the experience. The leader can share name, credentials for leading group, and a brief statement about experience. The leader should avoid self-disclosing personal information.

> **BOX 12.1**
>
> **Example of Group Guidelines**
>
> - Group sessions begin and end on time.
> - All views are heard and respected. Cell phones are silenced; there are no side conversations.
> - Only one person speaks at a time. No interrupting.
> - Emotion is acceptable; aggression is not. Disagreements should be expressed calmly and objectively.
> - Everyone is expected to stay for the entire meeting.
> - Who we see and what is said here stay here.

The first session is the time to explain the structure of group, including the purpose and group rules (Box 12.1). It is important the group starts and ends at scheduled times; otherwise, members who tend to be late will not change their behavior, and those who are on time will resent waiting for the others. The leader also explains when and if new members can join the group.

During the first session, the leader begins to assess the group dynamics or interactions—both verbal and nonverbal. During the course of the group sessions, these interactions will be important in understanding the group process and may determine the success of the group.

> **KEYCONCEPT Group dynamics** are the verbal and nonverbal interactions that occur in the group.

LEADING A GROUP

A group leader is responsible for monitoring and shaping the group process, as well as focusing on the group content. Although models of group development differ, most follow a pattern of a beginning, middle, and ending phase (Table 12.1) (Corey, Corey, & Corey, 2014). These stages should not be viewed as a linear progression with one preceding another but as a dynamic process that is constantly revisiting and reexamining group interactions and behaviors, as well as progressing forward. The group leader needs to be aware of the group's stage of development as well as leadership responsibilities.

> **KEYCONCEPT Group process** is the development and culmination of the session-to-session interactions of the members that move the group toward its goals.

Beginning Stage: The Honeymoon

In the beginning, the group leader acknowledges each member; constructs a working environment; develops

TABLE 12.1	COMPARISON OF MODELS OF GROUP DEVELOPMENT		
Phase	Robert Bales (1955)	William Schutz (1960)	Bruce Tuckman (1965)
Beginning	• *Orientation:* What is the problem?	• *Inclusion:* Deal with issues of belonging and being in and out of the group.	• *Forming:* Get to know one another and form a group.
Middle	• *Evaluation:* How do we feel about it?	• *Control:* Deal with issues of authority (who is in charge?), dependence, and autonomy.	• *Storming:* Tension and conflict occur; subgroups form and clash with one another. • *Norming:* Develop norms of how to work together.
Ending	• *Control:* What should we do about it?	• *Affection:* Deal with issues of intimacy, closeness, and caring versus dislike and distancing.	• *Performing:* Reach consensus and develop cooperative relationships.

From Bales, R. (1955). A set of categories for the analysis of small group interaction. *American Sociological Review*, 15, 257–263; Schutz, W. (1960). *FIRO: A three-dimensional theory of interpersonal behavior.* New York: Holt, Rinehart & Winston; Tuckman, B. (1965). Developmental sequence in small groups. *Psychological Bulletin*, 63(6), 384–399.

rapport with the members; begins to build a therapeutic relationship; and clarifies outcomes, processes, and skills related to the group's purpose (Corey et al., 2014). To carry out these functions, the leader processes group interactions by setting objectives and observing members' interactions as well as participating in the group. The leader reflects on, evaluates, and responds to interactions. The use of various techniques enhances the leader's ability to lead the group effectively and to help the group meet its goals (Table 12.2).

During beginning sessions, group members get to know one another and the group leader. The length of the beginning stage depends on the purpose of the group, the number of members, and the skill of the leader. It may last for only a few sessions or several. Members often exhibit polite, congenial behavior typical of those in new social situations. They are "good patients" and often intellectualize their problems; that is, these patients deal with emotional conflict or stress by excessively using abstract thinking or generalizations to minimize disturbing feelings. Members are usually anxious and sometimes display behavior that does not truly represent their feelings.

In this phase, members begin to test whether they can trust one another and the leader. Members may come late to group or try to extend group time. Sometime after the initial sessions, group members usually experience a period of conflict, either among themselves or with the leader. This conflict is a normal part of group development, and many believe that conflict is necessary to move into any working phase. Sometimes one or more group members become the scapegoat. Such situations challenge the leader to guide the group during this period by avoiding taking sides and treating all members respectfully.

Working Stage

The working stage of groups involves a real sharing of ideas and the development of closeness. A group personality may emerge that is distinct from the individual personalities of its members. The group develops norms, which are rules and standards that establish acceptable behaviors. Some norms are formalized, such as beginning group on time, but others are never really formalized, such as sitting in the same place each session. These normative standards encourage conformity and discourage behavioral deviations from the established norms. A member quickly learns the norms or is ostracized.

During this stage, the group realizes its purpose. If the purpose is education, the participants engage in learning new content or skills. If the aim of the group is to share feelings and experiences, these activities consume group meetings. During this phase, the group starts on time, and the leader often needs to remind members when it is time to stop.

Facilitating Group Communication

One of the responsibilities of the group leader is to facilitate both verbal and nonverbal communication to meet the treatment goals of the individual members and the entire group. Because of the number of people involved, developing trusting relationships within groups is more complicated than is developing a single relationship with a patient. The communication techniques used in establishing and maintaining individual relationships are the same for groups, but the leader also attends to the communication patterns among the members.

Encouraging Interaction

The nurse leads the group during this phase by encouraging interaction among members and being responsive to their comments. Active listening enables the leader to process events and track interactions. The nurse can then formulate responses based on a true understanding of the discussion. A group leader who listens also models

TABLE 12.2 TECHNIQUES IN LEADING GROUPS

Technique	Purpose	Example
Support: giving feedback that provides a climate of emotional support	Helps a person or group continue with ongoing activities Informs group about what the leader thinks is important Creates a climate for expressing unpopular ideas Helps the more quiet and fearful members speak up	"We really appreciate your sharing that experience with us. It looked like it was quite painful."
Confrontation: challenging a participant (needs to be done in a supportive environment)	Helps individuals learn something about themselves Helps reduce some forms of disruptive behavior Helps members deal more openly and directly with one another	"Tom, this is the third time you have changed the subject when we have talked about spouse abuse. Is something going on?"
Advice and suggestions: sharing expertise and knowledge that the members do not have	Provides information that members can use after they have examined and evaluated it Helps focus the group's task and goals	"The medication you are taking may be causing you to be sleepy."
Summarizing: statements at the end of sessions that highlight the session's discussion, any problem resolution, and unresolved problems	Provides continuity from one session to the next Brings to focus still unresolved issues Organizes the past in ways that clarify; brings into focus themes and patterns of interaction	"This session, we discussed Sharon's medication problems, and she will be following up with her physicians."
Clarification: restatement of an interaction	Checks on the meanings of the interaction and communication Avoids faulty communication Facilitates focus on substantive issues rather than allowing members to be sidetracked into misunderstandings	"What I heard you say was that you are feeling very sad right now. Is that correct?"
Probing and questioning: a technique for the experienced group leader that asks for more information	Helps members expand on what they were saying (when they are ready to) Gets at more extensive and wider range of information Invites members to explore their ideas in greater detail	"Could you tell us more about your relationship with your parents?"
Repeating, paraphrasing, highlighting: a simple act of repeating what was just said	Facilitates communication among group members Corrects inaccurate communication or emphasizes accurate communication	Member: "I forgot about my wife's birthday." Leader: "You forgot your wife's birthday."
Reflecting feelings: identifying feelings that are being expressed	Orients members to the feelings that may lie behind what is being said or done Helps members deal with issues they might otherwise avoid or miss	"You sound upset."
Reflecting behavior: identifying behaviors that are occurring	Gives members an opportunity to see how their behavior appears to others and to evaluate its consequences Helps members to understand others' perceptions and responses to them	"I notice that when the topic of sex is brought up, you look down and shift in your chair."

listening behavior for others, helping them improve their skills. Members may need to learn to listen to one another, track discussions without changing the subject, and not speak while others are talking. At the end of the session, the nurse summarizes the work of the session and projects the work for the next meeting.

The leader maintains a neutral, nonjudgmental style and avoids showing preference to one member over another. This may be difficult because some members may naturally seek out the leader's attention or ask for special favors. These behaviors are divisive to the group, and the leader should discourage them. Other important skills include providing everyone with an opportunity to contribute and respecting everyone's ideas. A leader who truly wants group participation and decision making does not reveal his or her beliefs.

Monitoring Verbal Communication

Group interaction can be viewed as a communication network that becomes patterned and predictable. In a group, verbal comments are linked in a chain formation. Monitoring verbal interactions and leading a group at the same time is difficult for one person. If there are two leaders, one may be the active leader of the group, and the other may sit outside the group and observe and record rather than participating. If all members agree, the leader can use an audio or video recorder for reviewing interaction after the group session.

Interesting interaction patterns can be observed and analyzed (Fig. 12.1). By analyzing the content and patterns, the leader can determine the existence of **communication pathways**—who is most liked in the group, who occupies a position of power, what subgroups have formed, and who is isolated from the group. People who sit next to each other tend to communicate among themselves. Usually, those who are well liked or display leadership abilities tend to be chosen for interactions more often than do those who are not. The leader can also determine if there is a change of subject when a sensitive topic is introduced.

Deciphering Content Themes

Group themes are the collective conceptual underpinnings of a group and express the members' underlying concerns or feelings regardless of the group's purpose. Themes that emerge in groups help members to understand group dynamics. Different groups have different themes. A grief group most likely would have a theme of loss or new beginnings and an adolescent group may

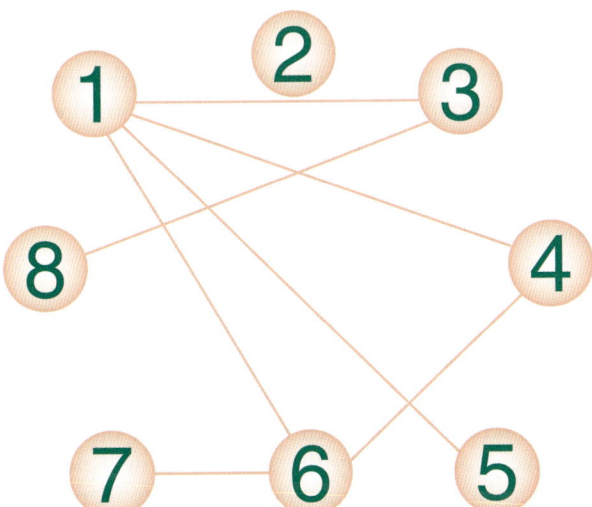

FIGURE 12.1 Sociometric analysis of group behavior. In this sociometric structure, response pattern was recorded during member interaction. Group members interacted with number 1 the most. Therefore, number 1 is the overchosen person. Numbers 5 and 7 are underchosen. Number 2 is never chosen and is determined to be the isolate.

BOX 12.2
Group Themes

A large symptom management group is ongoing at a psychiatric facility. It is coled by two nurses who are skilled in directing large groups and knowledgeable about the symptoms of mental disorders. Usually 12 people attend. The usual focus of the group is on identifying symptoms that indicate an impending reemergence of psychotic symptoms, medication side effects, and managing the numerous symptoms that medication is not controlling.

The nurses identified the appearance of the theme of powerlessness based on the following observations:

- **Session 1:** T. L. expressed his frustration at being unable to keep a job because of his symptoms. The rest of the group offered their own experiences of being unable to work.
- **Session 2:** C. R. is late to group and announces that she was late because the bus driver forgot to tell her when to get off, and she missed her stop. She is irritated with the new driver.
- **Session 3:** N. T. is out of medication and says that he cannot get more because he is out of money again. He asks the nurses to lend him some money and make arrangements to get free medication.
- **Session 4:** G. M. relies on his family for all transportation and refuses to use public transportation.

In all of these sessions, participants expressed feelings that are consistent with loss of power.

---

have a theme of independence. Although some predictable themes occur in groups, the obvious or assumed themes at the beginning may actually wind up differing from reality as the process continues. In one hospice support group, the members seemed to be focusing on the memories of their loved ones. However, upon examination of the content of their interactions, discussions were revolving around financial planning for the future (Box 12.2).

Monitoring Nonverbal Communication

Observing nonverbal communication contributes to understanding the group dynamics. Members communicate nonverbally with each other, not only the group leader. Eye contact, posture, and body gestures of one member impact other members. For example, if one member is explaining a painful experience and another member looks away and tries to engage still another, the self-disclosing member may feel devalued and rejected because the disruptive behavior is interpreted as disinterest. However, if the leader interprets the disruptive behavior as anxiety over the topic, he or she may try to engage the other member in discussing the source of the anxiety.

The leaders should monitor the nonverbal behavior of group members during each session. Often, one or two people can set the overall mood of the group. Someone who comes to a session very sad or angry can set a tone of sadness or anger for the whole group. An astute group leader recognizes the effects of an individual's mood on the total group. If the purpose of the group is to deal with emotions, the group leader may choose to discuss the member's problem at the beginning of the session. The leader, thus, limits the mood to the one person experiencing it. If the group's purpose is inconsistent with self-disclosure of personal problems, the nurse should acknowledge the individual member's distress and offer a private session after the group. In this instance, the nurse would not encourage repeated episodes of self-disclosure from that member or others.

Tracking Group Communication

The leader tracks the verbal and nonverbal interactions throughout the group sessions. Depending on the group's purpose, the leader may or may not share the observations with the group. For example, if the purpose of the group is psychoeducation, the leader may incorporate the information into a lesson plan without identifying any one individual. If the purpose of the group is to improve the self-awareness and interaction skills of members, the leader may point out the observations. The leader needs to be clear about the purpose of the group and tailor leadership strategies accordingly.

Determining Roles of Group Members

There are two official or **formal group roles**, the leader and the members; however, there are also important **informal group roles** or positions with implicit rights and duties that can either help or hinder the group's process. Ideally, one or more members assume **task roles** or functions. These individuals are concerned about the purpose of the group and "keeping things on task." For example, *information seeker* is the member who asks for clarification, the *coordinator* spells out relationships among ideas, and the *recorder* keeps the minutes.

Maintenance roles or functions are assumed by those who help keep the group together. Other members assume maintenance roles and make sure that the group members get along with each other and try to make peace if conflict erupts. These individuals are as interested in maintaining the group's cohesiveness as focusing on the group's tasks. The *harmonizer, compromiser,* and *standard setter* are examples of maintenance roles.

Both task and maintenance functions are needed in an effective group. In selecting members and analyzing the progress of the group, the leader pays attention to the balance between the task and maintenance functions. If too many group members assume task functions and too few assume maintenance functions, the group may have difficulty developing **cohesion**, or sticking together. If too many members assume maintenance functions, the group may never finish its work.

Individual roles are played by members to meet personal needs, such as feeling important or being an expert on a subject. These roles have nothing to do with the group's purpose or cohesion and can detract from the group's functioning (Box 12.3). If individual roles predominate, the group may be ineffective.

Dealing With Challenging Group Behaviors

Problematic behaviors occur in all groups. They can be challenging to the most experienced group leaders and frustrating to new leaders. In dealing with any problematic behavior or situation, the leader must remember to support the integrity of the individual members and the group as a whole.

Monopolizer

Some people tend to monopolize a group by constantly talking or interrupting others. This behavior is common in the beginning stages of group formation and usually represents anxiety that the member displaying such behavior is experiencing. Within a few sessions, this person usually relaxes and no longer attempts to monopolize the group. However, for some people, monopolizing discussions is part of their normal personality and will continue. Other group members usually find the behavior mildly irritating in the beginning and extremely annoying as time passes. Members may drop out of the group to avoid that person. The leader needs to decide if, how, and when to intervene. The best-case scenario is when savvy group members remind the monopolizer to let others speak. The leader can then support the group in establishing rules that allow everyone the opportunity to participate. However, the group often waits for the leader to manage the situation. There are a couple of ways to deal with the situation. The leader can interrupt the monopolizer by acknowledging the member's contribution but redirecting the discussion to others, or the leader can become more directive and limit the discussion time per member.

"Yes, But ..."

Some people have a patterned response to any suggestions from others. Initially, they agree with suggestions others offer them, but then they add "yes, but ..." and give several reasons why the suggestions will not work for them. Leaders and members can easily identify this patterned response. In such situations, it is best to avoid problem solving for the member and encourage the person to develop his or her own solutions. The leader can serve as a role model of the problem-solving behavior for the other members and encourage them to let the

> **BOX 12.3**
> **Roles and Functions of Group Members**
>
> **TASK ROLES**
> - *Initiator-contributor* suggests or proposes new ideas or a new view of the problem or goal.
> - *Information seeker* asks for clarification of the values pertinent to the group activity.
> - *Information giver* offers "authoritative" facts or generalizations or gives own experiences.
> - *Opinion giver* states belief or opinions with emphasis on what should be the group's values.
> - *Elaborator* spells out suggestions in terms of examples, develops meanings of ideas and rationales, and tries to deduce how an idea would work.
> - *Coordinator* shows or clarifies the relationships among various ideas and suggestions.
> - *Orienter* defines the position of the group with respect to its goals.
> - *Evaluator-critic* measures the outcome of the group against some standard.
> - *Energizer* attempts to stimulate the group to action or decision.
> - *Procedural technician* expedites group movement by doing things for the group such as distributing copies and arranging seating.
> - *Recorder* writes suggestions, keeps minutes, and serves as group memory.
>
> **MAINTENANCE ROLES**
> - *Encourager* praises, agrees with, and accepts the contributions of others.
> - *Harmonizer* mediates differences among members and relieves tension in conflict situations.
> - *Compromiser* operates from within a conflict and may yield status or admit error to maintain group harmony.
> - *Gatekeeper* attempts to keep communication channels open by encouraging or facilitating the participation of others or proposes regulation of the flow of communication through limiting time.
> - *Standard setter* expresses standards for the group to achieve.
> - *Group observer* keeps records of various aspects of group processes and interprets data to group.
> - *Follower* goes along with the movement of the group.
>
> **INDIVIDUAL ROLES**
> - *Aggressor* deflates the status of others; expresses disapproval of the values, acts, or feelings of others; attacks the group or problem; jokes aggressively; and tries to take credit for the work.
> - *Blocker* tends to be negative and resistant, disagrees and opposes without or beyond "reason," and attempts to bring back an issue after group has rejected it.
> - *Recognition seeker* calls attention to self through activities such as boasting, reporting on personal achievements, or acting in unusual ways.
> - *Self-confessor* uses group setting to express personal, non–group-oriented feelings or insights.
> - *Playboy* makes a display of lack of involvement in group's processes.
> - *Dominator* tries to assert authority or superiority in manipulating the group or certain members of the group through flattery, being directive, or interrupting others.
> - *Help-seeker* attempts to call forth sympathy from other group members through expressing insecurity, personal confusion, or depreciation of self beyond reason.
> - *Special interest pleader* speaks for a special group, such as "grass roots," usually representing personal prejudices or biases.
>
> Benne, K., & Sheats, P. (1948). Functional roles of group members. *Journal of Social Issues*, 4(2), 41–49.

member develop a solution that would work specifically for him or her.

Disliked Member

In some groups, members clearly dislike one particular member. This situation can be challenging for the leader because it can result in considerable tension and conflict. This person could become the group's scapegoat. The group leader may have made a mistake by placing the person in this particular group, and another group may be a better match. One solution may be to move the person to a better matched group. Whether the person stays or leaves, the group leader must stay neutral and avoid displaying negative verbal and nonverbal behaviors that indicate that he or she too dislikes the group member or is displeased with the other members for their behavior. Often, the group leader can manage the situation by showing respect for the disliked member and acknowledging his or her contribution. In some instances, getting supervision from a more experienced group leader is useful. Defusing the situation may be possible by using conflict resolution strategies and discussing the underlying issues.

The Silent Member

The engagement of a member who does not participate in group discussion can be challenging. This member has had a lifetime of being "the quiet one" and is usually comfortable in the silent role. The leader should respect the person's silent nature. Like all the other group members, the silent member often gains a considerable amount of information and support without verbally participating. It is best for the group leader to get to know the member and understand the meaning of the silence before encouraging interaction.

Group Conflict

Most groups experience periods of conflict. The leader first needs to decide whether the conflict is a natural part of the group process or whether the group needs to address some issues. Member-to-member conflict can be handled through conflict resolution. Leader-to-member conflict is more complicated because the leader has the formal position of power. In this instance, the leader can use conflict resolution strategies but should be sensitive to the power differential between the leader's role and the member's role.

Termination Stage or Saying Good-Bye

Termination can be difficult for a group, especially an effective one. During the final stages, members begin to grieve for the loss of the group's closeness and begin to reestablish themselves as individuals. Individuals terminate from groups as they do from any relationship. One person may not show up at the last session, another person may bring up issues that the group has already addressed, and others may demonstrate anger or hostility. Most members of successful groups are sad as the group terminates. During the last meetings, members may make arrangements for meeting after group. These plans rarely materialize or continue. Leaders should recognize these plans as part of the farewell process—saying good-bye to the group.

In terminating a group, the nurse discusses and summarizes the work of the group, including the accomplishments of members and their future plans. The nurse focuses on ending the group and avoids being pulled into working stage issues. For example, when a patient brings up an issue that was once resolved, the nurse reinforces the skills and then reminds the member of the actions that will be taken after the group has ended.

TYPES OF GROUPS

This section discusses the types of groups nurses commonly lead.

Psychoeducation Groups

The purposes of psychoeducation groups are to enhance knowledge, improve skills, and solve problems. The intervention strategies used in psychoeducation groups focus on transmission of information necessary for making some type of change and providing a process for making the change. Psychoeducation groups are formally planned, and members are purposefully selected. The group leader develops a lesson plan for each session that usually includes objectives, content outline, references, and evaluation tools. These groups are time limited and usually last for only a few sessions. If the group lasts longer than a few sessions, cohesiveness usually enhances outcomes, especially in those that teach health maintenance behaviors such as exercise and weight control (Brown, 2018).

There are a variety of psychoeducation groups, including recovery-oriented and mindfulness groups. Recovery-oriented groups facilitate consumer involvement in the educational process and build on the recovery principles (see Chapters 1 and 7). Examples of recovery-oriented groups include those that focus on how to manage a medication regimen or control angry outbursts. Group psychoeducation has changed perception of illness in persons with bipolar disorder, leading to an improvement in social functioning and improved self-esteem (Etain et al., 2018). Mindfulness groups are helpful in stress reduction (Chien, Bressington, Yip, & Karatzias, 2017).

Task Groups

Task groups focus on completion of specific activities, such as planning a week's menu. When members are strongly committed to completing a task and the leader encourages equal participation, cohesiveness promotes satisfaction and higher performance (Lockhart, 2017). To complete a task, group cohesiveness is especially important. Leaders can encourage cohesiveness by placing participants in situations that promote social interaction with minimal supervision, such as refreshment periods and team-building exercises.

Without cohesiveness, the group's true existence is questionable. In cohesive groups, members are committed to the existence of the group. In large groups, cohesiveness tends to be decreased, with subsequent poorer performance among group members in completing tasks. However, cohesiveness can be a double-edged sword. In very-cohesive groups, members are more likely to transgress personal boundaries. Dysfunctional relationships may develop that are destructive to the group process and ultimately not in the best interests of individual members.

Decision-Making Groups

The psychiatric nurse often leads decision-making groups that plan activities, develop unit rules, and select learning materials. The nurse who is leading a decision-making group should observe the process for any signs of **groupthink**, the tendency of group members to avoid conflict and adopt a normative pattern of thinking that is often consistent with the ideas of the group leader (Janis, 1972; 1982). Group members form opinions consistent with the group consensus rather than critically evaluating the situation. Groupthink is more likely to occur if the leader is respected or persuasive. It can also occur if a closed leadership style is used and external threat is present, particularly with time pressure (Goncalo, Polman, & Maslach, 2010). Many catastrophes, such as the *Challenger* explosion and Bay of Pigs invasion, have been attributed to groupthink.

There may be instances in which groupthink can lead to a reasonable decision: for example, a group decides to arrange a going-away party for another patient. In other situations, groupthink may inhibit individual thinking and problem solving: for example, a team is displaying groupthink if it decides that a patient should lose privileges based on the assumption that the patient is deliberately exhibiting bizarre behaviors. In this case, the team is failing to consider or examine other evidence that suggests the bizarre behavior is really an indication of psychosis. Another commonly occurring instance of groupthink occurs when a decision is made that is recommended by a charismatic leader who is held in high regard by staff members without the evidence to support the approach (Mannion & Thompson, 2014).

> **Concept Mastery Alert**
>
> Groupthink is the tendency of group members to avoid conflict and adopt a normative pattern of thinking that is often consistent with the ideas of the group leader. Group cohesion is the ability of the group to stick together.

Support Groups

Support groups are usually less intense than psychotherapy groups and focus on helping individuals cope with their illnesses and problems. Implementing support groups is one of the basic functions of the psychiatric nurse. In conducting this type of group, the nurse focuses on helping members cope with situations that are common for other group members. Counseling strategies are used. Leadership of the group requires group management, understanding the impact of the group process, role modeling, awareness, willingness, agreeableness, and openness (Pomery, Schofield, Xhilaga, & Gough, 2016). For example, a group of patients with bipolar illness whose illness is stable may discuss at a monthly meeting how to tell other people about the illness or how to cope with a family member who seems insensitive to the illness. Family caregivers of persons with mental illnesses benefit from the support of the group, as well as additional information about providing care for an ill family member.

Psychotherapy Groups

Psychotherapy groups treat individuals' emotional problems and can be implemented from various theoretic perspectives, including psychoanalytic, behavioral, and cognitive. These groups focus on examining emotions and helping individuals face their life situations. At times, these groups can be extremely intense. Psychotherapy groups provide an opportunity for patients to examine and resolve psychological and interpersonal issues within a safe environment. Mental health specialists who have a minimum of a master's degree and are trained in group psychotherapy lead such groups. Patients can be treated in psychotherapy and still be members of other nursing groups. Communication with the therapists is important for continuity of care.

One of the most respected approaches is Irvin D. Yalom's model of group psychotherapy. According to Yalom and Leszcz (2005), there are 11 primary factors through which therapeutic changes occur (Table 12.3). In this model, interpersonal relationships are very important because change occurs through a corrective emotional experience within the context of the group. The group is viewed as a social microcosm of the patients' psychosocial environment (Yalom & Leszcz, 2005).

TABLE 12.3 YALOM'S THERAPEUTIC FACTORS

Therapeutic Factors	Definition
Instillation of hope	Hope is required to keep patients in therapy
Universality	Finding out that others have similar problems
Imparting information	Didactic instruction about mental health, mental illness, and so on
Altruism	Learning to give to others
Corrective recapitulation of the primary family group	Reliving and correcting early family conflicts within the group
Development of socializing techniques	Learning basic social skills
Imitative behavior	Assuming some of the behaviors and characteristics of the therapist
Interpersonal learning	Analog of therapeutic factors in individual therapy, such as insight, working through the transference, and corrective emotional experience
Group cohesiveness	Group members' relationship to the therapist and other group members
Catharsis	Open expression of affect to purge or "cleanse" self
Existential factors	Patients' ultimate concerns of existence: death, isolation, freedom, and meaninglessness

From Yalom, I., & Leszcz, M. (2005). *The theory and practice of group psychotherapy.* New York: Basic Books.

Self-Help Groups

Self-help groups are led by people who are concerned about coping with a specific problem or life crisis. These groups do not explore psychodynamic issues in depth. Professionals usually do not attend these groups or serve as consultants. Alcoholics Anonymous, Overeaters Anonymous, and One Day at a Time (a grief group) are examples of self-help groups.

Age-Related Groups

Group interventions for specific age groups require attention to the developmental needs of the group members, any physical and mental impairments, social ability, and cognitive level. Children's groups should be structured to accommodate their intellectual and developmental functioning. Groups for older people should be adapted for age-related changes of the members (Box 12.4).

BOX 12.4

Working With Older People in Groups

SELF-ASSESSMENT
Because most group leaders do not have personal experience with the issues faced by older adults, the leaders should sensitize themselves to the positive and negative aspects of aging and the developmental issues facing older adults. Leaders need to be aware of their own negative reactions to aging and how this might affect their work.

COHORT EXPERIENCES
There is a wide variation in the experiences and history of older adults. Current 80- to 90-year-old adults grew up in the Great Depression of the 1930s, 65- to 80-year-old adults commonly experienced growing up during World War II, and the Baby Boomers (ages 55 to 65 years) were teenagers or young adults during the political and sexual revolution of the 1960s.

TYPICAL THEMES IN GROUP MEETINGS
- **Continuity with the past:** Older adults enjoy recalling, reliving, and reminiscing about past accomplishments.
- **Understanding the modern world:** They often use groups to understand and adapt to the modern world.
- **Independence:** They worry about becoming dependent. Physical and cognitive impairments are threats to independence. Loss of family members and friends are also threats. Leaders should be familiar with the grieving processes.
- **Changes in family relationships:** Family relationships, especially with children and grandchildren, are increasingly important as social roles change.
- **Changes in resources and environment:** Living on a fixed income focuses older people on the importance of their disposable income. They are more vulnerable to community and neighborhood changes because of their physical and financial limitations.

GROUP LEADERSHIP
- The pace of group meetings should be slowed.
- Greater emphasis should be placed on using wisdom and experience rather than learning new information.
- The group should be encouraged to use life review strategies such as autobiography and reminiscence.
- Teaching new coping skills should be placed within the context of previous attempts to resolve issues and problems (Toseland & Rizzo, 2004).

BOX 12.5

Medication Group Protocol

PURPOSE: Develop strategies that reinforce a self-medication routine.

DESCRIPTION: The medication group is an open, ongoing group that meets once a week to discuss topics germane to self-administration of medication. Members will not be asked to disclose the names of their medications.

MEMBER SELECTION: The group is open to any person taking medication for a mental illness or emotional problem who would like more information about medication, side effects, and staying on a regimen. Referrals from mental health providers are encouraged. Each person will meet with the group leader before attending the group to determine if the group will meet the individual's learning needs.

STRUCTURE: The format is a small group, with no more than eight members and one psychiatric nurse group leader facilitating a discussion about the issues. Topics are rotated.

TIME AND LOCATION: 2:00 to 3:00 PM, every Wednesday at the Mental Health Center.

COST: No charge for attending.

TOPICS
- How Do I Know If My Medications Are Working?
- Side Effect Management: Is It Worth It?
- Hints for Taking Medications Without Missing Doses!
- Health Problems That Medications Affect
- (Other topics will be developed to meet the needs of group members.)

EVALUATION: Short pretest and posttest for instructor's use only.

COMMON NURSING INTERVENTION GROUPS

Nurses lead groups of varying types that are geared toward a specific content area such as medication management, symptom management, anger management, and self-care skills. In addition, nurses' groups focus on other issues such as stress management, relaxation, and women's issues. A competent leader integrates group leadership, knowledge, and skills with nursing interventions that fit a selected group.

Medication Groups

Nurse-led medication groups are common in psychiatric nursing. Not all medication groups are alike, so the nurse must be clear regarding the purpose of each specific medication group (Box 12.5). A medication group can be used primarily to transmit information about medications, such as action, dosage, and side effects, or it can focus on issues related to medications, such as compliance, management of side effects, and lifestyle adjustments. Many nurses incorporate both perspectives.

Assessing a member's medication knowledge is important before he or she joins the group to determine what the individual would like to learn. People with mental illness may have difficulty remembering new information, so assessment of cognitive abilities is important. Assessing attention span, memory, and problem-solving skills gives valuable information that nurses can use in designing the group. The nurse should determine the members' reading and writing skills to select effective patient education materials.

An ideal group is one in which all members use the same medication. In reality, this situation is rare. Usually, the group members are using various medications. The nurse should know which medications each member is taking, but to avoid violating patient confidentiality, the nurse needs to be careful not to divulge that information to other patients. If group members choose, they can share the names of their medications with one another. A small group format works best, and the more interaction, the better. Using a lecture method of teaching is less effective than involving the members in the learning process. The nurse should expose the members to various audio and visual educational materials, including workbooks, videotapes, and handouts. The nurse should ask members to write down information to help them remember and learn through various modes. Evaluation of the learning outcomes begins with the first class. Nurses can develop and give pretests and posttests, which in combination can measure learning outcomes.

Symptom Management Groups

Nurses often lead recovery-oriented groups that focus on helping patients deal with a severe and persistent mental illness. Handling hallucinations, being socially appropriate, and staying motivated to complete activities of daily living are a few common topics. In symptom management groups, members also learn when a symptom indicates that relapse is imminent and what to do about it. Within the context of a symptom management group, patients can learn how to avoid relapse.

Anger Management Groups

Anger management is another common topic for a nurse-led group, often in the inpatient setting. The purposes of an anger management group are to discuss the concept of anger, identify antecedents to aggressive behavior, and develop new strategies to deal with anger other than verbal and physical aggression (see Chapter 14). The treatment team refers individuals with histories of being verbally and physically abusive, usually to family members, to these groups to help them better understand their emotions and behavioral responses. Impulsiveness and emotional lability are problems for many of the group members. Anger management usually includes a discussion of associated stressful situations, events that trigger anger, feelings about the situation, and unmet personal needs.

Self-Care Groups

Another common nurse-led recovery-oriented psychiatric group is a self-care group. People with psychiatric illnesses often have self-care deficits and benefit from the structure that a group provides. These groups are challenging because members usually know how to perform these daily tasks (e.g., bathing, grooming, performing personal hygiene), but their illnesses cause them to lose the motivation to complete them. The leader not only reinforces the basic self-care skills but also, more importantly, helps identify strategies that can motivate the patients and provide structure to their daily lives.

Reminiscence Groups

Reminiscence therapy has been shown to be a valuable intervention for older clients. In this type of group, members are encouraged to remember events from past years.

Such a group is easily implemented. Usually, a simple question about an important family event will spark memories. Reminiscence groups are usually associated with patients who have dementia who are having difficulty with recent memory. Reminiscence groups can also be used as an intergenerational intervention with healthy older adults and children. These groups can also reduce symptoms of depression, and improve aspects of quality of life, negative attitudes toward old age (Siverová & Bužgová, 2018).

SUMMARY OF KEY POINTS

- The definition of group can vary according to theoretic orientation. A general definition is that a group is two or more people who have at least one common goal or issue. Group dynamics are the interactions within a group that influence the group's development and process.

- Groups can be open, with new members joining at any time, or closed, with members admitted only once. Either small or large groups can be effective, but dynamics change in different size groups.

- The process of group development occurs in phases: beginning, middle, and termination. These stages are not fixed but dynamic. The process challenges the leader to guide the group. During the working stage, the group addresses its purpose.

- Leading a group involves many different functions, from obtaining and receiving information to testing and evaluating decisions. The leader should explain the rules of the group at the beginning of the group.

- Verbal communication includes the communication network and group themes. Nonverbal communication is more complex and involves eye contact, body posture, and the mood of the group. Decision-making groups can be victims of groupthink, which can have positive or negative outcomes. Groupthink research is ongoing.

- Seating arrangements can affect group interaction. The fewer physical barriers there are, such as tables, the better the communication. Everyone should be a part of the group, and no one should sit outside of it. In the most interactive groups, members face one another in a circle.

- Leadership skills involve listening; tracking verbal and nonverbal behaviors; and maintaining a neutral, nonjudgmental style.

- Although there are only two formal group roles, leader and member, there are many informal group roles. These roles are usually categorized according to purpose—task functions, maintenance functions, and individual roles. Members who assume task functions encourage the group members to stay focused on the group's task. Those who assume maintenance functions worry more about the group working together than the actual task itself. Individual roles can either enhance or detract from the work of the group.

- The leader should address behaviors that challenge the leadership, group process, or other members to determine whether to intervene. In some instances, the leader redirects a monopolizing member; at other times, the leader lets the group deal with the behavior. Group conflict occurs in most groups.

- There are many different types of groups. Psychiatric nurses lead psychoeducation and support groups. Mental health specialists who are trained to provide intensive therapy lead psychotherapy groups. Consumers lead self-help groups, and professionals assist only as requested. Leading age-related groups requires attention to the developmental, physical, social, and intellectual abilities of the participants. Themes of older adult groups include continuity with the past, understanding the modern world, independence, and changes in family and resources. Group leadership for older adult groups builds on participants' previous experiences and coping abilities in developing new coping skills.

- Medication, symptom management, anger management, and self-care groups are common nurse-led groups focused on specific interventions.

CRITICAL THINKING CHALLENGES

1. Group members are very polite to one another and are superficially discussing topics. You would assess the group as being in which phase? Explain your answer.
2. After three sessions of a support group, two members begin to share their frustration with having a mental illness. The group is moving into which phase of group development? Explain your answer.
3. Define the roles of the task and maintenance functions in groups. Observe your clinical group and identify classmates who are assuming task functions and maintenance functions.
4. Observe a patient group for at least five sessions. Discuss the seating pattern that emerges. Identify the communication network and the group themes. Then identify the group's norms and standards.
5. Discuss the conditions that lead to groupthink. When is groupthink positive? When is groupthink negative? Explain.
6. List at least six behaviors that are important for a group leader, including one for age-related groups. Justify your answers.
7. During the first meeting, one member seems very anxious and tends to monopolize the conversation. Discuss how you would assess the situation and whether you would intervene.
8. At the end of the fourth meeting, one group member angrily accuses another of asking too many questions. The other members look on quietly. How would you assess the situation? Would you intervene? Explain.

1998: *12 Angry Men*

In this excellent film, a young man stands accused of fatally stabbing his father. A jury of his "peers" is deciding his fate. This jury is portrayed by an excellent cast, including Jack Lemmon, George C. Scott, Tony Danza, and Ossie Davis. At first, the case appears to be "open and shut." This film depicts an intense struggle to reach a verdict and is an excellent study of group process and group dynamics.

Viewing Points: Identify the leaders in the group. How does leadership change throughout the film? Do you find any evidence of groupthink? How does the group handle conflict?

REFERENCES

Brown, N. W. (2018). *Psychoeducational groups: Process and practice* (4th ed.). New York: Taylor & Frances Group.

Cahill, K., & Lancaster, T. (2014). Workplace interventions for smoking cessation. (Review). *The Cochrane Collaborative, 2*, CD003440.

Chien, W. T., Bressington, D., Yip, A., & Karatzias, T. (2017). An international multi-site, randomized controlled trial of a mindfulness-based psychoeducation group programme for people with schizophrenia. *Psychological Medicine, 47*(12), 2018–2096.

Corey, M. S., Corey, G., & Corey, C. (2014). *Group process and practice* (9th ed.). Belmont, CA: Brooks Cole.

Etain, B., Scott, J., Cochet, B., Bellivier, F., Boudebesse, C., Drancourt, N., et al. (2018). A study of the real-world effectiveness of group psychoeducation for bipolar disorders: is change in illness perception a key mediator of benefit. *Journal of Affective Disorders, 227*, 714–720.

Goncalo, J. A., Polman, E., & Maslach, C. (2010). Can confidence come too soon? Collective efficacy, conflict and group performance over time. *Organizational Behavior & Human Decision Processes, 113*(1), 13–24.

Janis, I. (1972). *Victims of groupthink*. Boston, MA: Houghton Mifflin.

Janis, I. (1982). *Groupthink* (2nd ed.). Boston, MA: Houghton Mifflin.

Lockhart, N. C. (2017). Social network analysis as an analytic tool for task group research: A case study of an interdisciplinary community of practice. *The Journal for Specialists in Group Work, 62*(3), 152–175.

LoCoco, G., Gullo, S., Lo Verso, G., & Kivlighan, D. M. Jr. (2013). Sex composition and group climate: A group actor-partner interdependence analysis. *Group Dynamics: Theory, Research, and Practice, 17*(4), 270–280.

Mannion, R., & Thompson, C. (2014). Systematic biases in group decision-making: Implications for patient safety. *International Journal for Quality in Health Care, 26*(6), 606–612.

Pomery, A., Schofield, P., Xhilaga, M., & Gough, K. (2016). Skills, knowledge and attributes of support group leaders: A systematic review. *Patient Education and Counseling, 99*, 672–688.

Siverová, J., & Bužgová, R. (2018). The effect of reminiscence therapy of quality of life, attitudes to ageing, and depressive symptoms on institutionalized elder adults with cognitive impairment: A quasi-experimental study. *International Journal of Mental Health Nursing, 27*(5), 1430–1439.

Toseland, R. W., & Rizzo, V. M. (2004). What's different about working with older people in groups? *Journal of Gerontological Social Work, 44*(1/2), 5–23.

Yalom, I., & Leszcz, M. (2005). *The theory and practice of group psychotherapy*. New York: Basic Books.

UNIT IV
PREVENTION OF MENTAL DISORDERS

13
Stress and Mental Health

Mary Ann Boyd

KEY CONCEPTS
- adaptation
- allostatic load
- appraisal
- coping
- stress

LEARNING OBJECTIVES

After studying this chapter, you will be able to:

1. Discuss the concept of stress as it relates to mental health and mental illness.
2. Differentiate acute stress from chronic stress.
3. Discuss the factors that lead to allostatic load.
4. Discuss psychosocial factors that influence the experience of stress.
5. Discuss the variety of stress responses experienced by individuals.
6. Explain the role of coping and adaptation in maintaining and promoting mental health.
7. Apply critical thinking skills to the nursing process for a person experiencing stress.

KEY TERMS

- acute stress • allostasis • chronic stress • diathesis • emotion-focused coping • emotions • general adaptation syndrome • homeostasis • problem-focused coping • reappraisal • social functioning • social network • social support • stress response • Transactional Stress Model

---

Stress is a natural part of life, yet it is one of the most complex concepts in health and nursing. Although often thought of as negative, stress can be a positive experience when an individual approaches it with successful coping skills. For example, children learn to cope with stressful situations in preparation for adulthood. During severe stress, some people draw on resources that they never realized they had and grow from those experiences. However, early childhood stress and trauma, unresolved stress, or chronic stress can have negative mental and physical health consequences.

Stress is also associated with the development or exacerbation of symptoms of mental illness. For example, a stressful event may precipitate a psychosis. Family caregivers can develop depression as they continually monitor their family member, cope with illness-related behaviors, and often witness deterioration of their significant other (Gilhooly et al., 2016).

Stress is approached from several overlapping theoretical perspectives—physiologic, psychological, and social. Consequently, there are many definitions of stress depending on the theoretical perspective. This chapter provides an overview of the major evidence-based theories of stress and describes the applicability of the models in the practice of nursing.

BIOLOGIC PERSPECTIVES OF STRESS

Physiologic responses to stress are automatic and differ based on the event, duration, and intensity. Concepts, homeostasis, and allostasis are the foundation of the physiologic responses to stressful events.

Homeostasis versus Allostasis

The concept of **homeostasis**, which is the body's tendency to resist physiologic change and hold bodily functions relatively consistent, well-coordinated, and usually stable, was introduced by Walter Cannon in the 1930s. The body's internal equilibrium is regulated by physiologic processes such as blood glucose, pH, and oxygen. Set points (normal reference ranges of physiologic parameters) are maintained (Cannon, 1932).

Allostasis is a term used to describe the dynamic regulatory process that maintains homeostasis through a process of adaptation. Physiologic stability is achieved when the autonomic nervous system; the HPA; and the cardiovascular, metabolic, and immune systems respond to internal and external stimuli (McEwen, Gray, & Nasca, 2015).

Acute Stress

Acute stress, an intense biopsychosocial reaction to a threatening event, is time limited (usually less than a month), but can occur repeatedly. It can lead to physiologic overload, which in turn can have a negative impact on a person's health.

Acute stress is associated with the "fight-or-flight" response. When the brain (amygdala and hippocampus) interprets an event as a threat, the hypothalamus and autonomic nervous system are signaled to secrete adrenaline, cortisol, and epinephrine. These hormones activate the sympathetic nervous system and physiologic stability is challenged. A "fight-or-flight" response occurs when the heart rate, blood pressure, and blood sugar increase. Energy is mobilized for survival. As the sympathetic system is activated, the parasympathetic is muted (Table 13.1). After there is no longer a need for more energy and the threat is over, the body returns to a state of homeostasis.

Chronic Stress

Chronic stress is an ongoing physiologic reaction to events resulting in "wear and tear" on the body and negatively impacts health and well-being. The adaptive physiologic changes that occur during acute stress become maladaptive when prolonged and contribute to the risk for illness. The relationship between chronic stress and illness was identified many years ago with the introduction of the **general adaptation syndrome** (GAS).

General Adaptation Syndrome

Hans Selye, who is credited with initiation of the study of stress, defined stress as a nonspecific response to an

TABLE 13.1	FIGHT AND FLIGHT: PHYSIOLOGIC CHANGES	
Sympathetic Nervous System Effect	**Purpose**	**Parasympathetic Nervous System Conservation of Energy**
Increased serum glucose	Increased energy	Decreased sexual and sex hormone activity
Increased cardiac output and blood pressure (increase in renin and angiotensin)	Increased blood flow	Decreased growth, repair, and maturation
Increased oxygen tension and hematocrit	Increased supply of oxygen in blood	Decreased digestion, assimilation, and whole-food distribution
Other Physiologic Changes		
Effect	**Purpose**	
Increased immune responses	Reduced risk of infections	
Heightened vigilance in the brain	Increased decision-making attention and memory	
Hyperactivation of the hemostatic and coagulation systems	Prevention of excessive bleeding from wounds	

Adapted from Diamond, J. W. (2009). Allostatic medicine: Bringing stress, coping, and chronic disease into focus. Part 1. *Integrative Medicine*, 8(6), 40–44.

irritant, a perceived danger, or a life threat. He called stress evoked by positive emotions or events *eustress* and stress evoked by negative feelings and events *distress*. He showed that corticosteroid secretion from the pituitary gland increased during stress and contributed to development of illnesses. Selye described this process as GAS (Selye, 1956; 1974). This early work set the stage for our understanding of the role of the hypothalamic–pituitary–adrenal (HPA) in chronic stress.

We now understand that the sympathetic nervous system activates the HPA axis. When the hypothalamus secretes corticotropin-releasing hormone (CRH), the pituitary gland increases secretion of adrenocorticotropic hormone (corticotropin), which in turn stimulates the adrenocortical secretion of cortisol. Over time, excessive exposure of cortisol contributes to the dysregulation of the autonomic nervous system.

Allostatic Load

Today, chronic stress is associated with an allostatic load (AL), the cumulative changes of the biologic regulatory systems (cardiovascular, metabolic, and immune) as indicated by abnormal laboratory values. As wear and tear on the brain and body occurs, there is a corresponding increase in the AL (Fig. 13.1). The greater the AL, the greater the state of chronic stress and ultimately, the more negative changes in health (Duong, Bingham, Aldana, Chung, & Sumner, 2016; McEwen, 2015)

> **KEYCONCEPT** Allostatic load is the consequence of the wear and tear on the body and brain and leads to ill health.

Paradoxically, the same systems that are protective in acute stress can damage the body when activated by chronic stress. The benefits of the increase in circulating cortisol to the human body are initially adaptive, but if it continues, it can be quite damaging to both mental (depression) and physical (immune, cardiovascular, and metabolic) health (McVicar, Ravalier, & Greenwood, 2013; Sterling, 2012).

Consequences of Chronic Stress

In chronic stress, the immune system is suppressed. Cortisol is primarily immunosuppressive and contributes to reduction in lymphocyte numbers and function (primarily T-lymphocyte and monocyte subsets) and natural killer (NK) activities. The immune cells have receptors for cortisol and catecholamines that can bind with lymphatic cells and suppress the immune system. The continuous sustained activation of the sympathetic nervous system; HPA axis; cardiovascular, metabolic, and immune systems contributes to a hormonal overload, leading to impairment in memory, immunity, cardiovascular, and metabolic functions (McEwen, 2017).

Over time, chronic stress compromises health and increases susceptibility to illnesses. For instance, children who have suffered psychological neglect, abuse, or parental loss are more likely to display mood or anxiety disorders during adulthood (Benjet, Borges, & Medina-Mora, 2010). Elevation of white blood cell counts and lower counts of T, B, and NK cells are found in those who face academic examinations, job strain, caregiving for a family member with dementia, marital conflict, and daily stress. Altered parameters of immune function are present in those with negative moods (chronic hostility, depression, and anxiety), social isolation, and marital disagreement. Antibody titers to Epstein–Barr and herpes simplex viruses are also elevated in stressed populations. If the stress is long term, the immune alteration continues (McEwen, 2017).

Health disparities found in lower socioeconomic groups, racial and ethnic minorities, and older adults may be partly explained by the chronic stress they tend to experience. Elevated AL has been shown to exist in these groups and in relatively young women with histories of high stress and especially those with posttraumatic stress disorder (PTSD) and depression (Clark, Bond, & Hecker, 2007; Duong et al., 2016; Glover, Stuber, & Poland, 2006; Juruena, 2014; McEwen, 2017; Peek et al., 2010; Seeman, Epel, Gruenewald, Karlamangla, & McEwen, 2010) (see Box 13.1).

FIGURE 13.1 The development of allostatic load in response to stress. (Redrawn with permission from McEwen, B. S. [1998]. Protective and damaging effects of stress and stress mediators. *New England Journal of Medicine*, 3[38], 171–179. Copyright 1998 Massachusetts Medical Society. Reprinted with permission from Massachusetts Medical Society.)

BOX 13.1
Research for Best Practice: Allostatic Load

Chyu, L., & Upchurch, D. M. (2018). A longitudinal analysis of allostatic load among a multi-ethnic sample of midlife women: Findings from the study of women's health across the nation. Women's Health Issues, 28(3), 258–266.

THE QUESTION: Does AL increase over time (reflecting health declines and physiologic aging) in midlife women (42–52 years old)? Is lower socioeconomic status associated with higher AL?

METHODS: A community-based, multisite, prospective study examined biopsychosocial changes during menopausal transition among a cohort of midlife women (N = 1,932; 13,391 observations). Ten biomarkers were used to represent AL across cardiovascular, inflammatory, metabolic, and neuroendocrine systems. AL scores were calculated at baseline and at annual visits at seven time points. Higher AL scores indicated poorer health.

FINDINGS: Older age at baseline, lower household income, African American race, and speaking and reading English only were significant predictors of higher AL scores.

IMPLICATIONS FOR NURSING: AL can be used to identify high-risk women and begin early prevention and intervention to reduce disease burden and disparities at the population level.

Chronic Stress and Mental Illness

When stress is associated with the development or exacerbation of a mental illness, the diathesis–stress model can be applied. In this model, a **diathesis** or a genetic predisposition increases susceptibility of developing a disorder. As a result, adverse events during childhood increase the risk of alcohol and drug dependence, eating disorders, affective disorders, PTSD, and suicidal behavior. For example, a woman whose mother had a long history of depression (indicating a genetic predisposition to mental disorders for the daughter) and who was assaulted as she was leaving work and sustained multiple injuries. Her first manic episode occurred within 2 months (see Chapter 22).

No one lives in a stress-free environment, yet stress reduction leads to positive mental health. Conversely, many patients attribute their first illness episode to a stressful event such as an assault, rape, or family tragedy.

PSYCHOSOCIAL PERSPECTIVES OF STRESS

The **Transactional Stress Model** describes the psychological experience of stress. This model views stress as an interactive process arising from real or perceived internal or external environmental demands that are appraised as threatening or benign (Fig. 13.2) (Lazarus & Folkman, 1984). The external environment includes physical aspects such as air quality, cleanliness of food and water, temperature, and noise and social aspects such as living arrangements and personal contacts.

> **KEYCONCEPT** **Stress** is a process arising from real or perceived internal or external environmental demands that are appraised as threatening or benign (Lazarus & Folkman, 1984).

Appraisal

Appraisal, a key psychological concept, is the perception that an event or situation is a threat. One situation may be extremely perceived as threatening to one person but not to another (Box 13.2). The more important or meaningful the event, the more vulnerable the person is to stress. For example, chest pain is threatening not only because of the immediate pain and incapacitation, but the pain may mean a heart attack is occurring. The individual is afraid that he or she may not have the physiologic resources to survive the attack.

> **KEYCONCEPT** **Appraisal** is the process where potentially stressful events are evaluated for meaning and significance to individual well-being (Lazarus & Folkman, 1984).

BOX 13.2 CLINICAL VIGNETTE
Stress Responses to an Examination

Two students are preparing for the same examination. Susan is genuinely interested in the subject, prepares by studying throughout the semester, and reviews the content 2 days before test day. The night before the examination, she goes to bed early, gets a good night's sleep, and wakes refreshed but is slightly nervous about the test. She wants to do well and expects a difficult test but knows that she can retake it at a later date if she does poorly.

In contrast, Joanne is not interested in the subject matter and does not study throughout the semester. She "crams" 2 days before the test date and does an "all nighter" the night before. This is the last time that Joanne can take the examination, but she believes that she will pass because she has already taken it twice and is familiar with the questions. If she does not pass, she will not be able to return to school. On entering the room, Joanne is physically tired and somewhat fearful of not passing the test. As she looks at the test, she instantly realizes that it is not the examination she expected. The questions are new. She begins hyperventilating and tremoring. After yelling obscenities at the teacher, she storms out of the room. She is very distressed and describes herself as "being in a panic."

What Do You Think?
- How are the students' experiences different? Are there any similarities?
- Are there any nursing diagnoses that apply to Joanne's situation?

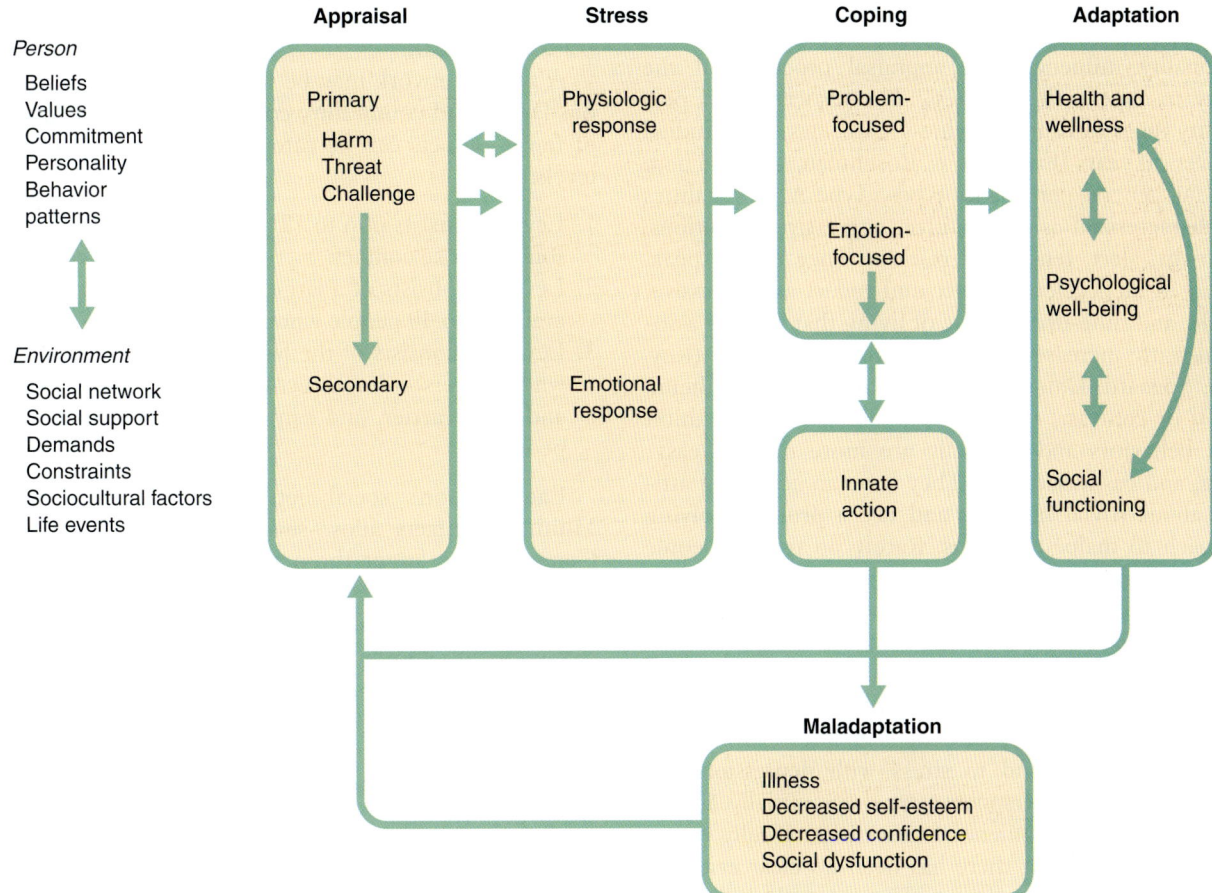

FIGURE 13.2 Stress, coping, and adaptation model.

Appraisal is a complex process that includes many aspects—the demands, constraints, and resources are balanced with personal goals and beliefs. A critical factor is the risk of the event to a person's well-being (Carpenter, 2016; Lazarus, 2001).

The appraisal process has two levels: primary and secondary. In a primary appraisal, a person evaluates the events occurring in his or her life as a threat, harm, or challenge. During primary appraisal of a goal, the person determines whether (1) the goal is relevant, (2) the goal is consistent with his or her values and beliefs, and (3) whether a personal commitment is present. In the vignette, Susan's commitment to the goal of doing well on the test was consistent with her valuing the content, which in turn motivated her to study regularly and prepare carefully for the examination. She believed that the test would be difficult. Joanne had a commitment to pass the test but did not value the content. Unlike Susan, Joanne believed that the test would be relatively easy because she expected the questions to be the same as those on the previous examination.

In a secondary appraisal, the person explains the outcome of events. There may be blame or credit given for the outcome. In the example, Susan was nervous but took the test. Joanne's secondary appraisal of the test-taking situation began with the realization that she might not pass the test because the questions were different. She acted impulsively by blaming the teacher for giving a different examination and by storming out of the room. She clearly did not cope effectively with a difficult situation.

Values and Goals

Cultural, ethnic, family, and religious values shape the significance of the event. What is important to one person may not be to another. For example, one person may value a high-paying salary and another may value the freedom to move around without the boundaries of material things.

If a goal (such as maintaining an important position) is important, a person is more likely to do what it takes to reach the goal. The more important the goal or the more difficult the goal is to obtain, the greater the likelihood of stress. For example, students who earn mostly or all As often feel more stress about examinations than do students who earn Bs and Cs because the higher grade is more difficult to obtain.

Personality Types

Personality influences the appraisal process and the ability to cope with the stress. The association of personality types to health or illness status has been studied for over 50 years (Friedman & Rosenman, 1974). There are four general personality types. Type A personalities are characterized as competitive, aggressive, ambitious, impatient, alert, tense, and restless. They think, speak, and act at an accelerated pace and reflect an aggressive, hostile, and time-urgent style of living that is often associated with increased psychophysiologic arousal (Roy, 2018; Sogaard, Dalgard, Holme, Røysamb, & Håheim, 2008). In contrast, type B personalities do not exhibit these behaviors and generally are more relaxed, easygoing, and easily satisfied. They have an accepting attitude about trivial mistakes and use a problem-solving approach to major problems. Rarely do type B people push themselves to obtain excesses from the environment or try to accomplish too much in too little time (Tishler, Bartholomae, & Rhodes, 2005).

Type C personalities are described as having difficulty expressing emotion and are introverted, respectful, conforming, compliant, and eager to please and avoid conflict. They respond to stress with depression and hopelessness. This personality type was initially associated with the development of cancer, specifically breast cancer in women, but there has been no clear evidence that the stress associated with this personality type has a role in the etiology of cancer (Bryant-Lukosius, 2003; Lală, Bobîrnac, & Tipa, 2010). It is more likely that this personality type will experience more depression and difficult marital adjustment (Bozo, Yagmur, & Eldoğan, 2017).

Type D (distressed) personalities experience increased negative emotion (depression) and pessimism and are unlikely to show their emotions to others. There is mixed research support for an association between a type D personality and mental health disorder and poor physical health status (Marchesi et al., 2014; Stevenson & Williams, 2014). Emerging data suggest that type D personality is related to the severity of acute coronary syndrome and diabetes (Conti, Carrozzino, Patierno, Vitacolonna, & Fulcheri, 2016; Garcia-Retamero, Petrova, Arrebola-Moreno, Catena, & Ramírez-Hernández, 2016).

Social Networks

A **social network** consists of linkages among a defined set of people with whom an individual has personal contacts. A social identity develops within this network (Azmitia, Syed, & Radmacher, 2008). Emotional support, material aid, services, information, and new social contacts increase personal resources, enhance the ability to cope with change, and influence the course of illnesses (Li & Wu, 2010).

A social network may be large, consisting of numerous family and community contacts, or small, consisting of few. Contacts can be categorized according to three levels:

1. Level I consists of 6 to 12 people with whom the person has close contact.
2. Level II consists of a larger number of contacts, generally 30 to 40 people whom the person sees regularly.
3. Level III consists of the large number of people with whom a person has direct contact, such as the grocer and mail carrier, and can represent several hundred people.

Each person's social network is slightly different. Multiple contacts allow several networks to interact. Generally, the larger the network, the more support is available. An ideal network structure is fairly dense and interconnected; people within the network are in contact with one another. Dense networks are better able to respond in times of stress and crisis and to provide emotional support to those in distress. For example, residents of a small town are more likely to provide food and shelter to fire victims than neighbors in a large urban area who have little contact with each other.

Ideally, a balance between intense and less intense relationships exists in a social network. When relationships are intense and include only one or two people, the opportunity to interact with other network members is limited. On the other hand, isolation can occur without at least a few intense relationships.

Social networks provide opportunities for give and take. Network members both provide and receive support, aid, services, and information. Reciprocity is particularly important because most friendships do not last without the give and take of support and services. A person who is always on the receiving end eventually becomes isolated from others.

Social Support

One of the important functions of the social network is to provide **social support** in the form of positive interpersonal interactions as part of a dynamic process that is in constant flux and varies with life events and health status (Whatley, Dilorio, & Yeager, 2010). Not all interpersonal interactions within a network are supportive. A person can have a large, complex social network but little social support. Some life events, such as marriage, divorce, and bereavement, actually change the level of social support by adding to or subtracting from a person's social network.

Social support serves three functions:

1. Emotional support contributes to a person's feelings of being cared for or loved.

TABLE 13.2	EXAMPLES OF FUNCTIONS OF SOCIAL SUPPORT
Function	Example
Emotional support	Attachment, reassurance, being able to rely on and confide in a person
Tangible support	Direct aid such as loans or gifts, services such as taking care of someone who is ill, doing a job or chore
Informational support	Providing information or advice, giving feedback about how a person is doing

Reprinted with permission from Schaefer, C., Coyne, J., & Lazarus, R. (1982). The health-related functions of social support. *Journal of Behavioral Medicine, 4*(4), 381–406.

2. Tangible support provides a person with additional resources.
3. Informational support helps a person view situations in a new light (Table 13.2).

Social support enhances health outcomes and reduces mortality by helping members make needed behavior changes and buffering stressful life events. In a supportive social environment, members feel helped, valued, and in personal control. Healthy people are likely to have strong support systems that help them cope with undesirable life events.

Cultural Factors

Cultural expectations and role strain serve as both demands and constraints in the experience of stress. If a person violates cultural group values to meet role expectations, stress occurs; for example, a person may stay in an abusive relationship to avoid the stress of violating a cultural norm that values lifelong marriage, no matter what the circumstances. The potential guilt associated with norm violation and the anticipated isolation from being ostracized seem worse than the physical and psychological pain caused by the abusive situation.

Employment Factors

Employment is another highly valued cultural norm and provides social, psychological, and financial benefits. In all cultures, work is assigned significance beyond economic compensation. It is often the central focus of adulthood and, for many, a source of personal identity. Even if employment brings little real happiness, being employed implies financial needs are being met. Work offers status, regulates life activities, permits association with others, and provides a meaningful life experience. Although work is demanding, unemployment can actually be more stressful because of the associated isolation and loss of social status.

Gender Influences

Gender expectations often become an additional source of demands and constraints for women, who assume multiple roles. In most cultures, women who work outside the home are expected to assume primary responsibility for care of the children and household duties. Most women are adept at separating these roles and can compartmentalize problems at work from those at home. When there is a healthy balance between work and home, women experience a low level of psychological stress. However, when the balance is disturbed, daily stress contributes to health problems (Low, Thurston, & Matthews, 2010).

Life Events

In 1967, Holmes and Rahe (1967) presented a psychosocial view of illness by pointing out the complex relationship between life changes and the development of illnesses. They hypothesized that people become ill after they experience major life events, such as marriage, divorce, and bereavement. The more frequent the changes, the greater the possibility of becoming sick. The investigators cited the events that they believed partially accounted for the onset of illnesses and began testing whether these life changes were actual precursors to illness. It soon became clear that not all events have the same effects. For example, the death of a spouse is usually much more devastating and stressful than a change in residence. From their research, the investigators were able to assign relative weights to various life events according to the degree of associated stress. Rahe (1994) devised the Recent Life Changes Questionnaire (Table 13.3) to evaluate the frequency and significance of life-changing events. Numerous research studies subsequently demonstrated the relationship between a recent life change and the severity of near-future illness (Rahe, 1994; Rahe et al., 2002). Recent studies show that life changes in older adults that resulted in feeling helpless or fearing for their life reported higher body mass index and more chronic illnesses (Seib et al., 2014). If several life changes occur within a short period, the likelihood that an illness will appear is even greater (Tamers et al., 2014).

RESPONSES TO STRESS

A **stress response** includes simultaneous physiologic and emotional responses. The physiologic stress responses were previously discussed. Emotional responses to stress depend on the significance of the event experience. It is now known that people experience stress differently depending on their gender. Whereas males are more likely to respond to stress with a fight-or-flight response, females have less aggressive responses; they "tend and befriend" (McEwen, 2005).

TABLE 13.3 RECENT LIFE CHANGES QUESTIONNAIRE

Life Changes	LCU Values[a]	Life Changes	LCU Values[a]
Family		Change in sleeping habits	31
Death of spouse	105	Revision of personal habits	31
Marital separation	65	Change in eating habits	29
Death of close family member	65	Change in church activities	29
Divorce	62	Vacation	29
Pregnancy	60	Change in school	28
Change in health of family member	52	Change in recreation	28
Marriage	50	Christmas	26
Gain of new family member	50	*Work*	
Marital reconciliation	42	Fired at work	64
Spouse begins or stops work	37	Retirement from work	49
Son or daughter leaves home	29	Trouble with boss	39
In-law trouble	29	Business readjustment	38
Change in number of family get-togethers	26	Change to different line of work	38
Personal		Change in work responsibilities	33
Jail term	56	Change in work hours or conditions	30
Sex difficulties	49	*Financial*	
Death of a close friend	46	Foreclosure of mortgage or loan	57
Personal injury or illness	42	Change in financial state	43
Change in living conditions	39	Mortgage (e.g., home, car)	39
Outstanding personal achievement	33	Mortgage or loan less than $10,000 (e.g., stereo)	26
Change in residence	33		
Minor violations of the law	32		
Begin or end school	32		

Directions: Sum the life-change units (LCUs) for your life-changing events during the past 12 months.
250–400 LCUs per year: Minor life crisis.
Over 400 LCUs per year: Major life crisis.
[a]LCU, life-change unit. The number of LCUs reflects the average degree or intensity of the life change.
Reprinted with permission from Rahe, R. H. (2000). Recent Life Changes Questionnaire (RLCQ).

Emotional Responses

Emotions (psychophysiologic reactions that define a person's mood) are usually ones of excitement or distress marked by strong feelings and usually accompanied by an impulse toward definite action. If the emotions are intense, a disturbance in intellectual functions occurs. When the situation is viewed as a challenge, emotions are more likely to be positive. If the event is evaluated as threatening or harmful, negative emotions are elicited. Emotions can be categorized as follows:

- *Negative emotions* occur when there is a threat to, delay in, or thwarting of a goal or a conflict between goals: anger, fright, anxiety, guilt, shame, sadness, envy, jealousy, and disgust.
- *Positive emotions* occur when there is movement toward or attainment of a goal: happiness, pride, relief, and love.
- *Borderline emotions* are somewhat ambiguous: hope, compassion, empathy, sympathy, and contentment.
- *Nonemotions* connote emotional reactions but are too ambiguous to fit into any of the preceding categories: confidence, awe, confusion, and excitement (Lazarus, 2006).

Emotions are expressed as themes that summarize dangers or benefits of each stressful situation. For instance, physical danger provokes fear; a loss leads to feelings of sadness (Table 13.4). Emotions have their own innate responses that are automatic and unique; for example, anger may automatically provoke tremors in one person but both tremors and perspiration in another. Emotions often provoke impulsive behavior. For example, the first impulse of a young musician facing his first performance at Carnegie Hall who experiences stage fright is to run home. As he resists this impulse, he begins coping with his fears in order to perform.

COPING

Coping is a deliberate, planned, and psychological effort to manage stressful demands. The coping process may

TABLE 13.4	CORE RELATIONAL THEMES FOR EACH EMOTION
Emotion	Relational Meaning
Anger	A demeaning offense against me and mine
Anxiety	Facing an uncertain, existential threat
Fright	Facing an immediate, concrete, and overwhelming physical danger
Guilt	Having transgressed a moral imperative
Shame	Having failed to live up to an ego ideal
Sadness	Having experienced an irrevocable loss
Envy	Wanting what someone else has
Jealousy	Resenting a third party for the loss of or a threat to another's affection
Disgust	Taking in or being too close to an indigestible object or idea (metaphorically speaking)
Happiness	Making reasonable progress toward the realization of a goal
Pride	Enhancement of one's ego identity by taking credit for a valued object or achievement, either our own or that of someone or a group with whom we identify
Relief	A distressing goal/incongruent condition that has changed for the better or gone away
Hope	Fearing the worst but yearning for better
Love	Desiring or participating in affection, usually but not necessarily reciprocated
Compassion	Being moved by another's suffering and wanting to help

Adapted from Lazarus, R. S. (2006). *Stress and emotion: A new synthesis.* New York: Springer. By permission of Oxford University Press, USA.

inhibit or override the innate urge to act. Positive coping leads to adaptation, which is characterized by a balance between health and illness, a sense of well-being, and maximum social functioning. When a person does not cope well, maladaptations occur that can shift the balance toward illness, a diminished self-concept, and deterioration in social functioning.

KEYCONCEPT **Coping** is a deliberate, planned, and psychological effort to manage stressful demands.

There are two types of coping. In **problem-focused coping**, the person attacks the source of stress and solves the problem (eliminating it or changing its effects), which changes the person–environment relationship. In **emotion-focused coping**, the person reduces the stress by reinterpreting the situation to change its meaning (Boxes 13.3 and 13.4).

No one coping strategy is best for all situations. Coping strategies work best in particular situations. Over time, these strategies become automatic and develop into patterns for each person. Hopefully, the strategies are effective. Some situations require a combination of strategies and activities. Ideally, a stressful situation is matched with the needed resources as the events are unfolding. Social support can be critical in helping people cope with difficult situations. Successful coping with life stresses is linked to quality of life and to physical and mental health (Lazarus, 2001).

BOX 13.3

Ways of Coping: Examples of Problem- versus Emotion-Focused Coping

PROBLEM-FOCUSED COPING
- When noise from the television interrupts a student's studying and causes the student to be stressed, the student turns off the television and eliminates the noise.
- An abused spouse is finally able to leave her husband because she realizes that the abuse will not stop even though he promises never to hit her again.

EMOTION-FOCUSED COPING
- A husband is adamantly opposed to visiting his wife's relatives because they keep dogs in their house. Even though the dogs are well cared for, their presence in the relative's home violates his need for an orderly, clean house and causes the husband sufficient stress that he copes with by refusing to visit. This becomes a source of marital conflict. One holiday, the husband is given a puppy and immediately becomes attached to the dog, who soon becomes a valued family member. The husband then begins to view his wife's relatives differently and willingly visits their house more often.
- A mother is afraid that her teenage daughter has been in an accident because she did not come home after a party. Then the woman remembers that she gave her daughter permission to stay at a friend's house. She immediately feels better.

BOX 13.4

Research for Best Practice: Emotion- versus Problem-Focused Coping for Health Threats

del-Pino-Casado, R., Pérez-Cruz, M., & Frías-Osuna, A. (2014). Coping, subjective burden and anxiety among family caregivers of older dependent. Journal of Clinical Nursing, 23, 3335–3344.

THE QUESTION: Do stressors, coping, and subjective burden contribute to anxiety in caregivers?

METHODS: Data from 140 family caregivers were analyzed using descriptive statistics, correlation coefficients, and path analysis. Sociodemographic data and several scales were used to collect data.

FINDINGS: Stressors, coping, emotion-focused coping, dysfunctional coping, and subjective burden were related to greater anxiety.

IMPLICATIONS FOR NURSING: Stressors, dysfunctional coping, and subjective burden can be used in clinical practice for early detection of and early intervention for anxiety. Problem solving, positive reappraisal, assertiveness, and control of negative thoughts may not be as effective in reducing anxiety.

As a part of the coping process, reappraisal is important because of the changing nature of the stressful situation. **Reappraisal**, which is the same as appraisal except that it happens after coping, provides feedback about the outcomes and allows for continual adjustment to new information.

ADAPTATION

Adaptation can be conceptualized as a person's capacity to survive and flourish (Lazarus, 2006). Adaptation or lack of it affects three important areas: health, psychological well-being, and social functioning. A period of stress may compromise any or all of these areas. If a person copes successfully with stress, he or she returns to a previous level of adaptation. Successful coping results in an improvement in health, well-being, and social functioning. Unfortunately, at times, maladaptation occurs.

> **KEYCONCEPT Adaptation** is a person's capacity to survive and flourish. Adaptation affects three important areas: health, psychological well-being, and social functioning.

It is impossible to separate completely the adaptation areas of health, well-being, and social functioning. A maladaptation in any one area can negatively affect the others. For instance, the appearance of psychiatric symptoms can cause problems in performance in the work environment that in turn elicit a negative self-concept. Although each area will be discussed separately, the reader should realize that when one area is affected, most likely all three areas are affected.

Healthy Coping

Health can be negatively affected by stress when coping is ineffective and the damaging condition or situation is not ameliorated or the emotional distress is not regulated. Examples of ineffective coping include using emotion-focused coping when a problem-focused approach is appropriate, such as if a woman reinterprets an abusive situation as her fault instead of getting help to remove herself from the environment. In addition, if a coping strategy violates cultural norms and lifestyle, stress is often exaggerated. Some coping strategies actually increase the risk for mortality and morbidity, such as the excessive use of alcohol, drugs, or tobacco. Many people use overeating, smoking, or drinking to reduce stress. They may feel better temporarily but are actually increasing their risk for illness. For people whose behaviors exacerbate their illnesses, learning new behaviors becomes important. Healthy coping strategies such as exercising and obtaining adequate sleep and nutrition contribute to stress reduction and the promotion of long-term health.

Psychological Well-Being

An ideal outcome to a stress response is feeling good about how stress is handled. Of course, outcome satisfaction for one person does not necessarily represent outcome satisfaction for another. For instance, suppose that two students receive the same passing score on an examination. One may feel a sense of relief, but the other may feel anxious because he appraises the score as too low. Understanding a person's emotional response to an outcome is essential to analyzing its personal meaning. People who consistently have positive outcomes from stressful experiences are more likely to have positive self-esteem and self-confidence. Unsatisfactory outcomes from stressful experiences are associated with negative mood states, such as depression, anger, guilt leading to decreased self-esteem, and feelings of helplessness. Likewise, if the situation was appraised as challenging rather than harmful or threatening, increased self-confidence and a sense of well-being are likely to follow. If the situation was accurately appraised as harmful or threatening but viewed as manageable, the outcome may also be positive.

Social Functioning

Social functioning, the performance of daily activities within the context of interpersonal relations and family and community roles, can be seriously impaired during stressful episodes. For instance, a person who is experiencing the stress of a divorce may not be able to carry out job responsibilities satisfactorily. Social functioning continues to be impaired if the person views the outcome as unsuccessful and experiences negative emotions. If successful coping with a stressful encounter leads to a positive outcome, social functioning returns to normal or is improved.

NURSING CARE FOR THE PERSON EXPERIENCING STRESS

The overall goals in the nursing care of the person experiencing stress are to resolve the stressful person–environment situation, reduce the stress response, and develop positive coping skills. The goals for those who are at high risk for stress (experiencing recent life changes, vulnerable to stress, or have limited coping mechanisms) are to recognize the potential for stressful situations and strengthen positive coping skills through education and practice.

Stress responses vary from one person to another. Acute stress is easier to recognize than chronic stress. In many instances, living with chronic stress has become a way of life and is no longer recognized. If there are significant emotional or behavioral symptoms in response to an identifiable stressful situation, a diagnosis of adjustment disorder may be made (American Psychiatric Association, 2013). From the assessment data, the nurse can determine any illnesses, the intensity of the stress response, and the effectiveness of coping strategies. Nurses typically identify stress responses in people or family members who are receiving treatment for other health problems.

Mental Health Nursing Assessment

The assessment of a person experiencing stress should include a careful health history, current stressful event, and coping resources. If a psychiatric disorder is present, symptoms may spontaneously reappear even when no alteration has occurred in the patient's treatment regimen.

Physical Assessment

Review of Systems

A systems review can elicit the person's own unique physiologic response to stress and can also provide important data on the effect of chronic illnesses. These data are useful for understanding the person–environment situation and the person's stress reactions, coping responses, and adaptation.

Physical Functioning

Physical functioning usually changes during a stress response. Typically, sleep is disturbed, appetite either increases or decreases, body weight fluctuates, and sexual activity changes. Physical appearance may be uncharacteristically disheveled—a projection of the person's feelings. Body language expresses muscle tension, which conveys a state of anxiety not usually present. Because exercise is an important strategy in stress reduction, the nurse should assess the amount of physical activity, tolerance for exercise, and usual exercise patterns. Determining the details of the person's exercise pattern and any recent changes can help in formulating reasonable interventions.

Pharmacologic Assessment

In assessing a person's coping strategies, the nurse needs to ask about the use of alcohol, tobacco, marijuana, and any other addictive substances. Many people begin or increase the frequency of using these substances as a way of coping with stress. In turn, substance abuse contributes to the stress behavior. Knowing details about the person's use of these substances (number of times a day or week, amount, circumstances, side effects) helps in determining the role these substances play in overall stress reduction or management. The more important the substances are in the person's handling of stress, the more difficult it will be to change the addictive behavior.

Stress also often prompts people to use antianxiety medication without supervision. Use of over-the-counter and herbal medications is also common. The nurse should carefully assess the use of any drugs to manage stress symptoms. If drugs are the primary coping strategy, further evaluation is needed with a possible referral to a mental health specialist. If a psychiatric disorder is present, the nurse should assess medication compliance, especially if the psychiatric symptoms are reappearing.

Psychosocial Assessment

Unlike assessment for other mental health problems, psychological assessment of the person under stress does not ordinarily include a mental status examination. Instead, psychological assessment focuses on the person's emotions and their severity, as well as his or her coping strategies. The assessment elicits the person's appraisal of risks and benefits, the personal meaning of the situation, and the person's commitment to a particular outcome. The nurse can then understand how vulnerable the person is to stress.

Using therapeutic communication techniques, a person's emotional state is assessed in a nurse–patient interview. By beginning the interview with a statement such as, "Let's talk about what you have been feeling," the nurse can elicit the feelings that the person has been experiencing. Identifying the person's emotions can be helpful in assessing the intensity of the stress being experienced. Negative emotions (anger, fright, anxiety, guilt, shame, sadness, envy, jealousy, and disgust) are usually associated with an inability to cope and experiencing severe stress.

After identifying the person's emotions, the nurse determines how the person reacts initially to them. For example, does the person who is angry respond by carrying out the innate urge to attack someone whom the person blames for the situation? Or does that person respond by thinking through the situation and overriding the initial innate urge to act? The person who tends to act impulsively has few real coping skills. For the person who can resist the innate urge to act and has developed coping skills, the focus of the assessment becomes determining their effectiveness.

In an assessment interview, it can be determined whether the person uses problem- or emotion-focused coping strategies effectively. Problem-focused coping is effective when the person can accurately assess the situation. In this case, the person sets goals, seeks information, masters new skills, and seeks help as needed. Emotion-focused coping is effective when the person has inaccurately assessed the situation and coping corrects the false interpretation.

Social assessment data are invaluable in determining the person's resources for positive coping. The ability to make healthy lifestyle changes is strongly influenced by the person's health beliefs and family support system. Even the expression of stress is related to social factors, particularly cultural expectations and values.

Assessment could include the use of the Recent Life Changes Questionnaire (refer to Table 13.3) to determine the number and importance of life changes that the patient has experienced within the past year. If several recent life changes have occurred, the person–environment relationship has changed. The person is likely to be either at high risk for or already experiencing stress.

The assessment should include identification of the person's social network. Because employment is the mainstay of adulthood and the source of many personal contacts, assessment of any recent changes in employment status is important. If a person is unemployed, the nurse should determine the significance of the unemployment and its effects on the person's social network. For children and adolescents, nurses should note any recent changes in their attendance at school. The nurse should elicit the following data:

- Size and extent of the patient's social network, both relatives and nonrelatives, professional and nonprofessional, and how long known
- Functions that the network serves (e.g., intimacy, social integration, nurturance, reassurance of worth, guidance and advice, access to new contacts)
- Degree of reciprocity between the patient and other network members; that is, who provides support to the patient and who the patient supports
- Degree of interconnectedness; that is, how many of the network members know one another and are in contact

Priority of Nursing Care

There are several possible priorities of nursing care depending on the individual's response to stress. For patients with changes in eating, sleeping, or activity, the priorities of care can focus on reestablishing these functional patterns. For other patients, the priorities may focus on psychological issues such as low self-esteem, fear, and hopelessness. Other patients may not have the psychological resources to cope with the situation, which will lead to a focus on coping skills.

Nursing Interventions

People under stress can usually benefit from approaches to supporting healthy behaviors. Activities of daily living are usually interrupted, and the affected individuals often feel that they have no time for themselves. The stressed person who is normally fastidiously groomed and dressed may appear disheveled and unkempt. Simply reinstating the daily routine of shaving (for a man) or applying makeup (for a woman) can improve the person's outlook on life and ability to cope with the stress.

Stress is commonly manifested in the areas of nutrition and activity. During stressful periods, a person's eating patterns change. To cope with stress, a person may either overeat or become anorexic. Both are ineffective coping behaviors and actually contribute to stress. Educating the patient about the importance of maintaining an adequate diet during the period of stress will highlight its importance. It will also allow the nurse to help the person decide how eating behaviors can be changed.

Exercise can reduce the emotional and behavioral responses to stress. In addition to the physical benefits of exercise, a regular exercise routine can provide structure to a person's life, enhance self-confidence, and increase feelings of well-being. People who are stressed are often not receptive to the idea of exercise, particularly if it has not been a part of their routine. Exploring the patient's personal beliefs about the value of activity will help to determine whether exercise is a reasonable activity for that person.

The person under stress tends to be tense, nervous, and on edge. Simple relaxation techniques help the person relax and may improve coping skills. If these techniques do not help the patient relax, distraction or guided imagery may be taught to the patient (see Chapter 10). In some instances, a patient should be referred to a mental health specialist for hypnosis or biofeedback should be considered for patients who have severe stress responses.

Psychosocial Nursing Interventions

Numerous interventions help reduce stress and support coping efforts. All of the interventions are best carried out within the framework of a supportive nurse–patient relationship.

Problem Solving

Assisting patients to develop appropriate problem-solving strategies based on personal strengths and previous experiences is important in understanding and coping with stressful situations. Some aspects of any situation cannot be changed, such as a family member's illness or death of a loved one, but usually there are areas within the patient's control that can be changed. For example, a caregiver cannot reverse the family member's disability, but she can arrange for short-term respite.

Encouraging patients to examine times when coping has been successful and examine aspects of that situation can help in identifying strengths and strategies for the current problem. For example, a young mother was completely overwhelmed with feelings of inadequacy after the birth of her third child. Further assessment revealed that the patient's mother had helped during the 6 weeks after the other children had been born. The patient's mother was not available for the third birth. First, the nurse validated that having three children could be overwhelming for anyone. The nurse also explained the postpartum hormonal may be contributing to the patient's feelings and that many mothers experience similar feelings. Finally, together, the nurse and the patient identified resources in her environment that could support her during the postpartum period.

Family Interventions

People who are coping with stressful situations can often benefit from interventions that facilitate family unit functioning and promote the health and welfare of all family members. To intervene with the total family, the stressed person must agree for the family members to be involved. If the data gathered from the assessment of supportive and unsupportive factors indicate that the family members are not supportive, the nurse should assist the patient to consider expanding his or her social network. If the family is the major source of support, the nurse should design interventions that support the functioning of the family unit. Parent education can also be effective in supporting family unit functioning. If family therapy is needed, the nurse should refer the family to an advanced practice specialist.

Evaluation and Treatment Outcomes

The treatment outcomes established in the initial plan of care guide the evaluation. Individual outcomes relate to improved health, well-being, and social function. Depending on the level of intervention, there can also be family and network outcomes. Family outcomes may be related to improved communication or social support; for instance, caregiver stress is reduced when other members of the family help in the care of the ill member. Social network outcomes focus on modifying the social network to increase support for the individual.

SUMMARY OF KEY POINTS

- Stress affects everyone. Coping with stress can produce positive and negative outcomes. The person can learn and grow from the experience or maladaptation can occur.
- The concept of homeostasis is the body's tendency to resist physiologic change and hold bodily functions relatively consistent, well-coordinated, and usually stable.
- When the brain interprets an event as a threat, physiologic stability is challenged, and a "fight-or-flight" response occurs.
- Allostasis describes a dynamic regulatory process that maintains homeostasis through a process of adaptation. Physiologic stability is achieved when the autonomic nervous system; the HPA; and the cardiovascular, metabolic, and immune systems respond to internal and external stimuli. As wear and tear on the brain and body occur, there is a corresponding increase in the number of abnormal biologic parameters called the AL. AL is an indication of chronic stress.
- Stress is defined as an environmental pressure or force that puts strain on a person's system. Acute stress can lead to physiologic overload, which in turn can have a negative impact on a person's health, well-being, and social functioning. Chronic stress is associated with AL that can lead to negative health outcomes.
- Stress responses are determined by the interaction with environment and the individual's cognitive appraisal of the risks and benefits of a situation. Stress responses are simultaneously emotional and physiologic, leading to an innate tendency to act.
- Many personal factors, such as personality patterns, beliefs, values, and commitment to an outcome, interact with environmental demands and constraints that produce a person–environment relationship.
- Effective coping can be either problem or emotion focused. The outcome of successful coping is adaptation through enhanced health, psychological well-being, and social functioning.
- Within the social network, social support can help a person cope with stress.
- The overall goals in the nursing management of stress are to resolve the stressful person–environment situation, reduce the stress response, and develop positive coping skills.

CRITICAL THINKING CHALLENGES

1. Compare and contrast the concepts of homeostasis and allostasis.
2. Discuss the impact of acute stress versus chronic stress. Why is chronic stress of more concern than acute stress?

3. Explain why one person may experience the stress of losing a job differently from another.
4. A man is overweight, has hypertension and insomnia, and was recently widowed. The doctor has told him to lose weight and quit smoking. He seeks your advice. Would you recommend a problem- or an emotion-focused approach?
5. A woman at the local shelter announced to her group that she was returning to her husband because it was partly her fault that her husband beat her. Is this an example of problem- or emotion-focused coping? Justify your answer.
6. Using the Stress Coping and Adaptation Model (see Fig. 13.2), assess a patient and determine the cognitive appraisal of significant events.

2007: *Noise*

David Owen (Tim Robbins) copes with the stressful noises of the city, specifically car alarms, by becoming aggressive and destructive. At first, the noise is merely an irritant. Later, he interprets the noise as an assault on everyone. He becomes an activist, protecting others and gradually becomes very grandiose. As his grandiosity increases, he becomes more and more driven to damage vehicles with active care alarms.

Viewing Points: What is the relationship between the physiologic response to the noise and his eventual grandiose behavior? How would you help him reduce the stressful experience and cope positively? Observe your own feelings throughout the movie. Did you experience stress?

UNFOLDING PATIENT STORIES FOR UNIT IV

Unfolding Patient Stories: David Carter • Part 2

Recall from Unit III 28-year-old **David Carter,** with schizophrenia, who was hospitalized after a violent outburst involving paranoid delusions and auditory hallucinations. He lives with his mother and previously worked as a grocery clerk. What could be influencing his increased social isolation? What factors should the nurse consider when developing a plan of care for discharge to promote David's social functioning and lessen his isolation?

Care for David and other patients in a realistic virtual environment: ***vSim** for Nursing* (thepoint.lww.com/vSimMentalHealth). Practice documenting these patients' care in DocuCare (thepoint.lww.com/DocuCareEHR).

Unfolding Patient Stories: George Palo • Part 1

George Palo, 90 years old, was diagnosed 6 months ago with mild neurocognitive disorder, Alzheimer type. He lives independently in an apartment within a retirement community. His wife of 65 years died 3 years ago. He was managing well until the recent loss of his 13-year-old dog. What responses and behaviors associated with bereavement should the nurse consider when assessing George? How can his cognitive disorder complicate the process of grieving? How can the nurse guide his progression through grief and bereavement? (George Palo's story continues in Unit VI.)

Care for George and other patients in a realistic virtual environment: ***vSim** for Nursing* (thepoint.lww.com/vSimMentalHealth). Practice documenting these patients' care in DocuCare (thepoint.lww.com/DocuCareEHR).

Unfolding Patient Stories: Sandra Littlefield • Part 2

Recall from Unit I **Sandra Littlefield,** with borderline personality disorder. She has a history of unstable relationships, several divorces, prostitution, poor impulse control, drug and alcohol abuse, anxiety, cutting, and suicide attempts. The nurse ascertains that she was sexually abused as a child. What factors in her history are suggestive of abuse? Describe areas of a psychosocial assessment associated with her behaviors. What nursing interventions and education can help promote Sandra's mental health stability?

Care for Sandra and other patients in a realisticvirtual environment: ***vSim** for Nursing* (thepoint.lww.com/vSimMentalHealth). Practice documenting these patients' care in DocuCare (thepoint.lww.com/DocuCareEHR).

REFERENCES

American Psychiatric Association. (2013). *Diagnostic and statistical manual of mental disorders* (5th ed.). Arlington, VA: Author.

Azmitia, M., Syed, M., & Radmacher, K. (2008). On the intersection of personal and social identities: Introduction and evidence from a longitudinal study of emerging adults. *New Directions for Child & Adolescent Development*, 120, 1–16.

Benjet, C., Borges, G., & Medina-Mora, M. E. (2010). Chronic childhood adversity and onset of psychopathology during three life stages: Childhood, adolescence and adulthood. *Journal of Psychiatric Research*, 44(11), 732–740.

Bozo, Ö., Yagmur, A., & Eldoğan, D. (2017). Does marital adjustment mediate type C personality-depressive symptoms relation? A comparison between breast cancer patients and cancer-free women. *Current Psychology*, 1–8. Retrieved December 23, 2017, from https://doi-org.libproxy.siue.edu/10.1007/s12144-017-9693-6

Bryant-Lukosius, D. (2003). Review: Limited evidence exists on the effect of psychological coping styles on cancer survival or recurrence. *Evidence Based Nursing*, 6(3), 88.

Cannon W. B. (1932). *The wisdom of the body*. New York: Norton.

Carpenter, R. (2016). A review of instruments on cognitive appraisal of stress. *Archives of Psychiatric Nursing*, 30(2), 271–279.

Clark, J. S., Bond, M. J., & Hecker, J. R. (2007). Environmental stress, psychological stress and allostatic load. *Psychology, Health & Medicine*, 12(1), 18–30.

Conti, C., Carrozzino, D., Patierno, C., Vitacolonna, E., & Fulcheri, M. (2016). The clinical link between type D personality and diabetes. *Frontiers in Psychiatry*, 7, 113.

Duong, M. T., Bingham, B. A., Aldana, P. C., Chung, S. T., & Sumner, A. E. (2016). Variation in the calculation of allostatic load score: 21 examples from HNANES. *Journal of Racial and Ethnic Health Disparities*, 4(3):455–461.

Friedman, M., & Rosenman, R. (1974). *Type A and your heart*. New York: Knopf.

Garcia-Retamero, R., Petrova, D., Arrebola-Moreno, A., Catena, A., & Ramírez-Hernández, J. A. (2016). Type D personality is related to severity of acute coronary syndrome in patients with recurrent cardiovascular disease. *British Journal of Health Psychology*, 21(3), 694–711.

Gilhooly, K. J., Gilhooly, M. L., Sullivan, M. P., McIntyre, A., Wilson, L., Harding, E., et al. (2016). A meta-review of stress, coping and interventions in dementia and dementia caregiving. *BMC Geriatrics*, 16, 106.

Glover, D. A., Stuber, M., & Poland, R. E. (2006). Allostatic load in women with and without PTSD symptoms. *Psychiatry*, 69(3), 191–203.

Holmes, T., & Rahe, R. (1967). The Social Readjustment Patient Scale. *Journal of Psychosomatic Research*, 11(2), 213–218.

Juruena, M. F. (2014). Early-life stress and HPA axis trigger recurrent adulthood depression. *Epilepsy & Behavior*, 38, 148–159.

Lalâ A., Bobîrnac, G., & Tipa, R. (2010). Stress levels, alexithymia, type A and type C personality patterns in undergraduate students. *Journal of Medicine & Life*, 3(2), 200–205.

Lazarus, R. S. (2001). Relational meaning and discrete emotions. In K. R. Scherer, A. Schorr, & T. Johnstone (Eds.). *Appraisal processes in emotion: Theory, methods, research* (pp. 37–67). New York: Oxford University Press.

Lazarus, R. S. (2006). *Stress and emotion: A new synthesis*. New York: Springer.

Lazarus, R., & Folkman, S. (1984). *Stress, appraisal, and coping*. New York: Springer.

Li, Y., & Wu, S. (2010). Social networks and health among rural-urban migrants in China: A channel or a constraint? *Health Promotion International*, 25(3), 371–380.

Low, C. A., Thurston, R. C., & Matthews, K. A. (2010). Psychosocial factors in the development of heart disease in women: Current research and future directions. *Psychosomatic Medicine*, 72(9), 842–854.

Marchesi, C., Ossola, P., Scagnelli, F., Paglia, F., Aprile, S., Monici, A., et al. (2014). Type D personality in never-depressed patients and the development of major and minor depression after acute coronary syndrome. *Journal of Affective Disorders*, 155, 194–199.

McEwen, B. S. (2005). Stressed or stressed out: What is the difference? *Journal of Psychiatry Neuroscience*, 30(5), 315–318.

McEwen, B. S. (2015). Biomarkers for assessing population and individual health and disease related to stress and adaptation. *Metabolism*, 64(3), S1–S10.

McEwen, B. S. (2017). Neurobiological and systemic effects of chronic stress. *Chronic Stress*, 1(1), 1–11.

McEwen, B. S., Gray, J., & Nasca, C. (2015). Recognizing resilience: Learning from the effects of stress on the brain. *Neurobiology of Stress*, 1, 1–11.

McVicar, A., Ravalier, J. M., & Greenwood, C. (2013). Biology of stress revisited: Intracellular mechanisms and the conceptualization of stress. *Stress & Health*, 30(4), 272–279.

Peek, M. K., Cutchin, M. P., Salinas, J. J., Sheffield, K. M., Eschbach, K., Stowe, R. P., et al. (2010). Allostatic load among non-Hispanic whites, non-Hispanic blacks, and people of Mexican origin: Effects of ethnicity, nativity, and acculturation. *American Journal of Public Health*, 100(5), 940–946.

Rahe, R. H. (1994). The more things change. *Psychosomatic Medicine*, 56(4), 306–307.

Rahe, R. H., Taylor, C. B., Tolles, R. L., Newhall, L. M., Veach, T. L., & Bryson, S. (2002). A novel stress and coping workplace program reduces illness and healthcare utilization. *Psychosomatic Medicine*, 64(2), 278–286.

Roy, B. (2018). Socio-economic variables: A contributing factor for the development of aggressive behaviour among the students with type A and type B personality. *Indian Journal of community Psychology*, 14(1), 125–132.

Seeman, T., Epel, E., Gruenewald, T., Karlamangla, A., & McEwen, B. S. (2010). Socio-economic differentials in peripheral biology: Cumulative allostatic load. *Annals of the New York Academy of Sciences*, 1186, 223–239.

Seib, C., Whiteside, E., Lee, K., Humphreys, J., Tran, T. H., Chopin, L., et al. (2014). Stress, lifestyle, and quality of life in midlife and older Australian women: Results from the Stress and the Health of Women Study. *Women's Health Issues*, 24(1), e43–e52.

Selye, H. (1956). *The stress of life*. New York: McGraw-Hill.

Selye, H. (1974). *Stress without distress*. Philadelphia, PA: J. B. Lippincott.

Sogaard, A. J., Dalgard, O. S., Holme, I., Røysamb, E., & Håheim, L. L. (2008). Associations between type A behavior pattern and psychological distress: 28 years of follow-up in the Oslo Study 1972/1973. *Social Psychiatry & Psychiatric Epidemiology*, 43(3), 216–223.

Sterling, P. (2012). Allostasis: A model of predictive regulation. *Physiology & Behavior*, 106, 5–15.

Stevenson, C., & Williams, L. (2014). Type D personality, quality of life and physical symptoms in the general population: A dimensional analysis. *Psychology & Health*, 29(3), 365–373.

Tamers, S. L., Okechukwu, C., Bohl, A. A., Guéguen, A., Goldberg, M., & Zins, M. (2014). The impact of stressful life events on excessive alcohol consumption in the French population: Findings from the GAZEL Cohort Study. *PLOS ONE*, 9(1), e87653.

Tishler, C. L., Bartholomae, S., & Rhodes, A. R. (2005). Personality profiles of normal healthy research volunteers: A potential concern for clinical drug trial investigators? *Medical Hypotheses*, 65(1), 1–7.

Whatley, A. D., Dilorio, C. K., & Yeager, K. (2010). Examining the relationships of depressive symptoms, stigma, social support and regimen-specific support on quality of life in adult patients with epilepsy. *Health Education Research*, 25(4), 575–584.

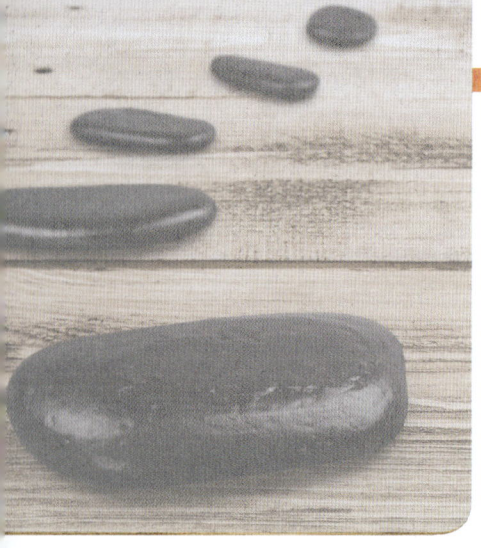

14
Management of Anger, Aggression, and Violence

Sandra P. Thomas

KEY CONCEPTS
- anger
- aggression
- gender, culture, and ethnic differences
- intervention fit
- violence

LEARNING OBJECTIVES

After studying this chapter, you will be able to:

1. Explore the difference between healthy and maladaptive styles of anger.
2. Discuss the principles of anger management as a psychoeducational intervention to promote wellness.
3. Discuss the factors that influence aggressive and violent behaviors.
4. Discuss the theories used to explain anger, aggression, and violence.
5. Identify the behaviors or actions that escalate and de-escalate violent behavior.
6. Recognize the risk for verbal and physical attacks on nurses.
7. Generate options for responding to the expression of anger, aggression, and violent behaviors in clinical nursing practice.
8. Apply the nursing process to the management of anger, aggression, and violence in patients.

KEY TERMS

- anger management • catharsis • instrumental aggression • inwardly directed anger • maladaptive anger • outwardly directed anger

Maladaptive anger and potentially lethal violent behavior are increasingly evident in contemporary Western society. Temper tantrums of athletes, episodes of road rage, and school shootings often dominate the evening news. Clearly, mismanagement of angry emotion is a serious social problem.

Language pertaining to anger is imprecise and confusing. Some of the words used interchangeably with anger include *annoyance*, *frustration*, *temper*, *resentment*, *hostility*, *hatred*, and *rage*. To avoid perpetuating the confusion, three key concepts were selected for use in this chapter: *anger*, *aggression*, and *violence*. Anger, aggression, and violence should not be viewed as a continuum because one does not necessarily lead to another. That is a myth. In fact, cultural myths about anger abound (Table 14.1).

One goal of this chapter is to dispel confusion between anger as a normal, healthy response to violation of one's integrity and maladaptive anger that is detrimental to one's mental and physical health. Understanding this distinction is an important aspect of emotional intelligence.

A second goal of this chapter is to outline risk factors for aggression and violence and describe preventive interventions, particularly as they pertain to the psychiatric nursing care environment. Verbal and physical aggression and violence also occur across a wide spectrum of other health care settings, including emergency departments, medical-surgical facilities, and primary care. All nurses must develop expertise in prevention and management of aggression. Contrary to a popular misconception, patients who have psychiatric problems are

TABLE 14.1	CULTURAL MYTHS ABOUT ANGER
Myth	Truth
Anger is a knee-jerk reaction to external events.	Humans can choose to slow down their reactions and to think and behave differently in response to events.
Anger can be uncontrollable, resulting in crimes of passion such as "involuntary manslaughter."	In societies that believe anger can be controlled, there are far fewer violent crimes than in the United States. Compare the statistics of Japan and the United States.
Anger behavior in adulthood is determined by temperament and childhood experiences.	Although temperament and early experiences are important, emotional development continues throughout life. Adults can acquire knowledge and skills to handle emotions more effectively.
Men are angrier than women.	Women experience anger as frequently as men, but societal constraints may inhibit their expression of it.
People must behave aggressively to get what they want.	Making an assertive request is more likely to lead to the desired outcome.

not more violent than other patients, but astute clinicians need to know which patients *might* become aggressive given a combination of known risk factors with specific environmental conditions.

ANGER

Anger is an internal affective state, usually temporary rather than an enduring negative attitude. If expressed outwardly, anger behavior can be constructive or destructive. Whereas destructive anger alienates other people and invites retaliation, constructive anger can be a powerful force for asserting one's rights and achieving social justice.

Anger is a signal that something is wrong in a situation; thus, the angry individual has the urge to act. The situation is more distressing than a minor annoyance such as a slow grocery line. An interpersonal offense such as unjust or disrespectful treatment (a spouse lying, a coworker taking advantage) often provokes anger. The meaning of an angry episode depends on the relational context. For example, anger is more intense and intermingled with considerable hurt when loved ones violate the implicit relational contract ("If he loved me, how could he lie about that? How can I trust him again?") (Thomas, 2006).

> **KEYCONCEPT** **Anger** is "a strong, uncomfortable emotional response to a provocation that is unwanted and incongruent with one's values, beliefs, or rights" (Thomas, 2001).

Maladaptive anger (excessive outwardly directed anger or suppressed anger) is linked to psychiatric conditions, such as depression (Perugi, Fornaro, & Akiskal, 2011), as well as a plethora of medical conditions. For example, anger and hostility are associated with hospitalizations in patients with heart failure (Keith et al., 2017), and *excessive outwardly directed anger* is linked to coronary heart disease (Ketterer et al., 2011), metabolic syndrome (Boylan & Ryff, 2015), and myocardial infarction (Mostofsky, Maclure, Tofler, Muller, & Mittleman, 2013).

Suppressed anger is related to arthritis, breast and colorectal cancer, chronic pain, and hypertension (Burns, Quartana, & Bruehl, 2011; Thomas, 2009). Furthermore, suppressed anger was a predictor of early mortality for both men and women in a large 17-year study (Potpara & Lip, 2011).

In contrast to these maladaptive anger management styles, research shows that anger discussed with other people in a constructive way has a beneficial effect on blood pressure (Everson-Rose & Lewis, 2005; Thomas, 1997a), as well as statistically significant associations with better general health, a higher sense of self-efficacy, less depression, and a lower likelihood of obesity (Thomas, 1997b). Anger controlled through calming strategies is associated with faster wound healing and other health benefits (Gouin, Kiecolt-Glaser, Malarkey, & Glaser, 2008; Gross, Groer, & Thomas, 2014). Thus, effective anger management is important in maintenance of emotional wellness and holistic health (Trost et al., 2017).

Skillful anger control is also essential to social and occupational success. People with poor anger control have more conflict at work, change jobs more frequently, take more unwise risks, and have more accidents than people with adaptive anger behavior (Halperin & Tagar, 2017).

The Experience of Anger

When you are angry, your heart pounds, your blood pressure rises, you breathe faster, your muscles tense, and you clench your jaw or fists as you experience an impulse to do something with this physical energy. Some individuals experience anger arousal as pleasurable, but others find its strong physical manifestations scary and unpleasant. People who were taught that anger is a sin may immediately try to ban it from awareness and deny its existence. However, suppression actually results in greater, more prolonged physiologic arousal. A better option is finding a way to safely release the physical energy, either through vigorous physical activity (e.g., jogging) or through a calming activity (e.g., deep breathing). Later, at an

> **BOX 14.1**
>
> **Self-Awareness Exercise: Personal Experience of Anger**
>
> People's reactions differ when they experience anger. Some people report a sense of power, control, and calmness different from their usual experience; others report feeling shaky, tearful, and on the verge of collapse. Still others describe physical sensations of nausea and dizziness.
>
> Think about the last time you felt angry. List the body sensations and other emotions that you experienced. Now ask a friend, colleague, or family member to do the same. Compare lists. What are the similarities and differences between you? How will awareness of these differences help you in your clinical practice?

opportune time, calmly discussing the incident with the provocateur permits clarification of misunderstandings and resolution of grievances. Box 14.1 invites the reader to explore variations in anger experience.

The physiology of anger involves the cerebral cortex, the sympathetic nervous system, the adrenal medulla (which secretes adrenaline and noradrenaline), the adrenal cortex (which secretes cortisol), the cardiovascular system, and even the immune system. From a biologic viewpoint, angry episodes may partially originate from developmental deficits, anoxia, malnutrition, toxins, tumors, neurodegenerative diseases, or trauma affecting the brain.

The Expression of Anger

While the physiologic arousal of anger is similar in all people, ways of expressing anger differ. The most common modes, or styles, of anger expression are listed in Table 14.2.

In Western culture, control of anger was the dominant stance from Greco-Roman times to the 20th century. Anger was viewed as sinful, dangerous, and destructive—an irrational emotion to be contained, controlled, and denied. This pejorative view contributed to the development of a powerful taboo against feeling and expressing anger. People who have accepted this persistent taboo may have difficulty even knowing when they are angry. They may use euphemisms such as "a little upset."

In contrast to the denial or containment of angry emotion, some mental health care providers began to advocate the use of **catharsis** during the early 20th century, based on the animal research of ethologists and on Freud's conceptualization of "strangulated affect"; rather than holding in their anger, people were urged to "vent it," lest there be a dangerous "slush fund" of unexpressed anger building up in the body (Rubin, 1970). The legacy of the ill-advised "ventilationist movement" is still with us, visible in rude, uncivil behavior in the nation's classrooms, offices, roadways, and other public places, as well as in countless homes where loud arguments are a daily occurrence.

More ideally, the clear expression of honest anger may prevent aggression and help to resolve a situation (Thomas, 2009). Suppression of anger, prolonged rumination about the grievance, and malevolent fantasies of revenge do not resolve a problem and may result in negative consequences later. Likewise, antagonistic anger toward an intimate partner or coworker only exacerbates the conflict (Sommer, Iyican, & Babcock, 2016). In contrast, if anger is expressed assertively, beneficial outcomes are possible. In Averill's classic study (1983) of everyday anger, 76% of those who were on the receiving end of

TABLE 14.2	STYLES OF ANGER EXPRESSION	
Style	**Characteristic Behaviors**	**Gender Socialization Issues**
Anger suppression	Feeling anxious when anger is aroused Acting as though nothing happened Withdrawing from people when angry Conveying anger nonverbally by body language Sulking, pouting, or ruminating	In North America, girls are often discouraged from openly expressing anger, lest they hurt someone's feelings. Females are more likely than males to engage in passive-aggressive tactics; to ruminate about unresolved conflict; and to have somatic anger symptoms, such as headaches.
Unhealthy outward anger expression	Flying off the handle Expressing anger in an attacking or blaming way Yelling, saying nasty things Calling the other person names or using profanity Using fists rather than words to express angry feelings	In North America, boys are encouraged to be aggressive and competitive, to express their anger in "manly" ways. Throughout life, males are more likely to express anger physically than females are.
Constructive anger discussion	Discussing the anger with a friend or family member even if the provocateur cannot be confronted at the time Approaching the person with whom one is angry and discussing the concern directly Using "I" language to describe feelings and request changes in another's behavior	Most research shows that females, more so than males, prefer to talk through anger episodes and restore relationship harmony. Both men and women may benefit from assertiveness training, problem-solving skills training, and conflict resolution workshops.

someone else's anger reported that they recognized their own faults as a result of the anger incident. Contrary to popular misconception, the relationship with the angry person was strengthened, not weakened.

Special Issues in the Nurse–Patient Relationship

Nurses may withdraw from angry patients and try to hide their own anger because "good nurses" do not get angry at patients. Coldness and distancing on the part of staff are acutely painful to patients (Jalil & Dickens, 2018). What patients want are steady, dependable, confident caregivers who will remain connected with them when they are angry.

Nurses' perceptions and beliefs about themselves as individuals and professionals influence their response to aggressive behaviors. For example, a nurse who considers any expression of anger inappropriate will approach an agitated patient differently from a nurse who considers agitated behavior to be meaningful. Understandably, nurses often shrink from patient anger when their own family backgrounds have been characterized by out-of-control anger or abuse. A nurse who has previously been assaulted by a patient is also more likely to have difficulty dealing with subsequent episodes of aggression (Box 14.2).

BOX 14.2

Research for Best Practice: Mental Health Nurses' Emotions and Exposure to Patient Aggression

Jalil, R., Huber, J. W., Sixsmith, J., & Dickens, G. S. (2017). Mental health nurses' emotions, exposure to patient aggression, attitudes to and use of coercive measures: Cross sectional questionnaire survey. International Journal of Nursing Studies, 75: 130–138.

THE QUESTION: What are the relationships between mental health nurses' exposure to patient aggression and their emotions/attitudes toward coercive containment measures and involvement in patient seclusion and restraint?

METHODS: Sixty-eight mental health nurses completed a questionnaire about their exposure to aggression, their attitudes towards seclusion and restraint, and their emotions.

FINDINGS: Verbal aggression that is targeted, demeaning, or humiliating is associated with higher experienced anger provocation and approval of restraints or seclusion, but anger did not predict involvement in the use of restraints or seclusion.

IMPLICATIONS FOR NURSING: Nurses may benefit from interventions that improve their skill and coping strategies for dealing with verbal aggression. Nurses should be sufficiently self-aware to avoid using restraints or seclusion when experiencing anger.

Some patients have an uncanny ability to target a nurse's vulnerable characteristics. Although it is normal to become defensive when feeling vulnerable, maintaining personal control is a must. If not, the potential for punitive interventions is greater. Threatening an agitated patient (e.g., "You are going to get an injection if you don't calm down") will only worsen a volatile situation. Nurses must collaborate with other members of the treatment team when interacting with particularly challenging patients, obtaining consultation from supervisors if necessary.

Assessment of Anger

Both **outwardly directed anger** (particularly the hostile, attacking forms) and **inwardly directed anger** (i.e., anger that is stifled despite strong arousal) produce adverse consequences, indicating a need for anger management intervention. Complicating matters, however, most people's anger styles cannot be neatly categorized as "anger-in" or "anger-out" because they behave differently in different environments (e.g., yelling at secretaries in the office, stifling anger at spouse). Therefore, it is necessary to conduct a careful assessment of a patient's behavior pattern across various situations.

The manner of anger expression is not the only important aspect of assessment. The difficulty in regulating the frequency and intensity of anger must also be assessed. Intense anger, evident in clenched fists and readiness to burst when arguing with others, can even trigger a heart attack (Buckley et al., 2015). Having an episode of intense anger caused an 8.5-fold increase in risk of acute coronary occlusion within the next 2 hours. The extent to which anger is creating problems at work or intimate relationships should be evaluated, as well as the presence or absence of coping techniques such as calming or diffusion through vigorous exercise. Given the current climate of evidence-based practice, it may be advantageous to administer a questionnaire that has been extensively used with thousands of people, permitting comparison of a client with established norms. The Spielberger State-Trait Anger Expression Inventory (STAXI) is one such tool (Spielberger, 1999). This instrument measures the general proneness to be aroused to anger (trait anger) as well as current feelings (state anger) and several styles of anger expression, including control through calming techniques.

Because anger and aggression can be symptomatic of many underlying psychiatric or medical disorders, from posttraumatic stress disorder (PTSD) and bipolar disorder to toxicities and head injuries, first any underlying disorder must be properly evaluated. At present, only one anger-related disorder, intermittent explosive disorder (IED), appears in the *Diagnostic and Statistical Manual of Mental Disorders* (*DSM-5*) (American Psychiatric

Association [APA], 2013). This diagnosis is used when recurring aggressive outbursts cannot be attributed to any other condition. People with IED display aggressive behavior that is disproportionate to the precipitating event, usually a minor provocation by a family member or other close associate (APA, 2013).

Once thought to be rare, more recent research has shown that IED is as common as many other psychiatric disorders (Coccaro, 2012). The disorder usually appears during the teen years and persists over the life course. A national study indicates that the average number of lifetime anger attacks per person is large (43 per person). Because the disorder involves inadequate production or functioning of serotonin, IED is commonly treated with selective serotonin reuptake inhibitors (SSRIs) (Coccaro et al., 2015). However, behavior therapy should also be included. Only 28.8% of patients with IED ever receive treatment for their anger (Kessler et al., 2006) although the IED population is responsive to treatment (Galbraith et al., 2018).

Culture and Gender Considerations in Assessment

Anger is one of the six universal emotions with identifiable facial features and emotionally inflected speech. People across the globe experience the emotion of anger, along with the impulse to act, but culture is perhaps the most important determinant of what angry individuals actually do. Thus, in Japan, a wife might indicate anger to her husband by creating a disorderly flower arrangement. Such a subtle nonverbal cue is unlikely to be understood (or even noticed) by a husband from another culture.

Cultural differences in anger behavior can emanate from the historical trajectories, religions, languages, and customs of a group of people (Thomas, 2006). The same event can provoke very different emotional responses in culturally different persons (e.g., a random act by a stranger could be perceived as insulting by one individual but dismissed with a laugh by someone from another culture).

> **KEYCONCEPT** Gender, culture, and ethnic differences in the experience and expression of anger must be taken into consideration before planning interventions.

Gender role socialization influences beliefs about the appropriateness of "owning" angry emotionality and revealing it to others. In Western cultures, aggressive behavior is expected in males and more conciliatory behavior in females (see Table 14.2). However, these generalizations may not apply to marginalized individuals, such as ethnic minorities. Some clients from Eastern cultures disapprove of anger for both genders, particularly cultures emphasizing connectedness rather than individualism (e.g., Japanese). Therefore, clients in such cultures may ruminate for lengthy periods about anger episodes rather than verbalizing their feelings. A more extensive discussion of culture and gender factors can be found in Thomas (2006).

The essential element in a cultural assessment is exploration of what the client learned about anger and its display in his or her culture and family of origin (the primary bearer of that culture). Adult clients can be encouraged to transcend cultural imperatives and childhood admonitions when these no longer serve them well. For example, research has shown that using anger to cope with racism has a negative effect on African-American well-being (Gerrard, Gibbons, Fleischli, Cutrona, & Stock, 2018). Reflecting on negative outcomes of anger behaviors can motivate client adoption of new strategies. Referral to an anger management course or therapy may be useful.

Anger Interventions

There are communication techniques that promote the expression of anger in nondestructive ways. However, most people lack skill in handling anger constructively. Few people have healthy role models to observe while growing up. Therefore, education in anger management can be valuable, both for psychological growth and improved interpersonal relations (Trost et al., 2017).

Anger Management: A Psychoeducational Intervention to Promote Wellness

Anger management is an effective intervention that nurses can deliver to persons whose anger behavior is maladaptive in some way (i.e., interfering with success in work or relationships) but *not violent*. In recent years, there has been an increase in court-mandated "anger management" for persons whose behavior is violent as opposed to angry. When these individuals do not greatly benefit, a conclusion may be drawn that anger management is ineffective. However, psychoeducational anger management courses cannot be expected to modify *violent* behavior (interventions designed for aggressive and violent individuals are presented later in the chapter).

The desired outcomes of any anger management intervention are to teach people to (1) effectively modulate the physiologic arousal of anger, (2) alter any irrational thoughts fueling the anger, and (3) modify maladaptive anger behaviors (e.g., blaming, attacking, or suppressing) that prevent problem-solving in daily living. Group work is valuable to anger management clients because they need to practice new behaviors in an interpersonal context that offers feedback and support. The leader of an anger management group functions as a teacher and coach, not a therapist. Therefore, potential participants should be screened and referred to individual counseling or psychotherapy if their anger is deep seated and chronic. Exclusion criteria are paranoia, organic disorders, and severe personality disorders (Thomas, 2001). Candidates for psychoeducational anger management classes must have some insight that their behavior is problematic and some desire to enlarge their behavioral repertoire.

Anger management includes both didactic and experiential components. Educational handouts, videos, and workbooks are usually used. Ideally, participants commit to attendance for a series of weekly meetings, ranging from 4 to 10 weeks. Between the group meetings, participants are given homework assignments such as keeping an anger diary and applying the lessons of the class in their homes and work sites. Fresh anger incidents can be brought to the class for role-plays and group discussion. It may be useful to conduct gender-specific or culturally specific groups (Thomas, 2001).

Individuals can successfully reduce anger and foster forgiveness for an offender through religious/spiritual anger management strategies such as prayer, meditation, or yoga (Smith-MacDonald, Norris, Raffin-Bouchal, & Sinclair, 2017).

Effectiveness of anger management has been demonstrated in studies of college students, angry drivers, angry veterans, various medical and psychiatric outpatients, and parents who have difficulty controlling anger toward their children (Kusmierska, 2011). Family members of patients with alcohol use disorders can also benefit from anger management.

Cognitive-Behavioral Therapy for Anger

Cognitive-behavioral therapy (CBT) is often recommended for the treatment of uncontrollable anger. The first step is establishing a therapeutic alliance because some angry individuals are not in a stage of readiness to change their behavior. CBT involves avoidance of provoking stimuli, self-monitoring regarding cues of anger arousal, stimulus control, response disruption, and guided practice of more effective anger behaviors. Relaxation training is often introduced early in the treatment because it strengthens the therapeutic alliance and convinces clients that they can indeed learn to calm themselves when angry. When the body relaxes, there is less physical impetus to act impulsively in a way that one will later regret.

AGGRESSION AND VIOLENCE

Aggression and violence command the attention of the criminal justice system as well as the mental health care system. During periods when people are a danger to others, they may be separated from the larger society and confined in prisons or locked psychiatric units. Because nurses frequently practice in these settings, management of aggressive and violent behavior is an essential skill.

Factors That Influence Aggressive and Violent Behavior

The violent individual may feel trapped, frightened, or desperate, perhaps at the end of his or her rope. The nurse must remember that many violent individuals have experienced childhood abandonment, physical brutality, or sexual abuse. Confinement that replicates earlier experiences of degrading treatment may provoke aggressive response, but humane care may kindle hope of recovery and rehabilitation. The response of the nurse may be critical in determining whether aggression escalates or diminishes. Aggressive or violent behavior does not occur in a vacuum. Both the patient and the context must be considered. Therefore, a multidimensional framework is essential for understanding and responding to these behaviors.

> **KEYCONCEPT** **Aggression** involves overt behavior intended to hurt, belittle, take revenge, or achieve domination and control. Aggression can be verbal (sarcasm, insults, threats) or physical (property damage, slapping, hitting). Mentally healthy people stop themselves from aggression by realizing the negative consequences to themselves or their relationships.

Impulsive aggression occurs in situations of anger and anxiety when the individual lashes out. **Instrumental aggression** is a goal-directed aggressive behavior that is premeditated and unrelated to immediate feelings of frustration or threat. It is a means to secure a goal or reward.

> **KEYCONCEPT** **Violence** is extreme aggression and involves the use of strong force or weapons to inflict bodily harm to another person and in some cases to kill. Violence connotes greater intensity and destruction than aggression. All violence is aggressive, but not all aggression is violent.

Theories of Aggression and Violence

This section discusses some of the main theoretical explanations for aggression and violence. A single model or theory cannot fully explain aggression and violence; instead, choose the most useful theories for explaining a patient's experience and for planning interventions.

Biologic Theories

The brain structures most frequently associated with aggressive behavior are the limbic system and the cerebral cortex, particularly the frontal and temporal lobes. Patients with a history of damage to the cerebral cortex are more likely to exhibit increased impulsivity, decreased

> **BOX 14.3**
>
> **Self-Awareness Exercise: Intensity of Anger**
>
> Imagine this scene:
>   You are coming home late at night. You've been at the library studying for midterm examinations and are tired. As you come up the front walk, you trip over a skateboard, probably left by one of the neighborhood children. Before you know it, you are sprawled across the front step.
>   What emotions threaten to overwhelm you at that moment? What contributes to the intensity of the anger that you feel?
>
> - The pain where you scraped your leg across the cement?
> - Your general state of tiredness?
> - The fact that you skipped dinner?
> - The five cups of coffee you had today?
> - The careless children who left a toy in your way?
>
>   If the same thing had happened when you were well rested and feeling good, would the feeling and the intensity be the same?

inhibition, and decreased judgment than are those who have not experienced such damage. The interaction of neurocognitive impairment and social history of abuse or family violence increases the risk for violent behavior, particularly for boys (Golding & Fitzgerald, 2019).

There is increasing evidence that activity of monoamine oxidase A (MAO A) is related to the development of impulsivity and aggression. Inhibition of this enzyme affects the activity of norepinephrine, serotonin, and dopamine, may play a significant role in the violence enacted by abused children, especially boys. Low serotonin levels are also associated with irritability, increased pain sensitivity, impulsiveness, and aggression (Burke, Fillion, Mejia, Ervin, & Palmour, 2018).

Gender differences in aggressive behavior can partially be explained by neurobiology. Activation of the amygdala is correlated with higher anger scores in men but not in women. When provoked, men also have more activation in the orbitofrontal cortex, rectal gyrus, and anterior cingulate cortex than women. Activation of these areas is associated with aggression (Repple et al., 2018). Sex hormones also play a role in some aggressive behavior, with testosterone associated with aggression (Been, Gibbon, & Meisel, 2018). Before reading additional research evidence, try the anger exercise in Box 14.3. What does daily experience suggest about biologically based aspects of the experience and expression of anger?

> **NCLEXNOTE** In caring for a potentially aggressive patient, the nurse should recognize that biochemical imbalance contributes to the person's inability to control aggression.

Psychological Theories

Several psychological explanations exist for aggressive and violent behaviors. This section discusses these theories and their treatment approaches.

Psychoanalytic Theories

Psychoanalytic theorists view emotions as instinctual drives. They view suppression of these drives as unhealthy and possible contributors to the development of psychosomatic or psychological disorders. Some psychoanalysts recommended the use of cathartic approaches to release patients' pent-up anger. Nurses in the mid-20th century often used interventions that directed the patient to "let it out" by pounding a pillow or ripping up telephone books. However, studies did not support the theory that catharsis reduces aggression.

Contemporary psychoanalysts do not adhere to any single explanatory model of aggression, often focusing on patients' tendencies to reenact old childhood conflicts or their defensive attempts to deny vulnerability. In working with angry patients, they focus on issues such as improved control over outbursts, heightened empathy for others, and repair of deficits in the personality structure. During analytic therapy, patients gradually achieve greater insight into unconscious processes (Feindler & Byers, 2006). Thus, they become aware of the reasons they developed maladaptive anger behaviors.

Behavioral Theories

As behavioral theories came into prominence, anger was viewed as a learned response to a stimulus rather than an instinctual drive. In the 1930s, the frustration-aggression hypothesis was advanced in which a person may experience anger and act violently in response to interference with or blocking of a goal. Laboratory experiments and the reality of everyday experience have proved the limitations of this theory (Thomas, 1990). Not all situations in which one's goal is blocked lead to anger or violence.

Social Learning Theory

In Bandura's social learning theory, he focuses on the role of learning and rewards in the expression of aggression and violence (Bandura, 2001). Children's observations of aggressive behaviors among family members and violence in their communities foster a context for learning that aggressive behavior is an acceptable way of getting what they want. According to this view, people develop aggressive and violent behaviors by participating in an environment that rewards aggression (Teng et al., 2019).

General Aggression Model

The general aggression model (GAM) is a framework that accounts for the interaction of cognition, affect, and arousal during an aggressive episode (Allen, Anderson, Bushman, 2018) (Fig. 14.1). In this model, an episode consists of *person and situation factors* in an ongoing *social interaction*. The episode is mediated through a person's

Chapter 14 • Management of Anger, Aggression, and Violence

similar episodes). Mood, emotion, and expressive motor responses (automatic reactions to specific emotions) represent the *affect component*. *Arousal* can be physiologic, psychological, or both.

PROMOTING SAFETY AND PREVENTING VIOLENCE

Paramount aims of psychiatric nurses, particularly those staffing inpatient facilities, are promoting safety and preventing violence. The nurse works toward these goals by establishing therapeutic nurse–patient relationships and creating a therapeutic milieu. Intervening with a potentially violent patient begins with assessment of the history and the predictive factors outlined in the next section.

Assessment for Aggression and Violence

The patient's history is the most important predictor of potential for aggression and violence. Schizophrenia, young age, alcohol use, drug misuse, and hostile-dominant interpersonal styles are also predictors of patient violence (d'Ettorre & Pellicani, 2017). Early life adverse circumstances, such as inadequate maternal nutrition, birth complications, traumatic brain injury, and lead exposure can contribute to risk for aggressive and criminal behaviors in adulthood (Golding & Fitzgerald, 2019). Important markers in the patient's history include previous episodes of rage and violent behavior, escalating irritability, intruding angry thoughts, and fear of losing control.

Characteristics Predictive of Aggression and Violence

The age, gender, and race of patients are *not* good predictors, but several research reports suggest that particular characteristics are predictive of violent behaviors. Usually, but not always, there are some observable precursors to aggression and violence: staring or glaring in an intimating manner, raising voice tone or volume, making sarcastic or demanding comments, and pacing.

Impaired Communication

Impaired communication (including hearing loss and reduced visual acuity), disorientation, and depression have been found to be consistently associated with aggressive behavior among nursing home residents with dementia (Bora, Velakoulis, & Walterfang, 2016).

In patients with cognitive impairments, the nurse needs to know when the patient last voided and the pattern of bowel movements. The urge to void can be a powerful stimulus to agitated behavior. Regular toileting routines are not just interventions to prevent incontinence.

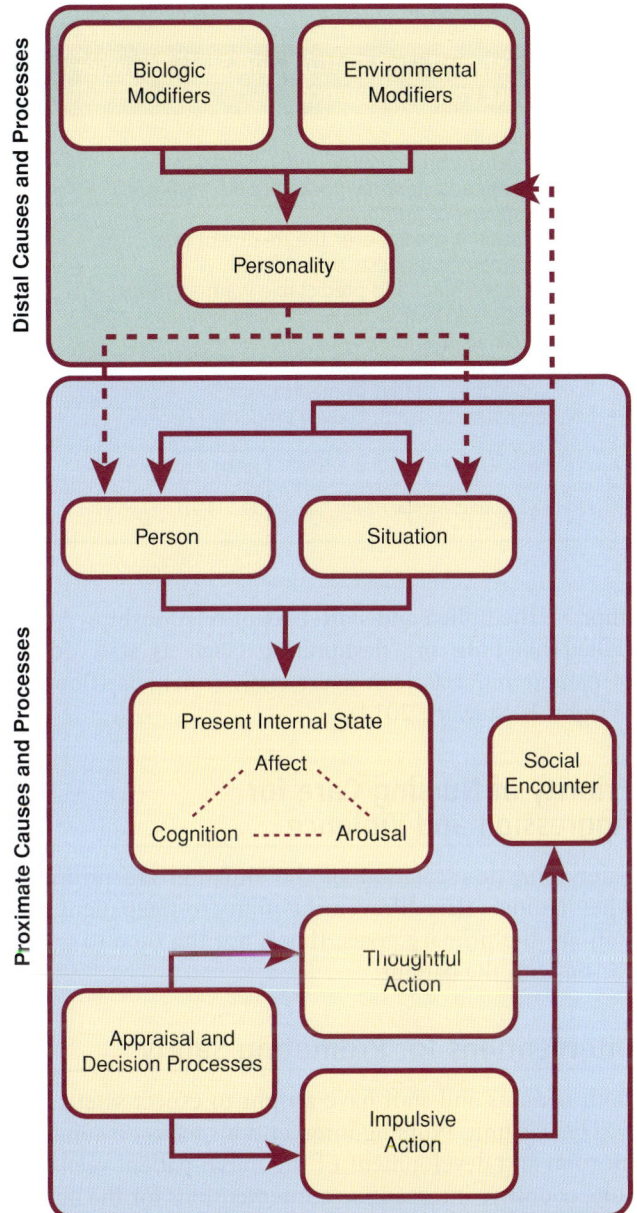

FIGURE 14.1 General aggression model overview. (Redrawn with permission from Anderson, C. A., & Anderson, K. B. (2008). Men who target women: Specificity of target, generality of aggressive behavior. *Aggressive Behavior, 34*(6), 605–622.)

thoughts, feelings, and intensity of arousal. Within this context, the individual appraises the episode and then decides about a follow-up action. The outcome is either thoughtful or impulsive action. The *person factors* include characteristics such as gender, personality traits, beliefs and attitudes, values, goals, and behavior patterns. *Situational factors* include the actual provocation (insults, slights, verbal and physical aggression, interference with achieving goals) and cues that trigger memories of similar situations. *Cognition* includes hostile thoughts and scripts (previous behavior patterns and responses to

Similarly, the anticipation of basic needs such as thirst and hunger is important, especially when working with adults and children who cannot readily express their needs. Other discomforts can arise from such conditions as ingrown toenails and adverse medication reactions.

Physical Condition

The patient's physical condition contributes to the likelihood of aggression. Patients with longstanding poor dietary habits (e.g., indigent patients, patients with alcoholism) often have deficiencies of thiamine and niacin. Increased irritability, disorientation, and paranoia may result. Assessing overall dietary intake is relevant, particularly of good tryptophan sources, such as wheat, flour, corn, milk, and eggs. Intake of caffeine, a potent stimulant, should be assessed and limited as necessary.

Social Factors

The nurse should evaluate social factors, such as crisis conditions in the patient's home, family, or community that could lead to aggression or violent episodes. If assessment reveals stressful actions by family members, such as evicting the patient from the home, attention must be devoted to mobilizing resources for family and community support and alternative housing.

Are financial or legal troubles placing increased stress on the patient? Is the patient experiencing conflict with other patients on the unit or with certain staff? People reenact in new relationships the same behaviors that created problems in old ones. Thus, behavior in a mental health facility provides important clues to a patient's habitual responses to authority figures, opposite-sex peers, and same-sex peers. Assessment data provide direction for interventions such as reassigning roommates or caregivers.

Milieu and Environmental Factors

Angry or out-of-control behavior is highly influenced by contextual factors. Successful psychiatric stabilization and treatment in a hospital often depend on the nature of the unit itself. A busy, noisy hospital unit can quickly provoke an aggressive episode. A rude comment or staff denial of a patient request can trigger physical assault. Documented times of increased violence include meals, medication, and shift change (Bader, Evans, & Welsh, 2014). Crowding and density during times of high patient census are also associated with patient aggression. Inadequate staffing has been identified as a contributing factor in units with a high incidence of assault.

Many characteristics of the unit culture and staff behavior, such as rigid rules and violation of boundaries, predict patient violence (Box 14.4). In units with a high incidence of violence, nurses should take steps to improve the milieu and staff–patient relationships. More skilled handling of "flashpoints," such as staff denial of patient requests, can avert crisis situations (Bowers, Wright, & Stewart, 2014).

> **BOX 14.4**
>
> **Characteristics of Unit Culture and Staff Behavior That Predict Patient Violence**
>
> - Rigid unit rules
> - Lack of patient privacy or boundary violations
> - Lack of patient autonomy (locked doors, restraints)
> - Strict hierarchy of authority
> - Lack of patient control over the treatment plan
> - Denial of patient requests or privileges
> - Lack of meaningful and predictable ward activities
> - Insufficient help with activities of daily living and other needs from staff
> - Patronizing behavior of staff
> - Power struggles related to medications
> - Failure of staff to listen, convey empathy
>
> *Source:* Hamrin, V., Iennaco, J., & Olsen, D. (2009). A review of ecological factors affecting inpatient psychiatric unit violence: Implications for relational and unit cultural improvements. *Issues in Mental Health Nursing, 30,* 214–226.

Priority of Nursing Care for Aggression and Violence

Safety and de-escalation of the situation are priorities when tempers flare. Preventing injury to the patient and staff are the primary goals; this is not the time to try to reason with the patient.

Interventions for Promoting Safety

Both patients and staff have a right to expect safety in a psychiatric unit. Nursing interventions focus on communication and development of the nurse–patient relationship, cognitive interventions, interventions for the milieu and environment, and violence prevention.

Communication and Development of the Therapeutic Nurse–Patient Relationship

Communicating with a patient who has the potential for aggression or violence follows the same principles discussed in Chapter 8. Aggressive behavior can be a patient's way to communicate a need, especially if there are communication deficits. The patient who behaves aggressively may receive rewards such as more frequent observation and more opportunities to discuss concerns with nurses.

Listening to the Patient's Illness Experience and Concerns

Development of the therapeutic nurse–patient relationship begins with listening. Many patients with persistent

> BOX 14.5 • THERAPEUTIC DIALOGUE • The Potentially Aggressive Patient
>
> *Paul is a 23-year-old patient in the high observation area of an inpatient unit. He is pacing back and forth. He is pounding one fist into his other hand. In the past 24 hours, Paul has been more cooperative and less agitated. The behavior the nurse observes now is more like the behavior that Paul displayed 2 days ago. Yesterday, the psychiatrist told Paul that he would be granted more freedom in the unit if his behavior improved. The psychiatrist has just seen Paul and refused to change the restrictions on Paul's activities.*
>
> **INEFFECTIVE APPROACH**
>
> **Nurse:** Paul, I can understand this is frustrating for you.
>
> **Paul:** How can you understand? Have you ever been held like a prisoner?
>
> **Nurse:** I do understand, Paul. Now you must calm down or more privileges will be removed.
>
> **Paul:** [voice gets louder] But I was told that calm behavior would mean more privileges. Now you are telling me calm behavior only gets me what I have got! Can't you talk to the doctor for me?
>
> **Nurse:** No, Paul, I can't talk to the doctor. [Paul appears more frustrated and agitated as the conversation continues.]
>
> **EFFECTIVE APPROACH**
>
> **Nurse:** Paul, you look upset (observation). What happened in your conversation with the psychiatrist? (seeking information)
>
> **Paul:** Yesterday he said calmer behavior would mean more freedom in the unit. I have tried to be calmer and not to swear. You said you noticed the difference. But today he says "no" to more freedom.
>
> **Nurse:** Some people might feel cheated if this happened to them. (validation). Is that how you feel?
>
> **Paul:** Yeah, I feel real cheated. Nothing I do makes a difference. That's the way it is here, and that's the way it is when I am out of the hospital.
>
> **Nurse:** Sounds like experiences like this leave you feeling powerless. (validation)
>
> **Paul:** I don't have any power, anywhere. Sometimes when I have no power I get mean. At least then people pay attention to me.
>
> **Nurse:** In this situation with your doctor, what would help you feel that you had some power? (inviting patient partnership)
>
> **Paul:** Well, if he would listen to me; If he would read my chart.
>
> **Nurse:** I am a bit confused by the psychiatrist's decision. I won't make promises that your privileges will change, but would it be okay with you if I talk with him?
>
> **Paul:** That would make me feel like someone is on my side.
>
> **CRITICAL THINKING CHALLENGE**
>
> - In the first scenario, how did the nurse escalate the situation?
> - Compare the first scenario with the second. How are they different?

mental illness have had traumatic experiences related to previous hospitalizations. Understandably, they may harbor distrust of mental health clinicians and resent being hospitalized again. Inviting patients and families to talk about their experiences with the health care system may highlight both their concerns and resources. Simply listening to patients' concerns and "being with" them is often as significant as "doing for" them (Thomas & Pollio, 2002) (Box 14.5).

Validating

Patients who experience intense anger and rage can feel isolated and anxious. The nurse can acknowledge these intense feelings by reflecting "This must be scary for you." Empathic responding can reduce emotional arousal because the patient feels understood and supported (see Chapter 8). By drawing on experience with other patients, the nurse can also reassure the patient that others have felt the same way.

Providing Choices

When possible, the nurse should provide the patient with choices, particularly patients who have little control over their situation because of their condition. Offering concrete choices is better than offering open-ended options. For example, a patient who is experiencing a manic episode and is confined to her room may have few options in her daily schedule. However, she may be allowed to make choices about food, personal hygiene, and which pajamas to wear.

Cognitive Interventions to Address Aggression

Cognitive interventions are very useful in interacting with a potentially aggressive patient (see Chapter 12). These interventions are useful when the patient is in a nonaggressive state and willing to discuss the irrational thought process underlying aggressive episodes. These periods of interaction allow exploration of the patient's beliefs, and provision of reassurance, support, and education.

> **NCLEXNOTE** The best time to teach the patient techniques for managing anger and aggression is when the patient is not experiencing the provoking event. Cognitive therapy approaches are useful and can be prioritized according to responses.

Providing Patient Education

Inpatient hospitalization offers opportunities for education of patients and families about a variety of topics. Nurses can seize "teachable moments" to convey important principles of anger management. For example, after an outburst of loud cursing by John, who mistakenly thought another patient (Jim) had stolen his cigarettes, the nurse helped him consider what he could have done differently in the situation. John was more amenable to learning about calming techniques and problem-solving strategies at this time because his behavior had resulted in adverse consequences (estrangement from Jim, disruption of the dayroom during a popular bingo game, and cancellation of his weekend pass). This incident could also be used for teaching in a subsequent group meeting of inpatients. Many units have daily meetings that permit processing of such conflicts. Jim could be invited to express his feelings about being falsely accused of stealing. Other patients may reveal how distressed they were when John was cursing loudly, providing John useful peer feedback about his outburst. Together, group members could generate ideas for more appropriate behavior.

Developing Prevention Strategies

Although patients are not always aware of it, escalation of feelings, thoughts, and behavior from calmness to violence may follow a pattern. Disruption of the pattern can sometimes be a useful means for preventing escalation and helping the patient regain composure. Patients can identify their own personal warning signs of aggression and develop aggression-prevention strategies. Nurses can suggest strategies to interrupt patterns:

- Counting to 10
- Using a relaxation or breathing technique (see Chapter 9)
- Removing oneself from interactions or stimuli that may contribute to increased distress (voluntarily taking "time-out")
- Doing something different (e.g., reading, listening to quiet music, watching television)

Milieu and Environmental Interventions

The inpatient environment can be modified proactively to decrease the potential of aggressive and violent behaviors (Box 14.6).

BOX 14.6
Environmental Management: Maintaining Patient Safety

DEFINITION
Maintaining patient safety includes identifying and eliminating environmental risks for persons who are at risk of injuring self or others.

ACTIVITIES
- Search the environment routinely to maintain it as hazard free.
- Remove potential weapons (e.g., sharps, ropelike objects) from the environment.
- Search the patient and belongings for weapons or potential weapons during inpatient admission procedures as appropriate.
- Monitor the safety of items that visitors bring to the environment.
- Instruct visitors and other caregivers about relevant patient safety issues.
- Limit patient use of potential weapons (e.g., sharps, ropelike objects).
- Monitor patient during use of potential weapons (e.g., razors).
- Place the patient with potential for self-harm with a roommate to decrease isolation and opportunity to act on self-harm thoughts, as appropriate.
- Assign a single room to the patient with potential for violence toward others.
- Place the patient in a bedroom located near a nursing station.
- Limit access to windows unless they are locked and shatterproof, as appropriate.
- Lock utility and storage rooms.
- Provide paper dishes and plastic utensils at meals.
- Place the patient in the least restrictive environment that still allows for the necessary level of observation.
- Provide ongoing surveillance of all patient access areas to maintain patient safety and therapeutically intervene, as needed.
- Remove other individuals from the vicinity of a violent or potentially violent patient.
- Maintain a designated safe area (e.g., seclusion room) for patient to be placed when violent.
- Provide plastic, rather than metal, clothes hangers, as appropriate.

Adapted from the Mental Health Environment of Care Checklist. VHA National Center for Patient Safety, Department of Veterans Affairs. Version 06-01-2015. Retrieved January 27, 2018, from http://www.patientsafety.va.gov/professionals/onthejob/mentalhealth.asp

Reducing Stimulation

For people whose perceptions or thoughts are disordered from brain damage, degeneration, or other thought-processing difficulties, modification of the environment may be one of the main interventions. The patient with a brain injury, progressive dementia, or distorted vision may be experiencing intense and highly confusing stimulation even though the environment, from the nurse or family's perspective, seems calm and orderly.

Likewise, introducing more structure into a chaotic environment can help decrease the risk for aggressive behavior. It is possible to make stimuli meaningful or to simplify and interpret the environment in many practical ways, such as by identifying people or equipment that may be unfamiliar, providing cues as to what is expected (e.g., posting signs with directions, putting a toothbrush and toothpaste by the sink), and removing or silencing unnecessary stimuli (e.g., turning off paging systems).

Considering the environment from the patient's viewpoint is essential. For instance, if the surroundings are unfamiliar, the patient will need to process more information. Lack of a recognizable pattern or structure further taxes the patient's capacity to encode information. Appropriate interventions include clarifying the meaning and purpose of people and objects in the environment, enhancing the patient's sense of control and the predictability of the environment, and reducing other stimuli as much as possible.

Interventions for Managing Imminent Aggression and Violence

De-escalation

Authentic engagement with the patient is the core component in a therapeutic de-escalation by the nurse. Creative, patient-centered strategies, not techniques of physical restraint, are of paramount importance. Individualizing interventions is important. In some patients, loudness and pacing can be ignored; in others, these behaviors indicate an escalation of agitation.

De-escalating potential aggression is always preferable to challenging or provoking a patient. De-escalating (commonly known as "talking the person down") is a skill that every nurse can develop. Trying to clarify what has upset the patient is important although not all patients are capable of articulating what provoked them, and some analyses will have to take place after a crisis has been diffused. The nurse can use therapeutic communication techniques to prevent a crisis or diffuse a critical situation (see Box 14.5).

The nurse who works with potentially aggressive patients should do so with respect and concern. The goal is to work with patients to find solutions, approaching these patients calmly, empathizing with the patient's perspective, and avoiding a power struggle. In dealing with aggression, as in other aspects of nursing practice, at times the best intervention is silence. It is easy to equate intervention with activity, the sense that "I must do something." But offering quiet calmness may be enough to help a patient regain control of his or her behavior.

> **KEYCONCEPT Intervention fit** The nurse who intervenes from within the context of the therapeutic relationship must be cognizant of the fit of a particular intervention.

Interventions that are appropriate in early phases of escalation differ from those used when the patient's agitation is greater. The patient's affective, behavioral, and cognitive response to an intervention provides information about its effects and guides the nurse's next response. The following approaches are important in caring for patients who are aggressive or violent:

- Using nonthreatening body language
- Respecting the patient's personal space and boundaries
- Having immediate access to the door of the room in case you need to leave the room
- Choosing to leave the door open to an office while talking to a patient
- Knowing where colleagues are and making sure those colleagues know where you are
- Removing or not wearing clothing or accessories that could be used to harm you, such as scarves, necklaces, or dangling earrings

Administering and Monitoring PRN Medications

Patients with potential for aggression and violence usually have a PRN (as-needed) medication order for agitation and aggression. Administering a PRN medication is left to the discretion of the nurse, who makes a judgment about the patient after careful assessment. Patients often recognize when a PRN medication is needed.

Avoiding the Use of Seclusion and Restraint

Seclusion and restraint have been used by nurses when patients need to be separated from other patients on the unit. The decision to use seclusion and restraint is a dynamic process involving evaluation of the risks to all who are present, as well as the need to maintain a therapeutic milieu. The decision is usually an interdisciplinary decision that follows accrediting guidelines.

The use of seclusion and restraint is now recognized as a traumatic experience for patients. Most patients with a mental disorder have already experienced traumas, usually in childhood. The act of placing an individual in seclusion or restraints retraumatizes the individual. Many hospitals no longer use restraints as a form of behavioral management. In instances where seclusion and restraint are used, they should be the last resort to protect the patient or the staff. De-escalation interventions should be tried first and clearly documented in the patient's record.

American institutions that receive Medicare or Medicaid reimbursement must adhere to guidelines issued by the Center for Medicare and Medicaid Services. These guidelines specify that a registered nurse must verify the need for restraint or seclusion and then contact the physician or other licensed practitioner; within 1 hour, that practitioner must examine the patient. Individual states have also enacted laws to regulate the use of restraints, and professional organizations released position statements on restraints as the last resort in an emergency (American Psychiatric Nurses Association, 2014).

Restraint-related injuries and deaths have prompted many facilities to ban their use entirely and train staff in alternative techniques. Comfort or sensory rooms are becoming more widespread, providing an appealing alternative to coercive interventions by unit staff. These rooms can provide stimulation for sight, smell, hearing, touch, and taste in a demand-free environment that is controlled by the patient. The rooms may reduce patients' distress and agitation and reduce the need for seclusion and restraint (Björkdahl, Perseius, Samuelsson, & Lindberg, 2016).

Evaluation and Treatment Outcomes

Treatment outcomes can be considered at both individual and aggregate levels. The desired outcome at the individual level is for the patient to regain or maintain control over aggressive or potentially aggressive thoughts, feelings, and actions. The nurse may observe that the patient shows decreased psychomotor activity (e.g., less pacing), has a more relaxed posture, speaks more directly about feelings of anger and personal needs, requires less sedating medication, shows increased tolerance for frustration and the ability to consider alternatives, and makes effective use of other coping strategies.

Evidence of a reduction in risk factors in the treatment setting includes decreased noise and confusion in the immediate environment; calmness on the part of nursing staff and others; and a climate of safety, clear expectations, and mutual acceptance and respect. In units, day hospitals, or group home settings, indicators of positive treatment outcomes include a reduction in the number and severity of assaults on staff and other patients, fewer incident reports, and increased staff competency in de-escalating potentially violent situations.

Following restraints and seclusion, a debriefing occurs with the persons involved in the incident, including the patient. This approach allows for a collaborative, community approach to preventing patient violence and avoids blaming one assailant for incidents that are provoked by a variety of contextual and interpersonal factors.

Responding to Assault on Nurses

Because nurses have extended contact with patients during highly stressful circumstances, there is always the risk that they may be the recipients of patient aggression. Nurses and nurses' aides are the targets of patient. Psychiatric nurses are assaulted more often than medical-surgical nurses, but physical violence and mental abuse occur more often in the emergency room than in the mental health unit (Pekurinen et al., 2017).

Assaults on nurses by patients can have both immediate and long-term consequences (see Table 14.3). Reported assaults range from verbal abuse or threats and minor altercations to severe injuries, rape, and murder. Any assault can produce severe consequences for the victim including PTSD. After a violent incident, the nurse may avoid the patient or watch for any signs of patient remorse; the nurse's response differs depending on the nurse's feelings of safety and comfort with the patient. The nurse's interpretation of the assaultive behavior will depend on many factors such as experience with assault, the type of assault (impulsive or instrumental), and the nurse's injury.

TABLE 14.3	NURSES' RESPONSES TO ASSAULT	
Response Type	Personal	Professional
Affective	• Irritability • Depression • Anger • Anxiety • Apathy	• Erosion of feelings of competence, leading to increased anxiety and fear • Feelings of guilt or self-blame • Fear of potentially violent patients
Cognitive	• Suppressed or intrusive thoughts of assault	• Reduced confidence in judgment • Consideration of job change
Behavioral	• Social withdrawal	• Possible hesitation in responding to other violent situations • Possible overcontrolling • Possible hesitation to report future assaults • Possible withdrawal from colleagues • Questioning of capabilities by coworkers
Physiologic	• Disturbed sleep • Headaches • Stomach aches • Tension	• Increased absenteeism because of somatic complaints

Unfortunately, patient aggression directed toward nurses is often downplayed or tolerated by nurses as "part of the job." Nurses seldom report attacks to the police or prosecute their attackers, but such incidents should be reported to supervisors and possibly to legal authorities, depending on the circumstances. Aggression by patients must be addressed vigorously because it can threaten the other patients, other health care professionals, family members, and visitors, as well as the nursing staff. Reporting violent attacks increases public awareness and the likelihood that protective legislation will be enacted. The environment should be modified with the addition of security alarms, video monitors, and de-escalation teams.

All nurses must be provided with training programs in the prevention and management of aggressive behavior. These programs, similar to courses on cardiopulmonary resuscitation (CPR), impart both knowledge and skills, lessening the likelihood of emotional freezing in the presence of violent patient behavior. Similar to CPR training, the courses need to be made available to nurses regularly, so that they have opportunities to reinforce and update what they have learned. Some states have enacted legislation mandating workplace violence prevention programs, but the curricula vary, and the quality of training lacks systematic evaluation. Commercially marketed training programs have been criticized because they fail to consider the predatory aspect of some patients' violence and fail to cite nursing research.

RESEARCH AND POLICY INITIATIVES

Additional understanding of the phenomena of anger, aggression, and violence as they occur in the clinical setting is needed. Nurses must research the effectiveness of particular anger and aggression management interventions. Although much of this chapter focused on individuals who need to *down*regulate anger, the reader must remember that anger suppressors have a need to *up*regulate their anger and express it more assertively. Treatments should be tailored based on assessment data and patients' progress.

There is a moral imperative for nurses to be involved in combating violence in the larger community. Lessening anger and violence in the workplace and the home demands involvement of all mental health professionals. Nurses can share their expertise with parents, children, teachers, and community agencies. Nurses are well positioned to teach health-promoting anger management classes in diverse practice settings, such as outpatient clinics, schools, and corporate sites. Classes for children and adolescents can be of great benefit because young people are forming the anger habits that will continue into adulthood.

SUMMARY OF KEY POINTS

- Anger is an emotional state, usually temporary, that can be expressed constructively or destructively. Destructive anger alienates other people and invites retaliation.
- Anger, aggression, and violence should not be viewed as a continuum. The anger of ordinary people seldom progresses to aggression or violence. Anger does not necessarily lead to aggression or violence.
- Anger management is a useful psychoeducational intervention that is effective with a wide variety of nonviolent individuals. However, anger management is not designed to modify violent behavior.
- Several theories explain anger, aggression, and violence and include neurobiologic and psychosocial theories. These theories serve as the basis of assessment and interventions.
- The GAM accounts for the interaction of cognition, affect, and arousal during an aggressive episode.
- There is no one factor that predicts aggression or violence. Factors that have been observed to be precursors are staring and eye contact, tone and volume of voice, anxiety, mumbling, and pacing.
- Nursing interventions can be affective, cognitive, behavioral, or sociocultural. A therapeutic milieu supports a nonviolent culture.
- Nurses who experience assault may experience changes in affective, cognitive, behavioral, and physiologic areas.
- Seclusion or restraints should be used only as a last resort.
- Patient aggression and violence are serious concerns for nurses in all areas of clinical practice. Training in and policies and procedures for the prevention and management of aggressive episodes should be available in all work settings.

CRITICAL THINKING CHALLENGES

1. Mary Jane, a 24-year-old single woman, has just been admitted to an inpatient psychiatry unit. She was transferred to the unit from the emergency department where she was treated for a drug overdose. She is sullen when she is introduced to her roommate and refuses to answer the questions the nurse has that are part of the admission procedure. The nurse tells Mary Jane that he will come back later to see how she is. A

few minutes later, Mary Jane approaches the nursing station and asks in a demanding tone to talk with someone and complains that she has been completely ignored since she came into the unit.
   a. What frameworks can the nurse use to understand Mary Jane's behavior?
   b. At this point in time, what data does he have to develop a plan of care?
   c. What interventions might the nurse choose to use to help Mary Jane behave in a manner that is consistent with the norms of this inpatient unit?

2. Discuss the influence of gender and cultural norms on the expression of anger. When a nurse is caring for a patient from a culture that the nurse is not familiar with, what could the nurse ask to ensure that his or her expectations of the patient's behavior are consistent with the gender and cultural norms of the patient?

3. Under what circumstances should people who are aggressive or violent be held accountable for their behavior? Are there any exceptions?

4. When a nurse minimizes verbally abusive behavior by a patient, family member, or health care colleague, what implicit message does he or she send?

2013: Mandela: Long Walk to Freedom

South African icon Nelson Mandela displays the gamut of angry behaviors in this biographic epic: (1) righteous anger on behalf of his clients when he was a young lawyer; (2) fiery anger at the cruel persecution of blacks during apartheid; and (3) violence against the government after the failure of nonviolent protests to achieve freedom from oppression. Bomb throwing at government buildings results in 27 years of imprisonment, which could have created lasting bitterness against his oppressors. Yet after his release Mandela forgives those who had imprisoned him, becomes the first black president of his country, and receives the Nobel Peace Prize. This remarkable true story provides many lessons for all of us.

Viewing Points: Although most of us will never be forced to endure such intolerable conditions, we all experience times of unfair or unkind treatment. How can we learn to use our anger productively or learn to let it go by forgiving those who wronged us?

REFERENCES

Allen, J. J., Anderson, C. A., & Bushman, B. J. (2018). The general aggression model. *Current Opinions in Psychology, 19*, 75–80.

American Psychiatric Association (APA). (2013). *Diagnostic and statistical manual of mental disorders (DSM-5)*. Arlington, VA: Author.

American Psychiatric Nurses Association. (2014). *2014 Position statement on the use of seclusion and restraint*. Falls Church, VA: Author.

Averill, J. R. (1983). Studies on anger and aggression: implications for theories of emotion. *American Psychologist, 38*(11), 1145–1160.

Bader, S., Evans, S., & Welsh, E. (2014). Aggression among psychiatric inpatients: the relationship between time, place, victims, and severity ratings. *Journal of the American Psychiatric Nurses Association, 20*(3), 179–186.

Bandura, A. (2001). Social cognitive theory: an agentic perspective. *Annual Review of Psychology, 52*, 1–26.

Been, L. E., Gibbons, A. V., & Meisel, R. L. (2018). Towards a neurobiology of female aggression. *Neuropharmacology*. doi: 10.1016/j.neuropharm.2018.11.039

Björkdahl, A., Perseius, K. I., Samuelsson, M., & Lindberg, M. H. (2016). Sensory rooms in psychiatric inpatient care: Staff experiences. *International Journal of Mental Health Nursing, 25*(5), 472–479.

Bora, E., Velakoulis, D., & Walterfang, M. (2016). Meta-analysis of facial emotion recognition in behavioral variant frontotemporal dementia: comparison with Alzheimer Disease and healthy controls. *Journal of Geriatric Psychiatry and Neurology, 29*(4), 201–211.

Bowers, L., Wright, S., & Stewart, D. (2014). Patients subject to high levels of coercion: staff's understanding. *Issues in Mental Health Nursing, 35*(5), 364–371.

Boylan, J. M., & Ryff, C. D. (2015). High anger expression exacerbates the relationship between age and metabolic syndrome. *Journals of Gerontology, Series B: Psychological Sciences and Social Sciences, 70*(1), 77–82.

Buckley, T., Hoo, S. Y., Fethney, J., Shaw, E., Hanson, P. S., & Tofler, G. H. (2015). Triggering of acute coronary occlusion by episodes of anger. *European Heart Journal: Acute Cardiovascular Care, 4*(6), 493–498.

Burke, M. W., Fillion, M., Mejia, J., Ervin, F. R., & Palmour, R. M. (2018). Perinatal MAO inhibition produces long-lasting impairment of serotonin function in offspring. *Brain Sciences, 8*(6). pii, E106.

Burns, J. W., Quartana, P., & Bruehl, S. (2011). Anger suppression and subsequent pain behaviors among chronic low back pain patients: moderating effects of anger regulation style. *Annals of Behavioral Medicine, 42*(1), 42–54.

Coccaro, E. F. (2012). Intermittent explosive disorder as a disorder of impulsive aggression for DSM-5. *American Journal of Psychiatry, 169*(6), 577–588.

Coccaro, E., Fanning, J., Phan, K., & Lee, R. (2015). Serotonin and impulsive aggression. *CNS Spectrums, 20*(3), 295–302.

d'Ettorre, G., & Pellicani, V. (2017). Workplace violence toward mental healthcare workers employed in psychiatric wards. *Safety and Health at Work, 8*(4), 337–342.

Everson-Rose, S. A., & Lewis, T. T. (2005). Psychosocial factors and cardiovascular diseases. *Annual Review of Public Health, 26*, 469–500.

Feindler, E. L., & Byers, A. (2006). Multiple perspectives on the conceptualization and treatment of anger-related disorders. In E. L. Feindler (Ed.). *Anger-related disorders: A practitioner's guide to comparative treatments* (pp. 303–320). New York: Springer.

Galbraith, T., Carliner, H., Keyes, K. M., McLaughlin, K. A., McCloskey, M. S., & Heimberg, R. G. (2018). The co-occurrence and correlates of anxiety disorders among adolescents diagnosed with intermittent explosive disorder. *Aggressive Behavior, 44*(6), 581–590.

Gerrard, M., Gibbons, F. X., Fleischli, M. E., Cutrona, C. E., & Stock, M. L. (2018). Moderation of the effects of discrimination-induced affective responses on health outcomes. *Psychology & Health, 33*(2), 193–212.

Golding, P., & Fitzgerald, H. E. (2019). The early biopsychosocial development of boys and the origins of violence in males. *Infant Mental Health Journal, 40*(1), 5–22.

Gouin, J., Kiecolt-Glaser, J. K., Malarkey, W. B., & Glaser, R. (2008). The influence of anger expression on wound healing. *Brain, Behavior, and Immunity, 22*(5), 699–708.

Gross, R., Groer, M., & Thomas, S. P. (2014). Relationship of trait anger and anger expression to C-reactive protein in post-menopausal women. *Health Care for Women International, 35*(5), 580–595.

Halperin, E., & Tagar, M. R. (2017). Emotions in conflicts: Understanding emotional processes sheds light on the nature and potential resolution of intractable conflicts. *Current Opinion in Psychology, 17*, 94–98.

Jalil, R., & Dickens, G. L. (2018). Systematic review of studies of mental health nurses' experience of anger and its relationships with their attitudes and practice. *Journal of Psychiatric Mental Health Nursing, 25*(3), 201–213.

Keith, F., Krantz, D. S., Chen, R., Harris, K. M., Ware, C. M., & Lee, A. K., et al. (2017). Anger, hostility, and hospitalizations in patients with heart failure. *Health Psychology, 36*(9), 829–838.

Kessler, R., Coccaro, E., Fava, M., Jaeger, S., Jin, R., & Walters, E. (2006). The prevalence and correlates of DSM-IV intermittent explosive disorder in the National Comorbidity Survey replication. *Archives of General Psychiatry, 63*(3), 669–678.

Ketterer, M., Rose, B., Knysz, W., Farha, A., Deveshwar, S., Schairer, J., et al. (2011). Is social isolation/alienation confounded with, and non-independent of emotional distress in its association with early onset of coronary artery disease? *Psychology, Health, & Medicine, 16*(2), 238–247.

Kusmierska, G. (2011). *Do anger management treatments help angry adults? A meta-analytic answer.* New York: City University of New York.

Mostofsky, E., Maclure, M., Tofler, G., Muller, J. E., & Mittleman, M. A. (2013). Relation of outbursts of anger and risk of acute myocardial infarction. *American Journal of Cardiology, 112*(3), 343–348.

Pekurinen, V., Willman, L., Virtanen, M., Kivimäki, M., Vahtera, J., & Välimäki, M. (2017). Patient aggression and the wellbeing of nurses: A cross-sectional survey study in psychiatric and non-psychiatric settings. *International Journal of Environmental Research and Public Health, 14*(10), 1245.

Perugi, G., Fornaro, M., & Akiskal, H. S. (2011). Are atypical depression, borderline personality disorder and bipolar II disorder overlapping manifestations of a common cyclothymic diathesis. *World Psychiatry, 10*(1), 45–51.

Potpara, T. S., & Lip, G. Y. (2011). Lone atrial fibrillation: what is known and what is to come. *International Journal Clinical Practice, 65*(4), 446–457.

Repple, J., Habel, U., Wagels, L., Pawliczek, C. M., Schneider, F., & Kohn, N. (2018). Sex differences in the neural correlates of aggression. *Brain Structure & Function, 223*(9):4115–4124.

Rubin, T. I. (1970). *The angry book.* New York: Collier.

Smith-MacDonald, L., Norris, J. M., Raffin-Bouchal, S., & Sinclair, S. (2017). Spirituality and mental well-being in combat veterans: A systematic review. *Military Medicine, 182*(11), e1920–e1940.

Sommer, J., Iyican, S., & Babcock, J. (2016). The relation between contempt, anger, and intimate partner violence: A dyadic approach. *Journal of Interpersonal Violence.* doi: 10.1177/0886260516665107

Spielberger, C. D. (1999). *Manual for the State Trait Anger Expression Inventory-2.* Odessa, FL: Psychological Assessment Resources.

Teng, Z., Nie, Q., Guo, C., Zhang, Q., Liu, Y., & Bushman, B. J. (2019). A longitudinal study of link between exposure to violent video games and aggression in Chines adolescents: The mediating role of moral disengagement. *Developmental Psychology, 55*(1), 184–195.

Thomas, S. P. (1990). Theoretical and empirical perspectives on anger. *Issues in Mental Health Nursing, 11*(3), 203–216.

Thomas, S. P. (1997a). Women's anger: relationship of suppression to blood pressure. *Nursing Research, 46*(6), 324–330.

Thomas, S. P. (1997b). Angry? Let's talk about it! *Applied Nursing Research, 10*(2), 80–85.

Thomas, S. P. (2001). Teaching healthy anger management. *Perspectives in Psychiatric Care, 37*(2), 41–48.

Thomas, S. P. (2006). Cultural and gender considerations in the assessment and treatment of anger-related disorders. In E. L. Feindler (Ed.). *Anger-related disorders: A practitioner's guide to comparative treatments* (pp. 71–95). New York: Springer.

Thomas, S. P. (2009). *Transforming nurses' stress and anger.* (3rd ed.). New York: Springer.

Thomas, S. P., & Pollio, H. R. (2002). *Listening to patients.* New York: Springer.

Trost, Z., Scott, W., Buelow, M. T., Nowlin, L., Turan, B., Boals, A., et al. (2017). The association between injustice perception and psychological outcomes in an inpatient spinal cord injury sample: The mediating effects of anger. *Spinal Cord, 55*(10), 898–905.

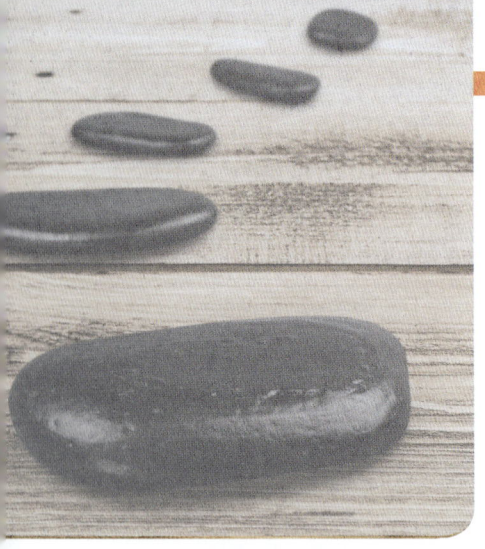

15

Crisis, Loss, Grief Response, Bereavement, and Disaster Management

Sara Rich Wheeler and Mary Ann Boyd

KEY CONCEPTS
- bereavement
- crisis
- disaster
- grief responses
- loss

LEARNING OBJECTIVES

After studying this chapter, you will be able to:

1. Describe the types of crises and losses.
2. Differentiate between grief responses and bereavement process.
3. Discuss theoretical models explaining grief responses, uncomplicated bereavement, and complicated bereavement.
4. Discuss nursing care for persons experiencing crises, loss, grief, bereavement, and disaster.
5. Evaluate the effects of crises, losses, and disasters on lifestyle and survival.
6. Explain the psychological impact of crises, losses, and disasters on survivors of catastrophic events.

KEY TERMS

- ABCs of psychological first aid • complicated bereavement • debriefing • developmental crisis • dual process model
- integrated bereavement theory • loss-oriented coping • oscillation • restoration-oriented coping • situational crisis
- traumatic crisis • uncomplicated bereavement

Successfully surviving crises, loss, and disaster may make a difference between being mentally healthy or mentally ill. This chapter explores the concepts of crisis, loss, grief responses, bereavement, and disaster management; broadens the scope and understanding of the responses of persons to crisis, loss, and disaster situations; and describes how the nursing process can be used to care for persons experiencing these events.

CRISIS

Adaptation and coping are a natural part of life (see Chapter 13). Crisis occurs when there is a perceived challenge or threat that overwhelms the capacity of the individual to cope effectively with the event at any age. Life is disrupted, and unexpected emotional (e.g., sadness, depression, anxiety) and biologic (e.g., nausea, vomiting, diarrhea, headaches) responses occur (see Box 15.1). Functioning can be severely impaired.

KEYCONCEPT Crisis is a time-limited event that triggers adaptive or nonadaptive responses to maturational, situational, or traumatic experiences. A crisis results from stressful events for which previous coping mechanisms fail to provide adequate adaptive skills to address the perceived challenge or threat. Adaptation to crisis typically occurs in 6 weeks.

A crisis occurs when an individual is at a breaking point. A crisis can have either positive or negative outcomes. If positive, there is an opportunity for growth and change as new ways of coping are learned. If negative, suicide, homelessness, or depression can result. A crisis

BOX 15.1
Grief Responses

Physical: stunned, weight gain/loss, insomnia, anorexia, exhausted, restless, aching arms, sleep difficulties, headaches, feels ill, palpitations, breathlessness, sighing, lack of strength, blurred vision

Emotional: crying, sobbing, sadness, guilt, anger, sense of failure, irritability, resentment, bitterness, denial, frustration, shame, fear of own death, oversensitivity to environment, senses the presence of the deceased

Social: social withdrawal from normal activity, isolation from others

Cognitive: forgetful, difficulty in making decisions, disorganized, concentration is difficult, preoccupation with thoughts of the deceased, time confusion, short attention span, think they are going crazy

---

generally lasts no more than 4 to 6 weeks. At the end of that time, the person in crisis should have begun to come to grip with the event and begun to harness resources to cope with its long-term consequences. By definition, there is no such thing as a chronic crisis. People who live in constant turmoil are not in crisis but in chaos.

Many events evoke a crisis, such as natural disasters (e.g., floods, tornadoes, earthquakes) and human-made disasters (e.g., wars, bombings, airplane crashes) as well as traumatic experiences (e.g., rape, sexual abuse, assault). In addition, interpersonal events (marriage, birth of a child) create crises in the lives of any person.

Feelings of fear, desperation, and being out of control are common during a crisis, but the precipitating event and circumstances are unusual or rare, perceived as a threat, and specific to the individual. For example, a disagreement with a family member may escalate into a crisis for one person, but not another. If the person is significantly distressed or social functioning is impaired, a diagnosis of acute stress disorder should be considered (American Psychiatric Association [APA], 2013). The person with an acute stress disorder has dissociative symptoms and persistently reexperiences the event (APA; see Chapter 27).

Historical Perspectives of Crisis

The psychiatrist Caplan (1961) defined a crisis as occurring when a person faces a problem that cannot be solved by customary problem-solving methods. When the usual problem-solving methods no longer work, a person's life balance or equilibrium is upset. During the period of disequilibrium, there is a rise in inner tension and anxiety followed by emotional upset and an inability to function. This conceptualization of phases of a crisis is used today (Fig. 15.1). According to Caplan, during a crisis, a person is open to learning new ways of coping to survive. The outcome of a crisis is governed by the kind of interaction that occurs between the person and available key social support systems.

Types of Crises

Research has focused on categorizing types of crisis events, understanding responses to a crisis, and developing intervention models that support people through a crisis.

Developmental Crisis

While Caplan was creating his crisis model, Erik Erikson was formulating ideas about crisis and development. He proposed that **maturational crises** are a normal part

---

A problem arises that contributes to increase in anxiety levels. The anxiety initiates the usual problem-solving techniques of the person.

↓

The usual problem-solving techniques are ineffective. Anxiety levels continue to rise. Trial-and-error attempts are made to restore balance.

↓

The trial-and-error attempts fail. The anxiety escalates to severe or panic levels. The person adopts automatic relief behaviors.

↓

When these measures do not reduce anxiety, anxiety can overwhelm the person and lead to serious personality disorganization, which signals the person is in crisis.

FIGURE 15.1 Phases of crisis.

of growth and development and successfully resolving a crisis at one stage allows one to move to the next. According to this model, the child develops positive characteristics after experiencing a crisis. If he or she develops less desirable traits, the crisis is not resolved (see Chapter 7). The concept of **developmental crisis** continues to be used today to describe significant maturational events, such as leaving home for the first time, completing school, and accepting the responsibility of adulthood.

Situational Crisis

A **situational crisis** occurs whenever a specific stressful event threatens a person's physical and psychosocial integrity and results in some degree of psychological disequilibrium. The event can be an internal one, such as a disease process, or any number of external threats. A move to another city, a job promotion, or graduation from high school can initiate a crisis even though they are positive events. Graduation from high school marks the end of an established routine of going to school, participating in school activities, and doing homework assignments. When starting a new job after graduation, the former student must learn an entirely different routine and acquire new knowledge and skills. If a person enters a new situation without adequate coping skills, a crisis may occur.

Traumatic Crisis

A **traumatic crisis** is initiated by unexpected, unusual events that can affect an individual or a multitude of people. In such situations, people face overwhelmingly hazardous events that entail injury, trauma, destruction, or sacrifice. Examples of events include national disasters (e.g., racial persecutions, riots, war), violent crimes (e.g., rape, murder, kidnappings, and assault and battery), and environmental disasters (e.g., earthquakes, floods, forest fires, hurricanes).

LOSS AND BEREAVEMENT

> **KEYCONCEPT** **Loss** can evoke minor to complex thoughts, feelings, and behaviors depending on the perceived relationship of the person with the lost loved object or person.

In death, the intensity of the loss is based on perceived relationship to the deceased. The interrelationship between internal and external factors influences the perception of loss. There are several types of losses. Death can occur suddenly, unexpectedly, be anticipated after a life-threatening event, or after a long-term, chronic illness. Stigmatic losses such as abortion, AIDS, homicide, and suicide can also affect coping with and healing after a loss. The first year after a loss is considered to be the most difficult as holidays, birthdays, anniversaries, and other important life events must be handled by the bereaved. Days surrounding the anniversary date of the death can be difficult for the bereaved. The terms *bereavement* and *mourning* are used interchangeably to describe the process of healing after a perceived loss. The outcomes of loss and bereavement can range from an increase in psychosocial functioning to maladaptation which can include death, illness, isolation, and/or mental illness.

> **KEYCONCEPT** **Grief responses** are intense, physical, emotional, social, cognitive, or social reactions to the death of a loved one. Spontaneous expressions to loss can include sobbing, crying, anger, and expressions of guilt.
> **Bereavement** is the process of healing and learning how to cope with the loss. It begins immediately after the loss, and can last months or years. Individual differences, age, religious and cultural practices, and social support influence grief responses and bereavement.

Theories of Bereavement

Stage Theories

There has been wide acceptance that grief and bereavement follow stages (Bowlby & Parkes, 1970; Kubler-Ross, 1969). Although over time, the stage theory of grief and bereavement has been challenged and remains unsupported by empirical evidence today, it continues to be used by health care professionals (Corr, 2018).

Integrative Bereavement Theory

The **integrated bereavement theory** consists of five stages (Sanders, 1998). See Box 15.2. Shock may be as brief as a few minutes to 2 weeks. When the rituals and customs of death are over, and social support begins to diminish the physical, emotional, and cognitive grief responses, bereavement begins in earnest during the phase of *Awareness of the loss*. Many environmental cues (i.e., bed, car, kitchen table, food in a grocery store) remind the bereaved of their loss. The bereaved may feel physical pain and deep emotions when faced with these cues. There are many emotional struggles during this time. These conflicts are hard to resolve because they usually involve change. Grief takes time and energy which can deplete the body's physical and emotional reserves. The immune system becomes impaired and the bereaved becomes more susceptible to illness. Physical and emotional exhaustion are paramount in this phase which motivates the bereaved to withdraw from others to conserve strength and energy.

The *conservation-withdrawal* phase closely resembles clinical depression. The bereaved feel as if they have

> **BOX 15.2**
> **Stages/Phases Bereavement Process**
>
> 1. *Shock and disbelief*
> 2. *Awareness of loss*
>   a. Separation anxiety predominates
>   b. Intense physical, emotional, social, and cognitive response
>   c. Identification with the deceased
> 3. *Conservation-withdrawal*
>   a. Social withdrawal
>   b. Consciously and unconsciously the bereaved understand his/her loved one has died
>   c. Little strength to do everyday activities
>   d. Closely resembles clinical depression
>   e. Turning point—a conscious process of deciding how the death is viewed and integrated into one's life
> 4. *Healing*
>   a. Acceptance of the loss intellectually
>   b. Acceptance of the loss emotionally
>   c. Change in the world view to match his/her reality
> 5. *Renewal*
>   a. Increase in self-esteem
>   b. Takes charge and is responsible for his/her life
>   c. New level of functioning and self-awareness
>   d. Renewed vitality
>
> Adapted from Sanders, C. M. (1998). *Grief: The mourning after. Dealing with adult bereavement.* New York: Wiley Interscience.

little strength to do everyday activities and need to rest. Despair prevails as he/she realizes their life with their loved one is over. They may feel helpless during this phase, especially if their role in life was defined by their loved one. For grief work to begin, the loss and changes created by the loss must be accepted. Extended family members and friends have gone on with their lives, and do not realize the bereaved are still grieving their loss. This leaves the bereaved feeling more alone. The *turning point* occurs for some in a dramatic turn of the mind; for others, it is a slow process of change in how the death is viewed and integrated in their life. Every day is not a bad day. There may be good moments in a bad day. Over time, the bereaved notice they are having more good days with a bad moment.

Healing begins to occur when internal perceptions begin to change from being bereaved to one who has experienced and survived a loss. Neither everyone heals after a loss, nor feels renewal. *Renewal* occurs when the bereaved has dealt with the social consequences of bereavement, experienced an increase in self-esteem, taken charge of, and are responsible for his/her life, and learned how to live again. New levels of functioning and awareness of self exist. As time goes by, remembering their loved one and surrounding life events (i.e., anniversary dates, birthdays, holidays, special memories, life's milestones) may trigger a "regrief." The bereaved may feel they have "dealt" with the loss, when all of a sudden, they experience grief responses. As the bereaved develop perspective on their loss and recognize this for what it is … bittersweet grief.

Throughout the bereavement process, the bereaved has searched for the meaning of the loss: What happened? Where are they? What did the death mean? How will the deceased be remembered? Who will remember them? and so on. This search continues until some conclusions have been reached. This is known as *loss integration*.

Dual Process Model

The **dual process model** (DPM) offers a nonlinear explanation of how grieving persons and families come to terms with their loss over time (Stroebe & Schut, 2015; Stroebe, Schut, & Boerner, 2010). According to DPM, the person adjusts to the loss by oscillating between **loss-oriented coping** (preoccupation with the deceased) and **restoration-oriented coping** (preoccupation with stressful events as a result of the death including financial issues, new identity as a widow[er]). **Oscillation** is the process of confronting (loss-oriented coping) and avoiding (restoration-oriented coping) the stresses associated with bereavement. At times, the bereaved person is confronted with the loss and memories, and at other times, the person will be distracted and the thoughts and memories will be avoided. The bereaved experiences relief from the intense emotion associated with the loss by focusing on other things. For example, the bereaved person may be recalling a special moment in the relationship such as a wedding or imagining what the person would say about a current event but then switches to thinking about completing tasks that the deceased had previously undertaken (e.g., paying bills, cooking meals). In the loss-oriented coping mode, emotions relate to the relationship with the deceased person; in the restoration-oriented coping, the bereaved person's emotions relate to the stressful events associated with the responsibilities and changes as a result of the loss. Over time, after repeated confrontation with the loss, there is no longer a need to think about certain aspects of the loss (Currie et al., 2018). See Figure 15.2.

Types of Bereavement

Uncomplicated Bereavement

Most bereaved people experience **uncomplicated bereavement** after the loss of a loved one. Uncomplicated bereavement grief is painful and disruptive, however, there is always movement. Questions surface such as "Why did the death happen?" "Why my loved one?" "Why me?" and, "Why did God allow this to happen?"

The bereavement process is often applied to other situations in which a loss occurs, not necessarily the death of a person. The "empty nest syndrome," divorce, birth of a handicapped child, and death of a pet are other examples of losses were there may be grief responses and bereavement.

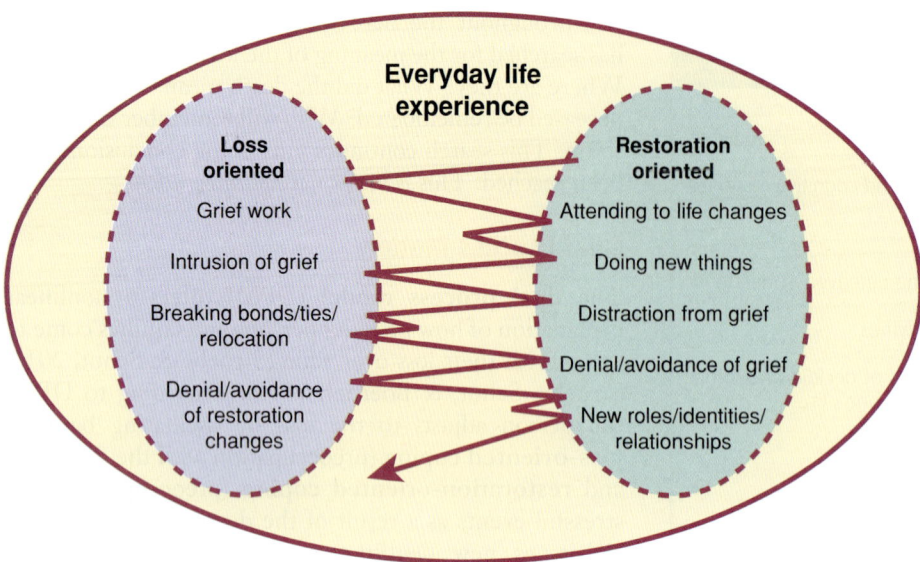

FIGURE 15.2 Dual process model of coping with bereavement. (Redrawn from Stroebe, M., & Schut, H. (1999). The dual process model of coping with bereavement: Rationale and description. *Death Studies, 23*, 213. Used with permission from Taylor & Francis Group.)

Most bereaved persons do not need clinical interventions and are able to find new meaning and purpose in their lives. Their self-esteem and sense of competency while threatened remain intact. They gradually accept the sense of loss as a reality and are able to move on with their lives. There is little evidence they need or benefit from counseling or therapy. Those who experience suicidal thoughts with a plan and/or suicidal gestures should be evaluated for depression and posttraumatic stress disorder (PTSD) (Bennett & Soulsby, 2012; Tol et al., 2014; Waller et al., 2016).

Traumatic Grief

Traumatic grief is a term that is used for a more difficult and prolonged grief. In traumatic grieving, external factors influence the reactions and potential long-term outcomes. For example, memories of the traumatic death of the deceased may lead to more traumatic memories including the violent death scene (Mutabaruka, Séjourné, Bui, Birmes, & Chabro, 2012). The external circumstances of death associated with traumatic grief include (1) suddenness and lack of anticipation; (2) violence, mutilation, and destruction; (3) degree of preventability or randomness of the death; (4) multiple deaths (bereavement overload); and (5) mourner's personal encounter with death involving a significant threat to personal survival or a massive and shocking confrontation with the death (or mutilation) of others (Zetumer et al., 2015).

Complicated Bereavement

Complicated bereavement or complicated grief disorder (CGD) occurs in about 10% to 20% of bereaved persons (Malgaroli, Maccallum, & Bonanno, 2018). The person is frozen or stuck in a state of chronic mourning which lasts for more than a month to 6 months after a loss. In other words, there is no movement in the bereaved's thought processes in how they view and experience their loss. The person may feel bitter over the loss and wish his or her life could revert to the time they were together. In complicated grief, there is an intense longing and yearning for the person who died that lasts for more than 6 months. Additionally, the person may have trouble accepting the death, an inability to trust others since the death, excessive bitterness related to the death, and feeling that life is meaningless without the deceased person (Claxton & Reynolds, 2012). Individuals who are more vulnerable for developing complicated bereavement are those who have experienced a sudden, unexpected loss, stigmatic loss, or death of a loved one after a long-term chronic illness as these situations have the potential to limit their social support. The lack of social support is a common denominator as the bereaved's social support system may not know what to say or do in these circumstances. Other reasons for the development of complicated bereavement may be other antecedents, such as having a pessimistic personality, and previous diagnosis of mental health disorder (Nielsen et al., 2017).

Teamwork and Collaboration: Working Toward Recovery

The goal for people experiencing a crisis is to return to the precrisis level of functioning. The role of the nurse is to provide a framework of support systems that guide the patient through the crisis and facilitate the development and use of positive coping skills.

BOX 15.3
Decision Tree for Determining Referral

Situation: A 35-year-old woman is being seen in a clinic because of minor burns she received during a house fire. Her home was completely destroyed. She is tearful and withdrawn, and she complains of a great deal of pain from her minor burns. Biopsychosocial assessment is completed.

ASSESSMENT RESULT	NURSING ACTION
Patient has psychological distress but believes that her social support is adequate. She would like to talk to a nurse when she returns for her follow-up visit.	Provide counseling and support for the patient during her visit. Make an appointment for her return visit to the clinic for follow-up.
The patient is severely distressed. She has no social support. She does not know how she will survive.	Refer the patient to a mental health specialist. The patient will need crisis intervention strategies provided by a mental health specialist.

EMERGENCY CARE ALERT ! It is important to be acutely aware that a person in crisis may be at high risk for suicide or homicide. To determine the level of effectiveness of coping capabilities of the person, the nurse should complete a careful assessment for suicidal or homicidal risk. If a person is at high risk for either, the nurse should consider referral for admission to the hospital.

NCLEXNOTE During a crisis, the behaviors and verbalizations of a person may provide data that are indicative of a mental illness. Nursing care should be prioritized according to the severity of responses. After the crisis has been resolved, assess whether the abnormal thoughts or feelings disappear.

During an environmental crisis (e.g., flood, hurricane, forest fire) that affects the well-being of many people, nursing interventions will be a part of the community's efforts to respond to the event. This is covered in more detail in the section of the chapter on disasters. On the other hand, when a personal crisis occurs, the person in crisis may have only the nurse to respond to his or her needs. After the assessment, the nurse must decide whether to provide the care needed or to refer the person to a mental health specialist. Box 15.3 offers guidance in making this decision.

EVIDENCE-BASED NURSING CARE OF PERSON IN CRISIS

Mental Health Nursing Assessment

The first priority is determining the extent of physical injury or trauma. The person should receive medical care for any injuries. Once medically stable, changes in health practices following the crisis provide clues to the severity of the disruption in functioning.

Physical Health

Maintaining health is important because a crisis can be physically exhausting. Disturbances in sleep and eating patterns and the reappearance of physical or psychiatric symptoms are common. Changes in body function may include tachycardia, tachypnea, profuse perspiration, nausea, vomiting, dilated pupils, and extreme shakiness. Some individuals may exhibit loss of control and have total disregard for their personal safety. These people are at high risk for injury, which may include infection, trauma, and head injuries (Betancourt et al., 2012). If sleep patterns are disturbed or nutrition is inadequate, the individual may not have the physical resources to deal with the crisis.

Emotional and Behavioral Responses

The mental health nursing assessment focuses on the individual's emotions and coping strengths. In the beginning of the crisis, the person may report feelings of numbness and shock. Responses to psychological distress should be differentiated from symptoms of psychiatric illnesses that may be present. Later, as the reality of the crisis sinks in, the person will be able to recognize and describe the felt emotions. The nurse should expect these emotions to be intense and be sure to provide some support during their expression.

Initially, the individual's thoughts and behaviors may be erratic and illogic. The nurse should assess for evidence of depression, confusion, uncontrolled weeping or screaming, disorientation, or aggression. The person may be suffering from a loss of feelings of well-being and safety. In addition, panic responses, anxiety, and fear may be present (Fischer, Postmes, Koeppl, Conway, & Fredriksson, 2011). The ability to cope by problem-solving may be disrupted. By assessing the person's ability to solve problems, the nurse can evaluate whether he or she can cognitively cope with the crisis situation and determine the kind and amount of support needed.

Social Functioning and Support

Assessment of the extent of disruption of normal daily activities and routines is essential. The person may not be shopping, paying bills, etc. The nurse should explore the presence of a social network of family and friends who are available to provide help and support during the crisis.

Priority Nursing Care

When assessing the coping ability of the client, the nurse should assess for unusual behaviors and determine the level of involvement of the person with the crisis. In addition, assess for evidence of self-mutilation activities that may indicate the use of self-preservation measures to avoid suicide. It is critical to assess the client's perception of the problem and the availability of support mechanisms (emotional and financial) for use by the person.

Any body system can be impacted by a crisis. Diarrhea and urinary incontinence can occur. Strengths related to physical health prior to the crisis should be considered. The person may have exercised regularly and is ready to use exercise as a way of dealing with the stress. Or the person may have had a healthy diet before the crisis and is now ready to reengage in healthier eating choices.

Survivors may experience post trauma syndrome, confusion, wanting to die, violence, anxiety, powerlessness, and difficulty coping with the loss. Because the response to a crisis is individual and differs from person to person, the nurse should make sure that a very complete assessment is done.

Therapeutic Relationship

A nurse is often meeting the person in crisis for the first time and will need to skillfully apply therapeutic communication techniques to meet the individual's immediate mental health needs. Patience, listening, and empathy are important tools that along with a calm, nurturing approach can help establish trust. In some instances, the nurse has a relationship with the patient who reaches out during a crisis. In that instance, the nurse will have already established the therapeutic relationship and can quickly provide meaningful support and interventions. Be careful not to give unrealistic or false reassurances of positive outcomes over which you have no control. For example, it is not a good idea to reassure the person that everything will be alright because things may get worse, not better.

> **NCLEXNOTE** Individual responses to a crisis can be best understood by assessing the usual responses of the person to stressful events. The response to the crisis will also depend on the meaning of the event to the person. The use of therapeutic communication principles is a priority when caring for a person who has experienced a crisis or disaster.

Mental Health Nursing Interventions

Immediate goals during a crisis may be preventing the person from committing suicide or homicide, arranging for food and shelter (if needed), and mobilizing social support. After safety needs are met, the individual can work toward recovery by addressing other goals such as reestablishing self-care routines and using positive coping strategies. Guidelines for crisis intervention and examples are presented in Table 15.1. Individuals should be encouraged to report any depression, anxiety, or interpersonal difficulties during the recovery period.

TABLE 15.1 GUIDELINES FOR CRISIS INTERVENTION

Approach	Rationale	Example
Support the expression (or nonexpression) of feelings according to cultural or ethnic practices.	Emotional support helps the person face reality. The emotional expression by the victim may be culturally driven.	Ask the person to actualize the loss using active and reflective listening. "Where you there when he/she died?" "Tell me how they died?" "What special remembrances do you have?" If the person is crying, sobbing, or angry; allow for the expression of his/her emotions. Sit quietly beside. When they are done you can say, "I can tell how terribly sad or angry you are." Try to avoid handing a tissue. Wait for them to look for a tissue before you hand them one.
Help the person think clearly and focus on one implication at a time.	Focusing on all the implications at once can be too overwhelming.	A woman left her husband because of abuse. At first, focus only on her living arrangements and safety. "You can say, there are several things we need to focus on now for your safety." At another time, discuss the other implications of the separation.
Avoid giving false reassurances, such as "It will be all right;" "It is for the best."	Giving false reassurances blocks communication. It may not be all right.	Patient: "My doctor told me that I have a terminal illness." Nurse: Restatement: "Your doctor told you, you have a terminal illness. What does that mean to you?"
Clarify fantasies with facts.	Accurate information is needed to solve problems.	A young mother is holding her child who has died. The mother expresses disbelief this has happened. Quietly sit beside her. The longer she holds her child, the realization this has occurred will settle within her. You do not need to point out the obvious.
Link the person and family with community resources, as needed.	Social support can ease the effect of the crisis or loss.	Provide information about a meeting of a support group such as that of the American Cancer Society, Alzheimer's Support Groups; compassionate friends; resolve through sharing or other local bereavement support groups.

Adapted from Lazarus, R. (1991). *Emotion and adaptation* (p. 122). New York: Oxford University Press; Worden, W. (1991). *Grief counseling and grief therapy: A handbook for the mental health practitioner*. New York: Springer.

Self-Care

A person needs to eat and sleep in order to have the energy to cope with a crisis. Personal hygiene may be suffering. The nurse should encourage the person to reestablish a healthy diet, practice sleep hygiene strategies, and attend to personal grooming. If the person is unable to function, a referral can be made to other health care clinicians. Medication may be needed to help maintain a high level of psychophysical functioning.

Medications

Medication cannot resolve a crisis, but the judicious use of these agents can help reduce its emotional intensity. For example, Mrs. Brown has just learned that both of her parents have perished in an airplane crash. When she arrives at the emergency department to identify their bodies, she is shaking, sobbing, and unable to answer questions. The emergency physician orders lorazepam (Ativan) (Box 15.4). The phases of treatment include initiation of treatment, assessment of stabilization from the treatment, and timeframe for maintenance of treatment.

1. **Initiation:** Because Mrs. Brown is overcome by grief and severe anxiety about seeing her parents' bodies, 2 mg of lorazepam is administered intramuscularly as ordered by the doctor. The nurse monitors the patient for onset of action and any side effects. If Mrs. Brown does not have some relief within 20 to 30 minutes, another injection can be given as ordered by the doctor.
2. **Stabilization:** During the next half hour, Mrs. Brown regains some of her composure. She is no longer shaking, and her crying is occasional. She is reluctant to identify her parents but can do so when accompanied by the nurse. After the paperwork is completed, Mrs. Brown is sent home with a prescription for lorazepam, 2 to 4 mg every 12 hours.
3. **Maintenance:** Mrs. Brown takes the medication during the next week as she plans and attends her parents' funeral and manages the affairs surrounding their deaths. The medication keeps her anxiety at a manageable level, enabling her to do the tasks required of her.
4. **Medication cessation:** Two weeks after the death of her parents, Mrs. Brown is no longer taking lorazepam. She is grieving normally and has periods of tearfulness and sadness about her loss, but she can cope. She visits with friends, reminisces with family members, and reads inspirational poems. All of these activities help her navigate the changes in her life brought about by her parents' sudden death.

This example demonstrates how a medication can be used to assist a person through a crisis. After that crisis has passed, the person can use his or her personal coping mechanisms to adapt.

BOX 15.4
Drug Profile: Lorazepam (Ativan)

DRUG CLASS: Benzodiazepine; antianxiety/sedative hypnotic agent

RECEPTOR AFFINITY: Acts mainly at the subcortical levels of the central nervous system (CNS), leaving the cortex relatively unaffected. Main sites of action may be the limbic system and reticular formation. It potentiates the effects of α-aminobutyric acid, an inhibitory neurotransmitter. The exact mechanism of action is unknown.

INDICATIONS: Management of anxiety disorders or for short-term relief of symptoms of anxiety or anxiety associated with depression (oral forms). Also used as preanesthetic medication in adults to produce sedation, relieve anxiety, and decrease recall of events related to surgery (parenteral form). Unlabeled parenteral uses for management of acute alcohol withdrawal.

ROUTE AND DOSAGE: Available in 0.5-, 1-, and 2-mg tablets; 2-mg/mL concentrated oral solution and 2- and 4-mg/mL solutions for injection.

Adults: Usually 2 to 6 mg/day orally, with a range of 1 to 10 mg/day in divided doses, with the largest dose given at night. 0.05 mg/kg intramuscularly (IM) up to a maximum of 4 mg administered at least 2 h before surgery. Initially 2 mg total or 0.044 mg/kg intravenously (IV) (whichever is smaller). Doses as high as 0.05 mg/kg up to a total of 4 mg may be given 15 to 20 min before the procedure to those benefiting by a greater lack of recall.

Geriatric patients: Dosage not to exceed adult IV dose. Orally, 1 to 2 mg/day in divided doses initially, adjusted as needed and tolerated.

Children: Drug should not be used in children younger than 12 years.

HALF-LIFE (PEAK EFFECT): 10 to 20 h (1 to 6 h [oral]; 60 to 90 min IM; 10 to 15 min IV).

SELECTED ADVERSE REACTIONS: Transient mild drowsiness, sedation, depression, lethargy, apathy, fatigue, light-headedness, disorientation, anger, hostility, restlessness, confusion, crying, headache, mild paradoxical excitatory reactions during first 2 weeks of treatment, constipation, dry mouth, diarrhea, nausea, bradycardia, hypotension, cardiovascular collapse, urinary retention, and drug dependence with withdrawal symptoms.

WARNINGS: Contraindicated in psychoses; acute narrow angle glaucoma; shock; acute alcoholic intoxication with depression of vital signs; and during pregnancy, labor and delivery, and while breastfeeding. Use cautiously in patients with impaired liver or kidney function and those who are debilitated. When given with theophylline, there is a decreased effect of lorazepam. When using the drug IV, it must be diluted immediately before use and administered by direct injection slowly or infused at a maximum rate of 2 mg/min. When giving narcotic analgesics, reduce its dose by at least half in patients who have received lorazepam.

SPECIFIC PATIENT AND FAMILY EDUCATION

- Take the drug exactly as prescribed; do not stop taking the drug abruptly.
- Avoid alcohol and other CNS depressants.
- Avoid driving and other activities that require alertness.
- Notify the prescriber before taking any other prescription or over-the-counter drug.
- Change your position slowly and sit at the edge of the bed for a few minutes before arising.
- Report to the prescriber any severe dizziness, weakness, drowsiness that persists, rash or skin lesions, palpitations, edema of the extremities, visual changes, or difficulty urinating.

Counseling

Counseling reinforces healthy coping behaviors and interaction patterns. Counseling, which focuses on identifying emotions and positive coping strategies, helps the person to integrate the effects of the crisis into a real life experience. Responses to crisis differ with individuals. Some may present with behaviors that indicate transient disruptions in their ability to cope. Others may be totally devastated. At times, telephone counseling may provide the person with enough help that face-to-face counseling is not necessary. If counseling strategies do not work, other stress reduction and coping enhancement interventions can be used (see Chapter 18). The nurse should refer anyone who cannot cope with a crisis to a mental health specialist for an evaluation.

Social Support Strategies

The nursing interventions for the social domain can focus on the individual, the family, and the community. A crisis often disrupts a person's social network, leading to changes in available social support. Development of a new social support network may help the person cope more effectively with the crisis. Supporting the development of new support contacts within the context of available social networks can be done by contacting available local and state agencies for assistance as well as specific private support groups and religious groups.

Telephone Hotlines

Public and private funding and the efforts of trained volunteers permit most communities to provide crisis services to the public. For example, telephone hotlines for problems ranging from child abuse to suicide are a part of health delivery systems of most communities. Crisis services permit immediate access to the mental health system for people who are experiencing an emergency (such as threatened suicide) or for those who need help with stress or a crisis.

Residential Crisis Services

Many communities provide, as part of the health care network, residential crisis services for people who need short-term housing. The specific residential crisis services available within a community reflect the problems that the community members judge as particularly important. For example, some communities provide shelter for teenage runaways; others offer shelter for abused spouses. Still others provide shelter for people who would otherwise require acute psychiatric hospitalization. These settings provide residents with a place to stay in a supportive, home-like atmosphere. The people who use these services are linked to other community services such as financial aid.

Evaluation and Treatment Outcomes

Outcomes developed in cooperation with the person experiencing the crisis guide the evaluation. Once assessment data are clustered and prioritized, the nursing priorities and the outcomes are determined. Once interventions are developed and implemented in cooperation with the individual in crisis, the person should come through the crisis with improved health, well-being, and social function. If complications occur, the nurse should make appropriate alterations in the entire nursing process or make appropriate referrals.

DISASTER AND TERRORISM

A disaster is a sudden ecologic or human-made phenomenon that is of sufficient magnitude to require external help to address the psychosocial needs as well as the physical needs of the victims. Acts of terrorism present situations that mimic disasters and can be categorized as a type of disaster.

> **KEYCONCEPT** A **disaster** is a sudden overwhelming catastrophic event that causes great damage and destruction that may involve mass casualties and human suffering requiring assistance from all available resources.

Although disasters can affect all members of a society, the most affected are the victims and survivors of the event, as well as nurses and others who are first to respond to the traumatic and life-threatening consequences of the event. The mental health of the survivors of disasters can be severely impacted by the event. Fear, anger, and distress elevate severe anxiety to the panic level, which can result in severe mental illnesses. Unresolved crisis or disastrous events can lead to disorganized thinking. Post-disaster depression is a real risk (North, Baron, & Chen, 2018). In addition, the victims may experience the development of acute stress disorder (which has a strong emphasis on dissociative symptoms) and PTSD.

Historical Perspectives of Disasters in the United States

Throughout history, disasters have been portrayed from a fatalistic perspective that humans have little control over catastrophic events. Some cultures contend that natural disasters are acts of God. Other cultures express their belief that natural disaster events can be attributed to gods dwelling within places such as volcanoes, with eruptions being an expression of the Gods' anger. Although often caused by nature, disasters can have human origins.

Wars and civil disturbances that destroy homelands and displace people are included among the causes of disasters. Other causes include a building collapse, blizzard, drought, earthquake, epidemic, explosion, famine, fire, flood, hazardous material or transportation incident (such as a chemical spill), hurricane, nuclear incident, terrorist attack, and tornado. Often, the unpredictability of such disasters causes fear, confusion, and stress that can have lasting effects on the health of affected communities and their sense of well-being.

In recent history, we have experienced several attacks of violence and terrorism that are unprecedented in North America. These include the destruction of the World Trade Center in New York on September 11, 2001, the Sandy Hook school tragedy in 2012, and the Boston Marathon bombing in 2013, all of which shattered North Americans' sense of safety and security.

Since September 11, 2001, the emergency response planning of federal, state, and local agencies has focused on possible terrorist attacks with chemical, biologic, radiologic, nuclear, or high-yield explosive weapons. Before September 11, 2001, government agencies and public health leaders had not incorporated mental health into their overall response plans to bioterrorism. But in the aftermath of the mass destruction of human life and property in 2001, government and health care leaders are recognizing the need for monumental mental health efforts to be implemented during episodes of terrorism and disaster. The psychological and behavioral consequences of a terrorist attack are now included in most disaster plans.

Hurricane Maria in Puerto Rico in 2018, Hurricane Harvey in Texas in 2017, and the earthquake and tsunami in Japan in 2011 highlight the importance of government preparedness for natural disasters as well as terrorism. In the United States, the lack of government response and breakdown in communication during Maria resulted in thousands of hurricane victims being displaced and injured. Many Puerto Ricans moved to Florida and experienced more emotional and psychological problems than those staying on the island (Scaramutti et al., 2019). The Japan disaster became a cascade of disasters, resulting in the death of thousands of residents and contamination from the damaged nuclear site. Consequences of these disasters will still be occurring months and years after the initial events.

Phases of Disaster

Natural and human-made disaster can be conceptualized in three phases:

1. *Prewarning of the disaster.* This phase entails preparing the community for possible evacuation of the environment, mobilization of resources, and review of community disaster plans. In some disasters, such as in the 2011 earthquake in Japan, there is very little warning.
2. *The disaster event occurs.* In this phase, the rescuers provide resources, assistance, and support as needed to preserve the biopsychosocial functioning and survival of the victims. In large disasters, the rescuers and health care professionals also experience the traumatic event as both residents and health care providers. The victims experience the initial trauma and threats that occur immediately after the disaster such as confusion (communication breakdown), lack of safety (no available law enforcement), and lack of health care services.
3. *Recuperative effort.* In the third phase, the focus is on implementing strategies for healing sick and injured people, preventing complications of health problems, repairing damages, and reconstructing the community. The disruption effects can be traumatic to the community residents. The debris, lack of trust of the government, fragmentation of families, financial problems, lack of adequate housing, inadequate temporary housing, and fear of another disaster contribute to the long-term negative effects of disasters.

Long-term mental health consequences are evident in most disasters. For example, in a follow-up study of alcohol use among survivors of 10 disasters, the majority of postdisaster alcohol-use disorders represented the continuation or recurrence of preexisting problems. Those with an alcohol-abuse disorder were four times more likely to cope by drinking alcohol than those who did not have a substance abuse problem, indicating that this group could benefit from mental health interventions (North, Ringwalt, Downs, Derzon, & Galvin, 2011).

Responses to Disaster or Terrorism

Psychiatric nurses encounter three different types of disaster victims. The first category is the victims who may or may not survive. If they survive, the victims often experience severe physical injuries. The more serious the physical injury, the more likely the victim will experience a mental health problem such as PTSD, depression, anxiety, or other mental health problems (Osofsky et al., 2018). Victims and families need ongoing health care to prevent complications related to both their physical and mental health (Sledge & Thomas, 2019).

The second category of victims includes the professional rescuers. These are persons who are less likely to experience physical injury but who often experience psychological stress. The professional rescuers, such as police officers, firefighters, nurses, and so on, have more effective coping skills than do volunteer rescuers who are not prepared for the emotional impact of a disaster.

However, many professional responders report experiencing PTSD for many months after the traumatic event in which they were involved (Haugen, Evces, & Weiss, 2012).

The third category includes everyone else involved in the disaster. Psychological effects may be experienced worldwide by millions of people as they experience terrorism or disaster vicariously or as direct victims of the terrorism/disaster event. After an act of terrorism, most people will experience some psychological stress, including an altered sense of safety, hypervigilance, sadness, anger, fear, decreased concentration, and difficulty sleeping. Others may alter their behavior by traveling less, staying at home, avoiding public events, keeping children out of school, or increasing smoking and alcohol use. After Hurricane Maria, most of Punta Santiago was without electrical power, and more than half of the households sustained severe damage. In the aftermath, schools were closed, jobs were lost. Families were subject to diseases, dependency on aid, and exposure to heat and humidity. Two-thirds of residents surveyed reported an increase in the significant symptoms associated with depression, generalized anxiety, or posttraumatic stress (Ferré et al., 2018). See Box 15.5.

BOX 15.5

Research for Best Practice: Posttraumatic Stress Disorder Following Disaster

Hu, X., Cao, X., Wang, H., Chen, Q., Liu, M., & Yamamoto, A. (2016). Probable post-traumatic stress disorder and its predictors in disaster-bereaved survivors: A longitudinal study after the Sichuan earthquake. Archives of Psychiatric Nursing, 30(2), 192–197.

THE QUESTION: What is trajectory of probable PTSD prevalence and severity and the predictors for PTSD severity in bereaved survivors at 6 months and 18 months after the 2008 Sichuan earthquake?

METHODS: A multistage stratified sampling included two cities randomly selected from the 10 hardest-hit cities in the earthquake. The sample included 226 bereaved survivors aged 18 and older who personally experienced the earthquake and lost biologic siblings, grandchildren, and grandparents. The symptoms of probable post-traumatic stress disorder were measured with a standardized scale.

FINDINGS: Prevalence of probable PTSD in bereaved survivors decreased significantly from 38.9% at 6 months to 16.8% at 18 months post-earthquake. Loss of a child, direct exposure to the death of family members, property loss, and mental health service utilization after the earthquake were significant predictors for PTSD severity.

IMPLICATIONS FOR NURSING: These findings support the importance of providing mental health nursing services following a major disaster.

Teamwork and Collaboration: Working Toward Recovery

The role of the behavioral health care worker in disasters, specifically a nuclear detonation in a US city is the support of lifesaving activities and the prevention of additional casualties from fallout. There are six broad categories of interventions including promoting appropriate protective actions, discouraging dangerous behaviors, managing patient/survivor flow to facilitate the best use of scarce resources, supporting first responders, assisting with triage, and delivering palliative care when appropriate (Dodgen, Norwood, Becker, Perez, & Hansen, 2011).

Priority Care Issues

Victims experiencing head injuries or psychic trauma after a disaster may have to be hospitalized. During a disaster, a victim with a mental illness may experience regression to his or her pretreatment condition. If community mental health facilities are available, they should be directed to seek assistance from mental health care professionals. The victims should receive follow-up care for the disaster response after they are discharged.

EVIDENCE-BASED NURSING CARE OF PERSONS EXPERIENCING DISASTERS

Mental Health Nursing Assessment

The nurse should assess the kind and severity of a natural or human-made disaster or terrorist act to determine the capability of individuals and communities to respond in a supportive way. Assessment includes the ages of the victims, gender, their capability to participate in problem-solving activities related to the devastation left by the disaster, and their level of self-confidence or self-esteem. The nurse should maintain a calm demeanor, obtain and distribute information about the disaster and the victims, and reunite victims and their families. In addition, there is a need to monitor the news media's impact on the mental health of the victims of the crisis. Sometimes, the persistence of the news media diminishes the ability of the survivors to achieve closure to the crisis. Constant rehashing of the disaster in the newspapers, television, and online can initiate feelings of anxiety and depression, or increase and prolong the severity of these feelings (Jones et al., 2016).

Women exhibit higher levels of distress than men after a disaster, especially pregnant women and older women. Children are especially vulnerable to disasters and respond according to their ages and family experiences. Traumatized children and adolescents are high-risk victims of a wide range of behavioral, psychological, and neurologic problems after experiencing various traumatic events (Osofsky & Osofsky, 2013; Pfefferbaum & North, 2013).

Physical Health

The nurse should assess physical reactions that may involve many changes in body functions, such as tachycardia, tachypnea, profuse perspiration, nausea, vomiting, dilated pupils, and extreme shakiness. Virtually any organ may be involved. Some victims may exhibit panic reactions and loss of control and have a total disregard for their personal safety. The victims may be suicidal or homicidal and are at high risk for injuries that may include infection, trauma, and head injuries. During the rescue, medical care is a priority. Any medical or psychiatric disorders should be assessed and information communicated to the rest of the health care team. Unexplained physical symptoms such as headache, fatigue, pain, chest pain, and gastrointestinal disturbances should be included in the assessment.

Mental Status

During a disaster, fear and hopelessness can immobilize victims. The victims may suffer from loss of feelings of well-being and various psychological problems, including panic responses, anxiety, and fear. Dissociation and fear are predictive of later developing PTSD and depressive symptoms. Victims witnessing others suffer are especially at high risk for future mental health problems and should be assessed for the details of the disaster (Benjet et al., 2016).

Emotional and Behavioral Responses

The survivors of the disaster may experience traumatic bereavement because of their feelings of guilt that they survived the disaster (Murray, 2018). Responses to psychological distress need to be differentiated from any psychiatric illness that the person may be experiencing. A response to a disaster may leave the person feeling overwhelmed, incapacitated, and disoriented.

The victims should be assessed for behaviors that indicate a depressed state, presence of confusion, uncontrolled weeping or screaming, disorientation, or aggressive behavior. Ideally, the nurse should assess the coping strategies the victim uses to normally manage stressful situations.

Social Support and Functioning

Cultural values and beliefs help define the significance and meaning of a disaster. In some instances, a disaster can slow development, but usually the customs, beliefs, and value systems remain the same. It is important that first responders and health care teams are sensitive to the cultural and religious beliefs of the community. In many instances, victims' spiritual beliefs and religious faith help them cope with the disaster.

In a disaster, the victims may experience economic distress because of job loss and loss of other resources. This may ultimately lead to psychological distress. In addition, acts of aggression and other mental health problems may emerge (Ozbay, Heyde, Reissman, & Sharma, 2013). Again, shelter, money, and food may not be available. The absence of basic human needs such as food, a place to live, or immediate transportation quickly becomes a priority that may precipitate acts of violence.

Priority of Nursing Care

Because the responses to disaster are so varied, a number of priorities can be generated from the assessment data. Priorities could be primarily physical issues, such as breathing or cardiac irregularities, or behavioral, such as self-injury.

Initially, fear and hopelessness can be expected. Depending on the long-term impact of the disaster and the type of disaster (e.g., terrorist attack or tsunami), there may be multiple deaths where grieving responses are a significant issue for survivors. Families may be displaced and property destroyed. Housing, shelter, and safety may emerge as top priorities.

Therapeutic Relationship

Therapeutic communication is key to understanding the extent of the psychological responses to a disaster and to establishing a bridge of trust that communicates respect, commitment, and acceptance. Developing rapport with the victim communicates reassurance and support.

Mental Health Nursing Interventions

The goals of care include helping the victims prioritize and match available resources with their needs, preventing further complications, monitoring the environment, disseminating information, and implementing disease control strategies (Centers for Disease Control and Prevention [CDC], 2016). The focus of nursing interventions is on the individual, family, and community.

Self-Care

Any physiologic problems or injuries should be treated quickly. During the emergency response, individuals will be triaged to the appropriate level of care. Victims who are primarily distressed and may have somatic symptoms will be treated after those suffering from exposure with critical injuries. The primary public health concern is clean drinking water, food, shelter, and medical care. In natural disasters, contaminated water and food and lack of shelter and medical care may worsen illnesses that already exist. All patients need to be reassured of the caring and commitment of the nurse to their safety, comfort, and well-being throughout the triage process. Ideally, a mental health specialist is an integral member of the triage team. Many of the same interventions used for persons experiencing stress or crisis will be used for these victims. See also Chapter 32 for discussion of somatization. Victims should be encouraged to do necessary chores and participate in decision-making.

Medications

During the treatment process, it may become necessary to administer an antianxiety medication or sedative, especially in the early phases of recovery.

Counseling

After the initial interventions, the nurse should support the development of resilience, coping, and recovery while providing technical assistance, training, and consultation. A useful model is the **ABCs of psychological first aid** that focuses on A (arousal), B (behavior), and C (cognition). When arousal is present, the intervention goal is to decrease excitement by providing safety, comfort, and consolation. When abnormal or irrational behavior is present, survivors should be assisted to function more effectively in the disaster, and when cognitive disorientation occurs, reality testing and clear information should be provided. In the initial phases, the nurse should assist the victim in focusing on the reality of problems that are immediate, with specific goals that are consistent with available resources as well as the culture and lifestyle of the victim.

Debriefing (the reconstruction of the traumatic events by the victim) may be helpful for some. Long a common practice, debriefing was believed to be necessary in order for the person to develop a healthy perspective of the event and ultimately prevent PTSD. However, debriefing is not useful for everyone. Additionally, cultural groups respond differently to traumatic events. Therefore, compulsory debriefing is not recommended. If the victim has symptoms of PTSD, referral to a mental health clinic for additional evaluation and treatment is important (see Chapter 27).

The nurse should prepare the victim for recovery by teaching about the effects of stress and helping the victim identify personal strengths and coping skills. Positive coping skills should be supported. The victims should be encouraged to report any depression, anxiety, or interpersonal difficulty during the recovery period. After most disasters, support groups are established that help victims and their families deal with the psychological effects of the disaster.

Psychoeducation

When the nurse explains anticipated reactions and behaviors, this helps the victims gain control and improve coping. For example, after a major disaster, they may have excessive worry, preoccupation with the event, and changes in eating and sleeping patterns. With time, counseling, and group work, these symptoms will lessen. Active coping strategies can be presented in multiple media forums, such as television and radio. After the initial shock, victims react by trying to do something to resolve the situation. When victims begin working to remedy the disaster situation, their physical responses become less exaggerated, and they are more able to work with less tension and fear.

Educating the public about the natural recovery process is important. Information gaps and rumors add to the anxiety and stress of the situation. Giving information and direction helps the public and victims to use the coping skills they already possess. Initially, the event may leave individuals and families in a stage of ambiguity with frantic, disorganized behavior. In addition, individuals and family members are concerned about their own physical and psychological responses to the disastrous event.

Community Care

Outreach is especially important because research shows that disaster victims do not access mental health systems. Peer-delivered mental health services are especially effective in identifying and connecting with victims, especially those with predisaster psychiatric problems (North & Pfefferbaum, 2013).

Family support systems may need to be reestablished. The health care community should actively reach out to the media and keep the press engaged. Direct attention to stories that inform and help the public respond should be encouraged. Some federal agencies assist victims of disasters. This assistance is available for individual, families, and communities. One of these agencies is the Federal Emergency Management Agency (FEMA). When a disaster occurs, FEMA sends a team of specialists who review the devastation of disaster. They provide counseling and mental health services and arrange for many of the victims to access other services needed for survival, including training programs. In addition, the Substance Abuse and Mental Health Services Administration (SAMHSA) of the Department of Health and Human Services is available to assist both victims of and responders to the disaster. When a disaster disrupts the victim's social network, other resources must be made available for social support.

The social support system provides an environment in which the victims experience respect and caring from the caregivers, the opportunity to ventilate and examine personal feelings regarding the tragedy, and the opportunity to begin the healing and recovery process. Supporting the development of more contacts within the social network can be done by organizing support groups within the area of the disaster that address grief and loss, trauma, psychoeducational needs, and substance abuse. In addition, the nurse may refer the victims to nearby support groups or religious groups that are appropriate to meet their needs.

Evaluation and Treatment Outcomes

To determine the effectiveness of nursing interventions, the nurse should evaluate the outcomes based on the success of resolution of the disaster. The outcomes will depend on the specific disaster and its meaning (appraisal) to the survivors. For example, are the survivors in a safe place? Are the victims able to cope with the disaster? Were the appropriate supports given, so the victims could draw upon their own strengths?

SUMMARY OF KEY POINTS

- A crisis is a time-limited event that occurs when coping mechanisms fail to provide adaptive skills to address a perceived challenge or threat.
- Grief responses are intense physical, emotional, social, and cognitive responses to loss, and bereavement is the process of healing after a loss. The variations in grief responses are influenced by the characteristics of the individual, perceived relationship to the deceased, and the type of loss.
- Stage theories propose that grief and bereavement follow stages/phases. Process models explain bereavement as nonlinear.
- For most persons, bereavement is uncomplicated and there is no need for counseling. Complicated grief occurs in about 10% to 20% of bereaved persons. Interventions such as medication, counseling, and/or a support group may be required for this group.
- Interventions are designed to support people through crises by helping them understand the process of recovery and identify the resources they need and how to get them.
- Disaster is a sudden, overwhelming catastrophic event that causes great damage and may cause mass casualties and human suffering that require assistance from all available resources.
- Depending on the disaster, interventions are provided to individuals, families, and communities.

CRITICAL THINKING CHALLENGES

1. Compare nursing interventions used for crises, bereavement, and disasters. What are the similarities? What are the differences?
2. After the death of his mother, a 24-year-old single man with bipolar disorder moves into an apartment. He continues to take his medication but feels sad about his mother's death. He is not adjusting well to living alone and tells his nurse that he no longer wants to go to work and feels he would be better off if he joined his mother. Identify priorities of nursing care and develop a plan of care for this young man.
3. Listen to people who have experienced a loss to determine where they are in the bereavement process. Discuss the role of medication and counseling when used in crisis or bereavement.
4. Compare uncomplicated bereavement to complicated bereavement. How would you recognize the difference? When would it be appropriate to refer a bereaved person to a support group or mental health specialist?
5. There is a terrorist threat in your community. A patient appears in the emergency department convinced he is going to die. How would you proceed with assessing this patient?

2007: *Grace is Gone*

Stanley Phillips (John Cusack) is a manager of a home-supply store and parent of two girls, 12-year-old Heidi (Shelan O'Keefe) and 8-year-old Dawn (Gracie Bednarczyk). His wife is a soldier in Iraq, but the viewers know her by her message left on the family answering machine. When an army captain and chaplain deliver the news that Grace had died bravely in combat, Stanley becomes numb. He impulsively takes his girls to wherever they desire—a theme park in Florida. Most of the movie follows the three on the trip and the father's attempt to delay and deny his wife's death.

Viewing Points: Describe Stanley's reaction when he receives the news of his wife's death. What clues are present that Heidi gradually understands that something terrible has happened?

REFERENCES

American Psychiatric Association. (2013). *Diagnostic and statistical manual of mental disorders* (5th ed.). Arlington, VA: Author.

Benjet, C., Bromet, E., Karam, E. G., Kessler, R. C., McLaughlin, K. A., Ruscio, A. M., et al. (2016). The epidemiology of traumatic event exposure worldwide: results from the World Mental Health Survey consortium. *Psychological Medicine, 46*(2), 327–343.

Bennett, K. M., & Soulsby, L. K. (2012). Wellbeing in bereavement and widowhood. *Illness, Crisis and Loss, 20*(4), 321–337.

Betancourt, T. S., Newnham, E. A., Layne, C. M., Kim, S., Steinberg, A. M., Ellis, H., et al. (2012). Trauma history and psychopathology in war-affected refugee children referred for trauma-related mental health services in the United States. *Journal of Traumatic Stress, 25*(6), 682–690.

Bowlby, J., & Parkes, C. M. (1970). Separation and loss within the family. In E. J. Anthony (Ed.). *The child in his family: International Yearbook of Child Psychiatry and Allied Professions* (pp. 197–216). New York: Wiley.

Caplan, G. (1961). *An Approach to community mental health*. New York: Grune & Stratton.

Centers for Disease Control and Prevention. (2016). Disaster mental health for states: Key principles, issues, and questions. Emergency preparedness and response. October 26, 2016. [Online]. Retrieved December 22, 2016 from https://emergency.cdc.gov/mentalhealth/states.asp

Claxton, R., & Reynolds, C. F. 3rd. (2012). Complicated grief #254. *Journal of Palliative Medicine, 15*(7), 829–830.

Corr, C. (2018). Elisabeth Kübler-Ross and the "Five Stages" Model in a sampling of recent American textbooks. *Omega, 15*:30222818809766.

Currie, E. R., Christian, B. J., Hinds, P. S., Perna, S. J., Robinson, C., Day, S., et al. (2018). Life after loss: Parent bereavement and coping experiences after infant death in the neonatal intensive care unit. *Death Studies*, 1–10. doi: 10.1080/07481187.2018.1474285.

Dodgen, D., Norwood, A. E., Becker, S. M., Perez, J. T., & Hansen, C. K. (2011). Social, psychological, and behavioral responses to a nuclear detonation in a U.S. city: Implications for health care planning and delivery. *Disaster Medicine & Public Health Preparedness, 5*(Suppl 1), S54–S64.

Ferré, I. M., Negrón, S., Shultz, J. M., Schwartz, S. J., Kossin, J. P., & Pantin, H. (2018). Hurricane Maria's impact on Punta Santiago, Puerto Rico: Community needs and mental health assessment six months postimpact. *Disaster Medicine and Public Health Preparedness*, 1–6. doi: 10.1017/dmp.2018.103.

Fischer, P., Postmes, T., Koeppl, J., Conway, L., & Fredriksson, T. (2011). The meaning of collective terrorist threat: Understanding the subjective causes of terrorism reduces its negative psychological impact. *Journal of Interpersonal Violence, 26*(7), 1432–1445.

Haugen, P. T., Evces, M., & Weiss, D. S. (2012). Treating posttraumatic stress disorder in first responders: A systematic review. *Clinical Psychology Review, 32*(5), 370–380.

Jones, N.M, Garfin, D. R., Holman, E. A., & Silver, R. C. (2016). Media use and exposure to graphic content in the week following the Boston Marathon Bombings. *American Journal of Community Psychology, 58*(1–2), 47–59.

Kubler-Ross, E. (1969). *On death and dying*. New York: Macmillan Publishing Company.

Malgaroli, M., Maccallum, F., & Bonanno, G. A. (2018). Symptoms of persistent complex bereavement disorder, depression, and PTSD in a conjugally bereaved sample: a network analysis. *Psychological Medicine, 48*(14), 2439–2448.

Murray, H. (2018). Survivor guilt in a posttraumatic stress disorder clinic sample. *Journal of Loss & Trauma, 23*(7), 600–607.

Mutabaruka, J., Séjourné, N., Bui, E., Birmes, P., & Chabrol, H. (2012). Traumatic grief and traumatic stress in survivors 12 years after the genocide in Rwanda. *Stress and Health, 28*(4), 289–296.

Nielsen, M. K., Neergaard, M. A., Jensen, A. B., Vedsted, P., Bro, F., & Guldin, M. B., (2017). Predictors of complicated grief and depression in bereaved caregivers: A nationwide prospective cohort study. *Journal of Pain and Symptom Management, 53*(3), 540–550.

North, C. S., & Pfefferbaum, B. (2013). Mental health response to community disasters: A systematic review. *JAMA, 310*(5), 507–518.

North, C. S., Ringwalt, C. L., Downs, D., Derzon, J., & Galvin, D. (2011). Postdisaster course of alcohol use disorders in systematically studied survivors of 10 disasters. *Archives of General Psychiatry, 68*(2), 173–180.

North, C. S., Baron, D., & Chen, A. F. (2018). Prevalence and predictors of postdisaster major depression. Convergence of evidence from 11 disaster studies using consistent methods. *Journal of Psychiatric Research, 102*, 96–101.

Osofsky, H. J., & Osofsky, J. D. (2013). Hurricane Katrina and the gulf oil spill: Lessons learned. *Psychiatric Clinics of North America, 36*(3), 371–382.

Osofsky, H. J., Weems, C. F., Graham, R. A., Osofsky, J. D., Hansel, T. C., & King, L. S. (2018). Perceptions of resilience and physical health symptom improvement following post disaster integrated health services. *Disaster Medicine and Public Health Preparedness*, 1–7. doi: 10.1017/dmp.2018.35

Ozbay, F., Auf der Heyde, T., Reissman, D., & Sharma, V. (2013). The enduring mental health impact of the September 11th terrorist attacks: Challenges and lessons learned. *Psychiatric Clinics of North America, 36*(3), 417–429.

Pfefferbaum, B., & North, C. S. (2013). Assessing children's disaster reactions and mental health needs: Screening and clinical evaluation. *Canadian Journal of Psychiatry, 58*(3), 135–142.

Sanders, C. M. (1998). *Grief: The mourning after: Dealing with adult bereavement* (2nd ed.). New York: Wiley Interscience.

Scaramutti, C., Salas-Wright, C. P., Vos, S. R., & Schwartz, S. J. (2019). The mental health impact of Hurricane Maria on Puerto Ricans in Puerto Rico and Florida. *Disaster Medicine and Public Health Preparedness, 13*(1), 24–27.

Sledge, D., & Thomas, H. F. (2019). From disaster response to community recovery: Nongovernmental entities, government, and public health. *American Journal of Public Health, 109*(3), 437–444.

Stroebe, M., & Schut, H. (2015). Family matters in bereavement: Toward an integrative intra-interpersonal coping model. *Perspective on Psychological Science, 10*(6), 873–879.

Stroebe, M., Schut, H., & Boerner, K. (2010). Continuing bonds in adaptation to bereavement: Toward theoretical integration. *Clinical Psychology Review, 30*(2), 259–268.

Tol, W. A., Barbui, C., Bisson, J., Cohen, J., Hijazi, Z., Jones, L., et al. (2014). World Health Organization Guidelines for management of acute stress, PTSD, and bereavement: Key challenges on the road ahead. *PLoS Medicine, 11*(12), e1001769.

Waller, A., Turon, H., Mansfield, E., Clark, K., Hobden, B., & Sanson-Fisher, R. (2016). Assisting the bereaved: A systematic review of the evidence for grief counselling. *Palliative Medicine, 30*(2), 132–148.

Zetumer, S., Young, I., Shear, M. K., Skritskaya, N., Lebowitz, B., Simon, N., et al. (2015). The impact of losing a child on the clinical presentation of complicated grief. *Journal of Affective Disorders, 170*, 15–21.

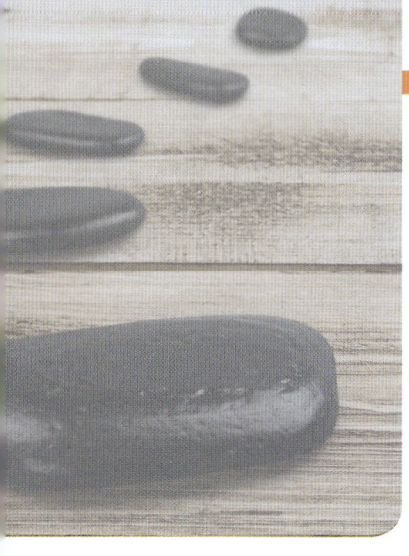

16
Suicide Prevention
Screening, Assessment, and Intervention

Rebecca Luebbert and Mary Ann Boyd

KEY CONCEPTS
- hopelessness
- lethality
- suicide

LEARNING OBJECTIVES

After studying this chapter, you will be able to:

1. Identify suicide as a major mental health problem in the United States.
2. Define *suicide, suicidality, suicide attempt, parasuicide,* and *suicidal ideation.*
3. Describe population groups that have high rates of suicide.
4. Describe risk factors associated with suicide completion.
5. Identify key factors associated with specific suicide acts.
6. Describe evidence-based interventions used to reduce imminent and ongoing suicide risk.
7. Explain the importance of documentation and reporting when caring for patients who may be at risk of suicide.

KEY TERMS
- acquired capability for suicide • case finding • commitment to treatment statement • ideation-to-action theories
- parasuicide • perceived burdensomeness • suicidal ideation • suicidality • suicide attempt • suicide contagion
- thwarted belongingness • volitional factors

Suicide is one of the major health problems in the United States, accounting for over 47,000 deaths in 2017 (AFSP, 2019). Suicide rates have increased in nearly every state in the past 20 years, an increase of 30% from 2000 to 2016. The public health problem of suicidal behavior is so important that several goals stated in *Healthy People 2010* and retained in *Healthy People 2020* directly target the reduction of deaths by suicide (Hedegaard, Curtin, & Warner, 2018; United States Department of Health and Human Services [U.S. DHHS], 2010).

Suicide is so rejected in contemporary society that people with strong suicidal thoughts do not seek treatment for fear of being stigmatized by others. Reports and portrayals of suicide in the popular media and television further stigmatize those who consider or attempt suicide. Society's unwillingness to talk openly about suicide also contributes to the common misperceptions resulting in many myths regarding suicide (Corrigan, Sheehan, & Al-Khouja, 2017; Sheehan, Corrigan, & Al-Khouja, 2016). Box 16.1 presents several myths and facts about suicide.

Suicides are preventable deaths when immediate friends and family and health care providers identify symptoms and use effective interventions. All practicing nurses will come into contact with patients who are thinking about suicide and often can prevent suicides by identifying and intervening with those at risk. Through individual and public education, nurses also can do much to demystify suicide and reduce stigma for those at risk. To reduce the devastating public impact of suicide on those at risk and their families, nurses must be knowledgeable about suicide and be able to implement effective preventive interventions. This chapter contains tools that can be used to reduce the broad effects of suicide and provide appropriate care for suicidal patients.

> **BOX 16.1**
>
> **Myths and Facts about Suicide**
>
> **Myth:** People who talk about suicide do not complete suicide.
> **Fact:** Many people who die by suicide have given definite warnings of their intentions. Always take any comment about suicide seriously.
> **Myth:** Suicide happens without warning.
> **Fact:** Most suicidal people give many clues and warning signs regarding their suicidal intention.
> **Myth:** Suicidal people are fully intent on dying.
> **Fact:** Most suicidal people are undecided about living or dying. A part of them wants to live; however, death seems like the only way out of their pain or situation. They may allow themselves to "gamble" with death, leaving it up to others to save them.
> **Myth:** When people become suicidal, they will always be suicidal.
> **Fact:** Most people are suicidal for a limited time, though these feelings could recur at a later time.
> **Myth:** You should never ask people if they are thinking about suicide, because doing so may put the idea in their heads.
> **Fact:** Asking about suicide does not give people the idea for suicide. It is important to ask the question so that you understand people's thoughts and intentions.
> **Myth:** When people who are suicidal feel better, they are no longer at risk.
> **Fact:** Sometimes suicidal people feel better because they have made a decision to die, and they may feel a sense of relief that their pain is ending.
>
> Adapted from Suicide.org. (2019). Suicide myths. Retrieved February 19, 2019, from http://www.suicide.org/suicide-myths.html

SUICIDE AND SUICIDE ATTEMPT

KEYCONCEPT **Suicide** is the voluntary act of killing oneself. It is a fatal, self-inflicted destructive act with explicit or inferred intent to die. It is sometimes called suicide completion.

This behavioral definition of suicide is limited and does not consider the complexity of a potential underlying mental illness, personal motivations, and situational and family factors that provoke the suicide act. Except for the very young, suicide occurs in all age groups, social classes, and cultures (NIMH, 2016).

The term **suicidality** refers to all suicide-related behaviors and thoughts of attempting or completing suicide and suicidal ideation. **Suicidal ideation** is thinking about and planning one's own death. Population studies show that suicidal ideation varies depending on characteristics of the participants and the way suicidal ideation is measured. Although suicidal ideation often does not progress, having recurrent suicidal thoughts is associated with poor mental health (Dugas, Low, O'Loughlin, & O'Loughlin, 2015).

A **suicide attempt** is a nonfatal, self-inflicted destructive act with explicit or implicit intent to die. Only recently have data on suicide attempts been compiled. In 2017 in the United States, an estimated 1.4 million adults attempted suicide, with adult females reporting an attempt 1.4 times more often than males (American Foundation for Suicide Prevention [AFSP], 2017). Suicidal ideation, previous psychiatric hospitalization, and a previous attempt are significant predictors of a completed suicide (Bostwick, Pabbati, Geske, & McKean, 2016).

Parasuicide is a voluntary, apparent attempt at suicide, commonly called a suicidal gesture, in which the aim is not death (e.g., taking a sublethal drug). Parasuicidal behavior varies by intent. Some people truly wish to die, but others simply wish to feel nothing for a while. Still others want to send a message about their emotional state. Parasuicide behavior is never normal and should always be taken seriously. Parasuicide occurs frequently in younger age groups but declines after the age of 44 years.

KEYCONCEPT **Lethality** refers to the probability that a person will successfully complete suicide. Lethality is determined by the seriousness of the person's intent and the likelihood that the planned method of death will succeed. A plan to use an accessible firearm to commit suicide has greater lethality than a suicide plan that involves superficial cuts of the wrist.

Suicide is ranked as the 10th leading cause of death and accounts for 14 deaths per 100,000 individuals. A suicide occurs approximately every 12 minutes in the United States, resulting in an average of 129 completed suicides per day. The suicide rate in the United States has been stable for several years despite a significant increase in the rate of suicide attempts. Mountain regions have the highest rate of suicide (Fig. 16.1). Its overall prevalence may be underestimated because suicide can be disguised as a vehicular accident or a homicide, especially in young people (AFSP, 2017; Centers of Disease Control and Prevention [CDC], National Center for Injury Prevention and Control, 2018).

Suicide Across the Life Span

Children, Adolescents, and Young Adults

Suicide is the second leading cause of death among those 10 to 34 years old (CDC, 2017). Mental disorders can lead to worse performance in school, alcohol or other drug abuse, family discord, violence, and suicide. Approximately 20% of US children and adolescents have mental disorders in their lifetime. The most recent Youth Risk and Behavior Survey found that in the preceding year among high school students: 17.2% seriously considered attempting suicide, 13.6% made a suicide plan, 7.4% attempted suicide, and 2.4% were injured in a suicide attempt. Female students were more likely to attempt suicide (9.3%) than male students (5.1%),

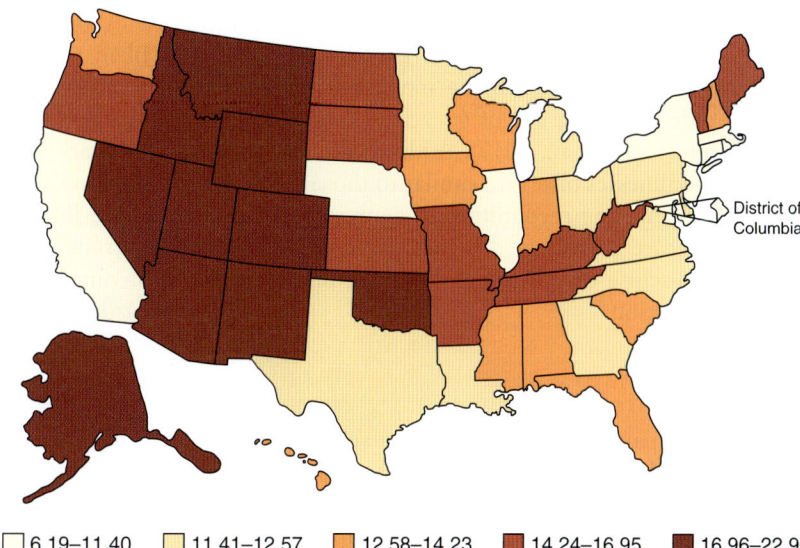

FIGURE 16.1 Number of deaths attributable to suicide in the United States per 100,000 population, 2008 to 2014. Data courtesy of CDC. (Retrieved from https://www.nimh.nih.gov/health/statistics/suicide.shtml)

though males were more likely to die by suicide than females. Suicide attempts vary according to racial and ethnic groups. Black students reported the highest rate of attempt (9.8%), whereas white students reported the fewest attempts (6.1%) (Kann et al., 2018).

Adults and Older Adults

In 2016, 15.6 deaths per 100,000 individuals in the United States were a result of suicide, with the highest rates occurring in the 45- to 54-year age group (Stone et al., 2018). Suicide rates peak during middle age, and a second peak occurs in those age 75 years and older. Alienation, loss, a sense of disconnectedness, physical illness, and financial difficulties are important precipitants to suicide in older adults (Wand, Peisah, Draper, & Brodaty, 2018; Winterrowd, Canetto, & Benoit, 2017).

Suicide rates in the military have been increasing for the last several years for both active duty and the National Guard. In 2015, over 600 service members died by suicide (Franklin, 2016). The suicide rate for veterans is estimated at 20 per day. There is considerable debate whether combat exposure or deployment is directly or indirectly responsible for this increase. As is the case with civilian suicide, suicide in the military seems to be related to mental health problems, intimate partner problems, alcohol or substance abuse problems, recent crises, and job problems (Logan et al., 2015). However, combat and deployment are associated with PTSD and depression, which are associated with suicide (Castro & Kintzle, 2014). Combat exposure is one of the leading factors for both men and women military members. For women, military sexual trauma also contributes to suicidal ideation and attempts (Kimerling, Makin-Byrd, Louzon, Ignacio, & McCarthy, 2016; Monteith et al., 2016).

Epidemiology and Risk Factors

Mental illness is an important factor contributing to suicide in adults. Many young adults who die by suicide also have a depressive disorder, and many others have personality disorders. Adolescents who have panic attacks are particularly at risk for suicide. Auditory hallucinations increase the risk for suicide because of the possibility of individuals impulsively responding to "voices" directing them to kill themselves. Substance abuse increases the likelihood that suicidal ideation will result in both parasuicidal and suicidal behaviors. Box 16.2 identifies risk factors for suicide (CDC, National Center for Injury Prevention and Control, 2019).

BOX 16.2
Factors Enhancing Suicide Risk

VULNERABILITY
Primary family member who has completed suicide
Psychiatric disorder
Previous attempt by the patient
Loss (e.g., death of significant other, divorce, job loss)
Unrelenting physical illness

RISK
White or Native American man
Older man
Adolescent non-Hispanic white or Native American male
Gay, lesbian, or bisexual orientation
Access to firearms
Middle-aged woman

INTENT
Suicide plan and means of executing it
Inability to commit to treatment

DISINHIBITION
Impulsivity
Isolation
Psychotic thoughts
Drug or alcohol use

Medical illness contributes to functional disability and also increases the likelihood of chronic depression, which in turn contributes to the increased suicide rate of those older than the age of 65 years (Fassberg et al., 2016; Winterrowd et al., 2017). Additionally, symptoms of comorbid illnesses often are similar to those of depressive disorder, making recognition of depressive disorder by primary care providers difficult. Patients are often reticent to disclose their suicidal thoughts, further complicating detection.

Psychological Risk Factors

Psychological pain, internal distress, low self-esteem, and interpersonal distress have long been associated with suicide (Ducasse et al., 2018). Childhood physical and sexual abuse are linked to suicide, suicidal ideation, and parasuicide. Cognitive risk factors include problem-solving deficits, impulsivity, rumination, and hopelessness. Impulsivity, anger, and reduced inhibition increase the risk of suicide. Recent purchase of a handgun increases the risk of self-harm (CDC, National Center for Injury Prevention and Control, 2019; Crifasi, Meyers, Vernick, & Webster, 2015; Wendell et al., 2016).

Social Risk Factors

Social isolation is a primary risk factor for suicide. Social distress leads to despair and can be caused by family discord, parental neglect, abuse, parental suicide, and divorce. Social distress can prevent the patient from accessing the support necessary to prevent suicidal acts. Other social factors associated with suicide risk include economic deprivation, unemployment, poverty, knowing someone who has died by suicide (especially if that person was a family member), and lack of access to behavioral health care (CDC, National Center for Injury Prevention and Control, 2019; Endo et al., 2017; Suicide Prevention Resource Center [SPRC], 2019b).

Gender

Males have a suicide completion rate nearly four times more than females. White males account for 78% of completed suicides, with middle-aged white men having the highest rate (AFSP, 2017). Men are more likely to use means that have a higher rate of success, with 56% of their suicide deaths by firearms (NIMH, 2016). Rural men have a much higher risk of suicide than urban men, and that gap is widening, perhaps attributable to the higher rates of gun ownership in rural areas (Logan et al., 2015). Substance abuse, aggression, hopelessness, emotion-focused coping, social isolation, and feeling little purpose in life have been associated with suicidal behavior in men.

Women across age and racial and ethnic groups are less likely to die from suicide than are men but are more likely to attempt suicide. Women make three attempts to every attempt by men. Adolescent girls and women ages 10 to 44 years have the highest rate of suicide attempts. Women are less likely to complete a suicide, partly because they are more likely to choose less lethal methods. Women with current or previous exposure to domestic violence are at an increased risk for suicidal behavior (Kavak, Atkturk, Ozdemir, & Abdurrezzak, 2018).

Sexuality

The lesbian, gay, bisexual, and transgender (LGBT) population is at increased risk for suicide (O'Brien, Putney, Hebert, Falk, & Aguinaldo, 2016). Other risk factors include early disclosure of their sexual orientation and early onset of sexual activity. A cross-national study meta-analysis showed that lifetime suicidal ideation was more common among gay men (40% to 55%) compared with heterosexual men (18% to 30%) as were lifetime suicide attempts (8% to 25% for gay men vs. 1% to 13% in heterosexual men) (Lewis, 2009). In lesbian, gay, and bisexual older adults, there are high levels of poor general health disability and mental distress (Fredriksen-Goldsen, Him, Shui, & Bryan, 2017).

Adolescents in sexual minority groups are often stigmatized and discriminated against. They have more suicidal ideation, more suicide attempts, and are more at risk for completed suicides than heterosexual adolescents (Yildiz, 2018). Individuals are more at risk for suicide when they experience conflict with family or friends because of their sexual identify, threat of violence, abuse, bullying, isolation, and other high-risk behaviors (American Association of Suicidology, 2019a). A nationwide study of youth health behaviors and experiences reported that a significantly higher percentage of lesbian, gay, or bisexual students (48%) seriously contemplated suicide as compared to 13% of heterosexual students, and 23% of lesbian, gay, or bisexual students attempted suicide as compared to 5% of heterosexual students (Kann et al., 2018).

There are alarming rates of suicidal ideation and suicide rates among transgender people. The suicide attempt rate among transgender persons ranges from 32% to 50%. Gender-based victimization, discrimination, bullying, violence, and rejection by family, friends, and communities are risk factors associated with suicidal behavior (Testa et al., 2017; Virupaksha, Muralidhar, & Ramakrishna, 2016).

Race and Ethnicity

There is considerable variation in the profile of suicide rates across racial groups, including the age when rates are at their peak and the duration of high rates across several age

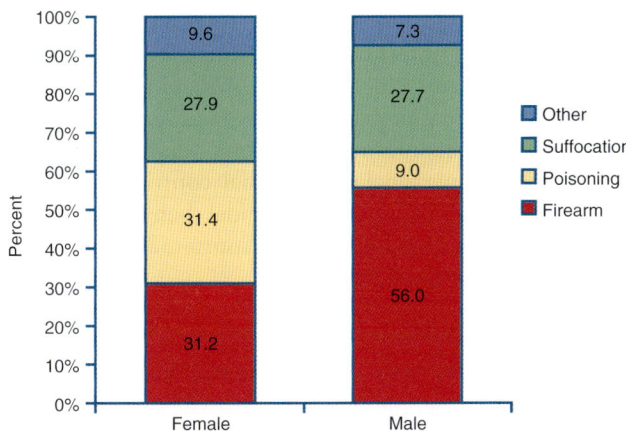

FIGURE 16.2 Suicide deaths by method in the United States (2015). Data courtesy of CDC. (Retrieved from https://www.nimh.nih.gov/health/statistics/suicide.shtml)

groups. Rates of suicide among American Indians/Alaska Natives and whites are highest, at 21.39 and 18.15 per 100,000, respectively. Lower suicide rates are found among Asian/Pacific Islanders (7.00 per 100,000), blacks (6.35 per 100,000), and Hispanics (6.38 per 100,000) (SPRC, 2019a).

The rate of suicides among Caucasians has steadily increased since 1999. Suicide rates are higher in males than in females for all groups, with a rate of 24.79 (males) and 7.16 (women) per 100,000. Completed suicides are highest for Caucasians between the ages of 40 and 64. Suicide rates among those older than 75 years are also high. The use of firearms is by far the most prominent method of suicide among Caucasians (CDC, 2017). Access to firearms contributes to the risk of completed suicides (Fig. 16.2). Firearm ownership in more prevalent in the United States than in any other country—approximately 35% to 39% of households have firearms (Anglemyer, Horvath, & Rutherford, 2014).

Family cohesion and social support in African-American families contribute to the lower rates of suicide in this group. In 2016, the suicide rate among African-American females was the lowest among men and women of all ethnicities. Although the overall suicide rate for African Americans is low, young African-American men take their lives at a rate considerably above that of other age groups. Higher rates of suicide in younger men is associated with being in foster care, early aggressive behavior, depression, and dissatisfaction with life (Liu et al., 2013; Wang, Lightsey, Tran, & Bonapart, 2013).

Even though the suicide rate for Hispanics (Latinos) is less than half of the overall US rate, suicide is the 12th leading cause of death for Hispanics of all ages and third leading cause of death for Hispanic males ages 15 to 34. Among Hispanic ethnic subgroups in the United States, Puerto Rican adults have the highest rates of suicide attempts. Hispanics born in the United States have higher rates of suicidal ideation and attempts than Hispanic immigrants (Suicide Prevention Resource Center [SPRC], 2013).

Suicide is the eighth leading cause of death for American Indians/Alaska Natives of all ages and the second leading cause of death among youth ages 10 to 24. Men and women ages 35 to 64 had a greater percentage increase in suicide rates between 1999 and 2013 than any other racial/ethnic group. Lifetime rates of having attempted suicide reported by adolescents ranged from 15.8% in girls to 11.8% in boys. Adolescent suicide attempts are significantly higher among youth (both sexes) raised on reservations (17.6%) compared to youth raised in urban areas (14.3%). Whereas exposure to suicide and access to alcohol and drugs contribute to suicide rates for Native Americans, family support and cultural and tribal orientation are protective (SPRC, 2013).

The scant literature on suicide among Asian populations shows that suicidal ideation, plans, and attempts are more common than popularly believed and vary within Asian ethnic groups. For example, Native Hawaiians living in Hawaii who were between the ages of 15 and 44 had a significantly higher suicide death rate than other racial/ethnic groups, but those over 45 had a much lower rate than Whites, the same rate as Japanese, and a higher rate than Filipinos. Asians who immigrated to the United States as children have higher rates of suicidal ideation and suicide attempts than US-born Asians. Cultural identification with the Asian culture (sense of belonging and affiliation with spiritual, material, intellectual, and emotional features) is associated with a 69% reduction in the risk of suicide attempt (SPRC, 2013).

The reasons for racial and ethnic variations are unclear. The rates of depressive disorder, a major risk factor for suicide, vary across racial group. Cultural stress, perceived discrimination, and vulnerability are thought to contribute to the risk of suicide. Additionally, use of mental health services is not consistent among various ethnic groups (Nestor, Cheek, & Kiu, 2016).

Etiology

The convergence of biologic, psychological, and social factors can be directly linked to suicidal behavior. In genetically and physiologically vulnerable individuals, thoughts, feelings, and personality factors can interfere with personal problem-solving, promote impulsivity, and support suicidal behavior. Poverty, unemployment, and social conflict also contribute to suicidal behavior in those at risk for suicide.

Biologic Theories

Depression and severe childhood trauma are linked to suicide. Those who complete suicide often have extremely low levels of the neurotransmitter serotonin.

Impairments in the serotonergic system contribute to suicidal behavior. Additionally, dysregulation in the hypothalamic–pituitary–adrenal (HPA) axis, abnormalities of neurotrophins and neurotrophin receptors, and abnormalities of neuroimmune functions may be associated with suicide risk (Pandey, 2013).

Genetic Factors

Suicide runs in families. First-degree relatives of individuals who have completed suicide have a two to eight times higher risk for suicide than do individuals in the general population. Suicide of a first-degree relative is highly predictive of a serious attempt in another first-degree relative. Children of depressed and suicidal parents have higher rates of suicidal behavior themselves. The genetic link to suicide is evident in twin studies. Suicidal behavior has a 50% concordance for completed suicide (Tidemalm et al., 2011).

There also appears to be a connection between early childhood sexual abuse and suicidality. Early childhood adverse experiences appear to lead to genetic changes that modify the expression of the neurologic system, impacting the biologic and psychological development. As a result, there is a propensity to react to stressors, increasing the likelihood of suicidal behavior (Brodsky, 2016).

Psychological Theories
Cognitive Theories

Most evidence on the psychological contributions to suicidal behavior point to cognitive, affective, behavioral, and personality factors that intensify the experience of hopelessness and disconnection from others. Aaron Beck first identified the cognitive triad of hopelessness, helplessness, and worthlessness as integral to the experience of depression (Beck, Rush, Shaw, & Emery, 1979). Since then, a significant evidence base has been established linking hopelessness, loneliness, and other cognitive symptoms to suicide (Klonsky, Qiu, & Saffer, 2017). Depressed persons who are hopeless are more likely to consider suicide than those who are depressed but hopeful about the future. Furthermore, it appears that lack of positive thoughts about the future is more likely to predict suicidal behavior than negative thoughts even though both contribute to hopelessness (Liu, Ahang, & Sun, 2017).

> **KEYCONCEPT** **Hopelessness** is the pervasive belief that undesirable events are likely to occur coupled with the belief that one's situation is unlikely to improve (Ellis & Rutherford, 2008).

Emotional and Personality Factors

Emotional factors and personality traits also play a role in suicidal behavior by enhancing perceptions of helplessness and hopelessness, contributing to poor self-esteem, and interfering with coping efforts. Shame, guilt, despair, and emotion-focused coping have been linked to suicidal behavior. Loss and grief are also important considerations. Emotional distress often is potentiated by personality traits that contribute to poor self-esteem, impulsivity, and suicidal behavior (Giner, Blaso-Fontecilla, De La Vega, & Courtet, 2016).

Ideation-to-Action Theories

Suicidal ideation does not necessarily lead to suicide attempts. Most people who think of suicide do not act on the idea, but the suicidal thoughts of those who do take lethal action are often indistinguishable from those who do not. **Ideation-to-action theories** examine factors that identify those who are most likely to attempt suicide. These emerging theories, which are supported by research, provide a basis for discriminating between those who are only thinking about suicide versus those who are likely to engage in suicidal acts.

The *Interpersonal Psychological Theory of Suicidal Behavior (IPTS)*, introduced by Thomas Joiner in 2005, proposes that three interacting factors indicate a high risk of suicide: thwarted belongingness, perceived burdensomeness, and acquired capability. The term **"thwarted belongingness"** is used to describe alienation from social relationships or experiences that is, the human need to belong is not being met. It refers to an individual's feelings of loneliness and isolation, as well as lack of reciprocal, caring, and meaningful relationships. **Perceived burdensomeness** is the perception that the individual is a burden to others. **Acquired capability for suicide**, which develops over time, involves a heightened sense of fearlessness and a high pain threshold (Joiner, 2005). IPTS views the act of suicide as being very difficult to carry out. When thwarted belongingness, perceived burdensomeness, and acquired capability come together in one person, these beliefs lead to the misperception that others would be better off without them and the idea that sacrificing themselves is the appropriate action to take. Researchers are testing the theory in a variety of clinical situations (Anestis et al., 2016; Ma, Batterham, Calear, & Han, 2016).

The *Integrated Motivational Volitional (IMV)* model proposes that motivational factors such as defeat and entrapment cause suicidal ideation. The progression from suicidal ideation to suicide attempt is explained by **volitional factors** such as acquired capability, access to lethal means, planning, and impulsivity (O'Connor & Kirtley, 2018). In a study differentiating between those thinking about suicide and those attempting suicide, those reporting a suicide attempt were found to have greater acquired capability, mental imagery about death, and impulsivity, and were more likely to know a friend who had made a previous suicide attempt (Weatherall et al., 2018).

The Three-Step Theory (3ST) explains progression from ideation to action in three steps. First, emotional pain and hopelessness cause the suicidal ideation. Second, thoughts of suicide become strong as the emotional pain exceeds connectedness. The third step involves the actual attempt, when the person has the knowledge and capacity to carry out the suicide (Klonsky et al., 2017). In this model, suicide prevention focuses on reducing pain, increasing hope, improving connections, and reducing capacity to carry out the suicide.

Social Theories

Before the turn of the 20th century, Emile Durkheim (1951 [1897]) linked suicide to the social conditions in which people live. Both a lack of social connectedness and social conditions contribute to suicidal behavior. People who are socially connected are less likely to engage in suicidal behavior. When an individual has others he or she can depend on, suicide can be prevented, even among those at significant risk. Even among people with social bonds, however, lack of community and social resources can interact with physiologic and psychological risk to increase the likelihood of suicide.

Social Distress

A lack of social connection contributes to suicidal ideation, attempts, and deaths across the life span. Among adults, those who are single, never married, separated, widowed, or living alone, and those reporting loneliness, alienation, and a lack of belongingness, are also more likely to engage in suicidal behavior (Calati et al., 2019). Being socially connected, however, does not in itself reduce risk. Interpersonal conflict and being a victim of bullying can contribute to suicidal behavior, especially in adolescents and young adults (John et al., 2018).

Suicide Contagion

Social exposure to suicide is associated with an increased personal risk for suicidal behavior, particularly among adolescents. Suicide behavior that occurs after the suicide death of a known other is called **suicide contagion** or cluster suicide. Suicide contagion seems to work through modeling and is more likely to occur when the individual contemplating suicide is of the same age, gender, and background as the person who died. Contagion can be prompted by the suicide of a friend, an acquaintance, online social networking, or an idolized celebrity. Actions of peer groups, media reports of suicide, and even billboards with content about suicide can trigger suicide behavior among adolescents (Colman, 2018); Zimmerman, Rees, Posick & Zimmerman, 2016). In the case of a celebrity suicide, the number of "copycat suicides" is proportional to the amount, duration, and prominence of media coverage (Ju, Young, Seok, & Yip, 2014). Evidence suggests that adolescents also can be influenced by simple individual and community suicide prevention efforts (Zimmerman et al., 2016).

Economic Disadvantage

Poverty and economic disadvantage are associated with depression, suicidal ideation, and suicide mortality. Individuals who are not employed, not married, and with low education and low income have a higher risk of suicide. Suicide risk is greater for adults in socially and materially deprived areas (Kerr et al., 2017). Adolescents from impoverished neighborhoods have more suicidal ideation and attempts, and suicides increase as the percentage of boarded-up buildings in a neighborhood increases, particularly if the individuals have a mental disorder (Page et al., 2014).

In impoverished communities, a lack of good schools and employment opportunities leads to unemployment and loss of meaningful social roles. Access to health care is limited in these communities, and there is an increased exposure to others exhibiting suicidal behavior that enhances suicide risk (Carpenter-Song & Snell-Rood, 2017).

Family Response to Suicide

Suicide has devastating effects on everyone it touches, especially family and close friends. One suicide is estimated to leave at least six survivors who are significantly impacted by the loss (Andriessen, Draper, Dudley, & Mitchell, 2016). In the aftermath of a family member's suicide, survivors experience more grief, anxiety and depression, guilt, shame, self-blame, and dysfunction than families whose loss was because of other reasons and the personal and familial disruption often lasts for years. Although recovery from a loved one's suicide is an ongoing task, survivors who are emotionally healthy before the suicide act and who have social support are able to manage the psychological trauma associated with suicide. Still, the intensity and duration of the post-suicide grief process for many survivors has led to the development of family intervention programs. Although the evidence base for these interventions is still small, strategies that support a positive sense of self, enhance problem-solving, promote the formation of a suicide story, encourage social reintegration, reduce stigma, use journaling, or permit the survivor to debrief may be effective in reducing subjective distress and to resolve grief (Andriessen et al., 2016). These strategies may be most effective delivered in survivor peer help groups.

Protective Factors

Protective factors buffer individuals from suicidal thoughts and behavior. Although identifying and understanding risk factors is very important, they have not been studied as extensively as risk factors. The Centers for Disease Control and Prevention identifies the following protective factors (CDC, National Center for Injury Prevention and Control, 2019).

- Effective clinical care for mental, physical, and substance abuse disorders
- Easy access to a variety of clinical interventions and support for help seeking
- Family and community support (connectedness)
- Support from ongoing medical and mental health care relationships
- Skills in problem-solving, conflict resolution, and nonviolent ways of handling disputes
- Cultural and religious beliefs that discourage suicide and support instincts for self-preservation

TREATMENT AND NURSING CARE FOR SUICIDE PREVENTION

Interdisciplinary Treatment and Recovery

The challenges of preventing suicides and promoting healthy coping belong to all disciplines. An interdisciplinary treatment or recovery approach along with peer support is needed for managing the threats of suicide.

Priority Care Issues

> **EMERGENCY CARE ALERT !** A true psychiatric emergency exists when an individual presents with one or more symptoms associated with imminent risk for suicidal behavior. Immediate and focused action is needed to prevent the patient's death.

The first priority is to provide for the patient's safety while initiating the *least* restrictive care possible. In contrast, an example of the *most* restrictive care is an outpatient who is admitted to a locked unit with one staff member who is assigned to observe the person at all times. Hospitalization should be reserved for those whose safety cannot be ensured in an outpatient environment.

Priority Care Issues: Preventing Suicide and Promoting Mental Health

Suicidal ideation, planning, and acts are not easily predicted and therefore are difficult to study. As a result, few evidence-based treatments exist that are known to prevent suicide and manage suicidal behavior. There is growing consensus that the suicidal act is part of a continuum of behaviors that extend long before and after a specific suicide behavioral incident. The beginning evidence points to four steps in preventing suicide and promoting long-term mental health: identification of those thinking about suicide (case finding), assessment to determine an imminent suicidal threat, intervening to change suicidal behavior associated with a specific suicidal threat, and institution of effective interventions to prevent future episodes of suicidal behavior.

Assessment

Case Finding

Case finding refers to identifying people who are at risk for suicide so proper treatment can be initiated. People who are contemplating suicide often do not share their ideation. This lack of disclosure often means that family, friends, and health professionals are unable to intervene until the suicidal ideation and planning have progressed. Yet early identification of suicidal ideation may reduce suicide deaths. Nurses can play important roles in suicide prevention by recognizing the warning signs. See Box 16.3 for the warning signs developed by the American Association of Suicidology (2019b); the mnemonic IS PATH WARM can serve as a useful memory aide for these signs.

Case finding requires careful and concerned questioning and listening that make the patient feel valued and cared about (Box 16.4). Most standardized health questionnaires have questions about suicide thoughts. Many nurses are concerned that asking patients about their suicidal thoughts will provoke a suicide attempt.

BOX 16.3

Warning Signs for Suicide

I—Ideation: Talking or writing about death, dying, or suicide
Threatening or talking of wanting to hurt or kill self
Looking for ways to kill self: seeking access to firearms, available pills, or other means
S—Substance abuse: Increased substance (alcohol or drug) use
P—Purposelessness: No perceived reason for living; no sense of purpose in life
A—Anxiety: Anxiety, agitation, unable to sleep or sleeping all the time
T—Trapped: Feeling trapped (like there is no way out)
H—Hopelessness
W—Withdrawal: Withdrawal from friends, family, and society
A—Anger: Rage, uncontrolled anger, seeking revenge
R—Recklessness: Acting reckless or engaging in risky activities, seemingly without thinking
M—Mood change: Dramatic mood changes

Adapted from American Association of Suicidology. (2019). Know the warning signs of suicide. Retrieved from http://www.suicidology.org/resources/warning-signs

BOX 16.4 • THERAPEUTIC DIALOGUE • Suicide

When Caroline sought medical care for a cold from her nurse practitioner, the nurse observed more than a cough and runny nose. Caroline appeared downcast and unusually sad. As the nurse and patient talked, the subject of family life came up, whereupon Caroline began to cry softly. As words tumbled out, she said she had been unhappy at home for a long time. When she was very young, she recalled being happy, but things changed when her brother was born, 4 years after her. Her father began to abuse her sexually, starting when Caroline was 5 years old and continuing until he moved out of the house when she was 12 years old. Caroline suspects her mother knew of the abuse, although she did nothing about it.

Two years ago, Caroline's father died by suicide. Caroline feels relieved about his death but frustrated that she never got a chance to tell him how angry she was with him. Caroline's relationship with her mother has not improved. Caroline says her mother favors her brother and is always telling her she won't amount to anything. Caroline begins to cry harder.

INEFFECTIVE APPROACH

Nurse: Clearly, many things are troubling you. Don't you think that things seem worse now because you have a cold?
Caroline: Well, that could be. What are you going to do to make me feel better?
Nurse: Give you some medicine to help you sleep and clear your nose. I think you should see a psychiatrist, too.
Caroline: I don't need a psychiatrist. I came here for my cold.
Nurse: I know you did, but you seem to be depressed.
Caroline: What are you, some kind of social worker? I am just tired.
Nurse: I am a nurse, and you seem down to me. Are you thinking about suicide?
Caroline: I don't think you know what you're talking about. I want to go now. Could you give me my medicine?

EFFECTIVE APPROACH

Nurse: It seems as though many things have been piling up on you. Does it seem that way to you, too?
Caroline: It sure does. I've just been trying to get through one day at a time, but now with this cold and no sleep, I feel like I can't go on.
Nurse: When you say you can't go on, what does that mean to you?
Caroline: Lately, I have been thinking about running away to some place where I can't be found and maybe starting over. But then I think, where would I go? Where would I stay? Who would take care of me?
Nurse: When you think that your plan for escape won't work, what happens?
Caroline: (Starting to cry again.) Then I think that maybe it would be better if I just did what my father did. I really don't think anyone would miss me.
Nurse: So you've thought about taking your life, like your Dad did?
Caroline: Yeah, and what really scares me is lately I have been thinking about that a lot. I keep saying to myself, "You're just tired," but I am so exhausted now that I can't chase the thoughts away.
Nurse: Do you think about suicide every day?
Caroline: It seems like I never stop thinking about it.
Nurse: Is there anything you can do to make the thoughts go away?
Caroline: Nothing. (Silence.)
Nurse: What would you do?
Caroline: I think I would get as many pills as I could find, drink a lot of alcohol, and maybe smoke some pot and just go to sleep.
Nurse: Do you have enough pills at home to kill yourself?
Caroline (wan smile): I was hoping that the sleeping medicine you would give me might do the job.
Nurse: It sounds like you need some help getting through this time in your life. Would you like some?
Caroline: I honestly don't know—I just want to sleep for a long time.

CRITICAL THINKING CHALLENGE

- In the first interaction, the nurse made two key blunders. What were they? What effect did they have on the patient? How did they interfere with the patient's care?
- What did Caroline do that might have contributed to the nurse's behavior in the first interaction?
- In the second interaction, the nurse did several things that ensured reporting of Caroline's suicidal ideation. What were they? What differences in attitude might differentiate the nurse in the first interaction from the nurse in the second?

This belief simply is not true. The patient expressing suicidal ideation often has had these thoughts for some time and may feel more socially connected when another recognizes the seriousness of the situation. Under no circumstances should a patient be promised secrecy about suicidal thoughts, plans, or acts. Instead, tell patients that disclosure of suicidal intent will be shared with other interdisciplinary team members so the safety of the patient can be ensured.

Assessing Risk

After suicidal ideation has been established, the next step is to determine the risk for a suicide attempt. Suicide risk assessment is difficult and whenever possible should proceed only with the assistance of other members of the interdisciplinary treatment team. Assessing for risk includes determining the seriousness of the suicidal ideation, degree of hopelessness, disorders, previous attempt, suicide planning and implementation, and availability and lethality of suicide method. Risk assessment also includes the patient's resources, including coping skills and social supports, that can be used to counter suicidal impulses. Box 16.5 lists some questions that might be asked in assessing the risk for suicide.

The greatest predictor of a future suicide attempt is a previous attempt, partly because the individual already has broken the "taboo" around suicidal behavior. Repeated episodes of self-harm with or without suicidal intent also increase immediate risk because they increase an individual's capacity to complete suicide. Other important signs of high risk are the presence of suicide planning behaviors (detailed plan, availability of means, opportunity, and capability) and engaging in final acts such as giving away prized possessions and saying goodbye to loved ones. Although the presence of a specific psychiatric disorder such as depression is an important consideration in risk assessment, anxiety, agitation, alcohol use, and impulsivity may be better indicators of immediate risk. On the other hand, support from important others, religious prohibitions, responsibility for young children, and employment may provide protection from suicidal impulses.

Ideally, an interdisciplinary team conducts suicide risk assessment in an emergency department or outpatient facility with multiple supports. Nurses practicing in more isolated situations should keep a list of contacts in settings that routinely conduct suicide risk assessments so the contacts may be consulted if a seriously suicidal individual appears in the nurse's setting.

> **NCLEXNOTE** Suicide assessment is always considered a priority. Practice by asking patients about suicidal thoughts and plans. Develop a plan with a suicidal patient that focuses on resisting the suicidal impulse. Apply the assessment process that delineates the (1) intent to die, (2) severity of ideation, (3) availability of means, and (4) degree of planning.

Interventions for Imminent, Intermediate, and Long-Term Suicide Prevention

Interventions for Those at Imminent Risk

There are three urgent priorities for care of a person who is at imminent risk for suicide: reconnecting the patient to other people and instilling hope, restoring emotional stability and reducing suicidal behavior, and ensuring safety. Reconnecting the patient interpersonally includes listening intently and without judgment to the patient's thoughts and feelings and validating his or her experience and suffering. This intervention directly challenges the patient's belief that no one cares. Using cognitive interventions can help the client to regain hope (see Chapter 10). These actions help reestablish links between the patient's presuicidal past and helps the patient begin establishing goals for the future (Gudmundsdottir & Thome, 2014).

Ensuring Patient Safety. Helping patients develop strategies for making safer choices when distressed is an important goal. Nurses caring for patients who are emerging from the initial hours and days of a suicide attempt can support the patient and focus on managing suicidal urges and developing protective strategies. As the nurse connects with the patient, together they can create a list of personal and professional resources that can be used when the individual is in crisis. With the nurse's help, the patient can

---

BOX 16.5

Assessment of Suicidal Episode

INTENT TO DIE
1. Have you been thinking about hurting or killing yourself?
2. How seriously do you want to die?
3. Have you attempted suicide before?
4. Are there people or things in your life who might keep you from killing yourself?

SEVERITY OF IDEATION
1. How often do you have these thoughts?
2. How long do they last?
3. How much do the thoughts distress you?
4. Can you dismiss them or do they tend to return?
5. Are they increasing in intensity and frequency?

DEGREE OF PLANNING
1. Have you made any plans to kill yourself? If yes, what are they?
2. Do you have access to the materials (e.g., gun, poison, pills) that you plan to use to kill yourself?
3. How likely is it that you could actually carry out the plan?
4. Have you done anything to put the plan into action?
5. Could you stop yourself from killing yourself?

visualize "emotional spaces that are safe places to go" when distressed.

Until recently, the no-suicide contract was a staple of psychiatric nursing practice and widely used across disciplines as a means of preventing suicide among those at risk. No-suicide contracts are verbal and written "contracts" between the individual at imminent risk for suicide and a health care provider that contain an agreement that the patient will not commit suicide during a specific time period. Careful evaluation of this practice has not established its efficacy in preventing suicidal behavior and suicide deaths. As a consequence, the nurse should avoid engaging in a no-suicide contract with a patient (Matarazzo, Homaifar, & Wortzel, 2014).

Inpatient Safety Considerations. When hospitalization is considered the best option to ensure the safety of the patient, the nurse has responsibility for providing a safe, therapeutic environment in which human connection, instilling hope, and changing suicidal behavior can occur. There are no evidence-based guidelines for preventing suicides in hospitals. Inpatient suicides do occur. One study reported an average of roughly 50 to 65 hospital inpatient suicides occurring per year in the United States, a rate that continues to present challenges for the inpatient nursing staff. The vast majority of inpatient suicides takes place in psychiatric facilities, and the method used in 70% of these events is hanging (Williams, Schmaltz, Castro, & Baker, 2018).

Removal of dangerous items and environmental hazards, continuous or intermittent observation of at-risk patients by hospital personnel trained in observation methods, and limitation of outpatient passes are the mainstays of hospital interventions. Observation procedures vary from facility to facility. For patients who require constant supervision, a staff member will be assigned only to the high-risk patient. For less risky patients, observation may entail close or intermittent observations.

Observation is not, in itself, therapeutic. An observation becomes therapeutic when interaction occurs with the patient. Psychiatric intensive care of this kind and restriction of freedom can be very upsetting to the patient who is withdrawn and isolated. Nurses can help patients reestablish personal control by including them in decisions about their care and restricting their behavior only as necessary. Nurses can also reduce the patient's stress while ensuring the patient's safety by intruding as little as possible on the person's exercise of free will. Observational periods can be used to help patients express a broad range of feelings and strengthen their belief in their own abilities to keep themselves safe. During observation, the nurse can help the patient describe feelings and identify ways to manage safety needs.

Interventions for Intermediate and Long-Term Risk

Patients who are suicidal may need ongoing preventive interventions. The risk varies with the genetic, psychiatric, and psychological profile of the patient and the extent of his or her social support. Discouragement and hopelessness often persist long past the suicidal episode. Episodes of hopelessness should be anticipated and planned for in the patient's care. Patients should be taught to expect setbacks and times when they are unable to see much of a future for themselves. They should be encouraged to think of times in their lives when they were not so hopeless and consider how they may feel similarly in the future. Helping patients review the goals they already have achieved and at the same time set goals that can be achieved in the immediate future can help them manage periods of discouragement and hopelessness.

Interventions for the Biologic Domain

Patients who have survived a suicide attempt often need physical care of their self-inflicted injury. Overdose, gunshot wounds, and skin wounds are common. For both groups, there will be biologic interventions for the underlying psychiatric disorder (see Unit 5).

Medication Management

Medication management focuses on treating the underlying psychiatric disorder. In schizophrenia and schizoaffective disorder, evidence suggests that antipsychotic use is related to decreased mortality compared with those not taking an antipsychotic, but currently clozapine is the only FDA-approved medication for suicide risk reduction in individuals with schizophrenia. Studies showing reduced suicide risk in patients with bipolar disorder or major depression taking lithium are not conclusive (AFSP, 2019). For depression, a nonlethal antidepressant, such as a selective serotonin reuptake inhibitor, usually is prescribed.

Electroconvulsive Therapy

Electroconvulsive therapy (ECT) has been used in both inpatient and outpatient settings to alleviate severe depression, especially in medically compromised groups such older adults, who may not tolerate conventional pharmacotherapy for depression (see Chapter 10). Rapid reduction in depression often leads to a decreased suicide drive. More research is needed to determine the role ECT may play in managing suicidal behavior. At this time, ECT is among several strategies used to decrease suicidal behavior over the long term (Kellner & Patel, 2018).

Interventions for the Psychological Domain

The goals of treatment in the psychological domain include reducing the capacity for suicidal behavior, increasing tolerance for distress, expanding coping abilities, and developing effective crisis management strategies. During the early part of a hospitalization, the most important way to reduce stress is to help the patient feel more secure and hopeful. As patients become more comfortable in their environment, the nurse can provide education about emotions, help patients explore and link pre-suicidal beliefs to a positive and hopeful future, support the application of new skills in managing negative thoughts, and help develop effective problem-solving skills.

Challenging the Suicidal Mindset

Teaching patients to distract themselves when thinking about suicide or engaging in negative self-evaluation can help to diminish suicidal ideation, dysfunctional thinking, and emotional reactivity. Simple distracting techniques such as reminding oneself to think of other things or engaging in other activities such as talking on the telephone, reading, or watching a movie are excellent temporary means of distracting the patient from negative cognitive states. See Box 16.6.

Validating the patient and teaching the patient to self-validate are powerful means of reducing suicidal thinking. Patients can learn that everyone experiences emotional distress and can begin to recognize it a routine event. To manage emotional distress and increase tolerance for it, patients can be taught simple anxiety management strategies such as relaxation and visualization. The patient can be encouraged to write about his or her emotional experiences.

When negative thoughts and emotions coexist, they reinforce each other and contribute to suicidal ideation. Individuals who are suicidal often believe they are a burden to their family, who would be better off without them. Nurses can challenge negative beliefs, especially the patient's idea that he or she is a burden to others. Ask the patient to describe the events that led to specific suicidal behavior so the patient can be engaged in developing alternative solutions. For each event, work with the patient to identify specific strategies that could be used to manage his or her distress, sense of disconnection, extreme focus on suicidal ideas, and other experiences that led the person to believe he or she had no option other than to die.

Developing New Coping Strategies

Preventing suicidal behavior requires that patients develop crisis management strategies, generate solutions to difficult life circumstances other than suicide, engage in effective interpersonal interactions, and maintain hope. The nurse can help the patient develop a written plan that can be used as a blueprint for action when the patient feels like he or she is losing control. The plan should include strategies that the patient can use to self-soothe; friends and family members that could be called, including multiple phone numbers where they can be reached; self-help groups and services such as suicide hotlines; and professional resources, including emergency departments and outpatient emergency psychiatric services.

Commitment to Treatment

Patients are usually ambivalent about wanting to die. The **commitment to treatment statement** (CTS) directly addresses ambivalence about treatment by asking the patient to engage in treatment by making a commitment to try new approaches. Different from the no-suicide contract, the CTS does not restrict the patient's rights regarding the option of suicide. Instead, the patient agrees to engage in treatment and access emergency service if needed. Underlying the CTS is the expectation that the patient will communicate openly and honestly about all aspects of treatment, including suicide. This commitment is written and signed by the patient. The efficacy of this approach has yet to be established by systematic research. Whether using the CTS or other means, be observant for lapses in the patient's participation in treatment and discuss them with the patient and other members of the interdisciplinary team.

Interventions for the Social Domain

Poor social skills may interfere with the patient's ability to engage others. The nurse should assess the patient's social capability early in treatment and make necessary provisions for social skills training. The interpersonal

---

BOX 16.6

Psychoeducation Checklist: Suicide Prevention

When teaching the patient and family about suicide and its prevention, be sure to address the following topics:
- Importance of emotional connections to family and friends
- Importance of instilling hope
- Discouraging suicidal ideation, rumination, self-harming behaviors
- Self-validation
- Emotional distress management
- Finding alternatives to suicidal behavior
- Establishing and using a crisis management plan
- Reestablishing the social network of the patient
- Information about treatment of underlying psychiatric disorders

relationship with the nurse is an ideal place to begin shaping social behaviors that will help the patient to establish a social network that will sustain him or her during periods of discouragement or crisis. Participation in support networks such as recovery groups, clubhouses, drop-in centers, self-help groups, or other therapeutic social engagement will help the patient become connected to others.

Patients need to anticipate that even some of the people closest to them will feel uncomfortable with their suicidal behavior. Helping the patient to anticipate the stigmatizing behavior of others and how to manage it will go far in reintegrating the patient into a supportive social community. The nurse can also explore the patient's participation in specific social activities such as attending church or community activities.

Evaluation and Treatment Outcomes

The most desirable treatment outcome is the patient's recovery with no future suicide attempts. Short-term outcomes include maintaining the patient's safety, averting suicide, and mobilizing the patient's resources. Whether the patient is hospitalized or cared for in the community, his or her emotional distress must be reduced. Long-term outcomes must focus on maintaining the patient in psychiatric treatment, enabling the patient and family to identify and manage suicidal crises effectively, and widening the patient's support network.

Continuum of Care

Whether the suicide prevention plan is instituted in the hospital or in an outpatient setting, the patient cannot be released to home until a workable plan of care is in place. The care plan includes scheduling an appointment for outpatient treatment, providing for continuing somatic treatments until the first outpatient treatment visit, ensuring post-release contact between the patient and significant other, providing for access to emergency psychiatric care, and arranging the patient's environment so it provides both structure and safety.

At the first follow-up visit, the patient and health care provider can establish a plan of care that specifies the intensity of outpatient care. Very unstable patients may need frequent supervision (e.g., telephone or face-to-face meetings or both) in the early days after hospitalization to maintain the patient's safety in the community. These contacts often can be short; their purpose is to convey the ongoing concern and caring of professionals involved in the patient's care. In arranging outpatient care, be certain to refer the patient to a provider who can provide the intensity of care the patient may need.

The patient's outpatient environment should be made as safe as possible before discharge. The nurse must share the care plan with family members so they can remove any objects in the patient's environment that could be used to engage in self-harm. The nurse should explain this measure to the patient to reinforce his or her sense of self-control. It is important to be reasonable in deciding what to remove from the environment. Patients who are truly determined to kill themselves after discharge will succeed in doing so, using whatever means are available.

Documentation and Reporting

The nurse must thoroughly document encounters with suicidal patients. This action is for the patient's ongoing treatment and the nurse's protection. Lawsuits for malpractice in psychiatric settings often involve completed suicides. The medical record must reflect that the nurse took every reasonable action to provide for the patient's safety.

The record should describe the patient's history, assessment, and interventions agreed upon by the patient and nurse. The nurse should document the presence or absence of suicidal thoughts, intent, plan, and available means to illustrate the patient's current and ongoing suicide risk. If the patient denies any suicidal ideation, it is important that the denial is documented. Documentation must include any use of drugs, alcohol, or prescription medications by the patient during the 6 hours before the assessment. It should include the use of antidepressants that are especially lethal (e.g., tricyclics), as well as any medication that might impair the patient's judgment (e.g., a sleep medication). Notes should reflect the level of the patient's judgment and ability to be a partner in treatment.

The documentation should reflect if any medications were prescribed, the dosages, and the number of pills dispensed. Notes should reflect the plan for ongoing treatment, including the time of the next appointment with the provider, instructions given to the patient about obtaining emergency care if needed, and the names of family members and friends who will act as supports if the patient needs them.

NURSES' REFLECTION

Caring for suicidal patients is highly stressful and can lead to secondary trauma for the nurse. Nurses who care for suicidal patients must regularly share their experiences and feelings with one another. Talking about how the situations or actions of patients make them feel will help alleviate symptoms of stress. Some nurses find outpatient therapy helpful because it enhances their understanding of what situations are most likely to trigger secondary trauma. By demonstrating how to manage effectively the stressors in their own lives, nurses can be powerful role models for their patients.

SUMMARY OF KEY POINTS

- Suicide is a common and major public health problem.
- Suicide completion is more common in white men, especially older men.
- Parasuicide is more common among women than men.
- People who attempt suicide and fail are likely to try again without treatment.
- Suicidal behavior has genetic and biologic origins.
- A suicide assessment focuses on the intention to die, hopelessness, available means, previous attempts and self-harm behavior, and degree of planning.
- Patients who are in crisis, depressed, or use substances are at risk for suicide.
- The major objectives of brief hospital care are to maintain the patient's safety, reestablish the patient's biologic equilibrium, help the patient reconnect to others, instill hope, strengthen the patient's cognitive coping skills, and develop an outpatient support system.
- The nurse who cares for suicidal patients is vulnerable to secondary trauma and must take steps to maintain personal mental health.

CRITICAL THINKING CHALLENGES

1. A religious African-American woman who lives with her three children, husband, and mother comes to her primary care provider. She is tearful and very depressed. What factors should be investigated to determine her risk for suicide and need for hospitalization?
2. A poor woman with no insurance is hospitalized after her third suicide attempt. Antidepressant medication is prescribed. What kinds of treatment will be most effective in preventing future suicidal behavior?
3. A young man enters his workplace inebriated and carrying a gun. He does not threaten anyone but says that he must end it all. Assuming that he can be disarmed, what civil rights must be considered in taking further action in managing his suicidal risk?
4. You are a nurse in a large outpatient primary care setting responsible for an impoverished population. You want to implement a case-finding program for suicide prevention. Discuss how you would proceed and some potential problems you might face.

1996 (Documentary): *Daughter of a Suicide*

This personal documentary is the story of a woman whose mother committed suicide when the daughter was 18 years old. The daughter recounts the emotional struggle and depression left as the lifelong legacy of suicide and explores her efforts to heal. Combining digital video, 16-mm, and super-8 film, *Daughter of a Suicide* uses interviews with family and friends to tell the story of both mother and daughter.

Viewing Points: How does this movie show that the effects of suicide do not end with a person's death?

1999: *The Virgin Suicides*

After the suicide death of their 13-year-old daughter Cecilia, the Lisbon family becomes recluses. The remaining daughters try to resume their life by defying the withdrawal of their parents. Unsuccessful, the movie climaxes with the suicide deaths of the three remaining teenage girls.

Viewing Points: What conditions in the girl's family led the girls to take their lives?

2005: *Paradise Now*

This movie traces the motivations of two suicide bombers in Palestine. It explores how the two young men came to the decision to kill themselves and others and their ambivalence about their impending deaths. Ultimately, one decides to live, and the movie ends with an ambiguous fate of the other. This movie provides insight into the background and troubled thoughts that precede a suicidal act.

Viewing Points: Can suicide be a political act? What other factors in these young men's lives might have contributed to their decision to volunteer as suicide bombers?

REFERENCES

American Foundation for Suicide Prevention (AFSP). (2017). Suicide Statistics. Retrieved February 16, 2019, from http://www.afsp.org/about-suicide/suicide-statistics

American Association of Suicidology. (2019a). Suicidal behavior among lesbian, gay, and bisexual youth. [Online]. Retrieved February 18, 2019, from https://www.suicidology.org/resources/facts-statistics

American Association of Suicidology. (2019b). Understanding and helping the suicidal individual. Fact sheet. [Online]. Retrieved February 16, 2019, from http://www.suicidology.org/resources/warning-signs

American Foundation for Suicide Prevention (2019). Treatment for suicide and suicide attempts. [Online]. Retrieved February 17, 2019, from https://afsp.org/about-suicide/preventing-suicide/

Andriessen, K., Draper, B., Dudley, M., & Mitchell, P. B. (2016). Pre- and post-loss features of adolescent suicide bereavement: A systematic review. *Death Studies, 40*(4), 229–246.

Anestis, J. C., Anestis, M. D., Rufino, K. A., Cramer, R. J., Miller, H., Khazen, L. R., et al. (2016). Understanding the relationship between suicidality and psychopathy: An examination of the Interpersonal-Psychological Theory of Suicidal Behavior. *Archives of Suicide Research, 20*(3), 349–368.

Anglemyer, A., Horvath, T., & Rutherford, G. (2014). The accessibility of firearms and risk for suicide and homicide victimization among household members. *Annals of Internal Medicine, 160*(2), 101–110.

Beck, A. T., Rush, A. J., Shaw, B. F., & Emery, G. F. (1979). *Cognitive therapy of depression*. New York: The Guildford Press.

Bostwick, J. M., Pabbati, C., Geske, J. R., & McKean, A. J. (2016). Suicide attempt as a risk factor for completed suicide: Even more lethal than we know. *American Journal of Psychiatry, 173*(11), 1094–1100.

Brodsky, B. S. (2016). Early childhood environment and genetic interactions: The diatheses for suicidal behavior. *Current Psychiatry Reports, 18*(9), 86.

Calati, R., Ferrari, C., Brittner, M., Oasi, O., Olie, E., Carvalho, A. F., et al. (2019). Suicidal thoughts and behaviors and social isolation: A narrative review of the literature. *Journal of Affective Disorders, 245*, 653–667.

Carpenter-Song, E., & Snell-Rood, C. (2017). The changing context of rural America: A call to examine the impact of social change on mental health and mental health care. *Psychiatric Services, 68*(5), 503–506.

Castro, C. A., & Kintzle, S. (2014). Suicides in the military: The post-modern combat veteran and the Hemingway effect. *Current Psychiatry Reports, 16*(8), 460.

Centers for Disease Control and Prevention (CDC). (2017). Fatal injury reports, national, regional and state, 1981–2016. Retrieved February 20, 2019, from https://webappa.cdc.gov/sasweb/ncipc/mortrate.html

Centers for Disease Control and Prevention (CDC), National Center for Injury Prevention and Control. (2018). Preventing suicide. Retrieved February 16, 2019, from http://www.cdc.gov/violenceprevention/suicide/index.html

Centers for Disease Control and Prevention (CDC), National Center for Injury Prevention and Control (2019). Suicide: Risk and protective factors. [Online]. Retrieved February 16, 2019, from https://www.cdc.gov/violenceprevention/suicide/riskprotectivefactors.html

Colman, I. (2018). Responsible reporting to prevent suicide contagion. *Canadian Medical Association Journal, 190*(30), E898–E899.

Corrigan, P. W., Sheehan, L., Al-Khouja, M. A., & Stigma of Suicide Research Team. (2017). Factor analysis of its stereotypes, prejudices, and discriminations. *Crisis, 38*(5), 351–359.

Crifasi, C. K., Meyers, J. S., Vernick, J. S., & Webster, D. W. (2015). Effects of changes in permit-to-purchase handgun laws in Connecticut and Missouri on suicide rates. *Preventative Medicine, 79*, 43–49.

Ducasse, D., Holden, R. R., Boyer, L., Artero, S., Calati, R., Guillaume, S., et al. (2018). Psychological pain in suicidality: A meta-analysis. *Journal of Clinical Psychiatry, 79*(3). Retrieved February 19, 2019, from https://www.psychiatrist.com/JCP/article/Pages/2017/v78n08/16r10732.aspx

Dugas, E. N., Low, N. C., O'Loughlin, E. K., & O'Loughlin, J. L. (2015). Recurrent suicidal ideation in young adults. *Canadian Journal of Public Health, 106*(5), e303–e307.

Durkheim, E. (1951 [1897]). *Suicide*. New York: Free Press.

Ellis, T. E., & Rutherford, B. (2008). Cognition and suicide: Two decades of progress. *International Journal of Cognitive Therapy, 1*(1), 47–68.

Endo, K., Ando, S., Shimodera, S., Yamasaki, S., Usami, S., Okazaki, Y., et al. (2017). Preference for solitude, social isolation, suicidal ideation, and self-harm in adolescents. *Journal of Adolescent Health, 61*(2), 187–191.

Fassberg, M. M., Cheung, G., Canetto, S. S., Erlangsen, A., Lapierre, S., Lindner, R., et al. (2016). A systematic review of physical illness, functional disability, and suicidal behavior among older adults. *Aging & Mental Health, 20*(2), 166–194.

Franklin, K. (2016). Department of Defense Quarterly Suicide Report Calendar Year 2016 2nd Quarter Defense Suicide Prevention Office (DSPO). [Online]. Retrieved on February 19, 2019, from https://www.dspo.mil/Portals/113/Documents/DoD%20Quarterly%20Suicide%20Report%20CY2016_Q4.pdf?ver=2017-04-24-112920-020

Fredriksen-Goldsen, K. I., Kim, H. J., Shui, C., & Bryan, A. E. B. (2017). Chronic health conditions and key health indicators among lesbian, gay, and bisexual older US adults, 2013–2014. *American Journal of Public Health, 107*(8), 1332–1338.

Giner, L., Blasco-Fontecilla, H., De La, Vega, D., & Courtet, P. (2016). Cognitive, emotional, temperament, and personality trait correlates of suicidal behavior. *Current Psychiatry Report, 18*(11), 102.

Gudmundsdottir, R. M., & Thome, M. (2014). Evaluation of the effects of individual and group cognitive behavioural therapy and of psychiatric rehabilitation on hopelessness of depressed adults: A comparative analysis. *Journal of Psychiatric & Mental Health Nursing, 21*(10), 866–872.

Hedegaard, H., Curtin, S. C., & Warner, M. (2018). Suicide rates in the United States continue to increase. *NCHS Data Brief*, (309), 1–8.

John, A., Glendenning, A. C., Marchant, A., Montgomery, P., Stewart, A., Wood, S, et al. (2018). Self-harm, suicidal behaviours, and cyberbullying in children and young people: Systematic review. *Journal of Medical Internet Research, 20*(4), e129.

Joiner, T. (2005). *Why people die by suicide*. Cambridge, MA: Harvard University.

Ju, J. N., Young, L. W., Seok, N. M., & Yip, P. S. (2014). The impact of indiscriminate media coverage of a celebrity suicide on a society with a high suicide rate: Epidemiological findings on copycat suicides from South Korea. *Journal of Affective Disorders, 156*, 56–61.

Kann, L., McManus, T., Harris, W. A., Shanklin, S. L., Flint, K. H., Queen, B., et al. (2018). Youth Risk Behavior Surveillance - United States, 2017. *Morbidity and Mortality Weekly Report (MMWR). Surveillance Summaries, 67*(8), 1–114.

Kavak, F., Akturk, U., Ozdemir, A., & Gultekin, A. (2018). The relationship between domestic violence against women and suicide risk. *Archives of Psychiatric Nursing, 32*(4), 574–579.

Kellner, C. H., & Patel, S. B. (2018). The role of ECT in the suicide epidemic. *Psychiatric Times, 35*(8), 23.

Kerr, W. C., Kaplan, M. S., Huguet, N., Caetano, R., Giesbrecht, N., & McFarland, B. H. (2017). Economic recession, alcohol, and suicide rates: Comparative effects of poverty, foreclosure, and job loss. *American Journal of Preventative Medicine, 52*(4), 469–475.

Kimerling, R., Makin-Byrd, K., Louzon, S., Ignacio, R. V., & McCarthy, J. F. (2016). Military sexual trauma and suicide mortality. *American Journal of Preventative Medicine, 50*(6), 684–691.

Klonsky, E. D., Qiu, T., & Saffer, B. Y. (2017). Recent advances in differentiating suicide attempters from suicide ideators. *Current Opinion Psychiatry, 30*(1), 15–20.

Lewis, N. M. (2009). Mental health in sexual minorities: Recent indicators, trends, and their relationship to place in North American and Europe. *Health & Place, 15*(4), 1029–1045.

Liu, R. T., Kraines, M. A., Puzia, M. E., Massing-Schaffer, M., & Kleiman, E. M. (2013). Sociodemographic predictors of suicide means in a population-based surveillance system: Findings from the national violent Death Reporting system. *Journal of Affective Disorders, 151*(2), 449–454.

Liu, Y., Zhang, J., & Sun, L. (2017). Who are more likely to attempt suicide again? A comparative study between the first and multiple timers. *Comprehensive Psychiatry, 78*, 54–60.

Logan, J. F., Skopp, N. A., Reger, M. A., Gladden, M., Smolenski, D. J., Floyd, F., et al. (2015). Precipitating circumstances of suicide among active duty U.S. Army Personnel versus U.S. civilians, 2005–2010. *Suicide and Life-Threatening Behavior, 45*(1), 65–77.

Ma, J., Batterham, P. J., Calear, A. L., & Han, J. (2016). A systematic review of the predictions of the Interpersonal-Psychological Theory of Suicidal Behavior. *Clinical Psychology Review, 46*, 34–45.

Matarazzo, B. B., Homaifar, B. Y., & Wortzel, H. S. (2014). Therapeutic risk management of the suicidal patient: Safety planning. *Journal of Psychiatric Practice, 20*(3), 220–224.

Monteith, L. L., Bahraini, N. H., Matarazzo, B. B., Gerber, H. R., Soberay, K. A., & Forster, J. E. (2016). The influence of gender on suicidal ideation following military sexual trauma among Veterans in the Veterans Health Administration. *Psychiatry Research, 244*, 257–265.

National Institute of Mental Health (NIMH). (2016). Suicide. Retrieved January 27, 2019, from https://www.nimh.nih.gov/health/statistics/suicide.shtml

Nestor, B. A., Cheek, S. M., & Liu, R.T. (2016). Ethnic and racial differences in mental health service utilization for suicidal ideation and behavior in a nationally representative sample of adolescents. *Journal of Affective Disorders, 202*, 197–202.

O'Brien, K. H., Putney, J. M., Hebert, N. W., Falk, A. M., & Aguinaldo, L. D. (2016). Sexual and gender minority youth suicide: Understanding subgroup differences to inform interventions. *LGBT Health, 3*(4), 248–251.

O'Connor, R. C., & Kirtley, O. J. (2018). The integrated motivational–volitional model of suicidal behaviour. *Philosophical Transactions of the Royal Society of London. Series B, Biological Sciences, 373*(1754), 20170268.

Page, A., Lewis, G., Kidger, J., Heron, J., Chittleborough, C., Evans, J., et al. (2014). Parental socio-economic position during childhood as a determinant of self-harm in adolescence. *Social Psychiatry & Psychiatric Epidemiology, 49*(2), 193–203.

Pandey, G. N. (2013). Biological basis of suicide and suicidal behavior. *Bipolar Disorder, 15*(5), 524–541.

Sheehan, L. L., Corrigan, P. W., & Al-Khouja, M. A., & Stigma of Suicide Research Team. (2016). Stakeholder perspectives on the stigma of suicide attempt survivors. *Crisis, 38*(2), 1–9.

Stone, D. M., Simon, T. R., Fowler, K. A., Kegler, S. R. Yuan, K., Holland, K.M... Crosby, A. E. (2018). Vital signs: trends in state suicide rates—United States, 1999–2016 and circumstances contributing to suicide—27 states, 2015. *Centers for Disease Control and Prevention, Morbidity and Mortality Weekly Report, 67*(22), 617–624.

Suicide Prevention Resource Center (SPRC). (2013). Suicide among racial/ethnic populations in the U.S. [Online]. Retrieved on February 20,

2019, from https://www.sprc.org/resources-programs/suicide-among-racialethnic-populations-us

Suicide Prevention Resource Center (SPRC). (2019a). Racial and ethnic disparities. [Online]. Retrieved on February 20, 2019, from https://www.sprc.org/racial-ethnic-disparities

Suicide Prevention Resource Center (SPRC). (2019b). Risk and protective factors. [Online]. Retrieved on February 18, 2019, from https://www.sprc.org/about-suicide/risk-protective-factors

Testa, R. J., Michaels, M. S., Bliss, W., Rogers, M. L., Balsam, K. F., & Joiner, T. (2017). Suicidal ideation in transgender people: Gender minority stress and interpersonal theory factors. *Journal of Abnormal Psychology*, *126*(1), 125–136.

Tidemalm, D., Runeson, B., Waern, M., Frisell, T., Carlstrom, E., Lichtenstein, P., et al. (2011). Familial clustering of suicide risk: A total population study of 11.4 million individuals. *Psychological Medicine*, *41*(12), 2527–2534.

United States Department of Health and Human Services [U.S. DHHS]. (2010). Healthy people 2020. Retrieved February 20, 2019, from http://www.healthypeople.gov

Virupaksha, H. G., Muralidhar, D., & Ramakrishna, J. (2016). Suicide and suicidal behavior among transgender persons. *Indian Journal of Psychological Medicine*, *38*(6), 505–509.

Wand, A. P. F., Peisah, C., Draper, B., & Brodaty, H. (2018). Understanding self-harm in older people: A systematic review of qualitative studies. *Aging & Mental Health*, *22*(3), 289–298.

Wang, M. C., Lightsey, O. R., Tran, K. K., & Bonaparte, T. S. (2013). Examining suicide protective factors among black college students. *Death Studies*, *37*(3), 228–247.

Wendell, J., Ratcliff, C. G., Price, E., Petersen, N. J., Dinapoli, E. A., & Cully, J. A. (2016). Factors associated with high frequency of suicidal ideation in medically ill Veterans. *Journal of Psychiatric Practice*, *22*(5), 389–397.

Wetherall, K., Cleare, S., Eschle, S., Ferguson, E., O'Connor, D. B., O'Carroll, R. E., et al. (2018). From ideation to action: Differentiating between those who think about suicide and those who attempt suicide in a national study of young adults. *Journal of Affective Disorders*, *241*, 475–483.

Williams, S. C., Schmaltz, S. P., Castro, G. M., & Baker, D. W. (2018). Incidence and method of suicide in hospitals in the United States. *Joint Commission Journal on Quality and Patient Safety*, *44*(11), 643–650.

Winterrowd, D., Canetto, S. S., & Benoit, K. (2017). Permissive beliefs and attitudes about older adult suicide: A suicide enabling script? *Aging & Mental Health*, *21*(2), 173–181.

Yildiz, E. (2018). Suicide in sexual minority populations: A systematic review of evidence-based studies. *Archives of Psychiatric Nursing*, *32*(4), 650–659.

Zimmerman, G. M., Rees, C., Posick, C., & Zimmerman, L. A. (2016). The power of (Mis)perception: rethinking suicide contagion in youth friendship networks. *Social Science and Medicine*, *157*, 31–38.

17
Mental Health Care for Survivors of Violence

Beverly Baliko

KEY CONCEPTS
- intimate partner violence
- psychological abuse
- sexual assault

LEARNING OBJECTIVES

After studying this chapter, you will be able to:

1. Describe types of violence and abuse, including intimate partner violence, stalking, rape and sexual assault, child abuse and neglect, and elder abuse.
2. Describe selected theories of violence.
3. Compare the reasons some people become abusive and why some victims remain in violent relationships.
4. Discuss the formation of a therapeutic relationship with a victim of violence.
5. Formulate nursing care plans for survivors of violence and abuse.
6. Describe treatment for perpetrators of abuse.

KEY TERMS

- child abuse • child neglect • cyberstalking • cycle of violence • elder abuse • intergenerational transmission of violence • lethality assessment • rape • revictimization • stalking

---

Violence in the form of abuse of intimate partners, children, and elders is a national health problem. This type of violence permanently changes the survivor's reality and meaning of life. It wounds deeply, endangering core beliefs about the self, others, and the world. It can damage or destroy the survivor's self-esteem.

Nurses encounter survivors of violence and abuse in all health care settings. For this reason, being knowledgeable about abuse risk factors, indicators, causes, assessment techniques, and effective nursing interventions is a must. This chapter presents evidence that can shape contemporary nursing practice in caring for persons and families who survive violence and abuse.

TYPES OF VIOLENCE AND ABUSE

The most common type of abuse occurs as a result of domestic (family) violence; that is, the perpetrator is or formerly was a loved and trusted partner or family member. When this kind of violence occurs, the world and home are no longer safe in the eyes of the survivor. This chapter includes a discussion of intimate partner violence (IPV), child abuse and neglect, and elder abuse with emphasis on IPV.

Intimate Partner Violence

IPV is a significant public health problem in the United States, and across the globe. Behaviors that constitute IPV include physical, sexual, and psychological (emotional) abuse or a combination of these perpetrated by a current or former spouse, significant other, or dating partner. The prevalence of IPV can only be estimated, because much abuse goes unreported. The most recent data available suggest that during their lifetimes, 1 in 4 women and nearly 1 in 10 men experience adverse psychological or physical consequences related to physical or sexual violence perpetrated by an intimate partner (Smith et al., 2018). Costs of billions of dollars annually are associated with acute and chronic medical and mental health needs of survivors, lost productivity, and lost lives (Centers for Disease Control and Prevention [CDC], 2018a). Approximately 63% of female murder victims are killed by current or former intimate partners (Violence Policy Center, 2018).

> **KEYCONCEPT** **Intimate partner violence** involves physical violence, sexual violence, stalking and psychological aggression (including coercive acts) by a current or former intimate partner. IPV occurs on a continuum from psychological abuse to lethal violence.

Physical Abuse

Physical abuse involves any act of aggression with or without use of an object or weapon that results in injury, pain, or impairment to another. Examples include striking, kicking, shoving, choking, burning. Frequently, this behavior becomes a pattern that increases in severity over time. Physical abuse not only causes immediate injuries but contributes to health problems that may persist long after the abuse ends. Although anyone can be a victim of physical abuse, women are far more likely than men to be seriously injured or killed by an intimate partner.

> **KEYCONCEPT** **Psychological abuse** (also referred to as emotional abuse) involves threats, intimidation, or violence used as a means of asserting dominance and causing fear. Psychological abuse includes behaviors such as criticizing, insulting, humiliating, or ridiculing someone in private or in public. Abusers may destroy property, threaten or harm pets, control or monitor spending and daily activities, or isolate a person from family and friends. Gaslighting is a form of psychological abuse in which the victim is made to question his or her own judgment and perceptions. Perpetrators downplay the consequences of their behavior, deny abusive intent, or argue that actions are somehow justified. They often blame the victim for provoking or otherwise causing the abuse, leaving the victim with feelings of guilt or responsibility. About one third of adults report experiencing psychological abuse by an intimate partner during their lifetime (Smith et al., 2018).

Whereas physical violence may be episodic, psychological abuse is frequently more unrelenting. Over time, psychological abuse is devastating to an individual's self-esteem and self-confidence and can lead to psychiatric and physical disorders resulting from chronic stress. The varieties of abuse used to exert power and control over romantic partners are represented in Figure 17.1.

> **KEYCONCEPT** **Teen partner abuse** Teens and adults are often not aware of the frequency with which teen dating violence occurs. In a recent national survey of adolescents in the United States, 12% of girls and 7% of boys reported being struck or physically hurt on purpose by a boyfriend or girlfriend in the 12 months prior to the survey (CDC, 2018b). Conflict or relationship problems with parents and peers may be predictors of teen partner abuse. Teens who experience violence in intimate relationships are more likely to develop problems such as depression, substance abuse, eating disorders, and thoughts of suicide (CDC, 2018b). School performance may suffer.

Comorbidities

Besides injuries and death, survivors suffer multiple conditions directly caused by IPV or the chronic stress associated with it. Anxiety disorders, depression, posttraumatic stress disorder (PTSD), and substance use disorders are all associated with family violence. Examples of health problems associated with IPV include asthma, gastrointestinal conditions, cardiovascular problems, bladder infections, migraines, joint pain, gynecological disorders, and sexually transmitted diseases (STDs) (CDC, 2018a). Strangulation and blows to the head can cause traumatic brain injuries that have lasting effects on cognition and functioning.

Risk Factors for Intimate Partner Violence

IPV occurs across all demographics and socioeconomic levels. Younger women, women who are divorced or separated, and Native American and Alaska Native women are at highest risk (National Center for Victims of Crime, 2017). Although women are disproportionately affected, men can also be victims of IPV. Nonheterosexual couples experience IPV at rates similar to heterosexual couples, but victims often receive less support as a result of social stigma associated with nontraditional relationships. Within any type of relationship, frequent conflicts, jealousy, and possessiveness are associated with an increased risk of violence.

Individual characteristics such as low self-esteem, emotional insecurity, depression, antisocial or borderline personality traits, or a history of violence increase the likelihood of perpetration of violence (CDC, 2018c). There is a strong association of substance use, especially alcohol abuse, with family violence. The presence of firearms in the home increases the risk of lethal violence.

Personal stressors such as low income and unemployment, and external stressors such as natural disasters or economic crises, may challenge individual and family coping, resulting in violence (CDC, 2018c). In unstable families, violence sometimes begins or escalates when a pregnancy occurs. Abuse during pregnancy is a significant risk factor for several fetal and maternal complications, including miscarriages, low birth weight, low maternal weight gain, infections, and anemia (Alhusen, Sharps, & Bullock, 2015). Pregnancy is a window of opportunity for health care providers to screen women for IPV and refer them to the appropriate services.

Chapter 17 • Mental Health Care for Survivors of Violence 241

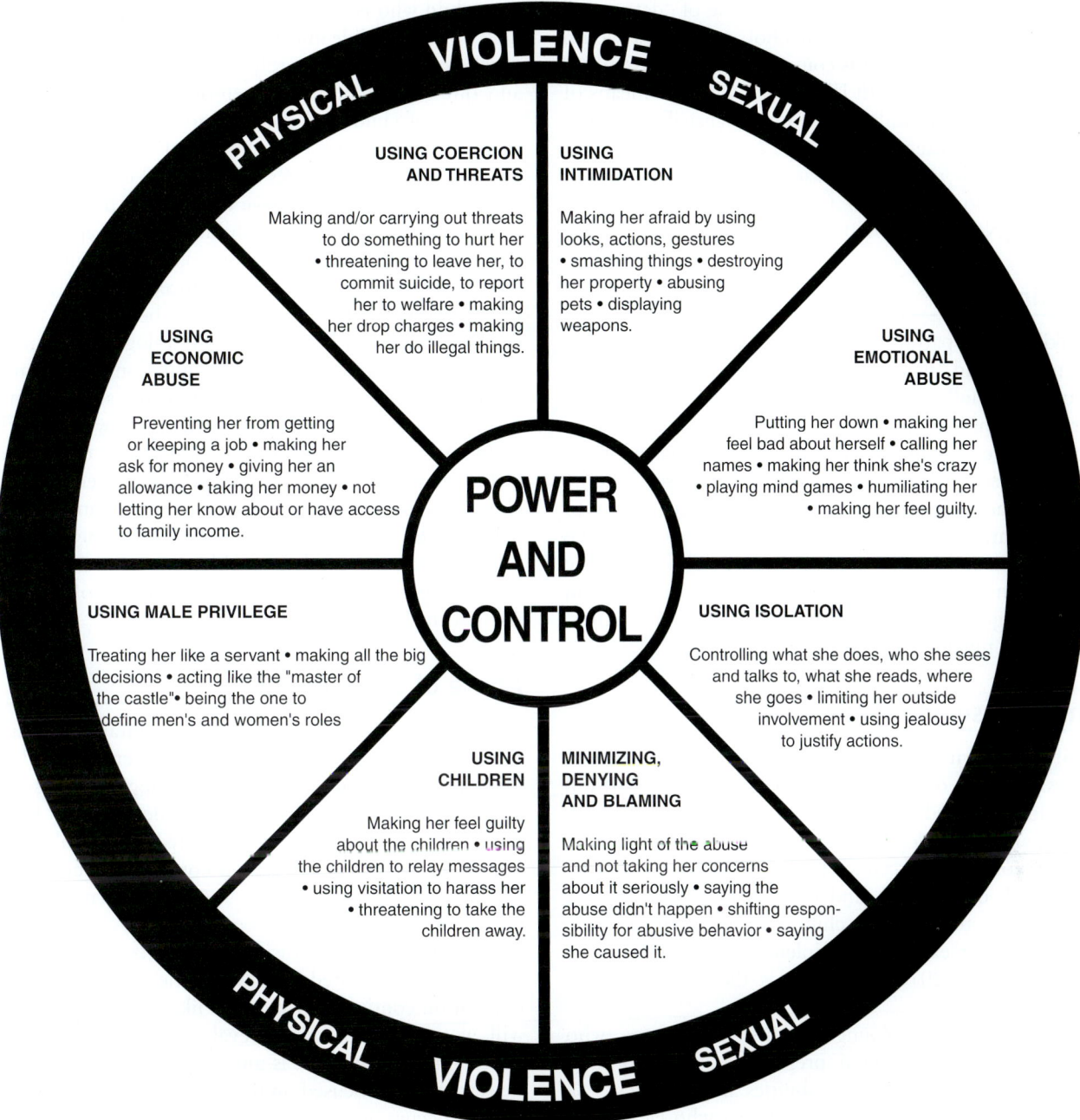

FIGURE 17.1 Power and control wheel. (Courtesy of Domestic Abuse Intervention Programs, 202 East Superior Street, Duluth, MN.)

> **KEYCONCEPT Sexual assault** includes any form of nonconsenting sexual activity, ranging from fondling to penetration.

Rape and Sexual Assault

Sexual assault is any type of sexual activity inflicted on a nonconsenting person or on someone who is unable to consent because of age, mental status, or impairment. Rape, the most severe form of sexual assault, refers to forced vaginal, oral, or anal penetration or attempted penetration by the offender, including use of a foreign object (Bureau of Justice Statistics, 2018). Perpetrators use physical force, coercion, or threats to gain control over their victims. **Rape** is a crime of violence and domination, with sexuality used as a weapon.

Most sexual assaults are perpetrated by someone known to the victim. Children are most likely to be sexually abused by family members or others close to them, as are elderly and disabled adults. Adolescents and young adults are especially vulnerable to drug-facilitated assault by acquaintances, which involves the use of "date-rape" drugs, often combined with alcohol, to make a victim incapable of resistance. It is common for sexual assault to occur in conjunction with IPV, as an additional means of intimidation and humiliation. Nonconsensual sex within a marriage was exempt from rape laws until the 1970s, and it was not until 1993 that all states had removed that exemption (National Coalition against Domestic Violence [NCADV], 2018).

Stalking

Stalking is a pattern of repeated unwanted contact, attention, and harassment that often increases in frequency. Stalkers harass and terrorize their victims through behavior that causes fear or substantial emotional distress. Stalking may include such behaviors as following someone, showing up at the person's home or workplace, vandalizing property, using technology to track or harass someone, or sending unwanted gifts. One in 6 women and 1 in 19 men experience stalking at some point in their lifetime (Smith et al., 2018). Stalking can be prolonged and takes a tremendous toll on victims' health and functioning.

Child Abuse and Neglect

Child abuse includes acts of commission and acts of omission. Acts of commission are intentional harmful behaviors directed toward a child and include physical, sexual, and psychological abuse. **Child neglect** is an act of omission, which occurs when a child's basic physical, emotional, educational, and health care needs are not met. Failure to protect a child from harm, inadequate supervision, or exposure to violence are other forms of neglect (CDC, 2018d). Neglect is the most common form of child abuse.

Children who are younger than 4 years of age, who are products of unwanted pregnancies, or who have developmental or physical disabilities are at highest risk of abuse (CDC, 2018d). Young parents who lack social support, resources, and knowledge of normal childhood development are at increased risk of abusing their children. Multiple stressors, emotional or substance abuse problems, and the use of harsh punishment are additional parental risk factors.

Children who are abused or neglected may develop physical, emotional, and behavioral problems (CDC, 2018d). Their cognitive development may be impaired and they may exhibit academic difficulties. Abuse leads to problems getting along with or trusting others. Survivors of child abuse are at increased risk for depression, anxiety, low self-esteem, and substance abuse. Adverse experiences in childhood have a negative impact on health and well-being throughout life.

A child who is emotionally or psychologically abused does not have visible injuries to alert others. Nevertheless, psychological abuse severely affects a child's self-esteem and often leaves permanent emotional scars. For many survivors of childhood abuse, emotional abuse is worse than physical abuse. Psychological abuse frequently co-occurs with other types of abuse and can take various forms. Children often believe the abuse is their fault.

Sexual abuse occurs to children of all ages and is frequently perpetrated by someone the child knows and trusts. To maintain their silence, children may be threatened or told that they will not be believed if they disclose the abuse. No child is psychologically prepared to cope with repeated sexual stimulation. A victim of prolonged sexual abuse will develop low self-esteem, a feeling of worthlessness, and a distorted view of sex. The child may become withdrawn, distrustful, or suicidal. Other characteristics of children who have been sexually abused include an unusual interest or avoidance of sexually related content, nightmares, seductiveness, refusal to go to school, conduct problems, secretiveness, and unusual aggressiveness (American Academy of Child & Adolescent Psychiatry [AACAP], 2018).

Abuse of Older Adults

Older adults and adults who have mental or physical disabilities are vulnerable to abuse. Elderly individuals may be victims of physical, psychological, or sexual abuse. The most common type of elder abuse is financial abuse, in which older adults may be manipulated by family or caregivers to give up control of their money and are vulnerable to scams and fraud perpetrated by outsiders.

Elder abuse is increasingly recognized as a serious problem in the United States and other countries. As the population continues to age, it is likely that the problem will worsen. The actual prevalence of elder abuse is uncertain, as most abuse is unreported, and relatively little research has focused on this population. The violence usually occurs at the hands of a caregiver or a person the older adult trusts, but is also a significant problem in nursing homes and assisted living facilities.

Individuals who are isolated, have poor support systems, or have mental or physical impairments that foster dependency on others are more vulnerable to harm. Older people may be reluctant to report maltreatment by those they love or on whom they depend, or cognitive deficits may prevent them from being able to articulate their situation. In addition to the obvious physical problems (e.g., injuries, pressure sores, malnutrition) that can result from abuse or neglect, older adults can experience worsening of existing medical conditions and emotional problems such as depression, anxiety, and fearfulness (CDC, 2016).

Costs of medical care related to abuse and neglect are estimated to be well over $5 billion annually; losses to elderly individuals associated with financial exploitation are similarly alarming (National Center on Elder Abuse [NCEA], n.d.). High-risk factors for those who are more likely to abuse older adults include using drugs or alcohol, high levels of stress, lack of social support, high emotional or financial dependence on the older adult, lack of training in taking care of older adults, and depression (CDC, 2016). Caring for a dependent older adult can be overwhelming. It is important for the nurse to listen to and assess both older adults and their caregivers to help prevent abuse and neglect in this population.

THEORIES OF VIOLENCE

No single cause is sufficient to explain the phenomenon of family violence. The neurobiologic and psychological factors that contribute to anger and poor impulse control (as outlined in Chapter 14) are relevant to the use of aggression in the home. However, the ability of many abusers to refrain from angry outbursts and violence in public settings suggests that their behavior toward family members is not solely attributable to poor self-control. The risk factors discussed in previous sections increase the likelihood of violence occurring but do not cause it. Many people share the same risks but do not engage in violence. Outlined below are a few prominent theories among the many researchers that attempt to explain IPV and other types of violence in the family. Individual characteristics likely intersect with risk factors to produce behavior that is learned and reinforced in families, communities, and society.

Social Learning Theory (Intergenerational Transmission of Violence)

Being a victim of childhood abuse is one of the strongest predictors of violence as an adult. Violent families create an atmosphere of tension, fear, intimidation, and confusion about intimate relationships. Children in violent homes learn that violent behavior is an approved and legitimate way to solve problems and to cope with difficulty. Social learning or **intergenerational transmission of violence** theory posits that children who witness or experience violence in their homes are more likely to perpetuate violent behavior within their own families (Copp, Giordano, Longmore, & Manning, 2016). Experiencing harsh physical discipline increases the risk of perpetrating family violence as an adult (Afifi, Mota, Sareen, & MacMillan, 2017). This learned behavior is reinforced when violence as a means of control or punishment is sanctioned within social systems or when there are inadequate social or legal constraints to discourage such behaviors.

Economic Disadvantage, Community Disorganization, and Attitudes Supportive of Violence

Neighborhoods that are more socially cohesive are more intolerant of deviant behavior. The presence of concentrated economic disadvantage (i.e., neighborhoods with the lowest incomes, high unemployment, and institutional disinvestment), racial or ethnic heterogeneity, and community instability is associated with community disorganization and weak social control, which leads to increased levels of crime and IPV. Within these disadvantaged communities, institutions that normally foster social control, such as churches, schools, and other community organizations, lose their ability to exercise social control over the community. Community disorganization, crime, and weak social control also foster individual acceptance of violence, which in turn is associated with increased rates of IPV, child abuse, and elder abuse (Copp et al., 2016).

Imbalances in Relationship Power

Another body of literature suggests that IPV is a manifestation of gender-based imbalances in relationship power. Usually, this perspective explains IPV as violence against women by their male romantic partners related to issues of gender, inequality, power and privilege, patriarchy, and the subordination of women (Namy et al., 2017). Patriarchal systems exist and are supported at the macro level (e.g., government, bureaucracies, religion) and at the micro level (e.g., families), and both levels have gender inequities. Within a patriarchal society, men often hold traditional gender role beliefs. For example, whereas men are heads of households and provide for their families, women are homemakers and mothers. When these beliefs are challenged, such as when a woman enters the workforce and earns more than her partner, men may feel threatened and respond with violence.

Historically, women and children had few or no rights in most cultures, and in many countries today, women's rights remain limited (Ramsey, 2011). Women and children were considered part of the household over which the male held absolute power and violence was accepted as a permissible way to exercise authority. Even after popular opinion changed and so-called "wife-beating" became formally illegal in all states in the United States by 1920, IPV was treated differently than other crimes and viewed as a private matter that rarely resulted in arrest or prosecution until the latter part of the 20th century. Until recently, men in the United States were able to use physical violence with relative impunity within the context of intimate relationships. In 1994, *The Violence Against Women Act* (VAWA) (*P.L. 103–122*) was the first US federal policy to combat interpersonal violence and other violence against women. This law declared civil

Phase 1. Tension Building
* Minor incidents
* Perpetrator establishes total control of victim by psychological and emotional means
* Perpetrator demands total acquiescence of victim. Verbal abuse and accusations follow
* Perpetrator isolates victim by approving/disapproving social contacts
* Perpetrator monitors victim's activities, phone calls, mail, and travels and demands explanations
* Perpetrator degrades and demoralizes victim by scrutinizing victim's physical and mental characteristics
  (unattractive, stupid) and functions and assaulting victim's self-esteem (worthless, "no good")

Phase 2. Violence Erupts
* Severe injury to victim and children
* Victim may incite violence as a way to control mounting terror
* Period of relative calm follows battering

Phase 3. Remorse Ensues
* Perpetrator becomes kind, contrite, and loving—begging for forgiveness and promising never to inflict abuse again (until the next time)
* Tension builds; the cycle repeats.

FIGURE 17.2 The cycle of violence.

rights for victim–survivors of gender-based violence and created new laws to protect them. Despite changes in laws, patriarchal attitudes continue to influence the dynamics of some families, sometimes bolstered by cultural and religious norms (Ogunsiji & Clisdell, 2017).

Cycle of Violence

Many, but not all, cases of IPV reflect a recognized **cycle of violence**. The cycle consists of three recurring phases that often increase in frequency and severity. The cycle is fully described in Figure 17.2.

Factors Influencing Leaving versus Staying in a Violent Relationship

Many women do not report abuse, fearing retaliation against themselves or their children. Often, they continue to hold strong feelings for their partners despite the abuse. When medical care is required, women may attribute their injuries to other causes; health care providers may be reluctant to inquire about abuse. Provision of assistance to women who are involved in violent intimate relationships can pose unique problems in that seeking support can be dangerous to the women if their activities are discovered by the abusive partner. Therefore, the challenge for health care providers is twofold—ensuring that support is both available and safely accessible, whether or not it is accepted at a given time. Even though it might be difficult to understand why a person would remain in an abusive relationship, it is critical to remain nonjudgmental and to realize that there are valid reasons for deciding to remain in a potentially harmful environment.

Leaving an abusive relationship is a process that can be quite complex. Many women leave and return several times as they learn new coping skills and build support networks before ending the relationship permanently. When abuse is intermittent, and strong emotional and psychological ties to the abusive partner remain, victims continue to hope that the behavior will change. Women who lack job skills, financial resources, and support systems may stay because of economic dependence on their partner. Some are concerned about losing custody of their children if they are unable to provide for them independently.

Fear is another important factor in deciding whether to leave or to stay in a violent relationship. Some women stay because of threats not only against themselves but against other family members or pets. Women recognize the valid concern that leaving may not stop the violence. If victims attempt to leave or actually do leave the relationship, perpetrators often escalate their violence, stalk their partners, and may even kill them, which makes leaving the time of greatest risk in an abusive relationship (NCADV, n.d.).

Safety Issues and Mandatory Reporting

Health care providers, including nurses, are mandated reporters. This means that they must report known or suspected abuse in specific circumstances. Some states require reporting of injuries sustained as a result of abuse. Mandatory reporting for IPV is controversial because it may act as a barrier to disclosure, especially in cases in which the victim fears that the abuser will retaliate (Buppert & Klein, 2008). All states require reporting of known or suspected abuse involving children and vulnerable adults. It is important for nurses to be familiar with the laws of the state in which they practice and with the policies of their organization. Removing children and older adults from their families or caregivers may be necessary to ensure their immediate safety. In most settings, nurses do not have to make this decision alone; rather, they involve other professionals to assist with assessment and alternate placement if the current living situation of an abused or neglected child or older adult cannot be made safe. When an older adult's decision making is not impaired (*competence* is the legal term), he or she must be allowed an appropriate degree of autonomy in deciding how to manage the problem even if he or she chooses to remain in the abusive situation (Pomerance, 2015). Forcing someone to do something against his or her wishes is itself a form of victimization by denying autonomous decision making.

ESTABLISHING A THERAPEUTIC RELATIONSHIP

Establishing a trusting nurse–patient relationship is one of the most important steps in caring for any person experiencing violence. When interviewing, to establish rapport and put the survivor at ease, start with the least sensitive areas and progress to more sensitive topics (Power, 2017). Survivors are unlikely to disclose sensitive information unless they perceive the nurse to be trustworthy and nonjudgmental. Important considerations in establishing open communication are ensuring confidentiality and providing a quiet, private place in which to interact. A supportive, empathetic approach is most effective. The nurse must continually monitor personal reactions to prevent negative feelings from influencing the nurse–patient relationship in a way that could retraumatize the survivor. Nurses must make clear during the assessment their responsibility for mandated reporting.

EVIDENCE-BASED NURSING CARE FOR PERSONS EXPERIENCING VIOLENCE

Nurses encounter survivors of violence and abuse in many health care settings, not just in mental health settings. Abuse may be disclosed or discovered by providers in urgent care clinics, primary care settings, obstetrics and gynecology settings, pediatric units, well-child clinics, geriatric units, schools, and nursing homes, among others.

Mental Health Nursing Assessment

Conducting a Safety Assessment First

Once physiologic stability is established, the nurse should determine whether the survivor is in danger for his or her life, either from homicide or suicide, and, if children are in the home, whether they are in danger. Trauma may trigger suicidal ideation or exacerbate pre-existing mental health conditions that place the survivor at risk. Suicide precautions should be initiated if indicated.

Children who are present during abusive episodes are at risk for emotional and developmental harm even if they are not direct recipients of abuse. Exposing a child to violence carries legal consequences in many states (Child Welfare Information Gateway, 2016).

The Danger Assessment Screen is a useful tool for assessing the risk that IPV will end in homicide (Campbell & Humphreys, 1993) (Box 17.1). This assessment may help survivors recognize the serious nature of the violence they routinely experience. An abbreviated version of this tool, the Danger Assessment-5 (Messing, Campbell, & Snider, 2017), can be used for brief screening.

Screening for Violence and Abuse

Because of the prevalence of IPV, the U.S. Preventive Services Task Force recommends universal screening for all women of child-bearing age (2016). However,

> **BOX 17.1**
> **Danger Assessment**
>
> Several risk factors have been associated with homicides (murders) of both batterers and victims in research that has been conducted after the killings have taken place. We cannot predict what will happen in your case, but we would like you to be aware of the danger of homicide in situations of severe battering and to see how many of the risk factors apply to your situation.
>
> 1. Has the physical violence increased in frequency during the past year?
> 2. Has the physical violence increased in severity during the past year or has a weapon or threat with weapon been used?
> 3. Does your partner ever try to choke you?
> 4. Is there a gun in the house?
> 5. Has your partner ever forced you to have sex when you did not wish to do so?
> 6. Does your partner use drugs? By drugs, I mean "uppers" or amphetamines, speed, angel dust, cocaine, "crack," street drugs, heroin, or mixtures.
> 7. Does your partner threaten to kill you, or do you believe he or she is capable of killing you?
> 8. Is your partner drunk every day or almost every day? (In terms of quantity of alcohol.)
> 9. Does your partner control most or all of your daily activities? For instance, does he or she tell you who you can be friends with, how much money you can take with you shopping, or when you can take the car?
> 10. Has your partner ever beaten you while you were pregnant? (If never pregnant by him, check here _____)
> 11. Is your partner violently and constantly jealous of you? (For instance, does he or she say, "If I can't have you, no one can.")
> 12. Have you ever threatened or tried to commit suicide?
> 13. Has he ever threatened or tried to commit suicide?
> 14. Is your partner violent toward the children?
> 15. Is your partner violent outside the home?
>
> TOTAL YES ANSWERS: _____
>
> Thank you. Please talk to your nurse, advocate, or counselor about what the danger assessment means in terms of your situation.
>
> Adapted from Campbell, J., & Humphreys, J. (Eds.). (1993). *Nursing care of survivors of family violence* (p. 259). St. Louis: Mosby.

> **BOX 17.2**
> **Abuse Assessment Screen**
>
> 1. Have you ever been emotionally or physically abused by your partner or someone important to you?   YES   NO
> 2. Within the past year, have you been hit, slapped, kicked, or otherwise physically hurt by someone?   YES   NO
>   If YES, by whom: _____
>   Number of times: _____
>   Mark the area of injury on body map.
> 3. Within the past year, has anyone forced you to have sexual activities?   YES   NO
>   If YES, who: _____
>   Number of times: _____
> 4. Are you afraid of your partner or anyone you listed above?   YES   NO

actual rates of screening in most settings are low. Most survivors do not report violence to health care workers without specifically being asked about it (Power, 2017). Survivors may be reluctant to report abuse because of shame, embarrassment, fear of not being believed, or fear of retaliation. Survivors who depend on the abuser for care or financial support may be concerned about consequences of disclosure. If the suspected abuser is present, it is important to speak to the survivor alone.

Validated screening tools are readily accessible (Basile, Hertz, & Back, 2007). Asking specific abuse screening questions substantially increases the detection of abuse. For that reason, nurses must develop a repertoire of age-appropriate, culturally sensitive abuse-related questions. Avoid using terms such as "abuse" and "rape," because those labels may not be consistent with an individual's perception of his or her experience (see Boxes 17.2 and 17.3).

Other questions that might be useful in eliciting disclosure are:

- "When there are fights at home, have you ever been hurt or afraid?"
- "It looks like someone has hurt you. Tell me about it."
- "Some women have described problems like yours. If this is happening to you, can we talk about it?"

When survivors are disclosing abuse, they need privacy and time to tell their story. The nurse should listen attentively without offering unsolicited advice or making judgmental remarks about the possible abuse or the perpetrator. Use validating messages to convey that the survivor is believed and that the nurse is concerned for his or her safety and well-being. Examples of such messages include:

- "I'm really sorry this happened to you."
- "I'm glad you told me."
- "It sounds like a frightening experience."
- "It was not your fault."

Survivors of IPV may deny the abuse, make excuses for the perpetrator's behavior, or attribute an injury to an unlikely cause. Avoid pressuring or confronting them, but carefully document a description of the survivor's account of how the injury happened, using the survivor's own words.

After assessment is completed in a health care agency and abuse is evident, the nurse should offer the adult survivor use of the telephone. This may be the only time that the survivor can make calls in private to family, who might offer support, or to the police, lawyers, or shelters. Scheduling future appointments may provide the survivor with a legitimate reason to leave the perpetrator and continue to explore options.

> **BOX 17.3**
>
> **Burgess-Partner Abuse Scale for Teens**
>
> Directions: During the past 12 months, you and one of your partners may have had a fight. Below is a list of things one of your partners may have done to you. Please circle the number of how often this partner did these things to you. This is not a test and there are no right or wrong answers. Remember, having a partner(s) does not mean you are having sex with the partner(s).
>
> *If you have not had a partner in the past 12 months, do not fill this form out.*
>
> | | Never | Once | A few times | More than a few times | Routinely or a lot |
> |---|---|---|---|---|---|
> | 1. My partner doesn't let me go out with my friends | 0 | 1 | 2 | 3 | 4 |
> | 2. My partner tells me what to wear | 0 | 1 | 2 | 3 | 4 |
> | 3. My partner says if I don't have sex with him/her then I don't love him/her | 0 | 1 | 2 | 3 | 4 |
> | 4. My partner says he/she will hurt me if I talk to another guy/girl | 0 | 1 | 2 | 3 | 4 |
> | 5. My partner calls me bad names like bitch | 0 | 1 | 2 | 3 | 4 |
> | 6. My partner says he/she will hurt me with a weapon | 0 | 1 | 2 | 3 | 4 |
> | 7. My partner forces me to have sex | 0 | 1 | 2 | 3 | 4 |
> | 8. My partner tells me I am stupid or dumb | | 1 | 2 | 3 | 4 |
> | 9. My partner follows me when I do things with my friends or family | 0 | 1 | 2 | 3 | 4 |
> | 10. My partner hits or kicks something when he/she gets mad at me | 0 | 1 | 2 | 3 | 4 |
> | 11. My partner kicks me | 0 | 1 | 2 | 3 | 4 |
> | 12. My partner says he/she can have sex with other people even though he/she said I can't | 0 | 1 | 2 | 3 | 4 |
> | 13. My partner gives me sexually transmitted infections | 0 | 1 | 2 | 3 | 4 |
> | 14. My partner hurts me using a weapon | 0 | 1 | 2 | 3 | 4 |
> | 15. My partner forces me to use drugs even though I don't want to | 0 | 1 | 2 | 3 | 4 |
> | 16. My partner beats me up so bad | 0 | 1 | 2 | 3 | 4 |
> | 17. My partner says he/she will hurt my family if don't do what he/she says | 0 | 1 | 2 | 3 | 4 |
> | 18. My partner tells me what school activities I can and can't do | 0 | 1 | 2 | 3 | 4 |
> | 19. My partner tells me what friends I can hang out with | 0 | 1 | 2 | 3 | 4 |
> | 20. My partner chokes me if he/she gets mad at me | 0 | 1 | 2 | 3 | 4 |
> | 21. My partner yells at me if he/she doesn't know where I am | 0 | 1 | 2 | 3 | 4 |
> | 22. My partner says we can't break up even though I want to | 0 | 1 | 2 | 3 | 4 |
>
> How many partners have you had in the past 12 months?_____
>
> Copyright 2002 & 2003 Stephanie E. Burgess; Permission is granted for use in research or clinical settings.
> Burgess, S., & Tavakoli, A. (2005). Psychometric assessment of the Burgess-Partner Abuse Scale for Teens (B-PAST). *Aquichan, 5,* 96–107.

Physical Health Assessment

Documentation of abuse or suspected abuse includes a complete history and physical examination. Note vital signs, sleep and appetite disturbances, exaggerated startle responses, flashbacks, and nightmares that may suggest PTSD or depression. Assess for injuries in need of immediate attention. Documentation should include a detailed history of how injuries occurred and a careful description of the injuries. A body map may be used to indicate location, size, and type of injuries. The nurse's documentation may become evidence if there are legal consequences related to the violence, even if the survivor declines to file a report at the time of the incident. Victims of violence experience mild to severe physical consequences. Mild injuries may include bruises and abrasions of the head, neck, face, trunk, and limbs. People who are chronically abused may have multiple bruises in various stages of healing. Severe injuries include multiple traumas, major fractures, major lacerations, and internal injuries (including chest and abdominal injuries and subdural hematomas). Loss of vision and hearing can result from blows to the head.

Physical or sexual violence may result in head injuries that can produce changes in cognition, affect, motivation, and behavior. Survivors of sexual abuse may have vaginal and perineal trauma. Anorectal injuries may also be present, including disruption of anal sphincters, retained foreign bodies, and mucosal lacerations. Examination for sexual abuse, acute or chronic events, may require

BOX 17.4

Special Concerns for Victims of Sexual Assault

ASSESSMENT FOCUS

The history and physical examination of the survivor of sexual assault differ significantly from other assessment routines because the evidence obtained may be used in prosecuting the perpetrator. Therefore, the purpose is twofold:

- To assess the patient for injuries
- To collect evidence for forensic evaluation and proceedings

Usually, someone with appropriate training, such as a nurse practitioner who has taken special courses, examines a victim of rape or sexual assault. Generalist nurses may be involved in treating the injuries that result from the assault, including genital trauma (e.g., vaginal and anal lacerations, and extragenital trauma (e.g., injury to the mouth, throat, wrists, arms, breasts, thighs).

KEY INTERVENTIONS

Nursing intervention to prevent short- or long-term psychopathology after sexual assault is crucial. Psychological trauma after rape and sexual assault includes immediate anxiety and distress and the development of PTSD, depression, panic, and substance abuse.

Key interventions include:

- Early treatment because initial levels of distress are strongly related to later levels of posttraumatic stress disorder, panic, and anxiety.
- Supportive, caring, and nonjudgmental nursing interventions during the forensic rape examination are also crucial. This examination often increases survivors' immediate distress because they must recount the assault in detail and submit to an invasive pelvic or anal examination.
- Anxiety-reducing education, counseling, and emotional support, particularly in regard to unwanted pregnancies and sexually transmitted infections, including HIV. All survivors should be tested for these possibilities. Treatment may include terminating a pregnancy; administering medications to treat gonorrhea, chlamydia, trichomoniasis, and syphilis; and administering medications that may decrease the likelihood of contracting HIV infection.
- Interventions that are helpful for survivors of domestic violence; these also apply to survivors of sexual assault.

---

referral to a trained registered nurse in sexual assault, known as a SANE (*s*exual *a*ssault *n*urse *e*xaminer) (Cole & Logan, 2008). Determine the need for emergency contraception, or prophylactic treatment for HIV or STDs (see Box 17.4 for additional considerations).

Healthy child development and deviations that may be related to abuse or neglect are critical components of the nursing assessment of children. Assessing developmental milestones, school history, and relationships with siblings and friends is important. Intracranial hemorrhage in an infant in the absence of an obvious cause, such as a motor vehicle accident, may suggest shaken baby syndrome. Infants do not begin to move or ambulate on their own prior to the age of 6 months, when they begin to crawl; therefore, any bruises on an infant before the age of 6 months is cause for suspicion. Any discrepancies between the history and physical examination and implausible explanations for injuries and other symptoms should be an alert to the possibility of abuse (Yaffe, 2010). Children and adolescents who wear clothing that covers parts of the body in a manner inconsistent with the season may be hiding bruises, abrasions, or burns caused by cigarettes or boiling water. Other circumstances that should heighten the suspicion of childhood abuse include multiple fractures or types of fractures (such as spiral fractures) that would only occur in an abusive situation. Other injuries such as bite marks or injuries to the genitals or anus always require further investigation.

For reference when assessing older adults, become familiar with normal aging and signs and symptoms of common illnesses to distinguish those conditions from abuse. Observe for signs of malnutrition or inattention to activities of daily living (ADLs). As with children, bruises, lacerations, and other injuries are suspicious if they are inconsistent with a description of how they occurred. Some older adults are unable to communicate effectively because of dementia or other cognitive impairment. Evidence that excessive medications or physical restraints are being used to control an older adult's behavior should be investigated. Box 17.5 lists indicators of actual or potential abuse that need to be thoroughly assessed for all survivors.

Psychosocial Assessment

Fear

Living with an abusive partner, parent, or caregiver means living with constant fear and uncertainty. Because victims never know what might precipitate an incident of violence, they are constantly hypervigilant and fearful. The back-and-forth nature of the relationship, that is, alternating between love and violence, is confusing, so the survivor may try to do everything possible to please the abuser in an effort to prevent another violent episode.

Low Self-Esteem

Being the victim of abuse is devastating to healthy self-esteem, or feelings of self-acceptance, self-worth, self-love, and self-nurturing. Emotional abuse may be particularly devastating. Victims are criticized, rejected, devaluated, and ignored. Feeling stupid was a recurring theme in a qualitative study of women who had left abusive relationships. Women consistently labeled themselves stupid for not recognizing abusive behaviors, allowing their partners to abuse them, and staying in an abusive relationship (Enander, 2010). Low self-esteem has been linked to physical and mental health problems, and problems with relationships, which may affect survivors' ability to achieve financial independence.

BOX 17.5
History and Physical Findings Suggestive of Abuse

PRESENTING PROBLEM
- Vague information about cause of problem
- Delay between occurrence of injury and seeking of treatment
- Inappropriate reactions of significant other or family
- Denial or minimizing of seriousness of injury
- Discrepancy between history and physical examination findings

FAMILY HISTORY
- Past family violence
- Physical punishment of children
- Children who are fearful of parent(s)
- Father or mother (or both) who demands unquestioning obedience
- Alcohol or drug abuse
- Violence outside the home
- Unemployment or underemployment
- Financial difficulties or poverty
- Use of older adult's finances for other family members
- Finances rigidly controlled by one member

HEALTH AND PSYCHIATRIC HISTORY
- Fractures at various stages of healing
- Spontaneous abortions
- Injuries during pregnancy
- Multiple visits to the emergency department
- Elimination disturbances (e.g., constipation, diarrhea)
- Multiple somatic complaints
- Eating disorders
- Substance abuse
- Depression
- Posttraumatic stress disorder
- Self-mutilation
- Suicide attempts
- Feelings of helplessness or hopelessness
- Low self esteem
- Chronic fatigue
- Apathy
- Sleep disturbances (e.g., hypersomnia, hyposomnia)
- Psychiatric hospitalizations

PERSONAL AND SOCIAL HISTORY
- Feelings of powerlessness
- Feelings of being trapped
- Lack of trust
- Traditional values about home, partner, and children's behavior
- Major decisions in family controlled by one person
- Few social supports (isolated from family, friends)
- Little activity outside the home
- Unwanted or unplanned pregnancy
- Dependency on caregivers
- Extreme jealousy by partner
- Difficulties at school or work
- Short attention span
- Running away
- Promiscuity
- Child who has knowledge of sexual matters beyond that appropriate for age
- Sexualized play with self, peers, dolls, toys
- Masturbation
- Excessive fears and clinging in children
- Verbal aggression
- Themes of violence in artwork and school work
- Distorted body image
- History of chronic physical or psychological disability
- Inability to perform activities of daily living
- Delayed language development

PHYSICAL EXAMINATION FINDINGS
General Appearance
- Fearful, anxious, hyperactive, hypoactive
- Watching partner, parent, or caregiver for approval of answers to your questions
- Poor grooming or inappropriate dress
- Malnourishment
- Signs of stress or fatigue
- Flinching when approached or touched
- Inappropriate or anxious nonverbal behavior
- Wearing clothing inappropriate to the season or occasion to cover body parts

Vital Statistics
- Elevated pulse or blood pressure
- Other signs of autonomic arousal (e.g., exaggerated startle response, excessive sweating)
- Underweight or overweight

Skin
- Bruises, welts, edema, or scars
- Burns (cigarette, immersion, friction from ropes, pattern like an electric iron or stove)
- Subdural hematoma
- Missing hair
- Poor skin integrity: dehydration, decubitus ulcers, untreated wounds, urine burns, or excoriation

Eyes
- Orbital swelling
- Conjunctival hemorrhage
- Retinal hemorrhage
- Black eyes
- No glasses to accommodate poor eyesight

Ears
- Hearing loss
- No prosthetic device to accommodate poor hearing

Mouth
- Bruising
- Lacerations
- Missing or broken teeth
- Untreated dental problems

Abdomen
- Abdominal injuries during pregnancy
- Intra-abdominal injuries

Genitourinary System or Rectum
- Bruising, lacerations, bleeding, edema, tenderness
- Untreated infections

Musculoskeletal System
- Recent fractures or old fractures in various stages of healing
- Dislocations
- Limited range of motion in extremities
- Contractures

Neurologic System
- Difficulty with speech or swallowing
- Hyperactive reflexes
- Developmental delays
- Areas of numbness
- Tremors

(Continued)

BOX 17.5
History and Physical Findings Suggestive of Abuse (Continued)

Mental Status
- Anxiety, fear
- Depression
- Suicidal ideation
- Difficulty concentrating
- Memory loss

Medications
- Medications that are not indicated by physical condition
- Overdose of drugs or medications (prescribed or over the counter)
- Medications not taken as prescribed

Communication Patterns and Relations
- Verbal hostility, arguments
- Negative nonverbal communication, lack of visible affection
- One person answers questions and looks to other person for approval
- Extreme dependency on family members

Guilt and Shame

A history of abuse is often associated with guilt and shame. Survivors are ashamed of being manipulated and violated and for having put themselves in such a situation. Abusive partners tell the survivors that the abuse is their fault and many victims believe them. Feelings of humiliation and shame prevent survivors from seeking medical care and other forms of support and reporting abuse to authorities. The experience of being battered is so degrading and humiliating that survivors are often afraid to disclose it to anyone. Many fear that they will not be taken seriously or will be blamed for inciting the abuse or for staying with their abusers. Keeping their circumstances secret and maintaining a front of normality places enormous tension and pressure on survivors.

Problems With Intimacy

Abused children, especially those who have experienced child sexual abuse, experience intrusion, abandonment, devaluation, or pain in the relationship with the abuser instead of the closeness and nurturing that are normal for intimate relationships (AACAP, 2018). Consequently, intimacy is associated with shame and fear rather than warmth and caring and with concerns about dominance and submission rather than mutuality. Shame in turn is associated with being submissive, feeling devalued, and the desire to retaliate against a person who is seen as the source of humiliation. In adulthood, unresolved feelings of shame as well as symptoms of PTSD or depression may disrupt the development of intimacy and lead to relationships characterized with dissatisfaction and poor relationship quality (Fering, Simon, & Cleland, 2009).

Conversely, some survivors of child abuse and child sexual abuse may engage in risky sexual behavior such as early sexual activity (before age 15 years), promiscuity, and prostitution (AACAP, 2018). These behaviors place survivors at risk for developing sexually transmitted diseases and HIV. Survivors who engage in this type of behavior may have learned that sexual activity is a means for securing affection, intimacy, or material rewards such as money or drugs.

Revictimization

Many survivors who experienced childhood trauma are revictimized later in life. Numerous factors are related to **revictimization**, including symptoms of PTSD, dissociation, boundary issues, and role reversal with both mothers and fathers (Enander, 2010). Excessive use of alcohol and other drugs by survivors makes them more vulnerable and less able to defend themselves. Survivors with substance use problems are more likely to enter a relationship with someone who also uses, placing them at risk for substance-related violence (Cole, Logan, & Shannon, 2008).

People with abuse histories frequently have difficulty with boundaries. During childhood abuse, they experienced frequent boundary violations and associate those violations with intimate relationships. Role reversal in childhood in which a child takes care of one or both parents may lead to difficulty with boundaries and may be associated with intrusiveness, boundary dissolution with a partner, and risk of IPV in adulthood (Enander, 2010).

Social Networks

An evaluation of social networks provides additional clues of psychological abuse and controlling behavior. Having supportive family or friends is crucial in short-term planning for developing a safety plan and is also important to long-term recovery. A survivor cannot leave an abusive situation with nowhere to go. Supportive family and friends may be willing to provide shelter and safety, as well as emotional support.

Social Isolation

Many perpetrators isolate their family from all social contacts, including other relatives. Some survivors isolate themselves because they are ashamed of the abuse or fear nonsupportive responses. Nurses can assess restrictions on freedom that may suggest abuse and control by asking such questions as: "Are you free to go where you want?" "Is staying home your choice?" and "Is there anything you would like to do that you cannot?"

Economic and Emotional Dependency

Women who have young children and depend on the perpetrator financially may believe that they cannot leave the abusive relationship. Those who are emotionally dependent on the perpetrator may experience an intense grief reaction that further complicates their leaving. Older adults and children often depend on the abuser and cannot leave the abusive situation without workable alternatives.

Priority of Nursing Care

Violence and abuse are critical situations that need to be addressed immediately. The nurse should focus on the individual's personal safety first and any injuries that have occurred.

Nursing Interventions

The goals of all nursing interventions in cases of violence are to prevent injury, stop the violence, ensure the survivor's safety, and restore health.

As appropriate concerning age and ability, nursing interventions should empower survivors to act on their own behalf. This must be done in a collaborative partnership. Nurses must be willing to offer support and information and not impose their own values on survivors by encouraging them to leave abusive relationships (Campbell, Webster, & Glass, 2009). Strong psychological and economic bonds tie many survivors to their perpetrators. Moreover, adult survivors who are capable of making decisions are the experts about their situations. They are the best judges to determine the appropriate time to leave a relationship.

Intervention strategies for older adults depend on whether the individual accepts or refuses assistance and whether he or she can make decisions. If the person refuses treatment, it is important to remain nonjudgmental and provide information about available services and emergency contact information. If the older adult appears incapable of making decisions, then guardianship, foster care, or nursing home placement may be needed. The nurse should initiate a referral to a case manager or other who can facilitate further intervention.

Safety Planning

One of the most important interventions when caring for individuals who are in an ongoing abusive relationship is to help survivors develop a safety plan (Domestic Violence Resource Center, 2018). The first step in developing such a plan is helping the survivor recognize the signs of danger. Changes in tone of voice, substance use, and increased criticism may indicate that the perpetrator is losing control. Detecting early warning signs helps survivors to escape before battering begins.

The next step is to devise the escape. For families at risk for violence, this may involve mapping the house for an escape route. The IPV survivor needs to have a bag packed and hidden but readily accessible that includes what is needed to get away. Important things to pack are clothes, a set of car and house keys, bank account numbers, birth certificate, insurance policies and numbers, marriage license, valuable jewelry, important telephone numbers, and money. If children are involved, the adult survivor should make arrangements to get them out safely. That might include arranging a signal to indicate when it is safe for them to leave the house and to meet at a prearranged place.

A safety plan for a child or dependent elder might include safe places to hide and important telephone numbers, including 911 and those of the police and fire departments and other family members and friends.

Physical Health Interventions

Treatment of trauma symptoms may include cleaning and dressing burns or other wounds and assisting with setting and casting broken bones. Malnourished and dehydrated children and older adults may require nursing interventions such as intravenous therapy or nutritional supplements that alleviate the alteration in nutrition and fluid and electrolyte imbalances. Victims of sexual assault require additional considerations (see Box 17.5).

> **KEYCONCEPT** Individuals who are experiencing IPV need their basic needs met (e.g., safety, housing, food, child care) before their psychological traumas can be addressed.

Promoting Healthy Daily Activity

Teaching sleep hygiene (i.e., practices conducive to healthy sleep patterns) and promoting exercise, leisure time, and nutrition will help battered survivors regain a healthy physical state and self-care activities. Taking care of themselves may be difficult for survivors who have spent years trying to separate themselves from their bodies (dissociate) to survive years of abuse. Techniques such as going to bed and arising at consistent times, avoiding naps and caffeine, and scheduling periods for relaxation just before retiring may be useful in promoting sleep (Pigeon, May, Perlis, Ward, Lu, & Talbot, 2009). Aerobic exercise is a useful technique for relieving anxiety and depression and promoting sleep.

Managing Care of Patients With Mental Health or Substance Abuse Issues

Survivors of abuse and sexual assault, and those in abusive relationships, may experience depression, anxiety, and posttraumatic stress. These disorders interfere with cognitive processes—including judgment, decision making, and problem solving—and impede healing even after the survivor is in a safe environment. Trauma-informed cognitive-behavioral therapy and interpersonal therapy specifically targeting psychological consequences of IPV are the most effective treatments for survivors (Arroyo, Lundahl, Butters, Vanderloo, & Wood, 2017). Refer the survivor to a qualified mental health provider for treatment.

Survivors who have a substance use disorder need referral to a treatment center for such disorders. The treatment center should have programs that address the special needs of survivors. Alcohol- and drug-dependent survivors frequently stop treatment and return to previous dysfunctional use patterns if their violence-related problems are not addressed appropriately (Ullman & Sigurvinsdottir, 2015). Survivors who are impaired by substances are at high risk for HIV infection and other infectious diseases. If survivors do not know their HIV status, they should be encouraged to get tested.

Psychosocial Interventions

Several issues must be addressed for survivors including guilt, shame, and stigmatization. These issues can be approached in several ways. Assisting survivors to verbalize their experience in an accepting nonjudgmental atmosphere is the first step. Directly challenging attributions of self-blame for the abuse and feelings of being dirty and different is another. Helping survivors to identify their strengths and validating thoughts and feelings may help to increase their self-esteem.

Working With Children

Children may need to learn a "violence vocabulary" that allows them to talk about their abuse and assign responsibility for abusive behavior. Children also need to learn that violence is not okay, and it is not their fault. Allowing children to discuss their abuse in the safety of a supportive, caring relationship may alleviate anxiety and fear. Respond to children's disclosures with sensitivity, belief, and a calm demeanor. Avoid pressuring children to talk or share details if they are uncomfortable (Ramamoorthy & Myers-Walls, 2013).

Reenacting the abuse through play is another technique that may be helpful in assisting children to express and work through their anxiety and fear. Play therapy uses dolls, human or animal figures, video games, or puppets to work through anxiety or fears. Other techniques include reading stories about recovery from abusive experiences (literal or metaphoric), using art or music to express feelings, and psychodrama. In addition, teaching strategies to manage fear and anxiety, such as relaxation techniques, coping skills, and imagery, may give the child an added sense of mastering his or her fear (National Child Traumatic Stress Network, n.d.).

Managing Anger

Anger and rage are part of the healing process for survivors. Expression of intense anger is uncomfortable for many nurses. However, anger expression should be expected from the survivor, so it is necessary to develop comfortable ways to respond. Moreover, an important nursing intervention is teaching and modeling anger expression appropriately. Inappropriate expressions of anger might drive supportive people away. Anger management techniques include appropriately recognizing and labeling anger and expressing it assertively rather than aggressively or passive-aggressively. Assertive ways of expressing anger include owning the feeling by using "I feel" statements and avoiding blaming others. Teaching anger management and conflict resolution may be especially important for children who have seen nothing but violence to resolve problems.

Coping With Anxiety

Anxiety management is a crucial intervention for all survivors. A high comorbidity exists involving trauma, PTSD, and anxiety disorders. During treatment, survivors experience situations and memories that provoke intense anxiety and must know how to soothe themselves when they experience painful feelings. Moreover, most survivors struggle with control issues, especially involving their bodies. Anxiety management skills offer one way to maintain some control over their bodies and choices (see Chapter 18).

Finding Strength and Hope

Providing hope and a sense of control is fundamental for survivors of trauma. Help survivors find hope by assisting them to identify specific strengths and aspects of their lives that are under their control. This type of intervention may empower survivors to find options other than remaining in an abusive relationship. Interventions that focus on empowerment encourage and create opportunities for survivors to make decisions about their lives, thereby restoring a sense of autonomy and competence lost in the abusive environment (Wood, 2015).

BOX 17.6

Psychoeducation Checklist: Abuse

When caring for the patient who has been abused, be sure to address the following topics in the teaching plan:

- Cycle of violence
- Access to shelters
- Legal services
- Government benefits
- Support network
- Symptoms of anxiety, dissociation, and PTSD
- Safety or escape plan
- Relaxation
- Adequate nutrition and exercise
- Sleep hygiene
- HIV testing and counseling

Psychoeducation

Other nursing interventions include teaching self-protection skills, healthy relationship skills, and healthy sexuality (Box 17.6). Again, this teaching may be especially important for children who have no role models for healthy relationships. Children also need to know what constitutes controlling and abusive behavior and how to get help for abuse. Survivors also need information about resources, such as shelters for battered women, legal services, government benefits, and support networks. Before giving the survivor any written material, first discuss the possibility that if the perpetrator were to find the information in the survivor's possession, he or she might use it as an excuse for further battering.

Family Interventions

Family interventions in cases of child abuse focus on behavioral approaches to improve parenting skills. A behavioral approach has multiple components. *Child management skills* help parents manage maladaptive behaviors and reward appropriate behaviors. *Parenting skills* teach parents how to be more effective and nurturing with their children. *Leisure skills* training is important to reduce stress in the household and promote healthy family time. *Household organization* training is another way to reduce stress by teaching effective ways to manage the multiple tasks that families have to perform. Such tasks include meal planning, cooking, shopping, keeping health care providers' appointments (e.g., dental care, health visits, counseling), and planning family activities (National Center for Parent, Family and Community Engagement, 2015).

Anger control and stress management skills are important parts of behavioral programs for families. Anger control programs teach parents to identify events that increase anger and stress and to replace anger-producing thoughts with more appropriate ones. Parents learn self-control skills to reduce the expression of uncontrolled anger. Stress-reduction techniques include relaxation techniques and methods for coping with stressful interactions with their children.

Community Involvement

Nurses may be involved in interventions to reduce violence at the community level. Many abusive caregivers, parents, and guardians as well as battered partners, older adults, and children are socially isolated. Developing support networks may help reduce stress and therefore reduce abuse. Community contacts vary for each abuser and survivor but might include crisis hot lines, support groups, and education classes.

Nurses may also make home visits. Home visits provide support to families and provide them with knowledge about stress and management. Abuse of any kind creates a volatile situation, so nurses may be putting themselves or the survivor in danger if they do make home visits. Carefully assess this possibility before proceeding. If necessary, arrange a safe place to meet the survivor instead.

Evaluation and Treatment Outcomes

Evaluation and outcome criteria depend on the setting for interventions. For instance, if a survivor is encountered in the emergency department, successful outcomes might be that injuries are appropriately managed and the patient's immediate safety is ensured. For long-term care, outcome criteria and evaluation might center on ending abusive relationships. Examples of other outcome criteria that would indicate successful nursing interventions are recognizing that one is not to blame for the violence, demonstrating knowledge of strengths and coping skills, and reestablishing social networks.

Evaluation of nursing care for abused children depends on attaining goals mutually set with the parents or guardians. An end to all violence is the optimal outcome criterion; however, attainment of smaller goals indicates progress toward that end. Outcomes such as increased problem-solving and communication skills within the family, increased self-esteem in both children and parents, and increased use of nonphysical forms of discipline may all indicate progress toward the total elimination of child abuse.

Follow-up efforts are important in evaluating the outcomes of elder abuse. The optimal outcome is to end all abuse and keep the older adult in his or her own living environment, if appropriate. Although the abuse may have been resolved temporarily, it may flare up again. Ongoing support for the caregiver and assistance with caregiving tasks may be necessary if the older adult is to remain at home. Nursing home or assisted living may be the only desirable option if the burden is too great for the family and the likelihood of ongoing abuse or neglect is high.

Another important outcome of nursing intervention with survivors is appropriate treatment of any disorder resulting from abuse (e.g., acute stress disorder, PTSD, anxiety disorders, dissociative identity disorder [DID], major depression, substance abuse). Follow-up nursing assessments should monitor symptom reduction or exacerbation, adherence to any medication regimen, and side effects of medication. The ultimate outcome is to end violence and enable the survivor to return to a more productive, safe, and nurturing life without being continually haunted by memories of the abuse.

Nurses must become accustomed to measuring gains in small steps when working with survivors. Making any changes in significant relationships has serious consequences and can be done only when the adult survivor is ready. It is easy to become angry or discouraged with survivors, so it is important not to communicate such feelings. Discussing such feelings with other staff provides a way of dealing with them appropriately. In such discussions with supervisors or other staff, it is imperative to protect the survivor's confidentiality by discussing feelings around issues, not particular individuals, in order to ensure that survivors cannot be identified.

TREATMENT FOR THE ABUSER

Participants in programs that treat abusers are usually present only because the court has mandated the treatment. Programs are often outpatient groups that meet weekly for an extended period of time, often 36 to 48 weeks. Some programs advocate longer programs, believing that chronic offenders require from 1 to 5 years of treatment to change abusive behavior. States vary on requiring that treatment programs for abusers contact partners.

Interventions must be culturally sensitive. Many factors can affect violence against others, including socioeconomic status, racial or ethnic identity, country of origin, and sexual orientation; those differences must be addressed. When applicable, intervention programs may require abusers to undergo substance abuse treatment concurrently, so patients are required to remain sober and to submit to random drug testing.

SUMMARY OF KEY POINTS

- The most common type of abuse results from domestic violence.
- IPV is a significant public health problem; it includes physical violence, sexual violence, stalking, and psychological aggression.
- IPV crosses all ethnic, racial, and socioeconomic lines. Women are more likely to be injured or killed by current or former intimate partners than by any other perpetrators.
- Stalking is repeated unwanted contact, attention, and harassment that increase in frequency.
- Child maltreatment includes child abuse (i.e., overt actions that cause harm, potential or threat of harm) and child neglect (i.e., failure to provide needs or to protect from harm or potential harm).
- Elders may also be physically, emotionally, and sexually abused or neglected. The most common type of elder abuse is economic.
- Among the many theories that have been proposed to explain violence are neurologic problems, psychopathology, alcohol and other drug abuse, intergenerational transmission of violence, and economic and community factors.
- A well-documented cycle of violence consists of three phases of increasing frequency and severity.
- Nurses need to be familiar with signs and symptoms of abuse and to be vigilant when assessing patients.
- Nurses need to be nonjudgmental when caring for a victim of abuse. Many reasons a person could cause a person to remain in an abusive situation.
- Nursing interventions include physical health interventions and psychosocial interventions that focus on helping victims identify their strengths and validating thoughts and feelings.

CRITICAL THINKING CHALLENGES

1. Abuse is a pervasive problem, in which anyone can be a victim (e.g., women, men, children, older adults, gays, lesbians). Why do so few nursing units and nurses make it routine to ask questions about abuse?
2. Abuse is not just a "women's issue." The prevalence of abuse might decrease if men make it a "men's issue" as well. What is preventing this from happening?
3. What are your thoughts and feelings about women who are victims of violence in which both partners (victim and perpetrator) abuse alcohol and other drugs?
4. What are your thoughts and feelings about women who will not leave an abusive relationship?
5. What are some reasons that people remain in abusive relationships?
6. Why do some survivors become involved in more than one abusive relationship?

7. How do you handle your feelings toward abusive parents or relatives who abuse older adults?
8. What are the issues in mandatory reporting of violence toward women, particularly violence?
9. Would your thoughts, feelings, and ability to intervene change if the violent relationship is between same sex partners?

1994: *Once Were Warriors*

A mother of 5 children reevaluates her 18-year marriage to her alcoholic, hot-tempered husband when his barroom violence tragically encroaches into their home life. Produced and filmed in New Zealand, this film also presents how urbanization has undermined the culture and strength of the indigenous Māori people.

Viewing Points: What evidence can you find in this film that may reflect intergenerational transmission of violence? In what ways do you think that culture can influence attitudes toward abuse (both positive and negative)? What are positive and negative cultural influences in this film?

1976: *Sybil*

Sally Field plays Sybil, a woman who experiences dissociative identity disorder after suffering horrible abuse during childhood. Help from a psychiatrist (Joanne Woodward) uncovers the memories that have led to the splitting of Sybil's personality. The movie contains harrowing scenes of the abuse Sybil experienced.

Viewing Points: What symptoms does Sybil show in the film? How does the psychiatrist work with Sybil's different personalities in this film?

2002: *Enough*

Jennifer Lopez stars as a blue-collar beauty (Slim Hiller) who marries the really wrong guy. Eventually, she discovers his philandering and spends the rest of the movie in a nomadic flight from his hot-tempered brutality. Bankrolled by her estranged father, she protects her young daughter. Knowing she must face the inevitable showdown, she turns to self-defense courses for empowerment.

Viewing Points: When did Slim and Mitch's relationship turn destructive? What are the characteristics of an abused partner displayed by Slim? What were Mitch Hiller's primary motives in stalking Slim?

REFERENCES

Afifi, T. O., Mota, N., Sareen, J., & MacMillan, H. L. (2017). The relationships between harsh physical punishment and child maltreatment in childhood and intimate partner violence in adulthood. *BMC Public Health, 17*(1), 493.

Alhusen, J. L., Sharps, R. E., & Bullock, L. (2015). Intimate partner violence during pregnancy: Maternal and neonatal outcomes. *Journal of Women's Health, 24*(1), 100–106.

American Academy of Child & Adolescent Psychiatry (AACAP) (2018). *Sexual abuse*. Retrieved June 18, 2019 from https://www.aacap.org/AACAP/Families_and_Youth/Facts_for_Families/FFF-Guide/Child-Sexual-Abuse-009.aspx

Arroyo, K., Lundahl, B., Butters, R., Vanderloo, M., & Wood, D. S. (2017). Short-term interventions for survivors of intimate partner violence: A systematic review and meta-analysis. *Trauma, Violence, & Abuse, 18*(2), 155–171.

Basile, K. C., Hertz, M. F., & Back, S. E. (2007). *Intimate Partner violence and sexual violence victimization assessment instruments for use in healthcare settings: Version 1*. Atlanta, GA: Centers for Disease Control and Prevention, National Center for Injury Prevention and Control.

Buppert, C., & Klein, T. A. (2008). Dilemmas in mandatory reporting for nurses. *Topics in Advanced Practice Nursing eJournal CME*. Retrieved June 18, 2019 from https://www.medscape.org/viewarticle/585562_1

Bureau of Justice Statistics. (2018). *Rape and sexual assault*. Retrieved June 18, 2018 from https://www.bjs.gov/index.cfm?ty=tp&tid=317

Burgess, S., & Tavakoli, A. (2005). Psychometric assessment of the Burgess-Partner Abuse Scale for Teens (B-PAST). *Aquichan, 5*(1), 96–107.

Campbell, J., & Humphreys, J. (Eds.). (1993). *Nursing care of survivors of family violence*. St. Louis: Mosby.

Campbell, J. C., Webster, D. W., & Glass, N. (2009). The danger assessment: Validation of a lethality risk assessment instrument for intimate partner femicide. *Journal of Interpersonal Violence, 24*(4), 653–674.

Centers for Disease Control and Prevention (CDC). (2016). *Understanding elder abuse. Fact sheet 2016*. Washington, DC: National Center for Injury Prevention and Control, Division of Prevention. Retrieved June 18, 2019 from https://www.ced.gov/violenceprevention/pdf/em-factsheet-a.pdf

Centers for Disease Control and Prevention (CDC). (2018a). *Intimate partner violence: Consequences*. Washington, DC: National Center for Injury Prevention and Control, Division of Prevention. Retrieved June 18, 2019 from https://www.cdc.gov/violenceprevention/intimatepartnerviolence/consequences.html

Centers for Disease Control and Prevention (CDC). (2018b). *Teen dating violence*. Washington, DC: National Center for Injury Prevention and Control, Division of Prevention. Retrieved June 18, 2019 from https://www.cdc.gov/violenceprevention/intimatepartnerviolence/teendatingviolence/fastfact.html

Centers for Disease Control and Prevention (CDC). (2018c). *Intimate partner violence: Risk and protective factors*. Washington, DC: National Center for Injury Prevention and Control, Division of Prevention. Retrieved June 18, 2019 from https://www.cdc.gov/violenceprevention/intimatepartnerviolence/riskprotectivefactors.html

Centers for Disease Control and Prevention (CDC). (2018d). *Child abuse and neglect*. Washington, DC: National Center for Injury Prevention and Control, Division of Prevention. Retrieved June 18, 2019 from https://www.cdc.gov/violenceprevention/childabuseandneglect/index.html

Child Welfare Information Gateway. (2016). *Child witnesses to domestic violence*. Washington, DC: U.S. Department of Health and Human Services, Children's Bureau.

Cole, J., & Logan, T. K. (2008). Negotiating the challenges of multidisciplinary responses to sexual assault victims: Sexual assault and victim advocacy programs. *Research in Nursing and Health, 31*(1), 76–85.

Cole, J., Logan, T. K., & Shannon, L. (2008). Women's risk for revictimization by a new abusive partner: For what should we be looking? *Violence & Victims, 23*(3), 315–330.

Copp, J. C., Giordano, P. C., Longmore, M. A., & Manning, W. D. (2016). The development of attitudes towards intimate partner violence: An examination of key correlates among a sample of young adults. *Journal of Interpersonal Violence*. Retrieved June 18, 2019 from https://doi.org/10.1177/0886260516651311

Domestic Violence Resource Center. (2018). *Safety planning*. Retrieved from https://www.dvrc-or.org/safety-planning

Enander, V. (2010). "A fool to keep staying": Battered women labeling themselves stupid as an expression of gendered shame. *Violence against Women, 16*(1), 5–31.

Fering, C., Simon, V. A., & Cleland, C. M. (2009). Childhood sexual abuse, stigmatization, internalizing symptoms, and the development of sexual difficulties and dating aggression. *Journal of Consulting and Clinical Psychology, 77*(1), 127–137.

Messing, J. T., Campbell, J. C., & Snider, C. (2017). Validation and adaptation of the Danger Assessment-5: A brief intimate partner violence risk assessment. *Journal of Advanced Nursing, 73*(12), 3220–3230.

Namy, S., Carlson, C., O'Hara, K., Nakuti, J., Bukuluki, P., Lwanyaaga, J., et al. (2017). Towards a feminist understanding of intersecting violence against women and children in the family. *Social Science & Medicine (1982), 184*, 40–48.

National Center for Parent, Family and Community Engagement. (2015). *Compendium of parenting interventions*. Washington, DC: National Center on Parent, Family, and Community Engagement, Office of Head Start, U.S. Department of Health & Human Services.

National Center for Victims of Crime. (2017). *2017 NCVRW Resource Guide: Intimate Partner Violence Fact Sheet*. Retrieved July 7, 2019 from https://ovc.ncjrs.gov/ncvrw2017/images/en artwork/Fact_Sheets/2017NCVRW_IPV_508.pdf

National Center on Elder Abuse. (n.d.). *Research*. Retrieved July 7, 2019 from https://ncea.acl.gov/whatwedo/research/statistics.html#defined

National Child Traumatic Stress Network. (n.d.). *Domestic violence: Interventions*. Retrieved July 7, 2019 from https://www.nctsn.org/what-is-child-trauma/trauma-types/domestic-violence/interventions

National Coalition Against Domestic Violence. (n.d.). *Why do victims stay?* Retrieved from https://ncadv.org/why-do-victims-stay

National Coalition Against Domestic Violence. (2018). *Marital rape*. Retrieved July 7, 2019 from https://ncadv.org/blog/posts/quick-guide-domestic-violence-and-sexual-abuse

Ogunsiji, O., & Clisdell, E. (2017). Intimate partner violence prevention and reduction: A review of literature. *Health Care for Women International*, *38*(5), 439–462.

Pigeon, W., May, P., Perlis, M., Ward, E., Lu, N., & Talbot, N. (2009). The effect of interpersonal psychotherapy for depression on insomnia symptoms in a cohort of women with sexual abuse histories. *Journal of Traumatic Stress*, *22*(6), 634–648.

Pomerance, B. (2015). Finding the middle ground on a slippery slope: Balancing autonomy and protection in mandatory reporting of elder abuse. *Marquette Benefits and Social Welfare Law Review*, *16*(2), 436–490.

Power, C. (2017). Domestic violence: What can nurses do? *Alabama Nurse*, *44*(4), 18–20.

Ramamoorthy, S., & Myers-Walls, J. A. (2013). Talking to a child who has been abused. Retrieved from https://www.extension.purdue.edu/provider-parent/Parent-Provider%20Relationships/Talking_Child_Been_Abused.htm

Ramsey, C. B. (2011). Domestic violence and state intervention in the American West and Australia, 1860–1930. *Indiana Law Journal*, *86*(185), 186–255.

Smith, S. G., Zhang, X., Basile, K. C., Merrick, M. T., Wang, J., Kresnow, M., et al. (2018). *National Intimate Partner and Sexual Violence Survey: 2015 Data Brief*. Retrieved July 7, 2019 from https://www.cdc.gov/violenceprevention/nisvs/2015NISVSdatabrief.html

Ullman, S. E., & Sigurvinsdottir, R. (2015). Intimate partner violence and drinking among victims of adult sexual assault. *Journal of Aggression, Maltreatment & Trauma*, *24*(2), 117–130.

U.S. Preventive Services Task Force. (2016). *Final Update Summary: Intimate partner violence and abuse of elderly and vulnerable adults: Screening*. Retrieved July 7, 2019 from https://www.uspreventiveservicestaskforce.org/Page/Document/UpdateSummaryFinal/intimate-partner-violence-and-abuse-of-elderly-and-vulnerable-adults-screening

Violence Policy Center. (2018). When men murder women: An analysis of 2016 homicide data. Retrieved from http://vpc.org/studies/wmmw2018.pdf

Wood, L. (2015). Hoping, empowering, strengthening: Theories used in intimate partner violence advocacy. *Journal of Women and Social Work*, *30*(3), 286–301.

Yaffe, M. (2010). Detection and reporting of elder abuse. *Family Medicine*, *42*(2), 481–486.

UNIT V

CARE AND RECOVERY FOR PERSONS WITH PSYCHIATRIC DISORDERS

18

Anxiety Disorders

Nursing Care of Patients With Anxiety, Phobia, and Panic

Mary Ann Boyd and Judith M. Erickson

KEY CONCEPTS
- anxiety
- panic
- phobia

LEARNING OBJECTIVES

After studying this chapter, you will be able to:

1. Differentiate normal anxiety responses from those suggestive of an anxiety disorder.
2. Identify indicators for the four levels of anxiety and nursing interventions appropriate for each level.
3. Describe the prevalence and incidence of anxiety disorders.
4. Analyze theories of anxiety disorders.
5. Apply nursing process with recovery-oriented interventions for persons with anxiety and anxiety disorders.
6. Develop wellness strategies for the person with anxiety and anxiety disorders.
7. Discuss the importance of integrated health care for persons with anxiety and anxiety disorders.

KEY TERMS

- agoraphobia • depersonalization • exposure therapy • flooding • implosive therapy • interoceptive conditioning • panic attacks • panic control treatment • positive self-talk • reframing • social anxiety disorder • specific phobia disorder • systematic desensitization

Case Study: Doug

Doug is a 50-year-old man who lives with his wife Norma and two sons; Greg, a sophomore in college and Leon, a high school student. Norma was recently laid off from her job and has been unable to find employment. The family is now experiencing financial and marital problems. Leon was recently expelled from school for drug and alcohol use. Doug had an argument with his boss and is afraid that he will lose his job. He appears at the emergency department for chest pain and is convinced he is having a heart attack. All lab test results are normal. Consider how the nurse can help Doug deal with his health issues.

Anxiety is part of many emotional problems and mental disorders. At one time, most mental conditions with anxiety aspects were categorized as "anxiety disorders," but today anxiety disorders have been redefined. Trauma–stressor-related disorder and obsessive–compulsive disorder (OCD), both previously identified as anxiety disorders, are now categorized as separate disorders (American Psychiatric Association [APA], 2013). Trauma- and stressor-related disorders, as well as dissociative disorders, are discussed in Chapter 19. OCDs are discussed in Chapter 20. In this chapter, panic disorder is also highlighted.

NORMAL VERSUS ABNORMAL ANXIETY RESPONSE

Anxiety is an unavoidable human condition that takes many forms and serves different purposes. Anxiety can be positive and can motivate one to act, or it can produce paralyzing fear, causing inaction. "Normal anxiety" is described as being of realistic intensity and duration for the situation and is followed by relief behaviors intended to reduce or prevent more anxiety (Peplau, 1989). A "normal anxiety response" is appropriate to the situation and can be used to help the individual identify which underlying problem has caused the anxiety.

> **KEYCONCEPT** **Anxiety** is an uncomfortable feeling of apprehension or dread that occurs in response to internal or external stimuli; it can result in physical, emotional, cognitive, and behavioral symptoms.

During a perceived threat, rising anxiety levels cause physical and emotional changes in all individuals. A normal emotional response to anxiety consists of three parts: physiologic arousal, cognitive processes, and coping strategies. Physiologic arousal, or the fight-or-flight response, is the signal that an individual is facing a threat. Cognitive processes decipher the situation and decide whether the perceived threat should be approached or avoided. Coping strategies are used to resolve the threat. Box 18.1 summarizes many physical, affective, cognitive, and behavioral symptoms associated with anxiety. The factors that determine whether anxiety is a symptom of a mental disorder include the intensity of anxiety relative to the situation, the trigger for the anxiety, and the particular symptom clusters that manifest the anxiety. Table 18.1 describes the four degrees of anxiety and associated perceptual changes and patterns of behavior. Anxiety is a component of all the disorders discussed in this chapter.

TABLE 18.1 DEGREES OF ANXIETY

Degree of Anxiety	Effects on Perceptual Field and on Ability to Focus Attention	Observable Behavior
Mild	Perceptual field widens slightly. Able to observe more than before and to see relationships (make connection among data). Learning is possible.	Is aware, alert, sees, hears, and grasps more than before. Usually able to recognize and identify anxiety easily.
Moderate	Perceptual field narrows slightly. Selective inattention: does not notice what goes on peripheral to the immediate focus but can do so if attention is directed there by another observer.	Sees, hears, and grasps less than previously. Can attend to more if directed to do so. Able to sustain attention on a particular focus; selectively inattentive to contents outside the focal area. Usually able to state, "I am anxious now."
Severe	Perceptual field is greatly reduced. Tendency toward dissociation: to not notice what is going on outside the current reduced focus of attention; largely unable to do so when another observer suggests it.	Sees, hears, and grasps far less than previously. Attention is focused on a small area of a given event. Inferences drawn may be distorted because of inadequacy of observed data. May be unaware of and unable to name anxiety. Relief behaviors generally used.
Panic (e.g., terror, horror, dread, uncanniness, awe)	Perceptual field is reduced to a detail, which is usually "blown up," i.e., elaborated by distortion (exaggeration), or the focus is on scattered details; the speed of the scattering tends to increase. Massive dissociation, especially of contents of self-system. Felt as enormous threat to survival. Learning is impossible.	Says, "I'm in a million pieces," "I'm gone," or "What is happening to me?" Perplexity, self-absorption. Feelings of unreality. Flights of ideas or confusion. Fear. Repeats a detail. Many relief behaviors used automatically (without thought). The enormous energy produced by panic must be used and may be mobilized as rage. May pace, run, or fight violently. With dissociation of contents of self-system, there may be a very rapid reorganization of the self, usually going along pathologic lines (e.g., a "psychotic break" is usually preceded by panic).

Adapted with permission from Peplau, H. (1989). Theoretic constructs: Anxiety, self, and hallucinations. In A. O'Toole & S. Welt (Eds.). *Interpersonal theory in nursing practice: Selected works of Hildegarde E. Peplau.* New York: Springer.

BOX 18.1
Symptoms of Anxiety

PHYSICAL SYMPTOMS

Cardiovascular
Sympathetic
Palpitations
Heart racing
Increased blood pressure

Parasympathetic
Actual fainting
Decreased blood pressure
Decreased pulse rate

Respiratory
Rapid breathing
Difficulty getting air
Shortness of breath
Pressure of chest
Shallow breathing
Lump in throat
Choking sensations
Gasping
Spasm of bronchi

Neuromuscular
Increased reflexes
Startle reaction
Eyelid twitching
Insomnia
Tremors
Rigidity
Spasm
Fidgeting
Pacing
Strained face
Unsteadiness
Generalized weakness
Wobbly legs
Clumsy motions

Skin
Flushed face
Pale face
Localized sweating (palm region)
Generalized sweating
Hot and cold spells
Itching

Gastrointestinal
Loss of appetite
Revulsion about food
Abdominal discomfort
Diarrhea
Abdominal pain
Nausea
Heartburn
Vomiting

Eyes
Dilated pupils

Urinary Tract Parasympathetic
Pressure to urinate
Increased frequency of urination

AFFECTIVE SYMPTOMS
Edgy
Impatient
Uneasy
Nervous
Tense
Wound-up
Anxious
Fearful
Apprehensive
Scared
Frightened
Alarmed
Terrified
Jittery
Jumpy

COGNITIVE SYMPTOMS

Sensory-Perceptual
Mind is hazy, cloudy, foggy, dazed
Objects seem blurred or distant
Environment seems different or unreal
Feelings of unreality
Self-consciousness
Hypervigilance

Thinking Difficulties
Cannot recall important things
Confused
Unable to control thinking
Difficulty concentrating
Difficulty focusing attention
Distractibility
Blocking
Difficulty reasoning
Loss of objectivity and perspective
Tunnel vision

Conceptual
Cognitive distortion
Fear of losing control
Fear of not being able to cope
Fear of physical injury or death
Fear of mental disorder
Fear of negative evaluations
Frightening visual images
Repetitive fearful ideation

BEHAVIORAL SYMPTOMS
Inhibited
Tonic immobility
Flight
Avoidance
Speech dysfluency
Impaired coordination
Restlessness
Postural collapse
Hyperventilation

Adapted from Beck, A. T., & Emery, C. (1985). *Anxiety disorders and phobias: A cognitive perspective* (pp. 23–27). New York: Basic Books.

PHOBIAS

KEY CONCEPT **Phobia** is an irrational fear of an object, person, or situation that leads to a compelling avoidance.

The development of a phobia may be the outcome of extreme anxiety. Phobias are often present in anxiety disorders but may also develop into a **specific phobia disorder** (discussed later).

Defense Mechanisms and Anxiety

Defense mechanisms are used to reduce anxiety by preventing or diminishing unwanted thoughts and feelings. See Chapter 8 for definitions. Defense mechanisms can be helpful in coping with everyday problems, but they become problematic when overused. The first step is identifying a person's use of defense mechanisms. The next step is determining whether the reasons the defense mechanisms are being used support healthy coping or are detrimental to a person's health. What may be healthy for one person may be unhealthy for another. See Box 18.2.

OVERVIEW OF ANXIETY DISORDERS

The primary symptoms of anxiety disorders are fear and anxiety. Even though symptoms of anxiety disorders can be found in healthy individuals, an anxiety disorder is diagnosed when the fear or anxiety is excessive or out of proportion to the situation. An individual's ability to work and interpersonal relationships may be impaired. Anxiety disorders are differentiated by the situation or objects that provoke fear, anxiety, or avoidance behavior and related cognitive thoughts (APA, 2013).

Anxiety disorders are the most common of the psychiatric illnesses treated by health care providers. Approximately 40 million American adults (older than 18 years) or about 18.1% of this age group within a given

---

BOX 18.2

Consequences of Decreasing Anxiety by Using Defense Mechanisms

DEFENSE MECHANISM	POSITIVE CONSEQUENCES	NEGATIVE CONSEQUENCES
Altruism	Satisfies internal needs through helping others.	Prevents examination of underlying fears or concerns.
Denial	Avoids feelings associated with recognizing a problem.	Avoidance of major problem that should be addressed.
Displacement	By taking out frustrations on an unsuspecting or vulnerable person, animal, or object, anxiety is reduced and the individual is protected from anticipated retaliation from the source of the frustration.	Does not deal with problem and inappropriately expresses feelings toward a more vulnerable person or object.
Intellectualization	Able to analyze events in a distant, objective, analytical way.	Inability to acknowledge feelings that may be interfering with relationships.
Projection	By assigning unwanted thoughts, feelings, or behaviors to another person or object, the individual does not have to acknowledge undesirable or unacceptable thoughts or feelings.	Does not acknowledge undesirable or unwanted feelings or thoughts and can act on inaccurate interpretation of the other person's thoughts and behaviors.
Rationalization	Avoids anxiety by explaining an unacceptable or disappointing behavior or feeling in a logical, rationale way. May protect self-esteem and self-concept.	Avoids the reality of a situation which may be detrimental to the individual.
Reaction Formation	Reduces anxiety by taking the opposite feeling. Hides true feelings, which may be appropriate in many situations.	Unable to acknowledge personal feelings about others, which leads to negative consequences.
Regression	When stressed, abandons effective coping strategies and reverts to behaviors used earlier in development. These strategies are comfortable and may be effective.	May reengage in detrimental behaviors such as smoking, drinking, or inappropriate interpersonal responses leading to ineffective coping.
Repression	Avoids unwanted thoughts and anxiety by blocking thoughts, experiences from conscious awareness.	Cannot recall traumatic events that should be addressed to be healthy (i.e., rape).
Sublimation	Avoids anxiety and channels maladaptive feelings or impulses into socially acceptable behaviors. Maintains socially acceptable behavior.	By not recognizing maladaptive feelings, the individual cannot address underlying feelings.
Suppression	Reduces anxiety by intentionally avoiding thinking about disturbing problems, wishes, feelings, or experiences. Useful in many situations such as test-taking situations.	Avoiding problem situation prevents finding a solution to the problem.

year have an anxiety disorder. Direct and indirect costs of treating anxiety disorders amount to tens of billions of dollars. Women experience anxiety disorders more often than men by a 2:1 ratio. Anxiety disorders may also be associated with other mental or physical comorbidities such as heart disease, respiratory disease, and mood disorders (Stein et al., 2018; Tully & Tzourio, 2017). The relationship between depression and anxiety disorders is particularly strong. A single patient may concurrently have more than one anxiety disorder or other psychiatric disorders as well.

Anxiety disorders tend to be chronic and persistent, with full recovery more likely among those who do not have other mental or physical disorders (Ayazi, Lien, Eide, Swartz, & Hauff, 2014). Three quarters of those with an anxiety disorder have their first episode by age 21.5 years.

Anxiety Disorders Across the Life Span

Prompt identification, diagnosis, and treatment of individuals with anxiety disorders may be difficult for special populations such as children and older adult patients. Often, the symptoms suggestive of anxiety disorders may go unnoticed by caregivers or are misdiagnosed because they mimic cardiac or pulmonary pathology rather than a psychological disturbance. Children and adolescents are discussed in Chapter 30; older adults are discussed in Chapter 31.

Children and Adolescents

Anxiety disorders are among the most common conditions of children and adolescents. If left untreated, symptoms persist and gradually worsen and sometimes lead to suicidal ideation and suicide attempts, early parenthood, drug and alcohol dependence, and educational underachievement later in life (Carballo et al., 2019).

Separation anxiety disorder (i.e., excessive fear or anxiety concerning separation from home or attachment figures) usually first occurs in childhood. Affected children experience extreme distress when separated from home or attachment figures, worry about them when separated from them, and worry about untoward events (i.e., getting lost) and what will happen to them. This disorder is discussed in Chapter 30.

A rare disorder typically seen in childhood is selective mutism in which children do not initiate speech or respond when spoken to by others (APA, 2013). Children with this disorder are often very anxious when asked to speak in school or read aloud. They may suffer academic impairment because of their inability to communicate with others.

Older Adults

Generally speaking, the prevalence of anxiety disorders declines with age. However, in the older adult population, rates of anxiety disorders are as high as mood disorders, which commonly co-occur. This combination of depressive and anxiety symptoms has been shown to decrease social functioning, increase somatic (physical) symptoms, and increase depressive symptoms (Grenier et al., 2018). In one study, nearly half of primary care patients with chronic pain had at least one attendant anxiety disorder. Detecting and treating anxiety is an important component of pain management (Kroenke et al., 2019). Because the older adult population is at risk for suicide, special assessment of anxiety symptoms is essential.

PANIC DISORDER

Panic is an extreme, overwhelming form of anxiety often experienced when an individual is placed in a real or perceived life-threatening situation. Panic is normal during periods of threat but is abnormal when it is continuously experienced in situations that pose no real physical or psychological threat. Some people experience heightened anxiety because they fear experiencing another panic attack. This type of panic interferes with the individual's ability to function in everyday life and is characteristic of panic disorder.

> **KEYCONCEPT** **Panic** is a normal but extremely overwhelming form of anxiety often experienced when an individual is placed in a real or perceived life-threatening situation.

Clinical Course

The onset of panic disorder is typically between 20 and 24 years of age. The disorder usually surfaces in childhood but may not be diagnosed until later. Panic disorder is treatable, but studies have shown that even after years of treatment, many people remain symptomatic. In some cases, symptoms may even worsen (APA, 2013).

Panic Attacks

Panic attacks are a major finding in panic disorder. A panic attack is a sudden, discrete period of intense fear or discomfort that reaches its peak within a few minutes and is accompanied by significant physical discomfort and cognitive distress (APA, 2013). Panic attacks usually peak in about 10 minutes but can last as long as 30 minutes before returning to normal functioning. The physical symptoms include palpitations, chest discomfort, rapid pulse, nausea, dizziness, sweating, paresthesias (burning, tickling, pricking of skin with no apparent reason), trembling or shaking, and a feeling of suffocation or shortness of breath. Cognitive symptoms include disorganized thinking, irrational fears, **depersonalization** (being detached from oneself), and a decreased ability to communicate. Usually, feelings of impending doom or death, fear of going crazy or losing control, and desperation ensue.

The physical symptoms can mimic those of a heart attack. Individuals often seek emergency medical care because they feel as if they are dying, but most have negative cardiac workup results. People experiencing panic attacks may also believe that the attacks stem from an underlying major medical illness (APA, 2013). Even with medical testing and assurance of no underlying disease, they often remain unconvinced.

Remember Doug? He had chest pains and believed he was having a heart attack. How can you help Doug recognize that even though he is not having a heart attack, his symptoms are serious and that his panic attack could indicate an underlying anxiety disorder? Why would you not tell him that everything is normal?

KEYCONCEPT Physical symptoms of panic attack are similar to cardiac emergencies. These symptoms are physically taxing and psychologically frightening to patients. Recognition of the seriousness of panic attacks should be communicated to the patient.

In a panic disorder, recurrent unexpected panic attacks are followed by persistent concern about experiencing subsequent panic attacks. Because of fear of future attacks, these affected individuals modify normal behaviors to avoid future attacks (APA, 2013). Panic attacks are either expected with an obvious cue or trigger or unexpected with no such obvious cue. The first panic attack is usually associated with an identifiable cue (e.g., anxiety-provoking medical conditions, such as asthma, or in initial trials of illicit substance use), but subsequent attacks are often unexpected without any obvious cue (Box 18.3). Panic attacks not only occur in panic disorder but can also occur in other mental disorders such as depression, bipolar disease, eating disorders, and some medical conditions such as cardiac or respiratory disorders (APA, 2013).

Diagnostic Criteria

Panic disorder is a chronic condition that has several exacerbations and remissions during the course of the disease. The disabling panic attacks often lead to other symptoms, such as phobias.

Other diagnostic symptoms include palpitations, sweating, shaking, shortness of breath or smothering, sensations of choking, chest pain, nausea or abdominal distress, dizziness, derealization or depersonalization, fear of going crazy, fear of dying, paresthesias, and chills or hot flashes (APA, 2013) (see Key Diagnostic Characteristics 18.1).

BOX 18.3 CLINICAL VIGNETTE

Panic Disorder

Susan, a 22-year-old female, has experienced several life changes, including a recent engagement, loss of her father to cancer and heart disease, graduation from college, and entrance to the workforce as a computer programmer in a large inner-city company. Because of her active lifestyle, her sleep habits have been poor. She frequently uses sleeping aids at night and now drinks a full pot of coffee to start each day. She continues to smoke to "relieve the stress." While sitting in heavy traffic on the way to work, she suddenly experienced chest tightness, sweating, shortness of breath, feelings of being "trapped," and foreboding that she was going to die. Fearing a heart attack, she went to an emergency department, where her discomfort subsided within half an hour. After several hours of testing, the doctor informed her that her heart was healthy. During the next few weeks, she experienced several episodes of feeling trapped and slight chest discomfort on her drive to work. She fears future "attacks" while sitting in traffic and while in her crowded office cubicle.

What Do You Think?
- What risk factors does Susan have that might contribute to the development of panic attacks?
- What lifestyle changes do you think would help Susan reduce stress?

Epidemiology and Risk Factors

Panic disorder has a moderately high lifetime prevalence in the general population with 1% to 2% 1-year prevalence rate and 4.8% lifetime rate (Olaya, Moneta, Miret, Ayuso-Mateos, & Haro, 2018). Increased risk is associated with being female; middle aged; of low socioeconomic status; and widowed, separated, or divorced. The estimates of isolated panic attacks may affect 22.7% of the population. Panic disorders occur in several cultures, but the panic symptoms may be experienced differently across racial/ethnic group (Assari, 2017).

Family history, substance and stimulant use or abuse, smoking tobacco, and severe stressors are risk factors for panic disorder. People who have several anxiety symptoms and those who experience separation anxiety during childhood often develop panic disorder later in life. Early life traumas, a history of physical or sexual abuse, socioeconomic or personal disadvantages, and behavioral inhibition by adults have also been associated with an increased risk for anxiety disorders in children (Bourdon et al., 2019).

Comorbidity

Patients may experience more than one anxiety disorder, depression, eating disorder, substance use or abuse, or schizophrenia (Mcuret, Kroll, Ritz, 2017).

> **KEY DIAGNOSTIC CHARACTERISTICS 18.1 • PANIC DISORDER**
>
> **Diagnostic Criteria**
> A. Recurrent unexpected panic attacks. A panic attack is an abrupt surge of intense fear or intense discomfort that reaches a peak within minutes, and during which time four (or more) of the following symptoms occur:
>   **Note:** The abrupt surge can occur from a calm state or an anxious state
>   1. Palpitations, pounding heart, or accelerated heart rate
>   2. Sweating
>   3. Trembling or shaking
>   4. Sensations of shortness of breath or smothering
>   5. Feelings of choking
>   6. Chest pain or discomfort
>   7. Nausea or abdominal distress
>   8. Feeling dizzy, unsteady, light-headed, or faint
>   9. Chills or heat sensations
>   10. Paresthesias (numbness or tingling sensations)
>   11. Derealization (feelings of unreality) or depersonalization (being detached from oneself)
>   12. Fear of losing control or "going crazy"
>   13. Fear of dying
>   **Note:** Culture-specific symptoms (e.g., tinnitus, neck soreness, headache, uncontrollable screaming or crying) may be seen. Such symptoms should not count as one of the four required symptoms
> B. At least one of the attacks has been followed by 1 month (or more) of one or both of the following:
>   1. Persistent concern or worry about additional panic attacks or their consequences (e.g., losing control, having a heart attack, "going crazy")
>   2. A significant maladaptive change in behavior related to the attacks (e.g., behaviors designed to avoid having panic attacks, such as avoidance of exercise or unfamiliar situations)
> C. The disturbance is not attributable to the physiologic effects of a substance (e.g., a drug of abuse, a medication) or another medical condition (e.g., hyperthyroidism, cardiopulmonary disorders)
> D. The disturbance is not better explained by another mental disorder (e.g., the panic attacks do not occur only in response to feared social situations, as in social anxiety disorder; in response to circumscribed phobic objects or situations, as in specific phobia; in response to obsessions, as in obsessive–compulsive disorder; in response to reminders of traumatic events, as in posttraumatic stress disorder; or in response to separation from attachment figures, as in separation anxiety disorder)
>
> **Target Symptoms**
> Discrete period of intense fear or discomfort with four (or more) of the following symptoms that develop abruptly and reach a peak within 10 minutes:
> - Palpitations, pounding heart, or accelerated heart rate
> - Sweating
> - Trembling or shaking
> - Sensations of shortness of breath or smothering
> - Feelings of choking
> - Chest pain or discomfort
> - Nausea or vomiting
> - Feeling dizzy, unsteady, light-headed, or faint
> - Derealization (feeling of unreality) or depersonalization (being detached from oneself)
> - Fear of losing control or going crazy
> - Fear of dying
> - Paresthesias (numbness or tingling sensations)
> - Chills or hot flushes
> - Great apprehension about the outcome of routine activities and experiences
> - Loss or disruption of important interpersonal relationships
> - Demoralization
> - Possible major depressive episode
>
> **Associated Findings**
> - Nocturnal panic attack (waking from sleep in a state of panic)
> - Constant or intermittent feelings of anxiety related to physical and mental health
> - Pervasive concerns about abilities to complete daily tasks or withstand daily stressors
> - Excessive use of drugs or other means to control panic attacks
>
> **Associated Physical Examination Findings**
> - Transient tachycardia
> - Moderate elevation of systolic blood pressure
>
> **Associated Laboratory Findings**
> - Compensated respiratory alkalosis (decreased carbon dioxide, decreased bicarbonate levels, almost normal pH)
>
> **Other Targets for Treatment**
> - Loss or disruption of important interpersonal or occupational activities
> - Demoralization
> - Possible major depressive episode
>
> Reprinted with permission from the *Diagnostic and statistical manual of mental disorders* (5th ed.). (Copyright © 2013). American Psychiatric Association. All Rights Reserved.

Although people with panic disorder are thought to have more somatic complaints than the general population, panic disorder does correlate with some medical conditions, including vertigo, cardiac disease, gastrointestinal disorders, asthma, and those related to cigarette smoking.

Etiology

Biologic Theories

There appears to be a substantial familial predisposition to panic disorder with an estimated heritability of 48% (Konishi et al., 2014). Studies show brain abnormalities in the "fear network" (amygdala, hippocampus, thalamus, midbrain, pons, medulla, and cerebellum) and changes in volume in different brain areas (Asok, Kandel, Rayman, 2019).

Serotonin and Norepinephrine

Serotonin and norepinephrine are both implicated in panic disorders. Norepinephrine effects act on those systems most affected by a panic attack—the cardiovascular, respiratory, and gastrointestinal systems. Serotonergic neurons are distributed in central autonomic and emotional motor control systems regulating anxiety states and anxiety-related physiologic and behavioral responses (Hornboll et al., 2018).

Gamma-Aminobutyric Acid

Gamma-aminobutyric acid (GABA) is the most abundant inhibitory neurotransmitter in the brain. GABA receptor stimulation causes several effects, including neurocognitive effects, reduction of anxiety, and sedation. GABA stimulation also results in increased seizure threshold. Abnormalities in the benzodiazepine–GABA–chloride ion channel complex have been implicated in panic disorder (Asok et al., 2019).

Hypothalamic–Pituitary–Adrenal Axis

Research implicates a role of the hypothalamic–pituitary–adrenal (HPA) axis in panic disorders (Quagliato & Nardi, 2018). A current explanation is that as stress hormones are activated, anxiety increases, which can lead to a panic attack. See Chapter 13.

Psychosocial Theories

Psychoanalytic and Psychodynamic Theories

Psychodynamic theories examine anxiety that develops after separation and loss. Many patients link their initial panic attack with recent personal losses. However, at this point the empirical evidence remains inadequate for a psychodynamic explanation. It remains unclear why some patients develop panic disorder whereas others with similar experiences develop other disorders (Pilecki, Arentoft, & McKay, 2011).

Cognitive Behavioral Theories

Learning theory underlies most cognitive behavioral explanations of panic disorder. Classic conditioning theory suggests that one learns a fear response by linking an adverse or fear-provoking event, such as a car accident, with a previously neutral event, such as crossing a bridge. One becomes conditioned to associate fear with crossing a bridge. Applying this theory to people with panic disorder has limitations. Phobic avoidance is not always developed secondary to an adverse event.

Further development of this theory led to an understanding of **interoceptive conditioning**, an association between physical discomfort, such as dizziness or palpitations, and an impending panic attack. For example, during a car accident, the individual may experience rapid heartbeat, dizziness, shortness of breath, and panic. Subsequent experiences of dizziness or palpitations, unrelated to an anxiety-provoking situation, incite anxiety and panic. Furthermore, people with panic disorder may misinterpret mild physical sensations (e.g., sweating, dizziness) as being catastrophic, causing panic as a result of learned fear (catastrophic interpretation). Some researchers hypothesize that individuals with a low sense of control over their environment or with a particular sensitivity to anxiety are vulnerable to misinterpreting normal stress. Controlled exposure to anxiety-provoking situations and cognitive countering techniques has proven successful in reducing the symptoms of panic.

Family Response to Disorder

Persons with a panic disorder may inadvertently cause excessive fears, phobias, or excessive worry in other family members. Families may limit social functions to prevent a panic attack. Those affected need a tremendous amount of support and encouragement from significant others.

Recovery-Oriented Care for Persons With Panic Disorder

Teamwork and Collaboration: Working Toward Recovery

Nurses are pivotal in providing a safe and therapeutic inpatient environment and teaching patients strategies for managing anxiety and fears. The nurse also administers prescribed medication, monitors its effects, and provides medication education. Advanced practice nurses, licensed clinical social workers, or licensed counselors provide individual psychotherapy sessions as needed. Often, a clinical psychologist gives psychological tests and interprets the results to assist in diagnosing and treating the panic disorder.

Panic Control Treatment

Panic control treatment involves intentional exposure (through exercise) to panic-invoking sensations such as dizziness, hyperventilation, tightness in the chest, and sweating. Identified patterns become targets for treatment. Patients are taught to use breathing training and cognitive restructuring to manage their responses and are instructed to practice these techniques between therapy sessions to adapt the skills to other situations.

Systematic Desensitization

Systematic desensitization, another exposure method used to desensitize patients, exposes the patient to a hierarchy of feared situations that the patient has rated from least to most feared. The patient is taught to use muscle relaxation as levels of anxiety increase through multisituational exposure. Planning and implementing **exposure therapy** require special training. Because of the multitude of outpatients in the treatment for panic disorder and **agoraphobia** (discussed later in the chapter), exposure therapy is a useful tool for home health psychiatric nurses. Outcomes of home-based exposure treatment are similar to clinic-based treatment outcomes.

Implosive Therapy

Implosive therapy is a provocative technique useful in treating panic disorder and agoraphobia in which the therapist identifies phobic stimuli for the patient and then presents highly anxiety-provoking imagery to the patient, describing the feared scene as dramatically and vividly as possible. **Flooding** is a technique used to desensitize the patient to the fear associated with a particular anxiety-provoking stimulus. Desensitizing is done by presenting feared objects or situations repeatedly without session breaks until the anxiety dissipates. For example, a patient with ophidiophobia (i.e., a morbid fear of snakes) might be presented with a real snake repeatedly until the patient's anxiety decreases.

Exposure Therapy

Many of the treatment approaches used for panic disorder are effective for phobias (discussed in later chapters). Exposure therapy is the treatment of choice for phobias. The patient is repeatedly exposed to real or simulated anxiety-provoking situations until he or she becomes desensitized and anxiety subsides.

Cognitive Behavioral Therapy

Cognitive behavioral therapy (CBT) is a highly effective tool for treating individuals with panic disorder. It has been considered the first-line treatment for those with panic and other anxiety disorders and is often used in conjunction with medications, including the selective serotonin reuptake inhibitors (SSRIs), in treating those with panic disorder (Bandelow et al., 2015). The goals of CBT include helping the patient to manage his or her anxiety and correcting anxiety-provoking thoughts through interventions, including cognitive restructuring, breathing training, and psychoeducation.

Integration With Primary Care

Coordination of care between mental health and primary leads to safer and management of anxiety disorders care services. Primary care providers are often asked to treat the physical consequences of anxiety such as hypertension and obesity (DeJesus et al., 2016). Anxiety can be caused by physical health issues such as immune, metabolic, and cardiovascular problems. Many prescription and nonprescription drugs can cause anxiety such as asthma, blood pressure, steroid, and thyroid medications. Without coordination of care, the clinicians will not be able to make a meaningful assessment which could lead to the wrong treatment.

Evidence-Based Nursing Care of Persons With Panic Disorder

Individuals often first seek help in the emergency department for their physical symptoms, but they are told that there are no life-threatening cardiac or neurologic causes for the severe physical symptoms. Although no laboratory tests exist to confirm anxiety disorders, a careful clinical assessment will reveal the presence of an anxiety disorder.

Mental Health Nursing Assessment

A comprehensive nursing assessment includes overall physical and mental status, suicidal tendencies and thoughts, cognitive thought patterns, avoidance behavior patterns, and family and cultural factors. Patients can be encouraged to keep a daily log of the severity of anxiety and the frequency, duration, and severity of panic episodes. This log will be a basic tool for monitoring progress as symptoms decrease.

Panic Attack Assessment

The assessment of the person with a panic disorder focuses on identifying the characteristics of the panic attack and the individual's strengths and problems. If the panic attack occurs in the presence of the nurse, direct assessment of the symptoms should be made and documented. Questions to ask the patient might include the following:

- What were you doing when the panic attack occurred?
- What did you experience before and during the panic episode, including physical symptoms, feelings, and thoughts?
- When did you begin to feel that way? How long did it last?
- Do you have an explanation for what caused you to feel and think that way?
- Have you experienced these symptoms in the past? If so, under what circumstances?

- Has anyone in your family ever had similar experiences?
- What do you do when you have these experiences to help you to feel safe?
- Have the feelings and sensations ever gone away on their own?

Physical Health Assessment

Key assessment areas of physical health include the use of legal or illegal substances that could have precipitated the panic attack, sleep patterns, activity levels, and health conditions.

Substance Use. Caffeine, pseudoephedrine, amphetamines, cocaine, or other stimulants are associated with panic disorder and may stimulate a panic attack. Tobacco use can also contribute to the risk for panic symptoms. Many individuals with panic disorder use alcohol or central nervous system (CNS) depressants in an effort to self-medicate anxiety symptoms; withdrawal from CNS depressants may produce symptoms of panic.

Sleep Patterns. Sleep is often disturbed in patients with panic disorder. In fact, panic attacks can occur during sleep, so the patient may fear sleep for this reason. Nurses should closely assess the impact of sleep disturbance because fatigue may increase anxiety and susceptibility to panic attacks.

Physical Activity. Panic disorder can be improved through active participation in a routine exercise program. If the patient does not exercise routinely, define the barriers to it. If exercise is avoided because of chronic muscle tension, poor muscle tone, muscle cramps, general fatigue, exhaustion, or shortness of breath, the symptoms may indicate poor physical health.

Medications. Several medications can cause anxiety. Bronchodilators, oral contraceptives, amphetamines (i.e., methylphenidate), steroids, thyroid medication, and several other medications can increase anxiety. Additionally, medicines that contain caffeine such as some pain and anti-inflammatory agents, decongestants (i.e., phenylephrine), and some illegal drugs (cocaine) also increase anxiety.

Other Physical Assessment Areas. Recent changes in physical status should be assessed. For example, pregnant patients should be assessed carefully for an underlying panic disorder. Although pregnancy may actually protect the mother from developing panic symptoms, postpartum onset of panic disorder requires particular attention.

During a time that tremendous effort is spent on family, postpartum onset of panic disorder negatively affects lifestyle and decreases self-esteem in affected women, leading to feelings of overwhelming personal disappointment.

Psychosocial Assessment

A psychosocial assessment includes the patient's report of the symptoms and a careful cognitive, behavioral, and social assessment.

Self-Report Scales. Self-evaluation is difficult in panic disorder. Often the memories of the attack and its triggers are irretrievable. Several tools are available to characterize and rate the patient's state of anxiety. Examples of these symptom and behavioral rating scales are provided in Box 18.4. All of these tools are self-report measures and as such are limited by the individual's self-awareness and openness. However, the Hamilton Rating Scale for Anxiety (HAM-A), provided in Table 18.2, is an example of a scale rated by the clinician (Hamilton, 1959). This 14-item scale reflects both psychological and somatic aspects of anxiety.

Mental Status Examination. During a mental status examination, individuals with panic disorder may exhibit anxiety symptoms, including restlessness, irritability, poor concentration, and apprehensive behavior. Disorganized thinking, irrational fears, and a decreased ability to communicate often occur during a panic attack. Assess by direct questioning whether the patient is experiencing suicidal thoughts, especially if he or she is abusing substances or is taking antidepressant medications.

Cognitive Thought Patterns. Catastrophic misinterpretations of trivial physical symptoms can trigger panic symptoms. After they have been identified, these thoughts should serve as a basis for individualizing patient education to counter such false beliefs. Table 18.3 presents a scale to assess catastrophic misinterpretations of the symptoms of panic.

Several studies have found that individuals who feel a sense of control have less severe panic attacks. Individuals who fear loss of control during a panic attack often make the following type of statements:

- "I feel trapped."
- "I'm afraid others will know or that I'll hurt someone."
- "I feel alone. I can't help myself."
- "I'm losing control."

These individuals also tend to show low self-esteem, feelings of helplessness, demoralization, and

> **BOX 18.4**
>
> ## Rating Scales for Assessment of Panic Disorder and Anxiety Disorders
>
> ### PANIC SYMPTOMS
>
> **Panic-Associated Symptom Scale (PASS)**
> Argyle, N., Delito, J., Allerup, P., Maier, W., Albus, M., Nutzinger, D., et al. (1991). The Panic-Associated Symptom Scale: Measuring the severity of panic disorder. *Acta Psychiatrica Scandinavica*, 83, 20–26.
>
> **Acute Panic Inventory**
> Dillon, D. J., Gorman, J. M., Liebowitz, M. R., Fyer, A. J., & Klein, D. F. (1987). Measurement of lactate-induced panic and anxiety. *Psychiatry Research*, 20, 97–105.
>
> **National Institute of Mental Health Panic Questionnaire (NIMH PQ)**
> Scupi, B. S., Maser, J. D., & Uhde, T. W. (1992). The National Institute of Mental Health Panic Questionnaire: An instrument for assessing clinical characteristics of panic disorder. *Journal of Nervous and Mental Disease*, 180, 566–572.
>
> ### COGNITIONS
>
> **Anxiety Sensitivity Index**
> Reiss, S., Peterson, R. A., & Gursky, D. M. (1986). Anxiety sensitivity, anxiety frequency, and the prediction of fearfulness. *Behaviour Research and Therapy*, 24, 1–8.
>
> **Agoraphobia Cognitions Questionnaire**
> Chambless, D. L., Caputo, G. C., Bright, P., & Gallagher, R. (1984). Assessment of fear in agoraphobics: The Body Sensations Questionnaire and the Agoraphobic Cognitions Questionnaire. *Journal of Consulting and Clinical Psychology*, 52, 1090–1097.
>
> **Body Sensations Questionnaire**
> Chambless, D. L., Caputo, G. C., Bright, P., & Gallagher, R. (1984). Assessment of fear in agoraphobics: The Body Sensations Questionnaire and the Agoraphobic Cognitions Questionnaire. *Journal of Consulting and Clinical Psychology*, 52, 1090–1097.
>
> ### PHOBIAS
>
> **Mobility Inventory for Agoraphobia**
> Chambless, D. L., Caputo, G. C., Jasin, S. E., Gracely, E., & Williams, C. (1985). *The mobility inventory for agoraphobia*. *Behavior Research and Therapy*, 23, 35–44.
>
> **Fear Questionnaire**
> Marks, I. M., & Matthews, A. M. (1979). Brief standard self-rating for phobic patients. *Behaviour Research and Therapy*, 17, 263–267.
>
> ### ANXIETY
>
> **State-Trait Anxiety Inventory (STAI)**
> Spielberger, C. D., Gorsuch, R. L., & Luchene, R. E. (1976). *Manual for the State-Trait Anxiety Inventory*. Palo Alto, CA: Consulting Psychologists Press.
>
> **Penn State Worry Questionnaire (PSWQ)**
> 16 items developed to assess the trait of worry.
> Meyer, T., Miller, M., Metzger, R., & Borkovec, T. (1990). Development and validation of the Penn State Worry Questionnaire. *Behaviour Research and Therapy*, 28(6), 487–495.
>
> **Beck Anxiety Inventory**
> 21 items rating the severity of symptoms on a 4-point scale.
> Beck, A., Epstein, N., Brown, G., & Steer, R. (1988). An inventory for measuring clinical anxiety: The Beck Anxiety Inventory. *Journal of Consulting and Clinical Psychology*, 56, 893–897.

overwhelming fears of experiencing panic attacks. They may have difficulty with assertiveness or expressing their feelings.

Family Factors. Marital and parental functioning can be adversely affected by panic disorder. During the assessment, the nurse should try to grasp the patient's understanding of how panic disorder with or without severe avoidance behavior has affected his or her life along with that of the family. Pertinent questions include the following:

- How has the disorder affected your family's social life?
- What limitations related to travel has the disorder placed on you or your family?
- What coping strategies have you used to manage symptoms?
- How has the disorder affected your family members or others?

Cultural Factors. Cultural competence calls for the understanding of cultural knowledge, cultural awareness, cultural assessment skills, and cultural practice. Therefore, cultural differences must be considered in the assessment of panic disorder. Different cultures interpret sensations, feelings, or understandings differently. For example, symptoms of anxiety might be seen as witchcraft or magic (APA, 2013). Several cultures do not have a word to describe "anxiety" or "anxious" and instead may use words or meanings to suggest physical complaints (Moitra, 2018). Many Asian over-the-counter (OTC) herbal remedies contain substances that may induce panic by increasing the heart rate, basal metabolic rate, blood pressure, and sweating (see Chapter 11).

Identifying Strengths. During the assessment, the patient's strengths will emerge. For example, a patient may tell you that he does not drink alcohol or use tobacco. Another may relate that he would like to exercise. Still another patient has a supportive partner or family member. The nurse can support these positive behaviors as the care plan is established.

Priority of Nursing Care

Suicide prevention is the first priority when caring for a person with a panic disorder. People with panic disorder

TABLE 18.2 HAMILTON RATING SCALE FOR ANXIETY

Max Hamilton designed this scale to help clinicians gather information about anxiety states. The symptom inventory provides scaled information that classifies anxiety behavior and assists the clinician in targeting behaviors and achieving outcome measures. Provide a rating for each indicator based on the following scale:

0 = None
1 = Mild
2 = Moderate
3 = Severe
4 = Severe, grossly disabling

Item	Symptoms	Rating
Anxious mood	Worries, anticipation of the worst, fearful anticipation, irritability	
Tension	Feelings of tension, fatigability, startle response, moved to tears easily, trembling, feelings of restlessness, inability to relax	
Fear	Of dark, strangers, being left alone, animals, traffic, crowds	
Insomnia	Difficulty in falling asleep, broken sleep, unsatisfying sleep and fatigue on waking; dreams, nightmares, night terrors	
Intellectual (cognitive)	Difficulty concentrating, poor memory	
Depressed mood	Loss of interest, lack of pleasure in hobbies, depression, early waking, diurnal swings	
Somatic (sensory)	Tinnitus, blurring of vision, hot and cold flushes, feelings of weakness, prickly sensation	
Somatic (muscular)	Pains and aches, twitching, stiffness, myoclonic jerks, grinding of teeth, unsteady voice, increased muscular tone	
Cardiovascular symptoms	Tachycardia, palpitations, pain in chest, throbbing of vessels, fainting feelings, missing beat	
Respiratory symptoms	Pressure or constriction in chest, choking feelings, sighing, dyspnea	
Gastrointestinal symptoms	Difficulty in swallowing, gas, abdominal pain, burning sensation, abdominal fullness, nausea, vomiting, looseness of bowels, loss of weight, constipation	
Genitourinary symptoms	Frequency of micturition, urgency of micturition, amenorrhea, menorrhagia, development of frigidity, premature ejaculation, loss of libido, impotence	
Autonomic symptoms	Dry mouth, flushing, pallor, tendency to sweat, giddiness, tension headache, raising of hair	
Behavior at interview	Fidgeting, restlessness or pacing, tremor of hands, furrowed brow, strained face, sighing or rapid respiration, facial pallor, swallowing, belching, brisk tendon jerks, dilated pupils, exophthalmos	

From Hamilton, M. (1959). The assessment of anxiety states by rating. *British Journal of Medical Psychology, 32*, 50–55.

---

are often depressed and consequently are at high risk for suicide. Adolescents with panic disorder may be at higher risk for suicidal thoughts or may attempt suicide more often than other adolescents (Lim, Ko, Shin, Shin, & Oh, 2015). As many as 15% of patients with panic disorder commit suicide; women with both panic disorder and depression or panic disorder and substance abuse are especially at risk (APA, 2013; Lim et al., 2015).

Once the nurse establishes that there is no indication of a risk for suicide, the nurse assesses whether the individual may be depressed, lonely, and socially isolated. Panic attacks may be unpredictable, leading the person to be fearful of another attack. Self-esteem may be low as feelings of powerlessness emerge. The patient may be experiencing physical panic symptoms such as dizziness and hyperventilation. Because the whole family is affected by one member's symptoms, the family's needs may need to be considered.

The patient's strengths should be considered in planning care. For example, the person may be motivated to gain more control through making lifestyle changes. There may be evidence of family support.

Outcomes will depend upon the particular health care issue and the interventions that are agreed upon by the patient and nurse.

Therapeutic Relationship

The therapeutic relationship is a critical aspect of helping the person work toward recovery. These individuals may appear to be very nervous or anxious throughout the interaction. The nurse should help the patient relax and be comfortable with discussing fears and anxiety. A calm, understanding approach in a comfortable environment will help the person relax and be willing to engage in a therapeutic relationship.

TABLE 18.3 PANIC ATTACK COGNITIONS QUESTIONNAIRE

Rate each of the following thoughts according to the degree to which you believe each thought contributes to your panic attack.

1 = Not at all
2 = Somewhat
3 = Quite a lot
4 = Very much

Thought	1	2	3	4
1. I'm going to die.	1	2	3	4
2. I'm going insane.	1	2	3	4
3. I'm losing control.	1	2	3	4
4. This will never end.	1	2	3	4
5. I'm really scared.	1	2	3	4
6. I'm having a heart attack.	1	2	3	4
7. I'm going to pass out.	1	2	3	4
8. I don't know what people will think.	1	2	3	4
9. I won't be able to get out of here.	1	2	3	4
10. I don't understand what is happening to me.	1	2	3	4
11. People will think I am crazy.	1	2	3	4
12. I'll always be this way.	1	2	3	4
13. I am going to throw up.	1	2	3	4
14. I must have a brain tumor.	1	2	3	4
15. I'll choke to death.	1	2	3	4
16. I'm going to act foolish.	1	2	3	4
17. I'm going blind.	1	2	3	4
18. I'll hurt someone.	1	2	3	4
19. I'm going to have a stroke.	1	2	3	4
20. I'm going to scream.	1	2	3	4
21. I'm going to babble or talk funny.	1	2	3	4
22. I'll be paralyzed by fear.	1	2	3	4
23. Something is physically wrong with me.	1	2	3	4
24. I won't be able to breathe.	1	2	3	4
25. Something terrible will happen.	1	2	3	4
26. I'm going to make a scene.	1	2	3	4

Adapted from Clum, G. A. (1990). *Panic attack cognitions questionnaire. Coping with panic: A drug-free approach to dealing with anxiety attacks.* Pacific Grove, CA: Brooks/Cole.

Mental Health Nursing Interventions

Establishing Mental Health and Wellness Goals

The course of panic disorder culminates in phobic avoidance as the affected person attempts to avoid situations that increase panic. Even though identifying and avoiding anxiety-provoking situations are important during therapy, drastically changing lifestyle to avoid situations does not aid recovery. Goals and interventions that focus on developing a healthy lifestyle, supporting a sense of accomplishment and control, and reducing anxiety and panic are particularly helpful in reducing the number and severity of the attacks.

Wellness Challenges. Many of the strategies that promote wellness are the same that are used to treat anxiety. For the person who is anxious or fearful, the individual may be more comfortable with a gradual incorporation of the strategies. Many wellness strategies for the person who is anxious should focus on physical health. See Box 18.5.

Teaching Breathing Control. Hyperventilation is common. Often, people are unaware that they take rapid shallow breaths when they become anxious.

Teaching patients breathing control can be helpful. Focus on the breathing and help them to identify the rate, pattern, and depth. If the breathing is rapid and shallow, reassure the patient that exercise and breathing practice can help change this breathing pattern. Then, assist the patient in practicing abdominal breathing by performing the following exercises:

- Instruct the patient to breathe deeply by inhaling slowly through the nose. Have him or her place a hand on the abdomen just beneath the rib cage.

BOX 18.5

Wellness Challenges for the Person With Anxiety

WELLNESS CHALLENGES
- Coping effectively with daily stresses without excessive worry
  - Strategies: Develop a daily schedule, allow time to relax, avoid trying to multitask, deep breathing, mindfulness
- Satisfying and enriching work
  - Strategies: Choose activities that are consistent with your skills and knowledge, consider other possibilities if job is too stressful
- Incorporate physical activity, healthy foods, and adequate sleep into daily life
  - Strategies: Schedule regular physical activity, make a weekly menu of healthy meals, establish healthy sleep hygiene routines
- Developing a sense of connection, belong, and a support system
  - Strategies: Join a support group, seek out recreational activities with friends and families
- Expanding a sense of purpose and meaning in life
  - Strategies: Focus on goals, values and beliefs, read inspiring stories or essays

---

- Instruct the patient to observe that when one is breathing deeply, the hand on the abdomen will actually rise.
- After the patient understands this process, ask him or her to inhale slowly through the nose while counting to five, pause, and then exhale slowly through pursed lips.
- While the patient exhales, direct attention to feeling the muscles relax, focusing on "letting go."
- Have the patient repeat the deep abdominal breathing for 10 breaths, pausing between each inhalation and exhalation. Count slowly. If the patient complains of light-headedness, reassure him or her that this is a normal feeling while deep breathing. Instruct the patient to stop for 30 seconds, breathe normally, and then start again.
- The patient should stop between each cycle of 10 breaths and monitor normal breathing for 30 seconds.
- This series of 10 slow abdominal breaths followed by 30 seconds of normal breathing should be repeated for 3 to 5 minutes.
- Help the patient to establish a time for daily practice of abdominal breathing.

Abdominal breathing may also be used to interrupt an episode of panic as it begins. After patients have learned to identify their own early signs of panic, they can learn the four-square method of breathing, which helps divert or decrease the severity of the attack. Patients should be instructed as follows:

- Advise the patient to practice during calm periods and to begin by inhaling slowly through the nose, count to four, and then hold the breath for a count of four.
- Direct the patient to exhale slowly through pursed lips to a count of four and then rest for a count of four (no breath).
- Finally, the patient may take two normal breaths and repeat the sequence.

After patients practice the skill, the nurse should assist them in identifying the physical cues that will alert them to use this calming technique.

Teaching Nutritional Planning. Maintaining regular and balanced eating habits reduces the likelihood of hypoglycemic episodes, light-headedness, and fatigue. To help teach the patient about healthful eating and ways to minimize physical factors contributing to anxiety:

- Advise the patient to reduce or eliminate substances in the diet that promote anxiety and panic, such as food coloring, monosodium glutamate, and caffeine (withdrawal from which may stimulate panic). Patients need to plan to reduce caffeine consumption and then eliminate it from their diet. Many OTC remedies are now used to boost energy or increase mental performance; some of these contain caffeine. A thorough assessment should be made of all OTC products used to assess the potential of anxiety-provoking ingredients.
- Instruct the patient to check each substance consumed and note whether symptoms of anxiety occur and whether the symptoms are relieved by not consuming the product.

Teaching Relaxation Techniques. Teaching the patient relaxation techniques is another way to help individuals with panic and anxiety disorders. Some are unaware of the tension in their bodies and first need to learn to monitor their own tension. Isometric exercises and progressive muscle relaxation are helpful methods to learn to differentiate muscle tension from muscle relaxation. This method of relaxation is also useful when patients have difficulty clearing the mind, focusing, or visualizing a scene, which are often required in other forms of relaxation, such as meditation. Box 18.6 provides one method of progressive muscle relaxation.

Promoting Increased Physical Activity. Physical exercise can effectively decrease the occurrence of panic attacks by reducing muscle tension, increasing metabolism, increasing serotonin levels, and relieving stress. Exercise programs reduce many of the precipitants of anxiety by improving circulation, digestion, endorphin stimulation, and tissue oxygenation. In addition, exercise lowers cholesterol levels, blood pressure, and weight. After assessing for contraindications to physical exercise, assist the patient in establishing a routine exercise

BOX 18.6

Teaching Progressive Muscle Relaxation

Choose a quiet, comfortable location where you will not be disturbed for 20 to 30 minutes. Your position may be lying or sitting, but all parts of your body should be supported, including your head. Wear loose clothing, taking off restrictive items, such as glasses and shoes.

Begin by closing your eyes and clearing your mind. Moving from head to toe, focus on each part or your body and assess the level of tension. Visualize each group of muscles as heavy and relaxed.

Take two or three slow abdominal breaths, pausing briefly between each breath. Imagine the tension flowing from your body.

Each muscle group listed below should be tightened (or tensed isometrically) for 5 to 10 seconds and then abruptly released; visualize this group of muscles as heavy, limp, and relaxed for 15 to 20 seconds before tightening the next group of muscles. There are several methods to tighten each muscle group and suggestions are provided below. Each muscle group may be tightened two to three times until relaxed. Do not overtighten or strain. You should not experience pain.

- Hands: tighten by making fists
- Biceps: tighten by drawing forearms up and "making a muscle"
- Triceps: extend forearms straight, locking elbows
- Face: grimace, tightly shutting mouth and eyes
- Face: open mouth wide and raise eyebrows
- Neck: pull head forward to chest and tighten neck muscles
- Shoulders: raise shoulders toward ears
- Shoulders: push shoulders back as if touching them together
- Chest: take a deep breath and hold for 10 seconds
- Stomach: suck in your abdominal muscles
- Buttocks: pull buttocks together
- Thighs: straighten legs and squeeze muscles in thighs and hips
- Calves: pull toes carefully toward you, avoid cramps
- Feet: curl toes downward and point toes away from your body

Finally, repeat several deep abdominal breaths and mentally check your body for tension. Rest comfortably for several minutes, breathing normally, and visualize your body as warm and relaxed. Get up slowly when you are finished.

---

program. Engaging in 10- to 20-minute sessions on treadmills or stationary bicycles two to three times weekly is ideal during the winter months. Casual walking or bike riding during warmer weather promotes health. Help the patient to identify community resources that promote exercise.

Pharmacologic Interventions

Some antidepressants (e.g., SSRIs and serotonin–norepinephrine reuptake inhibitors [SNRIs]) and antianxiety medication (e.g., benzodiazepines) are FDA approved for treating people with panic disorders (see Table 18.4).

Selective Serotonin Reuptake Inhibitors. The SSRIs are recommended as the first drug option in the treatment of patients with panic disorder. They have the best safety profile, and if side effects occur, they tend to be present early in treatment before the therapeutic effect takes place. Hence, the SSRIs should be started at low doses and titrated every 5 to 7 days. Antidepressant therapy is recommended for long-term treatment of the disorder and antianxiety as adjunctive treatment (Zugliani, Cabo, Nardi, Perna, & Freire, 2019). The SSRIs produce anxiolytic effects by increasing the transmission of serotonin by blocking serotonin reuptake at the presynaptic cleft. The initial increase in serotonergic activity with SSRIs

TABLE 18.4 MEDICATION FOR PANIC DISORDER

Medication	Starting Dose (mg/day)	Therapeutic Dose	Side Effects
Selective serotonin reuptake inhibitors (SSRIs)			Class effects: nausea, anorexia, tremors, anxiety, sexual dysfunction, jitteriness, insomnia, suicidality
Fluoxetine (Prozac)	10	20–60	Class effects
Sertraline (Zoloft)	25	50–200	Class effects, loose stools
Paroxetine (Paxil)	10	10–60	Class effects, drowsiness, fatigue
Paroxetine (controlled release) (Paxil CR)	12.5	12.5–75	Class effects
Serotonin–norepinephrine reuptake inhibitors (SNRIs)			Class effects: nausea, sweating, dry mouth, dizziness, insomnia, somnolence, sexual dysfunction, hypertension
Venlafaxine (extended release)	37.5	75–300	Class effects
Benzodiazepines			Class effects: sedation, cognitive slowing, physical dependence
Clonazepam (Klonopin)	0.25 tid	0.5–2.0 bid	Class effects
Alprazolam (Xanax)	0.25 tid	0.5–1.5 tid	Class effects

tid, three times a day; bid, two times a day.

BOX 18.7
Drug Profile: Alprazolam (Xanax)

DRUG CLASS: Antianxiety agent

RECEPTOR AFFINITY: Exact mechanism of action is unknown; believed to increase the effects of γ-aminobutyrate

INDICATIONS: Management of anxiety disorders, short-term relief of anxiety symptoms or depression-related anxiety, panic attacks with or without agoraphobia

ROUTES AND DOSAGES: Available in 0.25-, 0.5-, 1-, and 2-mg scored tablets

Adults: For anxiety: Initially, 0.25–0.5 mg PO tid titrated to a maximum daily dose of 4 mg in divided doses. For panic disorder: Initially, 0.5 mg PO tid increased at 3- to 4-day intervals in increments of no more than 1 mg/day

Geriatric Patients: Initially, 0.25 mg bid to tid, increased gradually as needed and tolerated

HALF-LIFE (PEAK EFFECT): 12–15 hours (1–2 hours)

SELECTED ADVERSE REACTIONS: Transient mild drowsiness, initially; sedation, depression, lethargy, apathy, fatigue, light-headedness, disorientation, anger, hostility, restlessness, headache, confusion, crying, constipation, diarrhea, dry mouth, nausea, and possible drug dependence

WARNINGS: Contraindicated in patients with psychosis, acute narrow-angle glaucoma, shock, acute alcoholic intoxication with depressed vital signs, pregnancy, labor and delivery, and breastfeeding. Use cautiously in patients with impaired hepatic or renal function and severe debilitating conditions. Risk for digitalis toxicity if given concurrently with digoxin. Increased CNS depression if taken with alcohol, other CNS depressants, and propoxyphene (Darvon).

SPECIFIC PATIENT AND FAMILY EDUCATION

- Avoid using alcohol, sleep-inducing drugs, and other OTC drugs
- Take the drug exactly as prescribed and do not stop taking the drug without consulting your primary health care provider
- Take the drug with food if gastrointestinal upset occurs
- Avoid driving a car or performing tasks that require alertness if drowsiness or dizziness occurs
- Report any signs and symptoms of adverse reactions
- Notify your primary health care provider if severe dizziness, weakness, or drowsiness persists or if rash or skin lesions, difficulty voiding, palpitations, or swelling of the extremities occurs

CNS, central nervous system; OTC, over-the-counter; PO, oral; tid, three times a day.

---

may cause temporary increases in panic symptoms and even panic attacks. After 4 to 6 weeks of treatment, anxiety subsides, and the antianxiety effect of the medications begins (see Chapter 11). Increased serotonin activity in the brain is believed to decrease norepinephrine activity. This decrease lessens cardiovascular symptoms of tachycardia and increased blood pressure that are associated with panic attacks. See Chapter 18 for administration and monitoring side effects.

NCLEXNOTE Psychopharmacologic treatment is almost always needed. Antidepressants are the medications of choice. Antianxiety medication is used only for short periods of time.

Serotonin–Norepinephrine Reuptake Inhibitors. The SNRIs increase levels of both serotonin and norepinephrine by blocking their reuptake presynaptically. Classified as antidepressants, the SNRIs are also used in anxiety disorders. Venlafaxine is the most commonly used SNRI (see Table 18.4). These medications have been shown to reduce the severity of panic and anticipatory anxiety. Similar to the SSRIs, they should not be abruptly discontinued (see Chapter 11).

Benzodiazepine Therapy. The high-potency benzodiazepines have produced antipanic effects; their therapeutic onset is much faster than that of antidepressants (see Table 18.4). Therefore, benzodiazepines are tremendously useful in treating intensely distressed patients. Alprazolam (Xanax), lorazepam (Ativan), and clonazepam (Klonopin) are widely used for panic disorder. They are well tolerated but carry the risk for withdrawal symptoms upon discontinuation of use (see Box 18.7). The benzodiazepines are still commonly used for panic disorder even though the SSRIs are recommended for first-line treatment of panic disorder (Quagliato, Freire, Nardi, 2018).

Administering and Monitoring Benzodiazepines. Treatment may include administering benzodiazepines concurrently with antidepressants for the first 4 weeks and then tapering the benzodiazepine to a maintenance dose. This strategy provides rapid symptom relief but avoids the complications of long-term benzodiazepine use. Benzodiazepines with short half-lives do not accumulate in the body, but benzodiazepines with half-lives of longer than 24 hours tend to accumulate with long-term treatment, are removed more slowly, and produce less intense symptoms on discontinuation of use (see Chapter 11).

Short-acting benzodiazepines, such as alprazolam, are associated with rebound anxiety, or anxiety that increases after the peak effects of the medication have decreased. Medications with short half-lives (alprazolam, lorazepam) should be given in three or four doses spaced throughout the day, with a higher dose at bedtime to allay anxiety-related insomnia. Clonazepam, a longer-acting benzodiazepine, requires less frequent dosing and has a lower risk for rebound anxiety.

Because of their depressive CNS effects, benzodiazepines should not be used to treat patients with comorbid sleep apnea. In fact, these drugs may actually decrease the rate and depth of respirations. Exercise caution in older adult patients for these reasons. Discontinuing medication use requires a slow taper during a period of several weeks to avoid rebound anxiety and serious withdrawal symptoms. Benzodiazepines are not indicated in the chronic treatment of patients with substance abuse but can be useful in quickly treating anxiety symptoms until other medications take effect.

Symptoms associated with withdrawal of benzodiazepine therapy are more likely to occur after high doses and long-term therapy. They can also occur after short-term therapy. Withdrawal symptoms manifest in several ways, including psychological (e.g., apprehension, irritability, agitation).

Monitoring for Drug Interactions. SSRIs should not be given with MAOIs because of potential drug interaction. Drugs that interact with benzodiazepines include the TCAs and digoxin; interaction may result in increased serum TCA or digoxin levels. Alcohol and other CNS depressants, when used with benzodiazepines, increase CNS depression. Their concomitant use is contraindicated. Histamine-2 blockers (e.g., cimetidine) used with benzodiazepines may potentiate sedative effects. Monitor closely for effectiveness in patients who smoke; cigarette smoking may increase the clearance of benzodiazepines.

Managing Side Effects. The side effects of benzodiazepine medications generally include headache, confusion, dizziness, disorientation, sedation, and visual disturbances. Sedation should be monitored after beginning medication use or increasing the dose. The patient should avoid operating heavy machinery until the sedative effects are known.

Concurrent use of SSRIs and the MAOIs is contraindicated. These antidepressants should not be given together.

Teaching Points. Warn patients to avoid alcohol because of the chance of CNS depression. In addition, warn them not to operate heavy machinery until the sedative effects of the medication are known.

Psychosocial Interventions

Therapeutic Interactions

Peplau (1989) devised general guidelines for nursing interventions that might be successful in treating patients with anxiety. These interventions help the patient attend to and react to input other than the subjective experience of anxiety. They are designed to help the patient focus on other stimuli and cope with anxiety in any form (Table 18.5). These general interventions apply to all anxiety disorders and therefore are not reiterated in subsequent sections.

Distraction

After patients can identify the early symptoms of panic, they may learn to implement distraction behaviors that take the focus off the physical sensations. Some activities include initiating conversation with a nearby person or engaging in physical activity (e.g., walking, gardening, or housecleaning). Performing simple repetitive activities such as snapping a rubber band against the wrist, counting backward from 100 by 3s, or counting objects along the roadway might also deter an attack.

Reframing

Reframing is a cognitive technique that can change the way a situation, event, or person is viewed and reduce the impact of anxiety-provoking thoughts. People with

TABLE 18.5	NURSING INTERVENTIONS BASED ON DEGREES OF ANXIETY
Degree of Anxiety	**Nursing Interventions**
Mild	Assist patient to use the energy anxiety provides to encourage learning.
Moderate	Encourage patient to talk: to focus on one experience, to describe it fully, and then to formulate the patient's generalizations about that experience.
Severe	Allow relief behaviors to be used but do not ask about them. Encourage the patient to talk: ventilation of random ideas is likely to reduce anxiety to a moderate level.
Panic	Stay with the patient. Allow pacing and walk with the patient. No content inputs to the patient's thinking should be made by the nurse. (They burden the patient, who will distort them.) Be direct with the fewest number of words: e.g., "Drink this" (give liquids to replace lost fluids and to relieve dry mouth); "Say what's happening to you," "Talk about yourself," or "Tell what you feel now" (to encourage ventilation and externalization of inner, frightening experience). Pick up on what the patient says, e.g., Patient: "What's happening to me—how did I get here?" Nurse: "Say what you notice." Use short phrases to the point of the patient's comment. Do not touch the patient; patients experiencing panic are very concerned about survival, are experiencing a grave threat to self, and usually distort intentions of all invasions of their personal space.

Adapted from Peplau, H. (1989). Theoretic constructs: Anxiety, self, and hallucinations. In A. O'Toole & S. Welt (Eds.). *Interpersonal theory in nursing practice: Selected works of Hildegarde E. Peplau.* New York: Springer.

anxiety disorders often view themselves negatively and use "should statements" and "negative labels." Should statements lead to rigid rules and unrealistic expectations. By encouraging patients to avoid the use of should statements and reframe their views, they can change their beliefs to be more realistic. For example, if a patient says, "I should be a better parent" or "I'm a useless failure," the nurse could ask the person to identify the positive aspects of parenting and other successes.

> **Consider This:**
> Could distraction and reframing help Doug reduce his anxiety and frequency of his panic attacks? What interventions would you recommend and why?

Positive Self-Talk

During states of increased anxiety and panic, individuals can learn to counter fearful or negative thoughts by using another cognitive approach. **Positive self-talk** involves planning and rehearsing positive coping statements "This is only anxiety, and it will pass," "I can handle these symptoms," and "I'll get through this" are examples of positive self-talk. These types of positive statements can give the individual a focal point and reduce fear when panic symptoms begin. Handheld cards that offer positive statements can be carried in a purse or wallet so the person can retrieve them quickly when panic symptoms are felt (Box 18.8).

NCLEXNOTE Cognitive interventions give patients with anxiety a sense of control over the recurring threats of panic and obsessions.

Psychoeducation

Psychoeducation programs help to teach patients and families about the symptoms of panic. Individuals with panic disorder legitimately fear going crazy, losing control, or dying because of their physical symptoms. Attempting to convince a patient that such fears are groundless only heightens anxiety and impedes communication. Information and physical evidence (e.g., electrocardiogram results, laboratory test results) should be presented in a caring and open manner that demonstrates acceptance and understanding of his or her situation.

Box 18.9 suggests topics for individual or small-group discussion. It is especially important to cover such topics as the differences between panic attacks and heart attacks, the difference between panic disorder and other psychiatric disorders, and the effectiveness of various treatment methods.

Wellness Strategies

Individuals with panic disorder, especially those with significant anxiety sensitivity, may need assistance in reevaluating their lifestyle. Time management can be a useful tool. In the workplace or at home, underestimating the time needed to complete a chore or being overly involved in several activities at once increases stress and anxiety. Procrastination, lack of assertiveness, and difficulties with prioritizing or delegating tasks intensify these problems.

Writing a list of chores to be completed and estimating time to complete them provide concrete feedback to the individual. Crossing out each activity as it is completed helps the patient to regain a sense of control and accomplishment. Large tasks should be broken into a series of smaller tasks to minimize stress and maximize sense of achievement. Rest, relaxation, and family time—frequently omitted from the daily schedule—must be included.

Evaluation and Treatment Outcomes

Although many researchers consider panic disorder a chronic, long-term condition, the positive results from outcome studies should be shared with patients to provide encouragement and optimism that patients can learn to manage these symptoms. Outcome studies have demonstrated success with panic control treatment, CBT therapy, exposure therapy, and various medications specific to certain symptoms.

Continuum of Care

As with any disorder, a continuum of patient care across multiple settings is crucial. Patients are treated in the least restrictive environment that will meet their safety needs. As the patient progresses through treatment, the environment of care changes from an emergency or inpatient setting to outpatient clinics or individual therapy sessions.

Integration With Primary Care

Some groups are more likely to seek out care in primary care rather than in mental health clinics. People with anxiety disorders are often treated in the primary care environment particularly those who experience panic disorder. Because panic attacks mimic cardiac difficulties, it is important that the patient continues to seek health care monitoring with medical clinicians.

Family Interventions

In addition to learning the symptoms of panic disorder, nurses should have information sheets or pamphlets

BOX 18.8 • THERAPEUTIC DIALOGUE • Panic Disorder

Doug is admitted to an inpatient unit following another severe panic attack. He had an argument with his high school son, who continues to use alcohol and marijuana. Financial problems are also escalating.

INEFFECTIVE APPROACH

Nurse: Oh…. Why are you crying?

Doug: (Looks up, gives a nervous chuckle.) Obviously, because I'm upset. I am tired of living this way. I just want to be normal again. I can't even remember what that feels like.

Nurse: You look normal to me. Everyone has bad days. It'll pass.

Doug: I've felt this way longer than you've been alive. I've tried everything, and nothing works.

Nurse: You're not the first depressed person that I've taken care of. You just need to go to groups and stay out of your room more. You'll start feeling better.

Doug: (Angrily) Oh, it's just that easy. You have no idea what I'm going through! You don't know me! You're just a kid.

Nurse: I can help you if you help yourself. A group starts in 5 minutes, and I'd like to see you there.

Doug: I'm not going to no damn group! I want to be alone so I can think!

Nurse: (Looks about anxiously.) Maybe I should come back after you've calmed down a little.

EFFECTIVE APPROACH

Nurse: Doug, I noticed that you are staying in your room more today. What's troubling you?

Doug: (Looks up) I feel like I've lost complete control of my life. I'm so anxious, and nothing helps. I'm tired of it.

Nurse: I see. That must be difficult. Can you tell me more about what you are feeling right now?

Doug: I feel like I'm going crazy. I worry all the time about having panic attacks. They make me scared I'm going to die. Sometimes I think I'd be better off dead.

Nurse: (Remains silent, continues to give eye contact.)

Doug: Do you know what it's like to be a prisoner to your emotions? I can't even go to work sometimes, and when I do, it's terrifying. I don't know what to think anymore.

Nurse: Doug, you have lived with this disorder for a long time. You say that the medications do not work to your liking, but what has helped you in the past?

Doug: Well, I learned in relaxation group that panic symptoms are probably caused by chemicals in my brain that are not working correctly. I learned that medications can help, but they don't work well for me. I tried an exposure plan and relaxation techniques to deal with my fears of leaving the house and my chronic anxiety. That did help some, but it's scary to do.

Nurse: It sounds like you have learned a lot about your illness, one that can be treated, so that you don't always have to feel this way.

Doug: This is easier to say right now when I'm here and can get help if I need it. It's hard to remember this when I'm in the middle of a panic attack and think I'm dying.

Nurse: It's harder when you're alone?

Doug: Much harder! And I'm alone so much of the time.

Nurse: Let's talk about some ways you can manage your panics when you're alone. Tell me some of the techniques you've learned.

CRITICAL THINKING CHALLENGE

- What tone is established by the nurse's opening question in the first scenario?
- Which therapeutic communication techniques did the nurse use in the second scenario to avoid the pitfalls encountered in the first scenario?
- What information was uncovered in the second scenario that was not touched on in the first?
- What predictions can you make about the interpersonal relationship likely to develop between the nurse and the patient in each scenario?

> **BOX 18.9**
>
> **Psychoeducation Checklist: Panic Disorder**
>
> When caring for the patient with panic disorder, be sure to include the following topic areas in the teaching plan:
> - Psychopharmacologic agents (anxiolytics or antidepressants) if ordered, including drug action, dosage, frequency, and possible adverse effects
> - Breathing control measures
> - Nutrition
> - Exercise
> - Progressive muscle relaxation
> - Distraction behaviors
> - Exposure therapy
> - Time management
> - Positive coping strategies

available concerning the disorder and any medications prescribed. Parents, especially single parents, will need assistance in child-rearing and may benefit from services designed to provide some respite. Moreover, the entire family will need support in adjusting to the disorder. A referral for family therapy is indicated, because involving the entire family in the therapy process is imperative. Families experience the symptoms, treatments, clinical setbacks, and recovery from chronic mental illnesses as a unit. Misunderstandings, misconceptions, false information, and the stigma of mental illness, singly or collectively, impede recovery efforts.

Emergency Care

Because individuals with panic disorder are likely to first present for treatment in an emergency department or primary care setting, nurses working in these settings should be involved in early recognition and referral. Consultation with a psychiatrist or mental health professional by the primary care physician can decrease both costs and overall patient symptoms. Several interventions may be useful in reducing the number of emergency department visits related to panic symptoms. Psychiatric consultation and nursing education can be provided in the emergency department to explore other avenues of treatment. Remembering that the patient experiencing a panic attack is in crisis, nurses can take several measures to help alleviate symptoms, including the following:

- Stay with the patient and maintain a calm demeanor. (Anxiety often produces more anxiety and a calm presence will help calm the patient.)
- Reassure the patient that you will not leave, that this episode will pass, and that he or she is in a safe place. (The patient often fears dying and cannot see beyond the panic attack.)
- Give clear concise directions using short sentences. Do not use medical jargon.
- Walk or pace with the patient to an environment with minimal stimulation. (The patient in panic has excessive energy.)
- Administer prn (i.e., as-needed) anxiolytic medications as ordered and appropriate. (Pharmacotherapy is effective in treating those patients with acute panic attack.)

After the panic attack has resolved, allow the patient to vent his or her feelings. This often helps the patient in clarifying his or her feelings.

Inpatient-Focused Care

Inpatient settings provide control for the stabilization of the acute panic symptoms and initiation of recovery-oriented strategies. Medication use is often initiated here because patients who show initial panic symptoms require in-depth assessment to determine the cause. As recovery begins, crisis stabilization, medication management, milieu therapy, and psychotherapies are introduced, and outpatient discharge linkage appointments are set. See Nursing Care Plan 18.1—which sets forth a plan of care for Tim, the case study patient in this chapter—is available at http://thepoint.lww.com/BoydEssentials2e.

Community Care

Most individuals with panic disorder are treated on an outpatient basis. Referral lists of community resources and support groups are useful in this setting. A discussion about the recovery and the importance of the 10 components helps healing begin (see Chapter 1 and 7). Nurses are more directly involved in treatment, conducting psychoeducation groups on relaxation and breathing techniques, symptom management, and anger management. Advanced practice nurses conduct CBT and individual and family psychotherapy. In addition, medication monitoring groups reemphasize the role of medications, monitor for side effects, and enhance treatment compliance overall.

GENERALIZED ANXIETY DISORDER

Generally speaking, patients with generalized anxiety disorder (GAD) feel frustrated, disgusted with life, demoralized, and hopeless. They may state that they cannot remember a time that they did not feel anxious. They experience a sense of ill-being and uneasiness and a fear of imminent disaster. Over time, they may recognize that their chronic tension and anxiety are unreasonable.

Clinical Course

The onset of GAD is insidious. Many patients complain of being chronic worriers. GAD affects individuals of all ages. About half of the individuals with GAD report an onset in childhood or adolescence, although onset after 20 years of age is also common. Adults with GAD often worry about matters such as their job, household finances, health of family members, or simple matters (e.g., household chores or being late for appointments). The intensity of the worry fluctuates and stress tends to intensify the worry and anxiety symptoms (APA, 2013).

Patients with GAD may exhibit mild depressive symptoms, such as dysphoria. They are also highly somatic, with complaints of multiple clusters of physical symptoms, including muscle aches, soreness, and gastrointestinal ailments. In addition to physical complaints, patients with GAD often experience poor sleep habits, irritability, trembling, twitching, poor concentration, and an exaggerated startle response. People with this disorder often are seen in a primary care setting with somatic symptoms (Metzler, Mahoney, & Freedy, 2016).

Diagnostic Criteria

GAD is characterized by excessive worry and anxiety (apprehensive expectation) for at least 6 months. The anxiety does not usually pertain to a specific situation; rather, it concerns several real-life activities or events. Ultimately, excessive worry and anxiety cause great distress and interfere with the patient's daily personal or social life.

Nursing Care

Nursing care for the person with GAD is similar to the care of the individual with a panic disorder. In many instances, antidepressants and an antianxiety agent will be prescribed. Nursing interventions should focus on helping the person target specific areas of anxiety and reducing the impact of the anxiety. See Box 18.10.

BOX 18.10

Psychoeducation Checklist: Generalized Anxiety Disorder

When caring for the patient with generalized anxiety disorder, be sure to include the following topic areas in the teaching plan:
- Psychopharmacologic agents (benzodiazepines, antidepressants, nonbenzodiazepine anxiolytics, β-blockers) if ordered, including drug action, dosage, frequency, and possible adverse effects
- Breathing control
- Nutrition and diet restriction
- Sleep measures
- Progressive muscle relaxation
- Time management
- Positive coping strategies

OTHER ANXIETY DISORDERS

Other disorders exist that have anxiety as their defining feature. These include generalized phobia, agoraphobia, specific phobias, and **social anxiety disorder**.

AGORAPHOBIA

Agoraphobia is fear or anxiety triggered by about two or more situations such as using public transportation, being in open spaces, being in enclosed places, standing in line, being in a crowd, or being outside of the home alone (APA, 2013). When these situations occur, the individual believes that something terrible might happen and that escape may be difficult. The individual may experience panic-like symptoms or other embarrassing symptoms (e.g., vomiting, diarrhea) (APA, 2013). Agoraphobia leads to avoidance behaviors. Such avoidance interferes with routine functioning and eventually renders the person afraid to leave the safety of home. Some affected individuals continue to face feared situations but with significant trepidation (i.e., going in public only to pay bills or to take children to school). Agoraphobia may occur with panic disorder but is considered a separate disorder.

SPECIFIC PHOBIA

Specific phobia disorder is marked by persistent fear of clearly discernible, circumscribed objects or situations, which often leads to avoidance behaviors. Phobic objects can include animals (e.g., spiders, snakes), natural environment (e.g., heights, storms), blood injection injury (e.g., fear of blood, injections), and situational (e.g., elevators, enclosed spaces). The lifetime prevalence rates range from 7% to 9%, and the disorder generally affects women twice as much as men (APA, 2013). It has a bimodal distribution, peaking in childhood and then again in the 20s. The focus of the fear in specific phobia may result from the anticipation of being harmed by the phobic object. For example, dogs are feared because of the chance of being bitten or automobiles are feared because of the potential of crashing. The focus of fear may likewise be associated with concerns about losing control, panicking, or fainting on exposure to the phobic object.

Anxiety is usually felt immediately on exposure to the phobic object; the level of anxiety is usually related to both the proximity of the object and the degree to which escape is possible. For example, anxiety heightens as a cat approaches a person who fears cats and lessens when the cat moves away. At times, the level of anxiety escalates to a full panic attack, particularly when the person must remain in a situation from which escape is deemed to be impossible. Fear of specific objects is fairly common and the diagnosis of specific phobia is not made unless the

> **BOX 18.11**
> **Common Phobias**
>
> - Acrophobia: fear of heights
> - Agoraphobia: fear of open spaces
> - Ailurophobia: fear of cats
> - Algophobia: fear of pain
> - Arachnophobia: fear of spiders
> - Brontophobia: fear of thunder
> - Claustrophobia: fear of closed spaces
> - Cynophobia: fear of dogs
> - Entomophobia: fear of insects
> - Hematophobia: fear of blood
> - Microphobia: fear of germs
> - Nyctophobia: fear of night or dark places
> - Ophidiophobia: fear of snakes
> - Phonophobia: fear of loud noises
> - Photophobia: fear of light
> - Pyrophobia: fear of fire
> - Topophobia: fear of a place, like a stage
> - Xenophobia: fear of strangers
> - Zoophobia: fear of animal or animals

> **BOX 18.12**
> **Research for Best Practice: Fever Phobia: A Cultural Trait?**
>
> Purssell, E., & Collin, J. (2016). Fever phobia: The impact of time and mortality–A systematic review and meta-analysis. International Journal of Nursing Studies, 56, 81–89.
>
> **THE QUESTION:** Is the heightened fear of fever a phenomenon that is learned on an individual basis or is it part of human culture?
>
> **METHODS:** There are multiple guidelines that suggest fever is not, in itself, dangerous. Through an extensive literature search, authors established that fever phobia, an exaggerated fear of fever by parents and care givers of children, is very common. This leads to over treatment and anxiety. After reviewing 200 papers, the authors found 40 papers that met an inclusion criterion and provided sufficient data for further analysis. They conducted a meta-analysis and cluster analysis using metaphor, meta, and Cluster in R.
>
> **FINDINGS:** Fear of brain damage, coma, convulsions, death, and dehydration was high in many studies. Mortality-related or geographic patterns do not support these fears. The fear of fever remains relatively high despite evidence that most febrile illnesses are relatively harmless and do not require treatment.
>
> **IMPLICATIONS FOR NURSING:** This study supports the difficulty in countering fearful beliefs with evidence. In this study, the authors concluded that the fever phobia is transmitted culturally and that individual education programs might not be effective. The authors suggest that febrile illness should be acknowledged as unpleasant and that antipyretic drugs should be rebranded as antipyretic analgesics and used primarily for pain control.

fear significantly interferes with functioning or causes marked distress. Assessment differentiates simple phobia from other diagnoses with overlapping symptoms. Box 18.11 lists a number of specific phobias. Among adult patients who are seen in clinical settings, the most-to-least common phobias are situational phobias, natural environment phobias, blood injection, injury phobia, and animal phobias (APA, 2013).

Blood injection injury phobia merits special consideration because the phobia involves medical treatments. The physiologic processes that are exhibited during phobic exposure include a strong vasovagal response, which significantly increases blood pressure and pulse, followed by deceleration of the pulse and lowering of blood pressure in the patient. Monitor closely when giving required injections or medical treatments.

About 75% of patients with blood injection injury phobia report fainting on exposure. Factors that may predispose individuals to specific phobias may include traumatic events; unexpected panic attacks in the presence of the phobic object or situation; observation of others experiencing a trauma; or repeated exposure to information warning of dangers, such as parents repeatedly warning young children that dogs bite.

Phobic content must be evaluated from an ethnic or cultural background. In many cultures, fears of spirits or magic are common. They should be considered part of a disorder only if the fear is excessive in the context of the culture, causes the individual significant distress, or impairs the ability to function. See Box 18.12.

Psychotropic drugs have not been effective in the treatment of specific phobia. Anxiolytics may give short-term relief of phobic anxiety, but no evidence confirms that they affect the course of the disorder. The treatment of choice for specific phobia is exposure therapy. Patients who are highly motivated can experience success with treatment (Barlow, Conklin, & Bentley, 2015).

SOCIAL ANXIETY DISORDER (SOCIAL PHOBIA)

Social anxiety disorder involves a persistent fear of social or performance situations in which embarrassment may occur. Exposure to a feared social or performance situation nearly always provokes immediate anxiety and may trigger panic attacks. People with social anxiety disorder fear that others will scrutinize their behavior and judge them negatively. They often do not speak up in crowds out of fear of embarrassment. They go to great lengths to avoid feared situations. If avoidance is not possible, they suffer through the situation with visible anxiety (APA, 2013).

People with social anxiety disorder appear to be highly sensitive to disapproval or criticism, tend to evaluate themselves negatively, have poor self-esteem, and a distorted view of their personal strengths and weaknesses.

They may magnify their personal flaws and underrate any talents. They often believe others would act with more assertiveness in a given social situation. Women are more likely to have social anxiety disorder, but both men and women tend to have difficulties with dating and with sexual relationships (Asher, Asnaani, Aderka, 2017). Children tend to underachieve in school because of test-taking anxiety. This is an important area that should be assessed in all patients.

Generalized social anxiety disorder is diagnosed when the individual experiences fears related to most social situations, including public performances and social interactions. These individuals are likely to demonstrate deficiencies in social skills and their phobias interfere with their ability to function (Asher et al., 2017).

People with social anxiety disorder fear and avoid only one or two social situations. Classic examples of such situations are eating, writing, speaking in public, or using public bathrooms. The most common fears for individuals with social anxiety disorder are public speaking, fear of meeting strangers, eating in public, writing in public, using public restrooms, and being stared at or being the center of attention.

Pharmacotherapy is a relatively new area of research in treating patients with social anxiety disorder. SSRIs are used to treat those with social anxiety disorder because they significantly reduce social anxiety and phobic avoidance. Benzodiazepines are also used to reduce anxiety caused by phobias. Providing referrals for appropriate psychiatric treatment is a critical nursing intervention.

SUMMARY OF KEY POINTS

- Anxiety-related disorders are the most common of all psychiatric disorders and comprise several disorders, including panic disorder.

- The anxiety disorders share the common symptom of recurring anxiety but differ in symptom profiles. Panic attacks can occur in many different disorders.

- Those experiencing anxiety disorders have a high level of physical and emotional illness and often experience dual diagnoses with other anxiety disorders, substance abuse, or depression. These disorders often render individuals unable to function effectively at home or at a job.

- Patients with panic disorder are often seen in various health care settings, frequently in hospital emergency departments or clinics, presenting with a confusing array of physical and emotional symptoms. Skillful assessment is required to eliminate possible life-threatening causes.

- Treatment approaches for all anxiety-related disorders are somewhat similar, including pharmacotherapy, psychological treatments, or often a combination of both.

- Nursing interventions include helping patients manage a panic attack, promoting healthy diet, exercise and sleep hygiene habits, medication administration and monitoring, psychoeducation, and cognitive interventions.

CRITICAL THINKING CHALLENGES

1. A patient is unable to focus on your directions. He does not seem to notice others in the room; instead he is intent on cutting his food into small pieces. Applying Peplau's stages of anxiety, what level of anxiety is he experiencing?
2. Compare and contrast the following treatment modalities for anxiety disorders: systematic desensitization, implosive therapy, exposure therapy, and CBT.
3. Identify the major nursing assessment areas for a person experiencing a panic disorder.
4. A patient asks you how to prevent hyperventilation. How would you answer her question?
5. Delineate the differences in treatment effects of antidepressants versus antianxiety medication in the treatment of panic disorder.
6. Compare the various phobias that people experience. What interventions should a nurse use for a person who has a blood injection injury phobia?
7. How might one differentiate shyness from social anxiety disorder?

A related Psychiatric–Mental Health Nursing video on the topic of Anxiety is available at http://thepoint.lww.com/BoydEssentials2e.

A Practice and Learn Interactive Case Study related to the video on the topic of Anxiety is available at http://thepoint.lww.com/BoydEssentials2e.

UNFOLDING PATIENT STORIES FOR UNIT V

Unfolding Patient Stories: Linda Waterfall • Part 2

Recall from Unit II **Linda Waterfall,** a 48-year-old Native American diagnosed with an aggressive form of breast cancer. The recommended treatment is a mastectomy followed by chemotherapy, which she refused. What is the association between her illness and episodes of severe anxiety since diagnosis? How can a secondary mental health disorder contribute to her physical decline from cancer? What psychosocial assessments and interventions should the nurse incorporate into the plan of care to manage her anxiety?

Care for Linda and other patients in a realistic virtual environment: **vSim** *for Nursing* (thepoint.lww.com/vSimMental Health). Practice documenting these patients' care in DocuCare (thepoint.lww.com/DocuCareEHR).

Unfolding Patient Stories: Li Na Chen • Part 2

Recall from Unit I **Li Na Chen** with major depressive disorder, who was hospitalized following her third suicide attempt with an overdose. She is transitioning to a partial hospitalization program before formal transition to home. Her husband is concerned about their two children, ages 12 and 14, and his ability to handle her after she is home. What questions can the nurse ask to clarify the husband's concerns? How can Li Na's depression and attempted suicide affect her husband and children? What psychosocial interventions can the nurse consider to support Li Na and her family after she is home?

Care for Li Na and other patients in a realistic virtual environment: **vSim** *for Nursing* (thepoint.lww.com/vSimMental Health). Practice documenting these patients' care in DocuCare (thepoint.lww.com/DocuCareEHR).

Unfolding Patient Stories: Sharon Cole • Part 2

Recall from Unit III **Sharon Cole,** diagnosed with bipolar disorder, who is admitted to the orthopedic unit following surgery for a fractured ankle from a fall during a manic episode. She is exhibiting manic behavior postoperatively with grandiose thoughts, irritability, and wanting to leave the hospital. What are the benefits of having a sitter at her bedside? What education would the nurse provide to a sitter without prior experience caring for a client with bipolar disorder and manic behavior? What instructions would promote safety for the patient and the sitter and deter a potentially volatile situation?

Care for Sharon and other patients in a realistic virtual environment: **vSim** *for Nursing* (thepoint.lww.com/vSimMental Health). Practice documenting these patients' care in DocuCare (thepoint.lww.com/DocuCareEHR).

Unfolding Patient Stories: Andrew Davis • Part 1

Andrew Davis is 56 years old and voluntarily admitted himself to an alcohol rehabilitation facility after his wife asked him to move out of their home. Of his three children, only his son will speak to him. He refuses to attend group therapy and an Alcoholics Anonymous (AA) meeting. How can the nurse establish a therapeutic relationship during the treatment stage of withdrawal and throughout recovery? Why is it important to cultivate trust between the nurse, Andrew, and his family? How can the nurse encourage Andrew to attend group therapy and the AA meeting? (Andrew Davis's story continues in Unit VI.)

Care for Andrew and other patients in a realistic virtual environment: **vSim** *for Nursing* (thepoint.lww.com/vSimMental Health). Practice documenting these patients' care in DocuCare (thepoint.lww.com/DocuCareEHR).

REFERENCES

American Psychiatric Association. (2013). *Diagnostic and statistical manual of mental disorders DSM-5* (5th ed.). Arlington, VA: Author.

Asher, M., Asnaani, A., & Aderka, I. M. (2017). Gender differences in social anxiety disorder: A review. *Clinical Psychology Review, 56,* 1–7.

Asok, A., Kandel, E. R., & Rayman, J. B. (2019). The neurobiology of fear generalization, *Frontiers in Behavioral Neuroscience, 2,* 329.

Assari, S. (2017). Psychiatric disorders differently correlate with physical self-rated health across ethnic groups. *Journal of Personalized Medicine, 7*(4), 6.

Ayazi, T., Lien, L., Eide, A., Swartz, L., & Hauff, E. (2014). Association between exposure to traumatic events and anxiety disorders in a post-conflict setting: A cross-sectional community study in South Sudan. *BMC Psychiatry, 14,* 6.

Bandelow, B., Reitt, M., Röver, C., Michaelis, S., Görlich, Y., & Wedekind, D. (2015). Efficacy of treatments for anxiety disorders: a meta-analysis. *International Clinical Psychopharmacology, 30*(4):183–192.

Barlow, D. H., Conklin, L. R, & Bentley, K. H. (2015). Psychological treatment for panic disorder, phobias, and social anxiety disorders. In P. E. Nathan & J. M. Gorman (Eds.). *A guide to treatments that work* (4th ed., pp. 409–463). New York: Oxford University Press.

Bourdon, J. L., Savage, J. E., Verhulst, B., Carney, D. M., Brotman, M. A., Pine, D. S., et al. (2019). The genetic and environmental relationship between childhood behavioral inhibition and preadolescent anxiety. *Twin Research and Human Genetics, 22*(1), 48–55.

Carballo, J. J., Llorente, C., Kehrmann, L., Flamarique, I., Zuddas, A., Purper-Ouakil, D., et al. (2019). Psychosocial risk factors for suicidality in children and adolescents. *European Child and Adolescent Psychiatry,* 1 8. https://doi-/10.1007/s00787-018-01270-9

DeJesus, R. S., Breitkopf, C. R., Ebbert, J. O., Rutten L. J., Jacobson, R. M., Jacobson, D. J., et al. (2016). Associations between anxiety diagnoses and body mass index differ by age, sex and race: A population based study. *Clinical Practice and Epidemiology in Mental Health, 12,* 67–74.

Grenier, S., Payette, M. C., Gunther, B., Askari, S., Desjardins, F. F., Raymond, B., et al. (2018). Association of age and gender with anxiety disorders in older adults: A systematic review and meta-analysis. *International Journal of Geriatric Psychiatry, 34*(3), 397–407.

Hamilton, M. (1959). The assessment of anxiety states by rating. *British Journal of Medical Psychology, 32*, 50–55.

Hornboll, B., Macoveanu, J., Nejad, A., Rowe, J., Elliott, R., Knudsen, G. M., et al. (2018). Neuroticism predicts the impact of serotonin challenges on fear processing in subgenual anterior cingulate cortex. *Scientific Reports, 8*, 17889.

Konishi, Y., Tanii, H., Otowa, T., Sasaki, T., Tochigi, M., Umekage, T., et al. (2014). Gene x gene x gender interaction of BDNF and COMT genotypes associated with panic disorder. *Progress in Neuro-Psychopharmacology and Biological Psychiatry, 51*, 199–125.

Kroenke, K., Krebs, E. E., Turk, D., Von Korff, M., Bair, M. J., Allen, K. D., et al. (2019). Core outcome measures for chronic musculoskeletal pain research: recommendations from a Veterans Health Administration work group. *Pain Medicine*, doi: 10.1093/pm/pny279.

Lim, S., Ko, E. M., Shin, D. W., Shin, Y. C., & Oh, K. S. (2015). Clinical symptoms associated with suicidality in patients with panic disorder. *Psychopathology, 48*(3), 137–144.

Metzler, D. H., Mahoney, D., & Freedy, J. R. (2016). Anxiety disorders in primary care. *Primary Care, 43*(2), 245–261.

Meuret, A.E., Kroll, J., Ritz, T. (2017). Panic disorder comorbidity with medical conditions and treatment implications. *Annual Review of Clinical Psychology, 13*, 209–240.

Moitra, E. (2018). Examination of ataque de nervios and ataque de nervios like events in a diverse sample of adults with anxiety disorders. *Depression and Anxiety, 35*(12), 1190–1197.

Olaya, B., Moneta, M. V., Miret, M., Ayuso-Mateos, J. L., & Haro, J. M. (2018). Epidemiology of panic attacks, panic disorder and the moderating role of age: Results from a population-based study. *Journal of Affective Disorders, 241*, 627–633.

Peplau, H. (1989). Theoretic constructs: Anxiety, self, and hallucinations. In A. O'Toole & S. Welt (Eds.). *Interpersonal theory in nursing practice: Selected works of Hildegarde E. Peplau*. New York: Springer.

Pilecki, B., Arentoft, A., & McKay, D. (2011). An evidence-based causal model of panic disorder. *Journal of Anxiety Disorders, 25*(3), 381–388.

Quagliato L. A., Freire R. C., Nardi A. E. (2018). Risks and benefits of medications for panic disorder: A comparison of SSRIs and benzodiazepines. *Expert Opinion on Drug Safety, 17*(3), 315–324.

Quagliato, L. A., & Nardi, A. E. (2018). Cytokine alterations in panic disorder: A systematic review. *Journal of Affective Disorders, 228*, 91–96.

Stein, L. A., Goldmann, E., Zamzam, A., Luciano, J. M., Messé, S. R., Cucchiara, B., et al. (2018). Association between anxiety, depression, and post-traumatic stress disorder and outcomes after ischemic stroke. *Frontiers in Neurology, 9*, 890.

Tully, P. J., & Tzourio, C. (2017). Psychiatric correlates of blood pressure variability in the elderly: The three city cohort study. *Physiology and Behavior, 168*, 91–97.

Zugliani M., Cabo, M. C., Nardi, A. E., Perna, G., & Freire, R. C. (2019). Pharmacological and neuromodulatory treatments for panic disorder: Clinical trials from 2010 to 2018. *Psychiatry Investigation, 16*(1), 50–58.

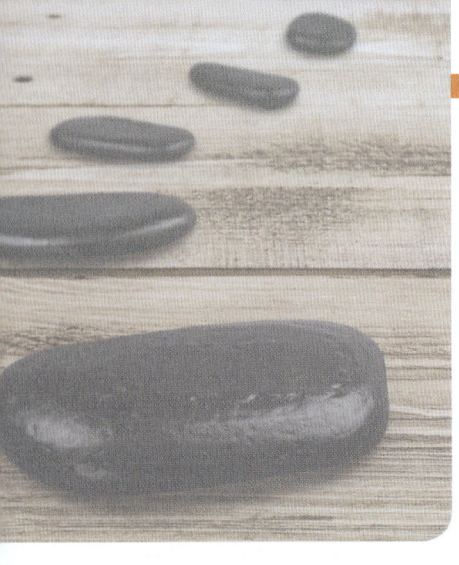

19

Trauma- and Stressor-Related Disorders

Nursing Care of Persons With Posttraumatic Stress and Other Trauma-Related Disorders

Mary Ann Boyd and William Jacobowitz

KEY CONCEPTS
- resilience
- psychological trauma
- traumatic event

LEARNING OBJECTIVES

After studying this chapter, you will be able to:

1. Discuss the role of psychological trauma in mental disorders.
2. Discuss the importance of resilience in prevention of mental disorders.
3. Describe the prevalence and incidence of posttraumatic stress disorder.
4. Delineate clinical symptoms and course of posttraumatic stress disorder.
5. Discuss theories related to posttraumatic stress disorder.
6. Apply nursing process with recovery-oriented interventions for persons with posttraumatic stress disorder.
7. Develop wellness strategies for persons with posttraumatic stress disorder.
8. Discuss the importance of integrated health care.
9. Describe dissociation and dissociative disorders.

KEY TERMS

- depersonalization • derealization • dissociation • emotional reactions • hyperarousal • intrusion • numbing
- posttraumatic stress disorder • psychological trauma • resilience • trauma-informed care • traumatic events

Case Study: Susan

Thirty-year-old Susan is admitted to an inpatient mental health unit following a suicide attempt. Her relationship with her husband has deteriorated since she returned from Iraq 6 months ago. She is overwhelmed by her responsibilities as a parent and wife. She has been diagnosed with posttraumatic stress disorder.

All of us experience stress in our daily lives, but our responses vary from person to person. One person may develop a severe **emotional reaction** (strong agitation of feelings) and another resilient individual is hardly aware of a traumatic event. While most stressful events do not lead to mental disorders, sometimes, emotional problems and mental disorders develop as the response to trauma. This chapter explains the role of **resilience** in buffering the mental health consequences of **psychological trauma** and the nursing care for those who develop trauma- and stressor-related disorders. **Posttraumatic stress disorder (PTSD)** is highlighted in this chapter.

TRAUMA AND RESILIENCE

Trauma can be viewed from several different perspectives. Physical trauma may result from bodily injury resulting from an accident, self-inflicted damage, or violence perpetrated by others. Falls are a leading cause of accidents in the home. Automobile accidents are a major threat to adolescents. Self-inflicted physical trauma is often associated with mental disorders. Physical abuse of intimate partners and elder abuse are nation-wide health problems. Rape and sexual abuse are physically traumatic, and frequently produce psychological trauma.

KEYCONCEPT Psychological trauma is an emotional injury caused by an overwhelmingly stressful event that threatens one's survival and sense of security.

Harassment, embarrassment, child abuse, sexual abuse, employment discrimination, police brutality, bullying, and domestic violence are examples of events that can lead to psychological trauma. Family violence, loss of family members, acts of terrorism, and natural disasters are all **traumatic events**. Exposure to war, natural disasters, and witnessing catastrophic events also may cause psychological trauma.

Not everyone who experiences a traumatic event will be emotionally injured. One explanation for the variability in experiencing psychological trauma is resilience.

Resilience reduces the impact of risk factors and enhances the ability to "bounce back" and recover from stressful experiences. The stronger the resilience, the less likely the individual will experience reactions that lead to maladaptive behaviors and outcomes (Naifeh et al., 2019). An important mental health promotion nursing strategy is enhancing resilience, especially for persons with mental and/or substance abuse problems. See Box 19.1.

Resilience develops in association with a positive self-concept and self-worth, a feeling of being in control of one's life, and a feeling of power. Resilience is acquired over time, beginning in early childhood, as positive problem-solving, communication, and coping skills are learned. Some children seem more resilient to trauma and are able to cope quite well with traumatic events (Mitra & Hodes, 2019). Positive family and community support also play a role in developing resilience.

BOX 19.1 CLINICAL VIGNETTE

Resilience

Joe, a 22-year-old college student, was a victim of an armed robbery. His companion was shot and killed when Joe refused to give the robbers his money. After the incident, he was preoccupied with thoughts of the murder and felt personally responsible for his friend's death.

Joe sought psychological help from the college counseling center. During weekly counseling sessions, Joe was able to reframe his experience. Although he still has brief periods of sadness, he no longer blames himself for his friend's death. He is now resuming his normal activities and is no longer having intrusive thoughts.

KEYCONCEPT Resilience is the capacity to withstand stress and catastrophe. It develops over time and is the culmination of multiple internal and external factors.

OVERVIEW OF TRAUMA- AND STRESSOR-RELATED DISORDERS

Exposure to a traumatic or otherwise stressful event can lead to a trauma- and stressor-related disorder such as reactive attachment disorder, disinhibited social engagement disorder, PTSD, acute stress disorder, and adjustment disorder. This chapter highlights PTSD.

Trauma- and Stressor-Related Disorders Across the Life Span

Trauma- and stressor-related disorders can develop at any time throughout a life span. In children, exposure to trauma can cause enduring emotional problems that lead to any one of these disorders. One of the most traumatic losses for children is an unexpected death of a loved one which can lead to multiple psychiatric disorders (see Chapter 30) (Atwoli et al., 2017).

Childhood psychological and physical abuse including sexual abuse can lead to a lifelong struggle with a trauma- and stressor-related disorder. Adverse childhood experiences are categorized by the CDC–Kaiser ACE study into three groups: abuse (emotional, physical, sexual); household challenges (mother treated violently, household substance abuse, mental illness in household, parental separation or divorce, criminal household member); and neglect (emotional, physical). In this study of 8,667 adult members of an HMO, childhood physical and sexual abuse, as well as witnessing of maternal battering was common. More than one third of the members experienced more than one type of maltreatment. The more frequent and severe the abuse as a child, the greater the PTSD symptoms as an adult (Chang, Jiang, Mkandarwire, & Shen, 2019; Oral et al, 2016).

Military violence is responsible for lifelong effects for deployed service members. There are many reports of older adults who served in World War II developing symptoms of PTSD in later life. There is a growing number of research studies that demonstrate the traumatic impact on children during military deployment and reintegration of their parents (Williamson, Stevelink, Da Silva, & Fear, 2018).

When an older adult experiences trauma, memories of a lifetime of previous traumas and abuse influence the current experience. Loss of partners, friends, and family members through death, marriage, or relocation can add to the trauma. Elder abuse is discussed in Chapter 31.

POSTTRAUMATIC STRESS DISORDER

PTSD occurs following exposure to an actual or threatened traumatic event such as death, serious injury, or sexual violence (National Institute of Mental Health [NIMH], 2019). Traumatic events include those that are directly experienced, witnessed, learned about from others, or due to repeated exposure to aversive events. Examples of traumatic events are violent personal assault, rape, military combat, natural disasters, terrorist attacks, being taken hostage, incarceration as a prisoner of war, torture, an automobile accident, or being diagnosed with a life-threatening illness.

> **KEYCONCEPT Traumatic events** include those that are directly experienced, witnessed, learned about from others, or repeated exposure to adverse events.

Clinical Course

Most people who experience a traumatic event do not develop PTSD. However, for those who do, the symptoms often develop within several days of the event and must persist for a minimum of 30 days in order for the criteria of the diagnosis to be met. In some cases, the symptoms may initially occur substantially after the event, sometimes up to 6 months later. This is known as delayed-onset PTSD (NIMH, 2019). About one third of the persons diagnosed with PTSD develop chronic symptoms. For these individuals, symptoms fluctuate in intensity with time and usually are worse during periods of stress. Children with PTSD may react differently than adults. See Box 19.2.

Diagnostic Criteria

PTSD is diagnosed following exposure to a traumatic event when symptoms in four general areas appear: (1) avoidance such as intrusive symptoms, avoidance of person(s), places, or objects that are a reminder of the traumatic event; (2) negative mood and cognitions or negative thoughts associated with the event; (3) **hyperarousal and reactivity** characterized by aggressive, reckless, or self-destructive behavior; and (4) sleep disturbances or hypervigilance for at least 1 month (NIMH, 2019).

Intrusion

In PTSD, **intrusion** is defined as involuntary appearance of thoughts, memories, or dreams of traumatic events that cause psychological and sometimes physiologic distress. Often the intrusive thoughts are associated with cues that symbolize or resemble the original event. Sometimes, the traumatic images, thoughts, or perceptions are reexperienced, known as flashbacks. Nightmares are common. Intrusive symptoms also include dissociative reactions (i.e., feeling or acting as if the event is reoccurring). Sleeping is difficult. Terrifying flashbacks and nightmares often include fragments of traumatic events exactly as they happened. Many stimuli (e.g., loud noises, odors) associated with the trauma cause flashbacks and dreams. Consequently, affected individuals avoid such stimuli (Brooks, Graham-Kevan, Robinson, & Lowe, 2019).

In children, older than six, repetitive play may occur that expresses the themes or aspects of the traumatic events. They may reenact the specific trauma. Nightmares of these children may not have content (NIMH, 2019).

> **Remember Susan?**
> She suffers from flashbacks of exploding helicopters when she hears loud noises. Her husband tells her she screams while sleeping. She reports frightening nightmares.

Avoidance and Numbing (Dissociative Symptoms)

Individuals with PTSD avoid reminders of the event including people, places, or activities associated with the event (e.g., fireworks may bring back memories of war). Many persons suffering with this disorder escape situations by altering their state of consciousness or **numbing**, by dissociating. **Dissociation** is a disruption in the normally occurring linkages among subjective awareness, feelings, thoughts, behavior, and memories (APA, 2013). A person who dissociates is making himself or herself "disappear." That is, the person has the feeling of leaving his or her body and observing what happens to him or her from a distance. During trauma, dissociation enables a person to observe the event while experiencing no pain or only limited pain and to protect himself or herself from awareness of the full impact of the traumatic event. See Box 19.3. Examples of dissociation include: (1) **derealization** (feelings of unreality) and **depersonalization** (the experience of self or the environment as strange or unreal); (2) periods of disengagement from the

---

BOX 19.2

PTSD Symptoms in Children and Adolescents

PTSD SYMPTOMS IN CHILDREN
- Bedwetting, after they had learned how to use a toilet
- Forgetting how or being unable to talk
- Acting out the scary event during playtime
- Being unusually clingy with a parent or other adults

PTSD SYMPTOMS IN ADOLESCENTS
- May show symptoms similar to adult
- Develop disruptive, disrespectful, or destructive behaviors
- Feel guilty for not preventing injury or death
- Thoughts of revenge

Source: U.S. Department of Health & Human Services (retrieved June 26, 2016, from www.nimh.nih.gov).

BOX 19.3 CLINICAL VIGNETTE

Dissociation

Carol, a 14-year-old high school student, was brutally raped by an older man. When the accused man was arrested, Carol could not recall any part of the attack. Her last memory was walking home after school and seeing a strange man parked on the street.

immediate environment during stress, such as "spacing out"; (3) alterations in bodily perceptions; (4) emotional numbing; (5) out-of-body experiences; and (6) amnesia about abuse-related memories.

Mood and Cognition

After a traumatic event, moods often become more irritable with episodes of explosive anger, fear, guilt, or shame. Individuals with PTSD often have difficulty experiencing positive emotions such as happiness or love. Consequently, they become estranged from loved ones who become frustrated with their family member's unpredictable moods and lack of emotional connection. In PTSD, the thought process becomes distorted with exaggerated negative beliefs or expectations about oneself, others, and the world. They may believe that no one can be trusted or that they are terrible people (NIMH, 2019).

Hyperarousal

After a traumatic experience, the stress system seems to go on permanent alert, as if the danger might return at any time. In this state of physiologic hyperarousal, the traumatized person is hypervigilant for signs of danger, startles easily, reacts irritably to small annoyances, and sleeps poorly. The state of hyperarousal causes other problems for family members. The affected individual is irritable and overreacts to others which cause others to avoid the person who in turn maintains a state of continual arousal (Marshall et al., 2019).

Susan and Her Family
Susan feels she does not fit into the family and no longer believes she has a role as a wife and mother. She is extremely irritable and argues with her husband constantly. She is suspicious of her neighbors and fearful that her children will be kidnapped.

Diagnostic Criteria for Children 6 Years and Younger

In children 6 years and younger, exposure to actual or threatened death, serious injury, or sexual violence may result in PTSD. The symptoms include recurrent, involuntary, and intrusive distressing memories of the events. These memories may not appear distressing and may be expressed as play. The child may not be able to explain or remember the content of the distressing dreams related to the event. For a child 6 years and under to be diagnosed with PTSD, one of the following symptoms must be present for at least 1 month and not related to physiologic changes caused by medication or illness: avoidance of stimuli or negative cognitions/mood associated with the traumatic event, irritable behavior and angry outbursts after the event with little or no provocation, or clinically significant distress (NIMH, 2019).

Epidemiology and Risk Factors

The lifetime prevalence of PTSD ranges from 6.1% to 9.2% in the United States and Canada. The type of trauma a person experiences is related to the probability of PTSD occurring. For example, in sexual relationship violence, there is a 33% probability that PTSD will occur compared to exposure to organized violence, such as a civilian in a war zone, of 3%. Risk factors for PTSD include a prior diagnosis of acute stress disorder; the extent, duration, and intensity of trauma involved; and environmental factors. High levels of anxiety, low self-esteem, and existing personality difficulties may increase the likelihood that PTSD will develop (Sareen, 2019).

PTSD varies among both genders. Women are approximately twice as likely as men to experience PTSD; the median time from onset to remission for women is 4 years compared with 1 year for men. Several factors may contribute to these differences. Men and women experience different types of traumatic events. More men report exposure to events such as fires or disasters, life-threatening accidents, physical assault, combat, being threatened with a weapon, and being held captive. More women report anxiety and depressive disorders, child abuse, sexual molestation, sexual assault, and traumatic events before the age of 18 years (Mota et al., 2019).

Consider This:
Susan was exposed to exploding improvised explosive devices (IEDs) while serving in Iraq. Between the ages of 6 to 9 years old, she was sexually abused by an uncle. She never told anyone.

PTSD symptoms in women who are sexually assaulted may vary based on their age at the time of the first sexual assault (Angelone, Marcantonio, Melillo, 2018). See Box 19.4. In a landmark study, childhood cancer survivors have been found to have four times the risk of developing

> **BOX 19.4**
>
> **Research for Best Practice: PTSD and Risky Sexual Behavior**
>
> Weiss et al. (2019). A longitudinal examination of posttraumatic stress disorder symptoms and risky sexual behavior: Evaluating emotion dysregulation dimensions as mediators. *Archives of Sexual Behavior, 48*(3), 975–986.
>
> **THE QUESTION:** Are PTSD symptoms a predictor of risky sexual behavior among trauma-exposed community women? Is emotional dysregulation a factor in risky sexual behavior?
>
> **METHODS:** A convenience sample of 491 women 18–25 recruited from four sites in the southern and midwestern United States completed 5 assessments every 4 months for a 16-month period. The assessments included: (1) traumatic exposure, (2) PTSD symptoms, (3) emotion dysregulation (inability to accept negative emotion ["When upset, I become angry at self for feeling that way"], difficulties engaging in goal-directed behaviors when distressed, difficulties controlling impulsive behaviors, limited strategies to regulate emotion, lack of emotional awareness and clarity), (4) risky sexual behavior (number of different vaginal sexual partners, number of instances of condomless sex, number of instance of risky/impulsive sexual behavior such as sex in exchange for money, drugs).
>
> **FINDINGS:** Women who were unable to accept their own negative feelings (i.e., they felt they should not be angry or upset) were more likely to be distressed and engage in risky sexual behavior to reduce the negative affect of the emotion and PTSD symptoms. Women who experienced difficulties controlling impulsive behavior would be more likely to engage in risky sexual behavior.
>
> **IMPLICATIONS FOR NURSING:** Early intervention in primary care and school settings for girls and women who are victims of sexual assault may prevent future revictimization and PTSD.

PTSD as their siblings (Oral et al., 2016). Similarly, high rates of PTSD have been reported among patients with alcohol and drug dependence who have experienced childhood abuse (Brown, Perera, Masho, Mezuk, & Cohen, 2015; Cavanaugh, Petras, & Martins, 2015).

However, high rates of PTSD in veterans returning from Iraq and Afghanistan are unprecedented in modern times. PTSD prevalence estimates range from 0% to 48% in males and from 2% to 68% in women (Ramchand, Rudavsky, Grant, Tanielian, & Jaycox, 2015). PTSD is more prevalent in the army, among enlisted personnel when compared to officers, and more common among health care occupations, combat specialists, and service and supply personnel. PTSD is predicted by prior stressors, childhood adversity and vulnerability, and predeployment symptoms. PTSD in veterans is associated with postdeployment violence and alcohol misuse. They are high risk for suicide (Ramchand et al., 2015).

Etiology

A growing body of research postulates that biologic factors, including neurobiology and genetics, interact with environmental factors, such as childhood experiences, and the severity and extent of the traumatic exposure, to affect susceptibility to PTSD. The amygdala and hippocampus appear to be important players in fear conditioning along with the thalamus, locus coeruleus, and sensory cortex. Interaction between the cortex and the amygdala may be necessary for specific stimuli to elicit traumatic memories (Lori et al., 2019).

Several neurochemical systems are involved in regulating fear conditioning, including norepinephrine, dopamine, opiate, and corticotropin-releasing systems. Hyperarousal symptoms are characteristic of increased noradrenergic function, particularly in the locus coeruleus and in the limbic system (hypothalamus, hippocampus, and amygdala), and of increased dopamine activity, particularly in the prefrontal–cortical systems (Malikowsa-Racia & Salat, 2019).

Behavioral sensitization may be one mechanism underlying the hyperarousal seen in PTSD. The sensitized person reacts with a magnified stress response to later, milder stressors. Research shows that traumatic exposure can alter neurotransmitter connectivity in the frontal areas resulting in severe reaction to a minor stressor. This finding would account for the fact that some individuals with PTSD experience intense fear, anxiety, and panic in response to minor stimuli. One example of behavioral sensitization is that PTSD after combat exposure is more likely to develop in veterans who are survivors of childhood abuse than in those who have not experienced prior trauma (Brown et al., 2015; Sadeh et al., 2015).

Recovery-Oriented Care for Persons With PTSD

Recovery from PTSD takes time and involves support and patience from the family and friends, as well as a team of health care providers. **Trauma-informed care** is important in supporting recovery and includes an understanding of trauma and an awareness of the impact it can have across settings, services, and populations (Substance Abuse and Mental Health Services Administration [SAMHSA], 2014). Early recognition of the symptoms and treatment lead to a more successful outcomes with less likelihood of major complications. It is important to understand that there are several paths to recovery.

Teamwork and Collaboration: Working Toward Recovery

Major approaches to the treatment of PTSD include pharmacotherapy and psychotherapy. The selection of treatment is guided by practice guidelines that recommend various interventions based on medical and functional status, pre-existing psychiatric and medical conditions, and current mental health assessment. The treatment guidelines, developed by the Department of Veterans Affairs and Department of Defense with the support of the Institute of Medicine, recommend education, brief psychotherapy sessions, and acute symptom management (sleep disturbance, hyperarousal, pain) for an acute reaction. During an acute reaction, psychological debriefing is not recommended. For treatment of more chronic symptoms, trauma-focused therapy and stress management are recommended along with medication (Department of VA & DOD, 2017).

The selective serotonin reuptake inhibitors (SSRIs), serotonin–norepinephrine reuptake inhibitors (SNRIs), benzodiazepines, and β-blockers may be effective in reducing the symptoms of PTSD. Recently, off-label use of prazosin, an alpha$_1$ inhibitor, has been shown to be effective in treating nightmares and improving sleep in PTSD (El-Solh, 2018). When prescribed in conjunction with psychotherapy, pharmacotherapy can minimize the excessive fear and anxiety of PTSD (Grasser & Javanbakht, 2019).

Psychotherapeutic approaches to the treatment of patients with PTSD include psychodynamic psychotherapy; cognitive behavioral therapy (CBT); and eye movement, desensitization, and reprocessing (EMDR). *Psychodynamic psychotherapy* focuses on different factors that may influence current PTSD symptoms such as early childhood experience and current relationships. There is emphasis on the unconscious mind. *CBTs* focus on the evaluation of situations, thoughts, feelings, and the problematic ways these evaluations cause a person to act. See Box 19.5.

EDMR is a process of reviewing and visualizing disturbing memories of traumatic or distressing experiences to reduce the long-term impact of the events. The patient is guided through images of the trauma, allowing for progressive desensitization. Under deep relaxation, the patient maintains an image of the traumatic event while focusing on the lateral movement of the clinician's finger. This recent approach has been successful in minimizing the fear response and avoidance pattern of those with PTSD (El-Solh, 2018). Virtual Reality Exposure Therapy (VRET), the use of a virtual environment to facilitate emotional process of memories related to the trauma, is being used in some treatment settings (Buck, Norr, Katz, Gahm, & Reger, 2018).

Group therapy and family therapy should also be considered in the treatment of those with PTSD. Sharing the traumatic experiences with family or with others who have experienced trauma can be both supportive and therapeutic. PTSD disrupts both the life of the patient and his or her significant others. Social support is a protective factor in the development of the disorder, and patients who have PTSD can benefit from tangible social support they receive from spouses, family, and friends (Han et al., 2018).

One of the greatest treatment challenges is avoiding secondary trauma. Hospitalization and restrictive treatment can retraumatize the patient. Being locked in a mental health unit or being restrained can be extremely traumatizing to the person who has already been traumatized.

BOX 19.5
Cognitive Behavioral Therapies

THERAPY	PURPOSE
Exposure Therapy	Helps people face and control their fear by exposing them to the trauma in a safe way. Strategies are mental imagery, writing, or visits to the place where the event happened.
Cognitive Restructuring	Helps people make sense of the bad memories by reframing their experiences in a more realistic way. They may feel guilt or shame about what is not their fault.
Cognitive Processing Therapy	Helps people understand why recovery from traumatic events has been difficult and how symptoms of PTSD affect daily life. Focus is on identifying how traumatic experiences changed thoughts and beliefs and influenced current feelings and behaviors.
Stress Inoculation Training	Teaches a person how to reduce anxiety. Like cognitive restructuring, this treatment helps people look at their memories in a healthy way.

Integration of Primary Care

The persons with PTSD may first seek help from a primary care provider. For example, sleep problems in adults and behavior problems of children are often treated in a nonmental health environment. Conversely, when mental health clinicians care for persons with PTSD, they must address the physical problems as well as their psychological problems. Because there is no one medication indicated for PTSD, there is a risk of multiple medications being prescribed to treat various physical and mental health problems. Ideally, individuals with PTSD should be treated in an integrated setting where close monitoring of all treatments is possible.

Safety Issues

PTSD is associated with an increased risk of suicide, suicide attempts, aggression, and substance abuse

(Ramchand et al., 2015). The first contact the nurse often has with the patient is after a suicide attempt or an aggressive episode. A careful assessment should include determination of the risk for self-injury or aggression toward others. These individuals are at high risk for substance abuse and suicide, so that a suicide risk assessment should be included in the nursing assessment. Safety measures such as suicide precautions may be needed, particularly if the person is hospitalized.

Evidence-Based Nursing Care for Persons With PTSD

Patients with PTSD receive nursing services in a variety of settings throughout the continuum of care. Many will access care through a primary care setting and others will seek out services in a mental health or primary health clinic. In many instances, the patient is reluctant to disclose information and has a difficult time trusting others. Distrust is especially common in persons whose trauma is associated with a violation of trust such as a rape. Gaining the patient's trust through a warm, empathic interaction, for example, offering the patient the opportunity to talk about the trauma without pressing them on the details, can lead to a meaningful therapeutic relationship.

Mental Health Nursing Assessment

After the physical health needs are met and suicidal/aggressive safety measures are established, the mental health nursing assessment targets specific areas. These include identification of the original trauma, specific physical symptoms, and the emotional and behavioral consequences of the patient's PTSD. The nursing assessment is best conducted through an interview to identify the impact of the trauma and the individual's physical and psychological strengths. The full assessment may need to take place over the course of one or more meetings, depending on the patient's capacity to discuss the traumatic events and sequelae without emotionally reexperiencing the trauma (retraumatization).

Trauma

Identifying the original trauma establishes the nature of the trauma and the length of time that the patient's PTSD has been present. However, if the person does not want to talk about the details of the trauma, the nurse should not pursue the topic. The meaning of the trauma to the individual is much more important than what happened. The survivor of trauma may be seeking help for the consequences of the trauma and is unable to discuss the original trauma. If the person wants to share information related to the traumatic experience, the following questions can be used in the assessment:

- In what ways has your life been different since the trauma?
- What does the trauma mean to you?
- Do you feel that you are the same person now as you were before the trauma? How are you the same? How are you different?
- Did anyone help you? Who are the supportive people in your life?
- Were you a survivor of trauma or abuse prior to the trauma associated with PTSD?

Physical Health Assessment

The assessment should not only focus on the physical problems, but also on healthy aspects. For example, nutrition, exercise, and self-care, such as hobbies and leisure activities may be the individual's strengths. The assessment process should be similar to the one described in Chapter 10.

Sleep: In PTSD, sleep is often disrupted or practically nonexistent. Disturbing nightmares are common. The nurse should compare sleep patterns before and after the trauma. Insomnia is typically characterized by difficulty falling asleep, fragmented sleep, or panic-like awakenings. The nurse should also assess for nightmares including frequency and intensity. Family members may be able to provide detailed information that is out of the patient's awareness.

Substance Use: Commonly, individuals with PTSD self-medicate to relieve the discomfort, anxiety, or pain caused by the trauma. The use of alcohol or other drugs is common. Assessment of the use of substances and the frequency will give direction for interventions.

> **Consider This:**
>
> Susan started drinking alcohol regularly in Iraq. After returning home, she continued to drink six to eight cans of beer every day.

Pain: The original trauma may result in chronic pain. For example, physical abuse or wartime injury may result in long-term physical treatment and pain. Prescribed pain medication is often used for reasons other than those for which it was prescribed. For example, a co-occurring traumatic brain injury may be present.

Other Somatic Responses: Patients with PTSD often have multiple unexplained physical problems (e.g., gastrointestinal, cardiovascular, neurologic, and musculoskeletal symptoms). Sometimes the patient is reluctant to admit a trauma such as a rape or domestic assault and instead seeks out medical care for physical problems.

> **BOX 19.6 CLINICAL VIGNETTE**
>
> **Survivor Guilt**
>
> A 92-year-old survivor of World War II concentration camps has suffered from depression most of his adult life. When admitted to a long-term care facility, his daughter told the nurse that her dad often had bouts of depression where he would bemoan the fact that he had lived and his parents and siblings had not. He often told his daughter that he felt guilty because he had survived the holocaust.

Obtaining a trauma history becomes very important when multiple physical symptoms are present.

Psychosocial Assessment

The focus of the psychosocial assessment is identifying the severity of the PTSD symptoms, the disruptions that these symptoms cause the affected individual and family and current coping approaches. The patient should be asked about intrusive thoughts, irritable moods, negative thoughts, avoidance behaviors, and arousal behaviors, and what impact they have on their daily lives.

In PTSD, guilt, shame, and depression are often present. Guilt may relate to feeling responsible for the events that led up to the trauma. Survivor guilt occurs when one person survives a traumatic event when others do not. See Box 19.6. Assessing self-esteem and self-concept will provide clues to the patient's resilience. See Chapter 10. A family assessment focusing on any changes in family dynamics that has occurred since the traumatic event should also be included.

The amount of daily stress can impact the ability of the person to manage PTSD symptoms. The individual may notice that the PTSD symptoms are worse on certain days or during certain circumstances. For example, one nurse noticed her hypervigilance was worse after working the night shift for several days. These stresses should be linked to the person's current coping skills which may be positive (meditation, relaxation) or negative (use of substances).

The nurse and the patient should discuss whether current coping skills are effective. Some coping skills may be effective immediately, but have negative consequences such as the use of substances. Developing new coping skills may be important in order to have both immediate relief and positive consequences.

Strengths Assessment

Throughout the assessment, the nurse should be listening for evidence of individual physical and psychosocial strengths. Was the patient physically healthy before the traumatic event occurred? How does the patient cope with the stress of the trauma? Does the patient have family or friends who can support the individual? Is the patient motivated to deal with PTSD symptoms, develop new coping strategies, and engage in a collaborative, therapeutic relationship? Are there financial or social resources available? This information can be used in helping patient develop a safety and recovery plan.

Priority of Nursing Care

The first priority is safety. If there is a risk for suicide, the nurse and patient should first begin to address these ideations and behaviors. For someone who has been traumatized and, as a result, developed PTSD, the nurse and patient can establish a recovery plan that addresses any areas that interfere with coping such as feelings of anxiety, hopelessness, and powerlessness. For some individuals, a loss of impulse control that results in angry outbursts or aggressive behavior characterizes their difficulty with their quality of life and well-being.

Therapeutic Relationship

Establishing a trusting relationship with a person with PTSD is the basis of nurse–patient collaboration. Needs and safety are defined by the survivor who chooses the help that is wanted. Developing a relationship may take time because many survivors have had their trust violated during the traumatic event. See Box 19.7. Trauma can have a lasting effect on the ability to trust others and form intimate relationships. Coping behaviors may be misinterpreted as being "noncompliant" and can lead to negative reactions by health care providers.

Mental Health Nursing Interventions

Trauma is linked to health challenges over the life span. Adverse childhood experiences can lead to physiologic changes that lead to long-term health and social problems. When caring for an individual with PTSD, the impact of the trauma should be considered. Survivors of trauma may respond to the present through the lenses of their past.

Establishing Mental Health and Wellness Goals

The nurse needs to guide the patient in prioritizing goals. It is unrealistic to expect the patient to work on all goals at a time. Trauma can leave people feeling powerless. For example, one place to start is with reestablishing reasonable eating and sleeping patterns. By introducing small changes, the patient will be able to determine which interventions are likely to be effective.

Wellness Strategies

Many of the wellness strategies are interventions to treatment the symptoms of PTSD. For example, sleep hygiene

BOX 19.7 • THERAPEUTIC DIALOGUE • Approaching Susan

Susan did not want to be admitted to the inpatient unit and reported that she did not want to live. Her husband wants Susan to forget about Iraq and return to her former self. When she arrived on the unit, she was asked several assessment questions. She did not want to tell her story again to the nurse. The nurse needed to complete the admission assessment.

INEFFECTIVE APPROACH

Nurse: Susan, I need to ask you some questions.
Susan: Can't it wait?
Nurse: Oh—unfortunately I have to ask questions.
Susan: I am tired of talking. Everyone is asking the same questions. For the record, I do not have a problem, I do not drink too much, and I wish my husband would go away.
Nurse: Your husband is a nice guy and is only trying to help.
Susan: You do not know what you are talking about. He wants to control me.
Nurse: If you just answer some questions, I can finish my assessment.
Susan: Not now. Go away.

EFFECTIVE APPROACH

Nurse: Hi Susan, my name is Jane, and I am your nurse today.
Susan: What do you want? I don't need a nurse.
Nurse: Well, we can just talk. What brought you here?
Susan: I am tired of talking. Everyone is asking the same questions. For the record, I do not have a problem, I do not drink too much, and I wish my husband would go away.
Nurse: Talking can be tiring. What questions have you been asked?
Susan: My whole life story—where I grew up, when I got married, how do I get along with my husband and children, what happened in Iraq?
Nurse: You have had a lot of questions since you have been here. How were you able to answer all those questions?
Susan: The worst questions were about abuse and Iraq. I don't think I can talk about that yet.
Nurse: Why don't we stick to the easier ones for now?
Susan: OK, I can try.

CRITICAL THINKING CHALLENGE

- What ineffective techniques did the nurse use in the first scenario? Whose needs was the nurse meeting?
- What effective techniques did the nurse use in the second scenario?

is important for those with sleep problems. Managing stress is very important for a person with this disorder. Practicing healthy stress management techniques are critical for handling the events related to hyperarousal. An innocent loud noise may be misinterpreted as a gunshot causing an aggressive response. Exercise helps reduce stress and supports healthy functioning.

Physical Health Interventions

Many of the same nursing interventions discussed in Chapter 18 are used with the person with PTSD. Proper nutrition and regular exercise can help fortify the resilience.

Sleep Enhancement. Sleep hygiene is also an important strategy because sleep disruption is common in PTSD. Early life adversity and PTSD severity are associated with fewer hours of resting and sleeping when compared to those who had lower early life adversity (see Chapter 28) (Gavrieli, Farr, Davis, Crowell, & Mantzoros, 2015). Nurses should collaborate with the patient in finding a strategy that will help the person sleep and manage nightmares. For example, the individual may want to sleep with the lights on because of the nightmares. However, light interferes with nighttime sleep for some people. It may be possible to go to sleep with the lights on, but to ask a family member to turn off the lights later. Some persons with PTSD find that they cannot sleep in their bed, but can sleep in a chair. Some of the following strategies may be helpful:

- Establish and maintain a regular bedtime and rising time.
- Avoid naps.
- Abstain from alcohol. Although alcohol may assist with sleep onset, an alerting effect occurs when it wears off.
- Refrain from caffeine after midafternoon. Avoid nicotine before bedtime and during the night. Caffeine and nicotine are strong stimulants and cause fragmented sleep.
- Avoid exercising 3 hours before bedtime.

Exercise and Yoga. Severe PTSD symptoms are associated with poor physical performance and physical function decrease (Hall et al., 2014). Yet, we know that exercise is associated with reduced PTSD symptoms (Ströhle, 2018). Nurses need to encourage patients with PTSD to engage in regular exercise, not only for health promotion, but also to reduce symptoms. Practicing yoga may motivate people with PTSD to increase physical activity along with enhancing self-efficacy. Simple stretching and breathing has shown to reduce abnormal cortisol levels and can be taught in many practice settings (Niles et al., 2018).

Nutrition Interventions. PTSD and early life adversity are associated with risk of obesity, diabetes, and cardiovascular disease. The greater the symptoms the higher the body weight and blood pressure and lower the insulin sensitivity (Farr et al., 2015). Poor diet quality including the consumption of *trans* fatty acids can be a major health issue with these individuals. Monitoring body weight and blood pressure should be included in the patient's plan of care. If these health issues are present, nurses should encourage patients to make different food choices and choosing healthy foods. Referral to a dietician may be necessary.

Smoking Cessation. Individuals with PTSD have higher smoking rates than others and fewer have quit than the general population. Smoking serves as a way of coping with the symptoms of PTSD. Smoking often co-occurs with alcohol use disorders and cannabis use. Nurses should discuss the health risks associated with these behaviors and encourage the patient to reduce their use. Smoking cessation programs are readily available in most communities (Homish, Hoopsick, Heavey, Homish, & Cornelius, 2019).

Medication Interventions

Two SSRI antidepressants, sertraline (Zoloft) and paroxetine (Paxil), are approved for PTSD and are used to treat symptoms such as sadness, worry, anger, and feeling numb inside. See Box 19.8.

Because the person with PTSD may take many different types of medication, the nurse needs to monitor for any drug interactions and teach the person about all the medications including expected therapeutic effect(s) and side effects. These individuals often take prescribed or over-the-counter (OTC) pain medications that may interact with mood stabilizers, antidepressants, antianxiety agents, or antipsychotic agents.

Substance Abuse Interventions. If the person has been using substances to dull the feelings associated with the trauma, the nurse should educate the individual about the addiction and make a referral to a substance abuse treatment team. It is important for the nurse to

---

BOX 19.8

Drug Profile: Sertraline (Zoloft)

DRUG CLASS: Antidepressant (selective serotonin reuptake inhibitor [SSRI])

RECEPTOR AFFINITY: Blocks the reuptake of serotonin

INDICATIONS: Major depressive disorder, obsessive–compulsive disorder, panic disorder, posttraumatic stress disorder, premenstrual dysphoric disorder, social anxiety disorder

ROUTES AND DOSAGES: Available in 25-mg, 50-mg, 100-mg tablets, 20 mg/mL

Adults: 50–200 mg PO once daily; start 50 mg PO once daily, may increase by 50 mg/day

HALF-LIFE (PEAK EFFECT): 62–104 hours

SELECTED ADVERSE REACTIONS: Nausea, headache, insomnia, diarrhea, dry mouth, ejaculatory dysfunction, somnolence, weakness, lack of energy, tremor, dyspepsia, anorexia, constipation, decrease in libido, nervousness, anxiety, rash, visual disturbance

WARNINGS: Increase suicidality risk in children, adolescents, and young adults with major depressive or other psychiatric disorders. Contradicted in persons being treated with monoamine oxidase inhibitors and pimozide, an antipsychotic. Risk for serotonin syndrome.

SPECIFIC PATIENT AND FAMILY EDUCATION

- Take exactly as prescribed
- Can be taken with or without food
- If a dose is missed, take missed dose as soon as patient remembers unless time for next dose; then skip missed dose
- Can cause sleepiness or may affect ability to make decisions, think clearly, or react quickly
- Do not drive, operate heavy machinery until patient knows how medication will affect him or her
- Do not drink alcohol while taking medication
- Report any signs and symptoms of adverse reactions, suicidal thoughts, or actions
- Notify your health care provider if severe agitation, hallucinations, coordination problems, muscle twitching, racing heartbeat, high or low blood pressure, muscle rigidity, sweating or fever, nausea, vomiting, diarrhea occur

use a nonjudgmental approach, recognizing the person is suffering from the trauma and is trying to cope with intrusive thoughts and pain. The nurse should emphasize that there are more effective coping mechanisms and offer hope that the person can find other means of alleviating the PTSD symptoms.

Psychosocial Nursing Interventions

Many of the same psychosocial interventions discussed in Chapter 18 can be used for persons with PTSD. Relaxation strategies and stress reduction techniques are particularly helpful for these individuals. Encouraging the person to participate in a support group can decrease the isolation that may be present and learn how others deal with their symptoms. Service and companion dogs are also helpful in helping the person address the stress of PTSD.

Trauma-Informed Care

When caring for persons with PTSD, we should assume that they have a history of traumatic stress. Extreme stress occurs when shocking or unexpected events overwhelm a person's ability to cope. Trauma-informed care considers the events and circumstances causing the trauma, the person's experience of these events, and the effects of the trauma (SAMHSA, 2014). The nurse should respect how and when a person chooses to talk about the trauma. Healing from trauma requires finding and maintaining a sense of safety, gaining a sense of control over one's life and environment.

The focus of the interactions should be on understanding "what happened," not on what is wrong with the person. The nurse seeks to understand the meaning of the experience to the individual. Similar events have different meanings to different people. When patients are describing traumatic events, it is important for the nurse to avoid responding in shock, dismay, or disgust. A welcoming approach creates a safe environment for the person to discuss the trauma. Within a collaborative relationship, coping strategies, not symptoms, are the focus. In safe environment, the person can develop positive coping skills and make sense of who they are.

Psychoeducation

PTSD impacts every aspect of a person's life. Trauma, genetic predisposition, brain changes, risk for multiple health problems, and risk for addiction are a part of PTSD. Education about the disorder, its consequences, health risks, and treatment become key topics for patient and family education. Psychoeducation should be individualized to the person's specific issues. There are general psychoeducation topics that should be considered for patient teaching. See Box 19.9.

> **BOX 19.9**
>
> **Psychoeducation Checklist: Posttraumatic Stress Disorder**
>
> When caring for a person with a PTSD, be sure to include the following topic areas in the teaching plan:
> - Identification of individual triggers and cues that lead to reexperiencing trauma
> - Safety plans for stressful periods
> - Recovery plans that focus on personal strengths
> - Risk factors for reoccurrence of symptoms
> - Various treatment options: if one does not help, others exist
> - Avoid substances such as alcohol and drugs
> - Nutrition
> - Exercise
> - Sleep hygiene
> - Follow-up appointments
> - Community services

Evaluation and Treatment Outcomes

The treatment of PTSD may last several years with changing goals. Early in treatment, the goals may be to reduce the intrusive thoughts and regulate sleep; later goals may include being able to establish a trusting relationship with a partner. The evaluation will be modified as the goals and interventions change.

Continuum of Care

The person with PTSD is primarily treated in the community rather than a medical facility as an inpatient. Short-term hospitalization for safety may be needed if suicidal or homicidal thoughts are strong or for an adjustment of medication.

Family Interventions

Families need support as they learn to cope with their family member with PTSD. Family members often feel hopeless in trying to understand the changes that their loved one is undergoing. In many instances, the member with PTSD is unable to share information about the trauma and the symptoms. If alcohol or other drugs are used to self-medicate, the family has additional challenges in dealing with the substance use. Support groups, education about PTSD, and family therapy are helpful.

Emergency Care

When individuals with PTSD need emergency care, they are usually having suicidal ideation or thoughts to hurt others. Safety interventions should be implemented. It is important for the nurse to know the nature of the trauma to be able to approach the patient. For example, a person previously exposed to combat may be sensitive to loud noises and is more likely to become aggressive when doors slam, whereas a woman who has been raped may not tolerate anyone touching her.

Inpatient-Focused Care

Inpatient settings provide a safe environment for the person who is tormented with frequent flashbacks, has become depressed and potentially suicidal, or is harboring thoughts about hurting others. Medications may be initiated or adjusted. See the Nursing Care Plan 19.1—which sets forth a plan of care for Susan, the case study patient in this chapter—is available at http://thepoint.lww.com/BoydEssentials2e.

Community Treatment

Treatment mostly occurs in the community with the individual attending group therapy, support groups, individual therapy, and medication management. Most appointments will occur after working hours. Nursing care can be delivered in all settings. The community setting is an excellent opportunity for patient and family education.

DISSOCIATIVE DISORDERS

Dissociative disorders are thought to be responses to extreme external or internal events or stressors where dissociation, or a splitting from the self, occurs as a way of coping with severe anxiety. Prevalence is higher among people who experience childhood physical or sexual abuse than among others. The onset of these disorders may be sudden or may occur gradually; the course of each may be long term or transient. Dissociative disorders include *dissociative amnesia*, the inability to recall important yet stressful information; *depersonalization/derealization disorder*, the feeling of being detached from one's mental processes; and *dissociative identity disorder* (DID) (formerly called multiple personality disorder), presence of at least two distinct personality or identity states.

The essential feature of these disorders involves a failure to integrate identity, memory, and consciousness. That is, unwanted intrusive thoughts disrupt one's contact with the here and now or memories that are normally accessible are lost. These disorders are closely related to the trauma- and stressor-related disorders but are categorized separately. Persons with dissociative disorders may also have comorbid substance abuse, mood disorders, personality disorders, or PTSD (APA, 2013).

DID has long been a controversial diagnosis, with many skeptics challenging the legitimacy of this disorder. Recent empirical evidence supports DID as a complex, posttraumatic developmental disorder. Once believed to be relatively rare, prevalence rates are reported at approximately 1.1% to 1.5% of community samples. The highest prevalence is found in groups highly exposed to trauma or cultural oppression (Brand et al., 2016). There is also emerging evidence that there are structural brain changes in persons with this disorder (Reinders et al., 2018).

Treatment options include the use of antidepressants to treat the patient's underlying mood and anxiety. Psychotherapy options include CBT, and psychodynamic psychotherapy to determine the triggers that lead to heightened anxiety and dissociation.

OTHER TRAUMA- AND STRESSOR-RELATED DISORDERS

Acute stress disorder is similar to PTSD except that it is resolved within 1 month of the traumatic event. Acute stress disorder can develop into PTSD if the symptoms last longer than 1 month. Two trauma- and stressor-related disorders typically occurring in childhood are reactive attachment disorder and disinhibited social engagement disorder. *Reactive attachment disorder* is characterized by inhibited, emotionally withdrawn behavior toward an adult caregiver. These children rarely seek or respond to comfort when distressed. This disorder usually occurs when the primary caregiver frequently changes. In *disinhibited social engagement disorder*, the child is overly familiar with others in ways uncharacteristic of cultural norms. For instance, the child does not hesitate to go somewhere with an unfamiliar adult.

One of the most common diagnoses for hospitalized persons is adjustment disorder (APA, 2013). These disorders occur within 3 months of the stressor. Affected individuals experience distress that seems out of proportion to the severity of the stressor and may be unable to function socially. After the situation is resolved, the symptoms subside.

SUMMARY OF KEY POINTS

- The development of psychological trauma depends on the meaning of the event and the resilience of the individual. The stronger the resilience, the more likely the individual will be able to withstand the negative impact of a potentially traumatic event.

- Resilience develops over time when there are positive self-concept and measured self-worth, and when problem-solving, communication, and coping skills have been learned.

- PTSD occurs after a traumatic event and is characterized by involuntary intrusive thoughts, avoidance and numbing, negative moods and thoughts, and hyperarousal.
- Women are twice as likely as men to experience PTSD. Service members returning from Iraq and Afghanistan have high rates of PTSD.
- There are several approaches to the treatment of PTSD including CBT, traditional psychotherapy, and medications.
- Nursing care focuses on assessing symptoms of PTSD, building strengths, and collaborating with the patient in counseling interventions, administration of medication, psychoeducation, and family support.

CRITICAL THINKING CHALLENGES

1. What are the various traumatic events that can lead to PTSD? Why do some people develop PTSD and others, who have experienced the same trauma, do not?
2. Identify strategies the nurse can use to support the development of resilience.
3. Differentiate intrusive thoughts from dissociative symptoms.
4. Give examples of derealization and depersonalization.
5. Compare trauma- and stressor-related disorders with dissociative disorders. How are they similar? How are they different?
6. How should a nurse approach a military veteran who is having intrusive thoughts, nightmares, and is unable to sleep?

2010: *The Dry Land*

James (Ryan O'Nan), an Iraq war veteran, returns to his small-town life in Texas. His family quickly realizes that he has changed and has PTSD. He is irritable, anxious, and considers suicide. He keeps a gun at his bedside. He drinks with his friends and is easily provoked into fights. His family cannot truly understand the pain he feels. An award-winning movie, it depicts a veteran's struggle with regaining his life.

Viewing Points: Identify the behaviors that are characteristic of PTSD. Identify the strengths that he demonstrated that represented resilience. Develop a plan of care that includes his family, friends, and community support.

REFERENCES

American Psychiatric Association. (2013). *Diagnostic and statistical manual of mental disorders DSM-5* (5th ed.). Arlington, VA: Author.

Angelone, D. J., Marcantonio, T., Melillo, J. (2018). An evaluation of adolescent and young adult (re)victimization experiences: Problematic substance use and negative consequences. *Violence Against Women*, 24(5), 586–602.

Atwoli, L., Stein, D. J., King, A., Petukhova, M., Aguilar-Gaxiola, S., Alonso, J., et al. (2017). Posttraumatic stress disorder associated with unexpected death of a loved one: Cross-national findings from the world mental health surveys. *Depression and Anxiety*, 34(4), 315–326.

Brand, B. L., Sar, V., Stavropoulos, P., Krüger, C., Korzekwa, M., Martínez-Taboas, A., et al. (2016). Separating fact from fiction: An empirical examination of six myths about dissociative identity disorder. *Harvard Review of Psychiatry*, 24(4), 257–270.

Brooks, M., Graham-Kevan, N., Robinson, S., & Lowe, M. (2019). Trauma characteristics and posttraumatic growth: The mediating role of avoidance coping, intrusive thoughts, and social support. *Psychological Trauma: Theory, Research, Practice, and Policy*, 11(2), 232–238.

Brown, M. J., Perera, R. A., Masho, S. W., Mezuk, B., & Cohen, S. A. (2015). Adverse childhood experiences and intimate partner aggression in the US: Sex differences and similarities in psychosocial mediation. *Social Science and Medicine*, 131, 48–57.

Buck, B., Norr, A., Katz, A., Gahm, G. A., & Reger, G. M. (2018). Reductions in reported persecutory ideation and psychotic-like experiences during exposure therapy for posttraumatic stress disorder. *Psychiatry Research*, 12, 272, 190–195.

Cavanaugh, C. E., Petras, H., & Martins, S. S. (2015). Gender-specific profiles of adverse childhood experiences, past year mental and substance use disorders, and their association among a national sample of adults in the United States. *Social Psychiatry and Psychiatric Epidemiology*, 50(8), 1257–1266.

Chang, X., Jiang, X., Mkandarwire, T., & Shen, M. (2019). Associations between adverse childhood experiences and health outcomes in adults aged 18–59 years. *PLoS One*, 14(2), e0211850.

Department of Veteran Affairs & Department of Defense. (2017). *VA/DoD clinical practice guideline for management of post-traumatic stress. Version 3.0.* Washington, DC: Quality, Safety and Value, VA, & Office of Evidence Based Practice, U.S. Army Medical Command. Retrieved February 18, 2019, from https://www.healthquality.va.gov/guidelines/MH/ptsd/VADoDPTSDCPGFinal012418.pdf

El-Solh, A. A. (2018). Management of nightmares in patients with post-traumatic stress disorder: Current perspectives. *Nature and Science of Sleep*, 10, 409–420.

Farr, O. M., Ko, B. J., Joung, K. E., Zaichenko, L., Usher, N., Tsoukas, M., et al. (2015). Posttraumatic stress disorder, alone or additively with early life adversity, is associated with obesity and cardiometabolic risk. *Nutrition, Metabolism, and Cardiovascular Diseases*, 25(5), 479–488.

Gavrieli, A., Farr, O. M., Davis, C. R., Crowell, J. A., & Mantzoros, C. S. (2015). Early life adversity and/or posttraumatic stress disorder severity are associated with poor diet quality, including consumption of trans fatty acids, and fewer hours of resting or sleeping in a US middle-aged population: A cross-sectional and prospective study. *Metabolism*, 64, 1597–1610.

Grasser, L. R., & Javanbakht, A. (2019). Treatments of posttraumatic stress disorder in civilian populations. *Current Psychiatry Reports*, 21(2):11.

Hall, K. S., Beckham, J. C., Bosworth, H. B., Sloane, R., Pieper, C. F., Morey, M. C., et al. (2014). PTSD is negatively associated with physical performance and physical function in older overweight military veterans. *Journal of Rehabilitation Research and Development*, 51(2), 285–296.

Han, K. M., Park, J. Y., Park, H. E., An, S. R., Lee, E. H., Yoon, H. K., et al. (2018). Social support moderates association between posttraumatic growth and trauma-related psychopathologies among victims of the Sewol Ferry Disaster. *Psychiatry Research*, 272, 507–514.

Homish, G. G., Hoopsick, R. A., Heavey, S. C., Homish, D. L., & Cornelius, J. R. (2019). Drug use and hazardous drinking are associated with PTSD symptoms and symptom clusters in US Army Reserve/National Guard Soldiers. *The American Journal on Addictions*, 28(1):22–28.

Lori, A., Maddox, S. A., Sharma, S., Andero, R., Ressler, K. J., & Smith, A. K. (2019). Dynamic patterns of threat-associated gene expression in the amygdala and blood. *Frontiers in Psychiatry*, 9, 778.

Malikowsa-Racia, N., & Salat, K. (2019). Recent advances in the neurobiology of posttraumatic stress disorder: A review of possible mechanisms underlying an effective pharmacotherapy. *Pharmacological Research*, 142, 30–49.

Marshall, G. N., Jaycox, L. H., Engel, C. C., Richardson, A. S., Dutra, S. J., Keane, T. M., et al. (2019). PTSD symptoms are differentially associated with general distress and physiological arousal: Implications for the conceptualization and measurement of PTSD. *Journal of Anxiety Disorders, 62*, 26–34.

Mitra, R., & Hodes, M. (2019). Prevention of psychological distress and promotion of resilience amongst unaccompanied refugee minors in resettlement countries. *Child: Care Health and Development, 45*(2), 198–215.

Mota, N. P., Turner, S., Taillieu, T., Garcés, I., Magid, K., Sethi, J., et al. (2019). Trauma exposure, DSM-5 post-traumatic stress disorder, and sexual risk outcomes. *American Journal of Preventive Medicine, 56*(2), 215–223.

Naifeh, J. A, Mash, H. B. H., Stein, M. B., Fullerton, C. S., Kessler, R. C., & Ursano, R. J. (2019). The Army Study to Assess Risk and Resilience in servicemembers (Army STARRS): Progress toward understanding suicide among soldiers. *Molecular Psychiatry, 24*(1), 34-48.

National Institute of Mental Health (NIMH) (2019). Post-traumatic stress disorder. U.S. Department of Health and Human Services, National Institutes of Health (NIH) Publication No. QF 16-6388.

Niles, B. L., Mori, D. L., Polizzi, C., Pless Kaiser, A., Weinstein, E. S., Gershkovich, M., et al. (2018). A systematic review of randomized trials of mind-body interventions for PTSD. *Journal of Clinical Psychology, 74*(9), 1485–1508.

Oral, R., Ramirez, M., Coohey, C., Nakada, S., Walz, A., Kuntz, A., et al. (2016). Adverse childhood experiences and trauma informed care: the future of health care. *Pediatric Research, 79*(1), 227–233.

Ramchand, R., Rudavsky, R., Grant, S., Tanielian, T., & Jaycox, L. (2015). Prevalence of, risk factors for, and consequences of posttraumatic stress disorder and other mental health problems in military populations deployed to Iraq and Afghanistan. *Current Psychiatry Reports, 17*(5), 37.

Reinders, A. A., Marquand, A. F., Schlumpf, Y. R., Chalavi, S., Vissia, E. M., Nijenhuis, E. R., et al. (2018). Aiding the diagnosis of dissociative identity disorder: Pattern recognition study of brain biomarkers. *British Journal of Psychiatry*, 1–9.

Sadeh, N., Spielberg J. M., Miller, M. W., Milberg, W. P., Salat, D. H., Amick, M. M., et al. (2015). Neurobiological indicators of disinhibition in posttraumatic stress disorder. *Human Brain Mapping, 36*(8), 3076–3086.

Saren, J. (2019). Posttraumatic stress disorder in adults: Epidemiology, pathophysiology, clinical manifestations, course, assessment, and diagnosis. In M.B. Stein & R. Hermann (Eds.). *Up to Date*. Retrieved February 15, 2019, from https://www.uptodate.com/contents/posttraumatic-stress-disorder-in-adults-epidemiology-pathophysiology-clinical-manifestations-course-assessment-and-diagnosis/print

Ströhle, A. (2018). Sports psychiatry: mental health and mental disorders in athletes and exercise treatment of mental disorders. *European Archives of Psychiatry and Clinical Neuroscience*, 1–14. Retrieved February 18, 2019, from https://doi.org/10.1007/s00406-018-0891-5

Substance Abuse and Mental Health Services Administration. (2014). *SAMHSA's concept of trauma and guidance for a trauma informed approach. HHS Publication No. (SMA) 14–4884*. Rockville, MD: Substance Abuse and Mental Health Services Administration.

Williamson, V., Stevelink, S. A., Da Silva, E., & Fear, N. T. (2018). A systematic review of wellbeing in children: A comparison of military and civilian families. *Child & Adolescent Mental Health and Psychiatry, 12*, 46.

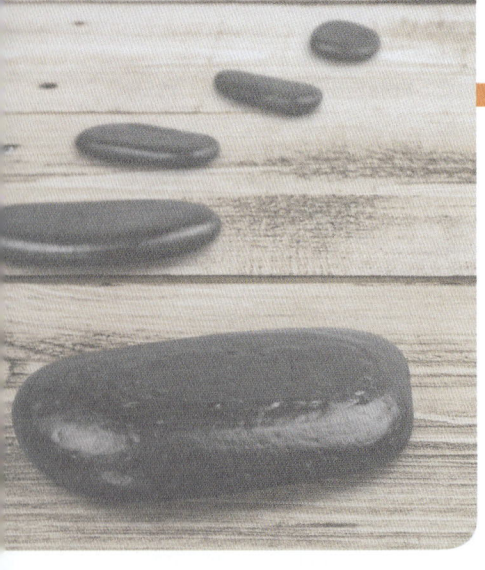

20
Obsessive–Compulsive and Related Disorders
Nursing Care of Persons With Obsessions and Compulsions

Patricia E. Freed

KEY CONCEPTS
- compulsions
- obsessions

LEARNING OBJECTIVES

After studying this chapter, you will be able to:

1. Discuss the role of obsessions and compulsions in mental disorders.
2. Describe the prevalence and incidence of obsessive–compulsive disorders.
3. Delineate clinical symptoms and course of obsessive–compulsive disorders.
4. Analyze theories of obsessive–compulsive disorders.
5. Apply nursing process with recovery-oriented interventions for persons with obsessive–compulsive disorders.
6. Differentiate other obsessive–compulsive disorders.

KEY TERMS

• Accommodation • Conditioned stimuli • Isolation • Obsessive–compulsive disorder • Reaction formation • Undoing

Case Study: Tim

Tim, a 32-year-old engineer, was diagnosed with OCD as a teenager when his obsession with cleanliness and compulsively washing his hands interfered with his friendships and school work.

Most of us experience times when we are preoccupied with specific thoughts or ideas. Many also find that routines or rituals are important in organizing our work and home life. When these preoccupations and rituals interfere with daily life, they become abnormal and may represent symptoms of a mental disorder. This chapter explains obsessions and compulsions and their role in **obsessive–compulsive disorders** (OCDs). OCD is highlighted in this chapter.

OBSESSIONS AND COMPULSIONS

When preoccupied thoughts become excessive, intrusive or unwanted, such thoughts are considered to be obsessions.

> **KEYCONCEPT Obsessions** are excessive, unwanted, intrusive, and persistent thoughts, impulses, or images that cause anxiety and distress.
>
> Obsessions are not under the person's control and are inconsistent with the person's usual thought patterns.

Common obsessions include fears of contamination, pathologic doubt, the need for symmetry and completion, thoughts of hurting someone, and thoughts of sexual images.

Routines are a part of everyday life. Getting up in the morning at the same time and going to work or school structures our lives and helps us be productive. When routines become ritualistic and interfere with normal daily activity, they become compulsions.

> **KEYCONCEPT** **Compulsions** are repetitive behaviors and mental acts performed in a ritualistic fashion with the goal of preventing or relieving anxiety and distress caused by obsessions.

For example, making sure a stove is turned off before leaving the house can be a safety routine, but being late for work because of making several trips to the stove before leaving the house is a compulsion. Common compulsions include handwashing, excessive cleaning, checking, arranging things, counting, ordering, and hoarding.

OVERVIEW OF OBSESSIVE–COMPULSIVE AND RELATED DISORDERS

Obsessions and compulsions are characteristic of obsessive–compulsive and related disorders. These disorders include OCD, body dysmorphic disorder (BDD), hoarding disorder, trichotillomania (i.e., compulsively pulling out one's hair), excoriation disorder, and substance/medication-induced OCD (see Table 20.1

TABLE 20.1	OBSESSIVE–COMPULSIVE AND RELATED DISORDERS
Disorder	**Description**
Obsessive–compulsive disorder	Distressful obsessions and compulsions that interfere with daily living and quality of life
Body dysmorphic disorder	Preoccupation with slight or imagined physical defects that are not apparent to others
Hoarding disorder	Difficulty discarding or parting with possessions with a strong need to save
Trichotillomania (hair-pulling disorder)	Inability to stop recurrent pulling out of hair with hair loss that is related to emotional release or anxiety release
Excoriation disorder (skin picking)	Inability to stop recurrent picking at skin for emotional release or anxiety release
Substance/medication-induced obsessive–compulsive disorder	OCD symptoms related to intoxication or withdrawal of substances

Source: American Psychiatric Association. (2013). *Diagnostic and statistical manual of mental disorders* (5th ed.). Arlington, VA: Author.

for a description of these disorders). These disorders are closely related to anxiety disorders (American Psychiatric Association [APA], 2013).

OBSESSIVE–COMPULSIVE DISORDER

In OCD, affected persons may have both obsessions and compulsions and believe that they have no control over them, which results in devastating consequences for affected individuals. Because of the nature of the disorder, nurses who work in settings other than psychiatric settings or in home health care may be among the first to identify an individual's symptoms as OCD and make the appropriate referrals. OCD is a separate disorder from obsessive–compulsive personality disorder discussed in Chapter 24.

Clinical Course

The average age of onset of OCD is preadolescence but can occur into the 20s to mid-30s (Substance Abuse and Mental Health Services Administration [SAMHSA], 2017). Symptoms of OCD often begin in childhood, but many persons receive treatment only after the disorder has significantly affected their lives. In preschool-age children, OCD is often misdiagnosed as separation anxiety disorder (Miyawaki et al., 2018). Symptom onset of the disorder is gradual, with some individuals showing a progressive decline in social and occupational functioning (APA, 2013). Men are affected more often as children and are most commonly affected by obsessions. Women have a higher incidence of checking-and-cleaning rituals, with onset typically in the early 20s. This chronic disorder is characterized by episodes of symptom diminution and exacerbation (APA, 2013). Predictors of poor outcomes include initial symptom onset during childhood, severe symptoms, long duration of illness, and male gender (Sharma, Thennarasu, & Reddy, 2014).

Obsessions create tremendous anxiety; individuals perform compulsions to relieve the anxiety temporarily. If the compensatory ritual is not performed, the person feels increased anxiety and distress. Compulsions are necessary, not pleasurable. They are often recognized as odd or strange to the individual. Initially, attempts are made to resist the compulsive behavior, but eventually, resistance fails, and the repetitive behaviors are incorporated into daily routines.

The most common obsession is fear of contamination and results in compulsive handwashing. Fear of contamination usually focuses on dirt or germs, but other materials may be feared as well, such as toxic chemicals, poison, radiation, and heavy metals. Individuals with contamination obsessions report anxiety as their most common effect, but shame and disgust, linked with embarrassment and guilt, also are experienced.

> **Remember Tim?**
> When Tim was in high school, he was unable to eat at the school cafeteria because he was afraid the other students' germs would contaminate his food. He avoided touching doorknobs and would wash his hands for 3 minutes if he inadvertently touched a doorknob.

Persons with OCD may become incapacitated by their symptoms and spend most of their waking hours locked in a cycle of obsessions and compulsions. They may even become unable to complete a task as simple as walking through a door without performing rituals. Interpersonal relationships suffer, and the person may actively isolate him- or herself. Individuals with OCD often engage in dissociative absorption, a tendency to become excessively absorbed in fantasy (movies, games) leading to decreased self-awareness and inattention to their surroundings. Dissociative absorption may predict the onset of obsessive–compulsive symptoms; this possible link is still being investigated (Soffer-Dudek, 2018).

Diagnostic Criteria

OCD is diagnosed when recurrent obsessions or compulsions (or both) cause considerable stress to the individual. These obsessions or compulsions are not caused by substance or medication use or other disorders. Some individuals recognize that these obsessions or compulsions are excessive and unrealistic; others have limited insight and are unsure whether the obsessive thoughts are true, but continue to have the thoughts and feel compelled to perform the actions. Another group of individuals are convinced that their obsessive thoughts are true. These thoughts and compulsive behaviors are stressful and interfere with normal daily routines (SAMHSA, 2016).

Obsessions

Some individuals have obsessions surrounding aggressive acts of hurting someone or themselves. After hitting a bump in the road, for example, they may obsess for hours over whether they have hit someone. Parents may have recurrent intrusive thoughts that they may hurt their child. Others obsess over the meaning of sins or whether they have followed the letter of the law. They tend to be hypermoral and have the need to confess. Their obsessions are seen as a form of religious suffering. These patients are often resistant to treatment. Religious obsessions are most common in persons who experience severe religious restrictions. Diagnosis is not made unless the thoughts or rituals clearly exceed cultural or religious norms, occur at inappropriate times as described by members of the same religion or culture, or interfere with social obligations (APA, 2013). Although it might be difficult to have a conversation centering on religious concerns and family practices, recent findings show that youth with religious obsessions benefit from treatment as much as their peers with OCD who do not experience religious obsessions (Wu et al., 2018).

Compulsions

Rituals are common compulsions in which objects must be in a certain order, motor activities are performed in a rigid fashion, or things are arranged in perfect symmetry. A ritual consumes a great deal of time to complete even the simplest task. Some individuals experience discontent, rather than anxiety, when things are not symmetrical or perfect. Others think magically and perform compulsive rituals to ward off an imagined disaster such as repeatedly turning on and off the alarm clock to prevent disaster. Those who hoard are compelled to check their belongings repeatedly to see that all is accounted for and check the garbage to make sure that nothing of value has been discarded.

 Concept Mastery Alert

> Certain actions, such as making sure that all doors are locked before going to bed, are safety considerations in which the associated anxiety is protective. This is a normal activity and concern, not a pathologic compulsion.

Obsessive–Compulsive Disorder Across the Life Span

Although OCD is relatively common, it is still under-recognized and undertreated. OCD affects people of all ages. Identification, diagnosis, and treatment of OCD are necessary for recovery and optimal functioning.

Children and Adolescents

OCD affects between 1% and 3% or more of children and adolescents (Jacob & Storch, 2013). Because children subscribe to myths, superstition, and magical thinking, obsessive and ritualistic behaviors may go unnoticed. Behaviors such as touching every third tree, avoiding cracks in the sidewalk, or consistently verbalizing fears of losing a parent in an accident may have some underlying pathology but are common behaviors in childhood. Typically, parents notice that a child's grades begin to fall as a result of decreased concentration and great amounts of time spent performing rituals. Children often have at least one other mental disorder and are less likely than adults to recognize the irrationality of their symptoms (Krebs & Heyman, 2015).

Older Adults

OCD is usually an early-onset disorder, and for some it can be a lifelong and debilitating condition. Among the elderly, OCD most likely began in late adulthood rather than childhood, and continuing symptoms are linked to higher rates of depression and poorer mental and social functioning (Dell'Osso et al., 2017). Elderly persons who engage in checking compulsions may have more thought disturbances and communication difficulties than those who engage in other types of compulsive behaviors (Klenfeldt et al., 2014). OCD seldom begins in late life; when these symptoms are noted after the age of 50, neurologic diseases should be excluded (Dell'Osso et al. 2017) (see Box 20.1).

Epidemiology and Risk Factors

OCD has a lifetime prevalence rate of 1.2% with females having a slightly higher rate than males (APA, 2013). First-degree relatives of people with OCD have a higher prevalence rate than the general population. Early-onset OCD increases the chances of OCD in relatives and predicts poorer treatment outcomes (Ruscio, Stein, Chiu, & Kessler, 2010).

Studies provide some support for a link between infection with β-hemolytic streptococci and OCD (Hachiya et al., 2013). High rates of OCD are found among individuals who are young, divorced or separated, and unemployed. OCD appears to be less common among African Americans than among non-Hispanic whites.

Comorbidity

It is estimated that one third of persons with OCD experience depression. Bipolar, cyclothymic, panic, mood, eating, and impulse control disorders commonly occur in those with OCD. Tourette syndrome, attention-deficit hyperactivity disorder (ADHD), and OCD frequently occur together, though symptom severity of each disorder decreases with age (Groth, Mol, Rask, Lange, & Skov, 2017). There are higher rates of both OCD and obsessive–compulsive symptoms in elderly persons who are depressed (Klenfeldt et al., 2014). OCD is more common in patients with schizophrenia when high anxiety, along with mood and psychotic symptoms, is present. Although OCD symptoms are treatable, they often remain unrecognized and untreated (Bener, Dafeeah, Abou-Saleh, Ghurgra, & Ventriglio, 2018).

Many individuals self-medicate to relieve the anxiety produced by obsessive thoughts. About one third experience substance abuse or dependence in their lifetime. In addition, some individuals may abuse benzodiazepines and other prescription medication. OCD and substance use disorder (SUD) are frequently comorbid, but there is a complex relationship between the severity of the illness and the use of substances. In fact, although further exploration is needed, severe OCD may actually protect against the development of SUD (Cuzen, Stein, Lochner, & Fineberg, 2014).

Somatic obsessions—such as persistent attention to normal bodily processes like breathing, blinking, and swallowing—can also be present and can become intrusive, terrifying thoughts, which can cause people to seek medical treatment, often just to get reassurance.

> **Consider This:**
>
>
>
> As a child, Tim frequently went to the school nurse about multiple physical symptoms. Later, he was unable to engage in sexual relations with a long-time girlfriend because the thought of the sex act made him feel nauseous, and twice he experienced severe vomiting. At the time, he sought emergency treatment, but ultimately no physical reason was discovered.

Etiology

During the 1990s, research evidence from neuroimaging studies, neurochemical studies, and treatment advances substantiated a predominantly neurobiologic basis for OCD. The following sections provide a brief overview of these findings and evidence pointing to genetic vulnerability. Psychological factors are also discussed because of their contributions to the disorder. Because no single explanation accounts for all aspects of OCD, a combination of factors will probably be found to produce the disorder.

BOX 20.1 CLINICAL VIGNETTE

Older Adult

Louise, a 76-year-old retired accountant, resides in an assisted living complex with her husband. Always very neat and organized, she recently began cleaning excessively, sometimes in the middle of the night. She developed a routine where she had to have everything cleaned before she could eat. Her husband expressed his concern to their primary care provider who referred them to a geriatric psychiatrist. A diagnosis of OCD was made. Louise recognizes that her behavior has changed and is interfering with her life but says she gets too nervous if she doesn't carry out her routine.

What Do You Think?
- Are there indications that she may have had subclinical OCD symptoms?
- What symptoms of OCD is Louise experiencing?

Biologic Theories

Genetic, neuropathologic, and biochemical research, reviewed in this section, suggests that OCD has a biologic basis involving several neuroanatomic structures.

Genetic Factors

OCD occurs more often in people who have first-degree relatives with OCD or with Tourette syndrome than it does in the general population. Some studies show an increased prevalence of anxiety and mood disorders in relatives of individuals who have OCD. Twin studies indicate that OCD occurs more frequently in siblings of twins. Further studies implicate specific genes and associate them with OCD (Shaw et al., 2014). These discoveries may lead to breakthroughs in pharmacologic treatments of OCD.

Neuropathologic Theories

Recent neuroimaging studies of individuals with OCD show hyperactivity in the orbitofrontal cortex, anterior cingulated cortex, and caudate nucleus, suggesting a causal role in the etiology of OCD (Tiago, Cooney, & Peterson, 2008).

Increased cerebral glucose metabolism is identified in various studies. There is particular interest in the underlying changes associated with compulsive behavior. Evidence suggests that abnormal repetitive behaviors are driven by dysfunction in cortico-striatal-thalamic-cortical circuits (Wood & Ahmari, 2015). A link between activity in specific brain circuits and reduction of OCD symptoms after successful pharmacologic or psychological treatment has been confirmed via meta-analysis (van der Straten, Denys, & van Wingen, 2017). Note that these studies don't confirm the neurologic etiology of OCD, but they make it possible to match responders to specific treatments.

Biochemical Theories

Serotonin plays a role in OCD. It has been studied through challenge tests in which serotonin agonists were administered to persons with OCD and with control subjects. The most convincing evidence for serotonin's role is that serotonin-specific antidepressants relieve the symptoms of OCD for most persons. A single neurotransmitter is unlikely to be entirely responsible for OCD.

Conventional and novel antipsychotic medications and mood stabilizers are used in conjunction with serotonin-targeting medications to treat refractory symptoms, indicating that other biochemical processes exist (Del Casale et al., 2018).

Psychological Theories

Although psychological theories of OCD have not been scientifically tested, the rich literature describing clinical examples and case histories helps us understand the symptoms and behaviors related to OCD. In addition, behavioral treatment of individuals with severe compulsions improves symptoms. Cognitive behavioral therapy (CBT), which should be considered in every treatment plan, is associated with lower relapse rates (Richter & Ramos, 2018).

Psychodynamic Factors

The psychodynamic theory hypothesizes that OCD symptoms and character traits arise from three unconscious defense mechanisms: **isolation** (separation of affect from a thought or impulse), **undoing** (an act performed with the goal of preventing consequences of a thought or impulse), and **reaction formation** (behavior and consciously stated attitudes that oppose underlying impulses). Classic psychoanalytic theory describes OCD as regression from the oedipal phase to the anal phase of development, which includes preoccupations with anger and dirt (see Chapter 5). This regression occurs when the patient becomes anxious about retaliation or loss of love.

Behavioral Factors

Behavioral explanations for OCD stem from learning theory. From this viewpoint, obsessions are seen as **conditioned stimuli**. Through being associated with noxious events, stimuli that are usually considered neutral become anxiety provoking. The individual then engages in activities to escape or avoid the anxiety. Compulsions develop as the individual discovers behaviors that successfully reduce the obsessional anxiety. As the principles of operant conditioning indicate, the more the behaviors decrease the anxiety, the more likely the individual is to continue using them. However, the rituals or behaviors preserve the fear response because the person avoids the initial stimuli and thus never extinguishes the compulsion. Interrupting this cycle is the focus of behavioral therapy in treating an individual with OCD.

Family Response to Disorder

OCD poses a considerable caregiving burden on families, which is heightened by severe symptoms, functional impairment, and comorbid psychopathologies in the child or caregiver (Wu et al., 2017). Severity of symptoms has been linked to family distress. Families often accommodate a family member's symptoms by taking part in rituals or by modifying their daily routines. Levels of **accommodation** should be carefully tracked and monitored, because reducing the family's involvement may improve treatment outcomes (La Buissonniere-Ariza et al., 2018)

Family assessment will reveal the amount of education and support needed and will begin the partnership among the individual, family, and treatment team. Evaluate the family's understanding of the disorder and of proposed treatments. Are they able and willing to help the individual practice cognitive and behavioral techniques? Are they knowledgeable about prescribed medicines? These questions offer a wonderful opportunity for individual and family education.

Family members offer a perspective on the severity of the individual's illness. Family members are experts in the patient's rituals and may observe subtle changes. Evaluate the family's response to changes in the individual's behavior as treatment progresses. You may have to discuss how the family will manage the changes brought about by a decrease in rituals. If obsessions and compulsions make it difficult for the individual to leave the home or function at work, financial difficulties may result. These factors should be assessed and appropriate assistance obtained through social services when necessary. Adverse family functioning is strongly associated with pediatric OCD, though its role remains unclear (Murphy & Flessner, 2015).

Tim's Family

Tim's parents recognized their son had unusual behaviors that interfered with his normal growth and development. When he was in high school, his parents took him to a psychiatrist who prescribed medication and offered brief counseling. Tim was able to successfully complete high school with honors and was accepted into a highly respected college. He was able to function when taking medications.

Recovery-Oriented Care for Persons With OCD

Teamwork and Collaboration: Working Toward Recovery

OCD can be difficult to treat because obsessions and compulsions consistently interfere with recovery efforts. OCD is treated with medications, CBT, and supportive therapy. The overall goal is for the patient to recover and to decrease the symptoms. Staff may have differing opinions about the amount of control the individual has over the behavior, but these differences of opinion must be resolved. All staff must be consistent in their expectations and acceptance of the patient's behaviors to keep these patients from becoming frustrated or confused regarding expectations during treatment (Box 20.2).

BOX 20.2 CLINICAL VIGNETTE

More Teamwork Needed

Robert, a 32-year-old man, is a new patient at a local psychiatric unit. He admitted himself to have his medicines evaluated because his obsessive thoughts and depression have worsened since his recent divorce. While in the hospital, he has quickly become viewed as a "problem patient" because he hoards linens and demands a new bar of soap for each of his five daily showers. He is compelled to open and close his door five times when he leaves or enters his room but does not know why. This behavior has led to arguments with his roommate. In an effort to "help him," the psychiatric technicians locked his bathroom door to prevent him from showering so frequently. He tried to enter his bathroom to shower and panicked when the technicians refused to allow him to shower, telling him, "You can live without it." After receiving PRN medication for extreme anxiety, Robert signed out of the hospital against medical advice because of embarrassment and anger toward the nursing staff.

What Do You Think?

- How could the technicians have handled the situation differently so as to not disrupt Robert's or the unit's clinical care?
- What nursing interventions might be appropriate in providing Robert's care?

Electroconvulsive Therapy

The effect of electroconvulsive therapy (ECT) on decreasing obsessions and compulsions cannot be confirmed or refuted. Authors who reviewed the literature concluded it may have no role in the routine treatment of OCD (Fontenelle et al., 2015). Previous reports of high success may have been compromised by poorly defined treatment resistance, less than optimal treatment, and other specific differences between the populations studied (Fontenelle et al., 2015). A recent case report described complete remission after a course of ECT in a patient with anorexia and disabling OCD, which did not recur during the first year of follow-up (Sağlam, Aksoy Poyraz, Poyraz, & Tosun, 2018). Although it is too early to draw a definite conclusion, future research may identify the effectiveness of ECT under certain circumstances or for those with specific comorbid conditions. Nursing's role in caring for the individual undergoing ECT is outlined in Chapter 11.

Transcranial Magnetic Stimulation

Transcranial magnetic stimulation (TMS), a noninvasive procedure that uses magnetic fields to stimulate brain cells, has recently been approved by the U.S. Food and Drug Administration (FDA) for the treatment of OCD. The procedure is contraindicated for patients with implanted metallic objects or implanted stimulator devices in or near the head. Those with a history of seizure disorder may be cautiously considered for treatment. During treatment, the patient wears earplugs to reduce exposure to the loud noises made by the device. Headache is the most commonly reported side effect of treatment, and other muscle discomforts or pain at the application site resolve shortly after treatment (FDA, 2018). There is emerging evidence that TMS may be effective in treatment-resistant cases of BDD (Hong, Nezgovorova, Uzunova, Schlussel, & Hollander, 2018).

Psychosurgery

Psychosurgery is sometimes used to treat extremely severe OCD that has not responded to prolonged and intensive drug treatment, behavioral therapy, or a combination of the two. Modern stereotactic surgical techniques that produce lesions of the cingulum bundle (a bundle of connective tissue) or anterior limb of the internal capsule (a region near the thalamus and part of the circuit connecting to the cortex) may bring about substantial clinical benefit in some individuals without causing significant morbidity (De Ridder et al., 2016). Other treatment options include radiotherapy and deep brain stimulation, in which electrical current is applied through an electrode inserted into the brain (Cleary, Ozpinar, Raslan, & Ko, 2015).

Safety Issues

As with any individual with a mental disorder, a suicide assessment must be completed. Although individuals with OCD do not usually become suicidal as a direct result of anxiety, the disorder greatly distresses the person, who realizes the pointlessness and absurdity of the behaviors. Often, the person has tolerated symptoms for quite some time before seeking treatment. The person may feel a sense of hopelessness and helplessness and may contemplate suicide to end the suffering. An additional risk for suicide is created by the high probability of major depression, which often accompanies OCD. Patients may feel a need to punish themselves for their intrusive thoughts (e.g., religious coupled with sexual obsessions). Some persons have aggressive obsessions, so that external limits may have to be imposed for the protection of others.

Evidence-Based Nursing Care of Persons With OCD

Persons with OCD may be any age; many have other disorders. Nursing care involves a careful assessment of the impact of the mental health disorder on individual and family. Nursing Care Plan 20.1—which sets forth a plan of care for Tim, the case study patient in this chapter—is available at http://thepoint.lww.com/BoydEssentials2e.

Mental Health Nursing Assessment

The nurse should assess the type and severity of the person's obsessions and compulsions. If the assessment occurs in a hospital, remember that some individuals with OCD experience a transient decrease in symptoms when admitted to a hospital; therefore, sufficient time must be allowed for an accurate assessment. If that time is unavailable, family members or significant others may provide an important source of information, with the individual's permission.

Physical Health Assessment

Individuals with OCD do not have a higher prevalence of physical disease than others. However, they may report multiple physical symptoms. With late-onset OCD (i.e., after 50 years of age) and with symptoms that occur with a febrile illness, cerebral pathology should be considered. Each person with OCD should be assessed for dermatologic lesions caused by repetitive handwashing, excessive cleaning with caustic agents, or bathing. Osteoarthritic joint damage secondary to cleaning rituals may also be observed. Undetected somatic compulsions, such as persistent nausea and vomiting, can contribute to diminished quality of life and pose diagnostic challenges for clinicians.

Most individuals appear neatly dressed and groomed, cooperative, and eager to answer questions. Speech should be at normal rate and volume, but often, individuals with an obsessional, ruminative style of thinking exhibit circumferential speech. This speech, loaded with irrelevant details, eventually addresses the question. Listening may be frustrating and require considerable patience, but remember that such speech, which expresses the individual's thinking, is part of the disorder and may be beyond the person's awareness. Continually interrupting and redirecting them can interfere with establishing a therapeutic relationship, especially in the initial assessment. Redirection should be done in a gentle and noncritical manner to allow the patient time to refocus.

Psychosocial Assessment

Identifying the degree to which the OCD symptoms interfere with the patient's daily functioning is important. Several rating scales can be used to identify symptoms and monitor improvement. Some of these scales are to be used by the nurse; others are self-rating scales for the patient, child, or family member. See Table 20.2 for more information about psychometrically valid scales, recommended as the cornerstone to evidence-based treatment (Rapp, Bergman, Piacentini, & McGuire, 2018).

TABLE 20.2	EVIDENCE-BASED ASSESSMENT TOOLS FOR OCD
Rating Scale	**Description**
Yale–Brown Obsessive Compulsive Scale Y-BOCS/Y-BOCS-II/CY-BOCS	A clinician-rated, 16-item scale with separate subtotals for the severity of obsessions and compulsions.
The Sheehan Disability Scale (SDS)	Brief, self-rated, 3-item, visual analog scale to assess disability. A global measure of functioning can be determined. Recommended for tracking functional changes over time.
Family Accommodation Scale for Obsessive-Compulsive Disorder (FAS-SR)	This self-rated, 19-item rating scale that can be used by the parent, child, or others to track and monitor the family's response to symptoms during treatment.
The Brown Assessment of Beliefs Scale (BABS)	A self-rated scale that scores on six dimensions: conviction, perception of others' views, explanation of differing views, idea fixity, attempts to reject beliefs, and insight. Helps rate the degree of conviction and insight, patients have concerning their obsessions.

Source: Rapp, A. M., Bergman, R. L., Piacentini, J., & McGuire, J. F. (2018) Evidence-based assessment of obsessive-compulsive disorder. *Journal of Central Nervous System Disease, 8,* 13–29.

Sociocultural factors are very important. At times, cultural or religious beliefs may be misunderstood and mistaken for obsessions or compulsions. These beliefs and actions must be evaluated in the context of the individual's culture. If these beliefs are consistent with the patient's social or cultural environment, are not harmful to the individual or others, and do not interfere with individual functioning in that environment, they should not be considered symptoms of OCD.

Strengths Assessment

The personal and social strengths of the person should emerge during the assessment interview. Does the child or adult enjoy good physical health? Is the person motivated for treatment? Does the person recognize that obsessions or compulsions are unusual or abnormal? Are there social supports? This information will be useful in establishing a recovery plan.

Priority of Nursing Care

Patients with OCD may present with various problems, depending on the particular obsession and the compulsions that have evolved to cope with that obsession. As a result, nursing priorities could run the gamut from psychological issues related to anxiety, poor self-concept, and loneliness to physical issues such as skin integrity. Outcomes are determined collaboratively after the issues have been identified.

Nursing Interventions

Establishing a therapeutic relationship with a person with OCD requires patience and active listening. The individual may go to great lengths to explain some minute aspect of her or his life. It is important not to interrupt or rush these explanations. Being unable to finish thoughts increases the patient's anxiety and frustration (see Box 20.3).

The nurse's interpersonal skills are crucial to successful intervention with the patient who has OCD. Nurses must control their own anxiety. The nurse should interact with the individual in a calm, nonauthoritarian fashion without exhibiting any disapproval of the patient or the patient's behaviors while demonstrating empathy about the distress that the disorder has caused. This approach is one of the most effective means available for communicating appreciation for the individual as separate from the illness.

Interventions focus on the physical consequences of the compulsion as well as the psychosocial aspects. The next section provides an overview of biopsychosocial interventions including medications.

Maintaining Skin Integrity

For the patient with cleaning or handwashing compulsions, attention to skin condition is necessary. Encourage the individual to use tepid water when washing and hand cream after washing. Remove harsh abrasive soaps and replace them with moisturizing soaps. Attempt to decrease the frequency of washing by agreeing on a time schedule and time-limited washing.

Medications

Selective serotonin reuptake inhibitors (SSRIs), including fluoxetine, fluvoxamine, paroxetine, and sertraline are recommended medications. Prolonged treatment with SSRIs at higher doses than are used for depression is recommended (Janardhan Reddy, Sundar, Narayanaswamy, & Math, 2017). A combination of medication and behavioral or CBT may produce better results (Del Casale et al., 2018). There is some question about the effectiveness of augmentation with antipsychotics, and if these medications are used, they should be prescribed in low doses, given an adequate trial of at least 8 weeks, and administered with careful consideration of the benefits and risks of long-term use (Janardhan Reddy et al., 2017) (see Box 20.4).

BOX 20.3 • THERAPEUTIC DIALOGUE • The Patient With Delusion

Tim is admitted to an inpatient unit; an initial assessment is currently being conducted.

INEFFECTIVE APPROACH

Nurse: Could you tell me what brings you here?

Tim: What? Oh, sorry I get distracted easily. What did you say?

Nurse: I said, why are you here? What do you hope to accomplish while you are here?

Tim: Well, this is how I see it. We need to make sure everyone is healthy, and I want to make sure…

Nurse: (interrupts) No, you don't understand what I am asking. WHY are you here?

Tim: Forget it. I want to see my wife.

EFFECTIVE APPROACH

Nurse: Tim, how can I help you?

Tim: Well, I am not sure. My wife thinks I am doing strange things. See, I want everyone to be protected and I think that it is important to stay healthy. There is an outbreak of staph infections and I want to make sure that my family is safe and I am just trying to figure things out.

Nurse: OK, it sounds like you are concerned about your family and you are trying to protect them.

Tim: Yes, it is all of the germs. They are everywhere.

Nurse: And you are trying to get rid of them?

Tim: Yes, my wife thinks I am going overboard and wants me to take my medication.

Nurse: Your medication?

Tim: Yes, I used to take medication when I felt like this.

Nurse: You don't take your medication anymore?

Tim: No, I don't need it.

Nurse: I see. But your wife thinks you do?

Tim: Yes, but I don't like the side effects.

Nurse: Such as?

Tim: Well, to tell you the truth, I'd rather not talk about it.

Nurse: OK. While you are here, we can look at different options to help you feel more comfortable.

CRITICAL THINKING CHALLENGE

- How did the first nurse's interaction block communication and increase Tim's frustration?
- What effective communication techniques did the nurse use in the second scenario?

BOX 20.4

Antidepressants FDA Approved for Obsessive–Compulsive Disorder

MEDICATIONS	CLASSIFICATION	DOSAGE	SIDE EFFECTS
Sertraline (Zoloft)	SSRI	Children (6–12 yrs old) 25 mg/day (13–17) 50 mg/day Adults 50 mg titrated to 200 mg/day	Sedation, dizziness, somnolence or insomnia, headache, sexual dysfunction, can cause excitability when initiated, weight gain (rare)
Fluvoxamine	SSRI	Children (8–17) 25–200 mg/day Adults 50–300 mg/day	
Fluoxetine (Prozac)	SSRI	Adolescents 20–60 mg/day Adults 20–60 mg/day	
Paroxetine (Paxil)	SSRI	Adults 20–60 mg/day	

Administering and Monitoring Medications. Antidepressants used to treat persons with OCD are often given in higher doses than those normally used to treat depressed patients (see Box 20.4). Aggressive treatment may be indicated to bring the symptoms under control. Thus, medication effects must be closely monitored, including signs of toxicity, to provide safe and adequate care. All antidepressants have a black box warning for suicidality in children, adolescents, and young adults. These medications often take several weeks or months to relieve compulsions and may take even longer to decrease obsessions.

Exposure and Response Prevention

An effective behavioral intervention for individuals with OCD who perform rituals is exposure and response prevention (ERP) (McGuire, Lewin, & Storch, 2014). The person is exposed to situations or objects that are known to induce anxiety but is asked to refrain from performing the ritualistic behaviors. One goal of this procedure is to help the person understand that resisting the rituals while exposed to the object of anxiety is less stressful and time-consuming than performing the rituals. Another goal is to confound the expectation of distressing outcomes and eventually extinguish the compulsive behaviors. Most individuals improve with ERP, but few become completely asymptomatic.

Thought Stopping

Thought stopping is used with individuals who have obsessional thoughts (Abramowitz et al., 2010). The person is taught to interrupt obsessional thoughts by saying, "Stop!" either aloud or silently. This activity interrupts and delays the uncontrollable spiral of obsessional thoughts. Research supporting this technique is scant; however, practitioners have found it useful in multimodal treatment with ERP, relaxation, and cognitive restructuring.

Relaxation Techniques

Individuals with OCD experience insomnia because of heightened anxiety levels. Relaxation exercises may be helpful in improving sleep patterns. These exercises do not affect OCD symptoms but they may be used to decrease anxiety. The nurse may also teach the person other relaxation measures, such as deep breathing, taking warm baths, practicing meditation, and music therapy, or other quiet activities.

Cognitive Restructuring

Cognitive restructuring is a method of teaching the person to restructure dysfunctional thought processes by defining and testing them. The goal of treatment is to alter the person's immediate, dysfunctional appraisal of a situation and perception of long term consequences. The individual is taught to monitor automatic thoughts and then to recognize the connection between thoughts, emotional response, and behaviors. The distorted thoughts are examined and tested by for-or-against evidence presented by the therapist, which helps the individual to realistically assess the likelihood that the feared event will happen if the compulsive behavior is not performed. The person begins to analyze his or her thoughts as incongruent with reality. For example, even if the alarm clock is not checked 30 times before going to bed, it will still go off in the morning, and the person will not be disciplined for tardiness at work. Maybe it needs to be checked only once or twice.

Interventions for Hospitalized Patients

Although most patients with OCD are treated in outpatient settings, some are hospitalized with comorbidities and are unable to care for themselves or pose a substantial risk of harm to self or others. Some suggestions for their care include:

- Unit routines must be carefully and clearly explained to decrease fear of the unknown.
- Assess and monitor the level of anxiety and disability.
- Monitor for psychiatric comorbidities and suicide risk.
- At least initially, do not prevent the individual from engaging in rituals because the person's anxiety level will increase.
- Recognize the significance of the rituals to the person and empathize with the person's need to perform them.
- Assist the individual in arranging a schedule of activities that incorporates some private time but also integrates the person into normal unit activities.
- Help the person recognize triggers to obsessive thoughts and ritualistic behaviors and the relationship between them.
- Give positive reinforcement for nonritualistic behavior.
- Reinforce the use of cognitive strategies, including constructive self-talk and cognitive restructuring.

Psychoeducation

Nurses play an important interdisciplinary role in managing medication for persons with OCD, which includes educating patients and families about medications. Because patients may become discouraged with a perceived lack of effect, they should be informed that these medications may take several weeks before their effects are realized. All patients should be warned not to stop taking prescribed medications abruptly (see Chapter 11).

Psychoeducation is a crucial nursing intervention for the person with OCD. Knowledge is power; the more the person knows about his or her disorder, the more

> **BOX 20.5**
>
> **Psychoeducation Checklist: Obsessive–Compulsive Disorder**
>
> When caring for the patient with OCD, be sure to include the patient's primary caregiver, if appropriate, and address the following topic areas in the teaching plan:
>
> - Psychopharmacologic agents if ordered, including drug action, dosage, frequency, and possible side effects
> - Skin care measures
> - Ritualistic behaviors and alternative activities
> - Thought stopping
> - Relaxation techniques
> - Cognitive restructuring
> - Recovery strategies
> - Community resources

control he or she will have over symptoms. The individual should be instructed not only about the biologic components of OCD but also about its treatments and disease course. Treatment is a shared responsibility between the individual and the health care provider; the individual should be included in the medication and treatment decision-making processes. If local support groups are available, the person should be referred to reduce feelings of uniqueness and embarrassment about the disease. Family education is also important so the individual will have help in practicing behavioral homework (Box 20.5).

Evaluation and Treatment Outcomes

Several methods can be used to measure the response to treatment (including nursing care): changes in Y-BOCS scores or other rating scales, remission of presenting symptoms, and the ability to complete activities of daily living. The individual should be able to participate in social or group activities with a degree of comfort and without self-harm or aggressive intent. He or she should also be able to demonstrate common knowledge of OCD by describing its symptoms, biologic basis, and treatments.

Continuum of Care

The symptoms of OCD can become debilitating. The symptoms wax and wane throughout treatment. As the focus of treatment shifts from inpatient to outpatient environments, individuals must be assessed continually to ensure favorable outcomes through early intervention if symptoms resurface.

Inpatient-Focused Care

In an inpatient setting, the presence of a person with severe OCD may present a nursing management challenge. These individuals require a significant amount of staff time. They may monopolize bathrooms or showers or have disruptive rituals involving eating. Nurses play an integral role in treating the person with OCD. The nurse should help the individual perform activities of daily living to ensure that they are completed. Monitoring medication effects, teaching psychoeducation groups, ensuring adequate caloric intake, and providing individual patient counseling are additional inpatient interventions.

Emergency Care

Individuals with OCD frequently use medical services long before they seek specialized psychiatric treatment. Therefore, early recognition of symptoms and referral are important concerns for nurses working in primary care and other medical settings. After individuals are referred, most psychiatric treatment of OCD occurs on an outpatient basis. Individuals with severe OCD and/or self-harming thoughts and behaviors are hospitalized for their own safety. In these settings, medications are the primary interventions (Patel et al., 2014).

Family Interventions

The families of persons with OCD need to be educated about the causes of the disorder. Understanding the biologic basis of the disorder should decrease some of the stigma and embarrassment they may feel about the bizarre nature of the patient's obsessions and compulsions. Education about both biologic and psychological treatment approaches should be provided.

Family assistance in monitoring symptom remission and side effects of the medication is invaluable. Family members can also assist the person with behavioral and cognitive interventions.

When caring for the person with OCD, be sure to include the individual's caregiver, if appropriate, and address the following topic areas in the teaching plan:

- Medications, including drug action, dosage, frequency, and possible side effects
- Skin care measures
- Ritualistic behaviors and alternative activities
- Thought stopping
- Relaxation techniques
- Cognitive restructuring
- Community resources

Community Treatment

Partial hospitalization programs and day treatment programs help individuals in their quest for recovery. These programs can support independence while individuals begin medications and behavioral therapies. Some patients require outpatient treatment daily when symptoms increase. Maintenance outpatient therapy may be scheduled weekly or twice weekly for several weeks until the symptoms are well controlled. Community agency visits are recommended to monitor medication.

TRICHOTILLOMANIA

Trichotillomania is chronic self-destructive hair pulling that results in noticeable hair loss, usually in the crown, occipital, or parietal areas of the head, although sometimes also involve the eyebrows and eyelashes. The individual has an increase in tension immediately before pulling out the hair or while attempting to resist the behavior. After the hair has been pulled, the person feels a sense of relief. Some would classify this disorder as one of self-mutilation. It becomes a problem when accompanied by significant distress or impairment in other areas of function. A hair-pulling session can last several hours, and the individual may either ritualistically eat the hairs or discard them. Hair ingestion may result in the development of a hairball, which can lead to anorexia, stomach pain, anemia, intestinal obstruction, and peritonitis. Other medical complications include infection at the hair-pulling site. Hair pulling is usually done alone and persons may deny it; for some there is little conscious awareness, and for others, active pulling may regulate negative feelings (Houghton et al., 2016).

Clinical Course

The onset of trichotillomania occurs among children before the age of 5 years and in adolescents. For the young child, distraction or redirection may successfully eliminate the behavior. The behavior in adolescents may begin a chronic course that may last well into adulthood.

Diagnostic Criteria

Trichotillomania is diagnosed when recurrent pulling out of hair with hair loss occurs. The individual is unable to decrease or stop such hair pulling, which causes considerable distress (APA, 2013).

Etiology and Treatment

This disorder is poorly understood. An etiologic relationship to OCD has not been established, but support is present for a familial connection (Keuthen, Altenburger, & Pauls, 2014). The prevalence of trichotillomania is estimated at 1% to 2% of the population (APA, 2013). No particular medication class demonstrates effectiveness in treatment. Studies of individual medications including olanzapine (antipsychotic) and clomipramine (tricyclic antidepressant) show treatment effectiveness (Rothbart et al., 2013). Cognitive behavior therapy and habit reversal training, a behavioral intervention, can improve the symptoms (Rogers et al., 2014).

Evidenced-Based Nursing Care of Persons With Trichotillomania

The assessment includes a review of current problems, developmental history (especially school conflicts and learning difficulties), family and social history, identification of support systems, previous psychiatric treatment, and general health history. The cultural context in which the trichotillomania occurs must be taken into consideration because in some cultures, this behavior may be viewed as socially acceptable. The hair-pulling history and pattern are also used to determine the duration and severity of the disorder. Within the therapeutic relationship, a cognitive behavioral approach can be used to help the person identify when hair pulling occurs, the precipitating events, and the details of the episode.

Individuals with trichotillomania report that anxiety, loneliness, anger, fatigue, guilt, frustration, and boredom can all trigger the hair-pulling behaviors. Current research has also shown that persons with chronic hair pulling typically avoid social activities and events (Tung, Flessner, Grant, & Keuthen, 2015). In addition, the economic impact of trichotillomania can be significant in relation to lost work or school days. Teaching about the disorder will help affected individuals understand that they are not alone and that others have also had this problem. The goal of treatment is to help the individual learn to substitute positive behaviors for the hair-pulling behavior through self-monitoring of events that precipitate the episodes.

EXCORIATION (SKIN-PICKING) DISORDER

Repetitive and compulsive picking of skin causing tissue damage characterizes **excoriation or skin-picking disorder** (APA, 2013). Although face, arms, or hands are the most common sites for picking, it can occur at other body sites. Most affected people pick with their fingers, but tweezers or pins are also sometimes used. Similar to other disorders, skin picking causes significant distress to individuals. Prevalence is estimated at 1.4%; it occurs more frequently in persons with OCD (APA, 2013). Treatment data are limited, but include behavioral and pharmacologic interventions. Lamotrigine (mood stabilizer/anticonvulsant agent) has been shown to be successful in one study (Grant, Odlaug, Chamberlain, & Kim, 2010). Nursing care is similar to caring for a person with trichotillomania.

BODY DYSMORPHIC DISORDER

Individuals with BDD focus on real (but slight) or imagined defects in appearance, such as a large nose, thinning hair, or small genitals. Preoccupation with the perceived defect causes significant distress and interferes with their ability to function socially. They feel so self-conscious that they avoid work or public situations. Some fear that their "ugly" body part will malfunction. Surgical correction of the problem by a plastic surgeon or a dermatologist does not correct their preoccupation and distress. BDD is an extremely debilitating disorder and can significantly impair an individual's quality of life. BDD usually begins in adolescence and continues throughout adulthood. These individuals are not usually seen in psychiatric settings unless they have a coexisting psychiatric disorder or a family member insists on psychiatric attention.

This disorder occurs in men and women, with a prevalence of 2.4% in the United States (APA, 2013). Prevalence of outpatients with OCD, social phobia, and other disorders ranges from 10% to 40% (Hong, Nezgovorova, & Hollander, 2018). The risk of depression, suicide ideation, and suicide is high. Individuals with BDD are four times more likely to exhibit high rates of suicidality compared to the general population and those with eating disorders, OCD, or any other anxiety disorder (Angelakis, Gooding, & Panagioti, 2016). No single theory explains the cause of BDD. Unrealistic cultural expectations and genetic predisposition most likely underlie this disorder (see Box 20.6).

HOARDING DISORDER

Difficulty parting with or discarding possessions, regardless of actual value, characterizes hoarding disorder. Individuals with this disorder have a need to save items and experience distress if their items are discarded. Most affected individuals with hoarding disorder also exhibit excessive acquisition (excessive purchasing of items or collecting free items).

The prevalence of this disorder is estimated 2% to 6% (APA, 2013). Hoarding may begin in childhood with an increase in severity throughout a life span. This disorder tends to be familial and present in different generations. Over 50% of the individuals have co-occurring depression or chronic anxiety. Treatment includes pharmacologic agents and CBT. There is some evidence that peer-led groups may be effective (Mathews et al., 2018).

Hoarding poses public health and safety risks for individuals, families, and communities. Excessive collection of items not only clutters living areas but can lead to being trapped in an inaccessible environment and one that is high risk for fire. Home health nurses are often the first health care providers that recognize the problem and so are a valuable resource in determining the safety hazards and helping the individual become aware of the problem and seek treatment…. Currently, treatment includes CBT and medication for co-occurring mental disorders (Mathews et al., 2016) (see Box 20.7).

BOX 20.6 CLINICAL VIGNETTE

Body Dysmorphic Disorder

K, a 16-year-old girl, for about 6 months has believed that her pubic bone is becoming increasingly dislocated and prominent. She believes that everyone stares at it and talks about it. She does not remember a particular event related to the appearance of the symptom but is absolutely convinced that she can be helped only by a surgical correction of her pubic bone.

She was treated recently for anorexia nervosa with marginal success. Although her weight is nearly normal, she continues to be preoccupied with the looks of her body. She spends almost the entire day in her bedroom, wearing excessively large pajamas and she refuses to leave the house. Once or twice a day, she lowers herself to the ground and measures, with her fingers, the distance between her pelvic girdle and the ground in order to check the position of the pubic bone.

In desperation, her parents called the clinic for help.

The family was referred to a home health agency and a psychiatric home health nurse who arranged for an assessment visit.

What Do You Think?

- How should the nurse approach K? Should an assessment begin immediately?
- From the vignette, identify nursing diagnoses, outcomes, and interventions.

Adapted from Sobanski, E., & Schmidt, M. H. (2000). "Everybody looks at my pubic bone"—a case report of an adolescent patient with body dysmorphic disorder. *Acta Psychiatrica Scandinavica, 101*, 80–82.

BOX 20.7

Research for Best Practice: Compulsive Hoarding Syndrome

Singh, S., & Jones, C. (2013). Compulsive hoarding syndrome: Engaging the patients in treatment. *Mental Health Practice, 17*(4), 16–20.

THE QUESTION: How can persons with hoarding disorder be engaged in treatment?

METHODS: A CBT treatment approach is described that has been adapted to include visual methods (photographs, videos) and imagery. The group approach encourages the individuals to be "in the moment" and experience the discomfort of their difficulties. Participants photographed cluttered areas in their home and determined what they would like to overcome, imagined life without all of the clutter, and identified how their life and relationships are affected by the problem. Then they identified what they would like to do about the problem. This exercise helped them recognize the problem and what to do about it. Psychoeducation is included in the group and is based on themes that emerge in the session.

FINDINGS: Using group processes, the group members became supportive of each other when undertaking changes. The group developed a buddy system where members supported each other outside the group. Through using the visual methods, the individuals were able to distance themselves from the problem and decrease the feeling of being overwhelmed. They were able to be more objective and develop an action plan.

IMPLICATIONS FOR NURSING: Helping individuals with this disorder will require creative, eclectic approaches using a combination of modalities.

SUMMARY OF KEY POINTS

- Obsessions are excessive, intrusive, or unwanted thoughts. Compulsions are repetitive behaviors performed in a ritualistic manner.
- The most common obsession is the fear of contamination.
- Compulsions relieve anxiety and should not be interrupted unless the behavior jeopardizes the safety of the person or others. Interrupting compulsive behavior increases the person's anxiety.
- OCD is characterized by obsessions, compulsion, or both. OCD can occur in children and adults.
- Medications and cognitive behavior therapy can help affected individuals to get through episodes and reduce the compulsive behavior.
- Nursing care focuses on motivating the person for change, administering and monitoring medication, providing psychoeducation, and supporting positive new behaviors.
- The primary characteristics of trichotillomania and excoriation disorders are compulsive behaviors that damage the hair or skin. Compulsive behaviors of both disorders cause significant distress to the person who cannot stop or decrease the behaviors. Medications and psychotherapy can reduce these behaviors.
- BDD involves excessive focus on slight or imagined defects in appearance. The person with these extremely distressing defects seeks treatment by plastic surgeons or dermatologists. Correction does not relieve the patient's preoccupation, which continues to interfere with his or her quality of life. These individuals are high risk for depression and suicide.
- Hoarding disorder can begin in childhood and last a lifetime. Individuals with this disorder need to save things and become very upset if items are removed. When excessive collection leads to extreme clutter, it becomes a safety issue.

CRITICAL THINKING CHALLENGES

1. Differentiate an obsession from a compulsion.
2. List common obsessions and their consequences to the individual and family.
3. Jane, a 35-year-old single mother, has been unable go to work because she fears her apartment will burn down. She is constantly checking the stove and furnace. Her family convinced her to be admitted to a mental health unit. Discuss how you would prioritize her assessment and develop a plan of care.
4. Jon, a 25-year-old man, is admitted to an inpatient unit for depression and extreme anxiety. He was diagnosed with OCD as a child and had been able to function with medication. He recently married and decided to stop taking his medication. When his symptoms recurred, his wife tried to prevent Jon's compulsive behaviors by removing the knobs from the stove. He became more anxious. As Jon's nurse, develop a teaching plan about OCD for his wife.
5. Explain the behaviors associated with trichotillomania, excoriation disorder, BDD, and hoarding disorder. What are the similarities and differences?

2004: *Aviator*

The movie starring Leonardo DiCaprio depicts the earlier years of film producer, industrialist, and aviator Howard Hughes who suffered from OCD. Hughes' perfectionism in his film making and his need for order related to his food and cleanliness eventually contributed to his functional decline. Several scenes illustrate his obsession and compulsion. Hughes' symptoms eventually take over his life and he retreats to a self-imposed solitary confinement.

Viewing Points: How does his early life contribute to the development of his OCD symptoms? Identify his obsessions and compulsions. If Howard Hughes were your patient, what nursing diagnoses and interventions would you want to implement? Identify teaching needs related to medication and the obsessions and compulsions.

REFERENCES

American Psychiatric Association (APA). (2013). *Diagnostic and statistical manual of mental disorders* (5th ed.). Arlington, VA: Author.

Abramowitz, J. S., Meltzer-Brody, S., Leserman, J., Killenberg, S., Rinaldi, K., Mahaffey, B. L., et al. (2010). Obsessional thoughts and compulsive behaviors in a sample of women with postpartum mood symptoms. *Archives of Women's Mental Health, 13*(6), 523–530.

Angelakis, I, Gooding, P. A., Panagioti, M. (2016). Suicidality in body dysmorphic disorder (BDD): A systematic review with meta-analysis. *Clinical Psychology Review, 49*, 55–66.

Bener, A., Dafeeah, E. E., Abou-Saleh, M. T., Ghurgra, D., & Ventriglio, A. (2018). Schizophrenia and co-morbid obsessive-compulsive disorder: Clinical characteristic. *Asian Journal of Psychiatry, 37*, 80–84.

Cleary, D. R., Ozpinar, A., Raslan, A. M., & Ko, A. L. (2015). Deep brain stimulation for psychiatric disorders: Where we are now. *Neurosurgical Focus, 38*(6), E2.

Cuzen, N. L., Stein, D. J., Lochner, C., & Fineberg, N. A. (2014). Comorbidity of obsessive-compulsive disorder and substance use disorder: A new heuristic. *Human Psychopharmacology: Clinical & Experimental, 29*(1), 89–93.

Del Casale, A., Sorice, S., Padovano, A., Simmaco, M., Ferracuti, S., Lamis, D. A., et al. (2018). Psychopharmacological treatment of obsessive-compulsive disorder (OCD). *Current Neuropharmacology, 16*(7). Retrieved from https://doi.org/10.2174/1570159X16666180813155017

Dell'Osso, B., Benatti, B., Rodriguez, C. I., Arici, C., Palazzo, C., Altamura, A. C., et al. (2017). Obsessive-compulsive disorder in the elderly: A report from the International College of Obsessive-Compulsive Spectrum Disorders. *European Psychiatry, 45*, 36–40.

De Ridder, D., Vanneste, S., Gillett, G., Manning, P., Glue, P., & Langguth, B. (2016). Psychosurgery reduces uncertainty and increases free will? A review. *Neuromodulation, 19*(3), 239–248.

Fontenelle, L. F., Coutinho, E. S., Lins-Martin, N. M., Fitzgerald, P. B., Fujiwara, H., & Yucel, M. (2015). Electroconvulsive therapy for obsessive-compulsive disorder: A systematic review. *Journal of Clinical Psychiatry, 76*(7), 949–957.

Grant, J. E., Odlaug, B. L., Chamberlain, M. D., & Kim, S. W. (2010). A double-blind, placebo-controlled trial of lamotrigine for pathologic skin picking: Treatment efficacy and neurocognitive predictors of response. *Journal of Clinical Psychopharmacology, 30*(4), 396–403.

Groth, C., Mol, D. N., Rask, C. U., Lange, T., & Skov, L. (2017). Course of Tourette Syndrome and comorbidities in a large prospective clinical study. *Journal of the American Academy of Child and Adolescent Psychiatry, 56*(4), 304–312.

Hachiya, Y., Miyata, R., Tanuma, N., Hongou, K., Tanaka, K., Shimoda, K., et al. (2013). Autoimmune neurological disorders associated with group-A beta-hemolytic streptococcal infection. *Brain & Development, 35*(7), 670–674.

Hong, K., Nezgovorova, V., & Hollander, E. (2018). New perspectives in the treatment of body dysmorphic disorder. Review. *F1000 Faculty Research, 7*, 361.

Hong, K., Nezgovorova, V., Uzunova, G., Schlussel, D., & Hollander, E. (2018). Pharmacological treatment of body dysmorphic disorder. *Current Neuropharmacology, 16*(1). doi: /10.2174/1570159X16666180426153940.

Houghton, D. C., Maas, J., Twohig, M. P., Saunders, S. M., Compton, S. N., Neal-Barnett, A. M., et al. (2016). Comorbidity and quality of life in adults with hair pulling disorder. *Psychiatry Research, 239*, 12–19.

Jacob, M. L., & Storch, E. A. (2013). Pediatric obsessive-compulsive disorder: A review for nursing professionals. *Journal of Child and Adolescent Psychiatric Nursing, 26*, 138–148.

Janardhan Reddy, Y. C., Sundar, A. S., Narayanaswamy, J. C., & Math, S. B. (2017). Clinical practice guidelines for obsessive-compulsive disorder. *Indian Journal of Psychiatry, 59*(Suppl 1), S74–S90.

Keuthen, N. J., Altenburger, E. M., & Pauls, D. (2014). A family study of trichotillomania and chronic hair pulling. *American Journal of Medical Genetics. Part B: Neuropsychiatric Genetics, 165*(2), 167–174.

Klenfeldt, I. F., Karlsson, B., Sigstsrom, R., Backman, K., Waern, M., Ostling, S., et al. (2014). Prevalence of obsessive-compulsive disorder in relation to depression and cognition in an elderly population. *The American Journal of Geriatric Psychiatry, 3*, 301–308.

Krebs, G., & Heyman, I. (2015). Obsessive-compulsive disorder in children and adolescents. *Archives of Disease in Childhood, 100*(5), 495–499.

La Buissonniere-Ariza, V., Schneider, S. C., Hojgaard, D., Kay, B. C., Riemann, B. C., Eken, S. C., et al. (2018). Family accommodation of anxiety symptoms in youth undergoing intensive multimodal treatment for anxiety disorders and obsessive-compulsive disorder: Nature, clinical correlates, and treatment response. *Comprehensive Psychiatry, 80*, 1–13.

Mathews, C. A., Mackin, R. S., Chou, C. Y., Uhm, S. Y., Bain, L. D., Stark, S. J. (2018). Randomised clinical trial of community-based peer-led and psychologist-led group treatment for hoarding disorders. *BJPsych Open, 7*, 361.

Mathews, C. A., Uhm, S., Chan, J., Gause, M., Franklin, J., Plumadore, J., et al. (2016). Treatment hoarding disorder in a real-world setting: Results from the Mental Health Association of San Francisco. *Psychiatry Research, 237*, 331–338.

McGuire, J. F., Lewin, A. B., & Storch, E. Q. (2014). Enhancing exposure therapy for anxiety disorders, obsessive-compulsive disorder and post-traumatic stress disorder. (Review). *Expert Review of Neurotherapeutics, 14*(8), 893–910.

Miyawaki, D., Goto, A., Iwakura, Y., Hirai, K., Miki, Y., Asada, N., et al. (2018). Preschool-onset obsessive compulsive disorder with complete remission. *Neuropsychiatric Disease Treatment, 14*, 1747–1753.

Murphy, Y. E., & Flessner, C. A. (2015). Family functioning in paediatric obsessive compulsive and related disorders. *British Journal of clinical Psychology, 54*(4), 414–434.

Patel, S. R., Humensky, J. L., Olfson, M., Simpson, H. B., Myers, R., & Dixon, L. B. (2014). Treatment of obsessive-compulsive disorder in a nationwide survey of office-based physician practice. *Psychiatric Services, 65*(5), 681–684.

Rapp, A. M., Bergman, R. L., Piacentini, J., & McGuire, J. F. (2018) Evidence-based assessment of obsessive-compulsive disorder. *Journal of Central Nervous System Disease, 8*, 13–29.

Richter, P. M., & Ramos, R. T. (2018). Obsessive-compulsive disorder. *Behavioral Neurology and Psychiatry, 25*(5), 828–844.

Rogers, K., Banis, M., Falkenstein, M. J., Malloy, E. J., McDonough, L., Nelson, S. O., et al. (2014). Stepped care in the treatment of trichotillomania. *Journal of Consulting and Clinical Psychology, 82*(2), 361–367.

Rothbart, R., Amos, T., Siegfried, N., Ipser, J. C., Fineberg, N, Chamberlain, S. R., et al. (2013). Pharmacotherapy for trichotillomania. *The Cochrane Database of Systematic Reviews,* (11):CD007662.

Ruscio, A. M., Stein, D. J., Chiu, W. T., & Kessler, R. C. (2010). The epidemiology of obsessive-compulsive disorder in the National Comorbidity Survey Replication. *Molecular Psychiatry, 15*(1), 53–63.

Sağlam, T., Aksoy Poyraz, C., Poyraz, B. Ç., & Tosun, M. (2018). Successful use of electroconvulsive therapy in a patient with anorexia nervosa and severe acute-onset obsessive-compulsive disorder. *International Journal of Eating Disorders, 51*(7), 1026–1028.

Shaw, P., Sharp, W., Sudre, G., Wharton, A., Greenstein, D., & Raznahan, A., (2014). Subcortical and cortical morphological anomalies as an endophenotype in obsessive-compulsive disorder. *Molecular Psychiatry, 20*(2), 224–231.

Sharma, E., Thennarasu, K., & Reddy, Y. C. (2014). Long-term outcome of obsessive-compulsive disorder in adults: A meta-analysis. *Journal of Clinical Psychiatry, 75*(9), 1019–1027.

Soffer-Dudek, N. (2018). Dissociative absorption, mind-wandering, and attention-deficit symptoms: Associations with obsessive-compulsive symptoms. *British Journal of Clinical Psychology, 58*(1), 51–69.

Substance Abuse and Mental Health Services Administration [SAMHSA]. (2017). *Understanding obsessive-compulsive disorder Young adults*. Retrieved October 24, 2018, from https://store.samhsa.gov/product/Understanding-Obsessive-Compulsive-Disorder-Young-Adults-/SMA16-5002

Substance Abuse and Mental Health Services Administration (SAMHSA). (2016). Obsessive-compulsive disorder and substance use disorders. *Advisory, 15*(3), 1–9.

Tiago, V. M., Cooney, R. E., & Peterson, B. S. (2008). The neural bases of obsessive-compulsive disorder in children and adults. *Developmental Psychopathology, 20*(4), 1251–1283.

Tung, E. S., Flessner, C. A., Grant, J. E., & Keuthen, N. J. (2015). Predictors of life disability in trichotillomania. *Comprehensive Psychiatry, 56*, 239–244.

U.S. Food & Drug Administration (FDA). (2018). FDA permits marketing of transcranial magnetic stimulation for treatment of obsessive compulsive disorder. Retrieved July 8, 2019 from https://www.fda.gov/newsevents/newsroom/pressannouncements/ucm617244.htm

van der Straten, A. Denys, D., & van Wingen, G. A. (2017). Impact of treatment on resting cerebral blood flow and metabolism in obsessive compulsive disorder: A meta analysis. *Scientific Reports, 7*(1), 17464.

Wood, J., & Ahmari, S. E. (2015). A framework for understanding the emerging role of corticolimbic-ventral striatal networks in OCD-associated repetitive behavior. *Frontiers in Systems Neuroscience, 9*, 171.

Wu, M. S., Hamblin, R., Nadeau, J., Simmons, J., Smith, A., Smith, A., et al. (2017). Quality of life and burden in caregivers of youth with obsessive-compulsive disorder presenting for intensive treatment. *Comprehensive Psychiatry, 80*, 46–56.

Wu, M. S., Rozenman, M., Peris, T. S., O'Neill, J., Bergman, R. L., Chang, S., et al. (2018). Comparing OCD-affected youth with and without religious symptoms: Clinical profiles and treatment response. *Comprehensive Psychiatry, 86*, 47–53.

21

Depression

Nursing Care of Persons With Depressive Moods and Suicidal Behavior

Barbara Jones Warren

KEY CONCEPTS
- mood
- depression
- suicidal behavior

LEARNING OBJECTIVES

After studying this chapter, you will be able to:

1. Discuss the role of mood and depression in mental disorders.
2. Describe the prevalence and incidence of major depressive disorder.
3. Delineate the clinical symptoms and course of major depressive disorder including suicidal behavior.
4. Discuss the primary theories of major depressive disorder and their relationship to suicidal behavior.
5. Apply the nursing process with recovery-oriented interventions for persons with major depressive disorder including those with suicidal behavior.
6. Discuss the need for integrated health care for persons with depression.
7. Develop wellness strategies for persons with depression.
8. Describe other depressive disorders.

KEY TERMS

- affect • anhedonia • cytokines • depression • depressive disorders • disruptive mood dysregulation disorder
- major depressive disorder • persistent depressive disorder • premenstrual dysphoric disorder • serotonin syndrome
- suicidality

Case Study: Louise

Louise is a 31-year-old woman who was admitted voluntarily to an inpatient mental health unit with depression with suicidal ideation. Louise and her husband Brian have three children ages 9, 5, and 3 years old.

Most people have bad days or times of feeling sad and overwhelmed. When depressed feelings interfere with daily activities and relationships, however, this mood can impair judgment and contribute to negative views of the world. In some instances, depression is a symptom of a depressive disorder. This chapter discusses mood and depression, depressive disorders, and the related serious issue of suicidal behavior. **Major depressive disorder** is highlighted.

MOOD AND DEPRESSION

Normal variations in mood occur in response to life events. Normal mood variations (e.g., sadness, euphoria, and anxiety) are time-limited and are not usually associated with significant functional impairment. Normal range of mood or affect, the expression of mood, varies considerably both within and among different cultures (Lin & Dmitrieva, 2019).

> **KEYCONCEPT** **Mood** is a pervasive and sustained emotion that influences one's perception of the world and how one functions.

Affect, or outward emotional expression, is related to the concept of mood. Affect provides clues to the person's mood. For example, in depression, people often have limited facial expression. Several terms are used to describe affect, including the following:

- *Blunted:* significantly reduced intensity of emotional expression
- *Bright:* smiling, projection of a positive attitude
- *Flat:* absent or nearly absent affective expression
- *Inappropriate:* discordant affective expression accompanying the content of speech or ideation
- *Labile:* varied, rapid, and abrupt shifts in affective expression
- *Restricted or constricted:* mildly reduced in the range and intensity of emotional expression

Depression is the primary mood of depressive disorders. Depression can be overwhelming. Unless appropriately treated, depression persists over time, has a significant negative effect on quality of life, and increases the risk of suicide (Lotfaliany et al., 2018; Tuithof et al., 2018).

> **KEYCONCEPT** **Depression** is a common mental state characterized by sadness, loss of interest or pleasure, feelings of guilt or low self-worth, disturbed sleep or appetite, low energy, and poor concentration (American Psychiatric Association [APA], 2013; World Health Organization [WHO], 2019).

OVERVIEW OF DEPRESSIVE DISORDERS

When a sad mood interferes with daily life, a **depressive disorder** may exist that will benefit from treatment. In depressive disorders, a sad, irritable, or empty mood is present with somatic and cognitive changes that interfere with functioning. Several depressive disorders vary according to duration, timing, or cause (APA, 2013). These include disruptive mood dysregulation, major depressive disorder, persistent depressive (dysthymia), premenstrual dysphoric, substance/medication-induced, other specified depressive and unspecified depressive disorders (APA, 2013). Disruptive mood dysregulation disorder is a new depressive disorder diagnostic category in the *DSM-5*.

The clinical symptoms and course of depressive phenomena are complex, dynamic, biopsychosocial processes involving life-span and cultural aspects. Persons with depressive disorders experience a lower quality of life and are at greater risk for development of physical health problems than those who are not depressed. Depressive disorders are so widespread that they are generally diagnosed and treated in the primary care setting. Every nurse will have an opportunity to impact this pandemic health concern (WHO, 2019).

Depressive disorders are characterized by severe and debilitating depressive episodes and are associated with high levels of impairment in occupational, social, and physical functioning. They cause as much disability and distress to patients as chronic medical disorders. Frequently, they are undetected and untreated. Because suicide is a significant risk, these disorders are associated with premature death, especially in those individuals who have been hospitalized for depression (Bachman, 2018).

Depressive Disorders Across the Life Span

Children and Adolescents

Children with depressive disorders have symptoms similar to those seen in adults with a few exceptions. They are more likely to have anxiety symptoms, such as fear of separation, and somatic symptoms, such as stomach aches and headaches. They may have less interaction with their peers and avoid play and recreational activities that they previously enjoyed. Mood may be irritable, rather than sad, especially in adolescents. See Chapter 30 for discussion of mental health disorders in children.

The risk of suicide, which peaks during the midadolescent years, is very real in children and adolescents. Mortality from suicide, which increases steadily through the teens, is the third leading cause of death for that age group. Findings from research indicate that chronic victimization increases the risk for depression and suicide ideation and attempts (Brunstein et al., 2019). The use of substances intensifies depressive symptomatology and the risk of suicide (Johns et al., 2018). See Chapter 16 for further discussion of suicide in children and adolescents.

Older Adults

Depression in older adults is often undetected or inadequately treated (Kok & Reynolds, 2017). However, it is estimated that 8% to 20% of older adults in the community and as many as 37% in primary care settings experience depressive symptoms (Blazer & Steffens, 2015). Treatment is successful in 60% to 80%, but response to treatment is slower than in younger adults. Depression in older adults is often associated with chronic illnesses, such as heart disease, stroke, and cancer; symptoms may have a more somatic focus. Depressive symptomatology in this group may be confused with symptoms of bipolar, dementia, or cerebrovascular accidents. Hence,

BOX 21.1 CLINICAL VIGNETTE

Depression in an Older Adult

Bob is a 75-year-old man who lost his wife to cancer 18 months ago. Since his wife's death, he continued to live in their family home with his dog. His dog died 2 weeks ago and he has been despondent since then. His children found him sitting on the side of his bed with a loaded gun. He had already written a note that he did not want to be a burden and that his children would be better off without him. His family brought him to the emergency department for evaluation.

What Do You Think?
- What is the likelihood that Bob would actually kill himself?
- What do you think the next recovery-oriented strategy should be for Bob and his family?

---

differential diagnosis may be required to ascertain the root and cause of symptoms. See Chapter 31 for further discussion of mental health disorders in older adults.

Suicide is a very serious risk for older adults, especially for men. Suicide rates peak during middle age, but a second peak occurs in those aged 75 years and older (Ivey-Stephenson, Crosby, Jack, Haileyesus, & Kresnow-Sedacca, 2017). See Box 21.1 and Chapter 31.

MAJOR DEPRESSIVE DISORDER

Clinical Course

Major depressive disorder is commonly a progressively recurrent illness. With time, episodes tend to occur more frequently, become more severe, and are of a longer duration. Onset of depression may occur at any age. However, the initial onset may occur in puberty; the highest onset occurs within persons in their 20s (APA, 2013). Recurrences of depression are related to age of onset, increased intensity and severity of symptoms, and presence of psychosis, anxiety, and/or personality features. The risk for relapse is higher in persons who have experienced initial symptoms at a younger age and incur other mental disorders (Hoertel et al., 2017).

Diagnostic Criteria

The primary diagnostic criterion for major depressive disorder is one or more moods, which is either a depressed mood or a loss of interest or pleasure in nearly all activities for at least 2 weeks. Four of seven additional symptoms must be present: disruption in sleep, appetite (or weight), concentration, or energy; psychomotor agitation or retardation; excessive guilt or feelings of worthlessness; and suicidal ideation (Key Diagnostic Characteristics 21.1).

The incidence of misdiagnosis is often greater for persons who are treated by someone from culturally and ethnically different populations. Their explanation of their symptomatology may be expressed using different terminology or the underrepresented group may feel uncomfortable with a clinician from a different culture (Hornberger, Medley-Proctor, Nettles, Cimporescu, & Howe, 2016).

Epidemiology and Risk Factors

The prevalence of major depressive disorder within the US population is approximately 10.4% within a 12-month time period, with a lifetime prevalence of 20.6%. Individuals between the ages of 18 and 29 years have a higher prevalence rate than those persons aged 65 and older. Episodes typically last more than 6 months. Females have a higher prevalence rate than males (13.4% vs. 7.2%). Depression is more prevalent in younger adults, white adults, and Native American adults than among African-American, Asian-American, and Hispanic adults (Hasin et al., 2018).

Data from the WHO indicate that depression is the leading cause of years lost because of disability. More than 50% of persons who recover from an initial episode of depression experience another episode within 5 to 10 years (WHO, 2019).

Risk factors for the development of depression include the following:

- Prior episode of depression
- Family history of depressive disorder
- Lack of social support
- Lack of coping abilities
- Presence of life and environmental stressors
- Current substance use or abuse
- Medical and/or mental illness comorbidity

Consider Louise

Her sister died as a result of drowning 2 months ago. She has been telling her husband that she just wants to go to sleep and not wake up. What risk factors do you recognize?

Ethnicity and Culture

Culture can influence the experience and communication of symptoms of depression. Persons from culturally and ethnically diverse populations may formulate and describe their depressive symptomatology differently

> **KEY DIAGNOSTIC CHARACTERISTICS 21.1 • MAJOR DEPRESSIVE DISORDER 296.XX**
>
> **296.2X MAJOR DEPRESSIVE DISORDER, SINGLE EPISODE**
> **296.3X MAJOR DEPRESSIVE DISORDER, RECURRENT**
>
> **Diagnostic Criteria**
>
> A. Five (or more) of the following symptoms have been present during the same 2-week period and represent a change from previous functioning; at least one of the symptoms is either (1) depressed mood or (2) loss of interest or pleasure.
>
> **Note:** Do not include symptoms that are clearly attributable to another medical condition.
>
> 1. Depressed mood most of the day, nearly every day, as indicated by either subjective report (e.g., feels sad, empty, hopeless) or observation made by others (e.g., appears tearful). (**Note:** In children and adolescents, can be irritable mood.)
> 2. Markedly diminished interest or pleasure in all, or almost all, activities most of the day, nearly every day (as indicated by either subjective account or observation).
> 3. Significant weight loss when not dieting or weight gain (e.g., a change of more than 5% of body weight in a month), or decrease or increase in appetite nearly every day. (**Note:** In children, consider failure to make expected weight gain.)
> 4. Insomnia or hypersomnia nearly every day.
> 5. Psychomotor agitation or retardation nearly every day (observable by others, not merely subjective feelings of restlessness or being slowed down).
> 6. Fatigue or loss of energy nearly every day.
> 7. Feelings of worthlessness or excessive or inappropriate guilt (which may be delusional) nearly every day (not merely self-reproach or guilt about being sick).
> 8. Diminished ability to think or concentrate, or indecisiveness, nearly every day (either by subjective account or as observed by others).
> 9. Recurrent thoughts of death (not just fear of dying), recurrent suicidal ideation without a specific plan, or a suicide attempt or a specific plan for committing suicide.
>
> The symptoms cause clinically significant distress or impairment in social, occupational, or other important areas of functioning.
>
> The episode is not attributable to the physiologic effects of a substance or to another medical condition.
>
> B. The symptoms cause clinically significant distress or impairment in social, occupational, or other important areas of functioning.
> C. The episode is not attributable to the physiologic effects of a substance or to another medical condition.
>
> **Note:** Criteria A to C represent a major depressive episode.
>
> **Note:** Responses to a significant loss (e.g., bereavement, financial ruin, losses from a natural disaster, a serious medical illness, or disability) may include the feelings of intense sadness, rumination about the loss, insomnia, poor appetite, and weight loss noted in Criterion A, which may resemble a depressive episode. Although such symptoms may be understandable or considered appropriate to the loss, the presence of a major depressive episode in addition to the normal response to a significant loss should also be carefully considered. This decision inevitably requires the exercise of clinical judgment based on the individual's history and the cultural norms for the expression of distress in the context of loss.
>
> The occurrence of the major depressive episode is not better explained by schizoaffective disorder, schizophrenia, schizophreniform disorder, delusional disorder, or other specified and unspecified schizophrenia spectrum and other psychotic disorders.
>
> There has never been a manic episode or a hypomanic episode.
>
> **Note:** This exclusion does not apply if all of the manic-like or hypomanic-like episodes are substance-induced or are attributable to the physiologic effects of another medical condition.
>
> Reprinted with permission from the *Diagnostic and statistical manual of mental disorders* (5th ed.) (Copyright © 2013). American Psychiatric Association. All Rights Reserved.

than in the clinical language used for diagnosis. For example, expressions such as "heartbrokenness" (Native American and Middle Eastern), "brain fog" (persons from the West Indies), "zar," and "running amok" may be used in place of such terms as "depressed," "sad," "hopeless," and "discouraged."

In some cultures, somatic symptoms, rather than sadness or guilt, may predominate. Individuals from various Asian cultural groups may have complaints of weakness, tiredness, or imbalance. "Problems of the heart" (in Middle Eastern cultures) or of being "heartbroken" (among Native Americans of the Hopi tribe) may be the way that persons from these cultural groups express their depressive experiences. Culturally distinctive experiences need to be assessed to ascertain any presence of depressive disorder from a "normal" cultural emotional response (Pedersen, Lonner, Draguus, & Trimble, 2016).

Comorbidity

Major depressive disorders often co-occur with other psychiatric disorders including those that are substance related. Depression often is associated with a variety of chronic medical conditions, particularly endocrine disorders, cardiovascular disease, and neurologic disorders (Lotfaliany et al., 2018).

Etiology

Biologic Theories

Genetic

Family, twin, and adoption studies demonstrate that genetic influences undoubtedly play a substantial role in the etiology of mood disorders. Major depressive disorder tends to run in families and has a heritable component.

Currently, a major research effort is focusing on developing a more accurate paradigm regarding the contribution of genetic factors to the development of mood disorders (Howard et al., 2019).

Neurobiologic Hypotheses

Neurobiologic theories of the etiology of depression emerged in the 1950s. These theories posit that major depression is caused by a deficiency or dysregulation in central nervous system (CNS) concentrations of the neurotransmitters norepinephrine, dopamine, and serotonin or in their receptor functions. These hypotheses arose in part from observations that some pharmacologic agents elevated mood; subsequent studies identified their mechanisms of action. All antidepressants currently available have their therapeutic effects on these neurotransmitters or receptors. Current research continues to focus on the role of neurotransmitters and the neurobiology of depression (Joca, Moreira, & Wegener, 2015).

Neuroendocrine and Neuropeptide Hypotheses

Major depressive disorder is associated with multiple endocrine alterations, specifically of the hypothalamic–pituitary–adrenal axis, the hypothalamic–pituitary–thyroid axis, the hypothalamic–growth hormone axis, and the hypothalamic–pituitary–gonadal axis. In addition, mounting evidence indicates that components of neuroendocrine axes (e.g., neuromodulatory peptides such as corticotropin-releasing factor) may themselves contribute to depressive symptoms. Evidence also suggests that the secretion of these hypothalamic and growth hormones is controlled by many of the neurotransmitters implicated in the pathophysiology of depression (Gong et al., 2019).

Psychoneuroimmunology

Psychoneuroimmunology is a recent area of research into a diverse group of proteins known as *chemical messengers* between immune cells. These messengers, called **cytokines**, signal the brain and serve as mediators between immune and nerve cells. The brain is capable of influencing immune processes, and conversely, immunologic response can result in changes in brain activity. Increased cytokine levels are associated with depression and cognitive impairment indicating that inflammatory reactions are involved in the development of some mental health disorders (Himmerich, Patsalos, Lichtblau, Ibrahim, & Dalton, 2019).

Psychological Theories

Psychological theories that serve as a basis for nursing practice for persons with a mental health disorder are explained in Chapter 5. Depression is one of the disorders treated from a psychological perspective. The following discussion identifies theoretical models often used in nursing care.

Psychodynamic Factors

Most psychodynamic theorists acknowledge some debt to Freud's original conceptualization of the psychodynamics of depression, which ascribes the cause to an early lack of love, care, warmth, and protection and resultant anger, guilt, helplessness, and fear regarding the loss of love. The ensuing conflict between wanting to be loved and fear of rejection engenders pathologic self-punishment (also conceptualized as aggression turned inward), self-rejection, low self-esteem, and depressive symptoms (see Chapter 5).

Behavioral Factors

The behavioral psychologists hold that depression primarily results from a severe reduction in rewarding activities or an increase in unpleasant events in one's life. The subsequent depression then leads to further restriction of activity, thereby decreasing the likelihood of experiencing pleasurable activities, which, in turn, intensifies the mood disturbance. Affected individuals often self-criticize and believe that they do not have the coping skills to deal with life's stresses. If family members believe that the person is "sick" and so lacks the necessary coping skills, they inadvertently reinforce the hopeless self-view of the depressed person.

Cognitive Factors

The cognitive approach maintains that irrational beliefs and negative distortions of thought about the self, the environment, and the future engender and perpetuate depressive effects (see Chapter 5). These depressive cognitions can be learned socially from family members or lack of experience in developing coping skills. These individuals think differently than nondepressed individuals and view their environment and themselves in negative ways. They blame themselves for any misfortunes that occur and see situations as being much worse than they are.

Developmental Factors

Developmental theorists posit that depression may result from the loss of a parent through death or separation or lack of emotionally adequate parenting. These factors may delay or prohibit the realization of appropriate developmental milestones.

Social Theories

Family Factors

Family theorists ascribe maladaptive patterns in family interactions as contributing to the onset of depression, particularly in the onset and occurrence of depression in younger individuals. A family becomes dysfunctional when interactions, decisions, or behaviors interfere with the positive development of the family and its individual members. Most families have periods of dysfunction, such as during a crisis or stressful situation when coping skills are not available. Unhealthy interactions within a family system can have a negative impact on one or more family members who do not have the coping skills to deal with the situation.

Environmental Factors

Depression has long been understood as a multifactorial disorder that occurs when environmental factors (e.g., death of family member) interact with the biologic and psychological makeup of the individual. Major depression may follow adverse or traumatic life events, especially those that involve the loss of an important human relationship or role in life. Social isolation, deprivation, and financial deprivation are associated with depression (Ge, Yap, Ong, & Heng, 2017).

Family Response to Disorder

Depression in one family member affects the whole family. Spouses, children, parents, siblings, and friends experience frustration, guilt, and anger when a family member is immobilized and cannot function. It is often hard for others to understand the depth of the mood and how disabling it can be. Financial hardship can occur when the affected family member cannot work and instead spends days in bed. The lack of understanding and difficulty of living with a depressed person can lead to abuse. Women between the ages of 18 and 45 years constitute the majority of those experiencing depression. This incidence may affect women's ability to not only have productive lives and take care of themselves but to also take care of their children or other family members for whom they may have responsibility. Moreover, research indicates that the incidence of depression may be higher in children whose mothers experience depression (Drury, Scaramella, & Zeanah, 2016).

>
> **Remember Louise?**
> According to her husband, Louise has neglected her self-care and that of her children since her sister's death. Brian is very understanding and supportive of Louise's need to grieve, but he is concerned that this is more than grief. Brian says that he is afraid to leave her alone and the children are suffering. What recommendations would you suggest to Louise's husband? Are there indications that Louise's grief is developing into depression?

Recovery-Oriented Care for Persons With Depressive Disorders

Teamwork and Collaboration: Working Toward Recovery

Depressive disorders are the most commonly occurring mental disorders, but they are usually treated within the primary care setting, rather than psychiatric setting. Nursing practice requires a coordinated ongoing interaction among patients, families, and health care providers to deliver comprehensive services. This includes using the complementary skills of both psychiatric and medical care colleagues for forming overall goals, plans, and decisions and for providing continuity of care as needed. Collaborative care between the primary care provider and mental health specialist is also key to achieving remission of symptoms and physical well-being, restoring baseline occupational and psychosocial functioning, and reducing the likelihood of relapse or recurrence.

Individuals with depression enter mental health settings when their symptoms become so severe that hospitalization is needed, usually after suicide attempts, or if they self-refer because of incapacitation. Antidepressants are indicated for depression and are discussed later in this chapter. Interdisciplinary treatment of these disorders, which is often lifelong, needs to include a wide array of health professionals in all areas. The specific goals of treatment are:

- Reduce or control symptoms and, if possible, eliminate signs and symptoms of the depressive syndrome.
- Improve occupational and psychosocial function as much as possible.
- Reduce the likelihood of relapse and recurrence through recovery-oriented strategies.

Cognitive and Interpersonal Therapies

Recent studies suggest that short-term cognitive and interpersonal therapies may be as effective as pharmacotherapy in milder depressions. In many instances, cognitive-behavioral therapy (CBT) is an effective strategy for preventing relapse in patients who have had only a partial response to pharmacotherapy alone (APA, 2013). CBT is implemented in individual or group therapy by a trained clinician.

Interpersonal therapy seeks to recognize, explore, and resolve the interpersonal losses, role confusion and transitions, social isolation, and deficits in social skills that may precipitate depressive states. It maintains that losses must be mourned and related affects appreciated, role confusion and transitions must be recognized and resolved, and social skills deficits must be overcome to acquire social supports.

Combination Therapies

For patients with severe or recurrent major depressive disorder, the combination of psychotherapy (including interpersonal, cognitive-behavioral, behavior, brief dynamic, or dialectical behavioral therapies) and pharmacotherapy has been found to be superior to treatment using a single modality. Clinical practice guidelines suggest that the combination of medication and psychotherapy is particularly useful in more complex situations (e.g., depression in the context of concurrent, chronic general-medical or other psychiatric disorders, or in patients who fail to experience complete response to either treatment alone). Psychotherapy in combination with medication is also used to address collateral issues, such as medication adherence or secondary psychosocial problems (Dunlop et al., 2019). If medications and psychotherapy are not effective, other options are available: electroconvulsive therapy (ECT), light therapy, and repetitive transcranial magnetic stimulation discussed later in the chapter.

Alternative Therapies

Alternative or complementary therapies are often used in the treatment of depression. Acupuncture, yoga or tai chi, meditation, guided imagery, and massage therapy are a few therapies that may be helpful to palliate depression. Music or art therapy is also used often in conjunction with medication or psychotherapy.

Integration With Primary Care

Depression is often treated in the primary care setting with readily available antidepressants. Unfortunately, the primary treatment for depression in this setting is medication. Many individuals need more than medication, but do not access mental health services for a variety of reasons such as stigma, fear of being labeled as mentally ill, and lack of resources. There are also several medical problems associated with depression such as hypothyroidism (Uhlenbusch et al., 2019). Pain is a common problem for individuals who are depressed (Zis et al., 2017). It is important to communicate with the primary care provider to coordinate care.

Safety Issues

The overriding concern for people with mood disorders is safety because these individuals may experience self-destructive thoughts and suicidal ideation. Hence, the assessment of possible suicide risk should be routinely conducted in any person who is depressed (see Chapter 16).

Evidence-Based Nursing Care of Persons With Depressive Disorder

An awareness of the risk factors for depression, a comprehensive and culturally competent mental health nursing assessment, history of illness, and past treatment are keys to formulating a treatment or recovery plan and to evaluating outcomes. Interviewing a family member or close friend about the patient's day-to-day functioning and specific symptoms may help determine the course of the illness, current symptoms, and level of functioning. The family's level of support and understanding of the disorder also need to be assessed. Nursing Care Plan 21.1—which sets forth a plan of care for Louise, the case study patient in this chapter—is available at http://thepoint.lww.com/BoydEssentials2e.

Mental Health Nursing Assessment

The mental health nursing assessment focuses on the physical consequences of the depression as well as the psychosocial aspects. The symptoms of depression are similar to those of some medical problems or medication side effects. Often, the mental health nurse is the only clinician who provides holistic care to a person with depression who is often treated by other disciplines.

Physical Health

The nursing assessment should include a physical systems review and thorough history of medical problems, with special attention to CNS function, endocrine function, anemia, chronic pain, autoimmune illness, diabetes mellitus, or menopause. Additional medical history includes surgeries; medical hospitalizations; head injuries; episodes of loss of consciousness; and pregnancies, childbirths, miscarriages, and abortions. A complete list of prescribed and over-the-counter (OTC) medications and herbal supplements should be compiled, including the reason a medication was prescribed or its use discontinued. A physical examination is recommended with baseline vital signs and baseline laboratory tests, including a comprehensive blood chemistry panel, complete blood counts, liver function tests, thyroid function tests, urinalysis, and electrocardiograms (see Chapter 9).

The following symptoms are characteristics of depression and should be assessed:

- *Appetite and weight changes:* In major depression, changes from baseline include a decrease or increase in appetite with or without significant weight loss or gain (i.e., a change of more than 5% of body weight in 1 month). Weight loss occurs when the person is not dieting. Older adults with moderate-to-severe depression need to be assessed for dehydration as well as weight changes.

- *Sleep disturbance:* The most common sleep disturbance associated with major depression is insomnia, which is broken into three categories: initial insomnia (difficulty falling asleep), middle insomnia (waking up during the night and having difficulty returning to sleep), and terminal insomnia (waking too early and being unable to return to sleep). Less frequently, the sleep disturbance is hypersomnia (i.e., prolonged sleep episodes at night or increased daytime sleep). The individual with either insomnia or hypersomnia complains of not feeling rested on awakening.
- *Tiredness, decreased energy, and fatigue:* Fatigue associated with depression is a subjective experience of feeling tired regardless of how much sleep or physical activity a person has had. Even the smallest tasks require substantial effort.

NCLEXNOTE In determining severity of depressive symptoms, nursing assessment should explore physical changes in appetite and sleep patterns and decreased energy. Remember these three major assessment categories. A question in the test may state several patient symptoms and expect the student to recognize that the patient being described is depressed.

Consider This:
Recall that Louise has not been eating because she is not hungry and has lost 15 lb over the last 6 weeks. She is also not sleeping well. She wakes up during the middle of the night and cannot go back to sleep. What symptoms of depression is Louise experiencing?

Medication Assessment

In addition to a physical assessment, an assessment of current medications should be completed. The frequency and dosage of prescribed medications, OTC medications, and use of herbal or culturally related medication treatments should be explored. In depression, the nurse must always assess the possible lethality of the medication the patient is taking. For example, if a patient has sleeping medications at home, the individual should be further queried about the number of pills in the bottle. Patients also need to be assessed for their use of alcohol, marijuana, and other mood-altering medications, as well as herbal substances because of the potential for drug–drug interactions. For example, patients taking antidepressants that affect serotonin regulation could also be taking St. John wort (*Hypericum perforatum*) to fight depression. The combined drug and herb could interact to cause serotonin syndrome (altered mental status, autonomic dysfunction, and neuromuscular abnormalities). SAMe (S-adenosyl-L-methionine) is another herbal preparation that patients may be taking. Patients need to be advised of possible adverse side effects of SAMe taken with any prescribed antidepressant because the exact action of this herb remains unclear.

Substance Use Assessment

A significant proportion of persons (40% to 60%) with a depressive disorder have a substance use disorder also. Conversely, alcohol use disorder increases the risk of a depressive disorder more than fourfold (Tolliver & Anton, 2015). These co-occurring disorders have an adverse impact on both mood and substance use outcomes. It is important that the nurse assesses the use of substances and consider the impact of co-occurring disorders. See Chapter 25.

Psychosocial Assessment

The psychosocial assessment for persons who have major depressive disorder includes the mental status (mood and affect, thought processes and content, cognition, memory, and attention), coping skills, developmental history, psychiatric family history, patterns of relationships, quality of support system, education, work history, and impact of physical or sexual abuse on interpersonal function. See Chapter 10. The nurse should identify the individual's strengths, as well as problem areas, by asking the patient to describe their thoughts, feelings, and behaviors before the current depressive episode. Including a family member or close friend in the assessment process can be helpful. The following discussion identifies key assessment areas for a depressed person.

Mood and Affect. The person with major depressive disorder has a sustained period of feeling depressed, sad, or hopeless and may experience **anhedonia** (loss of interest or pleasure). The patient may report "not caring any more" or not feeling any enjoyment in activities that were previously considered pleasurable. In some individuals, this may include a decrease in or loss of libido (i.e., sexual interest or desire) and sexual function. In others, irritability and anger are signs of depression, especially in those who deny being depressed. Individuals often describe themselves as depressed, sad, hopeless, discouraged, or "down in the dumps." If individuals complain of feeling "blah," having no feelings, constantly tired, or feeling anxious, a depressed mood can sometimes be inferred from their facial expression and demeanor (APA, 2013).

Numerous assessment scales are available for assessing depression. Easily administered self-report questionnaires can be valuable detection tools. These questionnaires cannot be the sole basis for making a diagnosis of major depressive episode, but they are sensitive to depressive symptoms. The following are five commonly used self-report scales:

- General Health Questionnaire (GHQ)
- Center for Epidemiological Studies Depression Scale (CES-D)
- Beck Depression Inventory (BDI)
- Zung Self-Rating Depression Scale (SDS)
- PRIME-MD

Clinician-completed rating scales may be more sensitive to improvement in the course of treatment, can assess symptoms in relationship to the depressive diagnostic criteria, and may have a slightly greater specificity than do self-report questionnaires in detecting depression. These include the following:

- Hamilton Rating Scale for Depression (HAM-D)
- Montgomery–Åsberg Depression Rating Scale (MADRS)
- National Institute of Mental Health Diagnostic Interview Schedule (DIS)

Thought Content. Depressed individuals often have an unrealistic negative evaluation of their worth or have guilty preoccupations or ruminations about minor past failings. Such individuals often misinterpret neutral or trivial day-to-day events as evidence of personal defects. They may also have an exaggerated sense of responsibility for untoward events. As a result, they feel hopeless, helpless, worthless, and powerless. The possibility of disorganized thought processes (e.g., tangential or circumstantial thinking) and perceptual disturbances (e.g., hallucinations, delusions) should also be included in the assessment.

Cognition and Memory. Many individuals with depression report an impaired ability to think, concentrate, or make decisions. They may appear easily distracted or complain of memory difficulties. In older adults with major depression, memory difficulties may be the chief complaint and may be mistaken for early signs of dementia (pseudodementia) (APA, 2013). When the depression is fully treated, the memory problem often improves or fully resolves.

Behavior

Changes in patterns of relating (especially social withdrawal) and changes in level of occupational functioning are commonly reported and may represent a significant deterioration from baseline behavior. Increased use of "sick days" may occur. For people who are depressed, special attention should be given to the individual's spiritual dimension and religious background.

Self-Concept

A positive self-esteem can be protective for the development of severe depression. A low self-esteem is associated with several health problems such as obesity, cardiovascular events, and depression (Bahrainian, Alizadeh, Raeisoon, Gorji, & Khazaee, 2014; Huang et al., 2015). Assessing self-esteem helps in establishing goals and direction for treatment.

Stress and Coping Patterns

The individual should be assessed for coping patterns. How does the person cope with the everyday stresses of life? How does the person cope with the depression and how does the depression impact the person's ability to cope with daily stressors? The nurse helps the patient identify positive coping patterns such as meditating, talking to a loved one and negative coping patterns such as overeating and using alcohol or nonprescribed drugs.

Suicidal Behavior. Patients with major depressive disorder are at increased risk for suicide. The development of suicide behavior is a complex phenomenon because symptoms are often hidden or veiled by somatic symptoms.

> **KEY CONCEPT** **Suicidal behavior** is the occurrence of persistent thought patterns and actions that indicate a person is thinking about, planning, or enacting suicide.

Suicidal ideation includes thoughts that range from a belief that others would be better off if the person were dead or thoughts of death (passive suicidal ideation) to actual specific plans for committing suicide (active suicidal ideation). See Chapter 16. The frequency, intensity, and lethality of these thoughts can vary and can help to determine the seriousness of intent. The more specific the plan and the more accessible the means, the more serious becomes the intent. The risk for suicide needs to be initially assessed in patients who incur depressive disorders as well as reassessed throughout the course of treatment.

Suicidal ideation is not a normal reaction to stress. Persons who express any suicidal ideation need immediate mental health assessment regarding the depth of their thoughts and intentions. Risk factors for suicide ideation include lack of availability and inadequacy of social supports; family violence, including physical or sexual abuse;

past history of suicidal ideation or behavior; presence of psychosis or substance use or abuse; and decreased ability to control suicidal impulses. See Chapter 16.

Ethnic and cultural differences exist regarding suicidal behavior. Men often use firearms. Women often use pills or other poisonous substances to commit suicide. Children often use suffocation. Data on suicide completion rates are reported highest in persons from Native Americans, Alaskan Natives, and those of non-Hispanic white descent. These rates are lowest for persons from Hispanic, non-Hispanic black, and Asian and Pacific Islander descent. Ongoing research regarding suicide in veterans indicates that they have a higher risk than persons in the general population (Dobscha et al., 2014). Psychological stress and previously diagnosed psychiatric disorders are major risk factors for veterans. Counseling and supportive services need to be provided to family and friends of persons who attempt or commit suicide because family and friends may experience feelings of grief, guilt, anger, and confusion (Linde, Treml, Steinig, Nagl, & Kersting, 2017).

> **NCLEXNOTE** The possibility of suicide should always be a priority with patients who are depressed. Assessment and documentation of suicide risk should always be included in patient care.

Strengths Assessment

Throughout the assessment, the nurse should be observing for strengths such as positive physical health status, coping skills, and social support. The following questions may be used to determine a person's strength:

- When you have been depressed before, how did you cope with the feelings?
- What do you do to relax?
- Do you reach out to anyone when you are feeling down?
- When you are not depressed, what makes you feel good?

Priority of Nursing Care

There are several symptoms and effects of depression that could potentially require nursing care. In collaboration with the individual, the nurse can establish priorities of care. Suicidal thoughts and behaviors are always the first priority. If a patient does not have suicidal thoughts, the nurse can focus on the physical impact of the depression such as lack of sleep, loss of appetite, and lack of energy to carry out daily routines. Feelings of hopelessness and low self-esteem are usually present and need attention. Many people who are depressed have difficulty making decisions. As the priorities are established, the results of the strength assessment should be identified. These strengths will help the person recover from the depressed state.

Therapeutic Relationship

One of the most effective tools for caring for any person with a mental disorder is the therapeutic relationship. For a person who is depressed, there are a number of effective approaches:

- Establishment and maintenance of a supportive relationship based on the incorporation of culturally competent interventions and strategies
- Availability in times of crisis
- Vigilance regarding danger to self and others
- Education about the illness and treatment goals
- Encouragement and feedback concerning progress
- Guidance regarding the patient's interactions with the personal and work environment
- Realistic goal setting and monitoring
- Support of individual strengths in treatment choices.

Interacting with individuals who are depressed is challenging because they tend to be withdrawn and have difficulty expressing feelings and engaging in interpersonal interactions. The therapeutic relationship can be strengthened through the use of cognitive interventions as well as the nurse's ability to win the patient's trust through the use of culturally competent strategies in the context of empathy (Box 21.2).

Cheerleading, or being overly cheerful to a person who is depressed, blocks communication and can be quite irritating to depressed patients. Nurses should avoid approaching patients with depression with an overly cheerful attitude. Instead, a calm, supportive empathic approach helps keep communication open.

> **NCLEXNOTE** Establishing the patient–nurse relationship with a person who is depressed requires an empathic quiet approach that is grounded in the nurse's understanding of the cultural needs of the patient.

Mental Health Nursing Interventions

Establishing Recovery and Wellness Goals

Nursing intervention selection is a collaborative process between the patient and the nurse. As goals and interventions are agreed by both the nurse and the patient, the person's strengths (e.g., motivation to get better, resources, family support) should be emphasized in making treatment choices.

Physical Care

Because weeks or months of disturbed sleep patterns and nutritional imbalance only worsen depression, one of the first nursing interventions is helping the person re-establish normal sleep patterns and healthy nutrition. Supporting self-care management by encouraging

> BOX 21.2 • THERAPEUTIC DIALOGUE • Approaching the Depressed Patient

Louise is severely depressed and has not left her hospital room since admission to the mental health unit. She has missed breakfast and is not interested in taking a shower or getting dressed.

INEFFECTIVE APPROACH

Nurse: Hello, Louise. My name is Sally. How are you feeling today?

Louise: I didn't sleep last night and need to rest. Please go away.

Nurse: Sorry, but it is time to get up. You have already missed breakfast. You have to take a quick shower now to get to group on time.

Louise: I have no interest in taking a shower or going to group.

Nurse: Why are you here if you don't want to be treated?

Louise: Go away. I don't want you in this room.

EFFECTIVE APPROACH

Nurse: Good morning. My name is Sally. I am your nurse today.

Louise: I didn't sleep last night and need to rest. Please go away.

Nurse: You didn't sleep well last night?

Louise: No, I can't remember when I was able to sleep through the night?

Nurse: Oh, I see. Is that why you missed breakfast?

Louise: I'm just not hungry. I have no energy.

Nurse: Lack of appetite and lack of energy are very common when people are depressed.

Louise: Really?

Nurse: Yes, so let's take one step at time. I'd like to help you get up.

Louise: Ok, I might be able to sit up.

Nurse: (Helps her sit up). Now, let's walk to the bathroom.

Louise: (Walks to the bathroom). Now what?

Nurse: Let's work on your AM care.

CRITICAL THINKING CHALLENGE

- What ineffective techniques did the nurse use in the first scenario and how did they impair communication?
- What effective techniques did the nurse use in the second scenario and how did they facilitate communication?

---

patients to practice positive sleep hygiene and eat well-balanced meals regularly helps the patient move toward remission or recovery.

Deep-breathing exercises three times a day have been shown to reduce self-reported depressive symptoms within 4 weeks in patients with coronary heart disease (Box 21.3). Activity and exercise are also important for improving depressed mood state. Most people find that regular exercise is hard to maintain. People who are depressed may find it impossible. When teaching about exercise, it is important to start with the current level of patient activity and increase it slowly. For example, if the patient is spending most of the time in bed, encouraging the patient to get dressed every day and walk for 5 or 10 minutes may be all that patient can tolerate. Gradually, patients should be encouraged to have a regular exercise program and to slowly increase their food intake. These activities are consistent with wellness goals.

Wellness Challenges

Depression robs the individual of energy to carry out simple activities. Previous wellness activities from physical activities, nutrition, and stress management often disappear during depression. The side effects of the antidepressants may actually interfere with normal wellness activities. The nurse should work with the individual to re-establish these activities. The individual may not feel like doing anything, but through the nurse–patient relationship, the nurse should seek commitment to gradually incorporate wellness activities. See Chapter 1 and Box 21.4.

Pharmacologic Interventions

Antidepressant medications have proved effective in all forms of major depression. To date, controlled trials have shown no single antidepressant drug to have greater

> **BOX 21.3**
>
> **Research for Best Practice: Breathing Exercise and Cognitive-Behavioral Interventions**
>
> Chien, H., Chung, Y., Yeh, M., et al. (2015). Breathing exercise combined with cognitive behavioural intervention improves sleep quality and heart rate variability in major depression. *Journal of Clinical Nursing, 24*(21–22), 3206–3214.
>
> **QUESTION:** Do cognitive-behavioral therapy and breathing exercises improve sleep quality and heart rate variability in major depression?
>
> **METHODS:** Eighty-nine participants completed this study. One group (n = 43) received cognitive-behavioral therapy combined with a breathing relaxation exercise for 4 weeks and the other group (n = 43) did not. Sleep quality and heart rate variability were measured at baseline, posttest 1 and 2, and follow-up.
>
> **FINDINGS:** The group using the cognitive-behavioral intervention with the breathing exercise improved sleep quality and variability of heart rate significantly more than the control group.
>
> **IMPLICATIONS FOR NURSING:** Nurses should consider using cognitive-behavioral interventions with breathing exercises for those who are depressed to improve their mood and reduce their depressive symptoms.

efficacy in the treatment of major depressive disorder. See Chapter 11 for a list of antidepressant medications, usual dosage range, half-life, and therapeutic blood levels.

An antidepressant is selected based primarily on an individual patient's target symptoms; genetic factors; responses related to cultural, racial, and ethnic influences; and a pharmacologic agent's side-effect profile. Other factors that may influence choice include prior medication response, drug interactions and contraindications, concurrent medical and psychiatric disorders, patient age, and cost of medication. Selecting medications on the basis of pharmacogenetic properties improves symptom remission (Bousman, Arandjelovic, Mancuso, Eyre, & Dunlop, 2019).

The newer antidepressants, selective serotonin reuptake inhibitors (SSRIs), serotonin-norepinephrine reuptake inhibitors (SNRIs), and the norepinephrine dopamine reuptake inhibitor (NDRI) are used most often because these drugs selectively target the neurotransmitters and receptors thought to be associated with depression and minimize side effects. See Box 21.5. Individualizing dosages is usually done by fine-tuning medication dosage based on patient feedback. The tricyclic antidepressants (TCAs) and monoamine oxidase inhibitors (MAOIs) are being used less often than the other agents. See Box 21.6. Given their dietary restrictions, MAOIs usually are reserved for patients whose depression fails to respond to other antidepressants or patients who cannot tolerate typical antidepressants.

> **NCLEXNOTE** Patients may be reluctant to take prescribed antidepressant medications or may self-treat depression based on their cultural beliefs and values (Leff et al., 2016; Sanchez, Ybarra, Chapa, & Martinez, 2016). A culturally competent nursing care and teaching plan needs to address the importance for adherence to a medication regimen and emphasize any potential drug–drug interactions.

> **BOX 21.4**
>
> **Wellness Challenges**
>
> - Coping effectively with lack of energy and sadness
>   - Strategies: Start with the easiest—take a walk after dinner; talk to a friend
> - Stress management
>   - Strategies: Say "no" to being a perfectionist; consider a massage; meditation
> - Decreasing feelings of worthlessness
>   - Strategies: Keep a list of accomplishments, help others; keep busy
> - Understanding the stigma of depression
>   - Strategies: Educate yourself and others about depression; join a support group
> - Recognizing the need for physical activity, healthy foods, and sleep
>   - Strategies: Track physical activity, diet, and sleep in a journal
> - Developing a sense of connection, belonging, and a support system
>   - Strategies: Contact at least one friend, attend religious service
> - Expanding a sense of purpose and meaning in life
>   - Strategies: Pray, meditate, help others, volunteer

Administering Medications. Antidepressants are available in oral form and should be taken as prescribed. See Box 21.7. Even after the first episode of major depression, medication should be continued for at least 6 months to 1 year after the patient achieves complete remission of symptoms. If the patient experiences a recurrence after tapering the first course of treatment, the regimen should be reinstituted for at least another year, and if the illness reoccurs, medication should be continued indefinitely (Schatzberg & DeBattista, 2015).

Monitoring Medications. Patients should be carefully observed for therapeutic and side effects of the antidepressants. In the depths of depression, saving medication for a later suicide attempt is quite common. During antidepressant treatment, the nurse should monitor and document vital signs, plasma drug levels (as appropriate), liver and thyroid function tests, complete blood counts, and blood chemistry to make sure that patients are receiving a therapeutic dosage and are adherent to the prescribed regimen. Results of these tests also help evaluate for toxicity (see Chapter 11 for therapeutic blood levels).

BOX 21.5
Drug Profile: Escitalopram Oxalate (Lexapro)

DRUG CLASS: Antidepressant

RECEPTOR AFFINITY: A highly selective serotonin reuptake inhibitor with low affinity for 5-HT 1–7 or α- and ß-adrenergic, dopamine D_{1-5}, histamine H_{1-3}, muscarinic M_{1-5}, and benzodiazepine receptors or for Na^+, K^+, Cl^-, and Ca^{++} ion channels that have been associated with various anticholinergic, sedative, and cardiovascular side effects.

INDICATIONS: Treatment of major depressive disorder, generalized anxiety disorder

ROUTES AND DOSAGES: Available as 5-, 10-, and 20-mg oral tablets

Adults: Initially 10 mg once a day. May increase to 20 mg after a minimum of 1 week. Trials have not shown greater benefit at the 20-mg dose

Geriatric: 10-mg dose is recommended. Adjust dosage related to the drug's longer half-life and the slower liver metabolism of older adult patients

Renal Impairment: No dosage adjustment is necessary for mild-to-moderate renal impairment

Children: Safety and efficacy have not been established in this population

HALF LIFE (PEAK EFFECT): 27 to 32 hours (4 to 7 hours)

SELECTED ADVERSE REACTIONS: Most common adverse events include insomnia, ejaculation disorder, diarrhea, nausea, fatigue, increased sweating, dry mouth, somnolence, dizziness, and constipation. Most serious adverse events include ejaculation disorder in men; fetal abnormalities and decreased fetal weight in pregnant patients; and serotonin syndrome if coadministered with MAOIs, St. John wort, or SSRIs, including citalopram (Celexa), of which escitalopram (Lexapro) is the active isomer.

BOXED WARNING: Suicidality in children, adolescents, and young adults

WARNING: There is potential for interaction with MAOIs. Lexapro should not be used in combination with an MAOI or within 14 days of discontinuing an MAOI.

SPECIFIC PATIENT AND FAMILY EDUCATION

- Do not take in combination with citalopram (Celexa) or other SSRIs or MAOIs. A 2-week washout period between escitalopram and SSRIs or MAOIs is recommended to avoid serotonin syndrome.
- Families and caregivers should be advised of the need for close observation and communication with the prescriber.
- Notify your prescriber if pregnancy is possible or being planned. Do not breast-feed while taking this medication.
- Use caution driving or operating machinery until you are certain that escitalopram does not alter your physical abilities or mental alertness.
- Notify your prescriber of any OTC medications, herbal supplements, and home remedies being used in combination with escitalopram.
- Ingestion of alcohol in combination with escitalopram is not recommended, although escitalopram does not seem to potentiate mental and motor impairments associated with alcohol.

MAOI, monoamine oxidase inhibitor; OTC, over-the-counter; SSRI, selective serotonin reuptake inhibitor.

Source: http://www.accessdata.fda.gov/drugsatfda_docs/label/2014/021323s044,021365s032lbl.pdf

BOX 21.6
Drug Profile: Mirtazapine (Remeron)

DRUG CLASS: Antidepressant

RECEPTOR AFFINITY: Believed to enhance central noradrenergic and serotonergic activity antagonizing central presynaptic α_2-adrenergic receptors. Mechanism of action is unknown

INDICATIONS: Treatment of depression

ROUTES AND DOSAGE: Available as 15- and 30-mg tablets

Adults: Initially, 15 mg/day as a single dose preferably in the evening before sleeping. Maximum dosage is 45 mg/day

Geriatric: Use with caution; reduced dosage may be needed.

Children: Safety and efficacy have not been established.

HALF-LIFE (PEAK EFFECT): 20 to 40 hours (2 hours)

SELECTED ADVERSE REACTIONS: Somnolence, increased appetite, dizziness, weight gain, elevated cholesterol or triglyceride and transaminase levels, malaise, abdominal pain, hypertension, vasodilation, vomiting, anorexia, thirst, myasthenia, arthralgia, hypoesthesia, apathy, depression, vertigo, twitching, agitation, anxiety, amnesia, increased cough, sinusitis, pruritus, rash, urinary tract infection, mania (rare), agranulocytosis (rare)

BOXED WARNING: Suicidality in children, adolescents, and young adults

WARNING: Contraindicated in patients with known hypersensitivity. Use with caution in older adults, patients who are breast-feeding, and patients with impaired hepatic function. Avoid concomitant use with alcohol or diazepam, which can cause additive impairment of cognitive and motor skills.

SPECIFIC PATIENT AND FAMILY EDUCATION

- Take the dose once a day in the evening before sleep.
- Families and caregivers should be advised of the need for dose observation and communication with the prescriber.
- Avoid driving and performing other tasks requiring alertness.
- Notify your prescriber before taking any OTC or other prescription drugs.
- Avoid alcohol and other CNS depressants.
- Notify your prescriber if pregnancy is possible or planned.
- Monitor temperature and report any fever, lethargy, weakness, sore throat, malaise, or other "flu-like" symptoms.
- Maintain medical follow-up, including any appointments for blood counts and liver studies.

CNS, central nervous system; OTC, over-the-counter.

Baseline orthostatic vital signs should be obtained before initiation of any medication, and in the case of medications known to have an impact on vital signs, such as TCAs, MAOIs, or SNRIs, they should be monitored on a regular basis. If these medications are administered to children or older adults, the dosage should be lowered to accommodate the physiologic state of the individual.

Managing Side Effects. Many people stop taking the prescribed antidepressants because of the side effects (see Box 21.8). Ideally, side effects are minimal and can

BOX 21.7

Guidelines for Administering and Monitoring Antidepressant Medications

Nurses should do the following in administering and monitoring antidepressant medications:

- Observe the patient for cheeking or saving medications for a later suicide attempt.
- Monitor vital signs (such as orthostatic vital signs and temperature): obtain baseline data before the initiation of medications.
- Monitor periodically results of liver and thyroid function tests, blood chemistry, and complete blood count as appropriate and compare with baseline values.
- Monitor the patient symptoms for therapeutic response and report inadequate response to prescriber.
- Monitor the patient for side effects and report to the prescriber serious side effects or those that are chronic and problematic for the patient. (Table 21.1 indicates pharmacologic and nonpharmacologic interventions for common side effects.)
- Monitor drug levels as appropriate. (Therapeutic drug levels for antidepressants are listed in Chapter 11.)
- Monitor dietary intake as appropriate, especially with regard to MAOI antidepressants.
- Inquire about patient use of other medications, alcohol, "street" drugs, OTC medications, and herbal supplements that might alter the desired effects of prescribed antidepressants.

MAOI, monoamine oxidase inhibitor; OTC, over-the-counter.

BOX 21.8

Antidepressants and Common Side Effects in Treating Depression

MEDICATIONS	COMMON SIDE EFFECTS	MEDICATIONS	COMMON SIDE EFFECTS
Selective Serotonin Reuptake Inhibitors (SSRIs)		**Other Antidepressants**	
Fluoxetine (Prozac)	Gastrointestinal distress	Trazadone (Oleptro)	Sedation
Sertraline (Zoloft)	Sedation		Anticholinergic effects
Paroxetine (Paxil)	Anticholinergic effects		Headache
Fluvoxamine (Luvox)	Weight gain or loss in some people		Dizziness
Citalopram (Celexa)			Nausea/vomiting
Escitalopram (Lexapro)	Sexual dysfunction	Vilazodone (Viibryd)	Diarrhea
	Dizziness		Nausea
	Diaphoresis		Dizziness
Serotonin Norepinephrine Reuptake Inhibitors (SNRIs)			Dry mouth
			Insomnia
Desvenlafaxine (Pristiq extended release)	Gastrointestinal distress		Abnormal dreams
	Anticholinergic effects	Vortioxetine (Brintellix)	Nausea
Duloxetine (Cymbalta)	Insomnia or sedation		Diarrhea
Levomilnacipran (Fetzima)	Decreased appetite		Dizziness
Venlafaxine (Effexor XR)	Sexual dysfunction		Dry mouth
	Abnormal dreams		Constipation
	Dizziness		Vomiting
	Jitteriness	**Tricyclic Antidepressants**	
	Hypertension	Amitriptyline	Drowsiness
	Irritability	Amoxapine	Anticholinergic effects
	Photosensitivity	Clomipramine (Anafranil)	Orthostatic hypotension
Norepinephrine Dopamine Reuptake Inhibitor (NDRI)		Imipramine (Tofranil)	Palpitations
Bupropion (Wellbutrin)	Anticholinergic effects	Desipramine (Norpramin)	Tachycardia
	Headache	Doxepin	Impaired coordination
	Agitation	Nortriptyline (Aventyl, Pamelor)	Increased appetite
	Gastrointestinal distress		Diaphoresis
	Insomnia	Protriptyline (Vivactil)	Weakness
	Anorexia		Disorientation
	Anxiety		Sexual side effects (impotence, changes in libido)
	Weight loss		
	Diarrhea and flatulence	**Tetracyclic Antidepressants**	
α₂ Antagonist		Maprotiline	Blurred vision
Mirtazapine (Remeron)	Sedation		Dizziness
	Anticholinergic effects		Lightheadedness
	Appetite increase		Sedation
	Weight gain		Dry mouth
	Hypercholesterolemia		Libido changes
	Weakness and lack of energy		Impotence
	Dizziness		Weight changes
	Hypertriglyceridemia		

BOX 21.8
Antidepressants and Common Side Effects in Treating Depression (Continued)

MEDICATIONS	COMMON SIDE EFFECTS	MEDICATIONS	COMMON SIDE EFFECTS
Monoamine Oxidase Inhibitors		Tranylcypromine (Parnate)	Orthostatic hypotension
Isocarboxazid (Marplan)	Dizziness		Dizziness
	Headache		Headache
	Nausea		Drowsiness
	Dry mouth		Sleep disturbance
	Constipation		Restlessness
	Drowsiness		Central nervous system stimulation
	Sleep disturbance		
	Orthostatic hypotension	Selegiline (Emsam)	Application site reaction
Phenelzine (Nardil)	Orthostatic hypotension		Headache
	Edema		Insomnia
	Dizziness		Diarrhea
	Headache		Dry mouth
	Drowsiness		Orthostatic hypotension
	Sleep disturbance		Dyspepsia

be alleviated by nonpharmacologic interventions. For example, if patient is having difficulty going to sleep, avoiding caffeinated products may help (Table 21.1). SSRIs tend to be safer and have fewer side effects than the older medications. The most common reason individuals stop taking their SSRIs are gastrointestinal side effects including diarrhea, cramping, and heartburn. The most common side effects associated with TCAs

TABLE 21.1 INTERVENTIONS TO RELIEVE SIDE EFFECTS OF ANTIDEPRESSANTS

Side Effect	Pharmacologic Intervention	Nonpharmacologic Intervention
Dry mouth, caries, inflammation of the mouth	Bethanechol 10–30 mg tid Pilocarpine drops	Sugarless gum Sugarless lozenges 6–8 cups of water per day Toothpaste for dry mouth
Nausea, vomiting	Change medication	Take medication with food Soda crackers, toast, tea
Weight gain	Change medication	Nutritionally balanced diet Daily exercise
Urinary hesitation Constipation	Bethanechol 10–30 mg tid Stool softener	6–8 cups of water per day Bulk laxative Daily exercise 6–8 cups of water per day Diet rich in fresh fruits, vegetables, and whole grains
Diarrhea	OTC antidiarrheal	Maintain fluid intake
Orthostatic hypotension		Increase hydration Sit or stand up slowly
Drowsiness	Shift dosing time Lower medication dose Change medication	One caffeinated beverage at strategic time Do not drive when drowsy No alcohol or other recreational drugs Plan for rest time
Fatigue	Lower medication dose Change medication	Daily exercise
Blurred vision	Bethanechol 10–30 mg tid Pilocarpine eye drops	Temporary use of magnifying lenses until body adjusts to medication
Flushing, sweating	Terazosin 1 mg once daily Lower medication dose Change medication	Frequent bathing Lightweight clothing
Tremor	β-blockers Lower medication dose	Reassure the patient that tremor may decrease as the patient adjusts to medication. Notify the caregiver if tremor interferes with daily functioning.

OTC, over-the-counter; tid, three times a day.

are the antihistaminic side effects (e.g., sedation weight gain) and anticholinergic side effects (potentiation of CNS drugs, blurred vision, dry mouth, constipation, urinary retention, sinus tachycardia, and decreased memory).

For the MAOIs, the most common side effects are headache, drowsiness, dry mouth and throat, constipation, blurred vision, and orthostatic hypotension. Additional selected adverse effects of MAOIs include insomnia, nausea, agitation, dizziness, asthenia, weight loss, and postural hypotension. Although priapism was not reported during clinical trials, the MAOIs are structurally similar to trazodone, which has been associated with priapism (prolonged painful erection). For those taking MAOIs, close attention to dietary restrictions should be given. See Chapter 11 for tyramine-restricted diets.

> **EMERGENCY CARE ALERT** ! If coadministered with food or other substances containing tyramine (e.g., aged cheese, beer, red wine), MAOIs can trigger a hypertensive crisis that may be life threatening. Symptoms include a sudden, severe pounding, or explosive headache in the back of the head or temples, racing pulse, flushing, stiff neck, chest pain, nausea and vomiting, and profuse sweating.

Managing Adverse Events

Suicidality. **Suicidality** is mentioned in a "black box" warning on all antidepressants indicating an increased risk of suicide exists in children, adolescents, and young adults with major depressive or other psychiatric disorders. After the age of 24 years, the suicidality risk does not increase and after 65, the risk of suicide actually decreases when taking an antidepressant. The SSRIs are the least lethal of the antidepressants, but fatalities have been reported (Schatzberg & DeBattisa, 2015).

> **EMERGENCY CARE ALERT** ! If possible, TCAs should not be prescribed for patients at risk for suicide. Lethal doses of TCAs are only three to five times the therapeutic dose, and more than 1 g of a TCA is often toxic and may be fatal. Death may result from cardiac arrhythmia, hypotension, or uncontrollable seizures.

Serum TCA levels should be evaluated when overdose is suspected. In acute overdose, almost all symptoms develop within 12 hours. Anticholinergic effects are prominent and include dry mucous membranes, warm and dry skin, blurred vision, decreased bowel motility, and urinary retention. CNS suppression (ranging from drowsiness to coma) or an agitated delirium may occur. Basic overdose treatment includes induction of emesis, gastric lavage, and cardiorespiratory supportive care.

MAOIs are more lethal in overdose than are the newer antidepressants and thus should be prescribed with caution if the patient's suicide potential is elevated

BOX 21.9

Serotonin Syndrome

CAUSE: Excessive intrasynaptic serotonin

HOW IT HAPPENS: Combining medications that increase CNS serotonin levels, such as SSRIs + MAOIs; SSRIs + St. John wort; or SSRIs + diet pills; dextromethorphan or alcohol, especially red wine; or SSRI + street drugs, such as LSD, MMDA, or ecstasy

SYMPTOMS: Mental status changes, agitation, ataxia, myoclonus, hyperreflexia, fever, shivering, diaphoresis, diarrhea

TREATMENT
- Assess all medications, supplements, foods, and recreational drugs ingested to determine the offending substances.
- Discontinue any substances that may be causative factors. If symptoms are mild, treat supportively on an outpatient basis with propranolol and lorazepam and follow-up with the prescriber.
- If symptoms are moderate to severe, hospitalization may be needed with monitoring of vital signs and treatment with intravenous fluids, antipyretics, and cooling blankets.

FURTHER USE: Assess on a case-by-case basis and minimize risk factors for further medication therapy.

CNS, central nervous system; LSD, lysergic acid diethylamide; MAOI, monoamine oxidase inhibitor; MMDA, 3-methoxy-4,5-methylenedioxyamphetamine; SSRI, selective serotonin reuptake inhibitor.

(see Chapter 11). An MAOI generally is given in divided doses to minimize side effects.

Serotonin Syndrome. **Serotonin syndrome** is a potentially serious side effect caused by drug-induced excess of intrasynaptic serotonin, 5-hydroxytryptamine (5-HT). See Box 21.9. First reported in the 1950s, it was relatively rare until the introduction of the SSRIs. Serotonin syndrome is most often reported in patients taking two or more medications that increase CNS serotonin levels by different mechanisms (Foong, Grindrod, Patel, & Kellar, 2018). The most common drug combinations associated with serotonin syndrome involve the MAOIs, the SSRIs, and the TCAs.

Although serotonin syndrome can cause death, it is mild in most patients, who usually recover with supportive care alone. Unlike neuroleptic malignant syndrome, which develops within 3 to 9 days after the introduction of neuroleptic medications (see Chapter 23), serotonin syndrome tends to develop within hours or days after starting or increasing the dose of serotonergic medication. Symptoms include altered mental status, autonomic dysfunction, and neuromuscular abnormalities. At least three of the following findings must be present for a diagnosis: mental status changes, agitation, myoclonus, hyperreflexia, fever, shivering, diaphoresis, ataxia, and diarrhea. In patients who also have peripheral vascular disease or atherosclerosis, severe vasospasm and hypertension may occur in the presence of elevated serotonin levels. In addition, in a patient who is a slow metabolizer of SSRIs, higher-than-normal levels of these antidepressants may circulate in the blood. Medications that are not usually considered serotonergic, such as dextromethorphan and meperidine have been associated with the syndrome (Dy, Arcega, Ghali, & Wolfe, 2017).

> **EMERGENCY CARE ALERT !** The most important emergency interventions are stopping use of the offending drug, notifying the prescriber, and providing necessary supportive care (e.g., intravenous fluids, antipyretics, cooling blanket). Severe symptoms have been successfully treated with antiserotonergic agents, such as cyproheptadine (Tormoehlen & Rusyniak, 2017).

Monitoring for Drug Interactions. Several potential drug interactions are associated with antidepressants. Alcohol consumption should be avoided when taking any antidepressant because SSRIs are metabolized in the liver, other medications that are also metabolized by the same enzyme can cause an increase in drug levels leading to toxicity and serotonin syndrome. For example, if migraine medications known as "triptans" are given with the SSRIs, serotonin syndrome can occur. Bupropion cannot be given at the same time as an MAOI. Grapefruit should not be consumed while taking trazodone. It is beyond the scope of this text to review drug–drug interactions in detail. Nurses should check with pharmacy resources for any drug–drug interactions when administering medications.

Teaching Points. If depression goes untreated or is inadequately treated, episodes can become more frequent, more severe, longer in duration, and can lead to suicide. Patient education involves explaining this pattern and the importance of continuing medication use after the acute phase of treatment to decrease the risk for future episodes. Patient concerns regarding long-term antidepressant therapy need to be assessed and addressed. All teaching points need to be developed and delivered using a culturally competent approach to enhance patient adherence.

Patients should also be advised not to take herbal substances such as St. John wort or SAMe if they are also taking prescribed antidepressants. St. John wort also should not be taken if the patient is taking nasal decongestants, hay fever and asthma medications containing monoamines, amino acid supplements containing phenylalanine, or tyrosine. The combination may cause hypertension.

Other Somatic Therapies

Electroconvulsive Therapy. Although its therapeutic mechanism of action is unknown, ECT is an effective treatment for patients with severe depression. It is generally reserved for patients whose disorder is refractory or intolerant to initial drug treatments and who are so severely ill that rapid treatment is required (e.g., patients with malnutrition, catatonia, or suicidality).

ECT is contraindicated for patients with increased intracranial pressure. Other high-risk patients include those with recent myocardial infarction, recent cerebrovascular accident, retinal detachment, or pheochromocytoma (a tumor in the cells of the adrenal gland) and those at risk for complications of anesthesia. Older age has been associated with a favorable response to ECT, but the effectiveness and safety in this group have not been shown. Because depression can increase the mortality risk for older adults, in particular, and some older adults do not respond well to medication, effective treatment is especially important for this age group (Dong et al., 2018).

The role of the nurse in the care of the patient undergoing ECT is to provide educational and emotional support for the patient and family, assess baseline or pretreatment levels of function, prepare the patient for the ECT process, monitor and evaluate the patient's response to ECT, provide assessment data with the ECT team, and modify treatment as needed (see Chapter 11 for more information). The actual procedure, possible therapeutic mechanisms of action, potential adverse effects, contraindications, and nursing interventions are described in detail in Chapter 11.

Light Therapy (Phototherapy). Light therapy is described in Chapter 11. Given current research, light therapy is an option for well-documented mild-to-moderate seasonal, nonpsychotic, winter depressive episodes in patients with recurrent major depressive disorders, including children and adolescents. Evidence also indicates that light therapy can modestly improve symptoms in nonseasonal depression, especially when administered during the first week of treatment in the morning for those experiencing sleep deprivation (Al-Karawi & Jubair, 2016).

Repetitive Transcranial Magnetic Stimulation. In 2008, the U.S. Food and Drug Administration approved repetitive transcranial magnetic stimulation (rTMS) for the treatment of patients with mild treatment-resistant depression. In rTMS, a magnetic coil placed on the scalp at the site of the left motor cortex releases small electrical pulses that stimulate the site of the left dorsolateral prefrontal cortex in the superficial cortex. This rapidly changing magnetic field stimulates the brain sufficiently to depolarize neurons and exert effects across synapses. These pulses (similar in type and strength as a magnetic resonance imaging machine) easily pass through the hair, skin, and skull, requiring much less electricity than

ECT. The patient is awake, reclining in an rTMS chair during the procedure, and can resume normal activities immediately after the procedure. Because anesthesia is not required, no risks are associated with sedation. Treatment of depression typically consists of 20 to 30 sessions, lasting 37 minutes each over 4 to 6 weeks. Depending on the level of practice and training, the nurse's role in the use of the rTMS varies from patient education, pre- and postprocedure care to performing the procedure (Sehatzadeh et al., 2019).

Psychosocial Interventions

Individuals experiencing depression have often withdrawn from daily activities, such as engaging in family activities, attending work, and participating in community functions. During hospitalization, patients often withdraw to their rooms and refuse to participate in unit activity. Nurses help the patient balance the need for privacy with the need to return to normal social functioning. Even though depressed patients should not be approached in an overly enthusiastic manner, they should be encouraged to set realistic goals to reconnect with their families and communities. Explain to patients that attending social activities, even though they do not feel like it, will promote the recovery process and help them achieve their goals.

Cognitive Interventions

Cognitive interventions such as thought stopping and positive self-talk can dispel irrational beliefs and distorted attitudes and in turn reduce depressive symptoms during the acute phase of major depression (see Chapter 10). Nurses should consider using cognitive approaches when caring for persons who are depressed. The use of cognitive interventions in the acute phase of treatment combined with medication is now considered first-line treatment for mildly to moderately depressed outpatients.

> **NCLEXNOTE** A cognitive therapy approach is recommended for helping persons restructure the negative thinking processes related to a person's concept of self, others, and the future. This approach should be included in most nursing care plans for patients with depression.

Behavioral Interventions

Behavioral interventions are effective in the acute treatment of patients with mildly to moderately severe depression, especially when combined with pharmacotherapy. Therapeutic techniques include activity scheduling, social skills training, and problem-solving. Behavioral therapy techniques are described in Chapter 5.

Group Interventions

Individuals who are depressed can receive emotional support in groups and learn how others deal with similar problems and issues. As group members serve as role models for new group members, they also benefit as their self-esteem increases, which strengthens their ability to address their issues (see Chapter 12). Group interventions are often used to help an individual cope with depression associated with bereavement or chronic medical illness. Group interventions are also commonly used to educate patients and families about their disorder and medications.

Psychoeducation

Patients with depression and their significant others often incorrectly believe that their illness is their own fault and that they should be able to "pull themselves up by their bootstraps and snap out of it." Persons from some cultural groups believe that the symptoms of depression may be a result of someone placing a hex on the affected person because the person has done something evil. It is vital to be culturally competent to be effective in teaching patients and their families about the treatment modalities for depression.

Patients need to know the full range of suitable treatment options before consenting to participate in treatment. Information empowers patients to ask questions, weigh risks and benefits, and make the best treatment choices. The nurse can provide opportunities for patients to question, discuss, and explore their feelings about past, current, and planned use of medications and other treatments. Developing strategies to enhance adherence and to raise awareness of early signs of relapse can be important aids to increasing treatment efficacy and promoting recovery (Box 21.10).

BOX 21.10

Psychoeducation Checklist: Major Depressive Disorder

When caring for the patient with a major depressive disorder, be sure to include the following topic areas in the teaching plan:
- Psychopharmacologic agents, including drug action, dosing frequency, and possible side effects
- Risk factors for recurrence; signs of recurrence
- Adherence to therapy and treatment program
- Recovery strategies
- Nutrition
- Sleep measures
- Self-care management
- Goal setting and problem-solving
- Social interaction skills
- Follow-up appointments
- Community support services

The family needs education and support during and after the treatment of family members. Because major depressive disorder is a recurring disorder, the family needs information about specific antecedents to a family member's depression and what therapeutic steps to take. For example, one patient may routinely become depressed during the fall of each year, with one of the first symptoms being excessive sleepiness. For another patient, a major loss, such as a child going to college or the death of a pet, may precipitate a depressive episode. Families of older adults need to be aware of the possibility of depression and related symptoms, which often occur after the deaths of friends and relatives. Families of children who are depressed often misinterpret depression as behavioral problems.

Milieu Therapy

While hospitalized, milieu therapy (see Chapter 10) helps depressed patients maintain socialization skills and continue to interact with others. When depressed, people are often unaware of the environment and withdraw into themselves. On a psychiatric unit, depressed patients should be encouraged to attend and participate in unit activities. These individuals have decreased energy levels and thus may be moving more slowly than others; however, their efforts should be praised.

Safety

In many cases, patients are admitted to the psychiatric hospital because of a suicide attempt. Suicidality should continually be evaluated, and the patient should be protected from self-harm (see Chapter 16). During the depths of depression, patients may not have the energy to complete a suicide. As patients begin to feel better and have increased energy, they therefore may be at a greater risk for suicide. If a previously depressed patient appears to have become energized overnight, he or she may have decided to commit suicide and thus may be relieved that the decision is finally made. The nurse may misinterpret the mood improvement as a positive move toward recovery; however, this patient may be very intent on suicide. These individuals should be carefully monitored to maintain their safety.

Family Interventions

Patients who perceive high family stress are at risk for greater future severity of illness, higher use of health services, and higher health care expense. Marital and family problems are common among patients with mood disorders; comprehensive treatment requires that these problems be assessed and addressed. They may be a consequence of the major depression but may also predispose persons to develop depressive symptoms or inhibit recovery and resilience processes. Research suggests that marital and family therapy may reduce depressive symptoms and the risk for relapse in patients with marital and family problems (Whisman & Beach, 2012). The depressed spouse's depression has marked impact on the marital adjustment of the nondepressed spouse. It is recommended that treatment approaches be designed to help couples be supportive of each other, to adapt, and to cope with the depressive symptoms within the framework of their ongoing marital relations. Many family nursing interventions may be used by the psychiatric nurse in providing targeted family-centered care. These include:

- Monitoring patient and family for indicators of stress
- Teaching stress management techniques
- Counseling family members on coping skills for their own use
- Providing necessary knowledge of options and support services
- Facilitating family routines and rituals
- Assisting the family to resolve feelings of guilt
- Assisting the family with conflict resolution
- Identifying family strengths and resources with family members
- Facilitating communication among family members

Support Groups

Nurses are exceptionally well positioned to engage patients and their families in the active process of improving daily functioning, increasing knowledge and skill acquisition, and increasing independent living. Consumer-oriented support groups can help to enhance the self-esteem and the support network of participating patients and their families. Advice, encouragement, and the sense of group camaraderie may make an important contribution to recovery (APA, 2013). Organizations providing support and information include the Depression and Bipolar Support Alliance (DBSA), National Alliance on Mental Illness (NAMI), and the Mental Health Association and Recovery, Inc. (a self-help group).

Evaluation and Treatment Outcomes

The major goals of treatment are to help the patient to be as independent as possible and to achieve stability, remission, and recovery from major depression. It is often a lifelong struggle for the individual. Ongoing evaluation of the patient's symptoms, functioning, and quality of life should be carefully documented in the patient's record in order to monitor outcomes of treatment.

Continuum of Care

Mild-to-moderate depression is often first recognized in primary care settings. Primary care nurses should be able to recognize depression in these patients and make appropriate interventions or referrals. Those with more severe depressive symptoms may be directly admitted to inpatient and outpatient mental health settings or emergency departments. The continuum of care beyond these settings may include partial hospitalization or day treatment programs; individual, family, or group psychotherapy; and home visits. Although most patients with major depression are treated in outpatient settings, brief hospitalization may be required if the patient is suicidal or psychotic (Mitchell, Kane, Kameg, Stark, & Kameg, 2017).

Nurses working on inpatient units provide a wide range of direct services, including administering and monitoring medications and target symptoms; conducting psychoeducational groups; and more generally, structuring and maintaining a therapeutic environment. Nurses providing home care have an excellent opportunity to detect undiagnosed depressive disorders and make appropriate referrals.

Integration With Primary Care

The medical home delivery model is becoming widely accepted in the United States. If a patient is cared within a medical home model, all of their health and mental health needs are coordinated by one health provider. Meaningful long-term relationships can be developed. The advantage of a medical home is a recognition and coordination of all health care needs. This model is helpful when many of the health disorders, associated with depression, occur. For example, substance abuse, obesity, and cardiovascular disorders are associated with depression and mood disorders (Berg et al., 2018).

OTHER DEPRESSIVE DISORDERS

Other depressive disorders with similar symptoms are treated similarly to the major depressive disorders. Nursing care should be individualized and based on their patients' mental health needs and strengths. A diagnosis of **persistent depressive disorder** (*dysthymia*) is made if major depressive disorder symptoms last for 2 years for an adult and 1 year for children and adolescents. These individuals are depressed for most of each day (APA, 2013). A major depressive disorder may precede the persistent depressive disorder or co-occur with it.

Premenstrual dysphoric disorder is characterized by recurring mood swings, feelings of sadness, or sensitivity to rejection in the final week before the onset of menses. The mood begins to improve a few days after menses begins. Stress, history of interpersonal trauma, and seasonal changes are associated with this disorder (APA, 2013).

Disruptive mood dysregulation disorder is characterized by severe irritability and outbursts of temper. The onset of disruptive mood dysregulation disorder begins before the age of 10 when children have verbal rages and/or are physically aggressive toward others or property. These outbursts are outside of the normal temper tantrums children display. They are more severe than what would be expected developmentally and occur frequently (i.e., two or three times a week). The behavior disrupts family functioning as well as the child's ability to succeed in school and social activities. This disorder can co-occur with attention-deficit/hyperactivity disorder. See Chapter 30.

Disruptive mood dysregulation disorder is similar to pediatric bipolar disorder, but the *DSM-5* differentiates it from bipolar disorder. Children with this disorder have similar deficits in recognition of emotion through facial expression, decision-making, and control as those with bipolar disorder. More research is needed in understanding this disorder.

SUMMARY OF KEY POINTS

- Moods influence perception of life events and functioning. Depressive disorders are characterized by persistent or recurring disturbances in mood that cause significant psychological distress and functional impairment (typified by feelings of sadness, hopelessness, loss of interest, and fatigue).

- Depressive disorders include both major depressive disorder, persistent depressive disorder (dysthymia), premenstrual dysphoric disorder, disruptive mood dysregulation disorder, and other related to medical conditions, medications, or substance use.

- Risk factors include a family history of depressive disorders, prior depressive episodes; lack of social support; stressful life events; substance use; and medical problems, particularly chronic or terminal illnesses.

- Treatment of major depressive disorder primarily includes antidepressant medication, psychotherapy, or a combination of both. ECT, light therapy, and repetitive transcranial magnetic stimulation are also used.

- Nurses must be knowledgeable regarding culturally competent strategies related to the use of antidepressant medications, pharmacologic therapeutic effects and associated side effects, toxicity, dosage ranges, and contraindications. Nurses must also be familiar with ECT protocols and associated interventions. Patient education and the provision of emotional support during the course of treatment are also nursing responsibilities.

- Many symptoms of depression (e.g., weight and appetite changes, sleep disturbance, decreased energy, fatigue) are similar to those of medical illnesses. Assessment includes a thorough medical history and physical examination to detect or rule out medical or psychiatric comorbidity.

- Mental health nursing assessment includes assessing mood; speech patterns; thought processes and content; suicidal or homicidal thoughts; cognition and memory; and social factors, such as patterns of relationships, quality of support systems, and changes in occupational functioning. Several self-report scales are helpful in evaluating depressive symptoms.

- Establishing and maintaining a therapeutic culturally competent nurse–patient relationship is key to successful outcomes. Nursing interventions that foster the therapeutic relationship include being available in times of crisis, providing understanding and education to patients and their families regarding goals of treatment, providing encouragement and feedback concerning the patient's progress, providing guidance in the patient's interpersonal interactions with others and work environment, and helping to set and monitor realistic goals.

- Psychosocial interventions for depressive disorders include self-care management, cognitive therapy, behavior therapy, interpersonal therapy, patient and family education regarding the nature of the disorder and treatment goals, marital and family interventions, and group interventions that include medication maintenance support groups and other consumer-oriented support groups.

CRITICAL THINKING CHALLENGES

1. Describe how you would do a suicide assessment on a patient who comes into a primary care office and is distraught and expressing concerns about her ability to cope with her current situation.
2. Describe how you would approach the patient who does not want to talk with you.
3. Describe how you would approach a patient who is expressing concern that the diagnosis of depressive disorder will negatively affect her social and work relationships.
4. Your depressed patient does not seem inclined to talk about his depression. Describe the measures you would take to initiate a therapeutic relationship with him.
5. Compare the side effects of the SSRIs, TCAs, and MAOIs.
6. Think about all the above situations and relate them to persons from culturally and ethnically diverse populations (e.g., African, Latino, or Asian descent; Jewish or Jehovah's Witness religions; across the life-span of individuals from children to older adult populations).

2002: *About Schmidt*

This movie is about a 67-year-old man, Warren Schmidt, played by Jack Nicholson, who retires from his job as an insurance company executive. He experiences work withdrawal and a lack of direction for his retirement. His wife, Helen, irritates him, and he has no idea what to do to fill his days. While watching television one day, he is moved to sponsor a child in Africa with whom he begins a long, one-sided correspondence. When his wife dies unexpectedly, he is initially numb, then sad, and finally angry when he discovers that she had an affair with his best friend many years ago. He is estranged from his only daughter, Jeanie, whose wedding to Randall, a man he thinks is beneath her, is imminent. The movie follows Warren as he searches for connection and meaning in his life.

Significance: Warren Schmidt demonstrates a common phenomenon among older adults when they retire. He also shows the impact of grief superimposed on initial dysthymia or depression.

Viewing Points: Look for the changes in Schmidt's manifestations of depression in different situations. Note how he experiences the various stages of grieving. What do you think about Schmidt's search for significance and meaning in his life?

1989: *Dead Poet's Society*

This film portrays John Keating, played by Robin Williams, as a charismatic English teacher in a conservative New England prep school for boys in 1959. John brings his love of poetry to the students and encourages them to follow their dreams and talents and make the most of every day. His efforts put him at odds with the administration of the school, particularly the headmaster, played by Norman Lloyd, as well as Tom Perry, the father of one of his students, played by Kurtwood Smith. Tom's son, Neil, played by Robert Sean Leonard, chooses to act in a school play despite the objection of his father to any extracurricular activities. When Neil cannot reconcile his love of theater and his father's expectations that he pursues a career in medicine, he kills himself. John Keating blames himself for the death, as does the school administration. He is fired by the administration but has a moment of pride when his students demonstrate their ability to think and act for themselves.

Significance: This film accurately portrays the sensitivity of adolescents and their longing for worthwhile role models. It also shows adolescent growth and development in a realistic manner. It demonstrates the combination of factors that accompany a decision to commit suicide. We can see how Neil feels caught between his desires and the demands of his father. In the cultural context of the late 1950s, few children or adolescents dared to challenge or defy their parents, especially such a domineering man as Tom Perry.

Viewing Points: Look for the differences in Neil's behavior with his peers and his father or other adults besides Mr. Keating. What, if any, clues do you get that Neil might attempt suicide? What actions by any of the main characters might have prevented his suicide?

 A related Psychiatric–Mental Health Nursing video on the topic of Depression is available at http://thepoint.lww.com/BoydEssentials2e.

 A Practice and Learn Interactive Case Study related to the video on the topic of Depression is available at http://thepoint.lww.com/BoydEssentials2e.

REFERENCES

Al-Karawi, D., & Jubair, L. (2016). Bright light therapy for nonseasonal depression: Meta-analysis of clinical trials. *Journal of Affective Disorders*, 198, 64–71.

American Psychiatric Association (APA). (2013). *Diagnostic and statistical manual of mental disorders DSM-5* (5th ed.). Arlington, VA: Author.

Bachman, S. (2018). Epidemiology of suicide and the psychiatric perspective. *International Journal of Environmental Research and Public Health*, 15(7), pii: E1425.

Bahrainian, S. A., Alizadeh, K. H., Raeisoon, M. R., Gorji, O. H., & Khazaee, A. (2014). Relationship of internet addiction with self-esteem and depression in university students. *Journal of Preventive Medicine & Hygiene*, 55(3), 86–89.

Berg, S.K., Rasmussen, T. B., Thrysoee, L., Thorup, C. B., Borregaard, B., Christensen, A. V., et al. (2018). Mental health is a risk factor for poor outcomes in cardiac patients: Findings from the national DenHeart survey. *Journal of Psychosomatic Research*, 112, 66–72.

Blazer, D. G., & Steffens, D. C. (2015). Depressive Disorders. In: D. G. Blazer, D. C. Steffens, & M. Thakur (Eds.). *The American psychiatric publishing textbook of geriatric psychiatry* (5th ed.). Arlington, VA: American Psychiatric Association. Retrieved February 27, 2019, from http://dx.doi.org/10.1176/appi.books.9781615370054.ds09

Bousman, C. A., Arandjelovic, K., Mancuso, S. G., Eyre, H. A., Dunlop, B. W., et al. (2019). Pharmacogenetic tests and depressive symptom remission: a meta-analysis of randomized controlled trials. *Pharmacogenomics*, 20(1), 37–47.

Brunstein, K. A., Barzilay, S., Apter, A., Carli, V., Hoven, C. W., Sarchiapone, M., et al. (2019). Bi-directional longitudinal associations between different types of bullying victimization, suicide ideation/attempts, and depression among a large sample of European adolescents. *Journal of Child Psychology and Psychiatry, and Allied Disciplines*, 60(2), 209–215.

Dobscha, S. K., Denneson, L. M., Kovas, A. E., Teo, A., Forsberg, C. W., Kaplan, M. S., et al. (2014). Correlates of suicide among veterans treated in primary care: Case-control study of a nationally representative sample. *Journal of General Internal Medicine*, 29(Suppl 4), 853–860.

Dong, M., Zhu X. H., Zheng W., Li X. H., Ng C. H., Ungvari G. S., et al. (2018). Electroconvulsive therapy for older adult patients with major depressive disorder: a systematic review of randomized controlled trials. *Psychogeriatrics*, 18(6), 468–475.

Drury, S. S., Scaramella, L., & Zeanah, C. H. (2016). The neurobiological impact of postpartum maternal depression: Prevention and intervention approaches. *Child Adolescent Psychiatric Clinics of North America*, 25, 179–200.

Dunlop, B. W., LoParo, D., Kinkead, B., Mletzko-Crowe, T., Cole, S. P., Nemeroff, C. B., et al. (2019). Benefits of sequentially adding cognitive-behavioral therapy or antidepressant medication for adults with nonremitting depression. *American Journal of Psychiatry*, 176(4), 275–286.

Dy, P., Arcega, V., Ghali, W., & Wolfe, W. (2017). Serotonin syndrome caused by drug to drug interaction between escitalopram and dextromethorphan. *BMJ Case Reports*, pii: bcr-2017-221486.

Foong, A. L., Grindrod, K. A., Patel, T., & Kellar, J. (2018). Demystifying serotonin syndrome (or serotonin toxicity). *Canadian Family Physician*, 64(10), 720–727.

Ge, L., Yap, C. W., Ong, R., Heng, B. H. (2017). Social isolation, loneliness and their relationships with depressive symptoms: a population-based study. *PLoS One*, 12(8): e0182145. doi: 10.1371/journal.pone.0182145.

Gong, C., Duan, X., Su, P., Wan, Y., Xu, Y., Tao, F., et al. (2019). Heightened HPA-axis stress reactivity and accelerated pubertal progression predicts depressive symptoms over 4-year follow up. *Psychoneuroendocrinology*, 103, 259–265.

Hasin, D. S., Sarvet, A. L., Meyers, J. L., Saha, T. D., Ruan, W. J., Stohl, M., et al. (2018). Epidemiology of adult DSM-5 major depressive disorder and its specifiers in the United States. *JAMA Psychiatry*, 75(4), 336–346.

Himmerich, H., Patsalos, O., Lichtblau, N., Ibrahim, M. A. A., Dalton, B. (2019). Cytokine research in depression: Principles, challenges, and open questions. *Frontiers in Psychiatry*, 10, 30.

Hoertel, N., Blanco, C., Oquendo, M. A., Wall, M. M., Olfson, M., Falissard, B., et al. (2017). A comprehensive model of predictors of persistence and recurrence in adults with major depression: Results from a national 3-year prospective study. *Journal of Psychiatric Research*, 95, 19–27.

Hornberger, A. P., Medley-Proctor, K., Nettles, C. D., Cimporescu, M. A., & Howe, G. W. (2016). The influence of the racial/ethnic match of interviewer and respondent on the measurement of couple's relationship quality and emotional functioning. *Couple and Family Psychology: Research and Practice*, 5(1), 12–26.

Howard, D. M., Adams, M. J., Clarke, T. K., Hafferty, J. D., Gibson, J., Shirali, M., et al. (2019). Genome-wide meta-analysis of depression identifies 102 independent variants and highlights the importance of the prefrontal brain regions. *Nature Neuroscience*, 22(3), 343–352.

Huang, C. Y., Chen, W. K., Lu, C. Y., Tsai, C. C., Lai, H. L., Lin, H. Y., et al. (2015). Mediating effects of social support and self-concept on depressive symptoms in adults with spinal cord injury. *Spinal Cord*, 53(5), 413–416.

Ivey-Stephenson, A. Z., Crosby, A. E., Jack, S. P., Haileyesus, T., & Kresnow-Sedacca, M. J. (2017). Suicide trends among and within urbanization levels by sex, race/ethnicity, age group, and mechanism of death—United States, 2001–2015. *MMWR Surveillance Summaries*, 66(18), 1–16.

Joca, S. R., Moreira, F. A., & Wegener, G. (2015). Atypical neurotransmitters and the neurobiology of depression. *CNS & Neurological Disorders Drug Targets*, 14(8), 1001–1011.

Johns, M. M., Lowry, R., Rasberry, C. N., Dunville, R., Robin, L., Pampati, S., et al. (2018). Violence victimization, substance use, and suicide risk among sexual minority high school students—United States, 2015–2017. *MMWR Morbidity Mortality Weekly Report*, 67(43), 1211–1215.

Kok, R. M., & Reynolds, C. F. 3rd (2017). Management of depression in older adults: A review. *JAMA*, 317(20), 2114–2122.

Leff, H. S., Chow, C., Wieman, D. Q., Ostrow, L., Cortés, D. E., & Harris, T. (2016). Measurement of perceived and technical quality of care for depression in racially and ethnically diverse groups. *Journal of Immigrant and Minority Health*, 18(4), 810–818.

Lin, J., & Dmitrieva, J. (2019). Cultural orientation moderates the association between desired affect and depressed mood among Chinese international students living in the United States. *Emotion*, 19(2), 371–375.

Linde, K., Treml, J., Steinig, J., Nagl, M., Kersting, A., et al. (2017) Grief interventions for people bereaved by suicide: A systematic review. *PLoS One*, 12(6), e0179496.

Lotfaliany, M., Bowe, S. J., Kowal, P., Orellana, L., Berk, M., & Mohebbi, M. (2108). Depression and chronic diseases: Co-occurrence and communality of risk factors. *Journal of Affective Disorders*, 241, 461–468.

Mitchell, A. M., Kane, I., Kameg, K. M., Stark, K. H., & Kameg, B. (2017). Integrated management of self-directed injury. In: K. R. Tusaie, & J. J. Fitzpatrick (Eds.). *Advanced practice psychiatric nursing: Integrating psychotherapy, psychopharmacology, and complementary and alternative approaches* (2nd ed.) (pp. 443–471). New York: Springer Publishing Company.

Pedersen, C. A., Lonner, W. J., Draguus, J. G., Trimble J. E., & Scharron-del Rio M. R. (2016). *Counseling across cultures* (7th ed.). Thousand Oaks, CA: Sage Publishing.

Sanchez, K., Ybarra, R., Chapa, T., & Martinez, O. N. (2016). Eliminating behavioral health disparities and improving outcomes for racial and ethnic minority populations. *Psychiatric Services*, 67(1), 13–15.

Schatzberg, A. F., & DeBattista, C. (2015). *Manual of clinical psychopharmacology* (8th ed.). Arlington, VA: American Psychiatric Publishing.

Sehatzadeh, S., Daskalakis, Z. J., Yap, B., Tu, H. A., Palimaka, S., Bowen, J. M., et al. (2019). Unilateral and bilateral repetitive transcranial magnetic stimulation for treatment-resistant depression: a meta-analysis of randomized controlled trials over 2 decades. *Journal of Psychiatry & Neuroscience, 44*(2), 1–13.

Stahl, S. M. (2017). *Stahl's essential psychopharmacology: The prescriber's guide* (6th ed.). New York: Cambridge University Press.

Tolliver, B. K., & Anton, R. F. (2015). Assessment and treatment of mood disorders in the context of substance abuse. *Dialogues in Clinical Neuroscience, 17*(2), 181–190.

Tormoehlen, L. M., & Rusyniak D. E. (2018). Neuroleptic malignant syndrome and serotonin syndrome. *Handbook of Clinical Neurology, 157*, 663–675.

Tuithof, M., Ten Have, M., van Dorsselaer, S., Kleinjan, M., Beekman, A., de Graaf, R., et al. (2018). Course of subthreshold depression into a depressive disorder and its risk factors. *Journal of Affective Disorders, 241*, 206–215.

Uhlenbusch, N., Löwe, B., Härter, M., Schramm, C., Weiler-Normann, C., & Depping, M. K. (2019). Depression and anxiety in patients with different rare chronic diseases: A cross-sectional study. *PLoS, 4*(2), e0211343.

Weintraub, M. J., Axelson, D. A., Kowatch, R. A., Schneck, C. D., & Miklowitz, D. J. (2019). Comorbid disorders as moderators of response to family interventions among adolescents with bipolar disorder. *Journal of Affective Disorders, 246*, 754–762.

Whisman, M. A., & Beach, S. R. (2012). Couple therapy for depression. *Journal of Clinical Psychology, 68*(5), 26–35. doi: 10.1002/jclp.21857.

World Health Organization (WHO). (2019). Evidence-based recommendations for management of depression in non-specialized health settings. Retrieved February 20, 2019, from http://www.who.int/mental_health/mhgap/evidence/depression/en/index.html

Zis, P., Daskalaki, A., Bountouni, I., Sykioti, P., Varrassi, G., & Paladini, A. (2017). Depression and chronic pain in the elderly: links and management challenges. *Clinical Interventions in Aging, 12*, 709–720.

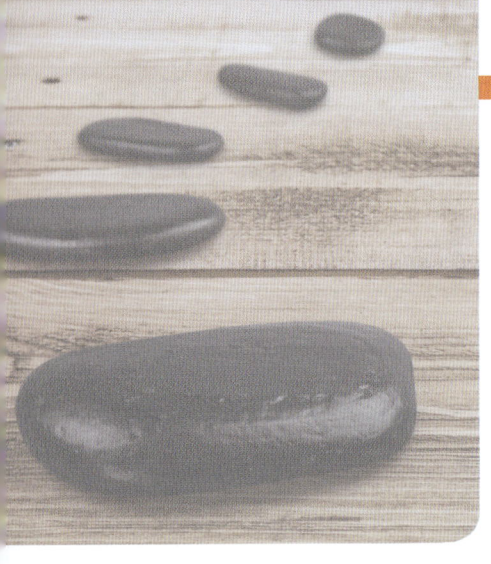

22
Bipolar Disorders
Nursing Care of Persons With Mood Lability

Mary Ann Boyd

KEY CONCEPTS
- mania
- mood lability

LEARNING OBJECTIVES

After studying this chapter, you will be able to:

1. Discuss the role of mania in mental disorders.
2. Describe the prevalence and incidence of bipolar disorders.
3. Delineate the clinical symptoms of bipolar disorders with emphasis on mood lability.
4. Describe the theories explaining bipolar disorder and mood lability.
5. Identify evidence-based interventions for patients diagnosed with bipolar disorders and for those who exhibit mood lability.
6. Develop recovery-oriented strategies that address the needs of persons diagnosed with bipolar disorders and for those who exhibit mood lability.
7. Develop wellness strategies for persons with bipolar disorder.
8. Identify the importance of coordinating mental health care with primary care.
9. Differentiate other bipolar and related disorders.

KEY TERMS

- bipolar I disorder • bipolar II disorder • cyclothymic disorder • elation • elevated mood • euphoria • expansive mood
- grandiosity • hypomania • mania • mood lability • rapid cycling • social rhythms

Case Study: Christine

Christine is a 34-year-old female who has a history of bipolar I disorder. She is brought to the emergency room by the police from the airport where she was demanding a plane ticket to Hawaii. She became very belligerent when she did not get her ticket. She is wearing an evening dress with several pieces of expensive jewelry. How would you document Christine's behavior and appearance? Was her belligerent behavior at the airport excessive considering the circumstances? How would you support her?

Everyone has ups and downs. Mood changes are a part of everyday life; expression of feeling is integral to communication. But when moods are so pervasive that they cloud reasoning and judgment, they become problematic and interfere with interpersonal relationships. In some instances, extreme moods such as **mania** are symptoms of mental disorders. This chapter discusses bipolar disorders that are characterized by severe mood changes with **bipolar I disorder** highlighted.

MANIA

Mania is one of the primary symptoms of bipolar disorders. It is recognized by an elevated, expansive, or irritable mood. Mania is easily recognized by the cognitive changes that occur. Elevated self-esteem is expressed as **grandiosity** (exaggerating personal importance) and may range from unusual self-confidence to grandiose delusions. Speech is pressured (push of speech); the person is more talkative than usual and at times is difficult to interrupt. There is often a flight of ideas (illogical connections between thoughts) or racing thoughts. Distractibility increases.

> **KEYCONCEPT** **Mania** is primarily characterized by an abnormally and persistently elevated, expansive, or irritable mood.

In mania, the need for sleep is decreased and energy is increased. The individual often remains awake for long periods or wakes up several times at night full of energy. Initially, there is an increase in goal-directed activity that is purposeful (e.g., cleaning the house), but it deteriorates into hyperactivity, agitation, and disorganized behavior. Social activities, occupational functioning, and interpersonal relationships are eventually impaired. There can be excessive involvement in pleasurable activities with little regard for painful consequences (e.g., excessive spending, risky sexual behavior, drug or alcohol abuse) (Box 22.1). Persons with mania are often hospitalized to prevent self-harm.

Even though mania is primarily associated with bipolar disorders, other psychiatric disorders, including schizophrenia, schizoaffective disorder, anxiety disorders, some personality disorders (borderline personality disorder and histrionic personality disorder), substance abuse involving stimulants, and adolescent conduct disorders, may have symptoms that mimic a manic episode. Mania can also be caused by medical disorders or their treatments, certain metabolic abnormalities, neurologic disorders, central nervous system (CNS) tumors, and medications.

Mood lability is the term used for the rapid shifts in moods that often occur in bipolar disorder. One month a person is happy and the next he or she is in the depths of depression. These mood shifts leave everyone around the person confused and interfere with social interaction.

BOX 22.1 CLINICAL VIGNETTE

The Patient With Mania

George was a day trader on the stock market. Initially, he was quite successful and, as a result, upgraded his lifestyle with a more expensive car; a larger, more luxurious house; and a boat. When the stock market declined dramatically, George continued to trade, saying that if he could just find the "right" stock he could earn back all of the money he had lost. He spent his days and nights in front of his computer screen, taking little or no time to eat or sleep. He defaulted on his mortgage and car and boat payments and was talking nonstop to his wife. She brought him to the hospital for evaluation.

What Do You Think?
- What behavioral symptoms of mania does George exhibit?
- What cognitive symptoms of mania does George exhibit?

> **KEYCONCEPT** **Mood lability** is alterations in moods with little or no change in external events.

Rapid cycling is an extreme form of mood lability that can occur in bipolar disorders. In its most severe form, rapid cycling includes continuous cycling between subthreshold mania and depression or **hypomania** and depression.

BIPOLAR DISORDERS

Bipolar and related disorders are characterized by periods of mania or hypomania that alternate with depression. These disorders are further classified as bipolar I, bipolar II, and **cyclothymic disorders**, depending on the severity of the manic and depressive symptoms. Bipolar disorder may also be related to substance abuse, prescription use, or a medical condition.

BIPOLAR I DISORDER

Bipolar I disorder is the classic manic-depressive disorder with mood swings alternating from depressed to manic. Although the depression component is similar to that experienced in a major depressive disorder, in this disorder there is also a distinct period (of at least 1 week or less if hospitalized) of abnormally and persistently elevated, expansive, or irritable mood with abnormally increased goal-directed behavior or energy (American Psychiatric Association [APA], 2013). An **elevated mood** can be expressed as **euphoria** (exaggerated feelings of well-being) or **elation** (feeling "high," "ecstatic," "on top of the world," or "up in the clouds"). An **expansive mood** is characterized by lack of restraint in expressing feelings; an overvalued sense of self-importance; and a constant and indiscriminate enthusiasm for interpersonal, sexual, or occupational interactions.

For some people, an irritable mood instead of an elevated mood is pervasive during mania. Such individuals are easily annoyed and provoked to anger, particularly when their wishes are challenged or thwarted. Maintaining social relationships during these episodes is difficult.

Consider Christine
When Christine is brought to the hospital, she is experiencing grandiose delusions. She believes that she is starting a business. She has spent a large amount of money over a short period of time on clothes and jewelry. Her neighbors reported that she was selling household goods in her yard. Her mood is labile. She is loud and condescending toward staff members. She has push of speech and flight of ideas. What behaviors are characteristic of bipolar disorder?

Clinical Course

Bipolar I disorder is a chronic multisystemic cyclic disorder. Those with an earlier onset have more frequent episodes than persons who develop the illness later in life. Bipolar disorder is a progressive condition with prodromal, symptomatic, and residual states. The progressive nature of this disorder can be arrested with an early diagnosis, proper treatment, and individually tailored management (Muneer & Mazommil, 2018). An early onset and a family history of illness are associated with multiple episodes or continuous symptoms. Symptoms of the illness can be unpredictable and variable. Bipolar I disorder can lead to severe functional impairment such as alienation from family, friends, and coworkers; indebtedness; job loss; divorce; and other problems of living (Dell'Osso et al., 2017).

Diagnostic Criteria

Consult the *Diagnostic and Statistical Manual of Mental Disorders*, 5th edition (APA, 2013) for diagnostic criteria for bipolar I disorder.

Bipolar I Disorder Across the Life-Span

Children and Adolescents

Bipolar disorder in children has been recognized only recently. Although it has not been well studied, depression usually appears first. Somewhat different than in adults, the hallmark of childhood bipolar disorder is intense rage. Children may display seemingly unprovoked rage episodes for as long as 2 to 3 hours. The symptoms of bipolar disorder reflect the developmental level of the child. Children younger than 9 years exhibit more irritability and emotional lability; older children exhibit more classic symptoms, such as euphoria and grandiosity. The first contact with the mental health system often occurs when the behavior becomes disruptive, possibly 5 to 10 years after its onset. These children often have other psychiatric disorders, such as attention deficit hyperactivity disorder or conduct disorder (Goldstein et al., 2017). See Chapter 30.

Older Adults

Older adults with bipolar disorder have more neurologic abnormalities and cognitive disturbances (confusion and disorientation) than younger patients. The incidence of mania decreases with age, but the onset of bipolar disorder can also occur in older adults. Symptoms are similar to the earlier onset bipolar disorder (Almeida, Hankey, Yeap, Golledge, & Flicker, 2018). See Chapter 31.

Epidemiology and Risk Factors

Risk factors for bipolar disorders include a family history of mood disorders; prior mood episodes; lack of social support; stressful life events; substance use; and medical problems, particularly chronic or terminal illnesses (Marangoni, Faedda, & Baldessarini, 2018; Marangoni, Hernandez, & Faedda, 2016).

Age of Onset

Bipolar disorder has an estimated lifetime prevalence of 1.1% for bipolar I and 1.4% for bipolar II (Angst et al., 2018; Kessler, Petukhova, Sampson, Zaslavsky, & Wittchen, 2012). Most patients with bipolar disorder experience significant symptoms between the ages of 15 and 24 years. Estimates of the prevalence of bipolar disorder in older adults decline with age (Baldessarini et al., 2012).

Gender

Although no significant gender differences have been found in the incidence of bipolar I and II disorders diagnoses, gender differences have been reported in phenomenology, course, and treatment response. In addition, some data show that female patients with bipolar disorder are at greater risk for depression than are male patients, but male patients may be at greater risk for manic episodes (Fellinger et al., 2019).

Ethnicity and Culture

Although there is a general belief that no significant racial and ethnic differences related to bipolar disorder exist, most of the research is based on Caucasians who have not experienced a disparity in access to healthcare. A lack of representation from ethnic/racial groups makes it difficult to determine the impact of race and ethnicity on the morbidity of people with bipolar disorder. Also, African Americans with bipolar disorder are more likely to be misdiagnosed as having schizophrenia, schizoaffective, or major depressive disorders, and older African Americans are more likely to use general medical service for treatment than mental health services (Akinhanmi et al., 2018; Byers et al., 2016; Fellinger et al., 2019).

Comorbidity

The two most common comorbid mental health conditions are anxiety disorders (panic disorder and social phobia are the most prevalent) and substance use (most commonly alcohol and marijuana). Individuals with a comorbid anxiety disorder are more likely to experience a more severe course. A history of substance use further complicates the course of illness and results in less chance for remission and poorer treatment compliance (Kessler et al., 2012; Spoorthy, Chakrabarti, & Grover, 2019). For health conditions, hyperlipidemia, hypertension, asthma, arthritis, and diabetes are more prevalent in serious mental disorders than in the general US population (Razzano et al., 2015).

Etiology

The etiology of mood disorders is unknown, but the current thinking is that bipolar disorder results when an interaction exists between the genetic predisposition and psychosocial stress such as abuse or trauma (Oliveira et al., 2018).

Biologic Theories

Chronobiologic Theories

Sleep disturbance is common in individuals with bipolar disorder, especially mania. Sleep patterns appear to be regulated by an internal biologic clock center in the hypothalamus. Artificially induced sleep deprivation is known to precipitate mania in some patients with bipolar disorder. It is possible that circadian dysregulation underlies the sleep–wake disturbances of bipolar disorder. Seasonal changes in light exposure also trigger affective episodes in some patients, typically depression in winter and hypomania in the summer in the northern hemisphere (Oliveira et al., 2018).

Genetic Factors

Results from family, adoption, and twin studies indicate that bipolar disorder is highly heritable. Studies of monozygotic twins show risks from 40% to 70% of acquiring the illness if their identical twin has the disorder range (Craddock & Sklar, 2013). No one gene or sequence of genes is responsible for the pathology of bipolar disorder. Evidence suggests that the genetic etiologies of schizophrenia and bipolar disorders overlap (Allardyce et al., 2018).

Chronic Stress, Inflammation, and Kindling

The role of an allostatic load or wear and tear on the body (see Chapter 13) is thought to contribute to cognitive impairment, comorbidity, and eventual mortality of those with bipolar disorder. As the allostatic load increases, the number of mood episodes increases, which in turn increases physical and mental health problems. An interaction between stress and brain development is viewed as dynamic; individuals have different kinds of stress adaptation depending on their neurobiologic responses (Muneer & Mazommil, 2018).

The characteristic mood dysregulation of bipolar I disorder is associated with a decrease in serum brain-derived neurotrophic factor (BDNF), oxidative stress resulting in DNA damage, and inflammation. Pro-inflammatory cytokines bind to neuronal death receptors leading to cell death. In some patients with repeated episodes, there is a decrease in hippocampal volume and reduction in prefrontal grey matter (Muneer & Mazommil, 2018).

A closely related concept is the kindling theory that posits that as genetically predisposed individuals experience repetitive subthreshold stressors at vulnerable times, mood symptoms of increasing intensity and duration occur. Eventually, a full-blown depressive or manic episode erupts. Each episode leaves a trace and increases the person's vulnerability or sensitizes the person to have another episode with less stimulation. In later episodes, there may be little or no stress occurring before the depression or mania. The disorder takes on a life of its own, and over time, the time between episodes decreases (Weiss et al., 2015).

Psychological and Social Theories

Psychosocial theories are useful in planning recovery-oriented interventions that focus on reducing environmental stress and trauma in genetically vulnerable individuals. It is now generally accepted that psychosocial and environmental events contribute to the severity of the disorder and the frequency of the mood episodes. Two promising theories are currently receiving research support.

The *behavioral approach system dysregulation* theory proposed that individuals with bipolar disorder are overly sensitive and overreact to relevant cues when approaching a reward. That is, the intensity of the goal-motivated behavior can lead to manic symptoms such as euphoria, decreased need for sleep, and excessive self-confidence. Conversely, the system can be deactivated and lead to depressive symptoms such as decreased energy, hopelessness, and sadness (Arfaie, Safikhanlou, Roodsari, Farnam, & Shafiee-Kandjani, 2018).

The *social rhythm disruption theory* is consistent with the research on the impact of the circadian rhythm dysregulation previously discussed. According to this theory, there are environmental factors that set the circadian clock such as the rising and setting of the sun. There are also social cues or **social rhythms** that can set the circadian clock such as the time we get out of bed, our first contact in the morning (person), when we start our day, have dinner, and go to bed.

These are patterned social events. Individuals with bipolar disorder have fewer regular social rhythms than those without bipolar disorder. This theory suggests that when patterned social events are disrupted, mood swings are more likely to appear (Crowe & Inder, 2018).

Family Response to Disorder

Bipolar disorder can devastate families, who often feel that they are on an emotional merry-go-round, particularly if they have difficulty understanding the mood shifts. A major problem for family members is dealing with the consequences of impulsive behavior during manic episodes, such as taking on excessive debt, assault charges, and sexual infidelities.

Remember Christine?
She has been married for 2 years to Karl, who was unaware of her bipolar disorder. He believed that she used to take antidepressants, but that she no longer needed them. Her episode at the airport occurred when he was out of town. He is concerned about her health and their new financial obligations. How do you explain that Karl was unaware of Christine's illness? How would you explain Christine's illness to her husband?

Recovery-Oriented Care of Persons With Bipolar Disorder

Teamwork and Collaboration: Working Toward Recovery

An important recovery goal is to minimize or prevent both manic and depressive episodes, which tend to accelerate over time. The fewer the episodes, the more likely the person can live a fully productive life. Three interconnected pathways can lead to relapse: stressful life events, medication nonadherence, and disruption in social rhythms (Crowe, Beaglehole, & Inder, 2016). Patients with bipolar disorder have a complex set of issues and have the best chance of recovery by working with an interdisciplinary team. Nurses, physicians, social workers, psychologists, and activity therapists all have valuable expertise. For children with bipolar disorder, schoolteachers and counselors are included in the team. For older adult patients, the primary care physician becomes part of the team. Helping the patient and family to learn about the disorder and manage it throughout a lifetime is critical for recovery.

The primary treatment modalities are medications, psychotherapy, education, and support. Mood stabilizers and antipsychotics are the mainstay medications in the treatment of bipolar disorders. Mood stabilizers are discussed later in this chapter. Antipsychotics are discussed in Chapter 23. Long-term psychotherapy may help prevent symptoms by reducing the stresses that trigger episodes and increasing the patient's acceptance of the need for medication. Patients should be encouraged to keep their appointments with the therapist, be honest and open, do the assigned homework, and give the therapist feedback on whether the treatment is effective.

Integration With Primary Care

There are several reasons that coordination of care is very important for persons with bipolar disorder. There is a large proportion of persons with bipolar disorder who are treated in the primary care setting. There may be an average of 6 to 8 years between onset of symptoms and diagnosis. Because there may be several episodes of depression before there is a manic episode, bipolar disorder is often misdiagnosed as depression in primary care leading to a delay in treatment. If antidepressants are prescribed for someone with a bipolar disorder, these medications may precipitate a manic episode. The need exists to improve the health of this population. Collaborative care of mental health with primary care increases the likelihood that a person would be screened for bipolar disorder resulting in an early diagnosis and effective treatment (Cerimele, Fortney, Pyne, & Curran, 2019). Patients with bipolar disorder frequently require primary care management for comorbidities such as cardiovascular and metabolic disorders.

Safety Issues

During a manic episode, patient safety is a priority. Risk of suicide is always present for those having a depressive or manic episode. During a depressive episode, the patient may believe that life is not worth living. During a manic episode, the patient may believe that he or she has supernatural powers, such as the ability to fly.

During a manic episode, poor judgment and impulsivity lead to risk-taking behaviors that can have dire consequences for the patient and family. For example, when one patient gambled all of his family's money away, he blamed his partner for letting him have access to the money. A physical confrontation with the partner resulted.

As patients recover from a manic episode, they may be so devastated by the consequences of their impulsive behavior and poor judgment during the episode that suicide seems like the only option.

> **Consider This:**
> Consider Christine's history of poor judgment during a manic episode. She left her first husband and their two children during her third manic episode. At that time, Christine went to Hawaii and stayed there for several months without informing her family of her whereabouts. She was homeless most of the time. Once Christine is stable, what interventions will support long-term remission of bipolar disorder?

Evidence-Based Nursing Care of Persons With Bipolar Disorder

The nursing care of patients with a bipolar disorder is one of the most interesting yet greatest challenges in psychiatric nursing. In general, the behavior of patients with bipolar disorder is normal between mood episodes. The nurse's first contact with the patient is usually during a manic or depressive episode.

Mental Health Nursing Assessment

Recovery-oriented nursing care begins with the initial assessment through engaging the patient in a partnership and empowering the person to make decisions in setting overall goals of care (Box 22.2). During acute episodes, the patient's judgment may be impaired, but as the manic or depressive symptoms subside, the person will be able to participate in care decisions.

Physical Health Assessment

The physical health assessment should follow the process explained in Chapter 9. Target assessment symptoms include the changes and severity of activity, eating, and sleep patterns. The patient may not sleep, resulting in irritability and physical exhaustion. Diet and body weight usually change during a manic or depressive episode. Laboratory studies, such as thyroid function and electrolytes, should be completed to detect evidence of malnutrition and fluid imbalance. Abnormal thyroid functioning can be responsible for the mood and behavioral disturbances. In mania, patients often become hypersexual and engage in risky sexual practices. Changes in sexual practices should be included in the assessment.

A careful assessment of current medications is important in determining physical status. Many times, manic or depressive episodes occur after patients stop taking their medication. Exploring reasons for discontinuing the medication will help in planning adherence strategies in the future. Some stop taking their medications because of side effects; others do not believe they have a mental disorder. The use of alcohol and other substances should be carefully assessed. Usually, a drug screen is ordered. In some instances, patients have been taking an antidepressant as prescribed for depression without realizing that a bipolar disorder existed.

Psychosocial Assessment

The psychosocial assessment should follow the process explained in Chapter 9. Individuals with bipolar disorder can usually participate fully in this part of the assessment.

Mood. By definition, bipolar disorder is a disturbance of mood. If the patient is depressed, using an assessment tool for depression may help determine the severity of depression. If mania predominates, evaluating the quality of the mood (e.g., elated, grandiose, irritated, or agitated) becomes important. Usually, mania is diagnosed by clinical observation.

Cognition. In a depressive episode, an individual may not be able to concentrate enough to complete cognitive tasks, such as those called for in a mental status assessment. During the acute phase of a manic or depressive episode, mental status may be abnormal, and in a manic phase, judgment is impaired by extremely rapid, disjointed, and distorted thinking. Moreover, feelings such as grandiosity can interfere with executive functioning. See Box 22.3.

BOX 22.2

Research for Best Practice: Promoting Personal Recovery

Crowe, M., & Inder, M. (2018). Staying well with bipolar disorder: A qualitative analysis of five-year follow-up interviews with young people. *Journal of Psychiatric and Mental Health Nursing, 25*(4), 236–244.

THE QUESTION: How do participants in psychotherapy for young people with bipolar disorder describe their experiences of the intervention and its impact on living with the disorder?

METHODS: A qualitative study was conducted 5 years after participants had completed a psychotherapy intervention in a randomized controlled trial for young people with bipolar disorder. Thirty people were recruited and interviewed regarding their experiences.

FINDINGS: Three themes were identified: self-awareness in the context of bipolar disorder, understanding bipolar disorder, and learning to stay well with bipolar disorder.

IMPLICATIONS FOR NURSING: Nurses can promote factors recognized by their patients as being helpful in learning to stay well including self-awareness, understanding the unique characteristics of their disorder, learning to take care of the self, and stabilization of social rhythms.

BOX 22.3 CLINICAL VIGNETTE

The Personal Experience of Mania

Sam is a 35-year-old man who was diagnosed with bipolar disorder 10 years ago. He is now being successfully treated and has insight into his disorder. In a recent discussion with his close friend, he describes his personal experience of mania.

At first, I started having more energy and felt happy most of the time. I decided to date a couple of women because I thought my girlfriend Jill was rather boring. Within a couple of weeks, I started sleeping less, but I thought that meant I could do more things. I decided to go back to school to be a scientist—thought I could save the world. I started to apply to graduate school and became very upset when I was told that I did not have the prerequisites for biochemistry. I was so mad that I started threatening the admissions counselor who in turn called the police. My family was called. They convinced the police that I would not bother the school again. After that I started drinking and smoking pot. I had periods of confusion and my family said I became disoriented. There is a lot I don't remember. Eventually, I was hospitalized and started on medication.

What Do You Think?
- At what point could have an early intervention prevented Sam from progressing to a major manic episode?
- Why does Sam not remember the complete manic episode?

Thought Disturbances. Psychosis commonly occurs in patients with bipolar disorder, especially during acute episodes of mania. Auditory hallucinations and delusional thinking are part of the clinical picture. In children and adolescents, however, psychosis is not so easily disclosed.

Stress and Coping. Stress and coping are critical assessment areas for a person with bipolar disorder. A stressful event often triggers a manic or depressive episode. In some instances, no particular stressors had preceded the episode, although it is important to discuss the possibility. Determining the patient's usual coping skills for stresses lays the groundwork for developing interventional strategies. Negative coping skills, such as substance use or aggression, should be identified because these skills need to be replaced with positive coping skills.

Risk Assessment. Persons with bipolar disorder are at high risk for injury to themselves and others, with 23% to 26% attempting suicide. People with bipolar disorder account for 3.4% to 14% of all suicide deaths with self-poisoning and hanging being the most common methods (Schaffer et al., 2015). Child abuse, spouse abuse, or other violent behaviors may occur during severe manic or depressive episodes; thus, patients should be assessed for suicidal or homicidal risk. In addition, they are at high risk for comorbid mental disorders such as substance abuse and anxiety disorders. Significant risks for cardiovascular and metabolic diseases are found in this group (Fornaro et al., 2015). Smoking is also a major health hazard (Li et al., 2017).

Social and Occupational Functioning

One of the tragedies of bipolar disorder is its effect on social and occupational functioning. Cultural views of mental illness influence the patient's acceptance of the disorder. During illness episodes, patients often behave in ways that jeopardize their social relationships. Losing a job and going through a divorce are common events. When performing an assessment of social function, the nurse should identify changes resulting from a manic or depressive episode.

Strengths Assessment

The nurse should always be listening for thoughts, feelings, or behaviors that could be identified as strengths. For example, one patient recognized an increase in drinking alcohol as a sign that he was beginning a manic episode and made an appointment with a health care provider. The following questions may be used to determine a person's strength.

- What healthy behaviors do you routinely practice?
- Are there any cues that a manic or depressive episode will occur?
- Who provides emotional support to you?
- What do you do to relax? Manage stress?
- What makes you feel good when you are on medication?
- How do you remember to take your medications?

Priority of Nursing Care

The priority of nursing care is always patient safety. Is the patient likely to self-injure or hurt another person (see Chapter 14)? After the patient's safety is established, the nurse analyzes the assessment data within the biopsychosocial priorities. For example, sleep deprivation, inadequate nutrition, and dehydration may be imminent needs. The person may be depressed or manic and unable to function socially. The person's coping skills may not be effective, and the person's job may be in jeopardy.

Mental Health Nursing Interventions

Therapeutic Relationship

Interacting with a person with mania is interesting and, at times, exhausting. The individual often quickly jumps

> **BOX 22.4**
> **Interacting With a Person With Mania**
> - Use a calm nonthreatening approach.
> - Be direct and use simple commands (e.g., time for lunch, let's go to group).
> - Avoid open-ended sentences; redirect conversation if flight of ideas occur; avoid confrontation and arguments.
> - Limit interaction time and recognize the patient's need for space and movement.
> - Do not place demands on patient that may be interpreted as excessive.

from subject to subject and is usually unable to sit still. When in a manic state, the individual can be very engaging and intense. Their stories may be very grandiose. The nurse should acknowledge the verbal content but recognize that many of the thoughts, feelings, and behaviors are symptomatic of mania and then try to re-focus the patient. If a person is in a depressive state, the nurse should use the same approach as when caring for a person with a depressed disorder as discussed in Chapter 21.

People with mania are typically impatient with others and may express irritability at someone's perceived incompetence and lack of understanding of their special powers. When interacting with a person with bipolar disorder, the nurse should remain calm and avoid any arguments. This is not the time to confront the person about his or her unrealistic perceptions of his or her status. For example, one agitated person was convinced that he owned a hotel. The nurse acknowledged how difficult it must be to have such responsibilities. He agreed with her and subsequently became less agitated. See Box 22.4.

In some instances, a person who has mania cannot sit still long enough to have a meaningful interaction. The nurse can initiate a conversation while walking with the patient, but there will be times when the nurse needs to give the patient space to avoid increasing agitation.

A therapeutic relationship can actually be instrumental in preventing a relapse. When a person is in the depths of a depression or the height of mania, therapeutic interaction is critical in helping the person take steps in recovery from either the depression or mania. However, often long periods of time pass when the affected person is living comfortably with bipolar disorder and attending to other issues. The periods of stable mental health are perfect times to focus on stress reduction, illness management, and relapse prevention.

Establishing Recovery and Wellness Goals

The person with a bipolar disorder has emotional ups and downs with periods of poor judgment and erratic behavior. However, there are many periods (months to years) where there are few symptoms. During these relatively quiet periods, it is possible to establish recovery and wellness goals. Goals focus on managing the long-term illness and supporting well-being. Recovery and wellness goals are interrelated. For example, preventing relapse includes managing stress (wellness dimension) that can trigger erratic behavior (mental health goals).

Self-Care

In a state of mania, the patient's physical needs are rest, adequate hydration and nutrition, and reestablishment of physical well-being. Self-care has usually deteriorated. For a patient unable to sit long enough to eat, snacks and high-energy foods that can be eaten while moving should be provided. Consumption of alcohol should be avoided. Sleep hygiene is a priority but may not be realistic until medications have taken effect. Limiting stimuli can be helpful in decreasing agitation and promoting sleep.

NCLEXNOTE Protection of patients with mania is always a priority. Ongoing assessment should focus on irritability, fatigue, and the potential for harming self or others.

After the patient's mood stabilizes, the nurse should focus on monitoring changes in physical functioning in sleep or eating behavior and teaching patients to identify antecedents to mood episodes such as a family argument or a financial problem. Strategies for dealing with future events can then be identified. The patient can begin to problem solve the best approach for future episodes.

A regular sleep routine should be maintained if possible. High-risk times for manic episodes, such as changes in work schedule (day to night), should be avoided if possible. Patients should be encouraged to monitor the amount of their sleep each night and report decreases in sleep of longer than 1 hour per night because this may be a precursor to a manic episode.

Highlighting the recovery concept of hope will support the person who has had multiple episodes and is frustrated with the impact of several episodes (Box 22.5). In educating persons with bipolar disorder, the nonlongitudinal nature of the disorders should be emphasized.

Wellness Challenges

Many self-care interventions that prevent or delay symptoms are also wellness strategies. For example, individuals with bipolar disorder who relapse often describe a stressful life event that led to the manic episode. These individuals appear to be more sensitive to life events than people without the disorder (Melo et al., 2016). The emotional dimension of wellness focuses on developing skills for coping with stress. If the individuals can strengthen their coping skills, they may be able to be less sensitive to stressful life events. See Box 22.6.

BOX 22.5 • THERAPEUTIC DIALOGUE • Instilling Hope

Christine is sitting in the dayroom of an inpatient unit with tears in her eyes. She acknowledges that she has bipolar disorder and wishes that she had been taking her medication and told her husband about her previous relapses.

INEFFECTIVE APPROACH

Nurse: Christine, I am glad that you realize that you have bipolar disorder and want to take your medication. You must commit to staying on your medicine or you will lose your second husband.

Christine: No one understands what it is like to have this problem. I don't quite understand how this little pill and seeing a shrink will help.

Nurse: Well, medication and therapy will help.

Christine: You don't know what I am talking about.

EFFECTIVE APPROACH

Nurse: Christine, I hope that you are feeling better.

Christine: No one understands what it is like to have this problem. I don't quite understand how this little pill and seeing a shrink will help.

Nurse: Let's talk about it. What does it feel like to have bipolar disorder?

Christine: Sometimes it is wonderful—on top of the world, but after the mood goes away, having this problem is terrible. The bad times outweigh the good feelings.

Nurse: Other people have said the same thing. Many people decide to take their medication and "check in" with a mental health provider in order to stay on track and avoid the bad times that can happen after a manic period.

Christine: Really?

Nurse: There are many successful people with bipolar disorder who find that taking medication helps keep order in their life. I can give you information about a support group.

Christine: Ok, I'm willing to try.

Nurse: Now, what about this medication. Are you willing to try it also? This medication is an effective treatment for bipolar disorder and has helped others to control moods.

Christine: Okay, but I want to know more about this medication.

Nurse: It's a deal. We can spend some time talking about your medications after dinner.

CRITICAL THINKING CHALLENGE

- How did the nurse block communication with Christine in the first scenario? Did she seem hopeful after the interaction?
- How did the nurse instill hope in Christine in the second scenario?

BOX 22.6
Wellness Challenges

- Reduce emotional responses to daily stresses
  - Strategies: Re-frame experiences, use problem-focused coping techniques, relaxation
- Support positive circadian rhythms consistent with relapse prevention needs
  - Establish sleep hygiene, eating routines
- Establish a healthy diet with reducing substance use
  - Eat at regular times, maintain a healthy diet
- Seeking pleasant environments that support well-being
  - Strategies: Seek comfortable, relaxing living arrangements, explore community resources that support people with bipolar disorder
- Satisfying current and future financial situations
  - Strategies: Seek financial counseling, protect resources during periods of relapses
- Satisfying and enriching work
  - Strategies: Select job opportunities that are consistent with health promotion activities
- Recognizing the need for physical activity, healthy foods, and sleep
  - Strategies: Encourage regular physical activity, discuss healthy diets, encourage establishing healthy sleep hygiene routines
- Developing a sense of connection, belonging, and a support system
  - Strategies: Explore expanding a positive support system
- Expanding a sense of purpose and meaning in life
  - Strategies: Focus on goals, values, and beliefs; read inspiring stories or essays

Medications

Medications are essential in bipolar disorder to achieve two goals: rapid control of symptoms and prevention of future episodes or, at least, reduction in their severity and frequency.

Mood-Stabilizing Drugs. The mainstays of pharmacotherapy are the mood-stabilizing drugs, including lithium carbonate (Lithium), divalproex sodium (Depakote), carbamazepine (Tegretol), and lamotrigine (Lamictal). Antidepressant therapy is not recommended in persons with bipolar depression because of a risk of switching from depression to mania.

Lithium Carbonate. Lithium is the most widely used mood stabilizer (Box 22.7). Combined response rates from five studies demonstrate that 70% of patients experienced at least partial improvement with lithium therapy. However, for many patients, lithium is not a fully adequate treatment for all phases of the illness, and particularly during the acute phase, supplemental use of antipsychotics and benzodiazepines is often beneficial.

> **NCLEXNOTE** Monitoring blood levels of lithium carbonate and divalproex sodium is an ongoing nursing assessment for patients receiving these medications. Side effects of mood stabilizers vary.

Lithium is a salt; the interaction between lithium levels and sodium levels in the body and the relationship between lithium levels and fluid volume in the body remain crucial issues in its safe, effective use. The higher the sodium levels, the lower the lithium level will be and vice versa. Thus, changes in dietary sodium intake can affect lithium blood levels that, in turn, may affect therapeutic results or increase the incidence and severity of side effects. The same principle applies to fluid volume. If body fluid decreases significantly because of hot weather, strenuous exercise, vomiting, diarrhea, or drastic reduction in fluid intake for any reason, then lithium levels can rise sharply, causing an increase in side effects, progressing to lethal lithium toxicity. The key is to start with a lower dose and then increase it slowly to maximize the therapeutic response and avoid overshooting the therapeutic window. See Table 22.1 for lithium interactions with other drugs. See Chapter 11 for further discussion of lithium's possible mechanisms of action, pharmacokinetics, side effects, and toxicity.

> **EMERGENCY CARE ALERT !** If symptoms of moderate or severe toxicity (e.g., cardiac arrhythmias, blackouts, tremors, seizures) are noted, withhold additional doses of lithium, immediately obtain a blood sample to analyze the lithium level, and push fluids if the patient can take fluids. Contact the physician for further direction about relieving the symptoms.

Mild side effects tend to subside or can be managed by nursing measures (Tables 22.2 and 22.3).

Concept Mastery Alert

Fine tremors are mild side effects of lithium. They are made worse by stress, so the nurse should assist the client in minimizing exposure to stressors. Lithium therapy can continue unless the tremors interfere with the client's quality of life.

Divalproex Sodium. Divalproex sodium (Depakote), an anticonvulsant, has a broader spectrum of efficacy and has about equal benefit for patients with pure mania as for those with other forms of bipolar disorder (i.e., mania, rapid cycling, comorbid substance abuse, and

---

BOX 22.7

Drug Profile: Lithium Carbonate

DRUG CLASS: Mood stabilizer

RECEPTOR AFFINITY: Alters sodium transport in nerve and muscle cells, increases norepinephrine uptake and serotonin receptor sensitivity, slightly increases intraneuronal stores of catecholamines, and delays some second messenger systems. Mechanism of action is unknown.

INDICATIONS: Treatment and prevention of manic episodes in bipolar affective disorder.

ROUTES AND DOSAGE: 150-, 300-, and 600-mg capsules. Lithobid, 300-mg slow-release tablets; Eskalith CR, 450-mg controlled-release tablets; lithium citrate, 300-mg/5 mL liquid form.

Adults: In acute mania, optimal response is usually 600 mg tid or 900 mg bid. Obtain serum levels twice weekly in acute phase. Do not rely on serum levels alone. Maintenance: Use lowest possible dose to alleviate symptoms and maintain serum level of 0.6 to 1.2 mEq/L. In uncomplicated maintenance, obtain serum levels every 2 to 3 months. Monitor patient's side effects.

Geriatric: Increased risk for toxic effects; use lower doses; monitor frequently.

Children: **6 to 12 years:** 15 to 60 mg/kg/day in 3 to 4 divided doses.

HALF-LIFE (PEAK EFFECT): Mean, 24 hours (peak serum levels in 1 to 4 hours). Steady state reached in 5 to 7 days.

SELECTED ADVERSE REACTIONS: Weight gain

WARNING: Avoid use during pregnancy or while breastfeeding. Hepatic or renal impairments increase plasma concentration.

SPECIFIC PATIENT/FAMILY EDUCATION

- Avoid alcohol and other CNS depressant drugs.
- Notify your prescriber if pregnancy is possible or planned. Do not breastfeed while taking this medication.
- Notify your prescriber before taking any other prescriptions, OTC medications, or herbal supplements.
- May impair judgment, thinking, or motor skills; avoid driving or other hazardous tasks.
- Do not abruptly discontinue use.

bid, twice a day; CNS, central nervous system; OTC, over-the-counter; tid, three times a day.

TABLE 22.1 LITHIUM INTERACTIONS WITH MEDICATIONS AND OTHER SUBSTANCES

Substance	Effect of Interaction
ACE inhibitors, such as: • Captopril • Lisinopril • Quinapril	Increase serum lithium; may cause toxicity and impaired kidney function
Acetazolamide	Increases renal excretion of lithium; decreases lithium levels
Alcohol	May increase serum lithium level
Caffeine	Increases lithium excretion; increases lithium tremor
Carbamazepine	Increases neurotoxicity despite normal serum levels and dosage
Fluoxetine	Increases serum lithium levels
Haloperidol	Increases neurotoxicity despite normal serum levels and dosage
Loop diuretics, such as furosemide	Increase lithium serum levels but may be safer than thiazide diuretics; potassium-sparing diuretics (e.g., amiloride, spironolactone) are safest
Methyldopa	Increases neurotoxicity without increasing serum lithium levels
NSAIDs, such as: • Diclofenac • Ibuprofen • Indomethacin • Piroxicam	Decrease renal clearance of lithium Increase serum lithium levels by 30%–60% in 3–10 days Aspirin and sulindac do not appear to have the same effect
Osmotic diuretics, such as: • Urea • Mannitol • Isosorbide	Increases renal excretion of lithium and decreases lithium levels
Sodium chloride	High sodium intake decreases lithium levels; low sodium diets may increase lithium levels and lead to toxicity
Thiazide diuretics, such as: • Chlorothiazide • Hydrochlorothiazide	Promote sodium and potassium excretion; increase lithium serum levels; may produce cardiotoxicity and neurotoxicity
TCAs	Increases tremor; potentiates pharmacologic effects of tricyclic antidepressants

ACE, angiotensin-converting enzyme; NSAID, nonsteroidal anti-inflammatory drug; TCA, tricyclic antidepressant.

secondary mania) (Box 22.8). The recommended initial dose in 750 mg daily, increases as rapidly as possible to achieve therapeutic response or desired plasma level. The maximum recommended dosage is 60 mg/kg/day (Depakote Prescribing Information, 2019). Divalproex is usually initiated at 250 mg twice a day or lower. In the inpatient setting, baseline liver function tests and a complete blood count with platelets should be obtained before starting therapy, and patients with known liver disease should not be given divalproex sodium. The black box warns of hepatotoxicity. Optimal blood levels appear to be in the range of 50 to 150 ng/mL. Levels should be obtained weekly until the patient is stable and then every 6 months. Divalproex sodium is associated with increased risk for birth defects. Cases of life-threatening pancreatitis have been reported in adults and children receiving valproate, both initially and after several years of use. Some cases were described as hemorrhagic, with a rapid progression from onset to death. If pancreatitis is diagnosed, valproate use should be discontinued (Depakote Prescribing Information, 2019).

Carbamazepine. Carbamazepine, an anticonvulsant, also has mood-stabilizing effects. Data from various studies suggest that it may be effective in patients who experience no response to lithium. The most common side effects of carbamazepine are dizziness, drowsiness, nausea, and vomiting, which may be avoided with slow incremental dosing. Carbamazepine has a boxed warning for aplastic anemia and agranulocytosis, but frequent clinically unimportant decreases in white blood cell counts also occur. Estimates of the rate of severe blood dyscrasias vary from 1 in 10,000 patients treated to a more recent estimate of 1 in 125,000 (Schatzberg & DeBattista, 2015). Mild, nonprogressive elevations of liver function test results are relatively common. Carbamazepine is associated with increased risk for birth defects.

In patients older than 12 years, carbamazepine is begun at 200 mg once or twice a day. The dosage is increased by no more than 200 mg every 2 to 4 days, to 800 to 1,000 mg a day or until therapeutic levels or effects are achieved. It is important to monitor for blood dyscrasias and liver damage. Liver function tests and complete blood counts with differential are the

TABLE 22.2 LITHIUM BLOOD LEVELS AND ASSOCIATED SIDE EFFECTS

Plasma Level	Side Effects or Symptoms of Toxicity
<1.5 mEq/L Mild side effects	Metallic taste in mouth Fine hand tremor (resting) Nausea Polyuria Polydipsia Diarrhea or loose stools Muscular weakness or fatigue Weight gain Edema Memory impairments
1.5–2.5 mEq/L Moderate toxicity	Severe diarrhea Dry mouth Nausea and vomiting Mild to moderate ataxia Incoordination Dizziness, sluggishness, giddiness, vertigo Slurred speech Tinnitus Blurred vision Increasing tremor Muscle irritability or twitching Asymmetric deep tendon reflexes Increased muscle tone
>2.5 mEq/L Severe toxicity	Cardiac arrhythmias Blackouts Nystagmus Coarse tremor Fasciculations Visual or tactile hallucinations Oliguria, renal failure Peripheral vascular collapse Confusion Seizures Coma and death

TABLE 22.3 INTERVENTIONS FOR LITHIUM SIDE EFFECTS

Side Effect	Intervention
Edema of feet or hands	Monitor intake and output of water; check for possible decreased urinary output. Monitor sodium intake. Patient should elevate legs when sitting or lying. Monitor weight.
Fine hand tremor	Provide support and reassurance if it does not interfere with daily activities. Tremor worsens with anxiety and intentional movements; minimize stressors. Notify prescriber if tremor interferes with patient's work so that compliance may be an issue. More frequent smaller doses of lithium may also help.
Mild diarrhea	Take lithium with meals. Provide for fluid replacement. Notify prescriber if it worsens; may need a change in medication preparation or may be early sign of toxicity.
Muscle weakness, fatigue, or memory and concentration difficulties	Provide support and reassurance; this side effect will usually pass after a few weeks of treatment. Short-term memory aids such as lists or reminder calls may be helpful. Notify prescriber if side effect becomes severe or interferes with the patient's desire to continue treatment.
Metallic taste	Suggest sugarless candies or throat lozenges. Encourage frequent oral hygiene.
Nausea or abdominal discomfort	Consider dividing the medication into smaller doses or giving it at more frequent intervals. Give medication with meals.
Polydipsia	Reassure patient that this is a normal mechanism to cope with polyuria.
Polyuria	Monitor intake and output. Provide reassurance and explain the nature of this side effect. Explain that this side effect causes no physical damage to the kidneys.
Toxicity	Withhold medication. Notify prescriber. Use symptomatic treatments.

minimal pretreatment laboratory tests and they should be repeated about 1 month after initiating treatment and at 3 months, 6 months, and yearly. Other yearly tests assessments should include electrolytes, blood urea nitrogen, thyroid function tests, urinalysis, and eye examinations. Carbamazepine levels are measured monthly until the patient is on a stable dosage. Studies suggest that blood levels in the range of 8 to 12 ng/mL correspond to therapeutic efficacy. See Table 22.4 for carbamazepine's interactions with other drugs. See Chapter 11 for further discussion of carbamazepine's possible mechanisms of action, pharmacokinetics, side effects, and toxicity.

EMERGENCY CARE ALERT ! Both valproate and carbamazepine may be lethal if high doses are ingested. Toxic symptoms appear in 1 to 3 hours and include neuromuscular disturbances, dizziness, stupor, agitation, disorientation, nystagmus, urinary retention, nausea and vomiting, tachycardia, hypotension or hypertension, cardiovascular shock, coma, and respiratory depression.

Lamotrigine. For a depressive episode, mood stabilizers such as lamotrigine (Lamictal), which requires a dose titration are frequently prescribed (Box 22.9). Lamotrigine is approved by the U.S. Food and Drug Administration (FDA) for the maintenance treatment of bipolar disorder. It may be particularly effective for rapid cycling and

BOX 22.8

Drug Profile: Divalproex Sodium (Depakote)

DRUG CLASS: Antimanic agent

RECEPTOR AFFINITY: Thought to increase level of inhibitory neurotransmitter, GABA, to brain neurons. Mechanism of action is unknown.

INDICATIONS: Mania, epilepsy, migraine.

ROUTES AND DOSAGE: Available in 125-mg delayed-release capsules, and 125-, 250-, and 500-mg enteric-coated tablets.

Adult Dosage: Dosage depends on symptoms and clinical picture presented; initially, the dosage is low and gradually increased depending on the clinical presentation.

HALF-LIFE (PEAK EFFECT): 6 to 16 hours (1 to 4 hours)

SELECTED ADVERSE REACTIONS: Sedation, tremor (may be dose related), nausea, vomiting, indigestion, abdominal cramps, anorexia with weight loss, slight elevations in liver enzymes, hepatic failure, thrombocytopenia, transient increases in hair loss.

BOXED WARNING: Hepatotoxicity, teratogenicity, pancreatitis

WARNING: Use cautiously during pregnancy and lactation. Contraindicated in patients with hepatic disease or significant hepatic dysfunction. Administer cautiously with salicylates; may increase serum levels and result in toxicity.

SPECIFIC PATIENT AND FAMILY EDUCATION

- Take with food if gastrointestinal upset occurs.
- Swallow tablets or capsules whole to prevent local irritation of mouth and throat.
- Notify your prescriber before taking any other prescription or OTC medications or herbal supplements.
- Avoid alcohol and sleep-inducing OTC products.
- Avoid driving or performing activities that require alertness.
- Do not abruptly discontinue use.
- Keep appointments for follow-up, including blood tests to monitor response.

GABA, gamma-aminobutyric acid; OTC, over-the-counter.

---

in the depressed phase of bipolar illness. If lamotrigine is given with valproic acid (Depakote), the dose should be reduced. Valproic acid decreases the clearance of lamotrigine. Lamotrigine does have an "FDA black box warning" for rash. Nurses should be especially vigilant for the appearance of any rash. If a rash does appear, it is most likely benign. However, it is not possible to predict whether the rash is benign or serious (Stevens–Johnson syndrome).

TABLE 22.4 SELECTED MEDICATION INTERACTIONS WITH CARBAMAZEPINE

Interaction	Drug Interacting With Carbamazepine
Increased carbamazepine levels	Erythromycin Cimetidine Propoxyphene Isoniazid Calcium channel blockers (verapamil) Fluoxetine Danazol Diltiazem Nicotinamide
Decreased carbamazepine levels	Phenobarbital Primidone Phenytoin
Drugs whose levels are decreased by carbamazepine	Oral contraceptives Warfarin, oral anticoagulants Doxycycline Theophylline Haloperidol Divalproex sodium Tricyclic antidepressants Acetaminophen: increased metabolism but also increased risk for hepatotoxicity

BOX 22.9

Drug Profile: Lamotrigine (Lamictal)

DRUG CLASS: Antiepileptic

RECEPTOR AFFINITY: Lamotrigine has a weak inhibitory effect on the serotonin 5-HT$_3$ receptor. It does not exhibit high-affinity binding: adenosine A$_1$ and A$_2$; adrenergic α_1, α_2, and β; dopamine D$_1$ and D$_2$; GABA-A and -B; histamine H$_1$; kappa opioid; muscarinic acetylcholine; and serotonin 5-HT$_2$.

INDICATIONS: Epilepsy, bipolar disorder (acute mood with standard therapy)

ROUTES AND DOSAGE: Available in tablets: 25 mg, 100 mg, 150 mg, and 200 mg scored

CHEWABLE DISPERSIBLE TABLETS: 2 mg, 5 mg, and 25 mg.

HALF-LIFE (PEAK EFFECT): 32 hours, but can be increased if taking valproate.

SELECTED ADVERSE REACTIONS: Dizziness, somnolence, and other symptoms and signs of CNS depression.

BOXED WARNING: Lamotrigine can cause serious rashes requiring hospitalization and discontinuation of treatment. The incidence of these rashes, which have included Stevens–Johnson syndrome, is approximately 0.3% to 0.8% in pediatric patients (aged 2 to 17 years) and 0.08% to 0.3% in adults receiving LAMICTAL.

WARNING: Hypersensitivity reaction, multiorgan failure, blood dyscrasias, and suicidal behavior and ideation have occurred.

SPECIFIC PATIENT AND FAMILY EDUCATION

- Do not drive a car or operate other complex machinery until you have gained sufficient experience taking lamotrigine.
- Lamotrigine may cause a serious rash that may cause you to be hospitalized or to stop taking lamotrigine; it may rarely cause death.

CNS, central nervous system; GABA, gamma-aminobutyric acid.

TABLE 22.5	FDA-APPROVED ANTIPSYCHOTICS FOR THE TREATMENT OF SYMPTOMS OF BIPOLAR DISORDER	
Antipsychotic Agent	FDA Indication for Bipolar Disorder	Adult Dosage
Aripiprazole (Abilify)	Acute treatment of manic episodes associated with bipolar disorder	10–30 mg per day
Aripiprazole (Abilify Maintena)	Maintenance monotherapy for treatment for bipolar I disorder in adults	300 mg monthly (extended release, injectable suspension)
Asenapine (Saphris)	Acute treatment of manic episodes associated with bipolar I disorder as monotherapy or adjunctive treatment to lithium or valproate	5–10 mg twice daily
Cariprazine (Vraylar)	Acute treatment of manic episodes associated with bipolar I disorder in adults	3–6 mg/day
Lurasidone (Latuda)	Depressive episodes associated with bipolar I disorder as monotherapy or as adjunctive treatment to lithium or valproate	20–120 mg daily with food (comprising 350 calories)
Olanzapine (Zyprexa)	Acute treatment of manic episodes associated with bipolar I disorder (monotherapy and in combination with lithium or valproate) and maintenance treatment of bipolar I disorder	10–15 mg daily
Quetiapine (Seroquel)	Bipolar I disorder, manic episodes; bipolar disorder, depressive episodes	300–800 mg daily
Risperidone (Risperdal)	Bipolar mania, combination of risperidone with lithium or valproate for short-term treatment of acute manic episodes associated with bipolar I disorder.	2–6 mg daily
Risperidone (Risperdal Consta)	Monotherapy or adjunctive to lithium or valproate for maintenance treatment of bipolar I disorder	25–50 mg every 2 weeks (extended release, injectable suspension)
Ziprasidone (Geodon)	Acute manic episodes associated with bipolar disorder, with or without psychotic features.	40–80 mg with food (comprising 500 calories)

FDA, U.S. Food and Drug Administration.

Antipsychotics. Several atypical antipsychotics that were primarily developed for the treatment of schizophrenia are also FDA approved for treatment of various symptoms of bipolar disorder. See Table 22.5. The dosages for the treatment of patients with bipolar disorder are generally lower than for those for schizophrenia. Recently, these agents have become a mainstay of treatment because they provide some of the broadest efficacy and are more likely used as the only medication to treat bipolar disorder than the mood stabilizers (Stahl, 2017). An overview of antipsychotics is presented in Chapter 11 and they are discussed in detail in Chapter 22.

Administering and Monitoring Medications. During acute mania, patients may not believe that they have a psychiatric disorder and may refuse to take medication. Because their energy level is still high, they can be very creative in avoiding medication. Through patience and the development of a trusting relationship, patients will more likely begin to participate in a shared decision-making process. It is important for patients to have a sense of empowerment and participation in treatment even during the most acute episodes. After patients begin to take medications, symptom improvement should be evident. If a patient is very agitated, a benzodiazepine may be given for a short period.

Managing Side Effects. Patients with bipolar disorder are usually treated with several medications. In addition, patients may be taking other "nonpsychiatric" medications. In some instances, one agent is used to augment the effects of another, such as supplemental thyroid hormone to boost antidepressant response in depression. Possible side effects for each medication should be listed and cross-referenced. When a side effect appears, the nurse should document the side effect and notify the prescriber, so that further evaluation can be made. In some instances, medications should be changed.

Monitoring for Drug Interactions. It is a well-established practice to combine mood stabilizers with antidepressants or antipsychotics. The previously discussed drug interactions should be considered when caring for a person with bipolar disorder. One big challenge is monitoring alcohol, drugs, over-the-counter (OTC) medications, and herbal supplements. A complete list of all medications should be maintained and evaluated for any potential interaction.

Promoting Adherence. Adherence to a complex medication regimen over months to years is difficult. Yet, one of the primary reasons that acute symptoms reappear is because of discontinuation of medications. It is important to recognize that taking medication as prescribed over time is difficult. Nurses can help patients and families incorporate taking medications into their lifestyles by developing realistic plans. The use of pill boxes, reminders, and other cues will increase the likelihood of adherence.

Teaching Points. For patients who are taking lithium, it is important to explain that a change in dietary salt intake can affect the therapeutic blood level. If salt intake is reduced, the body will naturally retain lithium to maintain homeostasis. This increase in lithium retention can lead to toxicity. After the patient has been stabilized on a lithium dose, salt intake should remain constant. This is fairly easy to do except during the summer, when excessive perspiration can occur. Patients should increase salt intake during periods of perspiration, increased exercise, and dehydration. Most mood stabilizers and antidepressants can cause weight gain. Patients should be alerted to this potential side effect and should be instructed to monitor any changes in eating, appetite, or weight. Weight reduction techniques may need to be instituted. Patients also should be clearly instructed to check with the nurse or physician before taking any OTC medications, herbal supplements, or any other complementary and alternative treatment approaches.

Other Somatic Therapies

Electroconvulsive therapy (ECT) may be a treatment alternative for patients with severe mania who exhibit unremitting, frenzied physical activity. Other indications for ECT are acute mania that is unresponsive to antimanic agents or high suicide risk. ECT is safe and effective in patients receiving antipsychotic drugs. Use of valproate or carbamazepine will elevate the seizure threshold, requiring some adjustments in treatment.

Psychosocial Interventions

Medications are necessary for treatment of bipolar disorder, but it is only one aspect of recovery. Psychosocial strategies are critical in successful treatment and prevention of relapse. Psychoeducation, individual cognitive behavioral therapy, individual interpersonal therapy, and adjunctive therapies (such as those for substance use) are all recommended psychotherapeutic approaches. There is emerging evidence supporting the use of interpersonal and social rhythm therapy and sleep/light manipulation targeting social rhythms promote mood stability (Crowe et al., 2016). See Box 22.10.

Several risk factors associated with bipolar disorders make patients more vulnerable to relapses and resistant to recovery. Among these are high rates of nonadherence to medication therapy, obesity, marital conflict, separation, divorce, unemployment, and underemployment. Even those who take their medication regularly are likely to experience recurrences and have difficulty keeping jobs and maintaining significant relationships.

Important goals of psychosocial interventions are identifying risk factors and developing strategies to address them. It is also important to help the patient understand the disorder and manage the mood lability and dysfunctional thoughts that are often precursors to a manic or depressive episode. The nurse partners with the patient in developing strategies to remember to take medications, identify therapeutic and side effects, and know when and how to contact a clinician. Particularly important are enhancing social and occupational functioning, improving quality of life, increasing the patient and family's acceptance of the disorder, and reducing the suicide (Crowe et al., 2016).

BOX 22.10

Research for Best Practice: Social Rhythm and Mental Health: A Cross-Cultural Comparison

Margraf, J., Lavallee, K., Zhang, X., & Schneider, S. (2016). Social rhythm and mental health: A cross-cultural comparison. PLoS One, 11(3), e0150312. doi: 10.137/journal.pone.0150312.

THE QUESTION: Are there relationships among social rhythms and various aspects of health, including physical health, negative mental health, and positive mental health?

METHODS: Questionnaire data were obtained from a large-scale multinational sample of 8,095 representative participants from the United States, Russia, and Germany.

FINDINGS: Social rhythm irregularity is related to increased reporting of health problems, depression, anxiety, and stress. Greater regularity is related to better overall health state, life satisfaction, and positive mental health.

IMPLICATIONS FOR NURSING: Social rhythm irregularity has a negative impact on mental health. Simple nursing interventions focusing on helping patients establish routines for social cues that impact circadian rhythms.

Teaching Patients and Family

Psychoeducation is designed to provide information on bipolar disorder and its successful treatment and recovery. The nurse can provide information about the illness and obstacles to recovery. Helping the patient recognize warning signs and symptoms of relapse and to cope with residual symptoms and functional impairment are important interventions. Watching for early warning signs and triggers can mean early treatment. Family members should be included in developing an emergency plan for recognizing and intervening if relapse symptoms occur. See Box 22.11.

In the interest of improved medication adherence, listening carefully to the patient's concerns about the medication, dosing schedules and dose changes, and side effects is helpful. Resistance to accepting the illness and to taking medication, the symbolic meaning of medication taking, and worries about the future can be discussed openly. Health teaching and weight management should be components of any psychoeducation program. In addition to individual variations in body weight, many of the medications (divalproex sodium, lithium, antidepressants, and atypical antipsychotics) are associated with weight gain. Monitoring weight and developing individual weight management plans can reduce the risk of relapse and increase the possibility of medication adherence. Box 22.12 provides a checklist for psychoeducation.

BOX 22.12

Psychoeducation Checklist: Bipolar I Disorder

When caring for the patient with a bipolar I disorder, be sure to include the following topic areas in the teaching plan:

- Psychopharmacologic agents, including drug action, dosage, frequency, and possible side effects
- Medication regimen adherence
- Recovery plan
- Relapse prevention plan
- Strategies to decrease agitation and restlessness
- Safety measures
- Self-care management
- Follow-up laboratory testing
- Support services

Support Groups

Support groups are helpful for people with this disorder. Participating in groups allows the person to meet others with the same disorder and to learn management and preventive strategies. Support groups also are helpful in dealing with the stigma associated with mental illness.

Interventions for Family Members

Marital and family interventions are often needed at different periods in the life of a person with bipolar disorder. For the family with a child with this disorder, additional parenting skills are needed to manage the behaviors. The goals of family interventions are to help the family understand and cope with the disorder. Interventions may range from occasional counseling sessions to intensive family therapy.

Family psychoeducation strategies have been shown to be particularly useful in decreasing the risk of relapse and hospitalization. The sooner the education is begun, the more effective this approach is (Sampogna et al., 2018).

Evaluation and Treatment Outcomes

Desired treatment outcomes are stabilization of mood and enhanced quality of life. Primary tools for evaluating outcomes are nursing observation and patient self-report. (Nursing Care Plan 22.1—which sets forth a plan of care for Christine, the case study patient in

---

BOX 22.11

Relapse Prevention and Emergency Plan

COMMON INDICATORS FOR RELAPSE

Mania
Reading several books or newspapers at once
Cannot concentrate on one topic
Talking faster than usual
Feeling irritable
Hungry all the time
Friends remark on changes in mood
More energy than usual

Depression
Quit cooking, cleaning, daily chores
Avoid people
Crave foods (e.g., chocolate)
Headaches
Do not care about other people
Sleeping more or restless sleep
People are irritating to be around

EMERGENCY PLAN
Keep a list of emergency contacts (primary health care provider, close family members)
Keep a current list of all medications, including their dosages
Information about other health problems
Symptoms that indicate others need to take responsibility for care
Treatment preferences (who, where, medications, advanced directive location)

this chapter—is available at http://thepoint.lww.com/BoydEssentials/2e)

Continuum of Care

Inpatient-Focused Care

Inpatient admission is the treatment setting of choice for patients who are severely psychotic or who are an immediate threat to themselves or others. In acute mania, nursing interventions focus on patient safety because patients are prone to injury because of hyperactivity and are often unaware of injuries they sustain. Distraction may also be effective when a patient is talking or acting inappropriately. Removal to a quieter environment may be necessary if other interventions have not been successful, but the patient should be carefully monitored. During acute mania, patients are often impulsive, disinhibited, and interpersonally inappropriate, so the nurse should avoid direct confrontations or challenges.

During manic phases, patients usually violate others' boundaries. For example, roommate selection for patients requiring hospital admittance needs to be carefully considered. If possible, a private room is ideal because patients with bipolar disorder tend to irritate others, who quickly tire of the intrusiveness. These patients may miss the cues indicating anger and aggression from others. The nurse should protect the patient who is manic from self-harm, as well as harm from other patients.

The length of stay in an inpatient unit will be relatively short, 3 to 5 days. The plan of care will focus on medication management, including control of side effects, initiation or revision of a recovery plan, psychoeducation, and promotion of self-care. Nurses should be familiar with drug–drug interactions and with interventions to help control side effects.

Intensive Outpatient Programs

Intensive outpatient programs for several weeks of acute-phase care during a manic or depressive episode are used when hospitalization is not necessary or to prevent or shorten hospitalization. These programs are usually called partial hospitalization. Close medication monitoring and milieu therapies that foster restoration of a patient's previous adaptive abilities are the major nursing responsibilities in these settings.

Setting up frequent office visits and crisis telephone calls are additional nursing interventions that can help to shorten or prevent hospitalization during the acute phase of a manic episode. Family sessions or psychoeducation that includes the patient are alternatives. Severely and persistently ill patients may need ongoing intensive treatment, but the frequency of visits can be decreased for patients whose conditions stabilize and who enter the continuation or the maintenance phase of treatment.

Spectrum of Care

In today's health care climate, with efforts to reduce hospitalization, most patients with bipolar disorder are treated in a community setting. Hospitalizations are usually brief; recovery is emphasized and medication regimen promote adherence. Psychoeducation helps in understanding and managing the disorder, and supportive psychotherapy helps these individuals move toward recovery. Patients need extended and continued follow-up to monitor medication trials and side effects, reinforce self-care management, and provide continued psychosocial support.

Mental Health Promotion

Mental health promotion activities should be the focus during remissions. During this period, patients have an opportunity to learn new coping skills that promote positive mental health. Stress management and relaxation techniques can be practiced for use when needed. A plan for managing emerging symptoms can also be developed during this period.

OTHER BIPOLAR AND RELATED DISORDERS

In **bipolar II disorder**, the individual is mostly depressed that this disorder can severely affect their social and occupational life. They have brief periods of elevated, expansive, or irritable moods, but bipolar II disorder is not as easily recognized as bipolar I disorder because the symptoms are less dramatic. Hypomania, a mild form of mania, is characteristic of bipolar II disorder. Judgment remains fundamentally intact.

In a cyclothymic disorder, hypomanic symptoms occur alternating with numerous periods of depressive symptoms. However, these symptoms are less severe than the bipolar disorders. To be diagnosed with this disorder, the symptoms have to be present for at least 2 years of numerous periods of hypomanic symptoms.

Illicit drug, prescription medications, and some medical conditions such as changes in thyroid functioning can be responsible for manic-like behavior. These symptoms cause significant distress and impairment in social functioning.

SUMMARY OF KEY POINTS

- Bipolar and related disorders are characterized by one or more manic episodes that cause marked impairment in social activities, occupational functioning, and interpersonal relationships and may require hospitalization to prevent self-harm.

- Bipolar and related disorders are characterized by periods of mania or hypomania that alternate with depression. These disorders are classified as bipolar I disorder, bipolar II disorder, or cyclothymic disorder, depending on the severity of the manic and depressive symptoms. Bipolar disorder may also be related to substance abuse, prescription drug use, or a medical condition.

- Manic episodes are periods in which the individual experiences abnormally and persistently elevated, expansive, or irritable mood characterized by inflated self-esteem, decreased need to sleep, excessive energy or hyperactivity, racing thoughts, easy distractibility, and an inability to stay focused. Other symptoms can include hypersexuality and impulsivity.

- Bipolar disorders are underreported and are often misdiagnosed. Bipolar I disorder is more dramatic than bipolar II disorder, so it is easier to diagnosis.

- Genetics play a role in the etiology of bipolar disorders. Risk factors include a family history of mood disorders; prior mood episodes; lack of social support; stressful life events; substance use; and medical problems, particularly chronic or terminal illnesses.

- Mental health nursing assessment includes assessing mood; speech patterns; thought processes and thought content; suicidal or homicidal thoughts; cognition and memory; and social factors, such as patterns of relationships, quality of support systems, and changes in occupational functioning. Several self-report scales are helpful in evaluating depressive symptoms.

- Many symptoms of bipolar depression, such as weight gain and appetite changes, sleep disturbance, decreased energy, and fatigue, are similar to those of medical illnesses. Assessment includes a thorough medical history and physical examination to detect or rule out medical or psychiatric comorbidity.

- Establishing and maintaining a therapeutic nurse–patient relationship is key to successful outcomes. Shared decision-making with the patient leads to positive outcomes. Recovery-oriented nursing interventions that foster the therapeutic relationship include being available in times of crisis, providing understanding and education to patients and their families regarding goals of treatment and recovery, providing encouragement and feedback concerning the patient's progress, providing guidance in the patient's interpersonal interactions with others and work environment, and helping to set and monitor realistic goals.

- Pharmacotherapy includes mood stabilizers used alone or in combination with antipsychotics or benzodiazepines to treat psychosis, agitation, or insomnia. Electroconvulsive therapy is a valuable alternative for patients with severe mania that does not respond to other treatment.

- Recent major advances in bipolar disorder treatment research validate the efficacy of integrated psychosocial and pharmacologic treatment involving family or couple therapies, psychoeducational programs, and individual cognitive behavioral or interpersonal therapies.

- Psychosocial interventions for bipolar disorders include self-care management, cognitive therapy, behavior therapy, interpersonal therapy, patient and family education regarding the nature of the disorder and treatment goals, marital and family therapy, and group therapy that includes medication maintenance support groups and other consumer-oriented support groups.

CRITICAL THINKING CHALLENGES

1. A patient tells you that he no longer needs medication because he has special powers that protect him from evil forces. He no longer needs sleep and can see things that others do not see. What approaches would you use to help the patient decide to take his medication?

2. Describe how you would approach a patient who is expressing concern that the diagnosis of bipolar disorder will negatively affect her social and work relationships.

3. Your patient with mania is experiencing physical hyperactivity that is interfering with his sleep and nutrition. Describe the actions you would take to meet the patient's needs for rest and nutrition.

4. Prepare a hypothetical discussion with a patient with potential bipolar disorder concerning the advantages

and disadvantages of lithium versus divalproex sodium for treatment of bipolar disorder.

5. Think about all of the above situations and relate them to persons from culturally and ethnically diverse populations (e.g., African American, Latino, or Asian descent; Jewish or Jehovah's Witness religions; across the life-span of individuals from children to older adult populations).

2007: *Michael Clayton*

Arthur Edens (Tom Wilkinson), a successful corporate lawyer, is experiencing the stress of a high-profile legal case and stops taking his medication. Consequently, he has a manic episode with delusions about one of the jurors, who he eventually contacts. The story traces the attempts by his colleague and friend Michael Clayton (George Clooney) to repair the damage Arthur's behavior has caused to the lawsuit and to get his friend treated before his mania further damages his life.

Significance: Viewers can gain insight into the devastating impact of mental illness on the successful career of a well-respected attorney. This film depicts the poor judgment, impulsivity, and consequences of a full-blown mania episode.

Viewing Points: Identify the mania symptoms that Arthur displays. What feelings are evoked when you see the strange behavior that he exhibits? If Arthur were your patient, how would you approach him, and what medication would you expect him to be prescribed?

A related Psychiatric–Mental Health Nursing video on the topic of Bipolar Disorders is available at http://thepoint.lww.com/BoydEssentials2e.

A Practice and Learn Interactive Case Study related to the video on the topic of Bipolar Disorders is available at http://thepoint.lww.com/BoydEssentials2e.

REFERENCES

Akinhanmi, M. O., Biernacka, J. M., Strakowski, S. M., McElroy, S. L., Balls Berry, J. E., Merikangas, K. R., et al. (2018). Racial disparities in bipolar disorder treatment and research: a call to action. *Bipolar Disorders, 20*(6), 506–514.

Allardyce, J., Leonenko, G., Hamshere, M., Pardiñas, A. F., Forty, L., Knott, S., et al. (2018). Association between schizophrenia-related polygenic liability and the occurrence and level of mood-incongruent psychotic symptoms in bipolar disorder. *JAMA Psychiatry, 75*(1), 28–35.

Almeida, O. P., Hankey, G. J., Yeap, B. B., Golledge, J., & Flicker, L. (2018). Older men with bipolar disorder diagnosed in early and later life: Physical health morbidity and general hospital service use. *Journal of Affective Disorders, 241*, 269–274.

American Psychiatric Association. (2013). *Diagnostic and statistical manual of mental disorders* (5th ed.). Arlington, VA: Author.

Angst, J., Rössler, W., Ajdacic-Gross, V., Angst, F., Wittchen, H. U., & Lieb, R., et al. (2018). Differences between unipolar mania and bipolar-I disorder: Evidence from nine epidemiological studies. *Bipolar Disorders*. doi: 10.1111/bdi.12732.

Arfaie, A., Safikhanlou, S., Roodsari, A. B., Farnam, A., & Shafiee-Kandjani, A. R. (2018). Assessment of behavioral approach and behavioral inhibition systems in mood disorders. *Basic and Clinical Neuroscience, 9*(4), 261–268.

Baldessarini, R. J., Tondo, L., Vázquez, G. H., Undurraga, J., Bolzani, L., Yildiz, A., et al. (2012). Age at onset versus family history and clinical outcomes in 1,665 international bipolar-I disorder patients. *World Psychiatry, 11*(1), 40–46.

Byers, A. L., Lai, A. X., Arean, P., Nelson, J. C., & Yaffe, K. (2016). Mental health service use across the life course among adults with psychiatric disorders and prior suicidal behavior. *Psychiatric Services, 67*(4), 452–455.

Cerimele, J. M., Fortney, J. C., Pyne, J. M., & Curran, G. M. (2019). Bipolar disorder in primary care: a qualitative study of clinician and patient experiences with diagnosis and treatment. *Family Practice, 36*(1):32–37.

Craddock, N., & Sklar, P. (2013). Genetics of bipolar disorder. *Lancet, 381*(9878), 1654–1662.

Crowe, M., Beaglehole, B., & Inder, M. (2016). Social rhythm interventions for bipolar disorder: A systematic review and rationale for practice. *Journal of Psychiatric and Mental Health Nursing, 23*(1), 3–11.

Crowe, M., & Inder, M. (2018). Staying well with bipolar disorder: A qualitative analysis of five-year follow-up interviews with young people. *Journal of Psychiatric and Mental Health Nursing, 25*(4), 236–244.

Dell'Osso, B., Camuri, G., Cremaschi, L., Dobrea, C., Buoli, M., Ketter, T. A., et al. (2017). Lifetime presence of psychotic symptoms in bipolar disorder is associated with less favorable socio-demographic and certain clinical features. *Comprehensive Psychiatry, 76*, 169–176.

Depakote Prescribing Information. (2019). [Online]. Accessed March, 2019. Available at: https://www.accessdata.fda.gov/drugsatfda_docs/label/2019/018723s061lbl.pdf

Fellinger, M., Waldhoer, T., König, D., Hinterbuchinger, B., Pruckner, N., Baumgartner, J., et al. (2019). Seasonality in bipolar disorder: Effect of sex and age. *Journal of Affective Disorders, 243*, 322–326.

Fornaro, M., Solmi, M., Veronese, N., De Berardis, D., Buonaguro, E. F., Tomasetti, C., et al. (2015). The burden of mood-disorder/cerebrovascular disease comorbidity: essential neurobiology, psychopharmacology, and physical activity interventions. *Journal of Affective Disorders, 29*(5):425–435.

Goldstein, B. I., Birmaher, B., Carlson, G. A., DelBello, M. P., Findling, R. L., Fristad, M., et al. (2017). The International Society for Bipolar Disorders Task Force report on pediatric bipolar disorder: Knowledge to date and directions for future research. *Bipolar Disorders, 19*(7):524–543.

Kessler, R. C., Petukhova, M., Sampson, N. A., Zaslavsky, A. M., & Wittchen, H. U. (2012). Twelve-month and lifetime prevalence and lifetime morbid risk of anxiety and mood disorders in the United States. *International Journal of Methods in Psychiatric Research, 21*(3), 169–184.

Li, X. H., An, F. R., Ungvari, G. S., Ng, C. H., Chiu, H. F., Wu, P. P., et al. (2017). Prevalence of smoking in patients with bipolar disorder, major depressive disorder and schizophrenia and their relationships with quality of life. *Scientific Reports, 7*(1):8430.

Marangoni, C., Faedda, G. L., Baldessarini, R. J. (2018). Clinical and environmental risk factors for bipolar disorder: Review of prospective studies. *Harvard Review of Psychiatry, 26*(1), 1–7.

Marangoni, C., Hernandez, M., Faedda, G. L. (2016). The role of environmental exposures as risk factors for bipolar disorder: A systematic review of longitudinal studies. *Journal of Affective Disorders, 193*, 165–74.

Melo, M. C., Garcia, R. F., Linhares Neto, V. B., Sá, M. B., de Mesquita, L. M., de Araújo, C. F., et al. (2016). Sleep and circadian alterations in people at risk for bipolar disorder: A systematic review. *Journal of Psychiatric Research, 83*, 211–219.

Muneer, A., & Mazommil, R. (2018). The staging of major mood disorders: clinical and neurobiological correlates. *Psychiatry Investigation, 15*(8), 747–758.

Oliveira, J., Marinho, V., Carvalho, V., Magalhães, F., Rocha, K., Ayres, C., et al. (2018). Genetic polymorphisms associated with circadian rhythm dysregulation provide new perspectives on bipolar disorder. *Bipolar Disorders, 20*(6):515–522.

Razzano, L. A., Cook, J. A., Yost, C., Jonikas, J. A., Swarbrick, M. A., Carter, T. M., et al. (2015). Factors associated with co occurring medical conditions among adults with serious mental disorders. *Schizophrenia Research, 161*(2–3), 458–464.

Sampogna, G., Luciano, M., Del Vecchio, V., Malangone, C., De Rosa, C., Giallonardo, V., et al. (2018). The effects of psychoeducational family intervention on coping strategies of relatives of patients with bipolar I disorder: results from a controlled, real-world, multicentric study. *Neuropsychiatric Disease and Treatment, 14*, 977–989.

Schaffer, A., Isometsä, E. T., Tondo, L., Moreno, D. H., Sinyor, M., Kessing, L. V., et al. (2015). Epidemiology, neurobiology and pharmacological interventions related to suicide deaths and suicide attempts in bipolar disorder: Part I of a report of the International Society for Bipolar Disorders Tasks Force on Suicide in Bipolar Disorder. *Australian & New Zealand Journal of Psychiatry, 49*(9), 785–802.

Schatzberg, A. F., & DeBattista, C. (2015). *Manual of clinical psychopharmacology* (8th ed.). Arlington, VA: American Psychiatric Publishing. [Online]. Accessed June 2016. Available at: http://psychiatryonline.org/doi/full/10.1176/appi.books.9781615370047.AS03.

Spoorthy, M. S., Chakrabarti, S., & Grover, S. (2019). Comorbidity of bipolar and anxiety disorders: An overview of trends in research. *World Journal of Psychiatry, 9*(1):7–29.

Stahl, S. M. (2017). *Stahl's essential psychopharmacology Prescriber's guide* (6th ed). New York: Cambridge University Press.

Weiss, R. B., Stange, J. P., Boland, E. M., Black, S. K., LaBelle, D. R., Abramson, L. Y., et al. (2015). Kindling of life stress in bipolar disorder: Comparison of sensitization and autonomy models. *Journal of Abnormal Psychology, 124*(1), 4–16.

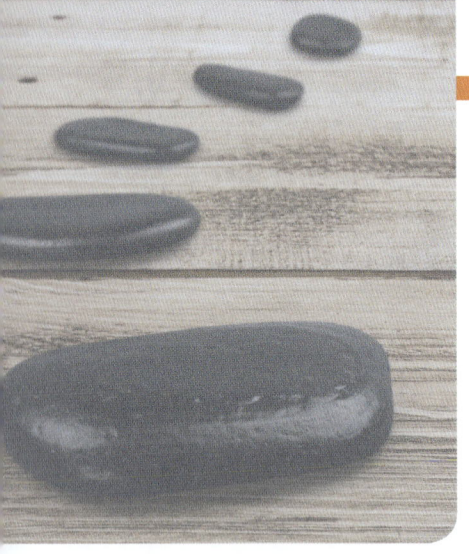

23

Schizophrenia and Related Disorders

Nursing Care of Persons With Thought Disorders

Andrea C. Bostrom

KEY CONCEPTS

- disorganized symptoms
- delusions
- hallucinations
- negative symptoms
- neurocognitive symptoms
- positive symptoms
- psychosis

LEARNING OBJECTIVES

After studying this chapter, you will be able to:

1. Identify key symptoms of schizophrenia.
2. Describe theories relevant to schizophrenia.
3. Develop strategies to establish a patient-centered, recovery-oriented therapeutic relationship with a person with schizophrenia.
4. Develop recovery-oriented nursing interventions for persons with schizophrenia.
5. Discuss medications used to treat people with schizophrenia and then evaluate their effectiveness.
6. Identify and evaluate expected outcomes of nursing care for persons with schizophrenia.
7. Discuss other common schizophrenia spectrum disorders.

KEY TERMS

- affective lability • aggression • agitation • agranulocytosis • akathisia • alogia • ambivalence • anhedonia • apathy
- autistic thinking • avolition • catatonia • catatonic excitement • cholinergic rebound • circumstantiality • clang association
- command hallucinations • concrete thinking • confused speech and thinking • delusions • diminished emotional expression
- echolalia • echopraxia • extrapyramidal side effects • flight of ideas • gut–brain axis • hallucinations • hypervigilance
- hypofrontality • illusions • loose associations • metonymic speech • neologisms • neuroleptic malignant syndrome
- oculogyric crisis • paranoia • pressured speech • prodromal • psychosis • referential thinking • regressed behavior
- retrocollis • stereotypy • stilted language • tangentiality • tardive dyskinesia • torticollis • verbigeration • waxy flexibility • word salad

Case Study: Arnold

Arnold, a 53-year-old man who was diagnosed with paranoid schizophrenia at an early age, had been living on the family farm for the last 30 years with his mother. After his mother's death, the farm was to be sold and divided among the siblings, who arranged for Arnold to move to town. Arnold became agitated and threatening and refused to believe that his parents had died and that he would have to leave the farm.

These fascinating schizophrenia spectrum disorders have confounded scientists and philosophers for centuries. Schizophrenia spectrum disorders are among the most severe mental illnesses; they are found in all cultures, races, and socioeconomic groups. Their symptoms have been attributed to possession by demons, considered punishment by gods for evils done, or accepted as evidence of the inhumanity of its sufferers. These explanations have resulted in enduring stigma for people diagnosed with these disorders. Today, the stigma persists, although it has less to do with demonic possession than with society's unwillingness to shoulder the costs associated with housing, treatment, and rehabilitation. All nurses need to understand these disorders.

SCHIZOPHRENIA SPECTRUM DISORDER

The schizophrenia spectrum disorders include schizophrenia, schizoaffective, delusional, and schizotypal disorders, brief psychotic disorder, schizophreniform disorder, and substance/medication-induced psychotic disorder (American Psychiatric Association [APA], 2013). Schizophrenia is the highlighted disorder in this chapter because it has a broad range of symptoms that are found in the other schizophrenia spectrum disorders. A discussion of the other disorders follows the content on schizophrenia. Schizotypal disorders will be discussed in the Personality Disorders chapter (see Chapter 24).

Central to understanding the problems of persons with schizophrenia spectrum disorders is the concept of **psychosis**, a term used to describe a state in which an individual experiences positive symptoms of schizophrenia, also known as psychotic symptoms (e.g., hallucinations; delusions; disorganized thoughts, speech, or behavior).

> **KEYCONCEPT** Psychosis, a state in which a person experiences hallucinations; delusions; or disorganized thoughts, speech, or behavior, is the key diagnostic factor in schizophrenia spectrum disorders.

SCHIZOPHRENIA

In the late 1800s, Emil Kraepelin first described the course of the disorder he called *dementia praecox* because of its early onset and notable changes in an individual's cognitive functioning. In the early 1900s, Eugen Bleuler renamed the disorder *schizophrenia*, meaning *split minds*, and began to determine that there was not just one type of schizophrenia but rather a group of schizophrenias. More recently, Kurt Schneider differentiated behaviors associated with schizophrenia as "first rank" symptoms (e.g., psychotic delusions, hallucinations) and "second rank" symptoms (i.e., all other experiences and behaviors associated with the disorder). These pioneering physicians had a great influence on the current diagnostic conceptualizations of schizophrenia that emphasize the heterogeneity of the disorder in terms of symptoms, course of illness, and positive and negative symptoms.

Clinical Course

Schizophrenia robs people of mental health and imposes social stigma. People with schizophrenia struggle to maintain control of their symptoms, which affect every aspect of their lives. The person with schizophrenia displays various interrelated symptoms and experiences and cognitive deficits in several areas.

Because schizophrenia is a disorder of thoughts, perceptions, and behavior, it is sometimes not recognized as an illness by the person experiencing the symptoms. Many people with thought disorders do not believe that they have a mental illness. Their denial of mental illness and the need for treatment poses problems for the family and clinicians. Ideally, in lucid moments, patients recognize that their thoughts are really delusions, that their perceptions are hallucinations, and that their behavior is disorganized. In reality, many patients do not believe that they have a mental illness but agree to treatment to please family and clinicians.

The natural progression of schizophrenia is usually described as a chronic illness that deteriorates over time and with an eventual plateau in the symptoms. Only for older adults with schizophrenia has it been suggested that improvement might occur. In reality, no one really knows what the course of schizophrenia would be if patients were able to adhere to a treatment regimen throughout their lives. Only recently have medications become relatively effective, with manageable side effects. The clinical picture of schizophrenia is complex; individuals differ from one another, and the experience for a single individual may vary from episode to episode.

Prodromal Period

A **prodromal period** (stage of early changes that are a precursor to the disorder) may begin in early childhood. More than half of patients report the following prodromal symptoms: tension and nervousness, lack of interest in eating, difficulty concentrating, disturbed sleep, decreased enjoyment and loss of interest, restlessness, forgetfulness, depression, social withdrawal from friends, feeling laughed at, more thinking about religion, feeling bad for no reason, feeling too excited, and hearing voices or seeing things (Liu, Wang, Jin, Lyu, et al, 2019; Racioppi et al., 2018). The benefit of discovering the presence of symptoms early, before they have solidified into a major disorder, is that treatment might be initiated earlier.

Acute Illness

Initially, the behaviors of this illness may be both confusing and frightening to the individual and the family. The symptoms of acute illness usually occur in late adolescence or early adulthood. The behaviors may be subtle; however, at some point they become so disruptive or bizarre that they can no longer be overlooked. These might include episodes of staying up all night for several nights, incoherent conversations, or aggressive acts against oneself or others. For example, one patient's parents reported their son walking around the apartment for several days holding his arms and hands as if they were a machine gun, pointing them at his parents and siblings, and saying "rat-a-tat-tat, you're dead." Another father described his son's first delusional–hallucinatory episode as so convincing that it was frightening. His son began visiting cemeteries and making "mind contact" with the deceased. He saw his deceased grandmother walking around in the home and was certain that pipe bombs were hidden in objects in his home.

As symptoms worsen, patients are less and less able to care for their basic needs (e.g., eating, sleeping, bathing). Substance use is common. Functioning at school or work deteriorates. Dependence on family and friends increases, so those individuals recognize the patients' need for treatment. In the acute phase, individuals afflicted by schizophrenia are at high risk for suicide. Patients may be hospitalized to protect themselves or others.

Initial treatment focuses on alleviation of symptoms through beginning therapy with medications, decreasing the risk of suicide through safety measures, normalizing sleep, and reducing substance use. Functional deficits persist during this period, so the patient and family must begin to learn to cope with these deficits. Emotional blunting diminishes the ability and desire to engage in hobbies, vocational activities, and relationships. Limited participation in social activities spirals into numerous skill deficits, such as difficulty engaging others interpersonally. Cognitive deficits lead to problems recognizing patterns in situations and transferring learning and behaviors from one circumstance to a similar one.

Stabilization

After the initial diagnosis of schizophrenia and initiation of treatment, stabilization of symptoms becomes the focus. Symptoms become less acute but may still be present. Treatment is intense during this period as medication regimens are established and patients and their families begin to adjust to the idea of a family member having a long-term severe mental illness. Ideally, the use of substances is eliminated. Socialization with others begins to increase, so that rehabilitation begins.

Recovery

The ultimate goal is recovery. Medication generally diminishes the symptoms and allows the person to work toward recovery. However, no medication will cure schizophrenia. As with any chronic illness, following a therapeutic regime, maintaining a healthy lifestyle, managing the stresses of life, and developing meaningful interpersonal relationships are important parts of the recovery. Family support and involvement are extremely important at this time. After the initial diagnosis has been made, patients and families must be educated to anticipate and expect relapse and know how to cope with it.

Relapses

Relapses can occur at any time during treatment and recovery. They are very detrimental to the successful management of this disorder. Relapse is not inevitable; however, it occurs with sufficient regularity to be a major concern in the treatment of schizophrenia. With each relapse, a longer period of time is needed to recover. Combining medications and psychosocial treatment greatly diminishes the severity and frequency of recurrent relapses (Lauriello, Perkins, 2019).

One major reason for relapse is failure to take medication consistently. Even with newer medications, adherence continues to be a challenge (Chang, Roh, & Kim, 2019). Discontinuing medications will almost certainly lead to a relapse (Dufort & Zipursky, 2019). Lower relapse rates are found, for the most part, among groups who carefully follow a treatment regimen.

Many other factors trigger relapse. Impairment in cognition and coping leaves patients vulnerable to stressors. Limited accessibility of community resources, such as public transportation, housing, entry-level and low-stress employment, and limited social services leaves individuals without access to social support. Income supports that can buffer the day-to-day stressors of living may be inadequate. The degree of stigmatization that the community holds for mental illness attacks the self-concept of patients. Social isolation and the level of responsiveness from family members, friends, and supportive others (e.g., peers and professionals) when patients need assistance also has an impact.

Consider Arnold
Recall that Arnold's relapse was triggered by his mother's death and being forced to leave the family farm.

Diagnostic Criteria

Schizophrenia is characterized by positive and negative symptoms that are present for a significant portion of a

> **KEY DIAGNOSTIC CHARACTERISTICS 23.1 • SCHIZOPHRENIA**
>
> **Diagnostic Criteria**
>
> A. Two (or more) of the following, each present for a significant portion of time during a 1-month period (or less if successfully treated). At least one of these must be (1), (2), or (3):
>   1. Delusions.
>   2. Hallucinations.
>   3. Disorganized speech (e.g., frequent derailment or incoherence).
>   4. Grossly disorganized or catatonic behavior.
>   5. Negative symptoms (i.e., diminished emotional expression or avolition).
>
> B. For a significant portion of the time since the onset of the disturbance, level of functioning in one or more major areas, such as work, interpersonal relations, or self-care, is markedly below the level achieved prior to the onset (or when the onset is in childhood or adolescence, there is failure to achieve expected level of interpersonal, academic, or occupational functioning).
>
> C. Continuous signs of the disturbance persist for at least 6 months. This 6-month period must include at least 1 month of symptoms (or less if successfully treated) that meet Criterion A (i.e., active-phase symptoms) and may include periods of prodromal or residual symptoms. During these prodromal or residual periods, the signs of the disturbance may be manifested by only negative symptoms or by two or more symptoms listed in Criterion A present in an attenuated form (e.g., odd beliefs, unusual perceptual experiences).
>
> D. Schizoaffective disorder and depressive or bipolar disorder with psychotic features have been ruled out because either (1) no major depressive or manic episodes have occurred concurrently with the active-phase symptoms, or (2) if mood episodes have occurred during active-phase symptoms, they have been present for a minority of the total duration of the active and residual periods of the illness.
>
> E. The disturbance is not attributable to the physiological effects of a substance (e.g., a drug of abuse, a medication) or another medical condition.
>
> F. If there is a history of autism spectrum disorder or a communication disorder of childhood onset, the additional diagnosis of schizophrenia is made only if prominent delusions or hallucinations, in addition to the other required symptoms of schizophrenia, are also present for at least 1 month (or less if successfully treated).
>
> **Target Symptoms and Associated Findings**
> - Inappropriate affect
> - Loss of interest or pleasure
> - Dysphoric mood (anger, anxiety, or depression)
> - Disturbed sleep patterns
> - Lack of interest in eating or refusal of food
> - Difficulty concentrating
> - Some cognitive dysfunction, such as confusion, disorientation, or memory impairment
> - Lack of insight
> - Depersonalization, derealization, and somatic concerns
> - Motor abnormalities
>
> **Associated Physical Examination Findings**
> - Physically awkward
> - Poor coordination or mirroring
> - Motor abnormalities
> - Cigarette-related pathologies, such as emphysema and other pulmonary and cardiac problems
>
> **Associated Laboratory Findings**
> - Enlarged ventricular system and prominent sulci in the brain cortex
> - Decreased temporal and hippocampal size
> - Increased size of basal ganglia
> - Decreased cerebral size
> - Slowed reaction times
> - Abnormalities in eye tracking
>
> Reprinted with permission from the *Diagnostic and Statistical Manual of Mental Disorders* (5th ed.) (Copyright ©2013). American Psychiatric Association. All Rights Reserved.

1-month period but with continuous signs of disturbance persisting for at least 6 months (APA, 2013). We define **positive symptoms** as hallucinations and delusions and **negative symptoms** as **diminished emotional expression** and **avolition** (lack of interest or motivation in goal-directed behavior, such as getting dressed, going to work or to school). See Key Diagnostic Characteristics 23.1.

Positive Symptoms of Schizophrenia

Positive symptoms can be thought of as excessive or distorted thoughts and perceptions that occur within the individual but are not experienced by others. Hallucinations and delusions are positive symptoms of schizophrenia. An easy way to remember the difference between hallucinations and delusions is that hallucinations involve one or more of the five senses. Delusions involve only thoughts.

A fairly common hallucination is a command hallucination, that is, an auditory hallucination instructing the patient to act in a certain way, because, voices are telling the person to do something. **Command hallucinations** range from innocuous (eat all of your dinner) to very serious (hurt someone or jump in front of a bus).

> **KEYCONCEPT Positive symptoms** reflect an excess or distortion of normal functions, including delusions and hallucinations (APA), 2013).

> **KEYCONCEPT Hallucinations** are perceptual experiences that occur without actual external sensory stimuli. They can involve any of the five senses, but they are usually *visual* or *auditory*. Auditory hallucinations are more common than visual ones. For example, the patient may hear voices carrying on a discussion about his or her own thoughts or behaviors.

> **KEYCONCEPT** Delusions are erroneous, fixed, false beliefs that cannot be changed by reasonable argument. They usually involve a misinterpretation of experience. For example, the patient believes someone is reading his or her thoughts or plotting against him or her. Various types of delusions include the following:
> - *Grandiose:* the belief that one has exceptional powers, wealth, skill, influence, or destiny
> - *Nihilistic:* the belief that one is dead or a calamity is impending
> - *Persecutory:* the belief that one is being watched, ridiculed, harmed, or plotted against
> - *Somatic:* beliefs about abnormalities in bodily functions or structures

Negative Symptoms of Schizophrenia

The term "negative symptoms" is used to describe emotions and behaviors that should be present but are diminished in persons with schizophrenia. Negative symptoms are not as dramatic as positive symptoms, but they can interfere greatly with the patient's ability to function day to day. Because expressing emotion is difficult for them, people with schizophrenia laugh, cry, and get angry less often. Their affect is flat; they show little or no emotion when personal loss occurs. They also experience ambivalence, which is the concurrent experience of equally strong opposing feelings so that it is impossible to make a decision. Avolition may be so profound that simple activities of daily living (ADLs), such as dressing or combing hair, may not get done. **Anhedonia** prevents the person with schizophrenia from enjoying activities. People with schizophrenia may have limited speech and difficulty saying anything new or carrying on a conversation. These negative symptoms cause the person with schizophrenia to withdraw and experience feelings of severe isolation.

> **KEYCONCEPT** **Negative symptoms** reflect a lessening or loss of normal functions, such as restriction or flattening in the range and intensity of emotion (diminished emotional expression), reduced fluency and productivity of thought and speech (**alogia**), withdrawal and inability to initiate and persist in goal-directed activity (avolition), and inability to experience pleasure (anhedonia).

Neurocognitive Impairment

Neurocognitive impairment exists in people with schizophrenia and may be independent of positive and negative symptoms. Neurocognition includes memory (short and long term); vigilance or sustained attention; verbal fluency or the ability to generate new words; and executive functioning, which includes volition, planning, purposeful action, and self-monitoring behavior. Working memory is a concept that includes short-term memory and the ability to store and process information.

> **KEYCONCEPT** **Neurocognitive impairment** in memory, vigilance, and executive functioning is related to poor functional outcomes in schizophrenia.

This impairment is independent of the positive symptoms. That is, cognitive dysfunction can exist even if the positive symptoms are in remission. Not all areas of cognitive functioning are impaired. Long-term memory and intellectual functioning are not necessarily affected. However, low intellectual functioning is common and may be related to a lack of educational experiences and opportunities due to the age of illness onset. Neurocognitive dysfunction is often manifested in disorganized symptoms (Vignapiano et al., 2019).

> **KEYCONCEPT** **Disorganized symptoms** of schizophrenia are findings that make it difficult for the person to understand and respond to the ordinary sights and sounds of daily living. These include **confused speech and thinking,** and disorganized behavior.

Disorganized Thinking

The following are examples of confused speech and thinking patterns:

- **Echolalia**—repetition of another's words that is parrot-like and inappropriate
- **Circumstantiality**—extremely detailed and lengthy discourse about a topic
- **Loose associations**—absence of the normal connectedness of thoughts, ideas, and topics; sudden shifts without apparent relationship to preceding topics
- **Tangentiality**—the topic of conversation is changed to an entirely different topic that is a logical progression but causes a permanent detour from the original focus
- **Flight of ideas**—the topic of conversation changes repeatedly and rapidly, generally after just one sentence or phrase
- **Word salad**—stringing together words that are not connected in any way
- **Neologisms**—words that are made up that have no common meaning and are not recognizable
- **Paranoia**—suspiciousness and guardedness that are unrealistic and often accompanied by grandiosity
- **Referential thinking**—a belief that neutral stimuli have special meaning to the individual, such as a television commentator who is speaking directly to the individual
- **Autistic thinking**—restricts thinking to the literal and immediate so that the individual has private rules of logic and reasoning that make no sense to anyone else
- **Concrete thinking**—lack of abstraction in thinking; inability to understand punch lines, metaphors, and analogies
- **Verbigeration**—purposeless repetition of words or phrases

- **Metonymic speech**—use of words with similar meanings interchangeably
- **Clang association**—repetition of words or phrases that are similar in sound but in no other way, for example, "right, light, sight, might"
- **Stilted language**—overly and inappropriately artificial formal language
- **Pressured speech**—speaking as if the words are being forced out

Disorganized perceptions often create oversensitivity to colors, shapes, and background activities. **Illusions** occur when the person misperceives or exaggerates stimuli that actually exist in the external environment. This is in contrast to hallucinations, which are perceptions in the absence of environmental stimuli. Ancillary symptoms that may accompany schizophrenia include anxiety, depression, and hostility.

Disorganized Behavior

Disorganized behavior (which may manifest as very slow, rhythmic, or ritualistic movement) coupled with disorganized speech make it difficult for the person to partake in daily activities. Examples of disorganized behavior include the following:

- **Aggression**—behaviors or attitudes that reflect rage, hostility, and the potential for physical or verbal destructiveness (usually comes about if the person believes someone is going to do him or her harm)
- **Agitation**—inability to sit still or attend to others, accompanied by heightened emotions and tension
- **Catatonia**—psychomotor disturbances such as stupor, mutism, posturing, or repetitive behavior
- **Catatonic excitement**—a hyperactivity characterized by purposeless activity and abnormal movements, such as grimacing and posturing
- **Echopraxia**—involuntary imitation of another person's movements and gestures
- **Regressed behavior**—behaving in a manner of a less mature life stage; childlike and immature behavior
- **Stereotypy**—repetitive purposeless movements that are idiosyncratic to the individual and to some degree outside of the individual's control
- **Hypervigilance**—sustained attention to external stimuli as if expecting something important or frightening to happen
- **Waxy flexibility**—posture held in an odd or unusual fixed position for extended periods of time

Disruption in Sense of Self

Many of the symptoms observed in schizophrenia may be attributable to brain deficiencies that affect the individual's experience of "self." The self is difficult to define but is often used to describe who we are: self-concept, self-consciousness, self-awareness, and, for people with schizophrenia, self-disturbance. This self-disturbance leads to significant difficulty determining what thoughts and experiences are internal versus external to the individual. Delusions and hallucinations can be explained by this, as can the person's failures of insight, self-awareness, and self-monitoring (Klaunig et al., 2019). Self-disturbance also suggests ways that adolescents and young adults may be identified during the prodromal period of the illness by their difficulties in integrating self-experiences. Treatment that focuses on self-disturbance aims to help clients to become active agents in their own care. This can be done by helping them to develop concepts of themselves in the world and creating narratives of how their experiences have developed and can be managed in the future in their own unique way (Lysaker & Roe, 2016). Treatment that helps to develop a sense of "self" is possible and integral to recovery (Davidson, 2019).

Schizophrenia Across the Life Span

Children

The diagnosis of schizophrenia is rare in children before adolescence. When it does occur in children aged 5 or 6 years, the symptoms are essentially the same as in adults. In this age group, hallucinations tend to be visual and delusions less developed. Because disorganized speech and behavior may be explained better by other disorders that are more common in childhood, those disorders should be considered before applying the diagnosis of schizophrenia to a child.

However, new studies suggest that the likelihood of children later experiencing schizophrenia can be predicted. Developmental abnormalities in childhood, including delays in attainment of speech and motor development, problems in social adjustment, and poorer academic and cognitive performance have been found to be present in individuals who experience schizophrenia in adulthood. Adults who had childhood cognitive, social, behavioral, and emotional impairments may be at higher risk of developing schizophrenia (Riglin, 2017).

Older Adults

People with schizophrenia usually get older and some people develop schizophrenia in late life. For older patients who have had schizophrenia since young adulthood, this may be a time in which they experience some improvement in symptoms or decrease in relapse fluctuations. There is some evidence that suggests that older adults with schizophrenia may be more likely to develop cognitive impairment than those without mental disorders (Shahab et al., 2019). However, their lifestyle is probably dependent on the effectiveness of earlier treatment, the support systems that are in place (including relationships with family members and professionals), and the interaction between environmental stressors and the patient's functional impairments. The cost of caring for older patients with schizophrenia remains high because many are no longer cared for in institutions and because community-based treatment has developed more slowly for this age group than for younger adults.

Epidemiology

Schizophrenia is found in all cultures and countries. It is prevalent in about 0.48% of the worldwide population (range from 0.34% to 0.85%) and is listed within the top 20 illnesses for life lost resulting from premature death and years lived in less than full health (Wu et al., 2018). Its economic costs are enormous. Direct costs include treatment expenses; indirect costs include lost wages, premature death, and involuntary commitment. In addition, employment among people with schizophrenia is one of the lowest of any group with disabilities. The costs of schizophrenia in terms of individual and family suffering are probably inestimable.

People with schizophrenia tend to cluster in the lowest social classes in industrialized countries and urban communities. The symptoms of the illness are so pervasive that it is difficult for these individuals to maintain any type of gainful employment. Homelessness is a problem for people with severe mental illness (e.g., schizophrenia or bipolar illness). People with schizophrenia are more likely to remain homeless with few opportunities for employment (Glick & Olfson, 2018).

Risk Factors

Genetic factors related to cognitive and brain function and brain structure are known risks for schizophrenia. Early neurologic problems, stressful life events, and nonhereditary genetic factors also contribute to the likelihood of developing the disorder. Environmental factors related to schizophrenia include migrant status, having an older father, *Toxoplasma gondii* antibodies, prenatal famine, lifetime cannabis use, obstetric complications, urban rearing, and winter or spring birth (Brown, 2011; Fan et al., 2018).

Age of Onset

Schizophrenia is usually diagnosed in late adolescence and early adulthood. Men tend to be diagnosed between the ages of 18 and 25 years and women between the ages of 25 and 35 years. The earlier the diagnosis and the longer the psychosis remains untreated, the more severe the disorder becomes (Shahab et al., 2019). Conversely, the earlier the psychosis is recognized and treated within an evidence-based comprehensive program, the better the outcomes (Dixon, Goldman, Srihari, & Kane, 2018).

Gender Differences

Men tend to be diagnosed earlier and have a poorer prognosis than women. This may be a sex-linked outcome, but it may also reflect the poorer prognosis for any individual who develops the disorder at an early age (Lewine, Martin, Hart, 2017).

Ethnic and Cultural Differences

Increasingly, efforts are being made to consider culture and ethnic origin when diagnosing and treating individuals with schizophrenia. Racial groups may have varying diagnostic rates of schizophrenia. However, it is not clear whether these findings represent correct diagnosis or misdiagnosis of the disorder based on the cultural bias of the clinician. For instance, schizophrenia has been consistently overdiagnosed among African Americans. African American and Hispanic individuals with bipolar disorder are more likely to have misdiagnoses of schizophrenia than are white individuals. Serious mental disorders may remain unrecognized in Asian Americans because of stereotypical beliefs that they are "problem free" (Maura & Weisman de Mamani, 2017).

Familial Differences

First-degree biologic relatives (e.g., children, siblings, parents) of an individual with schizophrenia have a 10 times estimated greater risk for schizophrenia than the general population. Other relatives may have an increased risk for related disorders such as schizoaffective disorder (SAD) and schizotypal personality disorder (Hilker et al., 2018).

Comorbidity

Several somatic and psychological disorders coexist with schizophrenia. This results in significant morbidity and mortality for people with schizophrenia, with individuals who have this diagnosis dying up to 20 years earlier than the general population. Physical health conditions and illnesses to which people with schizophrenia are particularly susceptible include tuberculosis, human immunodeficiency disease, hepatitis B and C, osteoporosis, poor dentition, impaired lung function, altered (reduced) pain sensitivity, sexual dysfunction, obstetric complications, cardiovascular problems, hyperpigmentation, obesity, diabetes mellitus (DM), metabolic syndrome with hyperlipidemia, polydipsia, thyroid dysfunction, and hyperprolactinemia (Kessler & Lev-Ran, 2019; Postolache, 2019).

Early mortality may be from natural causes (cardiovascular, cancer, chronic obstructive pulmonary disease, DM, and influenza and pneumonia) or unnatural causes (suicide, substance and alcohol abuse, and legal interventions) (Wu et al., 2018). Several health system factors contribute to this, including barriers to obtaining primary care, the insufficient preparation of mental health practitioners in managing physical illness, the tendency for mental health providers to fail to ask about physical health, and the absence of standards of care that include screening and monitoring medical issues.

Substance Use and Depression

Among the behavioral comorbidities, substance use is common. Depression may also be observed in patients with schizophrenia. This is an important symptom for several reasons. First, depression may be evidence that the diagnosis of a mood disorder is more appropriate. Second, depression is not unusual in chronic stages of schizophrenia and deserves attention. Third, 50% of people with schizophrenia attempt suicide, and 10% to 15% die by suicide. Risk factors for suicide are untreated psychosis, history of suicide attempt, age younger than 28 years, severity of depression, and substance abuse (Kim et al., 2019; Naguy & Al-Rabaie, 2017).

Diabetes Mellitus and Obesity

Interest has been renewed in the relationship between DM and schizophrenia. Years ago, an association was established between glucose regulation and psychiatric disorders, suggesting that people with schizophrenia may be more prone to type II DM than the general public (Franzen, 1970; Schimmelbusch, Mueller, & Sheps, 1971). Evidence that supports this view includes a higher rate of type II diabetes in first-degree relatives of people with schizophrenia and higher rates of impaired glucose tolerance and insulin resistance among people with schizophrenia. However, obesity, which is associated with type II diabetes, is a growing problem in the United States in general and is complicated in schizophrenia treatment by the tendency of individuals to gain weight after their disease is managed with medications. Weight gain in some individuals may be attributed to a return to a healthier living situation in which regular meals are available and symptoms that interfere with obtaining food regularly (e.g., delusions) are decreased. For others, weight gain may be a medication side effect (Kowalchuk et al., 2019).

Etiology

Schizophrenia is believed to be caused by the interaction of a biologic predisposition or vulnerability and environmental stressors (see the diathesis–stress model discussed

---

BOX 23.1

Deficits That Cause Vulnerability in Schizophrenia

COGNITIVE DEFICITS
- Deficits in processing complex information
- Deficits in maintaining a steady focus of attention
- Inability to distinguish between relevant and irrelevant stimuli
- Difficulty forming consistent abstractions
- Impaired memory

PSYCHOPHYSIOLOGIC DEFICITS
- Deficits in sensory inhibition
- Poor control of autonomic responsiveness

SOCIAL SKILLS DEFICITS
- Impairments in processing interpersonal stimuli, such as eye contact or assertiveness
- Deficits in conversational capacity
- Deficits in initiating activities
- Deficits in experiencing pleasure

COPING SKILLS DEFICITS
- Overassessment of threat
- Underassessment of personal resources
- Overuse of denial

Source: McGlashan, T. H. (1994). Psychosocial treatments of schizophrenia: The potential relationships. In N. C. Andreasen (Ed.), *Schizophrenia: From mind to molecule* (pp. 189–215). Washington, DC: American Psychiatric Press.

---

in Chapter 11). See Box 23.1 for deficits related to vulnerability in schizophrenia. Environmental stressors include pregnancy or obstetric complications and social adversity such as migration, unemployment, urban living, childhood abuse, and social isolation or absence of close friends (Fan et al., 2018).

Biologic Theories

Neuroanatomic Findings

The lateral and third ventricles are somewhat larger and total brain volume is somewhat less in persons with schizophrenia compared with those without schizophrenia. The thalamus and the medial temporal lobe structures, including the hippocampus, and superior temporal and prefrontal cortices, tend to be smaller also (Dietsche, Kircher, Falkenberg, 2017; Wang et al., 2019).

Genetic Associations

Genetic associations have been identified in a number of regions of the brain, and some have already been tied to neuropathways related to cognitive deficits. The future of treatment of schizophrenia will rely heavily on the outcome of ongoing research (Toulopoulou et al., 2019).

Neurodevelopment

The neurodevelopmental hypothesis explains the etiology of schizophrenia as pathologic processes caused by genetic and environmental factors that begin before the brain reaches its adult state. Evidence suggests that in utero during the first or second trimester, genes involved with cell migration, cell proliferation, axonal outgrowth, and myelination may be affected by neurologic insults such as viral infections. That is, early neurodevelopmental insults may lead to dysfunction of specific networks that become obvious at adolescence during the normal loss of some plasticity and synapse development (La Barbera, Vedele, Nobili, D'Amelio, & Krashia, 2019).

Neurotransmitters, Pathways, and Receptors

Positron emission tomography (PET) scan findings suggest that in schizophrenia, brain metabolism is generally reduced, with a relative hypermetabolism in the left side of the brain and in the left temporal lobe. Abnormalities exist in specific areas of the brain in the frontal, temporal, and cingulate regions. These findings support further exploration of differential brain hemisphere function in people with schizophrenia (Fig. 23.1). Other PET studies show **hypofrontality**, or a reduced cerebral blood flow and glucose metabolism in the prefrontal cortex of people with schizophrenia and hyperactivity in the limbic area (Buchsbaum, 1990; Hazlett, Vaccaro, Haznedar, & Goldstein, 2019) (Figs. 23.2 and 23.3).

Dopamine Dysregulation. A longstanding explanation of the neurobiological symptoms of schizophrenia is the dopamine hypothesis. Because conventional antipsychotics blocked dopamine and treated the positive symptoms of schizophrenia—specifically, hallucinations and delusions—it was reasoned that *hyperactivity* in the mesolimbic tract at the D2 receptor site in the striatal area (where memory and emotion are regulated) was responsible for these symptoms. Conversely, chronic low levels of dopamine in the prefrontal cortex were thought to underlie cognitive dysfunction in schizophrenia.

Today, research focuses on several of the molecular links to dopamine synthesis and increased release of dopamine. Dopamine has a role in the pathogenesis of schizophrenia, but it is more complicated than previously thought. Dopamine activity is related to other disorders, cortical functioning, and stress (Howes, McCutcheon, Owen, Murray, 2017).

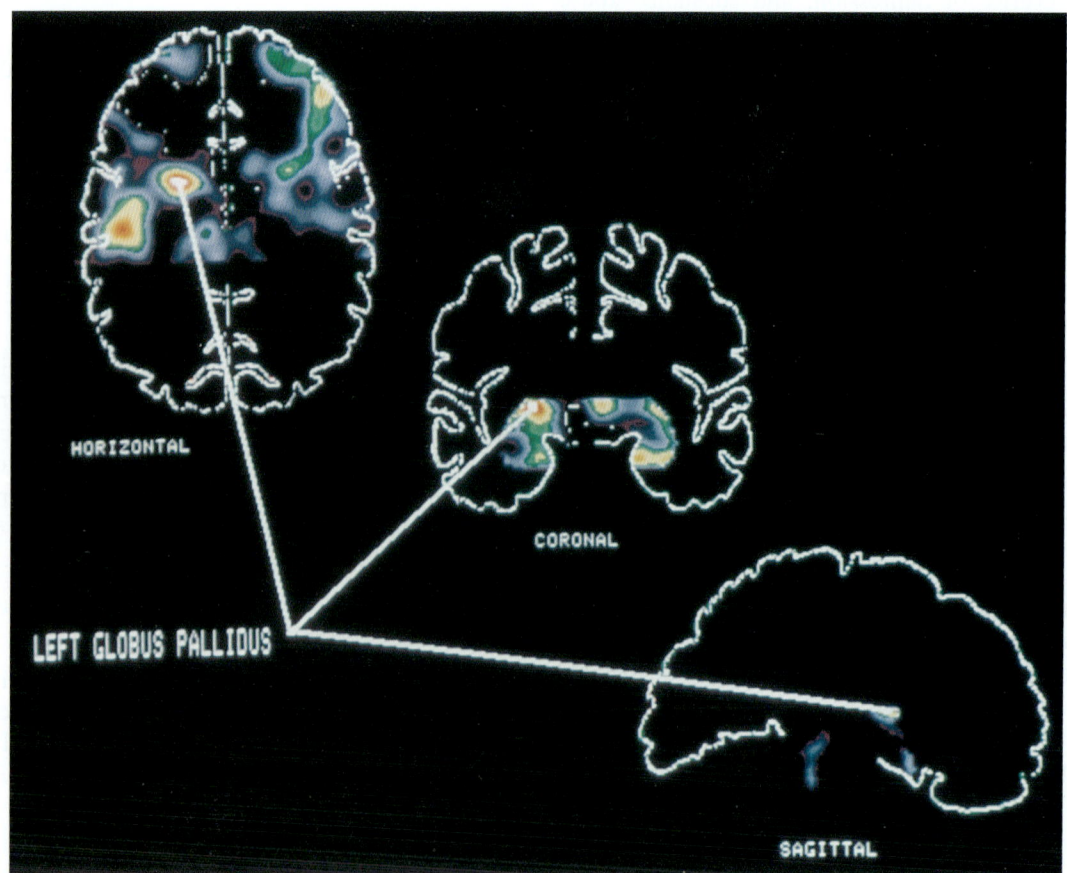

FIGURE 23.1 Area of abnormal functioning in a person with schizophrenia. These three views show the excessive neuronal activity in the left globus pallidus (portion of the basal ganglia next to the putamen). (Courtesy of John W. Haller PhD. *Departments of Psychiatry and Radiology*. St. Louis, MO: Washington University.)

FIGURE 23.2 Metabolic activity in a control subject (*left*), a subject with obsessive-compulsive disorder (*center*), and a subject with schizophrenia (*right*). (Courtesy of Monte S. Buchsbaum MD. *The Mount Sinai Medical Center and School of Medicine.* New York.)

FIGURE 23.3 Positron emission tomography scan with 18F-deoxyglucose shows metabolic activity in a horizontal section of the brain in a control subject (*left*) and in an unmedicated patient with schizophrenia (*right*). *Red* and *yellow* indicate areas of high metabolic activity in the cortex; *green* and *blue* indicate lower activity in the white matter areas of the brain. The frontal lobe is magnified to show reduced frontal activity in the prefrontal cortex of the patient with schizophrenia. (Courtesy of Monte S. Buchsbaum MD. *The Mount Sinai Medical Center and School of Medicine.* New York.)

Role of Other Receptors. Other receptors are also involved in dopamine neurotransmission, especially serotonergic receptors. It is becoming clear that schizophrenia does not result from dysregulation of a single neurotransmitter or biogenic amine (e.g., norepinephrine, dopamine, or serotonin). Investigators are also hypothesizing a role for glutamate and gamma-aminobutyric acid (GABA) because of the complex interconnections of neuronal transmission and the complexity and heterogeneity of schizophrenia symptoms. The N-methyl-D-aspartate (NMDA) class of glutamate receptors is being studied because of the actions of phencyclidine (PCP) at these sites and because of the similarity of the psychotic behaviors that are produced when someone takes PCP (see Figs. 23.1 to 23.3).

Gut Microbiota. Intestinal flora are necessary for brain development and overall health. Gut bacteria are involved in immune regulation and protect the body through the development of mucosal lymphoid tissue. The **gut–brain axis** (the two-way communication system that connects the gut with the brain) is involved with the intestinal microbiome, neuroendocrine (hypothalamus–pituitary–adrenal axis), immune, and nervous systems. The gut microbiota communicates with the CNS through the vagus nerve. Emerging research is linking the gut microbiota to the development of mental disorders through the gut–brain axis. It is hypothesized that abnormalities in the gut microbiota increase inflammatory cytokines that may cause neuronal damage, cell death, and abnormal brain development (Yuan, Kang, Zhuo, Huang, & Song, 2019).

Psychosocial Theories

Social factors can contribute to the changes in brain function that result in schizophrenia and add to the day-to-day challenges of living with a mental illness. Childhood trauma, living in an urban environment, and being a member of a minority are all associated with psychotic syndromes. They can also create barriers to obtaining necessary treatment and recovery (Fan et al., 2018; Mohammadzadeh, Azadi, King, Khosravani, & Sharifi Bastan, 2019). One of the major social stressors is the social stigma that surrounds all mental illnesses (see Chapter 1). The clinical vignette in Box 23.2 describes the impact of living with a stigmatizing illness. Another is the absence of good, affordable, and supportive housing in many communities. With 2010's enactment of insurance parity for mental illness in the Affordable Care Act, it is hoped that quality and continuity of care will be enhanced. Finally, the mental health service delivery system is fragmented; its quality and types of services vary from community to community, based in part on state legislative and mental health department funding differences.

BOX 23.2 CLINICAL VIGNETTE

Graduate Student in Peril

BGW, born in 1993, spent most of his teenage years using drugs and alcohol, behavior that started when he was 11 years old. He and his small group of friends spent their teenage years outside of school riding around on bicycles. He failed 8th grade, repeated it, and made it to 10th grade. He was removed permanently from school at the age of 16 years. His dress included a dirty denim jacket or Army fatigues, torn tee shirts with rock band logos, and tight-fitting jeans. At age 16, he was hospitalized for a psychotic episode initiated by lysergic acid diethylamide (LSD); it was the scariest moment of his life. His mind had been getting fuzzier every day; he had dabbled with black magic and Satanism. Later, he admitted that for years he had been trapped in a fantasy land, only partially explained by his drug use.

Years of treatment followed; even with abstinence from drugs, his mental status fluctuated. After antipsychotic agents were prescribed, he began to feel like himself. He was motivated to complete his GED and entered college. He kept his mental illness a secret. While in graduate school, his thoughts, feelings, and behaviors began to change. His thinking became delusional, his moods unpredictable, and his behaviors illogical. Finally, he was hospitalized again, and his condition was stabilized with medication. Currently, he is reapplying to graduate school and this time he vows to keep people close to him aware of his mental status.

What Do You Think?
- What role did stigma play in the treatment process?
- What information should BGW share with his social network about his mental illness and treatment?

Adapted from Graduate student in peril: A first person account of schizophrenia. (2002). *Schizophrenia Bulletin, 28*(4), 745–755.

Family Response to Disorder

Initially, families usually experience disbelief, shock, and fear along with concern for the family member. Families may attribute the episode to taking illicit drugs or to extraordinary stress or fatigue and hope that this is an isolated or transient event. They may be fearful of the behaviors and respond to patient anger and hostility with fear, confusion, and anxiety. They may deny the severity and chronicity of the illness and only partially engage in treatment. As families begin to acknowledge the disorder and the long-term care nature of recovery, they themselves may feel overwhelmed, angry, and depressed (McAuliffe, O'Connor, & Meagher, 2014). See Box 23.3 for discussion of recovery-oriented family interventions.

Recovery-Oriented Care of Persons With Schizophrenia

Teamwork and Collaboration: Working Toward Recovery

The most effective approach to treatment for individuals with schizophrenia involves various disciplines,

> **BOX 23.3**
>
> **Research for Best Practice: Family-Focused Recovery: Perspectives From Individuals With a Mental Illness**
>
> Waller, S., Reupert, A., Ward, B., McCormick, F., & Kidd, S. (2019). Family-focused recovery: Perspectives from individuals with a mental illness. International Journal of Mental Health Nursing, 28(1): 247–255.
>
> **THE QUESTION:** How do those with mental illness define "family" and the role of family in their recovery?
>
> **METHODS:** Purposive sampling and snowballing were used to recruit and conduct semistructured interviews with 12 people diagnosed with a severe mental illness.
>
> **FINDINGS:** Participants defined "family" in various ways, with some being very inclusive and others more selective. There was acknowledgement that family contributed to the individual's recovery in myriad ways, although the need for boundaries was stressed.
>
> **IMPLICATIONS FOR NURSING:** Nurses should recognize that there is not one definition of "family" and that it is important for the patient to define his or her family.

including nursing (both generalist and advanced practice psychiatric nurses), psychiatry, psychology, social work, occupational and recreational therapy, and pastoral counseling. Individuals with general education in psychology, sociology, and social work often serve as case managers, nursing aides, technicians, and other support personnel in hospitals and community treatment agencies.

Patients need help in accepting and understanding their illness, setting goals, and developing a support system that encourages their recovery. Recovery-oriented strategies can address any hopelessness associated with suicide attempts and encourage an independent lifestyle. Medication management is central to the treatment of schizophrenia and is the responsibility of the patient, physicians, nurses, and pharmacists. Psychosocial interventions can be implemented by all members of the mental health team and may include cognitive behavioral, music, vocational, mindfulness, and support therapies. These varied professionals and paraprofessionals are important because of the complex nature of the symptoms, the long-term nature of the disorder, and the need for health promotion support. Complementary and alternative therapies such as yoga, breathing exercises, relaxation, meditation, and aerobic exercise may be helpful as adjunctive to the usual care.

Integration With Primary Care

Traditionally, mental health problems were treated separately from medical needs. It was not uncommon for there to be little connection between the treatment of mental disorders and medical disorders. We now know that a person cannot successfully recover unless physical and mental health care are integrated. The medical needs of persons with schizophrenia are significant and require treatment. There should be a systematic coordination of general and behavior health. Ideally, the patient would have one record where all care would be documented.

Safety Issues

Several special concerns exist when working with people with schizophrenia. A suicide assessment always should be completed when a person is experiencing a psychotic episode. In an inpatient unit, patient safety concerns extend to potentially aggressive actions toward staff and other patients during episodes of psychosis. During times of acute illness, a priority of care is treatment with antipsychotic medications and, in some instances, hospitalization.

Nurses should assess the person's risk for suicide because of the high suicide and attempted suicide rates among persons with schizophrenia. See Chapter 16. One challenge is to distinguish among the displayed behaviors to determine if the person is displaying negative symptoms, side effects of antipsychotic medications, or actual depression and demoralization as a result of this illness. Does the patient speak of suicide, have delusional thinking that could lead to dangerous behavior, or have command hallucinations telling him or her to harm self or others? Does the patient have homicidal ideations? Does the patient lack social support and the skills to be meaningfully engaged with other people or a vocation? Does the patient express feelings of being a burden to loved ones? Substance-related disorders are also common among patients with schizophrenia, so that nurses should assess for substance use.

Evidence-Based Nursing Care of Persons With Schizophrenia

Recovery is a long-term journey requiring various nursing interventions at different times. During exacerbation of symptoms, many patients are hospitalized for safety and medication adjustment. During periods of relative stability, the nurse and patient collaborate in developing recovery-oriented strategies that include maintaining a healthy lifestyle, developing positive coping skills, and seeking meaningful relationships. Schizophrenia research is ongoing and the results are leading to new treatment approaches. It is critical that nurses continually seek out evidence-based strategies through accessing the best possible sources of evidence and formulating clinical questions. Nursing Care Plan 23.1—which sets forth a plan of care for Arnold, the case study patient in this chapter—is available at http://thepoint.lww.com/BoydEssentials2e.

Mental Health Nursing Assessment

The nursing assessment should include the biologic, psychological, and social aspects because schizophrenia affects all aspects of the person's life. Not only are symptoms assessed, but strengths are also important in the assessment process.

Physical Health

The nurse should first determine whether any underlying medical disorders are present, particularly those associated with schizophrenia such as DM, hypertension, and cardiac disease, or a family history of such disorders. Usually a medical examination is conducted by primary care providers prior to initiation of mental health care. People with schizophrenia have a higher mortality rate from physical illness and often have smoking-related illnesses, such as emphysema as well as other pulmonary and cardiac problems (Gimblett, 2015; Olfson et al., 2015).

Physical Functioning

Physical abilities can be a strength; the potential to maintain optimal physical health should be assessed. Self-care often deteriorates in schizophrenia; sleep may be nonexistent during acute phases. Information regarding physical functioning may best be collected from family members.

Nutrition

A nutritional history should be completed to determine baseline eating habits and preferences. Taking baseline measures for metabolic syndrome is highly recommended and should include weight, waist circumference, cholesterol, and blood sugar (Kioko, Williams, & Newhouse, 2016). A healthy diet is important in managing the illness. Medications can alter normal nutrition leading to excessive consumption of calories.

Medication

The nurse should obtain a complete list of medications that the patient is taking including over-the-counter (OTC) agents and herbal supplements. Before initiation of psychiatric medications, standardized assessment of abnormal motor movements should be conducted using one of several assessment tools designed for that purpose, such as the Abnormal Involuntary Movement Scale (AIMS) (see Appendix B), the Dyskinesia Identification System (DISCUS) (Sprague & Kalachnik, 1991), or the Simpson–Angus Rating Scale (Simpson & Angus, 1970), which is designed for Parkinson's symptoms.

Substance Use (Alcohol, Illicit Drugs, Tobacco)

The nurse should ask specific questions about alcohol, drug, and tobacco use. The use of these substances is quite common with people with schizophrenia and will significantly influence the treatment approach.

Psychosocial Assessment

The individual who is in an acute phase may be unable to provide an accurate history of early psychosocial issues. Family members' reports help in detailing occurrences of psychotic symptoms of delusions and hallucinations; however, onset of negative symptoms may be more difficult to date. In fact, negative symptoms vary from a slight deviation from normal to a clear impairment. Negative symptoms probably occur earlier than positive symptoms but are less easily recognized. Several assessment scales have been developed to help evaluate clusters of positive and negative symptoms. See Box 23.4.

Mental Status and Appearance

The patient may look eccentric or disheveled or have poor hygiene and bizarre dress. The patient's posture may suggest lethargy or stupor.

Mood and Affect

Patients with schizophrenia often display altered mood states. In some cases, they may show heightened emotional activity; others may display severely limited emotional responses. Affect, the outward expression of mood, is categorized on a continuum: flat (i.e., emotional expression entirely absent), blunted (i.e., expression of emotions present but greatly diminished), and full range of expression. Inappropriate affect is marked by incongruence between the emotional expression and the thoughts expressed (e.g., laughing when telling a sad story). Other common emotional symptoms include the following:

- **Affective lability**—abrupt, dramatic, unprovoked changes in type of emotions expressed
- **Ambivalence**—the presence and expression of two opposing feelings, leading to inaction
- **Apathy**—little emotional expression; diminished interest and desire

Speech

Thought content and other mental processes are expressed in speech. Both content and speech patterns should be assessed by the nurse. Speech content may include obvious obsessions or delusions, loose associations, or flight of ideas. In some instances, as already

BOX 23.4
Rating Scales for Use With Schizophrenia

SCALE FOR THE ASSESSMENT OF NEGATIVE SYMPTOMS (SANS)
Available from Nancy C. Andreasen, MD, PhD, Department of Psychiatry, College of Medicine, The University of Iowa, Iowa City, IA 52242. Copyright 1984.

SCALE FOR THE ASSESSMENT OF POSITIVE SYMPTOMS (SAPS)
Available from Nancy C. Andreasen (see above).

POSITIVE AND NEGATIVE SYNDROME SCALE (PANSS)
Kay, S. R., Fiszbein, A., & Opler, L. A. (1987). The Positive and Negative Syndrome Scale (PANSS) for Schizophrenia. *Schizophrenia Bulletin*, 13, 261–276. Available from first author.

ABNORMAL INVOLUNTARY MOVEMENT SCALE (AIMS)
Guy, W. (1976), *ECDEU: Assessment manual for psychopharmacology* (DHEW Publication No. 76–338). Washington, DC: Department of Health, Education, and Welfare, Psychopharmacology Branch.

BRIEF PSYCHIATRIC RATING SCALE (BPRS)
Overall, J. E., & Gorham, D. R. (1988). The Brief Psychiatric Rating Scale (BPRS): Recent developments in ascertainment and scaling. *Psychopharmacology Bulletin*, 24, 97–99.

DYSKINESIA IDENTIFICATION SYSTEM: CONDENSED USER SCALE (DISCUS)
Sprague, R. L., & Kalachnik, J. E. (1991). Reliability, validity, and a total score cutoff for the Dyskinesia Identification Scale System: Condensed User Scale (DISCUS) with mentally ill and mentally retarded populations. *Psychopharmacology Bulletin*, 27(1), 51–58.

SIMPSON–ANGUS RATING SCALE
Simpson, G. M., & Angus, J. W. S. L. (1970). A rating scale for extrapyramidal side effects. *Acta Psychiatrica Scandinavica*, 212(suppl), 11–19. Copyright 1970 Munksgaard International Publishers, Ltd.

noted, patients make up their own words (neologisms). Speech may be pressured (words seem to rapidly jump out without pauses) or slow. The nurse should note any difficulty in articulating words (dysarthria) or difficulty in swallowing (dysphagia) as indicators of medication-related side effects.

Thought Process Assessment

Thought process assessment includes determining if any hallucinations, delusions, disorganized communication, or cognitive impairments are present. Because thought process assessment is critical in the nursing assessment, each area is discussed separately below.

Hallucinations

Hallucinations are the most common example of disturbed sensory perception observed in patients with schizophrenia. Hallucinations are experienced in the sensory modalities (visual, auditory, gustatory, tactile, olfactory); however, auditory hallucinations are the most common type in schizophrenia. Some specific hallucinations may be sufficient to diagnose schizophrenia, such as hearing voices conversing with each other or carrying on a discussion with someone who is not there. Because most individuals will not spontaneously share their hallucinatory experiences with an interviewer, the nurse may need to rely on indirect evidence in the patient's behavior, such as (1) pauses during conversations in which the individual seems preoccupied or appears to be listening to someone other than the interviewer, (2) looking toward the perceived source of a voice, or (3) responding to the voices in some manner. Although patients may not spontaneously share their hallucinations, many validate observations of the examiner or admit to a history of hallucinations when asked. See Box 23.5. If a patient has command hallucinations, it is important for the safety of the person and others to know what the voices are telling the patient to do.

Delusions

Delusions are different from strongly held beliefs. Delusions do not change even though strong evidence contradicts the belief. The person continues to hold the belief despite contradictory evidence (APA, 2013). The person's culture must be considered when evaluating delusions. Delusional beliefs are those not sanctioned or held by a cultural or religious subgroup.

Bizarre delusions alone are sufficient to diagnose schizophrenia (APA, 2013). Bizarre delusions are those beliefs that are impossible, illogical, and not derived from ordinary life experiences. Bizarre delusions often include delusions of control (that some outside force controls thoughts and actions), thought broadcasting (that others can read or hear one's thoughts), thought insertion (that someone has placed thoughts into one's mind), and thought withdrawal (that someone is removing thoughts from one's mind). For example, a patient who has been seeing a hypnotist for 2 months reports that the hypnotist continued to read his mind and was "picking his brain away piece by piece." Another patient was convinced that a computer chip was placed in her vagina during a gynecologic examination and that this somehow directly influenced her physical movements and her thoughts.

Remember Arnold?
He believes that his parents are still alive and that they will return. He refuses to leave the farm and insists that everything be left as it is.

BOX 23.5 • THERAPEUTIC DIALOGUE • The Patient With Hallucinations

The following conversation took place in Arnold's room during the night checks. The nurse observed that Arnold was talking with someone, but no one else was in the room.

INEFFECTIVE APPROACH

Nurse: Arnold?
Arnold: Yeah?
Nurse: Who are you talking to?
Arnold: My mother visits me at night. I am telling her about my day.
Nurse: You know, Arnold, you are having an hallucination. Your mother died a few weeks ago.
Arnold: She did not. She is away for a while, but she will be back soon.
Nurse: Arnold. (Looks at nurse.) You are going to have to accept that your mother is gone.
Arnold: Oh yeah? What do you know?
Nurse: Well, we can talk about it in the morning.
Arnold: You don't know what you are talking about.

EFFECTIVE APPROACH

Nurse: Arnold?
Arnold: Yeah?
Nurse: Are you talking to someone?
Arnold: Yes, she visits me at night?
Nurse: Oh, does she talk to you?
Arnold: Yes, she asks me about my day. She visits in the evening?
Nurse: Is there anything else you talk about?
Arnold: No, she leaves after I tell her.
Nurse: OK, how do you feel when she visits you?
Arnold: A little sad, but I like to tell her about my day.
Nurse: A little sad?
Arnold: Yeah, I wish I could see her more.
Nurse: Sounds like you are lonely?
Arnold: Yea, it's nice when you talk with me.
Nurse: I can do that. If you are not asleep when I finish rounds, we can talk more.

CRITICAL THINKING CHALLENGE

- How did the nurse's impatience translate into Arnold's response in the first scenario?
- What effective communicating techniques did the nurse use in the second scenario?

Nonbizarre delusions generally have themes of jealousy and persecution and are derived from plausible life experiences. For example, a woman believes that her husband, from whom she has recently separated, is trying to poison her, or a man who believes that members of the Mafia are trying to kill him because, when he was in high school, he reported to the principal that several of his classmates were selling drugs at school (APA, 2013).

Assessing and judging the content of the delusion and exploring other aspects of the delusional experience are helpful in understanding the significance of these false beliefs. The underlying feeling that accompanies the delusion (i.e., fear or inflated self-esteem) should be explored. Other aspects to consider include the conviction with which the delusion is held; the extent to which other aspects of the individual's life are incorporated or affected by the delusion; the degree of internal consistency, organization, and logic evidenced in the delusion; and evaluating the amount of pressure (in terms of preoccupation and concern) individuals feel in their lives as a result of the delusion (Box 23.6).

Disorganized Communication

Abrupt shifts in the focus of conversation, which are often altered in schizophrenia, are typically symptomatic

BOX 23.6 • THERAPEUTIC DIALOGUE • The Patient With Delusions

John joined the nurse in a game of pool. The following conversation occurred as they played.

INEFFECTIVE APPROACH

John: The CIA put a transmitter in my molar, here (points to his right cheek).

Nurse: No one would put a transmitter in your tooth; come on, the CIA isn't looking for you.

John: Yeah, they want to monitor me while I'm here. I know that they have the real Osama bin Laden here in the hospital. They are trying to get the President to intervene with the Michigan Militia. Mark from Michigan told me that.

Nurse: Osama bin Laden can't possibly be here; he died years ago.

John: Maybe—but that was an imposter. They're just trying to keep people from knowing what they're doing.

Nurse: John, Osama bin Laden isn't in the hospital; if he were, I would know it because I work here.

John: (With anger) You don't know anything! You are probably working for the CIA too. I have nothing else to say to you.

EFFECTIVE APPROACH

John: The CIA put a transmitter in my molar, here (points to his right cheek).

Nurse: Oh. Which balls are mine?

John: You get the striped ones. Yeah, they want to monitor me while I'm here. I know that they have the real Osama bin Laden here in the hospital. They are trying to get the President to intervene with the Michigan Militia. Mark from Michigan told me that.

Nurse: Well, I don't know anything about that, but I want you to know that we will keep you safe.

John: Maybe…

Nurse: You sound a little overwhelmed with all the information you have.

John: No, no. I can handle it. The CIA can't do anything to me. I'll never talk.

Nurse: I thought they could hear you when you talk to me.

John: Huh? Oh, that transmitter is so that they can send me misinformation. They send a tower of babble to my brain. They are trying to confuse me so that I stay away from Osama Bin Laden. They all think they can keep me from my mission.

Nurse: Who are they?

John: Everyone in the government. The CIA, FBI, ATF, IRS—all those alphabets.

Nurse: So everyone in the government is trying to get to you?

John: Well, maybe not everybody. Just the ones that care about money and the militia. I don't think they care about me much in Commerce or Health and Human Services. Although they'd care too if they knew.

Nurse: I would think that's pretty frightening to have all these people out looking for you. You must be scared a lot.

John: It's scary, but I can handle it. I've handled it all my life.

Nurse: You've been in scary situations all your life?

John: Yeah. I don't know. Maybe not scary, just hard. I never seemed to be able to do as well as my parents wanted—or as I wanted.

CRITICAL THINKING CHALLENGE

- How did the nurse's argumentative responses cause the patient to react in the first scenario?
- What effective communication techniques did the nurse use in the second scenario?

---

of disorganized thinking. Impaired verbal fluency (i.e., ability to produce spontaneous speech) is commonly present. The most severe shifts in focus may occur after only one or two words (i.e., word salad), after one or two phrases or sentences (i.e., flight of ideas or loose associations), or somewhat less severely as a shift that occurs when a new topic is repeatedly suggested and pursued from the current topic (i.e., tangentiality).

Cognitive Impairments

Mental status assessment focuses on eliciting indications of cognitive impairments associated with schizophrenia. Although these impairments vary widely from patient to patient, several primary problems have been identified:

- Attention may be increased and sustained on external stimuli over a period of time (hypervigilance).

- The ability to distinguish and focus on relevant stimuli may be diminished.
- Familiar cues may go unrecognized or be improperly interpreted.
- Information processing may be diminished, leading to inappropriate or illogical conclusions from available observations and information (Dondé, Silipo, Dias, Javitt, 2018; John, Zikopoulos, Bullock, Barbas, 2018).

Cognitive impairments are not easy to recognize. By relying only on clinical assessment, the nurse can miss the extent of the impairment. Using a standardized instrument can provide a screening measurement of cognitive function. If impairment exists, neuropsychological testing by a qualified psychologist may be necessary.

Memory and Orientation. Impairment in orientation, memory, and abstract thinking is often present. Orientation to time, place, and person may remain relatively intact unless the patient is particularly preoccupied with delusions and hallucinations. Although all aspects of memory may be affected in schizophrenia, registration or the recall within seconds of newly learned information may be particularly diminished. This affects the individual's short- and long-term memory. The ability to engage in abstract thinking may be impaired. See Box 23.7.

BOX 23.7
Arnold's Cognitive Symptoms

Arnold's symptoms of schizophrenia began long before he was actually diagnosed. Throughout school he had difficulty learning new material. His teachers would describe him as being "slow" or "inattentive." Because he appeared to be functioning normally, his teachers and family attributed his poor academic behavior to lack of interest. His father would often get frustrated with him because he would spend many hours in his bedroom and would not help out on the farm. When prodded to complete school work or a household task, he would often get distracted before finishing the tasks. Family members and teachers quickly learned to provide several prompts for Arnold to complete a task. As he progressed to high school, he was labeled as a "slow learner" and assigned to less demanding classes.

The reality was that Arnold was experiencing unrecognized prodromal cognitive symptoms of schizophrenia. He was having difficulty remembering his assignments. He was having difficulty grasping concepts that other students seemed to easily understand. He was becoming frustrated with his difficulty and retreated to his room. He waited for specific directions that he could easily process. His thinking was concrete and he had difficulty expressing himself. When he was bombarded with several directions at once, he could not process any of the directions. In his frustration, he would throw objects, frightening others. His family was very concerned with the changes that were occurring with their once easy-going son.

Insight and Judgment. Insight and judgment are closely related to each other. Individuals display insight when they recognize that their hallucinations or delusions are symptoms of a mental disorder. Judgment is the ability to decide or act about a situation. If judgment is poor, the person may not recognize personal vulnerabilities and consequently engages in detrimental behavior. For example, the individual may be taken advantage by others or fail to realize a potentially dangerous situation.

Behavioral Responses

During periods of psychosis, unusual or bizarre behavior often occurs. These behaviors can usually be understood within the context of the patient's disturbed thinking. The nurse needs to understand the behavior means to the person. For example, one patient moved the family furniture into the yard because he thought that evil spirits were hiding in the furniture. His bizarre behavior was an attempt to protect his family. Another patient painted a sequence of numbers on his bedroom walls. He said that the numbers were the language of the angels. His delusional thoughts were the basis of his behavior.

Because of the negative symptoms, specifically avolition, patients may not seem interested or organized enough to complete normal daily activities. They may stay in bed most of the day or refuse to take a shower. Many times, they agree to get up in the morning and go to work, but they never get around to it. Several specific behaviors are associated with schizophrenia, including stereotypy (i.e., idiosyncratic, repetitive, purposeless movements), echopraxia (i.e., involuntary imitation of others' movements), and waxy flexibility (i.e., posture held in odd or unusual fixed positions for extended periods). In some cases, certain behaviors need to be evaluated carefully to distinguish them from movements that are associated with medication-related side effects, such as grimacing, stereotypical behavior, or agitation.

Self-Concept

In schizophrenia, self-concept is usually poor. Patients often are aware that they are hearing voices others do not hear. They recognize that they are different from others and are often scared of "going crazy." Many are aware of the loss of expectations for their future achievements. The pervasive stigma associated with having a mental illness contributes to the poor self-concept. Body image can be disturbed, especially during periods of hallucinations or delusions. For example, one patient believed that her body was infected with germs and she could feel them eating away her insides.

Stress and Coping Patterns

Stressful events are often linked to psychiatric symptoms. It is important to determine stresses from the patient's perspective because a stressful event for one may not be stressful for another. It is also important to determine typical coping patterns, especially negative coping strategies, such as the use of substances or showing aggressive behavior.

>
> **Consider This:**
> Recall Arnold's symptoms? They appeared after the stress of his parents' death.

Social Network

Several difficulties involving social functioning occur in schizophrenia. As the disorder progresses, individuals can become increasingly socially isolated. On a one-to-one basis, this occurs as the individual seems unable to connect with people in his or her environment. Several aspects of symptoms already discussed can contribute to this. For example, emotional blunting and anhedonia (the inability to experience pleasure) result in an experience of not being engaged in activities and relationships.

Interpretation of facial expressions and affect displayed by others is often problematic for people with schizophrenia. Cognitive deficits affect social relationships when individuals are unable to recall past interactions and have problems with decision making and judgment. Other behaviors that affect social relationships are poverty of speech and language and the inability to complete ADLs, which results in poor hygiene, malnutrition, and social isolation.

Functional Status

Functional status of patients with schizophrenia should be assessed initially and at regular intervals. Level of independence, ability to work, ability to maintain an independent living environment, and self-care should be evaluated.

Support Systems

In schizophrenia, support systems become very important in maintaining the patient in the community. The individual may become socially isolated if the treatment and management occur in long-term care facilities and group homes away from family and friends. One challenge is to identify and maintain the patient's links with family and significant others. Assessment of the formal support (e.g., family, health care providers) and informal support (e.g., neighbors, friends) should be conducted.

Quality of Life

People with schizophrenia often have a poor quality of life, especially older people, who may have spent many years in long-term hospitals. The nurse should assess the patient's quality of life and how it could be improved. Simple changes, such as arranging for a different roommate or improving access to social activities by meeting transportation needs, can greatly improve a patient's quality of life.

Strengths Assessment

An important part of recovery is identification of personal and family strengths. Because schizophrenia is usually diagnosed at a young age, the person may be physically fit with little evidence of chronic illness. As the assessment is completed, strengths will emerge. Family support is critical for a person with schizophrenia. Intellectual ability and coping with stress are areas that can be strengths. The following questions are examples that can be used in assessing strengths.

- What do you do for relaxation, fun?
- How do you manage stressful events?
- How do you cope with the voices, thoughts, or impulses?
- Who do you talk with when you are upset?
- Are you hopeful about the future, and if so, what gives you hope for the future?

Priority of Nursing Care

People with schizophrenia have a variety of nursing care needs that emerge at different times in the illness. For example, during an episode of psychosis, safety becomes a focus. Voices may be telling the individual to self-injure or injure others. Sleep may be a severe problem. Mood disturbances, specifically depression, may be a priority later in the course of the disorder. There may be hygiene issues that interfere with the person's ability to engage in social activities, or motivation may be an issue. A very careful and ongoing assessment of needs and issues is important throughout recovery.

> **NCLEXNOTE** When assessing a patient with schizophrenia, the nurse should prioritize the severity of the current responses to the disorder. If hallucinations are impairing functions, then managing hallucinations is a priority and medications are needed immediately. If hallucinations are not a problem, however, coping with negative symptoms becomes a priority.

Therapeutic Relationship

Development of the therapeutic nurse–patient relationship centers on developing trust, accepting the person as a worthy human being, and infusing the relationship with hope. People with schizophrenia are often reluctant to engage in any relationship because of previous rejection and, in some instances, an underlying suspiciousness, which is a part of the illness. They are often trying to trust their own thoughts and perceptions, so interactions with another human being may prove to be too overwhelming. If they are having hallucinations, their images of other people may be distorted and frightening as well.

The nurse should approach the patient in a calm and caring manner. Engaging the patient in a relationship may take time but it begins with the first encounter. Short time-limited interactions are best for a patient who is experiencing psychosis. Being consistent in interactions and following through on promises will help establish trust within the relationship.

Establishing a therapeutic relationship is crucial, especially with patients who deny that they are ill. Patients are more likely to agree to and continue treatment if these recommendations are made within the context of a safe, trusting relationship. Even if some patients deny having mental illness, they may take medication and attend treatment activities because they trust the nurse (Jaeger, Seiβhaupt, Flammer, Steinert, 2014).

Furthermore, for long-term care and outcomes, recovery-oriented relationships are important. Using the recovery model, all efforts should be made to individualize treatment. Care should be person centered through partnering with the patient in all aspects of care and encouraging self-direction. Treatment should be focused on strengths and the empowerment of the individual. Patients need encouragement to see that although their diagnosis may seem devastating, recovery is possible (Lean, et al., 2019).

Mental Health Nursing Interventions

Self-Care

For many people with schizophrenia, the plan of care will include specific interventions to enhance self-care, nutrition, and overall health knowledge. Negative symptoms commonly leave patients unable to initiate these seemingly simple activities. Developing a daily schedule of routine activities (e.g., showering, shaving) can help the patient structure the day. Most patients actually know how to perform self-care activities (e.g., hygiene, grooming) but lack motivation (avolition) to carry them out consistently. Interventions include developing a schedule with the patient for various hygiene-related activities and emphasizing the importance of maintaining appropriate self-care activities. Given the problems related to attention and memory in people with schizophrenia, education about these areas requires careful planning.

Activity, Exercise, and Nutritional Interventions

Encouraging activity and exercise is necessary, not only to maintain a healthy lifestyle but also to counteract the side effects of psychiatric medications that cause weight gain. Because the diagnosis is usually made in late adolescence or early adulthood, it is possible to establish solid exercise patterns early.

During episodes of acute psychosis, patients are sometimes unable to focus on eating. Often when patients begin antipsychotic medication, normal satiety and hunger responses change, and overeating or weight gain can become a problem. Patients report that their appetites increase and cravings for food develop when some medications are initiated. Promoting and maintaining healthy nutrition is a key intervention. Monitoring calorie intake is also important because of the effect many medications have on eating habits.

Weight gain is one of the reasons some patients stop taking their medications. Increased weight places patients at greater risk for several health problems, such as type II DM and early death. Monitoring for DM and managing weight are important activities for all health care providers. Patients should be screened for risk factors of DM, such as family history, obesity as indicated by a body mass index (BMI) exceeding or equal to 27, and age older than 45 years. Patients' weight should be measured at regular intervals and the BMI calculated. Blood pressure readings should be taken regularly. Laboratory findings for triglycerides, high-density lipoprotein cholesterol, and glucose level should be monitored and reviewed regularly. All health care providers should be alert to the development of hyperglycemia, particularly in patients known to have DM who begin taking second-generation antipsychotic agents. A program to address weight gain should be initiated at the earliest sign of weight gain (probably between 5 and 10 lb over desired body weight). Reduced caloric intake may be accomplished by increasing the patient's access to affordable, healthful, and easy-to-prepare foods. Behavioral management of weight gain includes keeping a food diary, diet teaching, and support groups (Manu et al., 2015). Setting small goals and offering a lot of encouragement can lead to some success.

Thermoregulation Interventions

Patients with schizophrenia may have disturbed body temperature regulation. In winter, they may seem to be oblivious to cold weather. In the heat of summer, they may dress for winter. Observing patients' responses to temperatures helps in identifying problems in this area. In patients who are taking psychiatric medications, body temperature needs to be monitored, and the patient needs to be protected from extremes in temperature.

Fluid Balance

Some persons with schizophrenia develop disturbed fluid and electrolyte balance. Nurses should observe for polydipsia (frequently drinking an excessive amount of fluids) or frequent incontinence. These individuals are obsessed with drinking water and compulsively consume fluids. For persons with schizophrenia who demonstrate polydipsia, regulation of their fluid intake is disturbed, resulting in an abnormally low serum sodium level, which can lead to severe water intoxication, a medical emergency.

Nursing interventions include teaching and assisting the patient to develop self-monitoring skills. Fluid intake and weight gain should be monitored to control fluid intake and reduce the likelihood of developing water intoxication. Patients with mild polydipsia are easily treated in outpatient settings and benefit from educational programs that teach them to monitor their own urine's specific gravity and daily weight gains. Patients with moderate polydipsia may respond well to education but still have a more difficult time controlling their own fluid intake, which requires more careful monitoring of intake and weight throughout the day. Patients with severe polydipsia require considerable assistance, probably in an inpatient unit, to restrict their continual water-seeking behavior. These patients may create disruption on the unit, so they are best managed by one-on-one observation to redirect their behavior.

Integration With Primary Care. Treatment interventions for mental disorders impact the general health status of the person. Frequent communication with primary care providers allows monitoring and adjustment of medical treatment. Medication interactions are a concern when patients are receiving medications from several different clinicians.

Medication Interventions: Antipsychotics

Antipsychotic medications are the treatment of choice for patients with psychosis. Antipsychotic drugs are used because they have the general effect of blocking dopamine transmission leading to a decrease in psychotic symptoms (see Chapter 11). Some medications also block other receptors of other neurotransmitters to varying degrees. See Table 23.1.

The prescription of first-generation antipsychotics (e.g., haloperidol, chlorpromazine) decreased dramatically with the introduction of second-generation antipsychotics. However, it is important that medication choice be individualized based on each patient's experience and preference as well as the side effect profiles of selected drugs rather than to limit drug selection to one type or class of antipsychotic medication. This is particularly true during the acute phase of the illness for people with schizophrenia who are known to respond to treatment.

TABLE 23.1 SELECTED ANTIPSYCHOTIC DRUGS

Generic Name	Trade Name	Dosage Range for Adults (mg/d)
Second-Generation Antipsychotics		
aripiprazole	Abilify	10–15
asenapine	Saphris	10–20
cariprazine	Vraylar	1.5–6 mg/d
clozapine	Clozaril	200–600
risperidone	Risperdal	4–16
olanzapine	Zyprexa	10–20
paliperidone	Invega	3–12
quetiapine	Seroquel	300–400
ziprasidone	Geodon	40–160
lurasidone	Latuda	40–80 mg
Selected First-Generation Antipsychotic Drugs Used to Treat Psychosis in the United States		
chlorpromazine	NA[a]	30–800
fluphenazine	NA	0.5–20
haloperidol	Haldol	1–15
loxapine	Loxitane	20–250
perphenazine	NA	4–32
pimozide	NA	1–10
thiothixene	Navane	5–25
trifluoperazine	NA	5–25

[a]Not applicable. No longer available as proprietary formulations.

Second-generation antipsychotic drugs including risperidone (Risperdal), olanzapine (Zyprexa), quetiapine (Seroquel), paliperidone (Invega), ziprasidone (Geodon), aripiprazole (Abilify), iloperidone (Fanapt), asenapine (Saphris), lurasidone (Latuda), and cariprazine (Vraylar) are available in a variety of formulations. See Box 23.8 for more information about risperidone. They are effective in treating both negative and positive symptoms. These newer drugs also target other neurotransmitter systems, such as serotonin. This is believed to contribute to their antipsychotic effectiveness.

Administering Medications

Nursing interventions during the initial acute phase of schizophrenia include prompt, safe, and informed administration of antipsychotic medications. Generally, it takes about 1 to 2 weeks for antipsychotic drugs to effect a change in symptoms. During the stabilization period, the selected drug should be given an adequate trial, generally 6 to 12 weeks, before considering a change in the drug prescription. For maximum absorption, ziprasidone and lurasidone should be given with food. Ziprasidone should be taken with a high-fat meal of 500 calories. For lurasidone, 350 calories should be eaten when administering this (Pfizer, 2019; U.S. Food and Drug Administration, 08/2015). If treatment

BOX 23.8
Drug Profile: Risperidone (Risperdal)

DRUG CLASS: Atypical antipsychotic

RECEPTOR AFFINITY: Antagonist with high affinity for D_2 and 5-HT2, also histamine (H1) and α_1-, α_2-adrenergic receptors, weak affinity for D1 and other serotonin receptor subtypes; no affinity for acetylcholine or β-adrenergic receptors

INDICATIONS: Treatment of schizophrenia; short-term treatment of acute manic episodes associated with bipolar I disorder; and irritability associated with autistic disorder in children and adolescents, including symptoms of aggression toward others, deliberate self-injuriousness, temper tantrums, and quickly changing moods

ROUTES AND DOSAGE: 0.25-, 0.5-, 1-, 2-, 3-, and 4-mg tablets and liquid concentrate (1 mg/mL); orally disintegrating tablets, 0.5-, 1-, 2-, 3-, and 4-mg

Adult: Schizophrenia: Initial dose: typically 1 mg bid. Maximal effect at 6 mg/d. Safety not established above 16 mg/d. Use lowest possible dose to alleviate symptoms

Bipolar mania: 2 to 3 mg/d

Geriatric: Initial dose, 0.5 mg/d; increase slowly as tolerated

Children: 0.25 mg per day for patients <20 kg and 0.5 mg per day for patients >20 kg

HALF-LIFE (PEAK EFFECT): Mean, 20 h (1 h; peak active metabolite = 3–17 h)

SELECT SIDE EFFECTS: Insomnia, agitation, anxiety, extrapyramidal symptoms, headache, rhinitis, somnolence, dizziness, headache, constipation, nausea, dyspepsia, vomiting, abdominal pain, hypersalivation, tachycardia, orthostatic hypotension, fever, chest pain, coughing, photosensitivity, weight gain

BOXED WARNING: Increased mortality in elderly patients with dementia-related psychosis

WARNING: Rare development of neuroleptic malignant syndrome. Observe frequently for early signs of **tardive dyskinesia**. Use caution with individuals who have cardiovascular disease; risperidone can cause electrocardiographic changes. Avoid use during pregnancy or while breast-feeding. Hepatic or renal impairments increase plasma concentration

SPECIFIC PATIENT/FAMILY EDUCATION

- Notify your prescriber if tremor, motor restlessness, abnormal movements, chest pain, or other unusual symptoms develop.
- Avoid alcohol and other CNS depressant drugs.
- Notify your prescriber if pregnancy is possible or if planning to become pregnant. Do not breastfeed while taking this medication.
- Notify your prescriber before taking any other prescription or OTC medication.
- May impair judgment, thinking, or motor skills; avoid driving or potentially other hazardous tasks.
- During titration, the individual may experience orthostatic hypotension and should change positions slowly.
- Do not abruptly discontinue.

bid, twice a day; CNS, central nervous system; OTC, over-the-counter.

Adherence to a prescribed medication regimen is the best approach to prevent relapse. Unfortunately, adherence to the second-generation antipsychotic agents is not improved from the first-generation antipsychotic. The use of long-acting injectables has improved compliance outcomes (Greene et al., 2018). Box 23.10 provides evidence related to interventions that promote medication adherence for patients with schizophrenia.

Patients with schizophrenia generally face a lifetime of taking antipsychotic medications. Rarely is discontinuation of medications prescribed; however, many patients stop taking medications on their own. Some conditions do require the cessation of medication use such as neuroleptic malignant syndrome (see later discussion), agranulocytosis (i.e., dangerously low level of circulating neutrophils), or drug reaction with eosinophilia and systemic symptoms (DRESS; i.e., fever with a rash and/or swollen lymph glands). Discontinuation is also an option when tardive dyskinesia develops. Discontinuation of medications, other than in the circumstances of a medical emergency, should be achieved by gradually lowering the dose over time. This diminishes the likelihood of withdrawal symptoms.

Monitoring Extrapyramidal Side Effects

Parkinsonism caused by antipsychotic drugs is identical in appearance to Parkinson disease and tends to occur in older patients. The symptoms are believed to be caused by the blockade of dopamine D_2 receptors in the basal ganglia, which throws off the normal balance between acetylcholine and dopamine in this area of the brain and effectively increases acetylcholine transmission. The symptoms are managed by reducing dosage and thereby increasing dopamine activity or adding an anticholinergic drug, thus decreasing acetylcholine activity, such as benztropine or trihexyphenidyl.

Dystonic reactions are also believed to result from the imbalance of dopamine and acetylcholine, with the latter dominant. Young men seem to be more vulnerable to this particular extrapyramidal side effect. This side effect, which develops rapidly and dramatically, can be very frightening for patients as their muscles tense and their body contorts. The experience often starts with **oculogyric crisis**, in which the muscles that control eye movements tense and pull the eyeball so that the patient is looking toward the ceiling. This may be followed rapidly by **torticollis**, in which the neck muscles pull the head to the side, or **retrocollis**, in which the head is pulled back, or oropharyngeal dysphagia, in which the patient has extreme difficulty in swallowing. The patient may also experience contorted limbs. These symptoms occur early in antipsychotic drug treatment, when the patient may still be enduring psychotic symptoms,

effects are not seen, a different antipsychotic agent may be tried. Clozapine is used when no other second-generation antipsychotic is effective; see Box 23.9 for more information about clozapine.

BOX 23.9

Drug Profile: Clozapine (Clozaril)

DRUG CLASS: Atypical antipsychotic

RECEPTOR AFFINITY: D1 and D2 blockade, antagonist for 5-HT2, histamine (H1), α-adrenergic, and acetylcholine. These additional antagonist effects may contribute to some of its therapeutic effects. Produces fewer extrapyramidal effects than standard antipsychotics with lower risk for tardive dyskinesia

INDICATIONS: Severely ill individuals who have schizophrenia and have not responded to standard antipsychotic treatment; reduction in risk of recurrent suicidal behavior in schizophrenia or schizoaffective disorders

ROUTES AND DOSAGE: Available only in tablet form, 25- and 100-mg doses

Adult Dosage: Initial dose 25 mg PO twice or 4 times daily, may gradually increase in 25–50 mg/d increments, if tolerated, to a dose of 300–450 mg/d by the end of the second week. Additional increases should occur no more than once or twice weekly. Do not exceed 900 mg/d. For maintenance, reduce dosage to lowest effective level

Children: Safety and efficacy with children younger than age 16 years have not been established

HALF-LIFE (PEAK EFFECT): 12 h (1–6 h)

SELECT ADVERSE REACTIONS: Drowsiness, dizziness, headache, hypersalivation, tachycardia, hypo- or hypertension, constipation, dry mouth, heartburn, nausea or vomiting, blurred vision, diaphoresis, fever, weight gain, hematologic changes, seizures, tremor, akathisia

BOXED WARNING: Agranulocytosis, defined as a granulocyte count of <500 mm^3, occurs at about a cumulative 1-year incidence of 1.3%, most often within 4–10 weeks of exposure, but may occur at any time; WBC count before initiation, and weekly WBC counts while taking the drug and for 4 weeks after discontinuation

Seizures, myocarditis, and other adverse cardiovascular and respiratory side effects (i.e., orthostatic hypotension)

WARNING: Increased mortality in elderly patients with dementia-related psychosis; rare development of NMS; *hyperglycemia and DM, tardive dyskinesia*, cases of sudden, unexplained death have been reported; avoid use during pregnancy and while breast-feeding

PRECAUTIONS: Fever, pulmonary embolism, hepatitis, anticholinergic toxicity, and interference with cognitive and motor functions

SPECIFIC PATIENT/FAMILY EDUCATION

- Need informed consent regarding risk for agranulocytosis. Weekly or biweekly blood draws are required. Notify your prescriber immediately if lethargy, weakness, sore throat, malaise, or other flu-like symptoms develop.
- You should not take clozapine if you are taking other medicines that may cause the same serious bone marrow side effects.
- Inform the patient of risk of seizures, hyperglycemia and diabetes, and orthostatic hypotension. It may potentiate the hypotensive effects of antihypertensive drugs and anticholinergic effects of atropine-like drugs.
- Administration of epinephrine should be avoided in the treatment of drug-induced hypotension.
- Notify your prescriber if pregnancy is possible or if you are planning to become pregnant. Do not breastfeed while taking this medication.
- Notify your prescriber before taking any other prescription or OTC medication. Avoid alcohol or other CNS depressant drugs.
- May cause drowsiness and seizures; avoid driving or other hazardous tasks.
- During titration, the individual may experience orthostatic hypotension and so should change positions slowly.
- Do not abruptly discontinue.

CNS, central nervous system; NMS, neuroleptic malignant syndrome; OTC, over-the-counter; WBC, white blood cell.

---

which compounds the patient's fear and anxiety and requires a quick response. The immediate treatment is to administer benztropine 1 to 2 mg, or diphenhydramine (Benadryl), 25 to 50 mg, intramuscularly or intravenously. This is followed by daily administration of anticholinergic drugs and, possibly, by a decrease in dosage antipsychotic medication. See Box 23.11 for more information about benztropine.

BOX 23.10

Research for Best Practice: Families and Medication Use and Adherence Among Latinos

Hernandez, M. & Barrio, C. (2017). Families and medication use and adherence among Latinos with schizophrenia. Journal of Mental Health, 26(1): 14–20.

THE QUESTION: What are the perceptions of treatment related to medication use among Latinos with schizophrenia and key family members?

METHODS: Purposive sampling was used to collect data from a total of 34 participants: 14 dyads (made up of 14 patients and 14 key family members) plus 6 key family members of other patients. These six family members, who were interviewed although the patient was not available, were included to provide additional information about family context. Semistructured interviews were conducted with participants in their preferred language.

FINDINGS: Concerns primarily centered on medication side effects. Patients expressed difficulty with low energy, lack of interest in desired activities, and weight gain, among other issues. Family members also noticed changes in patients' affect and behavior. Moreover, families worried about long-term medication use and its effect on patients' health.

IMPLICATIONS FOR NURSING: Family involvement in medication use is important and contributes to patient choices regarding treatment.

BOX 23.11
Drug Profile: Benztropine Mesylate

DRUG CLASS: Antiparkinsonism agent

RECEPTOR AFFINITY: Blocks cholinergic (acetylcholine) activity, which is believed to restore the balance of acetylcholine and dopamine in the basal ganglia

INDICATIONS: Used in psychiatry to reduce extrapyramidal symptoms (acute medication-related movement disorders), including pseudoparkinsonism, dystonia, and akathisia (but not tardive syndromes) caused by neuroleptic drugs such as haloperidol. Most effective with acute dystonia

ROUTES AND DOSAGE: Available in tablet form, 0.5-, 1-, and 2-mg doses, also injectable 1 mg/mL

Adult Dosage: For acute dystonia, 1–2 mg IM or IV usually provides rapid relief. No significant difference in onset of action after IM or IV injection. Treatment of emergent symptoms may be relieved in 1 or 2 days, with 1–2 mg PO 2–3 times/d. Maximum daily dose is 6 mg/d. After 1–2 weeks, withdraw drug to see if continued treatment is needed. Medication-related movement disorders that develop slowly may not respond to this treatment

Geriatric: Older adults and very thin patients cannot tolerate large doses

Children: Do not use in children younger than 3 years of age. Use with caution in older children

HALF-LIFE: 12–24 h; very little pharmacokinetic information is available

SELECT SIDE EFFECTS: Dry mouth, blurred vision, tachycardia, nausea, constipation, flushing or elevated temperature, decreased sweating, muscular weakness or cramping, urinary retention, urinary hesitancy, dizziness, headache, disorientation, confusion, memory loss, hallucinations, psychoses, and agitation in toxic reactions, which are more pronounced in elderly adults and occur at smaller doses

WARNING: Avoid use during pregnancy and while breast-feeding. Give with caution in hot weather because of possible heatstroke. Contraindicated with angle-closure glaucoma, pyloric or duodenal obstruction, stenosing peptic ulcers, prostatic hypertrophy or bladder neck obstructions, myasthenia gravis, megacolon, and megaesophagus. May aggravate the symptoms of tardive dyskinesia and other chronic forms of medication-related movement disorder. Concomitant use of other anticholinergic drugs may increase side effects and risk for toxicity. Coadministration of haloperidol or phenothiazines may reduce serum levels of these drugs

SPECIFIC PATIENT/FAMILY EDUCATION
- Take with meals to reduce dry mouth and gastric irritation.
- Dry mouth may also be alleviated by sucking sugarless candies, maintaining adequate fluid intake, and good oral hygiene; increase fiber and fluids in diet to avoid constipation; stool softeners may be required. Notify your prescriber if urinary hesitancy or constipation persists.
- Notify your prescriber if rapid or pounding heartbeat, confusion, eye pain, rash, or other side effects develop.
- May cause drowsiness, dizziness, or blurred vision; use caution driving or performing other hazardous tasks requiring alertness. Avoid alcohol and other CNS depressants.
- Do not abruptly stop this medication because a flu-like syndrome may develop.
- Use with caution in hot weather. Ensure adequate hydration. May increase susceptibility to heat stroke.

CNS, central nervous system; IM, intramuscular; IV, intravenous; PO, oral.

Akathisia appears to be caused by the same biologic mechanism as other extrapyramidal side effects. Patients are restless and report they feel driven to keep moving. They are extremely uncomfortable. Frequently, this response is misinterpreted as anxiety or increased psychotic symptoms, so that the patient may inappropriately be given increased dosages of an antipsychotic drug, which only perpetuates the side effect. If possible, the dose of antipsychotic drug should be reduced. A β-adrenergic blocker such as propranolol (Inderal), 20 to 120 mg, may be required. An anticholinergic medication may not be helpful. Failure to manage this side effect is a leading cause of patients ceasing to take antipsychotic medications (see Chapter 11).

Tardive dyskinesia, *tardive dystonia*, and *tardive akathisia* are less likely but still possible to appear in individuals taking second-generation, rather than first-generation, antipsychotics. Table 23.2 describes these and associated motor abnormalities. Tardive dyskinesia is late-appearing abnormal involuntary movements. It can be viewed as the opposite of parkinsonism both in observable movements and in etiology. Whereas muscle rigidity and absence of movement characterize parkinsonism, constant movement characterizes tardive dyskinesia. Typical movements involve the mouth, tongue, and jaw and include lip smacking, sucking, puckering, tongue protrusion, the "bonbon sign" (where the tongue rolls around in the mouth and protrudes into the cheek as if the patient is sucking on a piece of hard candy), athetoid (worm-like) movements of the tongue, and chewing. Other facial movements, such as grimacing and eye blinking, may also be present.

Movements in the trunk and limbs are frequently observable with tardive dyskinesia. These include rocking from the hips, athetoid movements of the fingers and toes, jerking movements of the fingers and toes, guitar strumming movements of the fingers, and foot tapping. The long-term health problems for people with tardive dyskinesia are choking associated with loss of control of muscles used for swallowing and compromised respiratory function leading to infections and possibly respiratory alkalosis.

Because the movements resemble the dyskinetic movements of some patients who have idiopathic Parkinson disease and who have received long-term treatment with L-DOPA (a direct-acting dopamine agonist that crosses the blood–brain barrier), the suggested hypothesis for tardive dyskinesia includes the supersensitivity of the dopamine receptors in the basal ganglia.

An effective treatment for tardive dyskinesia has been elusive. However, antipsychotic drugs mask the movements of tardive dyskinesia and have periodically been suggested as a treatment. This is counterintuitive because these drugs cause the disorder. Second-generation antipsychotic drugs, such as clozapine, may be less likely to

TABLE 23.2 EXTRAPYRAMIDAL SIDE EFFECTS OF ANTIPSYCHOTIC DRUGS

Side Effect	Period of Onset	Symptoms
Acute Motor Abnormalities		
Parkinsonism or pseudoparkinsonism	5–30 d	Resting tremor, rigidity, bradykinesia or akinesia, mask-like face, shuffling gait, decreased arm swing
Acute dystonia	1–5 d	Intermittent or fixed abnormal postures of the eyes, face, tongue, neck, trunk, and limbs
Akathisia	1–30 d	Obvious motor restlessness evidenced by pacing, rocking, shifting from foot to foot; subjective sense of not being able to sit or be still; these symptoms may occur together or separately
Late-Appearing Motor Abnormalities		
Tardive dyskinesia	Months to years	Abnormal dyskinetic movements of the face, mouth, and jaw; choreoathetoid movements of the legs, arms, and trunk
Tardive dystonia	Months to years	Persistent sustained abnormal postures in the face, eyes, tongue, neck, trunk, and limbs
Tardive akathisia	Months to years	Persistent unabating sense of subjective and objective restlessness

Adapted from Ferrando, S. J., Owen, J. A., Levenson, J. L. (2014). Psychopharmacology. In R. E. Hales, S. C. Ydofsky, & L. W. Roberts (Eds.). *The American Psychiatric Publishing Textbook of Psychiatry* (6th ed.). Arlington, VA: American Psychiatric Association. http://psychiatryonline.org/doi/full/10.1176/appi.books.9781585625031.rh27

cause it; however, recent interest suggests that the tardive dyskinesia is still prevalent but at a lesser rate (Misdrahi et al., 2019). Recently the medications deutetrabenazine and valbenazine have been approved by the FDA that appear to ameliorate the movements of tardive dyskinesia by decreasing the transport of dopamine to the synaptic cleft (via inhibition of vesicular monoamine transporter 2—VMAT2) (Ricciardi et al., 2019). However, the best management remains prevention through using the lowest possible dose of an antipsychotic drug over time that minimizes the symptoms of schizophrenia as well as regular evaluation of movements using tools like the DISCUS.

Monitoring Other Side Effects

Orthostatic hypotension is a common side effect of antipsychotic drugs. Primarily an antiadrenergic effect, decreased blood pressure may be generalized or orthostatic. Patients may be protected from falls by teaching them to rise slowly and by monitoring blood pressure before giving the medication. The nurse should monitor and document lying, sitting, and standing blood pressures when any antipsychotic drug therapy begins.

Hyperprolactinemia can occur. When dopamine is blocked in the tuberoinfundibular tract, it can no longer repress prolactin, the neurohormone that regulates lactation and mammary function. The prolactin level increases and, in some individuals, side effects appear. Gynecomastia (i.e., enlarged breasts) can occur in people of both sexes and is understandably distressing to individuals who may be experiencing delusional or hallucinatory body image disturbances. Galactorrhea (i.e., lactation) may also occur. Menstrual irregularities and sexual dysfunction are possible. If these symptoms appear, the medication should be reduced or changed to another antipsychotic agent. Hyperprolactinemia is associated with the use of haloperidol and risperidone.

Sedation is another possible side effect of antipsychotic medication and a frequent reason that patients discontinue medications. Patients should be monitored for the sedating effects of antipsychotic agents. In elderly patients, sedation can be associated with falls.

Weight gain is related to antipsychotic agents, especially olanzapine and clozapine. Patients may gain as much as 20 or 30 lb within 1 year. Such increased appetite and weight gain are distressing to patients. Diet teaching and monitoring may have some effect. Another solution is to increase the accessibility of healthful easy-to-prepare food. Simple exercise routines may be helpful.

New-onset DM should be assessed in patients taking antipsychotic drugs. An association has been found between new-onset DM and the administration of second-generation antipsychotic agents, especially after weight gain. Patients should be monitored for clinical symptoms of diabetes. Fasting blood glucose tests and hemoglobin A1C monitoring are commonly ordered for these individuals.

Cardiac arrhythmias may also occur. Prolongation of the QTc interval is associated with torsade de pointe (polymorphic ventricular tachycardia) or ventricular fibrillation. The potential for drug-induced prolonged QT interval is associated with many drugs. Ziprasidone (Geodon) is more likely than other second-generation antipsychotics to prolong the QT interval and thus change the heart rhythm. For these patients, baseline electrocardiograms may be ordered. Nurses should observe these patients for cardiac arrhythmias.

Agranulocytosis is a reduction in the number of circulating granulocytes and decreased production of granulocytes in the bone marrow, which limits one's ability to fight infection. Agranulocytosis can develop with the use of all antipsychotic drugs, but it is most likely to develop with clozapine use. Although laboratory values below 500 cells/mm^3 are indicative of agranulocytosis, often granulocyte counts drop to below 200 cells/mm^3 with this syndrome.

Patients taking clozapine should have regular blood tests. White blood cell and granulocyte counts should be measured before treatment is initiated and at least weekly or twice weekly after treatment begins. Initial white blood cell counts should be above 3,500 cells/mm^3 before treatment initiation; in patients with counts of 3,500 and 5,000 cells/mm^3, cell counts should be monitored three times a week if clozapine is prescribed. Any time the white blood cell count drops below 3,500 cells/mm^3 or granulocytes drop below 1,500 cells/mm^3, use of clozapine should be stopped, and the patient should be monitored for infection.

However, a faithfully implemented program of blood monitoring should not replace careful observation of the patient. It is not unusual for blood cell counts to drop precipitously over a period of 2 to 3 days. This may not be discovered when the patient is on a strict weekly blood monitoring schedule. Any reported symptoms that suggest a bacterial infection (e.g., fever, pharyngitis, weakness) should be cause for concern, so immediate evaluation of blood count status should be undertaken. Because patients are frequently discharged before the critical period of risk for agranulocytosis, patient education about these symptoms is also essential so that they will report these symptoms, obtain blood monitoring, and reduce their potential exposure to infections. In general, granulocyte levels return to normal within 2 to 4 weeks after discontinuation of use of the medication.

DRESS is a very rare, potentially life-threatening, drug-induced hypersensitivity reaction recently associated with ziprasidone therapy (Geodon). The FDA published a safety announcement related to ziprasidone's association to DRESS. Symptoms include skin eruption, hematologic abnormalities (e.g., eosinophilia, atypical lymphocytosis), lymphadenopathy, and internal organ involvement (e.g., liver, kidney, lung). DRESS has a mortality rate of 10% (U.S. Food and Drug Administration, 08/2015).

Preventing Drug–Drug Interactions

Antipsychotic medications have the potential to interact with other medications, nicotine, and grapefruit juice. For example, olanzapine and clozapine have the potential to interact with some antidepressants. Some antipsychotics are metabolized faster in smokers than nonsmokers (Huang, 2016). Conversely, problems with increased side effects from slower drug metabolism can occur when smoking cessation programs are initiated. Before giving a medication, the nurse should check all medications for potential interactions.

Teaching Points

Nonadherence to the medication regimen is an important factor in relapse; the family must be made aware of the importance of the patient's taking medications consistently. Medication education should cover the association between medications and the amelioration of symptoms, side effects and their management, and interpersonal skills that help the patient and family report medication effects.

Management of Complications

Neuroleptic Malignant Syndrome. Neuroleptic malignant syndrome (NMS) is a life-threatening condition that can develop in reaction to antipsychotic medications. The primary symptoms of NMS are: *mental status changes*, *severe muscle rigidity*, and *autonomic changes* including elevated temperature (usually between 101° and 103°F), tachycardia, and blood pressure lability. Mental status changes and severe muscle rigidity occur usually within the first week of initiation of antipsychotic therapy and can include two or more of the following: hypertension, tachycardia, tachypnea, prominent diaphoresis, incontinence, mutism, leukocytosis, and laboratory evidence of muscle injury (e.g., elevated creatinine phosphokinase). The incidence of NMS has decreased from 3% to 0.16%, probably because of increased awareness of symptoms, use of atypical antipsychotics and earlier interventions such as stopping the offending medication (Schneider et al., 2018). As many as 5 to 15% of affected patients may die as a result of the syndrome. In the past, NMS was probably underreported and may have accounted for unexplained emergency department deaths of patients taking these drugs because their symptoms did not seem serious.

The most important aspects of nursing care for patients with NMS relate to recognizing symptoms early, withholding any antipsychotic or any other dopamine antagonist (e.g., gastric reflux medications), and initiating supportive nursing care (Fig. 23.4). In any patient with muscle rigidity, fluctuating vital signs, abrupt changes in levels of consciousness, or any of the symptoms presented in Box 23.12, NMS should be suspected. The nurse should be especially alert for early signs and symptoms of NMS in high-risk patients, such as those who are agitated, physically exhausted, or dehydrated or who have an existing medical or neurologic illness. Patients receiving parenteral or higher doses of

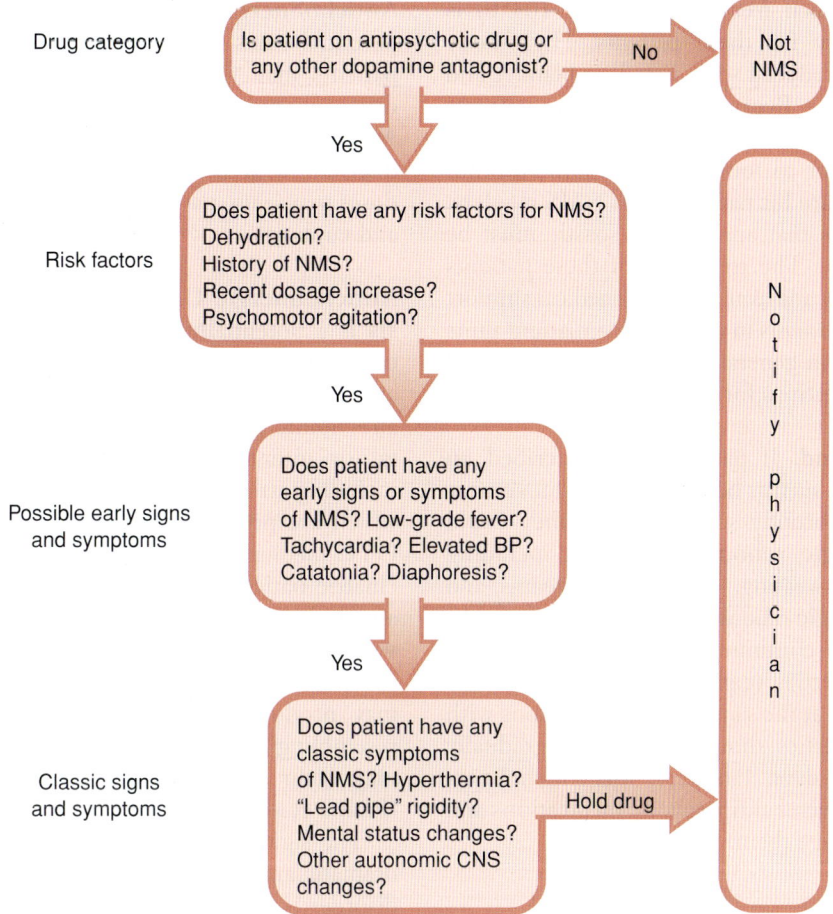

FIGURE 23.4 Action tree for "holding" an antipsychotic drug because of suspected neuroleptic malignant syndrome.

BOX 23.12

Recognizing Neuroleptic Malignant Syndrome

Onset: 2 weeks after initiation of antipsychotic treatment or change in dosage
Risk factors: Male gender, pre-existing medical or neurologic disorders, depot injection administration, and high ambient temperature

IMMINENT INDICATORS
- Mental status changes
- Muscle rigidity
- Hyperthermia
- Tachycardia
- Hypertension or hypotension
- Tachypnea or hypoxia
- Diaphoresis or sialorrhea
- Tremor
- Incontinence
- Creatinine phosphokinase elevation or myoglobinuria
- Leukocytosis
- Metabolic acidosis

Source: Neuroleptic malignant syndrome. https://rarediseases.org/rare-diseases/neuroleptic-malignant-syndrome/. Retrieved April 8, 2019.

---

neuroleptic drugs or lithium concurrently must also be carefully assessed. The nurse should carefully monitor fluid intake, and fluid and electrolyte status.

NCLEXNOTE Recognition of side effects, including movement disorders, tardive dyskinesia, and weight gain, should lead to interventions. NMS is a medical emergency.

Medical treatment focuses on symptom management and includes administering dopamine agonist drugs, such as bromocriptine (modest success), and muscle relaxants, such as dantrolene or benzodiazepine. Antiparkinsonism drugs are not particularly useful. Some patients experience improvement with electroconvulsive therapy (ECT).

The nurse must frequently monitor vital signs of the patient with symptoms of NMS. In addition, it is important to check the results of the patient's laboratory tests for increased creatine phosphokinase, an elevated white blood cell count, elevated liver enzymes, or myoglobinuria. The nurse must be prepared to initiate supportive measures or anticipate emergency transfer of the patient to a medical–surgical or an intensive care unit.

Treating fever (which frequently exceeds 103°F) is an important priority for these patients. High body temperature may be reduced with a cooling blanket and acetaminophen therapy. Because many of these patients experience diaphoresis, temperature elevation, or dysphagia, it is important to monitor hydration. Another important aspect of care for patients with NMS is safety. Joints and extremities that are rigid or spastic must be protected from injury. The treatment of these patients depends on the facility and availability of medical support services. In general, patients in psychiatric inpatient units that are separated from general hospitals are transferred to medical–surgical settings for treatment.

Cholinergic Rebound. If patients are prescribed an anticholinergic agent, such as benztropine, for movement disorders and they abruptly stop taking it, they could experience **cholinergic rebound** symptoms including vomiting, excessive sweating, and altered dreams and nightmares. Cholinergic rebound can be especially problematic if patients discontinue other medications with anticholinergic properties (e.g., antipsychotics, antidepressants, antibiotics) at the same time. Medications with anticholinergic properties should be reduced gradually (tapered) over several days. Table 23.3 lists anticholinergic side effects and several antipsychotic medications and interventions to manage them.

Anticholinergic Medication Effects and Abuse. The potential exists for abuse of anticholinergic drugs. Some patients may find the anticholinergic effects of these drugs on mood, memory, and perception pleasurable. Although at toxic dosages patients may experience a mild delirium with disorientation and hallucinations, lesser doses may cause patients to experience greater sociability and euphoria.

Anticholinergic Crisis. An **anticholinergic crisis** is a potentially life-threatening medical emergency caused by an overdose of or sensitivity to drugs with anticholinergic properties. This syndrome (also called anticholinergic delirium) may result from an accidental or intentional overdose of anticholinergic drugs, including atropine, scopolamine, or belladonna alkaloids, which are present in numerous prescription drugs and OTC medicines. The syndrome may also occur in psychiatric patients who are receiving therapeutic doses of anticholinergic drugs but who are also taking other drugs with anticholinergic properties. As a result of either drug overdose or sensitivity, these anticholinergic substances may produce acute delirium or a psychotic reaction resembling schizophrenia. Severe anticholinergic effects may occur in older patients, even at therapeutic levels (Pasina et al., 2019).

The signs and symptoms of anticholinergic crisis are dramatic and physically uncomfortable (Box 23.13). This disorder is characterized by fever; parched mouth; burning thirst; hot dry skin; decreased salivation; decreased bronchial and nasal secretions; widely dilated eyes (bright light becomes painful); decreased ability to accommodate visually; increased heart rate; constipation; difficulty urinating; and hypertension or hypotension. The face, neck, and upper arms may become flushed because of a reflexive blood vessel dilation. In addition to peripheral symptoms, patients with anticholinergic psychosis may experience neuropsychiatric symptoms of anxiety, agitation, delirium, hyperactivity, confusion, hallucinations (especially visual), speech difficulties, psychotic symptoms, or seizures.

TABLE 23.3 NURSING INTERVENTIONS FOR ANTICHOLINERGIC SIDE EFFECTS

Effect	Intervention
Dry mouth	Provide sips of water, hard candies, and chewing gum (preferably sugar free)
Blurred vision	Avoid dangerous tasks; teach patient that this side effect will diminish in a few weeks
Decreased lacrimation	Use artificial tears if necessary
Mydriasis	May aggravate glaucoma; teach patient to report eye pain
Photophobia	Wear sunglasses
Constipation	High-fiber diet; increased fluid intake; take laxatives as prescribed
Urinary hesitancy	Privacy; run water in sink; warm water over perineum
Urinary retention	Regular voiding (at least every 2–3 h) and whenever urge is present; catheterize for residual urine; record intake and output; evaluate for benign prostatic hypertrophy
Tachycardia	Evaluate for pre-existing cardiovascular disease

BOX 23.13

Signs and Symptoms of Anticholinergic Crisis

- **Neuropsychiatric signs:** confusion; recent memory loss; agitation; dysarthria; incoherent speech; pressured speech; delusions; ataxia; periods of hyperactivity alternating with somnolence, paranoia, anxiety, or coma
- **Hallucinations:** accompanied by "picking," plucking, or grasping motions; delusions; or disorientation
- **Physical signs:** nonreactive dilated pupils; blurred vision; hot, dry, flushed skin; facial flushing; dry mucous membranes; difficulty swallowing; fever; tachycardia; hypertension; decreased bowel sounds; urinary retention; nausea; vomiting; seizures; or coma

The acute psychotic reaction that is produced resembles schizophrenia. The classic description of anticholinergic crisis is summarized in the following mnemonic: "Hot as a hare, blind as a bat, mad as a hatter, dry as a bone."

In general, episodes of anticholinergic crisis are self-limiting, usually subsiding in 3 days. However, if left untreated, the associated fever and delirium may progress to coma or cardiac and respiratory depression. Although rare, death is generally caused by hyperpyrexia and brain stem depression. After use of the offending drug is discontinued, improvement usually occurs within 24 to 36 hours.

A specific and effective antidote, physostigmine, a reversible inhibitor of cholinesterase, is frequently used to treat and diagnose anticholinergic crisis. Administration of this drug rapidly reduces both behavioral and physiologic symptoms. However, the usual adult dose of physostigmine is 1 to 2 mg intravenously given slowly during a period of 5 minutes because rapid injection of physostigmine may cause seizures, profound bradycardia, or heart block. Physostigmine is relatively short acting, so it may need to be given several times during the course of treatment. This drug provides relief from symptoms for a period of 2 to 3 hours. In addition to receiving physostigmine, patients who intentionally overdose on large amounts of anticholinergic drugs are treated by gastric lavage, administration of charcoal, and catharsis. The dose may be given again after 20 or 30 minutes.

It is important for the nurse to be alert for signs and symptoms of anticholinergic crisis, especially in elderly and pediatric patients, who are much more sensitive to the anticholinergic effects of drugs, and in patients who are receiving multiple medications with anticholinergic effects. If signs and symptoms of the syndrome occur, the nurse should discontinue use of the offending drug and notify the physician immediately.

Electroconvulsive Therapy

ECT is suggested as a possible alternative when the patient's schizophrenia is not being successfully treated by medication alone. For the most part, this modality is not indicated unless the patient is catatonic or has depression that is not treatable by other means. In general, ECT is not used often for the treatment of schizophrenia, but it may be useful for those persons who are medication resistant, assaultive, and psychotic (Ward, Szabo, Rakesh, 2018).

Psychosocial Interventions

Psychosocial interventions, such as counseling, conflict resolution, behavior therapy, and cognitive interventions, are appropriate for patients with schizophrenia. The following discussion focuses on applying these interventions.

Therapeutic Interactions

Although antipsychotic medications may relieve positive symptoms, they do not always eliminate hallucinations and delusions. The nurse must continue helping the patient develop creative strategies for dealing with these sensory and thought disturbances. Information about the content of the hallucinations and delusions is necessary, not only to determine whether the medications are effective but also to assess safety and the meaning of these thoughts and perceptions to the patient. In caring for a patient who is experiencing hallucinations or delusions, nursing actions should be guided by three general patient outcomes:

- Decrease the frequency and intensity of hallucinations and delusions.
- Recognize that hallucinations and delusions are symptoms of a brain disorder.
- Develop strategies to manage the recurrence of hallucinations or delusions.

When interacting with a patient who is experiencing hallucinations or delusions, the nurse must remember that these experiences are real to the patient. It is important for the nurse to understand the content and meaning of the hallucinations, particularly those involving command hallucinations.

The nurse should never tell a patient that these experiences are not real. Discounting the experiences blocks communication. On the other hand, it is also dishonest for the nurse to tell the patient that the nurse is having the same hallucinatory experience. It is best to validate the patient's experiences and identify the meaning of these thoughts and feelings to the patient. For example, a patient who believes that he or she is under surveillance by the Federal Bureau of Investigation probably feels frightened and suspicious of everyone. By acknowledging how frightening it must be to always feel like you are being watched, the nurse focuses on the feelings that are generated by the delusion, not the delusion itself. The nurse can then offer to help the patient feel safe within this environment. The patient, in turn, begins to feel that someone understands him or her.

Enhancing Cognitive Functioning

After identifying deficits in cognitive functioning, the nurse and patient can develop interventions that target specific deficits. The most effective interventions usually involve the whole treatment team. If the ability to focus or maintain attention is an issue, patients can be encouraged to select activities that improve attention, such as computer games. For memory problems, patients can be encouraged to make lists and to write down important information.

Executive functioning problems are the most challenging for these patients. Patients who cannot manage daily problems may have planning and problem-solving impairments. For these patients, developing interventions that closely simulate real-world problems may help. Through coaching, the nurse can teach and support the development of problem-solving skills. For example, during hospitalizations, patients are given medications and reminded to take them on time. They are often instructed in a classroom setting but rarely have an opportunity to practice self-medication and figure out what to do if their prescription expires, the medications are lost, or they forget to take their medications. Even so, when discharged, patients are expected to take medication at the prescribed dose at the prescribed time. Interventions designed to have patients actively engage in problem-solving behavior with real problems are needed.

Other approaches to helping patients solve problems and learn new strategies for dealing with problems include solution-focused therapy, which focuses on the strengths and positive attributes that exist within each person, and cognitive behavioral therapy (Jones et al., 2019), which focuses directly on collaboratively determined symptoms and strategies to address them. These therapies involve years of training to master, but certain techniques can be used. For example, the nurse can ask patients to identify the most important problem from their perspective. This focuses the patient on an important issue for him or her.

Using Behavioral Interventions

Behavioral interventions can be very effective in helping patients improve motivation and organize routine, daily activities, such as maintaining a regular schedule and completing activities. Reinforcement of positive behaviors (getting up on time, completing hygiene, going to treatment activities) can easily be included in a treatment plan. In the hospital, patients gain unit privileges by following an agreed-on treatment plan. In the community, a behavioral intervention is more likely to be combined with other approaches or used for a specific behavior such as smoking (Wilson, 2019).

Psychoeducation

Teaching Strategies

Cognitive deficits (e.g., difficulty in processing complex information, maintaining steady focus of attention, distinguishing between relevant and irrelevant stimuli, and forming abstractions), may challenge the nurse planning educational activities. Evidence indicates that people with schizophrenia may learn best in an errorless learning environment (Kern et al., 2018). That is, they are directly given correct information and then encouraged to write it down. Errorless learning is an educational intervention based on the principle of operant conditioning that learning is stronger and more likely to last if it occurs in the absence of errors. Asking questions that encourage guessing is not as effective in helping patients retain information. Trial-and-error learning is avoided.

Teaching and explaining should occur in an environment with minimal distractions. Terminology should be clear and unambiguous. Visual aids can supplement verbal information, but these materials should have simple information stated in simple language. The nurse takes care not to overcrowd the visual material or incorporate images that draw attention away from important content. Teaching should occur in small segments with frequent reinforcement. Most importantly, teaching should occur when the patient is ready. Regular assessments of cognitive abilities with standardized instruments can help determine this readiness. These suggestions can be adapted for teaching during any phase of the illness.

Teaching About Symptoms

Teaching patients that hallucinations and delusions are part of the disorder becomes easier after the medication begins working. When patients believe and acknowledge that they have a mental illness and that some of their thoughts are delusions and some of their perceptions are hallucinations, they can develop strategies to manage their symptoms.

Patients benefit greatly by learning recovery strategies of self-regulation, symptom monitoring, and relapse prevention. By monitoring events, time, place, and stimuli surrounding the appearance of symptoms, the patient can begin to predict high-risk times for symptom recurrence. Cognitive behavioral therapy is often used in helping patients monitor and identify their emerging symptoms to prevent relapse (Liu, Yang, Gillespie, Guo, et al., 2019).

Another important nursing intervention is to help the patient identify to whom and where to talk about delusional or hallucinatory material. Because self-disclosure of these symptoms immediately labels someone as having a mental illness, patients should be encouraged to evaluate the environment for negative consequences of disclosing these symptoms. For example, it may be fine to talk about it at home but not at the grocery store.

Teaching How to Cope With Stress

Developing skills to cope with personal, social, and environmental stresses is important to everyone but particularly to those with a severe mental illness. Stresses can easily trigger symptoms that patients are trying to avoid. Establishing regular counseling sessions to support the development of positive coping skills is helpful for both hospitalized patients and those living in the community.

Social Skills Training

Social skills training, provided either individually or in groups, is also useful when working with patients who have schizophrenia (Vogel et al., 2019). This training teaches patients specific behaviors needed for social interactions. The skills are taught by lecture, demonstration, role-playing, and homework assignments. Nurses may be team members and be involved in case management or provision of services. Furthermore, efforts to offer supportive employment experiences (Carmona, Gómez-Benito, Rojo-Rodes, 2019) that incorporate patient preferences, rapid job search and employment, and ongoing job supports have shown effectiveness. Although long-term self-sufficiency has not necessarily been achieved, supportive employment has been the most effective vocational rehabilitation method.

Skill-training interventions should be designed to compensate for cognitive deficits. To help patients learn to process complex activities, such as catching a bus, preparing a meal, or shopping for food or clothing, nurses should break the activity into small parts or steps and list them for the patient's reference, for example:

- Leave your apartment with your keys in hand.
- Make sure you have correct bus fare in your pocket.
- Close the door.
- Walk to the corner.
- Turn right and walk three blocks to the bus stop.

Concept Mastery Alert

If the patient has active psychosis, with symptoms such as hallucinations and social withdrawal, wait until a lucid period to begin social skills training. When a patient is in active psychosis, it is not a good time to introduce additional stressors.

Providing Family Education

Because having a family member with schizophrenia is a life-changing event for the family and friends who provide care and support, educating patients and their families is crucial. It is a primary concern for the psychiatric–mental health nurse. Family support is crucial to help patients maintain treatment. Education should include information about the disease course, treatment regimens, support systems, and life management skills (Box 23.14). The most important factor to stress during patient and family education is the consistent taking of medication.

BOX 23.14

Psychoeducation Checklist: Schizophrenia

When caring for the patient with schizophrenia, be sure to include the caregiver during planning as appropriate and address the following topic areas in the teaching plan:
- Psychopharmacologic agents, including drug action, dosage, frequency, and possible side effects; stress the importance of adherence to the prescribed regimen
- Management of hallucinations
- Recovery strategies
- Coping strategies (e.g., self-talk, getting busy with something)
- Management of the environment
- Community resources

Promoting Patient Safety

Although violence is not a consistent behavior of people with schizophrenia, it is always a concern during the initial phase when hallucinations or delusions may put patients at risk for harming themselves or others. Nonviolent patients who are experiencing hallucinations and delusions can also be at risk for victimization by more aggressive patients. The patient who is hallucinating needs to be protected, which may include increased staff monitoring and, if necessary, a safer environment in a secluded area.

Identifying patient risk factors for violence, such as a history of violence, can alert the nursing staff of a potential for engaging in aggressive behavior, but careful assessment and management of the immediate environment and treating the psychiatric symptoms are more important in avoiding aggression. The nurse's best approach to avoiding violence or aggression is to demonstrate respect for the patient and the patient's personal space, assess and monitor for signs of fear and agitation, and use preventive interventions before the patient loses control. Patients should be encouraged to discuss their anger and to be involved in their treatment decisions. Medications should be administered as ordered. Because most antipsychotic and antidepressant medications take 1 to 2 weeks to begin moderating behavior, the nurse must be vigilant during the acute illness.

If the patient loses control and is a danger to self or others, restraints and seclusion may be used as a last resort. Health Care Financing Administration (HCFA) guidelines and hospital policy must be followed (see Chapter 3), and staff should be trained in the proper use of seclusion and restraints. In addition, staff need to have planned sessions after all incidents of violence or physical management to analyze the event. These sessions allow clinicians to learn how better to manage these situations and evaluate patients' cues. With sensitive leadership, these sessions can help health care workers to learn more about the interaction of patient and staff characteristics that can contribute to these incidents.

Convening Support Groups

People with mental illness benefit from support groups that focus on daily problems and the stress of dealing with a mental illness. These groups are useful throughout the continuum of care and help reduce the risk of suicide. In the hospital setting, the focus of the group can be simply sharing the experience of living with a mental illness. In the community, a regular support group can provide interaction with people with similar problems and issues. Friendships often develop from these groups. Using peer counseling and support groups is a component of recovery-oriented care, but research is needed to understand these groups' impact on care (Chien, Clifton, Zhao, & Lui, 2019).

Implementing Milieu Therapy

Individuals with schizophrenia may be hospitalized or may live in group homes for a long period of time. The challenge is helping people who are unable to live with family members to live harmoniously with strangers who have similar interpersonal difficulties. Arranging the treatment environment to maximize therapy is crucial to the rehabilitation of the patient.

Developing Recovery-Oriented Rehabilitation Strategies

Rehabilitation strategies are used to support the individual's recovery and integration into the community. See Box 23.15. Factors that have been shown to promote recovery include:

- Adjustment, coping, and reappraisal
- Responding to the illness
- Social support, close relationships, and belonging

Factors that have a negative impact on the process of recovery include: (1) negative interactions and isolation, (2) internal barriers, and (3) uncertainty and hopelessness (Soundy, et al., 2015).

Community-based psychosocial rehabilitation programs usually offer long-term intensive case management services to adults with schizophrenia. Programs provide a continuum of services to meet the changing needs of people with psychiatric disabilities. Patients set rehabilitation goals and services are then provided to help "clients" (most programs do not use the term "patients") reach their goals. Services range from daily home visits to providing transportation, occupational training and supported employment, and group support.

> **BOX 23.15**
>
> **A Brother's Perspective**
>
> A sibling describes his brother with schizophrenia and the importance of both medications and relationships.
>
> In 1998, at the age of 40 years, Robert was admitted to a psychiatric hospital. His brother was told at the time that he would never be able to live independently, and even if discharged, would only be repeatedly hospitalized. Robert had a long history of treatment and in 1998 he had received various types of antipsychotic medications, but he had not received any of the "new atypical variety." He was prescribed one of these drugs, and within months, the staff who had predicted the most discouraging of outcomes told Robert's brother that he was in the midst of a miraculous recovery—his thinking was clear and free from delusions and they were preparing Robert's discharge.
>
> A few weeks into the discharge planning, Robert called his brother; Robert was distressed because his social worker, whom Robert had known for years from a prior hospitalization, was leaving. The social worker had been abruptly transferred to another hospital. Robert deteriorated rapidly into tantrums, hallucinations, and dangerous behaviors. His discharge was put on hold. Robert's brother's rhetorical question was, "What was the difference between Robert on the same medication on Monday, when he was all right, and Tuesday, when he no longer was?" His answer to Robert's condition caused the loss of an important relationship.
>
> Robert is now living in a community-based home where the dedicated staff members have shown that they can maintain rehospitalization rates below 3%.
>
> Robert's brother has interviewed many former psychiatric patients for a book. He found that every one of his interviewees, while attributing their recovery to medications or finding God, or a particular program, also identified an important relationship with one human being who believed in their ability to recover. Most of the time, this person was a professional, such as a social worker, a nurse, or a doctor. Sometimes, however, it was a member of the clergy or family member. A believing relationship….
>
> Robert's brother concluded, "Let's provide a range of medications, and let's study their effectiveness, but let's remember that the pill is the ultimate downsizing. Let's find resources to give people afflicted with mental illness what all of us need: fellow human beings upon whom we can depend to help us through our dark times and, once through, to emerge into gloriously imperfect lives."
>
> For nurses, it is important to remember that it is not what we do *to* people, but rather, what we do *with* people: give hope, listen to their dreams, help them find ways to get as close as they can.
>
> Adapted from Neugeboren, J. (2006). Meds alone couldn't bring Robert back. *Newsweek*, from http://www.power2u.org/articles/recovery/meds.html. Retrieved April 6, 2019.

Assertive community treatment (ACT) is one example of these types of services and has a solid base of evidence to support its use (Aagaard, Tuszewski, Kølbæk, 2017).

Evaluation and Treatment Outcomes

Outcome research related to schizophrenia has redefined previous ways of thinking about the course of the disorder. Schizophrenia was formerly considered to have a progressively long-term and downward course, but it is now known that schizophrenia can be successfully treated and managed (Vita & Barlati, 2018). In one older but significant study, the researchers interviewed patients 20 to 25 years after diagnosis and found that 50% to 66% experienced significant improvement or recovery (Harding, Zubin, & Strauss, 1987). This study is important because it occurred before the development of second-generation antipsychotic agents. Today, we can be hopeful that even more people can experience improvement or recover from schizophrenia.

Continuum of Care

Continuity of care has been identified as a primary strategy for recovery because individuals with schizophrenia are at risk for becoming "lost" to services if left alone after discharge. Discharge planning encourages follow-up care in the community. In fact, many state mental health systems require an outpatient appointment before discharge. Treatment of people with schizophrenia occurs across a variety of settings. Not only inpatient hospitalization but also partial hospitalization, day treatment, and crisis stabilization can be used effectively.

Emergency Care

Emergency care ideally takes place in a hospital emergency department, but often the crisis occurs in the home. Patients are usually relapsing and do not recognize their bizarre or aggressive behaviors as symptoms. A specially trained crisis team is sent to assess the emergency and recommend further treatment. In the emergency department, patients are brought not only because of relapse but also because of medication side effects or water intoxication. Nurses should refer to the previous discussion for nursing management.

Inpatient-Focused Care

Inpatient hospitalizations are brief and focus on stabilization. Many times, patients are involuntarily admitted for a short period (see Chapter 3). During the stabilization period, the status is changed to voluntary admission, whereby the patient agrees to treatment.

Community Care

Most of the care of persons with schizophrenia is provided in the community through publicly supported recovery-oriented mental health delivery systems. The recovery journey can be long and require a variety of services such as ACT; outpatient therapy; case management; and psychosocial rehabilitation, including clubhouse programs. While the patient is in the community, his or her health care should be integrated with physical health care. Nurses should be especially vigilant that patients with mental illnesses receive proper primary and medical health care.

> **NCLEXNOTE** Priorities in the patient with acute symptoms of schizophrenia include managing psychosis and keeping the patient safe and free from harming him- or herself or others. In the community, the priorities are preventing relapse, maintaining psychosocial functioning, engaging in psychoeducation, improving quality of life, and instilling hope.

In some cases, it is not the disorder itself that threatens the mental health of the person with schizophrenia but the stresses of trying to receive care and services. Health care systems are complex and are often at the mercy of outdated policies. Development of assertiveness and conflict resolution skills can help the person in negotiating access to systems that will provide services. Developing a positive support system for stressful periods helps promote a positive outcome.

SCHIZOAFFECTIVE DISORDER

SAD, a complex and persistent psychiatric illness, is one of the schizophrenia spectrum disorders. SAD is characterized by periods of intense symptom exacerbation alternating with periods of adequate psychosocial functioning. This disorder is at times marked by psychosis; at other times, by mood disturbance. When psychosis and mood disturbance occur at the same time, a diagnosis of SAD is made (APA, 2013). Patients with SAD are more likely to exhibit persistent psychosis than are patients with a mood disorder. They feel that they are on a "chronic roller coaster ride" of symptoms that are often difficult to manage.

The long-term outcome of SAD is generally better than that of schizophrenia but worse than that of mood disorder. These patients resemble the mood disorder group in work function (see Chapter 21) and the schizophrenia group in social function. Persons with SAD usually have higher functioning than those with schizophrenia with severe negative symptoms and early onset of illness (Vardaxi, Gonda, Fountoulakis, 2018).

Patients with SAD are at risk for suicide. The risk for suicide in patients with psychosis is increased by the presence of depression. Risk factors for suicide increase with the use of alcohol or substances, cigarette smoking, previous suicide attempts and hospitalizations. Lack of regular social contact may be a factor that confers a long-term risk for suicidal behavior. This risk may be reduced by treatments designed to enhance social networks and contacts, and those focused on helping patients protect themselves against environmental stressors (Simon et al., 2019).

DELUSIONAL DISORDER

Delusional disorder is another schizophrenia spectrum disorder that is characterized by stable and well-systematized delusions that occur in the absence of other psychiatric disorders. A diagnosis of delusional disorder is based on the presence of one or more delusions for at least 1 month (APA, 2013). Delusions are the primary symptom of this disorder. Apart from the direct impact of the delusion, psychosocial functioning is not markedly impaired. Examples of delusions include being followed, poisoned, infected, loved at a distance, or deceived by a spouse or lover.

The course of delusional disorder varies. The onset can be acute, or the disorder can occur gradually and become chronic. Patients usually live with delusions for years, rarely receiving psychiatric treatment unless their delusion relates to their health (somatic delusion), or they act on the basis of their delusion and violate legal or social rules. Full remissions can be followed by relapses. Behavior is remarkably normal except when the patient focuses on the delusion. At that time, thinking, attitudes, and mood may change abruptly. Personality does not usually change, but the patient is gradually and progressively involved with the delusional concern (APA, 2013). Delusional disorder is relatively uncommon in clinical settings.

SCHIZOPHRENIFORM DISORDER

The essential features of schizophreniform disorder are identical to those of schizophrenia, with the exception of the duration of the illness, which can be less than 6 months. Symptoms must be present for at least 1 month to be classified as a schizophreniform disorder. About one third of the individuals recover with the other two thirds developing schizophrenia (APA, 2013).

BRIEF PSYCHOTIC DISORDER

In brief psychotic disorder, the length of the episode is at least 1 day but less than 1 month. The onset is sudden and includes at least one of the positive symptoms of schizophrenia. The person generally experiences emotional turmoil or overwhelming confusion and rapid, intense shifts of affect (APA, 2013). Although episodes are brief, impairment can be severe, and supervision may be required to protect the person. Suicide is a risk, especially in younger patients.

PSYCHOTIC DISORDERS ATTRIBUTABLE TO A SUBSTANCE

Patients with a psychotic disorder attributable to a substance present with prominent hallucinations or delusions that are the direct physiologic effects of a substance (e.g., drug use, toxin exposure) (APA, 2013). During intoxication, symptoms continue as long as the use of the substance continues. Withdrawal symptoms can last for as long as 4 weeks. Differential diagnosis is recommended.

SUMMARY OF KEY POINTS

- The schizophrenia spectrum disorders include schizophrenia, schizoaffective, delusional, and schizotypal disorders, brief psychotic disorder, schizophreniform disorder, and substance/medication–induced psychotic disorder (APA, 2013). Schizophrenia displays a complex of symptoms typically categorized as positive symptoms (i.e., those that exist but should not), such as delusions or hallucinations and disorganized thinking and behavior, and negative symptoms (characteristics that should be there but are lacking), such as alogia, avolition, anhedonia, and diminished emotional expression.

- The clinical course of schizophrenia begins with a prodromal period in childhood but is usually not recognized as a precursor to schizophrenia. An acute illness usually occurs in late adolescence and may require hospitalization when medication and recovery-oriented care are initiated. In recovery-oriented care, the nurse instills hope and partners with the person with schizophrenia to develop strategies to recover and lead a meaningful life.

- The cause of schizophrenia is thought to be related to genetic, neurodevelopmental, and neurotransmission dysfunction. Environmental stress can trigger acute episodes.

- Nursing assessment begins with the development of the therapeutic relationship and includes biologic, psychological, and social areas.

- Risk for self-injury or injury to others should always be included in the assessment. Establishment of

- baseline health information should be done before any medications are administered. Several standardized assessment tools are available to help assess characteristic abnormal motor movements.
- In general, the antipsychotic drugs used to treat patients with schizophrenia block dopamine transmission in the brain but also cause some troublesome and sometimes serious side effects, primarily anticholinergic side effects and extrapyramidal side effects (i.e., motor abnormalities). Newer second-generation antipsychotic agents block serotonin as well as dopamine. The nurse should be familiar with these drugs, their possible side effects, and the interventions required to manage or control side effects.
- **Extrapyramidal side effects** of antipsychotic drugs may appear early in drug treatment and include acute parkinsonism or pseudoparkinsonism, acute dystonia, and akathisia, but they may also appear later after months or years of treatment. The primary example of late-appearing extrapyramidal side effects is tardive dyskinesia, which is a severe syndrome involving abnormal motor movements of the mouth, tongue, jaw, trunk, fingers, and toes.
- Health promotion and wellness interventions are important for overall well-being. People with schizophrenia spectrum disorders have special challenges because their medications can produce a negative impact on their physical health. Nurses can provide education and guidance for positive activity, exercise, and nutrition strategies that can counteract the effect of the medications and symptoms.
- Because schizophrenia is a lifetime disorder and patients require the continued support and care of mental health professionals and family or friends, one of the primary nursing interventions is ensuring that patients and families are properly educated regarding the course of the disorder, importance of drug maintenance, and need for consistent care and support. Positive interaction between patients and their families is key to the success of long-term treatments and outcomes.
- Other schizophrenia spectrum disorders (e.g., schizoaffective, delusional, and schizotypal disorders, brief psychotic disorder, schizophreniform disorder, and substance/medication-induced psychotic disorder) have symptoms similar to those of schizophrenia. Nursing care should be individualized based on a nursing assessment and current evidence related to care.

CRITICAL THINKING CHALLENGES

1. Describe steps that a nurse should use to make sure an assessment considers the cultural basis of a patient's hallucination and delusions.
2. A patient asks you to explain the difference between "positive" and "negative" symptoms. Develop an answer in "lay" terms for the question.
3. What steps might the nurse take to develop trust in a patient who has hallucinations and delusions and is frightened of other people?
4. Given that a patient with mental illness requires extra efforts at confidentiality and that patients with schizophrenia are often suspicious of their family members, explain ways you can help families and patients develop positive interactions.
5. A patient tells you that she has nothing to live for and everyone would be better off without her. You recognize that she may be having suicidal thoughts. What assessment questions would you ask? How would you help her develop a safety plan?
6. Discuss how therapeutic communication might have to change when working with a person with schizophrenia who is displaying primarily negative symptoms. How will you deal with the person's diminished response to you (both verbally and emotionally) when you are teaching or giving instructions for activities? How will you help the person compensate for some of his or her cognitive deficits?
7. A person with schizophrenia is admitted during a relapse. He said that he did not want to take his haloperidol anymore because it made him shake. The physician prescribes olanzapine. Develop a medication education plan that includes a comparison between olanzapine and haloperidol.
8. Mr. J. has just received a diagnosis of schizophrenia. During a recent outpatient visit, he confides to a nurse that he just has stress and does not think that he really has any psychiatric problems. Identify assessment areas that should be pursued before the patient leaves his appointment. How would you confront the denial?
9. A patient says his medication is not working. He is taking ziprasidone (Geodon) 40 mg twice a day. He tells you that he takes 40 mg before breakfast and 40 mg before bed. What would interventions are needed to increase the effectiveness of the drug?
10. Ms. J. was prescribed olanzapine (Zyprexa) for schizophrenia 1 month ago. Since her last monthly visit, she has gained 15 lb. She is considering discontinuing her medication regimen because of the weight gain.

Develop a plan to address her weight gain and her intention to discontinue her medication regimen.

11. An older adult in a nursing home has a delusion that her husband is having an affair with her sister. Discuss nonpharmacologic nursing interventions that should be implemented with this patient. How would you explain her delusion to her husband? Develop a plan for clinical management, focusing on psychiatric nursing care, for a patient experiencing this condition.

12. Identify health promotion activities for a person with schizophrenia who is gaining weight while taking antipsychotics might pursue.

2001: *A Beautiful Mind*

This Academy Award–winning movie starring Russell Crowe is based on the biography by Sylvia Nasar of the mathematician and Nobel Laureate John Nash. It presents the life and experiences of this man as he dealt with schizophrenia. It shows how his life and work were altered and the effects on his relationships with family and colleagues. The movie depicts how this man came to terms with his illness.

Viewing Points: How does the treatment John Nash received in the 1950s differ from treatment today? How would you classify his symptoms according to the *DSM-5*? What is typical or problematic about Mr. Nash's relationship with the medications prescribed for him?

2009: *The Soloist*

Based on a true story, this movie portrays the experience of a reporter/novelist named Steve Lopez (played by Robert Downey, Jr.) when he befriends Nathaniel Anthony Ayers, "the soloist" (played by Jamie Fox), who has severe, persistent, and untreated schizophrenia—and more importantly, exceptional musical talent. Formerly a student at the prestigious Juilliard School of Music in New York City, Ayers now lives on the streets of Los Angeles playing his two-string violin. See also the book by the same title.

Viewing Points: What are the risks and rewards of taking on such a personal relationship? How best can nurses advocate for individuals with severe mental illness (and their family and friends) when community resources are inadequate?

 A related Psychiatric–Mental Health Nursing video on the topic of Schizophrenia is available at http://thepoint.lww.com/BoydEssentials2e.

 A Practice and Learn Interactive Case Study related to the video on the topic of Schizophrenia is available at http://thepoint.lww.com/BoydEssentials2e.

REFERENCES

Aagaard, J., Tuszewski, B., Kølbæk, P. (2017). Does assertive community treatment reduce the use of compulsory admissions? *Archives of Psychiatric Nursing*, 31(6), 641–646.

American Psychiatric Association. (2013). *Diagnostic and statistical manual of mental disorders* (5th ed.). Arlington, VA: Author.

Brown, A. S. (2011). The environment and susceptibility to schizophrenia. *Progress in Neurobiology*, 93(1), 23–58.

Buchsbaum, M. (1990). The frontal lobes, basal ganglia, and temporal lobes as a site for schizophrenia. *Schizophrenia Bulletin*, 16(3), 379–389.

Carmona, V. R., Gómez-Benito, J., Rojo-Rodes, J. (2019). Employment support needs of people with schizophrenia: A scoping study. *Journal of Occupational Rehabilitation*, 29(1), 1–10.

Chang, J. G., Roh, D., Kim, C. H. (2019). Association between therapeutic alliance and adherence in outpatient schizophrenia patients. *Clinical Psychopharmacology and Neuroscience*, 17(2), 273–278.

Chien, W. T., Clifton, A. V., Zhao, S., Lui, S. (2019). Peer support for people with schizophrenia or other serious mental illness. *Cochrane Database of Systematic Reviews*, 4, CD010880.

Davidson, L. (2019). Recovering a sense of self in schizophrenia. *Journal of Personality*, 23. doi: 10.1111/jopy.12471.

Dietsche, B., Kircher, T., Falkenberg, I. (2017). Structural brain changes in schizophrenia at different stages of the illness: A selective review of longitudinal magnetic resonance imaging studies. *Australian and New Zealand Journal of Psychiatry*, 51(5), 500–508.

Dixon, L. B., Goldman, H. H., Srihari, V. H., & Kane, J. M. (2018). Transforming the treatment of schizophrenia in the United States: The RAISE initiative. *Annual Review of Clinical Psychology*, 14, 237–258.

Dondé, C., Silipo, G., Dias, E. C., Javitt, D. C. (2018). Hierarchical deficits in auditory information processing in schizophrenia. *Schizophrenia Research*, 206—, 135–141.

Dufort, A., Zipursky, R. B. (2019). Understanding and managing treatment adherence in schizophrenia. *Clinical Schizophrenia & Related Psychoses*, doi: 10.3371/CSRP.ADRZ.121218.

Fan, C. C., McGrath, J. J., Appadurai, V., Buil, A., Gandal, M. J., Schork, A. J., et al. (2018). Spatial fine-mapping for gene-by-environment effects identifies risk hot spots for schizophrenia. *Nature Communications*, 9(1), 5296.

Franzen, G. (1970). Plasma free fatty acids before and after an intravenous insulin injection in acute schizophrenic men. *British Journal of Psychiatry*, 116(531), 173–177.

Gimblett, D. (2015). Monitoring physical health in patients with serious mental illness. *Mental Health Practice*, 18(5), 20–23.

Glick, I. D., Olfson, M. (2018). Psychiatric services and "the Homeless": Changing the paradigm. *Journal of Nervous and Mental Disorders*, 206(5), 378–379.

Greene, M., Yan, T., Chang, E., Hartry, A., Touya, M., Broder, M. S. (2018), Medication adherence and discontinuation of long-acting injectable versus oral antipsychotics in patients with schizophrenia or bipolar disorder. *Journal of Medical Economics*, 21(2), 127–134.

Harding, C., Zubin, J., & Strauss, J. (1987). Chronicity in schizophrenia: Fact, partial fact or artifact? *Hospital and Community Psychiatry*, 38(5), 477–486.

Hazlett, E. A., Vaccaro, D. H., Haznedar, M. M., Goldstein, K. E. (2019). F-18Fluorodeoxyglucose positron emission tomography studies of the schizophrenia spectrum: The legacy of Monte S. Buchsbaum, M.D. *Psychiatry Research*, 271, 535–540.

Hilker, R., Helenius, D., Fagerlund, B., Skytthe, A., Christensen, K., Werge, T. M., et al. (2018). Heritability of schizophrenia and schizophrenia spectrum based on the nationwide Danish twin register. *Biological Psychiatry*, 83(6), 492–498.

Howes, O. D., McCutcheon, R., Owen, M. J., Murray, R. M. (2017). The role of genes, stress, and dopamine in the development of schizophrenia. *Biological Psychiatry*, 81(1), 9–20.

Huang, H. C., Lua, A. C., Wu, L. S., Wu, B. J., Lee, S. M., Liu, C. Z. (2016). Cigarette smoking has a differential effect on the plasma level of clozapine in Taiwanese schizophrenic patients associated with the CYP1A2 gene -163A/C single nucleotide polymorphism. *Psychiatric Genetics*, 26(4), 172–177.

Jaeger, S., Weißhaupt, S., Flammer, E., & Steinert, T. (2014). Control beliefs, therapeutic relationship, and adherence in schizophrenia outpatients: A cross-sectional study. *American Journal of Health Behavior*, 38(6), 914–923.

John, Y. J., Zikopoulos, B., Bullock, D., Barbas, H. (2018). Visual attention deficits in schizophrenia can arise from inhibitory dysfunction in thalamus or cortex. *Computational Psychiatry, 2*, 223–257.

Jones, C., Hacker, D., Cormac, I., Meaden, A., Irving, C. B., Xia, J., et al. (2019). Cognitive behavioral therapy plus standard care versus standard care plus other psychosocial treatments for people with schizophrenia. *Schizophrenia Bulletin, 45*(2), 284–286.

Kay, S. R., Fiszbein, A., & Opler, L. A. (1987). The Positive and Negative Syndrome Scale (PANSS) for schizophrenia. *Schizophrenia Bulletin, 13*, 261–276.

Kern, R. S., Zarate, R., Glynn, S. M., Turner, L. R., Smith, K. M., Mitchell, S. S., et al. (2018). Improving work outcome in supported employment for serious mental illness: Results from 2 independent studies of errorless learning. *Schizophrenia Bulletin, 44*(1):38–45.

Kessler, T., Lev-Ran, S. (2019). The association between comorbid psychiatric diagnoses and hospitalization-related factors among individuals with schizophrenia. *Comprehensive Psychiatry, 89*, 7–15.

Kim, S. W., Kim, J. J., Lee, B. J., Yu, J. C., Lee, K. Y., Won, S. H., et al. (2019). Clinical and psychosocial factors associated with depression in patients with psychosis according to stage of illness. *Early Intervention in Psychiatry*, doi: 10.1111/eip.12806.

Kioko, E., Williams, K., & Newhouse, B. (2016). Improving metabolic syndrome screening on patients on second generation antipsychotic medication. *Archives of Psychiatric Nursing, 30*(6), 671–677.

Klaunig, M. J., Trask, C. L., Neis, A. M., Cohn, J. R., Chen, X., Berglund, A. M., et al. (2019). Associations among domains of self-disturbance in schizophrenia. *Psychiatry Research, 267*, 187–194.

Kowalchuk, C., Castellani, L. N., Chintoh, A., Remington, G., Giacca, A., Hahn, M. K. (2019). Antipsychotics and glucose metabolism: How brain and body collide. *American Journal of Physiology, Endocrinology and Metabolism. 316*(1), E1–E15.

La Barbera, L., Vedele, F., Nobili, A., D'Amelio, M., Krashia, P. (2019). Neurodevelopmental disorders: Functional role of Ambra1 in autism and schizophrenia. *Molecular Neurobiology*, doi: 10.1007/s12035-019-1557-7.

Lauriello, J., Perkins, D. O. (2019). Enhancing the treatment of patients with schizophrenia through continuous care. *Journal of Clinical Psychiatry, 80*(1), pii: al18010ah2c.

Lean, M., Fornells-Ambrojo, M., Milton, A., Lloyd-Evans, B., Harrison-Stewart, B., Yesufu-Udechuku, A., et al. (2019). Self-management interventions for people with severe mental illness: Systematic review and meta-analysis. *British Journal of Psychiatry, 214*(5), 260–268.

Lewine, R., Martin, M., Hart, M. (2017). Sex versus gender differences in schizophrenia: The case for normal personality differences. *Schizophrenia Research, 189*, 57–60.

Liu, Y., Wang, G., Jin, H., Lyu, H., Liu, Y., Guo, W., et al. (2019). Cognitive deficits in subjects at risk for psychosis, first-episode and chronic schizophrenia patients. *Psychiatry Research, 274*, 235–242.

Liu, Y., Yang, X., Gillespie, A., Guo, Z., Ma, Y., Chen, R., et al. (2019). Targeting relapse prevention and positive symptom in first-episode schizophrenia using brief cognitive behavioral therapy: A pilot randomized controlled study. *Psychiatry Research, 272*, 275–283.

Lysaker, P. H., & Roe, D. (2016). Integrative psychotherapy for schizophrenia: its potential for a central role in recovery oriented treatment. *Journal of Clinical Psychology: In Session, 72*(2), 117–122.

Manu, P., Dima, L., Shulman, M., Vancampfort, D., De Hert, M., Correll, C. U. (2015). Weight gain and obesity in schizophrenia: Epidemiology, pathobiology, and management. *Acta Psychiatrica Scandinavica, 132*(2):97–108.

Maura, J. & Weisman de Mamani. A. (2017). Mental health disparities, treatment engagement, and attrition among racial/ethnic minorities with severe mental illness: A review. *Journal of Clinical Psychology in Medical Settings. 24*(3-4), 187–210.

McAuliffe, R., O'Connor, L., & Meagher, D. (2014). Parents' experience of living with and caring for an adult son or daughter with schizophrenia at home in Ireland: A qualitative study. *Journal of Psychiatric & Mental Health Nursing, 21*(2), 145–153.

Misdrahi, D., Tessier, A., Daubigney, A., Meissner, W. G., Schurhoff, F., Boyer, L., et al. (2019). Prevalence of and risk factors for extrapyramidal side effects of antipsychotics: Results from the national FACE-SZ cohort. *Journal of Clinical Psychiatry. 80*(1), pii: 18m12246.

Mohammadzadeh, A., Azadi, M., King, S., Khosravani, V., Sharifi Bastan, F. (2019). Childhood trauma and the likelihood of increased suicidal risk in schizophrenia. *Psychiatry Research, 275*, 100–107.

Naguy, A., Al-Rabaie, A. (2017). Suicidality and survivability in schizophrenia. *Journal of Nervous and Mental Disorders, 205*(7), 585.

Neugeboren, J. (2006). Meds alone couldn't bring Robert back. *Newsweek*. Retrieved April 24, 2019 from http://www.power2u.org/articles/recovery/meds.html.

Olfson, M., Gerhard, T., Huang, C., Crystal, S., & Stroup, T. S. (2015). Premature mortality among adults with schizophrenia in the United States. *JAMA Psychiatry, 72*, 1172–1181.

Pasina, L., Colzani, L., Cortesi, L., Tettamanti, M., Zambon, A., Nobili, A., et al. (2019). Relation between delirium and anticholinergic drug burden in a cohort of hospitalized older patients: An observational study. *Drugs & Aging, 36*(1), 85–91.

Pfizer. (2019). GEODON U.S. Physician Prescribing Information including Patient Summary of Information. Retrieved April 4, 2019 from http://www.pfizer.com/products/product-detail/geodon.

Postolache, T. T., Del Bosque-Plata, L., Jabbour, S., Vergare, M., Wu, R., Gragnoli, C. (2019). Co-shared genetics and possible risk gene pathway partially explain the comorbidity of schizophrenia, major depressive disorder, type 2 diabetes, and metabolic syndrome. *American Journal of Medical Genetics B Neuropsychiatric Genetics. 180*(3), 186–203.

Racioppi, A., Sheinbaum, T., Gross, G. M., Ballespí, S., Kwapil, T. R., Barrantes-Vidal, N. (2018). Prediction of prodromal symptoms and schizophrenia-spectrum personality disorder traits by positive and negative schizotypy: A 3-year prospective study. *PLoS One. 13*(11), e0207150.

Ricciardi, L., Pringsheim, T., Barnes, T. R. E., Martino, D., Gardner, D., Remington, G., et al. (2019). Treatment recommendations for tardive dyskinesia. *Canadian Journal of Psychiatry*, 706743719828968. doi: 10.1177/0706743719828968.

Riglin, L., Collishaw, S., Richards, A., Thapar, A. K., Maughan, B., O'Donovan, M. C., et al. (2017). Schizophrenia risk alleles and neurodevelopmental outcomes in childhood: A population-based cohort study. *Lancet Psychiatry, 4*(1), 57–62.

Schimmelbusch, W. H., Mueller, P. S., & Sheps, J. (1971). The positive correlation between insulin resistance and duration of hospitalization in untreated schizophrenia. *British Journal of Psychiatry, 118*(545), 429–436.

Schneider, M., Regente, J., Greiner, T., Lensky, S., Bleich, S., Toto, S., et al. (2018). Neuroleptic malignant syndrome: Evaluation of drug safety data from the AMSP program during 1993–2015. *European Archives of Psychiatry and Clinical Neuroscience*. doi: 10.1007/s00406-018-0959-2.

Shahab, S., Mulsant, B. H., Levesque, M. L., Calarco, N., Nazeri, A., Wheeler, A. L., et al. (2019). Brain structure, cognition, and brain age in schizophrenia, bipolar disorder, and healthy controls. *Neuropsychopharmacology, 44*(5), 898–906.

Simon, G. E., Yarborough, B. J., Rossom, R. C., Lawrence, J. M., Lynch, F. L., Waitzfelder, B. E., et al. (2019). Self-reported suicidal ideation as a predictor of suicidal behavior among outpatients with diagnoses of psychotic disorders. *Psychiatric Services, 70*(3), 176–183.

Simpson, G. M., & Angus, J. W. (1970). A rating scale for extrapyramidal side effects. *Acta Psychiatrica Scandinavica, 212*(suppl), 11–19.

Soundy, A., Stubbs, B., Roskell, C., Williams, S. E., Fox, A., & Vancampfort, D. (2015). Identifying the facilitators and processes which influence recovery in individuals with schizophrenia: A systematic review and thematic synthesis. *Journal of Mental Health, 24*(2), 103–110.

Sprague, R. L., & Kalachnik, J. E. (1991). Reliability, validity, and a total score cutoff for the Dyskinesia Identification Scale System: Condensed User Scale (DISCUS) with mentally ill and mentally retarded populations. *Psychopharmacology Bulletin, 27*(1), 51–58.

Toulopoulou, T., Zhang, X., Cherny, S., Dickinson, D., Berman, K. F., Straub, R. E., et al. (2019). Polygenic risk score increases schizophrenia liability through cognition-relevant pathways. *Brain, 142*(2), 471–485.

U.S. Food and Drug Administration. (08/2015). Ziprasidone. (Geodon). Prescribing Information. Retrieved April 7, 2019 from www.fda.gov/Drugs/DrugSafety/ucm426391.htm?source=govdelivery&utm_medium=email&utm_source=govdelivery.

Vardaxi, C. C., Gonda, X., Fountoulakis, K. N. (2018). Life events in schizoaffective disorder: A systematic review. *Journal of Affective Disorders, 227*, 563–570.

Vignapiano, A., Koenig, T., Mucci, A., Giordano, G. M., Amodio, A., Altamura, M., et al. (2019). Disorganization and cognitive impairment in schizophrenia: New insights from electrophysiological findings. *International Journal of Psychophysiology*, S0167-8760(18), 30984-X.

Vita, A., Barlati, S. (2018). Recovery from schizophrenia: Is it possible? *Current Opinion in Psychiatry. 31*(3), 246–255.

Vogel, J. S., Swart, M., Slade, M., Bruins, J., van der Gaag, M., Castelein, S. (2019). Peer support and skills training through an eating club for people with psychotic disorders: A feasibility study. *Journal of Behavior Therapy and Experimental Psychiatry, 64*, 80–86.

Wang, X., Zhao, N., Shi, J., Wu, Y., Liu, J., Xiao, Q., et al. (2019). Discussion on the application of multi-modal magnetic resonance imaging fusion in schizophrenia. *Journal of Medical Systems, 43*(5), 131.

Ward, H. B., Szabo, S. T., Rakesh G. (2018). Maintenance ECT in schizophrenia: A systematic review. *Psychiatry Research, 264*, 131–142.

Wilson, S. M. (2019). Patient-informed treatment development of behavioral smoking cessation for people with schizophrenia. *Behavior Therapy. 50*(2), 395–409.

Wu Y., Kang, R., Yan, Y., Gao, K., Li, Z., Jiang, J., et al. (2018). Epidemiology of schizophrenia and risk factors of schizophrenia-associated aggression from 2011 to 2015. *Journal of International Medical Research, 46*(10): 4039–4049.

Yuan, X., Kang, Y., Zhuo, C., Huang, X. F., Song, X. (2019). The gut microbiota promotes the pathogenesis of schizophrenia via multiple pathways. *Biochemical Biophysical Research Communication*, S0006-291X(19), 30367–30365.

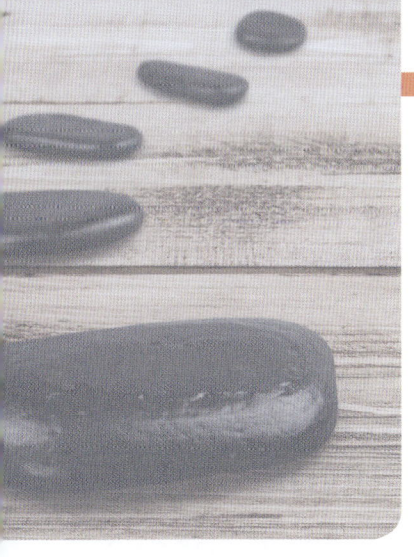

24
Personality and Impulse-Control Disorders

Nursing Care of Persons With Personality and Impulse-Control Disorders

Mary Ann Boyd and Kimberlee Hansen

KEY CONCEPTS

- antisocial personality disorder (ASPD)
- borderline personality disorder (BPD)
- difficult temperament
- emotional dysregulation
- impulse-control disorders
- impulsivity
- personality
- personality disorder
- self-harm
- temperament

LEARNING OBJECTIVES

After studying this chapter, you will be able to:

1. Describe the prevalence and incidence of personality disorders.
2. Delineate the clinical symptoms of borderline personality disorder and antisocial personality disorder with emphasis on emotional dysregulation, self-harm, temperament, and impulsivity.
3. Discuss the theories explaining personality disorders.
4. Identify evidence-based nursing interventions for persons with personality disorders.
5. Discuss communication strategies with persons with personality disorders.
6. Develop recovery-oriented strategies that address the needs of persons with personality disorders.
7. Compare and contrast disruptive impulse-control disorders.

KEY TERMS

- affective instability • avoidant personality disorder • cognitive schemata • conduct disorder • dependent personality disorder • dialectical behavior therapy (DBT) • dichotomous thinking • dissociation • emotional dysregulation • histrionic personality disorder • identity diffusion • impulse-control disorders • impulsivity • inhibited grieving • intermittent explosive disorder • invalidating environment • kleptomania • mentalization-based therapy (MBT) • mentalizing • narcissistic personality • obsessive-compulsive personality disorder • oppositional defiant disorder • paranoid personality disorder • parasuicidal behavior • personality disorder • personality traits • projective identification • pyromania • schizoid personality disorder • self-harm • schizotypy • schizotypal personality disorder • separation-individuation • splitting

Case Study: Rebecca

Rebecca is a 23-year-old single female who lives alone. She has few friends, but does attend regular psychotherapy sessions that help her understand her emotions and behaviors. She becomes very upset when her therapist leaves town for a planned vacation. Her family wants to help but are frustrated with Rebecca's inability to deal with every day stresses.

The concept of personality seems deceptively simple but instead is very complex. Historically, the term *personality* was derived from the Greek word *persona*, the theatrical mask used by dramatic players that had the connotation of a projected pretense or allusion. With time, the connotation changed from being an external surface representation to the internal traits of the individual.

> **KEYCONCEPT Personality** is a complex pattern of characteristics, largely outside of the person's awareness, which comprise the individual's distinctive pattern of perceiving, feeling, thinking, coping, and behaving.

Personality traits are prominent aspects of personality that are exhibited in a wide range of social and personal contexts. Intrinsic and pervasive, personality traits emerge from a complicated interaction of biologic dispositions, psychological experiences, and environmental situations that ultimately comprise a distinctive personality (Millon, 2011).

No sharp division exists between normal and abnormal personality functioning. Instead, personalities are viewed on a continuum from normal at one end to abnormal at the other. Many of the same processes involved in the development of a "normal" personality are responsible for the development of a personality disorder.

This chapter provides an overview of personality disorders with borderline personality disorder (BPD) explained in detail and antisocial personality disorder (ASPD) emphasized. Disruptive impulse-control and conduct disorders, a closely related group of disorders, are also discussed.

OVERVIEW OF PERSONALITY DISORDERS

A **personality disorder** is "an enduring pattern of inner experience and behavior that deviates markedly from the expectations of the individual's culture, is pervasive and inflexible, has an onset in adolescence or early adulthood, is stable over time, and leads to distress or impairment" (American Psychiatric Association [APA], 2013), p. 646).

> **KEYCONCEPT** A personality disorder diagnosis is based on abnormally inflexible behavior patterns of long duration, traced to adolescence or early adulthood that deviate from acceptable cultural norms.

The prevalence rate of any personality disorder in the adult population is estimated at 12.16% (Volkert, Gablonski, & Rabung, 2018). These rates are of public health significance because of the extreme social dysfunction and high health care use of persons with personality disorders. Many others do not seek treatment for the distress or impairment related to their personality disorder because they do not perceive themselves as having a problem. However, they frequently seek help for concurrent medical or mental health disorders.

At present, 10 personality disorders are recognized in the *DSM-5* within three clusters. Cluster A disorders are characterized by odd or eccentric behavior; Cluster B disorders are characterized by dramatic, emotional, or erratic behavior; and in Cluster C disorders, individuals appear anxious or fearful (APA, 2013).

CLUSTER A: PARANOID, SCHIZOID, AND SCHIZOTYPAL PERSONALITY DISORDERS

PARANOID PERSONALITY DISORDER

Clinical Course and Diagnostic Criteria

Paranoid personality disorder is characterized by a long-standing suspiciousness and mistrust of people in general. Individuals with these traits refuse to assume personal responsibility for their own feelings, assign responsibility to others, and avoid relationships in which they are not in control or power. These individuals are suspicious, guarded, and hostile. They are consistently mistrustful of others' motives, even those of relatives and close friends. Actions of others are often misinterpreted as deception, deprecation, and betrayal, especially regarding loyalty or trustworthiness of friends and associates (Birkeland, 2017).

People with paranoid personality disorder are unforgiving and hold grudges; their typical emotional responses are anger and hostility. They distance themselves from others and are outwardly argumentative and abrasive; internally, they feel powerless, fearful, and vulnerable. Other hallmark features of paranoid personality disorder are persistent ideas of self-importance and the tendency to be rigid and controlling. Blind to their own unattractive behaviors and characteristics, they often attribute these same traits to others. Their outward demeanor often seems cold, sullen, and humorless. They want to appear controlled and objective, yet often they react emotionally, displaying signs of nervousness, anger, envy, and jealousy. Orderly by nature, they are hypervigilant to any environmental changes that may loosen their control on the world. Occupational problems are common. In clinical populations, paranoid personality disorder is one of the strongest predictors of aggressive behavior, often associated with violence and stalking. People with this disorder do not seek mental health care until they have symptoms of comorbid disorders (Lee, 2017).

Epidemiology and Risk Factors

The prevalence estimates for paranoid personality range from 1.2% to 4.4%. Paranoid personality disorder is the second most prevalent personality disorder after obsessive-compulsive personality disorder (OCPD; Lee, 2017).

Etiology

The etiologic factors of paranoid personality remain unclear, but a genetic predisposition for an irregular maturation may be involved. As children, these individuals tend to be active and intrusive, difficult to manage, hyperactive, irritable, and have frequent outbursts of temper.

Evidence-Based Nursing Care for Persons With Paraniod Personality Disorder

Nurses most likely see these patients about other health problems but formulate nursing approaches based on the patient's underlying paranoia. Assessment of these individuals reveals disturbed or illogical thoughts that demonstrate misinterpretation of environmental stimuli. For example, a man was convinced that his wife was having an affair with the neighbor because his wife and the neighbor left their homes for work at the same time each morning. Although the man's beliefs were illogical, he never once considered that he was wrong. He frequently followed them but never caught them together. He continued to believe they were having an affair.

Because of their inability to develop relationships, these patients are often socially isolated and lack social support systems. Nursing interventions based on the establishment of a therapeutic relationship are difficult to implement because of the patient's mistrust. If a trusting relationship is established, the nurse helps the patient identify problematic areas, such as getting along with others or keeping a job. Through therapeutic techniques such as acceptance, confrontation, and reflection, the nurse and patient examine a problematic area to gain another view of the situation. Changing thought patterns takes time. Patient outcomes are evaluated in terms of small changes in thinking and behavior.

Continuum of Care

Individuals with paranoid personalities are unlikely to participate in treatment or recovery plans. If they have other comorbid disorders and are forced to seek treatment (through loss of their job or being ordered by a court in connection with an offense of a chargeable nature), they may seek help for depression or psychosis.

SCHIZOID PERSONALITY DISORDER
Clinical Course and Diagnostic Criteria

People with **schizoid personality disorder** are characterized as being expressively impassive and interpersonally disengaged (Millon, 2011). They tend to be unable to experience the joyful and pleasurable aspects of life. They are introverted, reclusive, and clinically seem distant, aloof, apathetic, and emotionally detached. Typically life-long loners, they have difficulty making friends, seem uninterested in social activities, and appear to gain little satisfaction in personal relationships. In fact, they appear to be incapable of forming social relationships. Their interests are directed at objects, things, and abstractions. They may do well at solitary jobs other people might find difficulty to tolerate. Often people with schizoid personality disorders may daydream excessively and become attached to animals, and they frequently do not marry or even form long-lasting romantic relationships. As children, they engage primarily in solitary activities, such as stamp collecting, computer games, electronic equipment, or academic pursuits such as mathematics or engineering. In addition, they seem to have a cognitive deficit characterized by obscure thought processes, particularly about social matters. Communication with others is confused and lacks focus. These individuals reveal minimum introspection and self-awareness, and interpersonal experiences are described in a very mechanical way.

Epidemiology

Schizoid personality disorder is rarely diagnosed in clinical settings. It is estimated that the prevalence is 3.1% (APA, 2013).

Etiology

The etiologic processes are speculative. There may be defects in either the limbic or reticular regions of the brain that may result in the development of the schizoid pattern (Millon, 2011). The defects of this personality may stem from an adrenergic–cholinergic imbalance in which the parasympathetic division of the autonomic nervous system is functionally dominant. Excesses or deficiencies in acetylcholine and norepinephrine may result in the proliferation and scattering of neural impulses that may be responsible for the cognitive "slippage" or affective deficits.

Evidence-Based Nursing Care for Persons With Schizoid Personality Disorder

Difficulty with social relations and low self-esteem are typical nursing priorities of patients with schizoid personality disorder. Major treatment goals are to enhance the experience of pleasure, prevent social isolation, and increase emotional responsiveness to others. Because these individuals often lack customary social skills, social skills training is useful in enhancing their ability to relate in interpersonal situations. The primary focus is to increase the patient's ability to feel pleasure. The nurse balances interventions between encouraging enough social activity to prevent the individual from retreating into a fantasy world and too much social activity that becomes intolerable to the patient.

The nurse may find working with such individuals unrewarding and as a result, the attending nurses may become frustrated, feel helpless, or become bored during the interactions. It is difficult to establish a therapeutic relationship with these individuals because they tend to shy away from interactions and are rarely motivated about treatment. Evaluation of outcomes should be in terms of increasing the patient's feelings of satisfaction with solitary activities.

Continuum of Care

People with schizoid personalities are rarely hospitalized unless they have a comorbid disorder. Family members may seek treatment for them in an outpatient setting.

SCHIZOTYPAL PERSONALITY DISORDER

Clinical Course and Diagnostic Criteria

Schizotypal personality disorder is characterized by a pattern of social and interpersonal deficits. The term **schizotypy** refers to traits that are similar to the symptoms of schizophrenia but are less severe. Cognitive perceptual symptoms are a primary characteristic and include magical beliefs (similar to delusions) and perceptual aberrations (similar to hallucinations). Other common symptoms include referential thinking (interpreting insignificant events as personally relevant) and paranoia (suspicion of others).

Schizotypal personality–disordered persons are more dramatically eccentric than those with schizoid personality disorder who are characteristically flat, colorless, and dull. These individuals are perceived as strikingly odd or strange in both appearance and behavior, even to laypersons. They may have unusual mannerisms, an unkempt manner of dress that does not quite "fit together," and inattention to usual social conventions (e.g., avoiding eye contact, wearing clothes that are stained or ill fitting, and being unable to join in the give-and-take banter of coworkers). Devoid of any close friends other than first-degree relatives, their mood is constricted or inappropriate, with excessive social anxieties. They usually exhibit an avoidant behavior pattern.

Persons with schizotypal personality disorder may respond to stress with transient psychotic episodes (lasting minutes to hours). Because of their short duration, the symptoms mirror but fall short of features that would justify the diagnosis of schizophrenia. Many individuals (30% to 50%) with schizotypal personality disorder also have a co-occurring major depressive disorder diagnosis when admitted to a hospital (APA, 2013; Racioppi et al., 2018). Schizotypal personality disorders may be slightly more common in males (APA, 2013).

Epidemiology and Risk Factors

The lifetime prevalence of schizotypal personality disorder is 3.9% with higher rates among men (4.2%) than women. There is cultural variation with black women and low-income individuals having a greater risk than others (Pulay et al., 2009).

Etiology

Magnetic resonance imaging (MRI) studies of individuals with schizotypal personality disorder show smaller gray matter volume, which are correlated with negative symptoms. Studies also show changes in temporal gyrus volume asymmetry and in the white matter tracts (Chan et al., 2018). There is also evidence that trauma-exposed individuals have a greater risk of developing schizotypal disorder (Quidé et al., 2018).

Evidence-Based Nursing Care for Persons With Schizotypal Personality Disorder

Depending on the amount of decompensation (i.e., deterioration of functioning and exacerbation of symptoms), the assessment of a patient with a schizotypal personality disorder can generate a range of nursing diagnoses. If a person has severe symptoms, such as delusional thinking or perceptual disturbances, the nursing priorities are similar to those for a person with schizophrenia (see Chapter 23). If symptoms are mild, social isolation, coping with stress and daily living, low self-esteem, and difficult social interactions are the focus of nursing care.

People with schizotypal personality disorder need help in developing recovery-oriented strategies to increase their sense of self-worth and recognize their positive attributes. They can benefit from social skills training and environmental management that increases their psychosocial functioning. Their eccentric thoughts and behaviors alienate them from others. Reinforcing socially appropriate dress and behavior can improve their overall appearance and ability to relate in the environment. Because they have a hard time generalizing from one situation to another, attention to cognitive skills is important.

Continuum of Care

Quality of life for a patient with schizotypal personality disorder can be improved with supportive psychotherapy, but their suspiciousness, lack of trust, or impaired social interactions make it difficult to establish a therapeutic relationship. These individuals do not usually seek treatment unless more serious symptoms appear, such as depression or anxiety. Medications are not generally used unless the individual has coexisting anxiety or depression.

Nursing care is often provided in a home or clinic setting, with the personality disorder being secondary to the purpose of the care. This means that nurses are focusing on other aspects of patient care and may miss the underlying psychiatric disorder. A psychiatric nursing consult may be needed for these patients to help identify the disorder.

CLUSTER B DISORDERS: BORDERLINE, ANTISOCIAL, HISTRIONIC, AND NARCISSISTIC PERSONALITY DISORDERS

BORDERLINE PERSONALITY DISORDER

People with **borderline personality disorder** (BPD) have problems regulating their moods, developing a self-identity, maintaining interpersonal relationships, maintaining reality-based thinking, and avoiding impulsive or destructive behavior. The severity and difficulty in treating the disorder leads to enormous public health costs from health care utilization and functional disability (Meuldijk, McCarthy, Bourke, & Grenyer, 2017).

> **KEYCONCEPT** **Borderline personality disorder** (BPD) is characterized by a disruptive pattern of instability related to self-identity, interpersonal relationships, and affect, combined with marked impulsivity and destructive behavior.

Clinical Course

Individuals with BPD appear more competent than they actually are and often set unrealistically high expectations for themselves. When these expectations are not met, they experience intense shame, self-hate, and self-directed anger. Their lives are like soap operas—one crisis after another. Some of the crises are caused by the individual's dysfunctional lifestyle or inadequate social milieu, but many are caused by fate—the death of a spouse or a diagnosis of an illness. They react emotionally with minimal coping skills. The intensity of their emotions often frightens them and others. Friends, family members, and coworkers limit their contact with the person, which furthers the sense of aloneness, abandonment, and self-hatred. It also diminishes opportunities for learning self-corrective measures.

Remissions from the acute symptoms (e.g., self-injurious behaviors, suicide attempts, or threats about suicide) are fairly common and the relapse rate is relatively low compared to other disorders. However, psychosocial functioning does not necessarily improve as symptoms decrease. Younger age and higher education levels predict higher functioning (Zanarini, Franken, Mioaurg, Reich, & Fitzmaurice, 2016).

Diagnostic Criteria

BPD is a "pervasive pattern of instability of interpersonal relationships, self-image, and affects, and marked impulsivity beginning by early adulthood and present in a variety of contexts" (APA, 2013), p. 663). See Key Diagnostic Characteristics 24.1. Individuals with BPD also exhibit related cognitive and behavioral dysfunctions.

KEY DIAGNOSTIC CHARACTERISTICS 24.1 • BORDERLINE PERSONALITY DISORDER 301.83

Diagnostic Criteria

A pervasive pattern of instability of interpersonal relationships, self-image, and diminished affect, and marked impulsivity, beginning by early adulthood and present in a variety of contexts, as indicated by five (or more) of the following:

1. Frantic efforts to avoid real or imagined abandonment. (Note: Do not include suicidal or self-mutilating behavior covered in Criterion 5.)
2. A pattern of unstable and intense interpersonal relationships characterized by alternating between extremes of idealization and devaluation.
3. Identity disturbance: markedly and persistently unstable self-image or sense of self.
4. Impulsivity in at least two areas that are potentially self-damaging (e.g., spending, sex, substance abuse, reckless driving, binge eating). (Note: Do not include suicidal or self-mutilating behavior covered in Criterion 5.)
5. Recurrent suicidal behavior, gestures, or threats, or self-mutilating behavior.
6. Affective instability due to a marked reactivity of mood (e.g., intense episodic dysphoria, irritability, or anxiety usually lasting a few hours and only rarely more than a few days).
7. Chronic feelings of emptiness.
8. Inappropriate intense anger or difficulty controlling anger (e.g., frequent displays of temper, constant anger, recurrent physical fights).
9. Transient stress-related paranoid ideation or severe dissociative symptoms.

Associated Behavioral Findings

- Pattern of undermining self at the moment a goal is to be realized
- Possible psychotic-like symptoms during times of stress
- Recurrent job losses, interrupted education, and broken marriages
- History of physical and sexual abuse, neglect, hostile conflict, and early parental loss or separation

Reprinted with permission from the American Psychiatric Association. (2013). *Diagnostic and statistical manual of mental disorders* (5th ed.). All Rights Reserved.

Unstable Interpersonal Relationships

People with BPD have an extreme fear of abandonment as well as a history of unstable or insecure attachments (Palihawadana, Broadbear, & Rao, 2019). Most have never experienced a consistently secure, nurturing relationship and are constantly seeking reassurance and validation. In an attempt to meet their interpersonal needs, they idealize others and establish intense relationships that violate others' interpersonal boundaries, which leads to rejection. When these relationships do not live up to their expectations, they devalue the person. Continually disappointed in relationships, these individuals, who are already intensely emotional and have a poor sense of self, feel estranged from others and inadequate in the face of perceived social standards. Intense shame and self-hate follow. These feelings often result in self-injurious behaviors, such as wrist cutting, self-burning, or head banging.

Consider Rebecca
Rebecca hates being alone, but her behaviors drive others away. When she feels rejected, anxious, or angry, she cuts her wrists, which decreases her anxiety.

Unstable Self-Image

These patients appear to have no sense of their own identity and direction; this becomes a source of great distress to them and is often manifested by chronic feelings of emptiness and boredom. It is not unusual for people with BPD to direct their actions in accord with the wishes of other people. For example, one woman with BPD describes herself: "I am a singer because my mother wanted me to be. I live in the city because my manager thought that I should. I become whatever anyone tells me to be. Whenever someone recommends a song, I wonder why I didn't think of that. My boyfriend tells me what to wear."

Unstable Affect

Affective instability (i.e., rapid and extreme shift in mood) is a core characteristic of BPD and is evidenced by erratic emotional responses to situations and intense sensitivity to criticism or perceived slights. For example, a person may greet a casual acquaintance with intense affection yet later be aloof with the same acquaintance. Friends describe individuals with BPD as moody, irresponsible, or intense. These individuals often fail to recognize their own emotional responses, thoughts, beliefs, and behaviors and have difficulty interpreting the facial affects of others. In this disorder recognizing emotions in others is altered (Santangelo et al., 2017).

Cognitive Dysfunctions

People with BPD often have **dichotomous thinking**. That is, they evaluate experiences, people, and objects in terms of mutually exclusive categories (e.g., good or bad, success or failure, trustworthy or deceitful). Their interpretation of normally occurring events is usually extremely positive or extremely negative. Sometimes their thinking becomes disorganized with irrelevant, bizarre notions and vague or scattered thought connections as well as delusions and hallucinations.

Another cognitive dysfunction common in BPD is **dissociation**, or times when thinking, feeling, or behaviors occur outside a person's awareness. It is a coping strategy for avoiding disturbing events. In dissociating, the person does not have to be aware of or remember traumatic events. There is evidence of functional changes in the frontolimbic regions (amygdala, anterior cingulate, inferior frontal gyrus, medial, and dorsolateral prefrontal cortices) and temporoparietal areas (Krause-Utz & Elzinga, 2018).

Impaired Problem Solving

In BPD, affected people often fail to engage in active problem solving. Instead, problem solving is attempted by soliciting help from others in a helplessly hopeless manner. Suggestions offered are rarely taken up.

Impulsivity

These individuals often have difficulty delaying gratification or thinking through the consequences before acting on their feelings; their actions are often unpredictable. Essentially, they act in the moment and clean up the mess afterward. Gambling, spending money irresponsibly, binge eating, engaging in unsafe sex, and abusing substances are typical of these individuals. They can also be physically or verbally aggressive. Job losses, interrupted education, and unsuccessful relationships are common.

Self-Harm Behaviors

The turmoil and unsuccessful interpersonal relationships and social experiences associated with BPD may lead the person to undermine him- or herself when a goal is about to be reached. The most serious consequences are suicide attempts or **parasuicidal behavior** (i.e., deliberate self-injury with intent to harm oneself).

KEYCONCEPT Self-harm is deliberate self-injurious behavior.

Self-harm behavior can be compulsive (e.g., hair pulling), episodic, or repetitive (e.g., cutting wrists, arms, other body parts) and is more likely to occur when the individual with BPD is depressed; has highly unstable interpersonal relationships, especially problems with intimacy and sociability; and is paranoid, hypervigilant (i.e., alert, watchful), and resentful. It is not unusual for persons with this disorder to self-harm in unusual ways such as swallowing pens, staples, and even razor blades, or banging one's head against a brick wall. All self-harm behaviors should be considered potentially life threatening and taken seriously.

Borderline Personality Disorder Across the Life Span

Many children and adolescents show symptoms similar to those of BPD, such as moodiness, self-destruction, impulsiveness, lack of temper control, and rejection sensitivity. If a family member has BPD, the adolescent should be carefully assessed for this disorder. Because symptoms of BPD begin in adolescence, it makes sense that some children and adolescents would meet the criteria for BPD even though it is not diagnosed before young adulthood. More likely, some personality traits, such as impulsivity and mood instability, in many adolescents should be recognized and treated whether or not BPD eventually develops.

Epidemiology and Risk Factors

The estimated prevalence of BPD is roughly 1.0% in community settings. In clinical settings, the prevalence of BPD is approximately 12% in outpatient mental health clinics and 22% in inpatient psychiatric settings, with a higher proportion of women. One possible explanation for more women being diagnosed more often is that it is more socially acceptable for women than men to seek help from the health care system. Another reason is that childhood sexual abuse, which more commonly affects girls, is one of the strongest risk factors for BPD. Another explanation is that because eating disorders are more common in women with BPD, they have a greater likelihood of also having a mood, anxiety, or posttraumatic stress disorder. Men with BPD are more likely to have a substance use problem and intermittent explosive disorder. Other studies cite parental loss and separation as risk factors. Clearly, more research is needed to identify risk factors for the development of BPD (Ellison, Rosenstein, Morgan, & Zimmerman, 2018).

Comorbidity

Ample clinical reports show the coexistence of personality disorders with other mental disorders such as mood, substance abuse, eating, dissociative, and anxiety disorders and other personality disorders. The coexistence of BPD with other disorders presents clinicians with the difficult choice of which disorder receives treatment priority. Symptoms associated with this disorder often provoke negative reactions on the part of clinicians, which interfere with clinicians' ability to provide effective care (Shah & Zanarini, 2018).

Etiology

Evidence supports a biopsychosocial etiology. Studies suggest that BPD traits are heritable, although the specific genetic factors remain unclear. There is clear evidence of differences in brain functioning between those with and without BPD. There is also clear evidence that psychological and social factors contribute to the development of the disorder (Meehan, Clarkin, & Lenzenweger, 2018). The following discussion highlights the leading explanations for BPD.

Biologic Theories

Evidence of central nervous system dysfunction in BPD is now clear, including possible structural changes. Biologic abnormalities are associated with three BPD characteristics: affective instability; transient psychotic episodes; and impulsive, aggressive, and suicidal behavior. Associated brain dysfunction occurs in the limbic system and frontal lobe and increases the behaviors of impulsiveness, parasuicide, and mood disturbance (Perez-Rodriguez et al., 2018).

Psychosocial Theories

Psychoanalytic Theories

Using psychoanalytic methodology suggests persons with BPD have not achieved the normal and healthy developmental stage of **separation-individuation**, during which a child develops a sense of self, a permanent sense of significant others (object constancy), and integration of seeing both bad and good components of oneself (Stern, Caligor, Horz-Sagstetter, & Clarkin, 2018). Those with BPD lack the ability to separate from the primary caregiver and develop a separate and distinct personality or self-identity. **Projective identification** is believed to play an important role in the development of BPD and is a defense mechanism by which people with BPD protect their fragile self-image. For example, when overwhelmed by anxiety or anger at being disregarded by another, they defend against the intensity of these feelings by unconsciously blaming others for what happens to them. They project their feelings onto a significant other with the unconscious hope that that person knows how to deal with it. Projective identification becomes a defensive way of interacting with the world, which leads to more rejection.

Maladaptive Cognitive Processes

Cognitive schemata are patterns of thought that determine how a person interprets events. Each person's cognitive schemata screen, code, and evaluate incoming stimuli. In personality disorders, maladaptive cognitive schemata cause misinterpretation of other people's actions or reactions and of events that result in dysfunctional ways of responding. Cognitive schemata are important in understanding BPD (and ASPD as well).

Individuals with BPD develop dysfunctional beliefs and maladaptive schemata early in life, leading them to misinterpret environmental stimuli continuously, which in turn leads to rigid and inflexible behavior patterns in response to new situations and people (Esmaeilian, Dehghani, Koster, & Hoorelbeke, 2019). Because those with BPD have been conditioned to anticipate rejection and disappointment in the past, they become entrenched in a pattern of fear and anxiety regarding encountering new people or situations. They have fears that disaster is going to strike at any minute. The work of cognitive therapists is to challenge distortions in thinking patterns and replace them with realistic ones.

Remember Rebecca?
Rebecca does not see herself as contributing to her problem but believes her misfortunes are caused by others. For example, when she encounters new people, she shares too much personal information and is disappointed when they do not respond with the same intensity. She interprets their response as rejection.

Social Theories: Biosocial Theories

The biosocial viewpoint proposed by Marsha Linehan and colleagues sees BPD as a multifaceted problem, a combination of innate emotional vulnerability (sensitivity and reactivity to environmental stress), emotional dysregulation (inability to control emotions in social interactions), and the environment (Linehan, 1993) (Box 24.1).

> **KEYCONCEPT Emotional dysregulation** is the inability to control emotions in social interactions and includes an instability of mood, marked shifts to or from depression, stress-related and transient mood crashes, rejection sensitivity, and inappropriate and intense outbursts of anger.

The emotional dysregulation and aggressive impulsivity entail both social learning and biologic regulation. Much of the neurobiologic research is directed at corticolimbic function and other cerebral function (Perez-Rodriguez et al., 2018). In fact, restoring balance in these systems permits more consistent neural firing between the limbic system and the frontal and prefrontal cortices. When these circuits are functional, the person has a greater capacity to think about his or her emotions and modulate behavior more responsibly.

The ability to control emotion is partly learned from private experiences and encounters with the social environment. BPD is believed to develop when emotionally vulnerable individuals interact with an **invalidating environment**, a social situation that negates private emotional responses and communication. When core emotional responses and communications are continuously dismissed, trivialized, devalued, punished, and discredited (invalidated) by respected or valued persons, the vulnerable individual becomes unsure about his or her feelings. A minor example of an invalidating environment or response follows: The parents of Emily, a 4-year-old girl, tell her that the family is going to grandmother's house for a family meal. The child responds, "I am not going to Gramma's. I hate Stevie (her cousin)." The parents reply, "You don't hate Stevie. He is a wonderful child. He is your cousin, and only a spoiled and selfish little girl would say such a thing." The parents have devalued Emily's feelings and discredited her comments, thereby invalidating her feelings and sense of personal worth.

BOX 24.1

Behavioral Patterns in Borderline Personality Disorder

1. *Emotional vulnerability.* Person experiences a pattern of pervasive difficulties in regulating negative emotions, including high sensitivity to negative emotional stimuli, high emotional intensity, and slow return to emotional baseline.
2. *Self-invalidation.* Person fails to recognize one's own emotional responses, thoughts, beliefs, and behaviors and sets unrealistically high standards and expectations for self. May include intense shame, self-hate, and self-directed anger. Person has no personal awareness and tends to blame social environment for unrealistic expectations and demands.
3. *Unrelenting crises.* Person experiences pattern of frequent, stressful, negative environmental events, disruptions, and roadblocks—some caused by the individual's dysfunctional lifestyle, others by an inadequate social milieu, and many by fate or chance.
4. *Inhibited grieving.* Person tries to inhibit and overcontrol negative emotional responses, especially those associated with grief and loss, including sadness, anger, guilt, shame, anxiety, and panic.
5. *Active passivity.* Person fails to engage actively in solving of own life problems but will actively seek problem solving from others in the environment; learned helplessness, hopelessness.
6. *Apparent competence.* Tendency for the individual to appear deceptively more competent than he or she actually is; usually because of failure of competencies to generalize across expected moods, situations, and time. Person fails to display adequate nonverbal cues of emotional distress.

Adapted from Linehan, M. (1993). *Cognitive-behavioral treatment of borderline personality disorder* (p. 10). New York: Guilford Press.

The most severe form of invalidation occurs in situations of child sexual abuse. Often, the abusing adult has told the child that this is a "special secret" between them. The child experiences feelings of fear, pain, and sadness, yet this trusted adult continuously dismisses the child's true feelings and tells the child what he or she should feel.

Family Response to Borderline Personality Disorder

Individuals with BPD are typically part of a chaotic family system, but their behavior adds to the chaos. Family members often feel captive to these patients. Family members are afraid to disagree with them or refuse to meet their multiple needs, fearing that self-destructive behavior will follow. During the course of the disorder, family members often get "burned out" and withdraw from the patient, only adding to the patient's fear of abandonment (Kay, Poggenpoel, Myburgh, & Downing, 2018).

Recovery-Oriented Care of Persons With Borderline Personality Disorder

Teamwork and Collaboration: Working Toward Recovery

BPD is a very complex disorder that requires collaboration of treatment by the entire mental health care team. Because BPD patients view the world in absolutes, nurses and other treatment team members are alternately categorized as all good or all bad. This defense is called **splitting** and presents clinicians with a challenge to work openly with each other as well as the patient until the issue can be resolved through team meetings and clinical supervision.

People with BPD are inadvertently highly stigmatized by many clinicians. Staff often accuse these individuals of "manipulation" to get attention and say so in a very derogatory manner. In reality, all of us want attention from significant people in our lives. Most of us have the necessary skills to successfully meet our need for closeness and attention without alienating the very people who are important to us. People with BPD are unsuccessful in developing long-term meaningful relationships or getting what they want because their approach alienates others. Their need for attention and closeness to others is very normal: it is how they seek attention that is problematic.

Psychotherapy is needed to help the individual with BPD manage the dysfunctional moods, impulsive behavior, and self-injurious behaviors. Specially trained therapists who are comfortable with the many demands of these patients are needed. These therapists represent a variety of mental health disciplines, including psychology, social work, and advanced practice nursing. This is a lifelong disorder requiring ongoing treatment as the individual copes with multiple interpersonal crises. Several types of medications are usually needed, including mood stabilizers, antidepressants, and anxiolytics; careful medication monitoring is necessary.

Dialectical behavior therapy (DBT) combines cognitive and behavior therapy strategies with acceptance-based practice drawn from Zen and humanistic approaches; it was developed for persons with BPD. Core interventions include problem solving, exposure techniques (i.e., gradual exposure to cues that set off aversive emotions), skills training, contingency management (i.e., reinforcement of positive behavior), and cognitive modification. Skills groups are an integral part of DBT and are taught in group settings in which patients practice emotional regulation, interpersonal effectiveness, distress tolerance, core mindfulness, and self-management skills. Weekly individual therapy sessions focus on enhancing motivation and improving competence (DeCou, Comtois, & Landes, 2019).

Mentalization-based therapy (MBT) is a psychodynamic psychotherapy that is used in both individual and group formats. In MBT, borderline personality symptoms are viewed as a result of distortion or reduction in **mentalizing**, which is the ability to understand the mental states of oneself and others, including thoughts, feelings, that lead to actions. The goal of MBT is to improve patients' capacity to accurately understand others' actions and develop self-awareness skills through a therapeutic relationship (Levy, McMain, Bateman, & Clouthier, 2018).

Safety Issues

Persons with BPD can be extremely volatile emotionally. Because they experience emotions so intensely, they are at high risk for self-harm and suicide. Self-harm threats should be taken very seriously.

Evidence-Based Nursing Care for Persons With Borderline Personality Disorder

Persons with BPD may enter the mental health system early (during young adulthood or even before) because of their chaotic lifestyles. Behavior includes unstable moods, problems with interpersonal relationships, low self-esteem, and self-identity issues. Thinking and behavior are dysregulated (Box 24.2). They have problems in daily living, including maintaining intimate relationships, keeping a job, and living within the law (Box 24.3). Nursing Care Plan 24.1—which sets forth a plan of care for Rebecca, the case study patient in this chapter—is available at http://thepoint.lww.com/BoydEssentials2e.

Mental Health Nursing Assessment

Physical Health Assessment

People with BPD are usually able to maintain personal hygiene and physical functioning. Because of the

BOX 24.2

Response Patterns of Persons With Borderline Personality Disorder

Affective (mood) dysregulation
Mood lability
Problems with anger
Interpersonal dysregulation
Chaotic relationships
Fears of abandonment
Self-dysregulation
Difficulties with sense of self
Sense of emptiness
Behavioral dysregulation
Parasuicidal behavior or threats
Impulsive behavior
Cognitive dysregulation
Dissociative responses
Paranoid ideation

Courtesy of M. Linehan, Department of Psychology, Box 351525, University of Washington, Seattle, WA 98195-1525, 1993.

---

comorbidity of BPD and eating disorders and substance abuse, however, a nutritional assessment may be needed. The assessment should also include the use of caffeinated beverages (e.g., coffee, tea, cola, energy drinks) and alcohol. In patients who engage in binging or purging, assessment should include examining the teeth for pitting and discoloration, as well as the hands and fingers for redness and calluses caused by inducing vomiting. The patient should be queried about physiologic responses of emotion. Sleep patterns also should be assessed because sleep alterations may suggest coexisting depression or mania.

Physical Indicators of Self-Injurious Behaviors

Patients with BPD should be assessed for self-injurious behavior or suicide attempts. It is important to ask the patient about specific self-abusive behaviors, such as cutting, scratching, or swallowing foreign objects. The patient may wear long sleeves to hide injury to the arms. Specifically, asking about thoughts of hurting oneself when experiencing a major upset provides an opportunity for prevention and for coaching the patient toward alternative self-soothing measures.

Medication Assessment

Patients with BPD may be taking several medications. For example, one patient may be taking a small dose of an antipsychotic and a mood stabilizer. Another may be taking a selective serotonin reuptake inhibitor (SSRI). Initially, patients may be reluctant to disclose all the medications they are taking because, for many of them, trial and error has led to repeated prescription. They are fearful of having medication taken away from them.

BOX 24.3 CLINICAL VIGNETTE

Borderline Personality Disorder

Joanne is a 22-year-old single woman who was recently fired from her job as a data entry clerk. She is living with her mother and stepfather, who brought her to the emergency department after finding her crouched in a fetal position in the bathroom, her wrists bleeding. She seemed to be in a daze. This is her first psychiatric admission although her mother and stepfather have suspected that she has "needed help" for a long time. In high school, she received brief treatment for a potential eating disorder. She remains very thin but is able to eat at least one meal per day. During periods of stress, she will go for days without eating. Joanne is the second of three children. Her parents divorced when she was 3 years old. She has not seen her father since he left. Although she has pleasant memories of her father, her mother has told her that he beat Joanne and her sisters when he was drinking. When Joanne was 6 years old, her older sister died as a result of an automobile accident. Joanne was in the car but was uninjured. As a child, Joanne was seen as a potential singing star. Her natural musical talent attracted her teachers' support, which encouraged her to develop her talent. She took singing lessons and entered statewide competitions in high school. Although she enjoyed the attention, she was never really comfortable in the limelight and felt "guilty" about having a talent that she sometimes resented. She was able to make friends but found that she was unable to keep them. They described her as "too intense" and emotional. She had one boyfriend in high school, but she was very uncomfortable with any physical closeness. After ending the relationship with the boyfriend, she concentrated on dieting to have a "perfect body." When her dieting attracted her parents' attention, she vowed to eat just enough to keep them "off her back about it." She spent much of her leisure time with her grandmother. She attended college briefly but was unable to concentrate. It was during college and after her grandmother's death that Joanne began cutting her wrists during periods of stress. It seemed to calm her.

After leaving college, Joanne returned home. She had several jobs and short-lived friendships. She was usually fired from her job because of "moodiness," and it took her several months before she would again find another. She spent days in her room listening to music. Her recent episode occurred after she was fired from work and spent 3 days in her bedroom.

What Do You Think?
- How would you describe Joanne's mood?
- Are Joanne's losses of her father and sister really severe enough to affect her ability to relate to others now? Do the losses seem to relate to the self-injury?
- What behaviors indicate problems with self-esteem and self-identity are present?

Development of rapport with special attention to a nonjudgmental approach is especially important when eliciting current medication practices. The effectiveness of the medication in relieving the target symptom needs to be determined. Use of alcohol, OTC medications, and street drugs should be carefully assessed to determine drug interactions.

Psychosocial Assessment

People with BPD have usually experienced significant losses in their lives that shape their view of the world. They experience **inhibited grieving**, "a pattern of repetitive, significant trauma and loss, together with an inability to fully experience and personally integrate or resolve these events" (Linehan, 1993). They have unresolved grief that can last for years and will avoid situations that evoke those feelings of separation and loss. During the assessment, the nurse can identify the losses (real or perceived) and explore the patient's experience during these losses, paying particular attention to whether the patient has reached resolution. A history of physical or sexual abuse and early separation from significant caregivers may provide important clues to the severity of the disturbances.

Mood fluctuations are common and can be assessed by any number of the depression and anxiety screening scales or by asking the following questions:

- What things or events bother you and make you feel sad or angry?
- Do these things or events trouble you more than they trouble other people?
- Do friends and family tell you that you are moody?
- Do you get angry easily?
- Do you have trouble with your temper?
- Do you think you were born with these feelings or did something happen to make you feel this way?

Appearance and activity level generally reflect the person's mood and psychomotor activity. Many of those with BPD have been physically or sexually abused and thus should be assessed for depression. A disheveled appearance can reflect depression or an agitated state. When feeling good, these patients can be very engaging; they tend to be dramatic in their style of dress and attract attention, such as by wearing an unusual hairstyle or heavy makeup. Because physical appearance reflects identity, patients may experiment with their appearance and seek affirmation and acceptance from others. Body piercing, tattoos, and other perceived adornments provide a mechanism to define self.

>
> **Rebecca's Assessment**
> Rebecca loves to project a dramatic appearance when she is feeling good. When she is in a good mood, she projects as an overly confident, engaging person. She has several body piercings. She refuses to discuss any childhood trauma or sexual abuse.

Impulsivity. Impulsivity can be identified by asking the patient whether he or she does things impulsively or spur of the moment. For example: "Have there been times when you were hurt by your actions or were sorry later that you acted in the way you did?" Direct questions about gambling, choices in sexual partners, sexual activities, fights, arguments, arrests, and habits related to consumption of alcohol can also help in identifying areas of impulsive behavior.

From a neurophysiologic perspective, impulsively acting before thinking seems to be mediated by rapid nerve firing in the mesolimbic area. This activates psychomotor responses before pathways reach the prefrontal cortex (Perez-Rodriquez, et al., 2018). Teaching the patient strategies to slow down automatic responses (e.g., deep breathing, counting to 10) buys time to think before acting.

Cognitive Disturbances. The mental status examination of those with BPD usually reveals normal thought processes that are not disorganized or confused except during periods of stress. Those with BPD usually exhibit dichotomous thinking, or a tendency to view things as absolute, either black or white, good or bad, with no perception of compromise. Dichotomous thinking can be assessed by asking patients how they view other people. Evidence of dichotomous thinking is indicated with responses of "good" or "bad," "wonderful" or "terrible."

Identity Disturbance. Unstable self-image is often manifested as an identity disturbance or **identity diffusion**, a loss of the capacity for self-definition and commitment to values, goals, or relationships. The nurse can recognize identity diffusion if the patient reports an ongoing "emptiness" or contradictory behavior. "I know I should not have gone out with him, but he wanted to see me." The person's thoughts and behavior will seem fragmented and superficial (Richetin, Preti, Costantini, & De Panfilis, 2017).

Dissociation and Transient Psychotic Episodes. With BPD, periods of dissociation and transient psychotic episodes may occur. Dissociation can be assessed by asking if there is ever a time when the patient does not remember events or has the feeling of being separate from his or her body. Some patients refer to this as "spacing out." By asking specific information about how often, how long, and when dissociation first was used, the nurse can get an idea of how important dissociation is as a coping skill. It is important to ask the person what is happening in the environment when dissociation occurs. Frequent dissociation indicates a highly habitual coping mechanism that is difficult to change. Because transient psychotic states occur, it is also important to elicit data regarding the presence of hallucinations or delusions and their frequency and circumstances.

Interpersonal Skills. Assessment of the person's ability to relate to others is important because interpersonal problems are linked to dissociation and self-injurious behavior. Information about friendships, frequency of contact, and intimate relationships provide data about the person's ability to relate to others. Patients with BPD often are sexually active and may have numerous sexual partners. Their need for closeness clouds their judgment about sexual partners, so it is not unusual to find these patients in abusive, destructive relationships with people with ASPD.

Self-Esteem and Coping Skills. Coping with stressful situations is one of the major problems of people with BPD. Assessment of their coping skills and their ability to deal with stressful situations is important. Self-esteem is closely related to identifying with health care workers. Patients with BPD perceive their families and friends as being weary of their numerous crises and their seeming unwillingness to break the vicious self-destructive cycle. Feeling rejected by their natural support system, these individuals create one within the health system. During periods of crisis, especially during the late evening, early morning, or on weekends, they may call or visit various psychiatric units asking to speak to specific personnel who formerly cared for them. They even know different nurses' scheduled days off and make the rounds to several hospitals and clinics. Sometimes they bring gifts to nurses or call them at home. Because their newly created social support system cannot provide the support that is needed, the patient continues to feel rejected. One of the treatment goals is to help the individual establish a more natural support network.

Functional Assessment. Some individuals with BPD can function very well except during periods when symptoms erupt. They hold jobs, are active in communities, and can perform well. During periods of stress, symptoms often appear. Conversely, some individuals with severe BPD function poorly; they seem to be always in a crisis, which often they have created.

Social Support Systems. Identification of social supports (e.g., family, friends, religious organizations) is the purpose in assessing resources. Knowing how the patient obtains social support is important in understanding the quality of interpersonal relationships. For example, some patients consider as their "best friends" nurses, physicians, and other health care personnel. Because these are false friendships (i.e., not reciprocated), they inevitably lead to frustration and disappointment. However, helping the patient find ways to meet other people and encouraging the patient's efforts are more realistic.

Risk Assessment: Suicide or Self-Injury

It is critical that patients with BPD be assessed for suicidal and self-damaging behavior, including alcohol and drug abuse (see Chapter 16). The assessment should include direct questions, such as asking whether the patient thinks about or engages in self-injurious behaviors. If so, the nurse should continue to explore the behaviors: what is done, how is it done, how frequently is it done, and what are the circumstances surrounding the self-injurious behavior. It is helpful to explain briefly to the patient that sometimes people cut, scratch, or pick at themselves as a way of bringing some relief and comfort. Although the behavior brings temporary relief, it also places the person at risk for infection. Approaching the assessment in this way conveys a sense of understanding and is more likely to invite the patient to disclose honestly.

Strengths Assessment

The strengths assessment is important because these positive thoughts, skills, and behaviors can be supported as the individuals replace self-defeating behaviors with positive ones. Many of these individuals are extremely resilient despite the trauma that they have often experienced. The person's strengths will emerge in the assessment and increase as the nurse gets to know the patient better. Some key questions include the following:

- How do you make yourself feel better?
- How do you resist the urge to hurt yourself?
- How do you make friends?
- What is the most positive thought, skill, or behavior that you have?

Priority of Care

The first priority in care is safety of the patient. Self-injury and suicide ideation should be considered when establishing recovery goals. If the patient is not experiencing suicidal or self-injury thoughts or behavior, the patient thought processes (dissociation) or ability to cope with everyday stress may emerge as priorities of care, especially if these interfere with daily living. If the individual copes with stressful situations by dissociating or hallucinating, the nurse should begin to help the patient identify other coping strategies. Patients who are very emotional sometimes find that they will be able to cope if they learn emotional regulation strategies. For other patients, identity issues, anxiety, or low self-esteem may become priorities of care.

Identified strengths should be included in the priorities. By including a person's strengths, such as being motivated to manage self-destructive thoughts, the nurse can channel these attributes to deal with the specific issues.

Evidence-Based Nursing Care for Persons With Borderline Personality Disorder

Therapeutic Relationship

Psychiatric–mental health registered nurses do not function as the patient's primary therapists, but they do need to establish a therapeutic relationship that strengthens the patient's coping skills and self-esteem and also supports individual psychotherapy. The therapeutic relationship helps the patient to experience a model of healthy interaction with consistency, limit setting, caring, and respect (both self-respect and respect for the patient). Patients who have low self-esteem need help in recognizing genuine respect from others and reciprocating with respect for others. In the therapeutic relationship, the nurse models self-respect by observing personal limits, being assertive, and clearly communicating expectations (Box 24.4). The nurse should always avoid using stigmatizing language, such as describing the person's behavior as manipulating instead of reporting or documenting specific behaviors.

Nurses should use their own self-awareness skills to examine their personal response to the patient. How the nurse responds to the patient can often be a clue to how others perceive and respond to the person. For example, if the nurse feels irritated or impatient during the interview that is a sign that others respond to this person in the same way; conversely, if the nurse feels empathy or closeness, chances are this patient can evoke these same feelings in others.

Nursing Interventions

Physical Care

Usually, the person can manage hydration and self-care fairly well. This section focuses on those areas that are more likely to be problematic.

BOX 24.4 • THERAPEUTIC DIALOGUE • Borderline Personality Disorder

INEFFECTIVE APPROACH

Rebecca: Hey, you know what? You are my favorite nurse. That night nurse sure doesn't understand me the way you do.
Nurse: Oh, I'm glad you are comfortable with me. Which night nurse?
Rebecca: You know, Sue.
Nurse: Did you have problems with her?
Rebecca: She is terrible. She sleeps all night or she is on the telephone.
Nurse: Oh, that doesn't sound very professional to me. Anything else?
Rebecca: Yeah, she said that you didn't know what you were doing. She said that you couldn't nurse your way out of a paper bag (smiling).
Nurse: She did, did she? (Getting angry.) She should talk.
Rebecca: Well, I gotta go to group. Where will you be? I feel so much better if I know where you are. I don't know how I can possibly be discharged tomorrow.

EFFECTIVE APPROACH

Rebecca: Hey, you know what? You are my favorite nurse. That night nurse sure doesn't understand me the way you do.
Nurse: I really like you, Rebecca. Tomorrow you will be discharged, and I'm glad that you will be able to return home. (Nurse avoided responding to "favorite nurse" statement. Redirected interaction to impending discharge.)
Rebecca: That night nurse slept all night.
Nurse: What was your night like? (Redirecting the interaction to Sara's experience.)
Rebecca: It was terrible. Couldn't sleep all night. I'm not sure that I'm ready to go home.
Nurse: Oh, so you are not quite sure about discharge? (reflection)
Rebecca: I get so, so lonely. Then, I want to hurt myself.
Nurse: Lonely feelings have started that chain of events that led to cutting, haven't they? (validation)
Rebecca: Yes, I'm very scared. I haven't cut myself for 1 week now.
Nurse: Do you have a plan for dealing with your lonely feelings when they occur?
Rebecca: I'm supposed to start thinking about something that is pleasant—like spring flowers in the meadow.
Nurse: Does that work for you?
Rebecca: Yes, sometimes.

CRITICAL THINKING CHALLENGE

- How did the nurse in the first scenario get sidetracked?
- How was the nurse in the second scenario able to keep the patient focused on herself and her impending discharge?

Sleep Hygiene. Disturbed sleep patterns are common in association with BPD. The nurse can intervene by helping the person establish a regular bedtime routine by teaching sleep hygiene strategies such avoiding foods and drinks that could interfere with sleep. If relaxation exercises are used, they should be adapted to the tolerance of the individual. Special consideration must be made for persons who have been physically and sexually abused and who may be unable to put themselves in a vulnerable position (e.g., lying down in a room with other people or closing their eyes). These patients may need additional safeguards to help them sleep, such as a night light or repositioning the furniture in the room to allow a quick exit.

Teaching Nutritional Balance. The nutritional status of the person with BPD can quickly become a priority, particularly if the patient has coexisting eating disorders, mood disorders, schizophrenia, or substance abuse. Eating is often a response to stress, so patients can quickly become overweight. This is especially a problem when the patient has also been taking medications that promote weight gain, such as antipsychotics, antidepressants, or mood stabilizers. Helping the patient learn the basics of nutrition, make reasonable choices, and develop other coping strategies are useful interventions. If patients are engaging in purging or severe dieting practices, teaching the patient about the dangers of both of these practices is important (see Chapter 26). Referral to an eating disorders specialist may be needed (Ripoll, 2012; Stoffers, Völlm, Rücker, Timmer, Huband, & Lieb, 2010).

Preventing and Treating Self-Harm. Patients with BPD are usually admitted to the inpatient setting because of threats of self-harm. Observing for antecedents of self-injurious behavior and intervening before an episode are important safety interventions. Patients can learn to identify situations leading to self-destructive behavior and develop preventive strategies.

> **Concept Mastery Alert**
>
> Because patients with BPD are impulsive and may respond to stress by harming themselves, observation of the patient's interactions and assessment of mood, level of distress, and agitation are important indicators of impending self-injury.

Remembering that self-harm is an effort to self-soothe by activating endogenous endorphins, the nurse can assist the patient to find more productive and enduring ways to find comfort. Linehan (1993) suggests using the Five Senses Exercise.

- Vision (e.g., go outside and look at the stars or flowers or autumn leaves)
- Hearing (e.g., listen to beautiful or invigorating music or the sounds of nature)
- Smell (e.g., light a scented candle, boil a cinnamon stick in water)
- Taste (e.g., drink a soothing, warm, nonalcoholic beverage)
- Touch (e.g., take a hot bubble bath, pet your dog or cat, get a massage)

Pharmacologic Interventions

Limiting medication is better for people with BPD. Patients should take medications only for target symptoms for a short time (e.g., an antidepressant for a bout with depression) because they may be taking many medications, particularly if they have a comorbid disorder, such as a mood disorder or substance abuse. Medications are used to control emotional dysregulation, impulsive aggression, cognitive disturbances, and anxiety as an adjunct to psychotherapy, but limited studies support the treatment of BPD with medication. Recent evidence shows some benefit from atypical antipsychotics but little recent evidence to support the use of mood stabilizers. The evidence to support or exclude SSRIs remains weak (Hancock-Johnson, Griffiths, & Picchioni, 2017).

Administering and Monitoring Medications. In inpatient settings, it is relatively easy to control medications; in other settings, however, patients must be aware that it is their responsibility to take their medication and monitor the number and type of drugs being taken. Patients who rely on medication to help them deal with stress and those who are periodically suicidal are at high risk for abuse of medications. Patients who experience unusual side effects are also at high risk for noncompliance. The nurse determines whether the patient is actually taking medication, whether the medication is being taken as prescribed, its effect on target symptoms, and the use of any OTC drugs (e.g., antihistamines, sleeping pills or herbal supplements with similar pharmacologic activity).

Managing Side Effects. Patients with BPD appear to be sensitive to many medications, so the dosage may need to be adjusted based on the side effects they experience. Listen carefully to the patient's description of the side effects. Any unusual side effects should be accurately documented and reported to the prescriber.

Teaching Points. Patients should be educated about the prescribed medications and their interactions with other drugs and substances, but they should be encouraged to avoid relying on medication alone. Interventions include teaching patients about the medication and how and where it acts in the brain and body, helping establish a routine for taking prescribed medication, reporting side effects, and facilitating the development of positive coping strategies to deal with daily stresses rather than relying on medications. Eliciting the patient's partnership in care improves adherence and thereby outcomes.

Psychosocial Interventions

Addressing Abandonment and Intimacy Fears

One key to helping patients with BPD is recognizing their fears of both abandonment and intimacy. Informing the patient of the length of the therapeutic relationship as much as possible allows the patient to engage in and prepare for termination with the least pain of abandonment. If the patient's hospitalization is time limited, it is important to acknowledge the limit overtly and remind the patient with each contact how many sessions remain.

In day treatment and outpatient settings, the duration of treatment may be indeterminate, but the nurse may not be available that entire time. The termination process cannot be casual; this would stimulate abandonment fears. However, some patients end prematurely when the nurse informs them of the impending end as a way to leave before being rejected. The best approach is to explore these anticipated feelings with the patient. After careful planning, the nurse and patient discuss how to cope with anticipated feelings, including the wish to run away, review the progress the patient has made, and summarize what the patient has learned from the relationship that can be generalized to future encounters.

Establishing Personal Boundaries and Limitations

Personal boundaries are highly context specific; for example, stroking the hair of a stranger on the bus would be inappropriate, but stroking the hair and face of one's intimate partner while sitting together would be appropriate. Clarifying limits requires making explicit what is usually implicit. This may mean having a standing time during each shift that the nurse will talk with the patient. The nurse should refrain from offering personal information, which is frequently confusing to the person with BPD. At times, the person may present in a somewhat arrogant and seemingly entitled way. It is important for the nurse to recognize such a presentation as reflective of internal confusion and dissonance. Responding in a very neutral manner avoids confrontation and a power struggle, which might also unwittingly reinforce the patient's internal sense of inferiority.

Some additional strategies for establishing the boundaries of the relationship include the following:

- Documenting in the patient's chart the agreed-on appointment expectations
- Sharing the treatment plan with the patient
- Confronting violations of the agreement in a nonpunitive way
- Discussing the purpose of limits in the therapeutic relationship and applicability to other relationships

When patients violate boundaries, it is important to respond right away but without taking the behavior personally. For example, if a patient is flirtatious, simply say something like, "X, I feel uncomfortable with your overly friendly behavior. It seems out of place because we have a professional relationship. That would be more fitting for an intimate relationship that we will never have."

Using Behavioral Interventions

The goal of behavioral interventions is to replace dysfunctional behaviors with positive ones. The nurse has an important role in helping patients control emotions and behaviors by acknowledging and validating desired behaviors and ignoring or confronting undesired behaviors. Patients often test the nurse for a response, so nurses must decide how to respond to particular behaviors. This can be tricky because even negative responses can be viewed as positive reinforcement by the patient. In some instances, if the behavior is irritating but not harmful or demeaning, it is best to ignore, rather than focus, on it. However, grossly inappropriate and disrespectful behaviors require confrontation. If a patient throws a glass of water on an assistant because she is angry at the treatment team for refusing to increase her hospital privileges, an appropriate intervention would include confronting the patient with her behavior and issuing the consequences, such as losing her privileges and apologizing to the assistant.

However, such an incident can be used to help the patient understand why such behavior is inappropriate and how it can be changed. The nurse should explore with the patient what happened, what events led up to the behavior, what the consequences were, and what feelings were aroused. Advanced practice nurses or other therapists explore the origins of the patient's behaviors and responses, but the generalist nurse needs to help the patient explore ways to change behaviors involved in the current situation. The laboriousness of this analytic process may be a sufficient incentive for the patient to abandon the dysfunctional behavior.

Challenging Dysfunctional Thinking

The nurse can often challenge the patient's dysfunctional ways of thinking and encourage the person to think about the event in a different way. When a patient engages in catastrophic thinking, the nurse can challenge by asking, "What is the worst that could happen?" and "How likely would that be to occur?" Or in dichotomous thinking, when the patient fixates on one extreme perception or

BOX 24.5 CLINICAL VIGNETTE

Challenging Dysfunctional Thinking

Ms. S had worked for the same company for 20 years with a good job record. After an accident, she made some minor mistakes in her work that she quickly corrected. She informed her company nurse that her work was "really slipping" and that she was fearful of her coworkers' disapproval and of getting fired from her job. The nurse asked her to keep a journal of coworkers' comments for the next week. At the next visit, the following dialogue occurred:

Nurse: I noticed that you received several compliments on your work. Even a close friend of your boss expressed appreciation for your work.

Ms. S: It was a light week at work. I really don't believe they meant what they said.

Nurse: I can see how you can believe that one or two comments are not genuine, but how do you account for four and five good reports on your work?

Ms. S: Well, I don't know.

Nurse: It looks like your beliefs are not supported by your journal entries. Now, what makes you think that your boss wants to fire you after 20 years of service?

alternates only between the extremes, the nurse should ask the patient to think about any examples of exceptions to the extreme. The point of the challenge is not to debate or argue with the patient but to provide different perspectives to consider. Encouraging patients to keep journals of real interactions to process with the nurse or therapist is another effective way of testing the reality of their thinking and anticipations, affording more choices and flexibility (Box 24.5).

In problem solving, the nurse might encourage the patient to debate both sides of the problem and then search for common ground. Practicing communication and negotiation skills through role-playing helps the patient make mistakes and correct them without harm to her or his self-esteem. The nurse also encourages patients to use these skills in their everyday lives and report back on the results, asking patients how they feel applying the skills and how doing so affects their self-perceptions. Success, even partial success, builds a sense of competence and self-esteem (Table 24.1).

Psychoeducation

Patient education within the context of a therapeutic relationship is one of the most important, empowering interventions for the generalist psychiatric–mental health nurse to use. Teaching patients skills to resist parasuicidal urges, improve emotional regulation, enhance interpersonal relationships, tolerate stress, and enhance overall quality of life provide the foundation for long-term behavioral changes. These skills can be taught in any treatment setting as a part of the overall facility program (Box 24.6). If nurses are practicing in a facility where DBT is the treatment model, they can be trained in DBT and can serve as group skills leaders.

Teaching Emotional Regulation. A major goal of cognitive therapeutic interventions is emotional regulation—recognizing and controlling the expression of feelings. Patients often fail even to recognize their feelings; instead, they respond quickly without thinking about the consequences. Remember, the time needed for

TABLE 24.1 THOUGHT DISTORTIONS AND CORRECTIVE STATEMENTS

Thought Distortion	Corrective Statement
Catastrophizing	
"This is the most awful thing that has ever happened to me"	"This is a sad thing but not the most awful."
"If I fail this course, my life is over."	"If you fail the course, you can take the course again. You can change your major."
Dichotomizing	
"No one ever listens to me."	"Your husband listened to you last night when you told him …"
"I never get what I want."	"You didn't get the promotion this year, but you did get a merit raise."
"I can't understand why everyone is so kind at first and then always dumps me when I need them the most."	"It is hard to remember those kind things and times when your friends have stayed with you when you needed them."
Self-Attribution Errors	
"If I had just found the right thing to say, she wouldn't have left me."	"There is not a single right thing to say, and she left you because she chose to."
"If I had not made him mad, he wouldn't have hit me."	"He has a lot of choices in how to respond, and he chose hitting. You are responsible for your feelings and actions."

BOX 24.6
Psychoeducation Checklist: Borderline Personality Disorder

When caring for the patient with borderline personality disorder, be sure to include the following topic areas in the teaching plan:

- Management of medication, if used, including drug action, dosage, frequency, and possible adverse effects
- Regular sleep routines
- Nutrition
- Safety measures
- Functional versus dysfunctional behaviors
- Cognitive strategies (e.g., distraction, communication skills, thought stopping)
- Structure and limit setting
- Social relationships
- Recovery strategies
- Community resources

---

taking action is shorter than the time needed for thinking before acting. Pausing makes up for the momentary lag between the limbic and autonomic response and the prefrontal response.

Another element of emotional regulation is learning to delay gratification. When the patient wants something that is not immediately available, the nurse can teach patients to distract themselves, find alternate ways of meeting the need, and think about what would happen if they have to wait to meet the need.

Teaching Effective Ways to Communicate. Another important area of patient education is teaching communication skills. Patients lack interpersonal skill in relating because they often had inadequate modeling and few opportunities to practice. The goals of relationship skill development are to identify problematic behavior that interferes with relationships and to use appropriate behaviors in improving relationships. The starting point is with communication. The nurse teaches the patient basic communication approaches, such as making "I" statements, paraphrasing what the other party says before responding, checking the accuracy of perceptions with others, compromising and seeking common ground, listening actively, and offering and accepting reactions. Besides modeling the behaviors, the nurse guides patients in practicing a variety of communication approaches for common situations. When role-playing, the nurse needs to discuss not only what the skills are and how to perform them but also the feelings patients have before, during, and after the role-play.

In day treatment and outpatient settings, the nurse can give the patient homework, such as keeping a journal, applying role-playing skills to actual situations, and observing behaviors in others. In the hospital, the patient can experience the same process, where the nurse is available to offer immediate feedback. Whatever the setting or whatever the specific problems addressed, the nurse must keep in mind and remind the patient that change occurs slowly. Thus, working on the problems occurs gradually, with severity of symptoms as the guide to deciding how fast and how much change to expect.

Building Social Skills and Self-Esteem. In the hospital, the nurse can use group therapy to discuss feelings and ways to cope with them. Women with BPD benefit from assertiveness classes and women's health issues classes. Many of the women are involved in abusive relationships and lack the ability to resolve these relationships because of their extreme anxiety regarding separating from those they love and their extreme need to feel connected. These women verbalize desires to do it, but they do not have the strength and self-confidence needed to leave. Exposing them to a different style of interaction as well as validation from other people increases their self-esteem and ability to get away from negative influences.

Evaluation and Treatment Outcomes

Evaluation and treatment outcomes vary depending on the severity of the disorder, the presence of comorbid disorders, and the availability of resources. For a patient with severe symptoms or continual self-injury, keeping the patient safe and alive may be a realistic outcome. Helping the patient resist parasuicidal urges may take years. In contrast, individuals who rarely need hospitalization and have adequate resources can expect to recover from the self-destructive impulses and learn positive interaction skills that promote a high-quality lifestyle. Most patients fall somewhere in between, with periods of symptom exacerbation and remission. In these patients, increasing the symptom-free time may be the best indicator of outcomes.

Continuum of Care

Treatment and recovery involve long-term therapy. Hospitalization is sometimes necessary during acute episodes involving parasuicidal behavior, but after this behavior is controlled, patients are discharged. It is important for these individuals to continue with treatment in the outpatient or day treatment setting. Because these individuals often appear more competent and in control than they are, nurses must not be deceived by these outward appearances. These individuals need continued follow-up and long-term therapy, including individual therapy, psychoeducation, and positive role models. (See Box 24.7.)

> **BOX 24.7**
>
> **Research For Best Practice: Brief Admissions During Prolonged Treatment**
>
> Helleman, M., Goossens, P. J., Kaasenbrood, A., & van Achterberg, T. (2016). Brief admissions during prolonged treatment in a case involving borderline personality disorder and posttraumatic stress disorder: Use and functions. *Journal of the American Psychiatric Nurses Association, 22*(3), 215–224.
>
> **THE QUESTION:** How can brief admissions be used during a long-term treatment process (7 years) for a person suffering from severe symptoms of borderline personality disorder and complex PTSD?
>
> **METHODS:** A descriptive qualitative case study design explored the usefulness of brief admissions to an acute care setting for a 37-year-old female with borderline personality disorder and PTSD. Multiple sources of data were triangulated to reach convergence on the functions and use of brief admissions across and extended treatment period. Semistructured interviews were conducted with the patient, her husband, psychiatric, community psychiatric nurse, and a clinical nurse involved in her care. Key concepts in the interview transcripts were identified, coded, and analyzed by two researchers.
>
> **FINDINGS:** Initially the main goal of the brief admission was to prevent suicide and self-harm. As treatment progressed, the brief admission served other functions such as prevention of long admissions, prevention of dropout from therapy, opportunities to exercise newly acquired skills, opportunities to expand autonomy and self-care, and to establish preconditions needed to maintain social roles.
>
> **IMPLICATIONS FOR NURSING:** Brief admission can positively influence the treatment course for a patient with diagnoses of borderline personality disorder and PTSD.

ANTISOCIAL PERSONALITY DISORDER

ASPD is defined as "a pervasive pattern of disregard for, and violation of, the rights of others occurring since age 15 years" (APA, 2013, p. 659). This diagnosis is given to individuals 18 years of age or older who fail to follow society's rules—that is, they do not believe that society's rules are made for them and so are consistently irresponsible. For many, evidence suggests a conduct disorder (introduced later in the chapter) before the age of 15 years. The term *psychopath*, or *sociopath*, a person with a tendency toward antisocial and criminal behavior with little regard for others, is often used in describing the behaviors of people with ASPD.

> **KEYCONCEPT Antisocial personality disorder** is characterized by a pervasive pattern of disregard for and violation of the rights of others.

Clinical Course and Diagnostic Criteria

ASPD has a chronic course, but the antisocial behaviors tend to diminish later in life, particularly after the age of 40 years (APA, 2013). Individuals with ASPD are arrogant and self-centered and feel privileged and entitled. They are self-serving, and they exploit and seek power over others. They can be interpersonally engaging and charming, which is often mistaken for a genuine sense of concern for other people. In reality, they lack empathy; are unable to express human compassion; and tend to be insensitive, callous, and contemptuous of others. Deceit and manipulation for personal profit or pleasure are central features associated with this disorder. They are behaviorally impulsive and interpersonally irresponsible. Many with this disorder repeatedly perform acts that are grounds for arrest (whether they are arrested or not), such as destroying property, harassing others, stealing, or pursuing other illegal occupations. They act hastily and spontaneously, are temperamentally aggressive and shortsighted, and fail to plan ahead or consider alternatives. They fail to adapt to the ethical and social standards of the community. They lack a sense of personal obligation to fulfill social and financial responsibilities, including those involved with being a spouse, parent, employee, friend, or member of the community. They lack remorse for their transgressions (APA, 2013).

Some of these individuals openly and flagrantly violate laws and end up in jail. But most people with ASPD never come in conflict with the law and instead find a niche in society, such as in business, the military, or politics that rewards their competitively tough behavior. Although ASPD is characterized by continual antisocial acts, the disorder is not synonymous with criminality. See Key Diagnostic Characteristics 24.2.

Epidemiology and Risk Factors

Twelve-month prevalence rates of ASPD are estimated between 0.2% and 3.3% (APA, 2013). Males with alcohol use disorder and those released from substance abuse clinics, prisons, or other forensic settings have the highest rates. Adverse socioeconomic (i.e., poverty) or sociocultural (i.e., migration) factors also are associated with higher prevalence (APA, 2013). Gender differences also exist in how symptoms are manifest (Key Diagnostic Characteristics 24.2).

Age of Onset

To be diagnosed with ASPD, the individual must be at least 18 years old and must have exhibited one or more childhood behavioral characteristics of conduct disorder before the age of 15 years, such as aggression to people or animals, destruction of property, deceitfulness or theft, or

> **KEY DIAGNOSTIC CHARACTERISTICS 24.2 • ANTISOCIAL PERSONALITY DISORDER 301.7**
>
> **Diagnostic Criteria**
> A. A pervasive pattern of disregard for and violation of the rights of others, occurring since age 15 years, as indicated by three (or more) of the following:
>   1. Failure to conform to social norms with respect to lawful behaviors, as indicated by repeatedly performing acts that are grounds for arrest.
>   2. Deceitfulness, as indicated by repeated lying, use of aliases, or conning others for personal profit or pleasure.
>   3. Impulsivity or failure to plan ahead.
>   4. Irritability and aggressiveness, as indicated by repeated physical fights or assaults.
>   5. Reckless disregard for safety of self or others.
>   6. Consistent irresponsibility, as indicated by repeated failure to sustain consistent work behavior or honor financial obligations.
>   7. Lack of remorse, as indicated by being indifferent to or rationalizing having hurt, mistreated, or stolen from another.
>
> B. The individual is at least 18 years of age.
> C. There is evidence of conduct disorder with onset before the age of 15 years.
> D. The occurrence of antisocial behavior is not exclusively during the course of schizophrenia or bipolar disorder.
>
> **Associated Findings**
> - Lacking empathy
> - Callous, cynical, and contemptuous of the feelings, rights, and suffering of others
> - Inflated and arrogant self-appraisal
> - Excessively opinionated, self-assured, or cocky
> - Glib, superficial charm; impressive verbal ability
> - Irresponsible and exploitative in sexual relationships; history of multiple sexual partners and lack of a sustained monogamous relationship
> - Possible dysphoria, including complaints of tension, inability to tolerate boredom, and depressed mood
>
> Reprinted with permission from the American Psychiatric Association. (2013). *Diagnostic and statistical manual of mental disorders* (5th ed.). All Rights Reserved.

serious violation of rules. The likelihood of developing adult ASPD is increased if onset of conduct disorder is seen before the age of 10 years as well as an accompanying childhood attention deficit hyperactivity disorder (ADHD) diagnosis (APA, 2013).

Comorbidity

ASPD is associated with several other psychiatric disorders, including mood, anxiety, and other personality disorders. ASPD is strongly associated with alcohol and drug abuse (Tielbeek et al., 2018). However, a diagnosis of ASPD is not warranted if the antisocial behavior occurs only in the context of substance abuse. For example, some people who misuse substances sometimes engage in criminal behavior, such as stealing or prostitution, only when in pursuit of drugs. Therefore, it is crucial to assess whether the person with possible ASPD has engaged in illegal activities at times other than when pursuing or using substances.

Etiology

Biologic Theories

Perhaps more than any other personality disorder, an extensive number of biologically oriented studies explore the genetic bases, neuropsychological factors, and arousal levels among this group of pathologies. Many of these studies show changes associated with personality disorders or characteristics, but we do not have evidence that these changes caused the disorder. These studies often overlap with studies of aggression, temperament, and substance use (Kolla, Dunlop, Meyer, & Downar, 2018; Tielbeek et al., 2017).

MRI studies demonstrate difference in the brain regions that are related to impulsivity and irresponsibility (Deming et al., 2018). These findings support the neural basis of fearlessness in these individuals. Impairment in moral judgment is associated with dysfunction of the prefrontal cortex (Taber-Thomas, Asp, Koenigs, Sutterer, Anderson, & Tranel, 2014). In adolescence, antisocial behavior is related to increased amygdala reactivity to interpersonal threats, which may lead to anger-related behavior (Dotterer, Hyde, Swartz, Hariri, & Williamson, 2017).

Psychosocial Theories

Temperament

Scientists believe temperament is neurobiologically determined, and many believe that it is central to understanding personality disorders. A temperament, the natural predisposition to express feelings and actions, is evident during the first few months of life and remains stable through development. For example, whereas some infants are more relaxed or calm and sleep a lot, others are extremely alert, startled by the slightest noise, cry more, and sleep less.

Difficult temperaments are common in ASPD and are often at the basis of their aggression and impulsivity.

> **KEYCONCEPT** **Temperament** comprises a person's characteristic intensity, rhythmicity, adaptability, energy expenditure, and mood. A **difficult temperament** is characterized by withdrawal from stimuli, low adaptability, and intense emotional reactions. Four key behaviors are present in a difficult temperament: aggression, inattention, hyperactivity, and impulsivity.

Temperaments consist of two behavioral dimensions that interact with each other. The activity spectrum varies from intense to passive. The adaptability spectrum varies from having a positive attitude about new stimuli with high flexibility to withdrawal from new stimuli and minimal flexibility in response to change. A strong relationship is found between difficult temperament and ASPD behaviors (Lennox & Dolan, 2014).

Attachment

One of the leading explanations of ASPD is that unsatisfactory attachments in early relationships lead to antisocial behavior in later life. Attachment, attaining and retaining interpersonal connection to a significant person, begins at birth. In a secure attachment, a child feels safe, loved, and valued and develops the self-confidence to interact with the rest of the world. Experiences within the context of secure relationships enable the child to develop trust in others. Strong attachments between parents and child may lower the risk of delinquency, assault, and other offenses that are characteristic of those who develop antisocial behavior (Christian, Sellbom, & Wilkinson, 2017).

In individuals with ASPD, a failure to make or sustain stable attachments in early childhood can lead to avoidance of future attachments. Risk factors for developing dysfunctional attachments include parental abandonment or neglect, loss of a parent or primary caregiver, and physical or sexual abuse. Parents who lacked secure attachment relationships in their own childhoods may be unable to form secure attachment relationships with their own children.

Family Issues

In many cases, individuals with ASPD come from chaotic families in which alcoholism and violence are the norm. Individuals who have been victims of abuse or neglect, live in a foster home, or had several primary caregivers are more likely to be victimized by antisocial behaviors, especially aggression. Child abuse and growing up in a home with domestic violence increase risk of antisocial behavior (Green & Browne, 2019). However, it is difficult to separate the influence of social factors on the development of the disorder because the symptoms of ASPD are expressed as social manifestations, including unemployment, multiple divorces and separations, and violence.

Family Response to Antisocial Personality Disorder

If family members are present in a patient's life, they have probably been abused, mistreated, or intimidated by these patients. For example, one patient sold his mother's possessions while she was at work. Another abused his wife after drinking. However, family members may be fiercely loyal to the patient and blame themselves for his or her shortcomings.

Recovery-Oriented Care of Persons With Antisocial Personality Disorder

Teamwork and Collaboration: Working Toward Recovery

People rarely seek mental health care for ASPD but rather for treatment of depression, substance abuse, uncontrolled anger, or forensic-related problems. Patients with psychiatric disorders who are admitted through the courts often have a comorbid diagnosis of ASPD. Antisocial personality–disordered patients usually present for treatment as a result of an ultimatum. Treatment is often a choice between losing a job, being expelled from school, ending a marriage or relationship with children, or giving up on a chance at probation and psychological treatment. Under these circumstances treatment is usually forced on them; most prisons and other correctional facilities require inmates to attend psychotherapy sessions. In either case working with people with ASPD is likely to be a frustrating and exasperating experience for the nurse due to the patient's clear lack of insight and/or motivation to change. Treatment is difficult and involves helping the patient alter his or her cognitive schemata. The overall treatment goals are to develop a nurturing sense of attachment and empathy for other people and situations and to live within the norms of society.

Safety Issues

Although they can be interpersonally charming, these patients can become verbally and physically abusive if their expectations are not met. Protection of other patients and staff is a priority.

Evidence-Based Nursing Care of Persons With Antisocial Personality Disorder

Mental Health Nursing Assessment

ASPD does not significantly impair physical functioning except in the presence of coexisting substance use disorder or another psychiatric diagnosis involved. Because substance abuse is a major problem with this population, the physical effects of chronic use of addictive substances must be considered. Conversely, someone who has health problems secondary to chronic substance misuse should also be assessed for concurrent personality disorders. Many patients with ASPD are committed to mental health care by the court system.

Eliciting psychosocial data from persons with ASPD may be difficult because of their basic mistrust about authority figures. They may not give an accurate history or may embellish aspects to project themselves in a more positive light. They often deny any criminal activity even if they are admitted in police custody.

Key areas of assessment are determining the quality of relationships, impulsivity, and the extent of aggression. These individuals do not assume responsibility for their own actions and often blame others for their misfortune. Their disregard for others is manifested in their interactions. For example, one patient with human immunodeficiency virus was engaging in unprotected sex with several different women because he wanted to "have fun as long as I can." He was completely unconcerned about the possibility of transmitting the virus. These individuals often make good first impressions. Self-awareness is especially important for the nurse because of the initial charming quality of many of these individuals. When these patients realize that the nurse cannot be used or manipulated, they lose interest in the nurse and revert to their normal, egocentric behaviors. Nursing Care Plan 24.2 is available at http://thepoint.lww.com/BoydEssentials2e.

Priority of Care

People with ASPD are often admitted to psychiatric units following a violent incident such as a physical confrontation or a suicide attempt. As with any patient, safety is a priority. One of the first priorities is to establish a safe environment for the patient and staff. After safety is established, other mutually agreed-upon priorities can be considered, such as improving interpersonal communication with family members or addressing anger issues.

Outcomes should be short term and relevant to a specific problem. For example, if a patient has been chronically unemployed, a reasonable short-term outcome is to set up job interviews rather than obtain a job.

Therapeutic Relationship

Therapeutic relationships are difficult to establish because these individuals do not attach themselves to others and are often unable to use a relationship to change behavior. The goal of the therapeutic relationship is to identify dysfunctional thinking patterns and develop new problem-solving behaviors. After the first few meetings with these patients, the nurse may believe that the relationship has a good start, but in reality, a superficial alliance is usually formed. Additional sessions reveal the lack of patient commitment to the relationship. These patients begin to revisit topics discussed in previous sessions or lose interest in trying to work on problems. By using self-awareness skills and accessing supervision regularly, the nurse can identify blocks in the development of a therapeutic relationship (or lack of) and his or her response to the relationship.

Mental Health Nursing Interventions

In instances in which there are concurrent disorders, the patient with ASPD may actually interfere with interventions aimed at improving physical functioning. For example, a patient with schizophrenia and ASPD may not develop enough trust within a relationship to examine his or her delusional thoughts or other aspects of dysfunction, such as alcohol or drug abuse.

Facilitating Self-Responsibility

Facilitating self-responsibility (i.e., encouraging a patient to assume more responsibility for personal behavior) is an important intervention. The nursing activities that are particularly helpful include holding the patient responsible for his or her behavior, monitoring the extent that self-responsibility is assumed, and discussing the consequences of not dealing with responsibilities. The nurse needs to refrain from arguing or bargaining about the unit rules, such as time for meals, use of the television room, and smoking. Instead, positive feedback is given to the patient for accepting additional responsibility or changing behavior.

Enhancing Self-Awareness

Enhancing self-awareness (i.e., exploring and understanding personal thoughts, feelings, motivation, and behaviors) is another nursing intervention that is helpful in developing an understanding about relating peacefully to the rest of the world. Encouraging patients to recognize and discuss their thoughts and feelings helps the nurse understand how the patient views the world. Some evidence indicates that substance misuse can be improved through cognitive behavioral treatment, but there is little evidence that the core problems of this disorder (aggression, reconviction, global functioning, and social functioning) are improved with psychological interventions (Brazil, van Dongen, Maes, Mars, & Baskin-Sommers, 2018).

Teaching Points

Patient education efforts have to be creative and thought provoking. In teaching a person with ASPD, a direct approach is best, but the nurse must avoid "lecturing,"

BOX 24.8 • THERAPEUTIC DIALOGUE • Antisocial Personality Disorder

INEFFECTIVE APPROACH

Danny: Hey, I need a light for my cigarette.
Nurse: Really? You know the rules—no smoking on the unit.
Danny: I'm not going to smoke here. I just need a light so that I can have a cigarette when I leave here.
Nurse: I also need your cigarettes. Cigarettes are contraband.
Danny: You are terrible – just like the bitch who kicked me out. Who do you think you are anyway?
Nurse: You need to quiet down.
Danny: Yeah, says who?
Nurse: I will call security if you don't quiet down.
Danny: Call them, I don't care.

EFFECTIVE APPROACH

Danny: Hey, I need a light for my cigarette.
Nurse: A light? I don't have a light.
Danny: I need a light so that I can smoke later.
Nurse: Oh, I see. Did you have a lighter when you were admitted?
Danny: Yea, they took everything away including my belt and shoe laces.
Nurse: The reason for storing everything is for the safety of everyone. When you are discharged you can retrieve everything. I also need to store any cigarettes you have.
Danny: What makes you think I have any cigarettes?
Nurse: Well, you asked for a light. Many patients manage to bring cigarettes into the unit. I need to put them with your things. You can retrieve them when you are discharged.
Danny: This place is something.
Nurse: I will put your cigarettes in a bag with your name on them.
Danny: This sucks. But here they are.

CRITICAL THINKING CHALLENGE

- How did the nurse in the first scenario get sidetracked?
- How was the nurse in the second scenario able to convince Danny to give up his cigarettes without escalating his anger?

---

which the patient will resent. In teaching the patient about positive health care practices, impulse control, and anger management, the best approach is to engage the patient in a discussion about the issue and then direct the topic to the major teaching points. These patients often take great delight in arguing or showing how the rules of life do not apply to them. A sense of humor is important, as are clear teaching goals and avoiding being sidetracked (see Boxes 24.8 and 24.9).

Group Interventions

Group interventions are more effective than individual modalities because other patients and staff can validate or challenge the patient's view of a situation. Problem-solving groups that focus on identifying a problem and developing a variety of alternative solutions are particularly helpful because patient self-responsibility

BOX 24.9

Psychoeducation Checklist: Antisocial Personality Disorder

When caring for the patient with antisocial personality disorder, be sure to include the following topic areas in the teaching plan:

- Positive health care practices, including substance abuse control
- Effective communication and interaction skills
- Impulse control
- Anger management
- Group experience to help develop self-awareness and impact of behavior on others
- Analyzing an issue from the other person's viewpoint
- Maintenance of employment
- Interpersonal relationships and social interactions

is reinforced when patients remind each other of better alternatives. Patients are likely to confront each other with dysfunctional schemata or thinking patterns. Teaching patients with ASPD the same communication techniques as those with BPD will also encourage self-responsibility. These patients often attend groups that focus on the development of empathy.

Milieu Interventions

Milieu interventions, such as providing a structured environment with rules that are consistently applied to patients who are responsible for their own behavior, are important. While living in close proximity to others, the individual with ASPD will demonstrate dysfunctional social patterns that can be identified and targeted for correction. For example, these patients often violate ward rules, such as no smoking or limitations on the number of visitors, and may bring contraband, such as illegal drugs, into the unit.

In an inpatient unit, interventions can be more intense and focus on helping the patient develop positive interaction skills and experience a consistent environment. For example, the focus of nursing interventions may be the patient's continual disregard of the rights of others. On one unit, a patient continually placed orders for pizzas in the name of another patient who had limited intelligence and was genuinely afraid of the person with ASPD. The victimized patient always paid for the pizza. When the nursing staff realized what was happening, they confronted the patient with ASPD about the behavior and revoked his unit privileges.

Anger Management

Aggressive behavior is often a problem for these individuals and their family members. Similar to patients with BPD, people with ASPD tend to be impulsive. Instead of self-injury, these individuals are more likely to strike out at those who are perceived to be interfering with their immediate gratification. Anger-control assistance (helping to express anger in an adaptive, nonviolent manner) becomes a priority intervention. Because the expression of anger and aggression develops during a lifetime, these individuals can benefit from anger management techniques.

Social Support

Social support for these individuals is often minimal, just as it is for individuals with BPD, but the reasons are different. These individuals have often taken advantage of friends and relatives who, in turn, no longer trust them. Helping the patient build a new support system after new skills are learned is usually the only option.

For these individuals to develop friends and re-engage family members, they must learn to interact in new ways, develop empathy, and risk an attachment. For many, this never truly becomes a reality.

Interventions for Family Members

Family members of patients with ASPD usually need help in establishing boundaries. Because there is a long-term pattern of interaction in which family members feel responsible for the patient's antisocial behavior, these patterns need to be stopped. Families need help in recognizing the patient's responsibility for his or her actions.

Evaluation and Treatment Outcomes

The outcomes of interventions for patients with ASPD need to be evaluated in terms of management of specific problems, such as maintaining employment or developing a meaningful interpersonal relationship. The nurse will most likely see these patients for other health care problems, so adherence to treatment recommendations and development of health care practices (e.g., reducing smoking and alcohol consumption) can also be factored into the evaluation of outcomes.

Continuum of Care

People with ASPD rarely seek mental health care unless there is a comorbid condition such as depression. Nurses are most likely to see these patients in medical–surgical settings for comorbid conditions. Consistency in interventions is necessary in treating the patient throughout the continuum of care.

HISTRIONIC PERSONALITY DISORDER
Clinical Course and Diagnostic Criteria

"Attention seeking," "excitable," and "emotional" are terms used to describe people with **histrionic personality disorder**. Histrionic personality disorder is more likely in women. Affected individuals are lively and dramatic and draw attention to themselves by their enthusiasm, dress, and apparent openness. They are the "life of the party" and, on the surface, seem interested in others. Their insatiable need for attention and approval quickly becomes obvious. Their need to be "center stage" arises in two ways: (1) their interests and topics of conversation focus on their own desires and activities, and (2) their behavior, including their speech pattern, continually calls attention to themselves. These needs are inflexible and persistent even after others attempt to meet them. Persons with histrionic personality disorders are quick to form new friendships and just as quick to become demanding. Because they are trusting and easily influenced by other opinions, their behavior often appears inconsistent. Their strong dependency need makes them overly trusting and gullible. They are moody and often experience a sense of helplessness when others are uninterested in them. They are sexually seductive in their attempts to gain attention and often are uncomfortable within a single relationship. Their appearance is provocative and their speech dramatic. They express strong opinions without supporting facts. Loyalty and fidelity are lacking (Hamlat, Young, & Hankin, 2019). Gender influences the manifestations of this disorder. Women dress seductively, may express dependency on selected men, and may "play" a submissive role. Men may dress in a very masculine manner and seek attention by bragging about athletic skills or successes in their jobs. Individuals with this disorder have difficulty achieving any true intimacy in interpersonal relationships. They seem to possess an innate sensitivity to the moods and thoughts of those they wish to please. This hyperalertness enables them to maneuver quickly to gain their attention. They then attempt to control relationships by their seductiveness at one level but become extremely dependent on their friends at another level. Their demand for constant attention quickly alienates their friends. They become depressed when they are not the center of attention.

Epidemiology and Risk Factors

The prevalence of histrionic personality disorder is estimated at 1.8% of the general population of the United States (Grant et al., 2004). No gender differences arise in the occurrence of this disorder; however, this diagnosis is seen more frequently in women than men clinically. Risk of occurrence of this disorder is greater among African Americans than whites. Low-income groups and less educated persons are also at higher risk for occurrence of histrionic personality disorder. Widowed, separated, divorced, or people who never married are at greater risk than married ones. This disorder occurs concurrently with other mental disorders; anxiety disorder, obsessive-compulsive syndromes, somatoform syndromes, substance use disorder, and mood disorders in which they overplay their feelings of dysthymia by expressing them through dramatic and eye-catching gestures (Millon, 2011).

Etiology

Research related to this personality disorder is minimal. Some speculate that there is a biologic component and that heredity may play a role but that the biologic influence is less than in some of the previously discussed personality problems. In infancy and early childhood, these individuals are extremely alert and emotionally responsive. The tendencies for sensory alertness may be traced to responses of the limbic and reticular systems. They demonstrate a high degree of dependence on others and a type of dissociation in which they have reduced awareness of their behavior in relation to others (Millon, 2011).

It is believed that these highly alert and responsive infants seek more gratification from external stimulation during their first few months of life. Depending on the responsiveness of caregivers to them, they develop behavior patterns in response to their caregivers. It is believed that these children experience brief, highly charged, and irregular reinforcement from multiple caregivers (parents, siblings, grandparents, foster parents) who are unable to provide consistent experiences.

Parental behavior and role modeling are also believed to contribute to the development of histrionic personality disorder. Many of the women with this disorder reported that they are just like their mother, who is emotionally labile, bored with the routines of home life, flirtatious with men, and clever in dealing with people. It is believed that through role modeling, these children learn and mimic the behaviors observed in caregivers or adults (Millon, 2011).

Evidence-Based Nursing Care for Persons With Histrionic Personality Disorder

The ultimate treatment goal for patients with histrionic personality disorder is to correct the tendency to expect others to fulfill all of their needs. When these individuals seek mental health care, they have usually experienced a period of social disapproval or deprivation. Their hope is that the mental health providers will help fulfill their needs. Specific goals are needed to protect the person from becoming dependent on a mental health system. In the nursing assessment, the nurse focuses on the quality of the individual's interpersonal relationships. It is common that the person is dissatisfied with his or her partner, and sexual relations may be nonexistent.

During the assessment, the patient will make statements that indicate low self-esteem. Because these individuals believe that they are incapable of handling life's demands and have been waiting for a truly competent person to take care of them, they have not developed a positive self-concept or adequate problem-solving abilities.

Priority of care areas for persons with this disorder include focusing on self-esteem and coping patterns. Outcomes focus on helping the patient develop autonomy, a positive self-concept, and mature problem-solving skills.

A variety of interventions support the outcomes. A nurse–patient relationship that allows the patient to explore positive personality characteristics and develop independent decision-making skills forms the basis of the interventions. Reinforcing personal strengths, conveying confidence in the patient's ability to handle situations, and examining the patient's negative perceptions of him- or herself can be done within the therapeutic relationship. Encouraging the patient to act autonomously can also improve the individual's sense of self-worth. Attending assertiveness groups can help increase the individual's self-confidence and improve self-esteem.

Continuum of Care

Patients with histrionic personality disorder do not seek mental health care unless they have a coexisting medical or mental disorder. They are likely to be treated within the community for most of their lives, with the exception of short hospitalizations for nonpsychiatric problems.

NARCISSISTIC PERSONALITY DISORDER

Clinical Course and Diagnostic Criteria

People with **narcissistic personality** disorder are grandiose, have an inexhaustible need for admiration, and lack empathy. Beginning in childhood, these individuals believe that they are superior, special, or unique and that others should recognize them in this way (Hamlat et al., 2019). They are often preoccupied with fantasies of unlimited success, power, beauty, or ideal love. They overvalue their personal worth, direct their affections toward themselves, and expect others to hold them in high esteem. They define the world through their own self-centered view. Their sense of entitlement is striking. People with narcissistic personality disorder are benignly arrogant and feel themselves above the conventions of their cultural group. They handle criticism poorly and may become enraged if someone dares to criticize them or else they may appear totally indifferent to criticism. They believe they are entitled to be served and that it is their inalienable right to receive special considerations. People with this disorder want to have their own way and are frequently ambitious for fame and fortune. These individuals are often successful in their jobs but may alienate their significant others, who grow tired of their narcissism. They cannot show empathy, and they feign sympathy only for their own benefit to achieve their selfish ends. Clinically, those with narcissistic personality disorder show overlapping characteristics of BPD and ASPD.

Epidemiology

The prevalence of narcissistic personality disorder is 6.2% of the U.S. general population with rates greater for men (7.7%) than for women (4.8%) according to a recent national epidemiologic survey (Stinson et al., 2008). Narcissistic personality disorder can be found in professionals who are highly respected such as those in law, medicine, and science and those associated with celebrity status. Persons with this disorder may impart an unrealistic sense of omnipotence, grandiosity, beauty, and talent to their children; therefore, children of parents with a narcissistic personality disorder have a higher than usual risk of developing the disorder themselves. It also commonly occurs in only children and among first-born boys in cultural groups in which males have special privileges (Millon, 2011).

Etiology

Limited evidence suggests biologic factors contribute to the development of this disorder. One notion about its development is that it is the result of parents' overvaluation and overindulgence of a child. These children are overly pampered and indulged, with every whim catered to. They learn to view themselves as special beings and to expect special treatment and subservience from others. They do not learn how to cooperate, share, or consider others' desires and interests. An alternate explanation is that the child never truly separated emotionally from his or her primary caregiver and therefore cannot envision functioning independently. According to another set of theories, these individuals try to avoid or reduce intense feelings of shame and engage in diverse strategies to gain attention for themselves (Roepke & Vater, 2014).

Evidence-Based Nursing Care for Persons With Narcissistic Personality Disorder

The nurse usually encounters persons with narcissism in medical settings and in psychiatric settings with a coexisting psychiatric disorder. They are difficult patients who often appear snobbish, condescending, and patronizing in their attitudes. It is unlikely that these individuals are motivated to develop sensitivity to others and socially cooperative attitudes and behaviors. Building a therapeutic relationship is a slow process because these patients avoid self-reflection and often reject the clinician's approaches. Nurses need to use their self-awareness skills in interacting with these patients. The nursing process focuses on the coexisting responses to other health care problems (Ronningstam & Weinberg, 2013).

Continuum of Care

Similar to patients with histrionic disorder, those with narcissistic personality disorder do not seek mental health care unless they have a coexisting medical or mental disorder. They are likely to be treated within the community for most of their lives, with the exception of short hospitalizations for nonpsychiatric problems.

CLUSTER C DISORDERS: AVOIDANT, DEPENDENT, AND OBSESSIVE-COMPULSIVE PERSONALITY DISORDERS

AVOIDANT PERSONALITY DISORDER

Clinical Course and Diagnostic Criteria

Avoidant personality disorder is characterized by staying out of social situations in which interpersonal contact with others may be expected. Individuals appear timid, shy, and hesitant; they also fear criticism and feel inadequate. These individuals are extremely sensitive to negative comments and disapproval and appraise situations more negatively than others do. This behavior becomes problematic when it restricts their social activities and work opportunities because of their extreme fear of rejection.

In childhood, they are shy, but instead of growing out of the shyness, it becomes worse in adulthood. They perceive themselves as socially inept, inadequate, and inferior, which in turn justifies their isolation and rejection by others. Vocationally, people with avoidant personality disorder often take jobs on the sidelines, rarely obtaining personal advancement or exercising much authority, but to employers, they seem shy and eager to please. They are reluctant to enter relationships unless they are given strong assurance of uncritical acceptances, so they consequently often have no close friends or confidants (Millon, 2011).

Epidemiology and Risk Factors

The prevalence of avoidant personality disorder is 2.4% in the general population (APA, 2013), but it has been reported in 10% of outpatients in mental health clinics (Grant et al., 2004). The problem with examining the epidemiology of avoidant personality disorder is its potential overlap with generalized social phobia. Several studies found that a significant portion of the patients with diagnoses of social phobia also met criteria for avoidant personality disorder (Carter & Wu, 2010; Cox, Pagura, Stein, & Sareen, 2009). More research is needed to clarify the relationship between avoidant personality and anxiety disorders.

Etiology

Experts speculate that individuals with avoidant personality disorder experience aversive stimuli more intensely and more frequently than others do because they may possess an overabundance of neurons in the aversive center of the limbic system (Millon, 2011).

Evidence-Based Nursing Care for Persons With Avoidant Personality Disorders

Assessment of these individuals reveals a lack of social contacts, a fear of being criticized, and evidence of chronic low self-esteem. The focus of nursing care will be issues of self-esteem and being socially isolated. The person's ability to cope with stress may need to be strengthened also. The establishment of a therapeutic relationship is necessary to be able to help these individuals meet their treatment outcomes. The development of the nurse–patient relationship is a slow process and requires an extreme amount of patience on the part of the nurse. These individuals may not have had positive interpersonal relationships and need time to be able to be sure that the nurse will not criticize and demean them. Interventions should focus on refraining from any negative criticism, assisting the patient to identify positive responses from others, exploring previous achievements of success, and exploring reasons for self-criticism. The patient's social dimension should be examined for activities that increase self-esteem and interventions focused on increasing these self-esteem–enhancing activities. Social skills training may help reduce symptoms.

Continuum of Care

Long-term therapy is ideal for patients with avoidant personality disorder because it takes time to make changes in one's behavior. Mental health nurses may initially see these individuals for other health problems. Encouraging the patient to continue with therapy and contacting the therapist when necessary are important in maintaining continuity of care. These patients are hospitalized only for a coexisting disorder.

DEPENDENT PERSONALITY DISORDER

Clinical Course and Diagnostic Criteria

People with **dependent personality disorder** cling to others in a desperate attempt to keep them close. Their need to be taken care of is so great that it leads to doing anything to maintain the closeness, including total submission and disregard for themselves.

Decision-making is difficult or nonexistent. They adapt their behavior to please those to whom they are attached. They lean on others to guide their lives. They ingratiate themselves with others and denigrate themselves and their accomplishments. Their self-esteem is determined by others. Behaviorally, they withdraw from adult responsibilities by acting helpless and seeking nurturance from others. In interpersonal relationships, they need excessive advice and reassurance. They are compliant, conciliatory, and placating. They rarely disagree with others and are easily persuaded. Friends describe them as gullible. They are warm, tender, and noncompetitive. They timidly avoid social tension and interpersonal conflicts (Hamlat et al., 2019). However, these individuals are at risk for suicide and parasuicide, perpetration of child abuse, perpetration of domestic violence (in men), and victimization by a partner (in women) (Bornstein, 2012).

Epidemiology and Risk Factors

A recent study estimates the prevalence at 0.49% (APA, 2013). The diagnosis is made more frequently in women than in men. This gender difference may represent a sex bias by clinicians because when standardized instruments are used, men and women receive diagnoses at equal rates. The risk of dependent personality disorder is greater for the least educated and for widowed, divorced, separated, and never married women (Disney, 2013).

Etiology

It is likely that a biologic predisposition exists to develop the dependency attachments of this disorder. However, no research studies support a biologic hypothesis. Dependent personality disorder is most often explained as a result of parents' genuine affection, extreme attachment, and overprotection. Children then learn to rely on others to meet their basic needs and do not learn the necessary skills for autonomous behavior. Persons with chronic physical illnesses in childhood may be prone to developing this disorder.

Evidence-Based Nursing Care for Persons With Dependent Personality Disorder

Nurses can determine the extent of dependency by assessment of self-worth, interpersonal relationships, and social behavior. They should determine whether there is currently someone on whom the person relies (parent, spouse) or whether there has been a separation from a significant relationship by death or divorce.

Priorities of care that are usually identified include low self-esteem, difficulties in social situations, and coping with stresses of everyday life. Home management skills may be a priority if the patient does not have these skills and has to make decisions related to finances, shopping, cooking, and cleaning. The challenge of caring for these patients is to help them recognize their dependent patterns; motivate them to want to change; and teach them adult skills that have not been developed, such as balancing a checkbook, planning a weekly menu, and paying bills when they are due. Occasionally, if a patient is extremely fatigued, lethargic, or anxious, the disorder interferes with efforts at developing greater independence, antidepressants or antianxiety agents may be used in therapy.

These patients readily engage in a nurse–patient relationship and initially look to the nurse to make all decisions. The nurse can support patients to make their own decisions by resisting the urge to tell them what to do. Ideally, these patients are in individual psychotherapy and working toward long-term personality changes. The nurse can encourage patients to stay in therapy and to practice the new skills that are being learned. Assertiveness training is helpful.

Continuum of Care

Individuals with dependent personality disorder readily seek out therapy and are likely to spend years seeking therapy. Hospitalization occurs for comorbid conditions such as depression.

OBSESSIVE-COMPULSIVE PERSONALITY DISORDER

Clinical Course and Diagnostic Criteria

Obsessive-compulsive personality disorder (OCPD) stands out because it bears close resemblance to obsessive-compulsive disorder (OCD), and is closely related to anxiety disorder. Although these disorders have similar names, the clinical manifestations are quite different. A distinguishing difference is that those with the OCD tend to use obsessive thoughts and compulsions when anxious but less so when anxiety decreases. Persons with OCPD do not demonstrate obsessions and compulsions but rather a pervasive pattern of preoccupation with orderliness, perfectionism, and control. They also have the capacity to delay rewards; whereas those with OCD do not (Pinto, Steinglass, Greene, Weber, & Simpson, 2013). Individuals with this disorder attempt to maintain control by careful attention to rules, trivial details, procedures, and lists (Thamby & Khanna, 2019). They may be completely devoted to work, which typically has a rigid character, such as maintaining financial records or tracking inventory. They are uncomfortable with unstructured leisure time, especially vacations. Their leisure activities are likely to be formalized (e.g., season tickets to sports, organized tour groups). Hobbies are approached seriously.

Behaviorally, individuals with OCPD are perfectionists, maintaining a regulated, highly structured, strictly organized life. A need to control others and situations is common in their personal and work lives. They are prone to repetition and have difficulty making decisions and completing tasks because they become so involved in the details. They can be overly conscientious about morality and ethics and value polite, formal, and correct interpersonal relationships. They also tend to be rigid, stubborn, and indecisive and are unable to accept new ideas and customs. Their mood is tense and joyless. Warm feelings are restrained, and they tightly control the expression of emotions (Tang, Chen, & Lung, 2018).

Epidemiology and Risk Factors

OCPD is one of the most prevalent personality disorders in the general population, with estimated prevalence ranging from 2.1% to 7.9% (APA, 2013). This disorder is associated with higher education, employment, and marriage. Subjects with the disorder had a higher income than did those without the disorder.

Etiology

As with some other personality disorders, evidence for a biologic formulation is scant. The basis of the compulsive patterns that characterize OCPD is parental overcontrol and overprotection that is consistently restrictive and sets distinct limits on the child's behavior. Parents teach these children a deep sense of responsibility to others and to feel guilty when these responsibilities are not met. Play is viewed as shameful, sinful, and irresponsible, leading to dire consequences. They are encouraged to resist the natural inclinations toward play and impulse gratification, and parents try to impose guilt on the child to control behavior.

Evidence-Based Nursing Care for Persons With OCPD

These individuals seek mental health care when they have attacks of anxiety, spells of immobilization, sexual impotence, and excessive fatigue. The nursing assessment focuses on the patient's physical symptoms (sleep, eating, sexual), interpersonal relationships, and social problems. There may be multiple nursing care priorities such as anxiety, loneliness, decision-making, sexual problems, insomnia, and interpersonal relationships. People with OCPD realize that they can improve their quality of life, but they find it extremely anxiety provoking to make the necessary changes. To change the compulsive pattern, psychotherapy is needed. There may be short-term pharmacologic intervention with an antidepressant or anxiolytic as an adjunct may take place. A supportive nurse–patient relationship based on acceptance of the patient's need for order and rigidity will help the person have enough confidence to try new behaviors. Examining the patient's belief that underlies the dysfunctional behaviors can set the stage for challenging the childhood thinking. Because the compulsive pattern was established in childhood, it will take a long time to modify the behavior.

Continuum of Care

People with OCPD are treated primarily in the community. If there is a coexisting disorder or the person experiences periods of depression, hospitalization may be useful for a short period of time.

DISRUPTIVE, IMPULSE-CONTROL, AND CONDUCT DISORDERS

OVERVIEW OF DISRUPTIVE, IMPULSE-CONTROL, AND CONDUCT DISORDERS

Disruptive, impulse-control, and **conduct disorders** are a group of mental conditions that have the essential feature of irresistible impulsivity. Behaviors associated with these disorders violate the rights of others and/or are in conflict with societal norms (APA, 2013). Disorders discussed include oppositional defiant disorder, conduct disorder, intermittent explosive disorder, kleptomania, and pyromania. ASPD was discussed earlier in this chapter.

> **KEYCONCEPT Impulsivity**, acting without considering consequences or alternative actions, results when neurobiologic overactivity is stimulated by psychological, personality, or social factors related to personal needs of the individual (Tansey, 2010).

> **KEYCONCEPT Impulse-control disorders** often coexist with other disorders and are characterized by an inability to resist an impulse or temptation to complete an activity that is considered harmful to oneself or others.

Tension increases before the individual commits the act and derives excitement or gratification when the act is committed. The release of tension is perceived as pleasurable, but remorse and regret usually follow the act. The disruptive behavior disorders, which include oppositional defiant disorder and conduct disorder, are a group of conditions marked by significant problems of conduct.

Oppositional defiant disorder is characterized by a persistent pattern of disobedience, argumentativeness, angry outbursts, low tolerance for frustration, and tendency to blame others for misfortunes, large and small. Children with oppositional defiant disorder have trouble making friends and often find themselves in conflict with adults. See Box 24.10.

Conduct disorder is characterized by more serious violations of social norms, including aggressive behavior, destruction of property, and cruelty to animals. Children and adolescents with conduct disorder often lie to achieve short-term ends, may be truant from school, may run away from home, and may engage in petty larceny or even mugging.

Epidemiology

Disruptive behavior disorders are more common in boys and are associated with lower socioeconomic status and urban living (Miranda-Mendizabal et al., 2019). These disorders are relatively common in school-aged children and are frequently presenting complaints in child psychiatric treatment settings.

The prevalence of conduct disorder estimates range from 2% up to 10% with a median of 4%. The disorder appears to be fairly consistent across various countries that differ in race and ethnicity. Prevalence rates rise from childhood to adolescence and are higher among males than among females. Males with conduct disorder frequently are involved in fighting, stealing, vandalism,

BOX 24.10 CLINICAL VIGNETTE

Leon (Conduct Disorder)

Leon, a 14-year-old Hispanic boy, was admitted to the child psychiatric inpatient service from the emergency department (ED) after a fight with his mother. His mother reported that she and Leon had argued earlier in the evening and that he stormed out of the house screaming and vowing he would never return. Several hours later, Leon came back, yelling and demanding entry into the apartment. Leon's father was working. While his mother was getting up to open the door, Leon continued to yell and scream, waking the neighbors. This led to further arguing between Leon and his mother. Before long, the police were called, and Leon was taken to the ED.

The admission interview revealed that Leon had run away on several occasions and had even stayed away overnight. Although he strongly denied drug use, he had gotten drunk on several occasions. He had also been in several fights, the latest of which resulted in an expulsion from school. Three months before admission, he was caught trying to steal a CD from a music store. More recently, he boasted that he and his friends had snatched a purse at an outdoor concert and had broken into a car to steal its contents. Leon's school performance has been declining; he was truant on several occasions and will probably have to repeat ninth grade.

Leon was born in Puerto Rico and is the oldest of three children. His family moved to the mainland shortly after his birth, and the primary language at home is Spanish. His father is employed as a janitor and speaks very little English. His mother works as a secretary and has achieved fairly good command of English. He has received no treatment except for consultation with the school social worker.

What Do You Think?
- When conducting a nursing assessment, what would you want to learn about Leon's school performance?
- What information could you provide Leon's parents about pharmacotherapy? About behavior management?

---

and school disciplinary problems. Females with the diagnosis are more likely to practice lying, truancy, running away, substance use, and prostitution. Whereas males tend to exhibit both physical aggression and relational aggression (i.e., behaviors that harm social relations of others), females tend to exhibit relatively more relational aggression (APA, 2013). Conduct disorder is one of the most frequently diagnosed disorders in children in mental health facilities. Individuals with conduct disorder are at greater risk for experiencing mood or anxiety disorders and substance-related disorders (APA, 2013).

Etiology

The etiologies of oppositional defiant disorder and conduct disorder are complex. More attention has been paid to conduct disorder, probably because it is the more serious of the two. Models used to understand aggressiveness (see Chapter 14) are useful in examining these childhood disorders, which appear to have both genetic and environmental components.

Evidence-Based Nursing Care for Persons With Disruptive, Impulse-Control, and Conduct Disorders

Mental Health Nursing Assessment

The nurse gathers data from multiple sources. Adolescents with these disorders are at high risk for physical injury as a result of fighting and impulsive behavior. Sexual promiscuity is common, resulting in an increased frequency of pregnancy and sexually transmitted diseases.

An important aspect of assessment is to rule out comorbid conditions that may partially explain or complicate the person's lack of behavioral control. These conditions include ADHD, learning disabilities, chemical dependency, depression, bipolar illness, or generalized anxiety disorder. Young people who are chronically depressed may be irritable and easily frustrated. Given the tendency of adolescents to act out their frustration, chronic depression may exacerbate their behavior. Conduct problems can also elevate the risk for depression because young people who regularly elicit negative attention from parents and teachers and are constantly at odds with their environment may become despondent.

Adolescents with conduct problems are usually brought or forced into the mental health system by family, school, or the court system because of fighting, truancy, speeding tickets, car accidents, petty crimes, substance abuse, or suicide attempts. These young people may be hostile, sarcastic, defensive, and provocative. At the same time, they may appear calm, outgoing, and engaging. Inconsistencies, distortions, and misrepresentations of the truth are common when interviewing these children, so obtaining a clear history may be difficult. Therefore, instead of asking whether an event or behavior occurred, it may be better to ask when it occurred. These adolescents are adept at changing the subject and diverting discussions from sensitive issues. They often use denial, projection, and externalization of anger as defense mechanisms when asked for self-disclosure. The assessment, which may take several sessions, should be conducted in a nonjudgmental fashion. High levels of marital conflict, parental substance abuse, and parental antisocial behavior often mark family history. In planning interventions for patients with oppositional defiant disorder or conduct disorder, the focus is on problem behaviors. Therapeutic progress may be slow, at least partly because these patients often lack trust in authority figures.

Priority of Care

After patient and staff safety are established, improving communication and coping skills should be the patient's priorities. The nurse can help the patient develop insight into the need for enhanced communication and positive coping.

Nursing Interventions

Children with oppositional defiant disorder or conduct disorder who also have specific neurodevelopmental disorders should be placed in appropriate programs for remediation. If a diagnosis of ADHD or depression emerges from the evaluation, appropriate pharmacotherapy should be considered (see previous discussion of ADHD and after the discussion regarding depression).

Social Skills Training

The nurse should communicate behavioral expectations clearly and enforce them consistently. Consequences of appropriate and inappropriate actions also should be clear. Specific approaches for improving social and problem-solving skills are fundamental features for school-aged children and adolescents. Insofar as children and adolescents with conduct problems fail to recognize the adverse effects of their verbal and nonverbal behavior, their deficit can be formulated as an interpersonal problem. Social skills training teaches adolescents with these behavior disorders to recognize the ways in which their actions affect others. Training involves techniques such as role-playing, modeling by the therapist, and giving positive reinforcement to improve interpersonal relationships and enhance social outcomes.

Problem-Solving Therapy

In contrast to social skills training, which proposes that problems of conduct are the result of poor interpersonal skills, problem-solving therapy conceptualizes conduct problems as the result of deficiencies in cognitive processes. These processes include assessment of situations, interpretation of events, and expectations of others that are congruent with behavior. These children often misinterpret the intentions of others and may perceive hostility with little or no cause. Problem-solving skills training teaches these children to generate alternative solutions to social situations, sharpen thinking concerning the consequences of those choices, and evaluate responses after interpersonal conflicts.

Parent Management Training and Education

Parent training begins with educating parents about disruptive behavior disorders, focusing particularly on impulsiveness, impaired judgment, and self-control. Children with long-standing problems in these areas often elicit punitive responses and negative attributions about their behavior from their parents. Ironically, because these parental responses focus on the child's failure, they may contribute to the child's behavior problems. An important second step is to clarify parental expectations and interpretation of the child's behavior. Parent management training may be offered to a group of parents or to individuals.

The aims of education are to provide parents with new ways of understanding their child's behavior and to promote improved interactions between parent and child. The most commonly presented techniques include the importance of positive reinforcement (praise and tangible rewards) for adaptive behavior, clear limits for unacceptable behavior, and use of mild punishment (e.g., a time out) (Box 24.11).

Referral to Family Therapy

Family therapy is directed at assisting the family with altering maladaptive patterns of interaction or improving adjustment to stressors, such as changes or loss in family membership. Multisystem family therapy, which considers the child in the context of multiple family and community systems, has shown promise in the treatment of adolescents with conduct disorder.

BOX 24.11

Time-Out Procedure

- *Labeling behavior:* Identify the behavior that the child is expected to perform or cease. The aim of this statement is to make clear what is required of the child. It typically takes the form of a simple declarative sentence: "Threatening is not acceptable."
- *Warning:* In this step, the child is informed that if he or she does not perform the expected behavior or stop the unacceptable behavior, he or she will be given a "time out." "This is a warning: if you continue threatening to hit people, you'll have a time out."
- *Time out:* If the child does not heed the warning, he or she is told to take a time out in simple straightforward terms: "Take a time out."
- *Duration:* The usual duration for a time out is 5 minutes for children 5 years of age or older.
- *Location:* The child sits in a designated time-out chair without toys and without talking. The chair should be located away from general activity but within view. A kitchen timer can be used to mark the time, but the clock does not start until the child sits quietly in the designated spot.
- *Follow-up:* The child is asked to recount why he or she was given the time out. The explanation need not be detailed, and no further discussion of the matter is required. Indeed, long discourse about the child's behavior is not helpful and should be avoided.

Evaluation and Treatment Outcomes

The nurse can review treatment goals and objectives to assess the child's progress with respect to verbal and physical aggression, socially appropriate resolution of conflicts, compliance with rules and expectations, and better management of frustration. As is true for the initial assessment, evaluation of treatment outcomes relies on input from parents, teachers, and other health care team members.

Continuum of Care

Children and adolescents with conduct disorders may be involved with many different agencies in the community, such as child welfare services, school authorities, and the legal system. Mental health services are requested when a child or adolescent's behavior is out of control or a when comorbid disorder is suspected. Helping the patient and family negotiate their way through this maze of services may be an essential part of the treatment plan.

INTERMITTENT EXPLOSIVE DISORDER

Episodes of aggressiveness that result in assault or destruction of property characterize people with **intermittent explosive disorder**. The severity of aggressiveness is out of proportion to the provocation. The episodes can have serious psychosocial consequences, including job loss, interpersonal relationship problems, school expulsion, divorce, automobile accidents, or jail. This diagnosis is given only after all other disorders with aggressive components (e.g., delirium, dementia, head injury, BPD, ASPD, substance abuse) have been excluded. Little is known about this disorder, but it is a more common condition than previously thought. The prevalence of intermittent explosive disorder in the United States is about 2.7%. The onset is most common in childhood or adolescence and rarely begins for the first time after the age 40 years. The mean age at onset is 14 years. It is more prevalent in individuals with a high school education or less (APA, 2013). The anger experience and expression of anger contribute to suicidality (McCloskey & Ammerman, 2018).

The treatment of this disorder is multifaceted. Psychopharmacologic agents are sometimes used as an adjunct to psychotherapeutic, behavioral, and social interventions. Serotonergic antidepressants and gamma-aminobutyric acid (GABA)-ergic mood stabilizers have been used. Anxiolytics are used to treat obsessive patients who experience tension states and explosive outbursts. Medication alone is insufficient, and anger management should be included in the treatment plan.

KLEPTOMANIA

In **kleptomania**, individuals cannot resist the urge to steal, so they independently steal items that they could easily afford. These items are not particularly useful or wanted. The underlying issue is the act of stealing. The term kleptomania was first used in 1838 to describe the behavior of several kings who stole worthless objects (Aboujoude & Koran, 2010). These individuals experience an increase in tension and then pleasure and relief at the time of the theft. Kleptomania occurs in about 4% to 22% of individuals arrested for shoplifting. Its prevalence in the general population however is very rare, at approximately 0.3% to 0.6%. Females outnumber males at a ratio of 3:1 (APA, 2013). Because it is considered a "secret" disorder, little is known about it, but it is believed to last for years despite numerous convictions for shoplifting. It appears that kleptomania often has its onset during adolescence (Grant & Kim, 2005).

Some shoplifting appears to be related to anxiety and stress in that it serves to relieve symptoms. In a few instances, brain damage has been associated with kleptomania (Blum, Odlaug, Redden, & Grant, 2018). Depression is the most common symptom identified in a compulsive shoplifter.

Kleptomania is difficult to detect and treat and means of treatment are little known. It appears that behavior therapy is frequently used. Medication that helps relieve the depression has been successful in some cases. More investigation is needed (Chamberlain & Grant, 2019).

PYROMANIA

Irresistible impulses to start fires characterize **pyromania**, repeated fire setting with tension or arousal before setting fires; fascination or attraction to the fires; and gratification when setting, witnessing, or participating in the aftermath of fire. These individuals often are regular "fire watchers" or even firefighters. They are not motivated by aggression, anger, suicidal ideation, or political ideology. Little is known about this disorder because only a small number of deliberate fire starters are apprehended, and of those individuals, only a few undergo a psychiatric evaluation. The prevalence of fire setting in the general population is about 1%, but most fire setting is not done by people with pyromania, which occurs infrequently, mostly in men. However, those with a history of fire setting are most likely male, young, and never married and are more likely to have other psychiatric issues such as ASPD, substance use, and impulsivity (Tanner, Hasking, & Martin, 2016). Prevalence rates are lower among African Americans and Hispanics (Vaughn et al., 2010).

Early research demonstrated low serotonin and norepinephrine levels associated with arson. Little is known about treatment, and as with the other impulse-control disorders, no approach is uniformly effective. Historically, fire starters generally possess poor interpersonal skills, exhibit low self-esteem, battle depression, and have difficulty managing anger. Education, parenting training, behavior contracting with token reinforcement, problem-solving skills training, and relaxation exercises may all be used in the management of the patient's responses (Tanner et al., 2016).

CONTINUUM OF CARE FOR DISRUPTIVE, IMPULSE-CONTROL DISORDERS

Impulse-control disorders require long-term treatment, usually in an outpatient setting. Group therapy is often a facet of treatment because patients can talk in a community where people share common experiences. Hospitalization is rare except when patients have comorbid psychiatric or medical disorders.

SUMMARY OF KEY POINTS

- A personality is a complex pattern of characteristics, largely outside of the person's awareness, that comprise the individual's distinctive pattern of perceiving, feeling, thinking, coping, and behaving.

- A personality disorder is an enduring pattern of inner experience and behavior that deviates markedly from the expectations of the individual's culture, is pervasive and inflexible, has an onset in adolescence or early adulthood, is stable over time, and leads to distress or impairment.

- For many patients with personality disorders, maintaining a therapeutic nurse–patient relationship can be one of the most helpful interventions. Through this therapeutic relationship, the patient experiences a model of healthy interaction, establishing trust, consistency, caring, boundaries, and limitations that help to build the patient's self-esteem and respect for self and others. In some personality disorders, nurses will find it more difficult to engage the patient in a true therapeutic relationship because of the patient's avoidance of interpersonal and emotional attachment (i.e., antisocial personality disorder or paranoid personality disorder).

- Patients with personality disorders are rarely treated in an inpatient facility except during periods of destructive behavior or self-injury. Treatment is delivered in the community and over time. Continuity of care is important in helping the individual change life-long personality patterns.

- People with borderline personality disorder have difficulties regulating emotion and have extreme fears of abandonment, leading to dysfunctional relationships; they often engage in self-injury.

- Medications, including mood stabilizers, antidepressants, and antipsychotics, are useful in regulating the symptoms. They should, however, only be taken for target symptoms for a short time because patients may already be taking other medications, particularly for a comorbid disorder.

- During hospitalizations, keeping the patients safe by preventing self-harm is priority. Open communication and use of dialectical behavior therapy techniques are important interventions.

- Recovery-oriented approaches are grounded in cognitive behavioral therapy. The interdisciplinary treatment or recovery team needs to maintain open communication to work effectively with a person with BPD.

- Antisocial personality disorder, often synonymous with psychopathy, includes people who have no regard for and refuse to conform to social rules.

- The primary characteristic of disruptive, impulse-control disorders is impulsivity, which leads to inappropriate social behaviors that are considered harmful to oneself or others and that give the patient excitement or gratification at the time the act is committed.

CRITICAL THINKING CHALLENGES

1. Define the concepts *personality* and *personality disorder*. When does a normal personality become a personality disorder?

2. Karen, a 36-year-old woman receiving inpatient care, was admitted for depression; she also has a diagnosis of borderline personality disorder. After a telephone argument with her husband, she approaches the nurse's station with her wrist dripping with blood from cutting. What nursing approach best fits this behavior? What interventions should the nurse use with the patient after the self-injury is treated?

3. A 22-year-old man with borderline personality disorder is being discharged from the mental health unit after a severe suicide attempt. As his primary psychiatric nurse, you have been able to establish a therapeutic relationship with him but are now terminating the relationship. He asks you to meet

with him "for just a few sessions" after his discharge because his therapist will be on vacation. What are the issues underlying this request? What should you do? Explain and justify.

4. Compare the biologic theory with the psychoanalytic and Linehan's biosocial theory. What are the primary differences between these theories?

5. Compare the characteristics, epidemiology, and etiologic theories of antisocial and borderline personality disorders.

6. Discuss the differences between histrionic and obsessive-compulsive personality disorder.

7. Compare and contrast antisocial personality disorder with narcissistic personality trait.

8. Define and summarize personality disorders. Compare the following among the Cluster A, B, and C disorders:
   a. Defining characteristics
   b. Epidemiology
   c. Biologic, psychological, and social theories
   d. Key nursing assessment data
   e. Priority of care and outcomes
   f. Specific issues related to a therapeutic relationship
   g. Interventions

9. Define and summarize the impulse-control disorders. Compare the following among kleptomania, pyromania, and conduct disorders:
   a. Defining characteristics
   b. Epidemiology
   c. Biologic, psychological, and social theories
   d. Key nursing assessment data
   e. Nursing care priorities
   f. Interventions

1987: *Fatal Attraction*

This award-winning film portrays the relationship between a married attorney, Dan Gallagher (played by Michael Douglas), and Alex Forest, a single woman (played by Glenn Close). Their one-night affair turns into a nightmare for the attorney and his family as Alex becomes increasingly possessive and aggressive, demonstrating behaviors characteristic of borderline personality disorder, including anger, impulsivity, emotional lability, fear of rejection and abandonment, vacillation between adoration and disgust, and self-mutilation.

Viewing Points: Identify the behaviors of Alex that are characteristics of borderline personality disorder. Identify the feelings that are generated by the movie. With which characters do you identify? For which characters do you feel sympathy? If Alex had lived and been admitted to your hospital, what would be your first priority?

1975: *Grey Gardens*

This documentary by Albert and David Maysles is the unbelievable true story of Mrs. Edith Bouvier Beale and her daughter Edie, who are the aunt and first cousin of Jacqueline Kennedy Onassis. The film depicts mother and daughter, known as "Big Edie" and "Little Edie," who have descended into a strange life of dependence and eccentricity.

Living in a world of their own in a decaying 28-room East Hampton mansion, their living conditions—infested by fleas, inhabited by numerous cats and raccoons, deprived of running water, and filled with garbage—give viewers a glimpse into schizotypal personality disorder.

Viewing Points: Identify the behaviors of Big Edie and Little Edie that are characteristic of schizotypal personality disorder. Do "Big Edie" and "Little Edie" exhibit a folie à deux (a shared psychotic disorder)? Why or why not?

Related Psychiatric–Mental Health Nursing videos on the topics of Antisocial Personality Disorder and Borderline Personality Disorder are available at http://thepoint.lww.com/BoydEssentials.

Related Psychiatric–Mental Health Nursing Practice and Learn Interactive Case Studies related to the videos on the topics of Antisocial Personality Disorder and Borderline Personality Disorder are available at http://thepoint.lww.com/BoydEssentials.

REFERENCES

Aboujaoude, E., & Koran, L. M. (2010). *Impulse control disorders*. New York: Cambridge University Press.

Alcorn, J. L., Gowin, J. L., Green, C. E., Swann, A. C., Moeller, F. G., & Lane, S. D; Aggression, American Psychiatric Association. (2013). *Diagnostic and statistical manual of mental disorders* (5th ed.). Washington, DC: Author.

Birkeland, S. F. (2017). Paranoigenic extremes—A reappraisal concerning paranoid personality disorder. *Current Psychiatry Reviews, 13*(1), 23–34.

Blum, A. W., Odlaug, B. L., Redden, S. A., & Grant, J. E. (2018). Stealing behavior and impulsivity in individuals with kleptomania who have been arrested for shoplifting. *Comprehensive Psychiatry, 80*, 186–191.

Bornstein, R. F. (2012). Illuminating a neglected clinical issue: Societal costs of interpersonal dependency and dependent personality disorder. *Journal of Clinical Psychology, 68*(7), 766–781.

Brazil, I. A., van Dongen, J. D. M., Maes, J. H. R., Mars, R. B., & Baskin-Sommers, A. R. (2018). Classification and treatment of antisocial individuals: From behavior to biocognition. *Neuroscience & Biobehavioral Reviews, 91*, 259–277.

Carter, S. A., & Wu, K. D. (2010). Relations among symptoms of social phobia subtypes, avoidant personality disorder, panic, and depression. *Behavior Therapy, 41*(1), 2–13.

Chamberlain, S. R., & Grant, J. E. (2019). Efficacy of pharmacological interventions in targeting decision-making impairments across substance and behavioral addictions. *Neuropsychology Review, 29*(1), 93–102.

Chan, C. C., Szeszko, P. R., Wong, E., Tang, C. Y., Kelliher, C., Penner, J. D., et al. (2018). Frontal and temporal cortical volume, white matter tract integrity, and hemispheric asymmetry in schizotypal personality disorder. *Schizophrenia Research*, pii: S0920-9964(18)30047-1. doi: 10.1016/j.schres.2018.01.025.

Christian, E., Sellbom, M., & Wilkinson, R. B. (2017). Clarifying the associations between individual differences in general attachment styles and psychopathy. *Personality Disorders, 8*(4):329–339.

Clarkin, J. F., & De Panfilis, C. (2013). Developing conceptualization of borderline personality disorder. *The Journal of Nervous and Mental Disease, 201*(2), 88–93.

Cox, B. J., Pagura, J., Stein, M. B., & Sareen, J. (2009). The relationship between generalized social phobia and avoidant personality disorder in a national mental health survey. *Depression and Anxiety, 26*(4), 354–362.

DeCou, C. R., Comtois, K. A., & Landes, S. J. (2019). Dialectical behavior therapy is effective for the treatment of suicidal behavior: A meta-analysis. *Behavior Therapy*, 50(1), 60–72.

Deming, P., Philippi, C. L., Wolf, R. C., Dargis, M., Kiehl, K. A., & Koenigs, M. (2018). Psychopathic traits linked to alterations in neural activity during personality judgments of self and others. *Neuroimage Clinical*, 18, 575–581.

Disney, K. L. (2013). Dependent personality disorder: A critical review. *Clinical Psychology Review*, 33, 1184–1196.

Dotterer, H. L., Hyde, L. W., Swartz, J. R., Hariri, A. R., & Williamson, D. E. (2017). Amygdala reactivity predicts adolescent antisocial behavior but not callous-unemotional traits. *Developmental Cognitive Neuroscience*, 24, 84–92.

Ellison, W. D., Rosenstein, L. K., Morgan, T. A., & Zimmerman, M. (2018). Community and clinical epidemiology of borderline personality disorder. *Psychiatric Clinics of North America*, 41, 561–573.

Esmaeilian, N., Dehghani, M., Koster, E. H. W., & Hoorelbeke, K. (2019). Early maladaptive schemas and borderline personality disorder features in a nonclinical sample: A network analysis. *Clinical Psychology & Psychotherapy*. doi: 10.1002/cpp.2360.

Grant, B. F., Hasin, D. S., Stinson, F. D., Dawson, D. A., Chou, S. P., Ruan, W. J., et al. (2004). Prevalence, correlates, and disability of personality disorders in the United States: Results from the national epidemiologic survey on alcohol and related conditions. *Journal of Clinical Psychiatry*, 65(7), 948–958.

Grant, J. E., & Kim, S. W. (2005). Quality of life in kleptomania and pathological gambling. *Comprehensive Psychiatry*, 46(1), 34–37.

Green, K., & Browne, K. (2019). Personality disorder traits, trauma, and risk in perpetrators of domestic violence. *International Journal of Offender Therapy and Comparative Criminology*, 8, 306624X19826516.

Hamlat, E. J., Young, J. F., & Hankin, B. L. (2019). Developmental course of personality disorder traits in childhood and adolescence. *Journal of Personality Disorders*, 14, 1–19.

Hancock-Johnson, E., Griffiths, C., & Picchioni, M. (2017). A focused systematic review of pharmacological treatment for borderline personality disorder. *CNS Drugs*, 31(5), 345–356.

Kay, M. L., Poggenpoel, M., Myburgh, C. P., & Downing, C. (2018). Experiences of family members who have a relative diagnosed with borderline personality disorder. *Curationis*, 41(1), e1–e9.

Kolla, N. J., Dunlop, K., Meyer, J. H., & Downar, J. (2018). Corticostriatal connectivity in antisocial personality disorder by MAO-A genotype and its relationship to aggressive behavior. *The International Journal of Neuropsychopharmacology*, 21(8), 725–733.

Krause-Utz, A., & Elzinga, B. (2018). Current understanding of the neural mechanisms of dissociation in borderline personality disorder. *Current Behavioral Neuroscience Reports*, 5(1), 113–123.

Lee, R. (2017). Mistrustful and misunderstood: A review of paranoid personality disorder. *Current Behavioral Neuroscience Reports*, 4(2): 151–165.

Lennox, C., & Dolan, M. (2014). Temperament and character and psychopathy in male conduct disordered offenders. *Psychiatry Research*, 215(3), 706–710.

Levy, K. N., McMain, S., Bateman, A., & Clouthier, T. (2018). Treatment of borderline personality disorder. *Psychiatric Clinics of North America*, 41, 711–728.

Linehan, M. (1993). *Cognitive-behavioral treatment of borderline personality disorder*. New York: Guilford Press.

McCloskey, M. S., & Ammerman, B. A. (2018). Suicidal behavior and aggression-related disorders. *Current Opinion in Psychology*, 22, 54–58.

Meehan, K. B., Clarkin, J. F., & Lenzenweger, M. F. (2018). Conceptual models of borderline personality disorder, Part 1. *Psychiatric Clinics of North America*, 41, 535–548.

Meuldijk, D., McCarthy, A., Bourke, M. E., & Grenyer, B. F. (2017). The value of psychological treatment for borderline personality disorder: Systematic review and cost offset analysis of economic evaluations. *PLoS One*, 12(3), e0171592.

Millon, T. (2011). *Disorders of personality: Introducing a DSM/ICD spectrum from normal to abnormal* (3rd ed.). Hoboken, NJ: John Wiley & Sons, Inc.

Miranda-Mendizabal, A., Castellví, P., Parés-Badell, O., Alayo, I., Almenara, J., Alonso, J., et al. (2019). Gender differences in suicidal behavior in adolescents and young adults: Systematic review and meta-analysis of longitudinal studies. *International Journal of Public Health*, 64(2), 265–283.

Palihawadana, V., Broadbear, J. H., & Rao, S. (2019). Reviewing the clinical significance of 'fear of abandonment' in borderline personality disorder. *Australasian Psychiatry*, 27(1), 60–63.

Perez-Rodriguez, M. M., Bulbena-Cabré, A., Bassir Nia, A., Zipursky, G., Goodman, M., & New, A. S. (2018). The neurobiology of borderline personality disorder. *Psychiatric Clinics of North America*, 41, 633–650.

Pinto, A., Steinglass, J. E., Greene, A. L., Weber, E. U., & Simpson, H. B. (2013). Capacity to delay reward differentiates obsessive-compulsive disorder and obsessive compulsive personality disorder. *Biological Psychiatry*, 75(8), 653–659.

Pulay, A. J., Stinson, F. S., Dawson, D. A., Goldstein, R. B., Chou, S. P., Huang, B., et al. (2009). Prevalence, correlates, disability, and comorbidity of DSM-IV schizotypal personality disorder: Results from the Wave 2 National Epidemiologic Survey on alcohol and related conditions. *Primary care companion to the Journal of Clinical Psychiatry*, 11(2), 53–67.

Quidé, Y., Cohen-Woods, S., O'Reilly, N., Carr, V. J., Elzinga, B. M., & Green, M. J. (2018). Schizotypal personality traits and social cognition are associated with childhood trauma exposure. *The British Journal of Clinical Psychology*, 57(4), 397–419.

Racioppi, A., Sheinbaum, T., Gross, G. M., Ballespí, S., Kwapil, T. R., & Barrantes-Vidal, N. (2018). Prediction of prodromal symptoms and schizophrenia-spectrum personality disorder traits by positive and negative schizotypy: A 3-year prospective study. *PLoS One*, 13(11), e0207150.

Richetin, J., Preti, E., Costantini, G., & De Panfilis, C. (2017). The centrality of affective instability and identity in Borderline Personality Disorder: Evidence from network analysis. *PLoS One*, 2(10), e0186695.

Ripoll, L. H. (2012). Clinical psychopharmacology of borderline personality disorder: An update on the available evidence in light of the Diagnostic and Statistical Manual of Mental Disorders-5. *Current Opinion in Psychiatry*, 25(1), 52–58.

Roepke, S., & Vater, A. (2014). Narcissistic personality disorder: An integrative review of recent empirical data and current definitions. *Current Psychiatry Reports*, 16(5), 445–453.

Ronningstam, E., & Weinberg, I. (2013). Narcissistic personality disorder: Progress in recognition and treatment. *Focus*, 11(2), 167–177.

Santangelo, P. S., Reinhard, I., Koudela-Hamila, S., Bohus, M., Holtmann, J., Eid, M., et al. (2017). The temporal interplay of self-esteem instability and affective instability in borderline personality disorder patients' everyday lives. *Journal of Abnormal Psychology*, 126(8), 1057–1065.

Shah, R., & Zanarini, M. C. (2018). Comorbidity of borderline personality disorder: Current status and future directions. *Psychiatric Clinics of North America*, 41, 583–593.

Stern, B. L., Caligor, E., Horz-Sagstetter, S., & Clarkin, J. F. (2018). An object-relations based model for the assessment of borderline psychopathology. *Psychiatric Clinics of North America*, 41, 595–611.

Stinson, F. S., Dawson, D. A., Goldstein, R. B., Chou, S. P., Huang, B., Smith, S. M., et al. (2008). Prevalence, correlates, disability, and comorbidity of DSM-IV narcissistic personality disorder: Results from the Wave 2 National Epidemiologic Survey on alcohol and related conditions. *Journal of Clinical Psychiatry*, 69(7), 1033–1045.

Stoffers, J., Völlm, B. A., Rücker, G., Timmer, A., Huband, N., & Lieb, K. (2010). Pharmacological interventions for people with borderline personality disorder. *Cochrane Database of Systematic Reviews*, (6), CD005653. doi: 10.1002/14651858.CD005653.pub2.

Taber-Thomas, B. C., Asp, E. W., Koenigs, M., Sutterer, M., Anderson, S. W., & Tranel, D. (2014). Arrested development: Early prefrontal lesions impair the maturation of moral judgement. *Brain*, 137(pt 4), 1254–1261.

Tang, H., Chen, P., Lung, F. (2018). Personality and alexithymic disparity in obsessive-compulsive disorder based on washing and checking. *Psychiatric Quarterly*, 89(2), 371–381.

Tanner, A., Hasking, P., & Martin, G. (2016). Co-occurring non-suicidal self-injury and firesetting among at-risk adolescents: Experiences of negative life events, mental health problems, substance use, and suicidality. *Archives of Suicide Research*, 20(2), 233–249.

Tansey, T. N. (2010). Impulsivity: An overview of a biopsychosocial model. *Journal of Rehabilitation*, 76(3), 3–9.

Thamby, A., & Khanna, S. (2019). The role of personality disorders in obsessive-compulsive disorder. *Indian Journal of Psychiatry*, 61(Suppl 1), S114–S118.

Tielbeek, J. J., Barnes, J. C., Popma, A., Polderman, T. J., Lee, J. J., Perry, J. R., et al. (2018). Exploring the genetic correlations of antisocial behaviour and life history traits, *BJPsych Open*, 4(6), 467–470.

Tielbeek, J. J., Johansson, A., Polderman, T. J., Rautiainen, M. R., Jansen, P., Taylor, M., et al. (2017). Genome-wide association studies of a broad spectrum of antisocial behavior. *JAMA Psychiatry*, 74(12), 1242–1250.

Vaughn, M. G., Fu, Q., DeLisi, M., Wright, J. P., Beaver, K. M., Perron, B. E., et al. (2010). Prevalence and correlates of fire-setting in the United States: Results from the national epidemiological survey on alcohol and related conditions. *Comprehensive Psychiatry*, 51(3), 217–223.

Volkert, J., Gablonski, T. C., & Rabung, S. (2018). Prevalence of personality disorders in the general adult population in Western countries: Systematic review and meta-analysis. *The British Journal of Psychiatry*, 213(6), 709–715.

Zanarini, M. C., Frankenburg, F. R., Reich, D. B., & Fitzmaurice, G. M. (2016). Fluidity of the subsyndromal phenomenology of borderline personality disorder over 16 years of prospective follow-up. *American Journal of Psychiatry*, 173(7), 688–694.

25
Addiction and Substance-Related Disorders

Nursing Care of Persons With Alcohol and Drug Use

Mary Ann Boyd

KEY CONCEPTS
- addiction
- denial
- motivation

LEARNING OBJECTIVES

After studying this chapter, you will be able to:

1. Differentiate the actions, effects, and withdrawal symptoms of alcohol, marijuana, stimulants, tobacco, hallucinogens, opioids, inhalants, and also gambling disorder.
2. Discuss the evidence that serves as a basis of care and treatment of persons with substance-related and non–substance-related disorders.
3. Implement the nursing process for a person with substance-related and non–substance-related disorders.

KEY TERMS

- alcohol withdrawal syndrome • Alcoholics Anonymous • brief interventions • codependence • confabulation • confrontation • craving • delirium tremens • denial • detoxification • gambling disorder • hallucinogen • harm reduction • inhalants • intoxication • Korsakoff's amnestic syndrome • methadone maintenance • motivation • motivational interviewing • opioids • recovery • relapse • substance-induced disorder • substance use disorder • sudden sniffing death • tolerance • Wernicke–Korsakoff syndrome • Wernicke encephalopathy • withdrawal

Case Study: Gladys

Gladys, a 68-year-old widow, lives by herself in a comfortable apartment. She spends her days with friends and visiting her grandchildren. At night, she frequently has an alcoholic drink to relax her and help her sleep. She denies that she has a drinking problem.

The human use and abuse of alcohol and other drugs has been around since the beginning of history; so too have the subsequent social and emotional problems that accompany substance use. This chapter reviews the concept of addiction, types of substance use, biologic and psychological effects, current theories of substance-related disorders, and interventions. **Gambling disorder** is a non–substance-related disorder that is also discussed in this chapter. Gambling behaviors and their consequences have similar characteristics to the behaviors associated with substance disorders. The nurse's role in helping persons with these disorders' recovery is discussed. Professional issues related to chemical dependency within the nursing profession are also examined.

OVERVIEW OF SUBSTANCE USE AND ABUSE

Alcohol, tobacco, marijuana, and illegal prescription drug use have reached epidemic proportions in the United States, with the incidence rising in younger age groups, particularly among adolescents and young adults. One of the goals of *Healthy People 2020* is "to reduce substance abuse to protect the health, safety, and quality of life for all, especially children" (U.S. Department of Health and Human Services, 2010). A major challenge facing our country is the opioid epidemic. The overriding concern about using mind-altering substances is that these substances compromise health, and the continued use will lead to addiction.

> **KEYCONCEPT Addiction** is a condition of continued use of substances (or reward-seeking behaviors) despite adverse consequences.

Many mind-altering substances are physiologically addicting and easily can lead to severe health and legal problems. Use by ingestion, smoking, sniffing, or injection of some mind-altering substances such as alcohol, pain medication, tobacco, or caffeine is legal for adults. Other substances such as cocaine and heroin are illegal in the United States. Abuse occurs when a person uses alcohol or drugs for the purpose of intoxication or, in the case of prescription drugs, for purposes other than their intended use. Substance-related disorders involve substances that are commonly abused.

Physiologic dependence can develop with many different types of medications such as β-blockers, antidepressants, opioids, antianxiety agents, and others. As long as medications are used for their intended purposes and under the supervision of qualified health care providers, physiologic dependence is a part of treatment. That is, dependence can be a normal response to some medications (American Psychiatric Association [APA], 2013).

Diagnostic Criteria

Substance-related disorders are categorized into two categories: substance use disorders and substance-induced disorders. **Substance-induced disorders** occur when medications used for other health problems or medical/mental health disorders causes **intoxication, withdrawal,** or other health-related problems. A **substance use disorder** occurs when an individual continues using substances despite cognitive, behavioral, and physiologic symptoms. The *DSM-National 5* identifies 10 diagnostic categories of substances including alcohol, caffeine, cannabis (marijuana), hallucinogens, inhalants, opioids, sedative–hypnotics, stimulants, tobacco, and others (APA, 2013). Gambling disorder is included within the substance use disorder category because gambling behaviors can activate the brain's reward system similar to the substance use disorders.

A substance use disorder occurs when there is an underlying change in brain circuitry that may persist after **detoxification**, the process of safely and effectively withdrawing a person from an addictive substance, usually under medical supervision. These brain changes lead to pathologic behaviors that occur with repeated relapses and intense drug cravings when exposed to the drug-related cues (e.g., a party, emotional experiences) (APA, 2013).

Epidemiology

Age of Onset

In the United States, alcohol is the most abused substance, followed by marijuana. Alcohol use is at historically low levels for adolescents. In 2018, 8.2% of 8th graders, 18.6% of 10th graders, and 30.2% of 12th graders reported getting drunk in the previous month. In 2018, less than 14% of high school seniors reported binge drinking—a drop of a more than one third since the late 1990s—but illicit drug use continues to be a concern. In 2018, 0.7% of 8th graders, 3.4% of 10th graders, and 5.8% of 12th graders used marijuana daily. Marijuana use reflects a change in attitude and perception that marijuana is a safe drug, especially in light of recent legalization of marijuana in some states (National Institute of Drug Abuse [NIDA], 2019a).

The nonmedical use of prescription and over-the-counter (OTC) medicines continues to represent a significant part of the adolescent drug use, but prescription opioids have significantly decreased over the last 5 years. Fewer teens smoke cigarettes (5.3% of middle school students and 16% high school students). The use of e-cigarettes remains high, with 9.10% of 8th graders, 16.0% of 10th graders, and 23.8% of seniors reporting use of e-cigarettes (National Institute of Drug Abuse [NIDA], 2019b).

Ethnicity and Culture

Use of illicit and legal substances among Asians is consistently lower than in the other ethnic groups. In 2013, current illicit drug use was 3.7% among Asians, 5.0% among Native Hawaiians or Other Pacific Islanders, 7.1% among Hispanics, 9.5% among whites, 8.1% among blacks or African Americans, 12.2% among American Indians or Alaska Natives, and 17.4% among persons of two or more races. These statistics have been relatively stable since 2003 except for whites (from 8.5% to 9.5%) and African Americans (from 8.7% to 10.5%) (Substance Abuse and Mental Health Services Administration [SAMHSA], 2018).

The highest use of alcohol is among whites (57.7%) and persons reporting two or more races (47.4%) followed by African Americans (43.6%), Hispanics (43%), Native Hawaiians or Other Pacific Islanders (38.4%), American Indians or Alaska Natives (37.3%), and Asians (34.5%). The highest tobacco use reported is among the American Indians or Alaska Natives (40.1%), followed by persons reporting two or more races (31.2%), whites (27.7%), African Americans (27.1%), Native Hawaiians and Other Pacific Islanders (25.4%), Hispanics (18.8%), and Asians (10.1%) (SAMHSA, 2014).

Comorbidity

Many people who abuse substances have other mental disorders. Some disorders are in part a byproduct of long-term substance use; others predispose the individual to alcohol or drug abuse. Whatever the reason, nurses should be aware that patients who abuse substances often have psychotic, anxiety, mood, or personality disorders (SAMHSA, 2018).

>
> **Consider Gladys**
> She is also depressed and spends many days in bed. During the last few months her alcohol consumption has increased significantly.

Individuals who abuse substances are at high risk for death from drug overdoses and are at increased risk for death from other causes, including homicide, suicide, and opportunistic infections (such as HIV) secondary to drug injection. Earlier studies have documented the connection between alcohol abuse and increased risk for diabetes mellitus (DM), gastrointestinal problems, hypertension, liver disease, and stroke (Winhusen, Theobald, Kaelber, & Lewis, 2019).

Etiology

Substance abuse encompasses the body, the mind, and society's influences. Human and animal studies confirm a genetic predisposition for drinking behaviors and self-administering mind-altering drugs, but as yet no precise genetic marker has been established. Temperament, self-concept, age, motivation for change, social consequences for problematic behaviors, parental and family relationships, and peer pressure all contribute to expression of substance abuse—a chronic and progressive disorder.

Family Responses to Substance Use and Abuse

Abuse of substances by one or more members has devastating effects on families, their functioning, and the community. Fetal alcohol syndrome (FAS) results from drinking alcohol during pregnancy. Addictions lead to loss of jobs and family relationships. Use of illegal substances can lead to arrest and prison.

Many families try to help their family member learn to abstain or reduce the use of substances. Support groups provide education and help in understanding the addiction. Conversely, some persons who recover from substance abuse find that they must distance themselves from families that are actively using and abusing alcohol and drugs.

Treatment and Recovery

The goal for persons abusing substances is to recover from the abuse. **Recovery** involves a partnership between health care providers and the individual and family. For many of the individuals, a period of intense treatment is necessary to safely manage the physical and psychological withdrawal symptoms that occur when a substance is no longer used. Specific withdrawal symptoms depend on the addictive substance and are explained below as the substances are discussed. The withdrawal process usually involves detoxification. After a person has safely withdrawn from the substance of abuse, the real work toward recovery can begin. A primary concern is relapse, the recurrence of alcohol- or drug-dependent behavior in an individual who has previously achieved and maintained abstinence for a significant time beyond the period of detoxification.

TYPES OF SUBSTANCES AND RELATED DISORDERS

Alcohol

Alcohol (or ethanol) found in various proportions in liquor, wine, and beer relaxes inhibitions and heightens emotions. Mood swings can range from bouts of gaiety to angry outbursts. Cognitive impairments can vary from reduced concentration or attention span to impaired judgment and memory. Alcohol ultimately produces a sedative effect by depressing the central nervous system (CNS). Depending on the amount of alcohol ingested, the effects can range from feelings of mild sedation and relaxation to confusion and serious impairment of motor functions and speech to severe intoxication that can result in coma, respiratory failure, and death.

Table 25.1 provides a summary of the effects of abused substances.

All patients should be screened not only for alcohol use disorders but also for drinking patterns or behaviors that may place them at increased risk for experiencing adverse health effects or alcoholism. A frequently used screening tool is the CAGE Questionnaire. This tool consists of four self-report responses to questions about respondents' beliefs of cutting down on their drinking, their experience of others criticizing their drinking, the presence of guilt about drinking, and early morning drinking (Ewing, 1984). People who abuse alcohol exhibit various patterns of use. Some engage in heavy drinking on a regular or daily basis, others may abstain from drinking during the week and engage in heavy drinking on the weekends, and still others experience longer periods of sobriety interspersed with bouts of binge drinking (several days of intoxication).

TABLE 25.1	SUMMARY OF EFFECTS OF ABUSED SUBSTANCES, OVERDOSE, WITHDRAWAL SYNDROMES, AND PROLONGED USE			
Substance	Route	Effects (E) and Overdose (O)	Withdrawal Syndrome	Prolonged Use
Alcohol	PO	E: Sedation, decreased inhibitions, relaxation, decreased coordination, slurred speech, nausea O: Respiratory depression, cardiac arrest	Tremors; seizures, elevated temperature, pulse, and blood pressure; delirium tremens	Affects all systems of the body. Can lead to other dependencies
Stimulants (e.g., amphetamines, cocaine)	PO, IV, inhalation, smoking	E: Euphoria, initial CNS stimulation and then depression, wakefulness, decreased appetite, insomnia, paranoia, aggressiveness, dilated pupils, tremors O: Cardiac arrhythmias or arrest, increased or lowered blood pressure, respiratory depression, chest pain, vomiting, seizures, psychosis, confusion, seizures, dyskinesias, dystonias, coma	Depression: psychomotor retardation at first and then agitation; fatigue and then insomnia; severe dysphoria and anxiety; cravings, vivid, unpleasant dreams; increased appetite. Amphetamine withdrawal is not as pronounced as cocaine withdrawal.	Often alternates with use of depressants. Weight loss and resulting malnutrition and increased susceptibility to infectious diseases. May produce schizophrenia-like syndrome with paranoid ideation, thought disturbance, hallucinations, and stereotyped movements
Cannabis (marijuana, hashish, THC)	Smoking, PO	E: Euphoria or dysphoria, relaxation and drowsiness, heightened perception of color and sound, poor physical coordination, spatial perception and time distortion, unusual body sensations (e.g., weightlessness, tingling), dry mouth, dysarthria, and cravings for particular foods O: Increased heart rate, reddened eyes, dysphoria, lability, disorientation		Can decrease motivation and cause cognitive deficits (e.g., inability to concentrate, impaired memory)
Hallucinogens (LSD, MDMA)	PO	E: Euphoria or dysphoria, altered body image, distorted or sharpened visual and auditory perceptions, depersonalization, bizarre behavior, confusion, incoordination, impaired judgment and memory, signs of sympathetic and parasympathetic stimulation, palpitations (blurred vision, dilated pupils, sweating) O: Paranoia, ideas of reference, fear of losing one's mind, depersonalization, derealization, illusions, hallucinations, synesthesia, self-destructive or aggressive behaviors, tremors	"Flashbacks" or HPPD may occur after termination of use.	
PCP	PO, inhalation, smoking	E: Feeling superhuman, decreased awareness of and detachment from the environment, stimulation of the respiratory and cardiovascular systems, ataxia, dysarthria, decreased pain perception O: Hallucinations, paranoia, psychosis, aggression, adrenergic crisis (cardiac failure, cerebrovascular accident, malignant hyperthermia, status epilepticus, severe muscle contractions)		"Flashbacks," HPPD, organic brain syndromes with recurrent psychotic behavior, which can last up to 6 months after not using the drug, numerous psychiatric hospitalizations and police arrests
Opioids (heroin, codeine)	PO, injection, smoking	E: Euphoria, sedation, reduced libido, memory and concentration difficulties, analgesia, constipation, constricted pupils O: Respiratory depression, stupor, coma	Abdominal cramps, rhinorrhea, watery eyes, dilated pupils, yawning, "goose flesh," diaphoresis, nausea, diarrhea, anorexia, insomnia, fever	Can lead to criminal behavior to get money for drugs, risk for infection-related to needle use (e.g., HIV, endocarditis, hepatitis)

TABLE 25.1 SUMMARY OF EFFECTS OF ABUSED SUBSTANCES, OVERDOSE, WITHDRAWAL SYNDROMES, AND PROLONGED USE (Continued)

Substance	Route	Effects (E) and Overdose (O)	Withdrawal Syndrome	Prolonged Use
Sedatives, hypnotics, anxiolytics	PO, injection	E: Euphoria, sedation, reduced libido, emotional lability, impaired judgment O: Respiratory depression, cardiac arrest	Anxiety rebound and agitation, hypertension, tachycardia, sweating, hyperpyrexia, sensory excitement, motor excitation, insomnia, possible tonic–clonic convulsions, nightmares, delirium, depersonalization, hallucinations	Often alternated with stimulants, use with alcohol enhances chance of overdose, risk for infection related to needle use
Inhalants (e.g., glue, lighter fluid)	Inhalation	E: Euphoria, giddiness, excitation O: CNS depression: ataxia, nystagmus, dysarthria, coma, and convulsions	Similar to findings with alcohol but milder, with anxiety, tremors, hallucinations, and sleep disturbance as the primary symptoms	Long-term use can lead to hepatic and renal failure, blood dyscrasias, damage to the lungs; CNS damage (e.g., OBS, peripheral neuropathies, cerebral and optic atrophy, parkinsonism)
Nicotine	Smoking	E: Stimulation, enhanced performance and alertness, and appetite suppression O: Anxiety	Mood changes (e.g., craving, anxiety) and physiologic changes (e.g., poor concentration, sleep disturbances, headaches, gastric distress, and increased appetite)	Increased chance for cardiac disease and lung disease
Caffeine	PO	E: Stimulation, increased mental acuity, inexhaustibility O: Restlessness, nervousness, excitement, insomnia, flushing, diuresis, gastrointestinal distress, muscle twitching, rambling flow of thought and speech, tachycardia or cardiac arrhythmia, agitation	Headache, drowsiness, fatigue, craving, impaired psychomotor performance, difficulty concentrating, yawning, nausea	Physical consequences are under investigation

CNS, central nervous system; HIV, human immunodeficiency virus; HPPD, hallucinogen persisting perceptual disorder; LSD, D-lysergic acid diethylamide; MDMA, 3,4-methylenedioxymethamphetamine; OBS, organic brain syndrome; PO, oral; PCP, phencyclidine; THC, D-9-tetrahydrocannabinol.

The level of CNS impairment while under the influence of alcohol depends on how much has been consumed in a given period of time and how rapidly the body metabolizes it. Intoxication is determined by the level of alcohol in the blood, called blood alcohol level (BAL). The body can metabolize 1 oz of liquor, a 5-oz glass of wine, or a 12-oz can of beer per hour without intoxication. Table 25.2 lists behavioral responses at various BALs.

Effects of Long-Term Abuse

People who use alcohol regularly usually develop alcohol **tolerance,** the ability to ingest an increasing amount of alcohol before they experience a "high" and show cognitive and motor effects. The locus coeruleus, which

TABLE 25.2 BLOOD ALCOHOL LEVELS AND BEHAVIOR

Number of Drinks	Blood Alcohol Levels (mg%)	Behavior
1–2	0.05	Impaired judgment, giddiness, mood changes
5–6	0.10	Difficulty driving and coordinating movements
10–12	0.20	Motor functions severely impaired, resulting in ataxia; emotional lability
15–20	0.30	Stupor, disorientation, and confusion
20–24	0.40	Coma
25	0.50	Respiratory failure, death

normally inhibits the action of ethanol, is believed to be instrumental in the development of alcohol tolerance. Even though these individuals do not appear intoxicated, their BALs reflect the increased amount of alcohol and are affecting their bodies as described in Table 25.1. Excessive or long-term abuse of alcohol can adversely affect all body systems; the effects can be serious and permanent. Box 25.1 lists the major physical complications of alcohol abuse for the major organ systems.

Alcohol Withdrawal and Detoxification

Withdrawal from alcohol presents many physiologic and psychological challenges. Because of physiologic addiction, abrupt cessation of alcohol ingestion can cause mild to severe physical withdrawal symptoms, depending on the length and amount of alcohol use. **Alcohol withdrawal syndrome** is characterized by an increased heart rate and blood pressure, diaphoresis, mild anxiety, restlessness, and hand tremors. The most severe symptoms are **delirium tremens** (autonomic hyperarousal, disorientation, hallucinations) and grand mal (tonic–clonic) seizures. These symptoms can be life threatening (Table 25.3). In patients with alcoholism and in chronic drinkers, the alcohol withdrawal syndrome usually begins within 12 hours after abrupt discontinuation or attempt to decrease consumption. If seizures occur, they usually do so within the first 48 hours of withdrawal.

Alcohol withdrawal can be accomplished safely without a person experiencing serious physical consequences. **Detoxification** is period of time where the patient is observed, usually in a hospital setting and given medication to avoid withdrawal symptoms. Uncomplicated alcohol withdrawal is usually completed within 48 to 96 hours. Assessing for vital sign changes, nausea, vomiting, tremors, perspiration, agitation, headache, and change in mental status are important nursing interventions. The Clinical Institute Withdrawal Assessment for Alcohol Scale (CIWA-Ar) is frequently used for assessment (Box 25.2). Close monitoring continues until there is no indication of withdrawal symptoms.

Several medications are used to prevent physiologic complications and provide a gradual withdrawal from alcohol. Antianxiety and sedating drugs, such as benzodiazepines, are titrated downwardly over several days as a

> **BOX 25.1**
> **Medical Complications of Alcohol Abuse**
>
> - **Cardiovascular system:** Cardiomyopathy, congestive heart failure, hypertension
> - **Respiratory system:** Increased rate of pneumonia and other respiratory infections
> - **Hematologic system:** Anemias, leukemia, hematomas
> - **Nervous system:** Withdrawal symptoms, irritability, depression, anxiety disorders, sleep disorders, phobias, paranoid feelings, diminished brain size and functioning, organic brain disorders, blackouts, cerebellar degeneration, neuropathies, palsies, gait disturbances, visual problems
> - **Digestive system and nutritional deficiencies:** Liver diseases (fatty liver, alcoholic hepatitis, cirrhosis), pancreatitis, ulcers, other inflammations of the gastrointestinal (GI) tract, ulcers and GI bleeds, esophageal varices, cancers of the upper GI tract, pellagra, alcohol amnestic disorder, dermatitis, stomatitis, cheilosis, scurvy
> - **Endocrine and metabolic systems:** Increased incidence of diabetes mellitus, hyperlipidemia, hyperuricemia, and gout
> - **Immune system:** Impaired immune functioning, higher incidence of infectious diseases, including tuberculosis and other bacterial infections
> - **Integumentary system:** Skin lesions, increased incidence of infection, burns, and other traumatic injury
> - **Musculoskeletal system:** Increased incidence of traumatic injury, myopathy
> - **Genitourinary system:** Hypogonadism, increased secondary female sexual characteristics in men (hypoandrogenization and hyperestrogenization), erectile dysfunction in men, electrolyte imbalances due to excess urinary secretion of potassium and magnesium

TABLE 25.3 ALCOHOL WITHDRAWAL SYNDROME

	Stage I: Mild	Stage II: Moderate	Stage III: Severe
Vital signs	Heart rate elevated, temperature elevated, normal or slightly elevated systolic blood pressure	Heart rate, 100–120 bpm; elevated systolic blood pressure and temperature	Heart rate, 120–140 bpm; elevated systolic and diastolic blood pressures; elevated temperature
Diaphoresis	Slight	Usually obvious	Marked
Central nervous system	Oriented; no confusion; no hallucinations Mild anxiety and restlessness Restless sleep Hand tremors; "shakes"; no convulsions	Intermittent confusion; transient visual and auditory hallucinations and illusions (mostly at night) Painful anxiety and motor restlessness Insomnia and nightmares Visible tremulousness, rare convulsions	Marked disorientation, confusion, disturbing visual and auditory hallucinations, misidentification of objects, delusions related to the hallucinations, delirium tremens, disturbances in consciousness Agitation, extreme restlessness, and panic states Unable to sleep Gross uncontrollable tremors, convulsions common
Gastrointestinal system	Impaired appetite, nausea	Anorexia, nausea, and vomiting	Rejecting all fluid and food

BOX 25.2

Clinical Institute Withdrawal Assessment of Alcohol Scale, Revised (CIWA-Ar)

Patient: _____ Date: _____ Time: _____ (24-hour clock, midnight = 00:00)

Pulse or heart rate, taken for 1 min: _____ Blood pressure: _____

NAUSEA AND VOMITING – Ask "Do you feel sick to your stomach? Have you vomited?" Observation.
0 no nausea and no vomiting
1 mild nausea with no vomiting
2
3
4 intermittent nausea with dry heaves
5
6
7 constant nausea, frequent dry heaves and vomiting

TREMOR – Arms extended and fingers spread apart. Observation.
0 no tremor
1 not visible but can be felt fingertip to fingertip
2
3
4 moderate, with patient's arms extended
5
6
7 severe, even with arms not extended

PAROXYSMAL SWEATS – Observation.
0 no sweat visible
1 barely perceptible sweating, palms moist
2
3
4 beads of sweat obvious on forehead
5
6
7 drenching sweats

ANXIETY – Ask "Do you feel nervous?" Observation.
0 no anxiety, at ease
1 mild anxious
2
3
4 moderately anxious, or guarded, so anxiety is inferred
5
6
7 equivalent to acute panic states as seen in severe delirium or acute schizophrenic reactions

AGITATION – Observation.
0 normal activity
1 somewhat more than normal activity
2
3
4 moderately fidgety and restless
5
6
7 paces back and forth during most of the interview, or constantly thrashes about

TACTILE DISTURBANCES – Ask "Have you any itching, pins and needles sensations, any burning, any numbness, or do you feel bugs crawling on or under your skin?" Observation.
0 none
1 very mild itching, pins and needles, burning or numbness
2 mild itching, pins and needles, burning or numbness
3 moderate itching, pins and needles, burning or numbness
4 moderately severe hallucinations
5 severe hallucinations
6 extremely severe hallucinations
7 continuous hallucinations

AUDITORY DISTURBANCES – Ask "Are you more aware of sounds around you? Are they harsh? Do they frighten you? Are you hearing anything that is disturbing to you? Are you hearing things you know are not there?" Observation.
0 not present
1 very mild harshness or ability to frighten
2 mild harshness or ability to frighten
3 moderate harshness or ability to frighten
4 moderately severe hallucinations
5 severe hallucinations
6 extremely severe hallucinations
7 continuous hallucinations

VISUAL DISTURBANCES – Ask "Does the light appear to be too bright? Is its color different? Does it hurt your eyes? Are you seeing anything that is disturbing to you? Are you seeing things you know are not there?" Observation.
0 not present
1 very mild sensitivity
2 mild sensitivity
3 moderate sensitivity
4 moderately severe hallucinations
5 severe hallucinations
6 extremely severe hallucinations
7 continuous hallucinations

HEADACHE, FULLNESS IN HEAD – Ask "Does your head feel different? Does it feel like there is a band around your head?" Do not rate for dizziness or lightheadedness. Otherwise, rate severity.
0 not present
1 very mild
2 mild
3 moderate
4 moderately severe
5 severe
6 very severe
7 extremely severe

ORIENTATION AND CLOUDING OF SENSORIUM – Ask "What day is this? Where are you? Who am I?"
0 oriented and can do serial additions
1 cannot do serial additions or is uncertain about date
2 disoriented for date by no more than 2 calendar days
3 disoriented for date by more than 2 calendar days
4 disoriented for place/or person

Total **CIWA-Ar** Score _____
Rater's Initials _____
Maximum Possible Score 67

The **CIWA-Ar** is not copyrighted and may be reproduced freely. This assessment for monitoring withdrawal symptoms requires approximately 5 minutes to administer. The maximum score is 67 (see instrument). Patients scoring less than 10 do not usually need additional medication for withdrawal.

Sullivan, J. T., Sykora, K., Schneiderman, J., Naranjo, C. A. N. Sellers, E. M. (1989). Assessment of alcohol withdrawal: The revised Clinical Institute Withdrawal Assessment for Alcohol scale (**CIWA-Ar**). British Journal of Addiction, 84, 1353–1357.

substitution for the alcohol. Chlordiazepoxide (Librium) and diazepam have longer half-lives and smoother tapers. Lorazepam (Ativan) is better for older adults and people with liver impairment. Antidepressants are usually initiated to treat mood states, and sleep medication is used to promote a regular sleep pattern. Antipsychotic medications are also used if needed.

Alcohol withdrawal symptoms can occur in any patient who abuses alcohol and is forced to stop drinking because of an admission to a hospital or any alcohol-free environment. Patients who abuse alcohol for long periods of time are at high risk for alcohol withdrawal syndrome. Observing for signs of seizure activity is a priority nursing intervention.

Remember Gladys?
Gladys abruptly stopped her alcohol intake when she was admitted to the hospital for depression and suicidal thoughts. She did not tell her primary care provider that her intake of alcohol was significant. She began to go through withdrawal.

Alcohol-Induced Amnestic Disorders

Although certain alcohol-related cognitive impairments are reversible with abstinence, long-term alcohol abuse can cause specific neurologic complications that lead to organic brain disorders, known as alcohol-induced amnestic disorders. Alcohol is directly toxic to the brain, causing atrophy of the frontal cortex and eventually chronic brain syndrome. Patients with alcohol-induced amnestic disorders usually have a history of many years of heavy alcohol use and are generally older than 40 years.

Wernicke encephalopathy, a degenerative brain disorder caused by thiamine deficiency, is characterized by vision impairment, ataxia, hypotension, confusion, and coma. **Korsakoff's amnestic syndrome**, associated with alcoholism, involves the heart and the vascular and nervous systems, but the primary problem is acquiring new information and retrieving memories. Symptoms include amnesia, **confabulation** (i.e., telling a plausible but imagined scenario to compensate for memory loss), attention deficit, disorientation, and vision impairment. Although Wernicke encephalopathy and Korsakoff's amnestic syndrome can appear as two different disorders, they are generally considered to be different stages of the same disorder called **Wernicke–Korsakoff syndrome**, with Wernicke encephalopathy representing the acute phase and Korsakoff's amnestic syndrome the chronic phase. Early symptoms can be reversed, but without long-term treatment, the prognosis is poor (Yoon, Gedzior, & DePry, 2019).

Prevention of Relapse

Relapse prevention is important in the recovery of people with substance-related disorders, and alcohol addiction is no exception. Psychosocial interventions such as self-help groups, psychoeducation, and cognitive behavioral therapy (CBT) are designed specifically for those with alcohol addictions. These interventions are discussed later in this chapter.

Other medications are used for those who are recovering. Disulfiram (Antabuse) is neither a treatment nor a cure for alcoholism, but it can be used as adjunct therapy to help deter some individuals from drinking while using other treatment modalities to teach new coping skills to alter abuse behaviors (Box 25.3). Disulfiram plus even small amounts of alcohol produces side effects. Severe reactions may include respiratory depression, cardiovascular collapse, arrhythmias, myocardial infarction, acute congestive heart failure, unconsciousness, convulsions, and death.

Acamprosate calcium is a delayed-release tablet that decreases alcohol intake and reduces the risk of returning to drink alcohol in the person who is alcohol-dependent. It is indicated for the maintenance of abstinence from alcohol in patients who are alcohol-dependent. Acamprosate is effective if the individual is abstinent from alcohol prior to its initiation (Donoghue et al., 2015).

Naltrexone was originally used as a treatment for heroin abuse, but it is now approved for the treatment of alcohol dependence (Box 25.4). Naltrexone is formulated in a once-daily pill and a monthly injection (Vivitrol). The precise mechanism of action for naltrexone's effect is unknown; however, reports from successfully treated patients suggest three kinds of effects: (1) it can reduce **craving** (the urge or desire to drink despite negative consequences), (2) it can help maintain abstinence, and (3) it can interfere with the tendency to want to drink more if a recovering patient slips and has a drink. Naltrexone may be particularly useful in patients who continue to drink heavily (Srivastava & Gold, 2018).

Promotion of Health: Adequate Nutrition and Supplemental Vitamins

Multivitamins and adequate nutrition are essential for patients who are withdrawing from alcohol. Because malnutrition is common, other vitamin replacement may be necessary for certain individuals. Thiamine (vitamin B_1) is initiated during detoxification, given to decrease ataxia and other symptoms of deficiency. It is usually given orally, 100 mg three to four times daily, but can be given intramuscularly or by intravenous infusion with glucose. Folic acid deficiency is corrected with administration of 1.0 mg orally four times daily. Magnesium deficiency also

BOX 25.3
Drug Profile: Disulfiram (Antabuse)

DRUG CLASS: Antialcoholic agent, enzyme inhibitor

RECEPTOR AFFINITY: Inhibits the enzyme aldehyde dehydrogenase, blocking oxidation of alcohol and allowing acetaldehyde to accumulate to concentrations 5 to 10 times higher than normal in the blood during alcohol metabolism. Believed to inhibit norepinephrine synthesis.

INDICATIONS: Management of selected patients with chronic alcohol use who want to remain in a state of enforced sobriety

ROUTE AND DOSAGE: Available in 250- and 500-mg tablets

Adults: Initially, a maximum dose of 500 mg/day PO in a single dose for 1 to 2 weeks. Maintenance dosage of 125 to 500 mg/day PO not to exceed 500 mg/day, continued until patient is fully recovered socially and a basis for permanent self-control is established.

HALF-LIFE (PEAK EFFECT): Unclear (12 hours)

SELECTED SIDE EFFECTS: Drowsiness, fatigue, headache, metallic or garlic-like aftertaste. If taken with alcohol: flushing, throbbing in head and neck, throbbing headaches, respiratory difficulty, nausea, copious vomiting, sweating, thirst, chest pain, palpitations, dyspnea, hyperventilation, tachycardia, hypotension, syncope, weakness, vertigo, blurred vision, confusion; severe reactions may include arrhythmias, cardiovascular collapse, acute congestive heart failure, and unconsciousness.

WARNINGS: Never administer to an intoxicated patient or without the patient's knowledge. Do not administer until patient has abstained from alcohol for at least 12 hours. Contraindicated in patients with severe myocardial disease, coronary occlusion, or psychoses and in patients receiving current or recent treatment with metronidazole, paraldehyde, alcohol, or alcohol-containing preparations. Use cautiously in patients with DM, hypothyroidism, epilepsy, cerebral damage, chronic and acute nephritis, cirrhosis or dysfunction.

POSSIBLE DRUG INTERACTIONS: Concomitant administration of phenytoin, diazepam, or chlordiazepoxide may increase serum levels and risk for drug toxicity. Increased prothrombin time caused by disulfiram may lead to a need to adjust dosage of oral anticoagulants.

SPECIFIC PATIENT AND FAMILY EDUCATION

- Take the drug daily; take it at bedtime if it makes you dizzy or tired. Crush or mix tablets with liquid if necessary.
- Do not take *any* form of alcohol (e.g., beer, wine, liquor, vinegar, cough mixtures, sauces containing alcohol, aftershave lotions, liniments, or cologne); doing so may cause a severely unpleasant reaction.
- Wear or carry medical identification with you at all times to alert any medical emergency personnel that you are taking this drug.
- Keep appointments for follow-up blood tests.
- Avoid driving or performing tasks that require alertness if drowsiness, fatigue, or blurred vision occur.
- Know that the metallic aftertaste is transient and will disappear after use of the drug is discontinued.

PO, oral.

BOX 25.4
Drug Profile: Naltrexone (Relistor)

DRUG CLASS: Narcotic antagonist

RECEPTOR AFFINITY: Binds to opioid receptors in the CNS and competitively inhibits the action of opioid drugs, including those with mixed narcotic agonist–antagonist properties

INDICATIONS: Adjunctive treatment of alcohol or narcotic dependence as part of a comprehensive treatment program

ROUTE AND DOSAGE: Available in 50-mg tablets

Adults: For alcoholism: 50 mg/day PO; for narcotic dependence: initial dose of 25 mg PO; if no signs or symptoms seen, complete dose with 25 mg. Usual maintenance dose is 50 mg/day PO.

Children: Safety has not been established for use in children younger than 18 years.

HALF-LIFE (PEAK EFFECT): 3.9 to 12.9 hours (60 minutes)

SELECTED SIDE EFFECTS: Difficulty sleeping, anxiety, nervousness, headache, low energy, abdominal pain or cramps, nausea, vomiting, delayed ejaculations, decreased potency, rash, chills, increased thirst, joint and muscle pain

WARNINGS: Contraindicated in pregnancy and patients allergic to narcotic antagonists. Use cautiously in narcotic addiction because may produce withdrawal symptoms. Do not administer unless patient has been opioid free for 7 to 10 days. Also, use cautiously in patients with acute hepatitis, liver failure, depression, or suicidal tendencies and in those who are breast-feeding. Must make certain patient is opioid free before administering naltrexone. Always give naloxone challenge test before using, except in patients showing clinical signs of opioid withdrawal.

SPECIFIC PATIENT AND FAMILY EDUCATION

- Understand that this drug will help facilitate abstinence from alcohol and block the effects of narcotics.
- Wear a medical identification tag to alert emergency personnel that you are taking this drug.
- Avoid use of heroin or other opioid drugs; small doses may have no effect, but large doses can cause death, serious injury, or coma.
- Report any signs and symptoms of adverse effects.
- Notify other health care providers that you are taking this drug.
- Keep appointments for follow-up blood tests and treatment program.

CNS, central nervous system; PO, oral.

is found in those with long-term alcohol dependence. Magnesium sulfate, which enhances the body's response to thiamine and reduces seizures, is given prophylactically for patients with histories of withdrawal seizures. The usual dose is 1.0 g intramuscularly, four times daily for 2 days.

Stimulants

Cocaine

Cocaine (also known as coke, snow, nose candy, flake, blow, big c, lady, white, or snowbirds) is made from the leaves of the *Erythroxylum coca* plant into a coca paste that is refined into cocaine hydrochloride, a crystalline form (thus the white powder appearance), which is commonly inhaled or "snorted" in the nose, injected intravenously (with water), or smoked. The smokeable form of cocaine, often called *free-base cocaine*, can be made by mixing the crystalline cocaine with ether or sodium hydroxide. Crack cocaine, often simply called "crack," is a form of free-base cocaine produced by mixing the crystal with water and baking soda or sodium bicarbonate, and boiling it until a rock precipitant remains. The hardened crystal is then broken into pieces ("cracked") and smoked in cigarettes or water pipes. This extremely potent form produces a rapid high with intense euphoria and a dramatic crash. It is extremely addictive because of the intense and rapid onset of euphoric effects, which leave users craving more.

After cocaine is inhaled or injected, the user experiences a sudden burst of mental alertness and energy ("cocaine rush") and feelings of self-confidence, being in control, and sociability, which last 10 to 20 minutes. This high is followed by an intense let-down effect ("cocaine crash") in which the person feels irritable, depressed, tired, and craves more of the drug. Users experience a serious psychological addiction and pattern of abuse. Although cocaine users typically report that the drug enhances their feelings of well-being and reduces anxiety, cocaine also is known to bring on panic attacks in some individuals. Long-term cocaine use leads to increased anxiety. Increased use of cocaine is associated with stress and drug craving (NIDA, 2018a).

Biologic Responses to Cocaine

Cocaine is absorbed rapidly through the blood–brain barrier and is also readily absorbed through skin and mucous membranes. Rapid intoxication occurs when cocaine is injected intravenously or inhaled. Cocaine increases dopaminergic and serotonergic activity by attaching to transport proteins and in turn by blocking neurotransmitter reuptake. Increased dopamine causes euphoria and psychotic symptoms. Cocaine increases norepinephrine levels in the blood, causing tachycardia, hypertension, dilated pupils, and rising body temperatures. Serotonin excess contributes to sleep disturbances and anorexia. With prolonged cocaine use, these neurotransmitters are eventually depleted.

Cocaine Intoxication

Intoxication causes CNS stimulation, the length of which depends on the dosage and route of administration. With steadily increasing doses, restlessness proceeds to tremors and agitation followed by convulsions and CNS depression. In lethal overdose, death generally results from respiratory failure. Toxic psychosis is also possible; it may be accompanied by physical signs of CNS stimulation (e.g., tachycardia, hypertension, cardiac arrhythmias, sweating, hyperpyrexia, convulsions).

Cocaine and alcohol taken together could cause a potentially dangerous reaction. Taken in combination, the two drugs are converted by the body to cocaethylene, which has a longer duration of action in the brain and is more toxic than either drug individually. Notably, this mixture of cocaine and alcohol is a common two-drug combination that frequently results in drug-related death (Singh, 2019).

Cocaine Withdrawal

Severe anxiety, along with restlessness and agitation, is among the major symptoms of cocaine withdrawal. Users quickly seek more cocaine or other drugs, such as alcohol, marijuana, or sleeping pills, to rid themselves of the terrible effects of crashing. Withdrawal causes intense depression, craving (i.e., a strong desire to use cocaine despite negative consequences), and drug-seeking behavior that may last for weeks. Individuals who discontinue cocaine use often relapse.

Long-term cocaine use depletes norepinephrine, resulting in a "crash" when use of the drug is discontinued that causes the user to sleep 12 to 18 hours. On awakening, withdrawal symptoms may occur, characterized by sleep disturbances with rebound rapid eye movement (REM) sleep, anergia (i.e., lack of energy), and decreased libido, depression with possible suicidality, anhedonia, poor concentration, and cocaine craving. Treating individuals with cocaine addiction is complex, because it involves assessing the psychobiologic, social, and pharmacologic aspects of abuse.

> **NCLEXNOTE** In cocaine withdrawal, patients are excessively sleepy because of norepinephrine depletion. Recovery is difficult because of the intense cravings. Nursing interventions should focus on helping patients solve problems related to managing these cravings.

Amphetamines

Amphetamines, known on the street as speed, uppers, ups, black beauties, pep pills, or copilots, were first synthesized for medical use in the 1880s. Amphetamines (Biphetamine, Delcobese, dextroamphetamine) and other stimulants, such as phenmetrazine and methylphenidate (Ritalin, Focalin), act on the CNS and peripheral nervous system. They are used to treat ADHD in children, narcolepsy, depression, and obesity (on a short-term basis). Some people abuse these drugs to achieve the effects of alertness, increased concentration, a sense of increased energy, euphoria, and appetite suppression. Amphetamines are indirect catecholamine agonists and cause the release of newly synthesized norepinephrine. Similar to cocaine, they block the reuptake of norepinephrine and dopamine, but they do not affect the serotonergic system as strongly. They also affect the peripheral nervous system and are powerful sympathomimetics, stimulating both α- and β-receptors. This stimulation results in tachycardia, arrhythmias, increased systolic and diastolic blood pressures, and peripheral hyperthermia. The effects of amphetamine use and the clinical course of an overdose are similar to those of cocaine.

Methamphetamine

Methamphetamine, also known as meth, speed, ice, chalk, crank, fire, glass, and crystal, is an illegal potent CNS stimulant that releases excess dopamine responsible for the drug's toxic effects, including damage to nerve terminals. Highly addictive, it comes in many forms and can be smoked, snorted, orally ingested, or injected. A brief intense sensation, or rush, is reported by those who smoke or inject methamphetamine. Oral ingestion or snorting produces a long-lasting high instead of a rush, which can continue for as long as half a day. This illegal substance is cheap, easy to make, and has devastating consequences.

High doses can elevate body temperature and stimulate seizures. Methamphetamine has a longer duration of action than cocaine and leads to prolonged stimulant effects. Long-term effects include dependence and addiction psychosis (e.g., paranoia, hallucinations), mood disturbances, violent behavior, repetitive motor activity, stroke, contracting HIV and hepatitis, intense itching leading to skin sores from scratching, weight loss, and extensive tooth decay (Fig. 25.1) (NIDA, 2018b). Methamphetamine is often used in a "binge and crash" pattern. Tolerance occurs within minutes, and the pleasurable effect disappears even before the drug concentration in the blood falls significantly. After being assessed, referral of the patient to a drug treatment program is necessary.

FIGURE 25.1 Severe tooth decay caused by abuse of methamphetamine.

MDMA and Other Club Drugs

The drug 3,4-methylenedioxymethamphetamine (MDMA), also known as Ecstasy or Molly, is known as a "club drug" because it is used by teens and young adults as part of the nightclub, bar, and rave scenes. MDMA, chemically similar to both stimulants and hallucinogens, causes activity of dopamine, norepinephrine, and serotonin to increase. It produces feelings of increased energy, pleasure, emotional warmth, and distorted sensory and time perception. MDMA can cause hallucinations, confusion, depression, paranoia, sleep problems, drug craving, severe anxiety, nausea, muscle cramping, involuntary teeth clenching, blurred vision, chills, and sweating. In higher doses, MDMA can sharply increase body temperature (i.e., malignant hyperthermia), leading to muscle breakdown, kidney and cardiovascular failure, and death. MDMA effects last about 3 to 6 hours (NIDA, 2018c).

Rohypnol gamma-hydroxybutyrate (GHB) and ketamine are predominantly CNS depressants but are also considered "club drugs." Often colorless, tasteless, and odorless, the drugs can be ingested unknowingly. Known also as "date rape" drugs when mixed with alcohol, they can be incapacitating, causing a euphoric, sedative-like effect and producing an "anterograde amnesia," which means that individuals may not remember events they experience while under the influence of these drugs. Ketamine is associated with an increased heart rate and blood pressure, impaired motor function, memory loss, numbness, and vomiting. At high doses, delirium, depression, respiratory depression, and cardiac arrest can occur. Ketamine is used as an anesthetic in veterinary practice (NIDA, 2018d).

Nicotine

Nicotine, the addictive chemical mainly responsible for the high prevalence of tobacco use, is the primary reason tobacco is named a public health menace. Smoking is more prevalent among people with alcoholism, polysubstance users, and persons with mental disorders than among the general population. Smoking is two to three times more prevalent in persons with mental illnesses than the general population and is five times higher among those with schizophrenia, bipolar disorder, post-traumatic stress disorder (PTSD), and alcohol/illicit drug use disorders (Prochaska, Das, & Young-Wolff, 2017).

Biologic Response to Nicotine

Nicotine stimulates the central, peripheral, and autonomic nervous systems, causing increased alertness, concentration, attention, and appetite suppression. Readily absorbed, it is carried in the bloodstream to the liver where it is partially metabolized. It is also metabolized by the kidneys and excreted in urine (NIDA, 2019b).

Nicotine acts as an agonist of the nicotinic cholinergic receptor sites and stimulates autonomic ganglia in both the parasympathetic and sympathetic nervous systems, resulting in increased release of norepinephrine or acetylcholine. The release of epinephrine by nicotine from the adrenal medulla increases fatty acids, glycerol, and lactate levels in the blood, thereby increasing the risk for atherosclerosis and cardiac muscle pathology.

Other medical complications of nicotine use are numerous. Smoking cigarettes and cigars causes respiratory problems, lung cancer, emphysema, heart problems, and peripheral vascular disease. In fact, smoking is the largest preventable cause of premature death and disability. Cigarette smoking kills at least 480,000 people in the United States each year and makes countless others ill. The use of smokeless tobacco is also associated with serious health problems (NIDA, 2018e).

Repeated use of nicotine produces both tolerance and addiction. Recent research has shown that nicotine addiction is extremely powerful and is at least as strong as addictions to other drugs, most of those who quit relapse within 1 year (NIDA, 2018e).

Nicotine Withdrawal and Smoking Cessation

Nicotine withdrawal is marked by mood changes (e.g., craving, anxiety, irritability, depression) and physiologic changes (difficulty in concentrating, sleep disturbances, headaches, gastric distress, increased appetite). Nicotine replacements such as nicotine transdermal patches, nicotine gum, nasal spray, and inhalers have been used successfully to assist in withdrawal by reducing the craving for tobacco. Patches are rotated on skin sites and help maintain a steady blood level of nicotine. They are used daily with the decrease in strength of nicotine occurring during a period of 6 to 12 weeks.

Successful smoking cessation usually requires more than one type of intervention, including social support and education. However, studies do show that even giving a brief instruction to patients about quitting smoking can be effective. Medications are often used as a smoking cessation strategy. The antidepressant bupropion is marketed as Zyban to help people quit smoking. Another medication, varenicline tartrate (Chantix) reduces the craving and rewarding effects of nicotine by preventing nicotine from accessing one of the acetylcholine receptor sites involved with nicotine dependence, but it can cause depression and related psychiatric symptoms in some people. This side effect may limit its usefulness for some people with psychiatric disorders (Piper et al., 2017; Zhang et al., 2016).

Auricular therapy, or ear acupressure, is being studied as a potential adjunctive treatment for nicotine addiction. Acupressure is based on the principles of an ancient Chinese system of medicine with a goal of returning the body to a harmonic balanced state. Through stimulating acupoints on the ear, endogenous endorphin levels and regulation of the sympathetic nervous system changes the taste for tobacco, suppressing nicotine addiction, decreasing nicotine withdrawal symptoms, reducing the desire to smoke, and promoting cessation for a short period of time. Emerging research into this therapy shows positive effects (Vieira, Reis, Matos, Machado, & Moreira, 2018).

Electronic cigarettes (e-cigarettes) were introduced as smoking cessation aids. They are smokeless, battery-operated devices designed to deliver nicotine with flavorings or other chemicals to the lungs without burning tobacco to do so. They resemble regular tobacco cigarettes, cigars, or pipes. More than 250 e-cigarette brands are on the market. E-cigarettes are designed to simulate the act of tobacco smoking without the toxic chemicals produced by burning tobacco leaves. Their safety and effectiveness in smoking cessation are being questioned because e-cigarettes deliver highly addictive nicotine into the lungs and the vapor of some of them contains known carcinogens and toxic chemicals. Additionally, adolescents are increasingly using e-cigarettes believing they are safe, but instead, they may instead serve as a gateway to try other tobacco products. On May 5, 2016, the FDA announced that nationwide tobacco regulations now extend to all tobacco products including e-cigarettes and their liquid solutions, cigars, hookah tobacco, and pipe tobacco (NIDA, 2018e).

Caffeine

Caffeine is a stimulant found in many drinks (coffee, tea, cocoa, soft drinks); chocolate; and OTC medications, including analgesics, stimulants, appetite suppressants, and cold relief preparations. Metabolism of caffeine is very complicated, involving more than 25 metabolites, and varies among different populations (Brosen, 2015). Recently, high-energy drinks, consisting of alcohol and caffeine, are being marketed to reduce the impairment caused by ingestion of alcohol. The reality is that these energy drinks give a false sense of physical and mental competence and decrease the awareness of impairment. Deaths have been associated with these drinks (Chrysant & Chrysant, 2015).

Symptoms of caffeine intoxication can include five or more of the following: restlessness, nervousness, excitement, insomnia, flushed face, diuresis, gastrointestinal disturbance, muscle twitching, rambling flow of thought and speech, tachycardia or cardiac arrhythmia, periods of inexhaustibility, and psychomotor agitation (Chrysant & Chrysant, 2015).

Caffeine withdrawal syndrome involves headache, drowsiness, and fatigue, sometimes with impaired psychomotor performance; difficulty concentrating; craving; and psychophysiologic complaints, such as yawning or nausea. Patients with caffeine dependence can be supported in their efforts at withdrawal by learning about the caffeine content of beverages and medication, using decaffeinated beverages, and managing individual withdrawal symptoms.

Cannabis

Marijuana is the common name for the plant *Cannabis sativa*, also known as hemp and many other names. Two main cannabinoids from the marijuana plant are well known: cannabidiol (CBD) and D-9-tetrahydrocannabinol (THC). Hashish, a resin found in flowers of the mature *C. sativa* plant, is its strongest form, containing 10% to 30% THC. Although there are other active ingredients in marijuana, THC gets the most attention because of its psychoactive properties.

Marijuana is fat soluble and is absorbed rapidly after being smoked or taken orally. After ingestion, THC binds with an opioid receptor in the brain—the μ-receptor. This action engages endogenous brain opioid receptors, which are associated with enhanced dopamine activity because THC blocks dopamine reuptake. THC can be stored for weeks in fat tissue and in the brain and is released extremely slowly. Long-term use leads to the accumulation of cannabinoids in the body, primarily the frontal cortex, the limbic areas, and the brain's auditory and visual perception centers. In other areas of the brain, it exerts cardiovascular effects, results in ataxia, and causes increased psychotropic effects. Marijuana use impairs the ability to form memories, recall events, and shift attention from one thing to another. It disrupts coordination of movement, balance, and reaction time. Contrary to popular belief, marijuana is addictive, is an irritant to the lungs, and can produce the same respiratory problems experienced by tobacco users (i.e., daily cough, phlegm). People who smoke marijuana miss work more often than those who do not smoke it, but it is not yet known whether marijuana smoke contributes to the risk of lung cancer (NIDA, 2015b).

Marijuana is usually smoked and causes relaxation, euphoria, at times dyscoria (i.e., abnormal pupillary reaction or shape), spatial misperception, time distortion, and food cravings. It also causes relaxation and drowsiness, unlike other hallucinogens, and is often associated with decreased motivation after long-term use. Effects begin immediately after the drug enters the brain and last from 1 to 3 hours.

The Food and Drug Administration (FDA) has approved drugs containing marijuana, such as dronabinol (Marinol) and nabilone (Cesamet), which contain THC and are used to treat nausea caused by chemotherapy. The known safety issues related to marijuana include impairment of short-term memory, altered judgment and decision-making, anxiety, and paranoia or psychosis especially in high dose (NIDA, 2018f). Marijuana is legal as a recreational drug in some states in the United States.

"Spice" and "K2" are terms used for synthetic cannabinoid compounds found in various herbal mixtures that produce an experience similar to that of marijuana. Spice mixtures of this type are illegal to sell in the United States because of their addictive properties. The effects of synthetic cannabinoids can be unpredictable and severe or even life threatening. Some of these compounds bind more strongly to the same receptors as THC and could produce a more powerful and unpredictable effect. Spice products are popular among young people and are second only to marijuana among illegal drugs used mostly by high school seniors. Emergency departments are seeing an alarming increase in adolescents being treated for severe adverse events related to synthetic cannabinoid use. Fatalities can occur and there is no antidote available (NIDA, 2018g).

Hallucinogens and Dissociative Drugs

The term **hallucinogen** refers to drugs that produce euphoria or dysphoria, altered body image, distorted or sharpened visual and auditory perception, confusion, lack of coordination, and impaired judgment and memory. Hallucinogens cause hallucinations and profound distortions in a person's perceptions of reality. These drugs can be made from plant sources and mushrooms or man-made. They are categorized as hallucinogens and dissociative drugs. When under the influence of either type of drug, people report rapid, intense emotional swings and seeing images, hearing sounds, and feeling sensations that seem real but are not. Severe reactions may cause paranoia, fear of losing one's mind, depersonalization, illusions, delusions, and hallucinations. Hallucinogens typically affect the autonomic and regulatory nervous systems first, increasing heart rate and body temperature, and slightly elevating blood pressure. The individual may experience a dry mouth, dizziness, and subjective feelings of being hot or cold. Gradually, these physiologic changes fade, but then perceptual distortions and hallucinations may become prominent. Intense mood and sexual behavior changes may occur; the user may feel unusually close to others or distant and isolated. Classic hallucinogens include LSD (d-lysergic acid diethylamide), psilocybin (4-phosphoryloxy-*N*,*N*-dimethyltryptamine), Peyote (Mescaline), DMT (dimethyltryptamine), and ayahuasca. Dissociative drugs include PCP (phencyclidine), DXM (dextromethorphan), *Salvia divinorum*, and ketamine (see below). Dextromethorphan is a cough suppressant and expectorant ingredient in some OTC cold and cough medicines and is commonly abused by adolescents and young adults (NIDA, 2018h).

The true content of hallucinogenic drugs purchased on the street is always in doubt; they are often misidentified or adulterated with other drugs. There are more than 100 different hallucinogens with substantially different molecular structures (NIDA, 2018h).

Patients in acute states of intoxication or in dissociated states may become combative. During the acute state, the primary intervention goals are to reduce stimuli, maintain a safe environment for the patient and others, manage behavior, and observe the patient carefully for medical and psychiatric complications. Instructions to the patient should be clear, short, and simple, and delivered in a firm but nonthreatening tone.

Prescription and Over-the-Counter Drugs

Use of prescription drugs for nonmedical purposes has escalated since 2002 with more than 15.2 million Americans taking a pain reliever, tranquilizer, stimulants, or sedative for nonmedical purposes. The United States is in the midst of an epidemic of prescription opioid overdose deaths. In 2017, the overdose rates from prescription opioids significantly increased among people more than 65 years of age. Overdose death rates from prescription opioids among men were 6.1 per 100,000; the rates among women were 4.2 per 100,000. The highest overdose death rates were in West Virginia, Maryland, Kentucky, and Utah (Centers for Disease control and Prevention [CDC], 2018\9). Abuse of prescription and OTC drugs occurs when one of the following criteria is met:

- Taking a medication that has been prescribed for someone else
- Taking a drug in higher quantity or in another manner than prescribed
- Taking a drug for another purpose than prescribed (NIDA, 2018i)

The **opioids** (e.g., oxycodone, hydrocodone, morphine, fentanyl, codeine) prescribed for pain are some of the more commonly abused prescription medications. The most commonly abused CNS depressants are the barbiturates (e.g., pentobarbital and benzodiazepines [diazepam, alprazolam, clonazepam, lorazepam]), which are prescribed for anxiety and sleep. The *DSM-5* diagnosis, *sedative, hypnotic, or anxiolytic use disorder* would be given when these drugs are abused. Amphetamines (Adderall, Dexedrine) and methylphenidate (Concerta, Ritalin) are stimulants prescribed for ADHD that are also frequently abused. Often, patients combine these drugs with alcohol, which is extremely dangerous and can put patients at risk for overdose, causing coma or death.

OTC cough medicine containing DXM can produce the same effects as those of ketamine or PCP, such as impaired motor function, numbness, nausea or vomiting, and increased heart rate and blood pressure. In some cases, severe respiratory depression and hypoxia have occurred (NIDA, 2018i).

Opioids and Morphine Derivatives

The term **opioid** refers to any substance that binds to an opioid receptor in the brain to produce an agonist action. Derived from poppies, opioids are powerful drugs that have been used for centuries to relieve pain. They include opium, heroin, morphine, and codeine. Even centuries after their discovery, opioids are still the most effective pain relievers. They also cause CNS depression, sleep, or stupor. Although heroin has no medicinal use, other opioids, such as morphine and codeine, are used to treat pain related to illnesses (e.g., cancer) and during medical and dental procedures. When used as directed by a clinician, opioids are safe and generally do not produce addiction. However, opioids also possess very strong reinforcing properties and can quickly trigger addiction when used improperly.

Two important effects produced by opioids are pleasure (or reward) and pain relief. The brain itself also produces substances known as endorphins that activate the opioid receptors. Opioids cause tolerance and physical dependence that appear to be specific for each receptor subtype. Tolerance develops, particularly to the analgesic, respiratory depression, and sedative actions of opioids. Often, a 100% increase in dose is used to achieve the same physical effects when tolerance exists. Physical dependence can develop rapidly. When the use of the drug is discontinued, after a period of continuous use, a rebound hyperexcitability withdrawal syndrome usually occurs. Table 25.4 describes the onset, duration, and symptoms of mild, moderate, and severe withdrawal symptoms.

Heroin is an illegal highly addictive drug that is mostly abused and the most rapidly acting of the opioids.

TABLE 25.4	SEVERITY OF OPIOID WITHDRAWAL SYNDROME		
Initial Onset and Duration	Mild Withdrawal	Moderate Withdrawal	Severe Withdrawal
Onset: 8–12 hours after last use of short-acting opioids. 1–3 days after the last use for longer-acting opioids, such as methadone	Physical: yawning, rhinorrhea, perspiration, restlessness, lacrimation, sleep disturbance	Physical: dilated pupils, bone and muscle aches, sensation of "goose flesh," hot and cold flashes	Nausea; vomiting; stomach cramps; diarrhea; weight loss; insomnia; twitching of muscles and kicking movements of legs; increased blood pressure, pulse, and respirations
Duration: Severe symptoms peak between 48 and 72 hours. Symptoms abate in 7–10 days for short-acting opioids. Methadone withdrawal symptoms can last several weeks	Emotional: increased craving, anxiety, dysphoria	Emotional: irritability, increased anxiety, and craving	Emotional: depression, increased anxiety, dysphoria, subjective sense of feeling "wretched"

Typically sold as a white or brownish powder or as the black sticky substance known as "black tar heroin" on the streets, it is frequently "cut" with other substances, such as sugar, starch, powdered milk, quinine, and strychnine or other poisons. It can be sniffed, snorted, and smoked but is most frequently injected, which poses risks for transmission of human immunodeficiency (HIV) devices and other diseases resulting from the sharing of needles or other injection equipment.

Naturally occurring neurotransmitters normally bind to the μ-opioid receptors which are involved in pain, hormonal release, and feelings of well-being. When heroin enters the brain, it is converted to morphine and immediately binds to the μ-opioid receptors stimulating the release of dopamine, which causes an intense pleasurable rush. Usually, the individual also experiences a warm flushing of the skin, dry mouth, and a heavy feeling in the limbs. Side effects include nausea, vomiting, and severe itching. Following these initial side effects, drowsiness, clouded mental function, slowing of the heart rate, and extreme slowing of breathing can occur (NIDA, 2018j).

One of the most detrimental long-term side effects of heroin is addiction itself, which causes neurochemical and molecular changes and profoundly alters brain structure and composition. Enlarged ventricular spaces and loss of frontal volume are reported. Heroin also produces profound degrees of tolerance and physical dependence, which are powerful motivating factors for compulsive use and abuse. After becoming addicted, heroin users gradually spend more and more time and energy obtaining and using the drug until these activities become their primary purpose in life (NIDA, 2018j).

Opioid Intoxication or Overdose

Emergency treatment of individuals with opioid intoxication is initiated with an assessment of CNS functioning, specifically arousal and respiratory functioning. Naloxone, an opioid antagonist, is given as a rescue drug when extreme drowsiness, slowed breathing, or loss of consciousness occurs. It reverses respiratory depression, sedation, and hypotension caused by the opioid agent. Administration of naloxone is life-saving. Naloxone is administered intravenously, intramuscularly, or intranasally. When administered intravenously, the pharmacologic effect is generally apparent within 2 minutes. When administered through other routes, the effect is more prolonged. Naloxone is active for 30 to 81 minutes. Depending upon the strength of the opiate, a second dose is often needed when reversing the overdose.

Initial Opioid Detoxification

Ideally, opioid detoxification is achieved by gradually reducing an opioid dose over several days or weeks. Many treatment programs include administering low doses of a substitute drug, such as methadone, which can help satisfy the drug craving without providing the same subjective high. If opioids are abruptly withdrawn ("cold turkey") from someone who is physically dependent on them, severe physical symptoms occur, including body aches, diarrhea, tachycardia, fever, runny nose, sneezing, sweating, yawning, nausea or vomiting, nervousness, restlessness or irritability, shivering or trembling, abdominal cramps, weakness, and elevated blood pressure.

Maintenance Treatment

Methadone maintenance is the treatment of people with opioid addiction with a daily stabilized dose of methadone. Methadone is used because of its long half-life of 15 to 30 hours. It is a potent opioid and is physiologically addicting, but it satisfies the opioid craving without producing the subjective high of heroin (Box 25.5).

> **BOX 25.5**
>
> ### Drug Profile: Methadone (Dolophine)
>
> **DRUG CLASS:** Narcotic agonist, analgesic
>
> **RECEPTOR AFFINITY:** Binds to opioid receptors in the CNS to produce analgesia, euphoria, sedation; the receptors mediating the effects of endogenous opioids, which are thought to be enkephalins, endorphins
>
> **INDICATIONS:** Detoxification and temporary maintenance treatment of narcotic addiction; relief of severe pain
>
> **ROUTE AND DOSAGE:** Available in 5-, 10-, and 40-mg tablets; oral concentrate
>
> **Adults:** Detoxification: Initially 15 to 30 mg. Increase dosage to suppress withdrawal signs. 40 mg/day in single or divided dose is usually an adequate stabilizing dose; continue stabilizing dose for 2 to 3 days; then gradually decrease dosage. Usual maintenance dose is 20 to 120 mg/day in single dosing.
>
> **HALF-LIFE (PEAK EFFECT):**
> PO 90 to 120 minutes
> IM 1 to 2 hours
> SC 1 to 2 hours
>
> **SELECTED SIDE EFFECTS:** Lightheadedness, dizziness, sedation, nausea, vomiting, facial flushing, peripheral circulatory collapse, arrhythmia, palpitations, urethral spasm, urinary retention, respiratory depression, circulatory depression, respiratory arrest, shock, cardiac arrest
>
> **WARNINGS:** Never administer in the presence of hypersensitivity to narcotics, diarrhea caused by poisoning (before toxins are eliminated), bronchial asthma, or chronic obstructive pulmonary disease. Use caution in the presence of acute abdominal conditions and cardiovascular disease. Increased effect and toxicity of methadone if taken concurrently with cimetidine and/or ranitidine. Methadone hydrochloride tablets are for PO administration only and *must not* be used for injection. It is recommended that methadone hydrochloride tablets, if dispensed, be packaged in child-resistant containers and kept out of the reach of children to prevent accidental injection.
>
> **SPECIFIC PATIENT AND FAMILY EDUCATION**
> - Take drug exactly as prescribed.
> - Avoid use of alcohol.
> - Take the drug with food while lying quietly; this should minimize nausea.
> - Eat small, frequent meals to treat nausea and loss of appetite.
> - If experiencing dizziness and drowsiness, avoid driving a car or performing other tasks that require alertness.
> - Administer mild laxative for constipation.
> - Report severe nausea, vomiting, constipation, shortness of breath, or difficulty breathing. Methadone products, when used for treatment of narcotic addiction, shall be dispensed only by approved hospital and community pharmacies and maintenance programs approved by the FDA and designated state authority.
>
> CNS, central nervous system; IM, intramuscular; FDA, Food and Drug Administration; PO, oral; SC, subcutaneous.

Detoxification is accomplished by setting the beginning methadone dose and then slowly reducing it during the next 21 days. Treatment programs determine the dose of methadone that will block subjective feelings of craving and will not cause somnolence or intoxication in patients. The initial dose of methadone is determined by the severity of withdrawal symptoms and is usually 20 to 30 mg orally. If symptoms persist after 1 to 2 hours, the dosage can be raised. Dosage should then be re-evaluated daily during the first few days of treatment. Initial doses of exceeding 40 mg can cause severe discomfort as the detoxification proceeds.

Patients receive this dose daily in conjunction with regular drug abuse counseling focused on the elimination of illicit drug use; lifestyle changes, such as finding friends who do not use drugs or achieving stability in one's living situation; strengthening social supports; and structuring time into pursuits that do not involve drug use. After illicit drug use ceases for a period of time, major lifestyle changes have been made, and social supports are in place, patients may gradually detoxify from methadone with continuing support through community support groups, such as Narcotics Anonymous.

The length of methadone treatment varies for each patient. The protocol for starting detoxification from methadone varies widely, depending on the patient's commitment to abstinence, lifestyle changes that have occurred, and strong peer group support, all of which are needed to sustain the patient during methadone detoxification when increased cravings often occur. Methadone treatment combined with behavioral therapy and counseling has been used effectively and safely to treat opioid addiction for more than 40 years. Combined with behavioral therapy and counseling, methadone enables patients to stop using heroin.

Naltrexone, similar to naloxone, has been used successfully to treat opioid addiction. It binds to opioid receptors in the CNS and competitively inhibits the action of opioid drugs, including those with mixed narcotic agonist–antagonist properties, thereby blocking the intoxicating effects. It differs from naloxone in that naltrexone is longer acting and is formulated as a 50-mg tablet given once daily. Naltrexone is not used as a rescue drug for respiratory depression associated with an opioid overdose. However, if an opioid-addicted individual takes naltrexone before he or she is fully detoxified from opioids, withdrawal symptoms may appear (see Table 25.4).

Buprenorphine is a long-acting partial agonist that acts on the same receptors as heroin and morphine, relieving drug cravings without producing the same intense "high" or dangerous side effects. At low doses, buprenorphine produces sufficient agonist effect to enable opioid-addicted individuals to discontinue the misuse of opioids without experiencing withdrawal symptoms. Buprenorphine carries a lower risk of abuse, addiction, and side effects compared with full opioid agonists. Buprenorphine is highly bound to plasma proteins and metabolized by the liver. The half-life of buprenorphine is 24 to 60 hours. Buprenorphine has poor oral bioavailability and moderate sublingual bioavailability. Formulations for opioid addiction treatment are given as sublingual tablets.

Buprenorphine and naloxone are combined into one formulation with a brand name of *Bunavail*, *Suboxone*, or *Zubsolv*, and is indicated for the maintenance treatment of opioid addiction. The medication is administered sublingually as a single dose. The purpose of adding the naloxone to the buprenorphine is to protect the patient from an overdose in case the patient has been misusing opiates. Otherwise, the naloxone has no beneficial purpose.

Inhalants

Inhalants are organic solvents, also known as *volatile substances* that are CNS depressants. When inhaled, they cause euphoria, sedation, emotional lability, and impaired judgment. Intoxication can result in respiratory depression, stupor, and coma. Inhalants are typically abused by young children with adolescents using less than younger children. Different inhalants tend to be used by various age groups. New users (ages 12 to 15) are more likely to abuse glue, shoe polish, spray paints, gasoline, and lighter fluids. The 16- to 17-year-olds most commonly abuse nitrous oxide or "whippets" and adults a class of nitrites such as amyl nitrites or "poppers." Addiction is rare, but inhalants can be intermediate between legal and illegal drugs and their use can be fatal (NIDA, 2017).

Most inhalants are common household or industrial products that give off mind-altering chemical fumes when sniffed. They include the following:

- *Volatile Solvents*: Liquids that vaporize at room temperature such as paint thinners or removers, degreasers, dry-cleaning fluids, gasoline, and lighter fluid. Office supply solvents include correction fluids, felt-tip marker fluid, electronic contact cleaners, and glue.
- *Aerosols*: Sprays that contain propellant and solvents such as spray paint, hair spray, fabric protector spray, aerosol computer cleaning products, vegetable oil spray, analgesics, asthma sprays, deodorants, and air fresheners.
- *Gases*: Household or commercial products such as butane lighters and propane tanks, whipped cream aerosols or dispensers, and refrigerant gases; medical anesthetics such as ether, chloroform, halothane, and nitrous oxide ("laughing gas").
- *Nitrites*: Organic nitrites include cyclohexyl, butyl, and amyl nitrites. When marketed for illicit uses, organic nitrates are sold in small brown bottles labeled "video head cleaner," "room odorizer," "leather cleaner," or "room deodorizer" (NIDA, 2017).

Most inhalants other than nitrites depress the CNS in a manner similar to alcohol (e.g., slurred speech, lack of coordination, euphoria, dizziness). They may cause lightheadedness, hallucinations, and delusions. The nitrites enhance sexual pleasure by dilating and relaxing blood vessels. They are thought to be antagonistic at the NMDA receptor and may cause neuronal damage in the mesolimbic system (Cruz, Torres-Flores, & Galván, 2019).

Inhalant Intoxication

Inhalants are easily absorbed through the lungs and are widely distributed in the body, reaching the highest concentrations in fat tissue and the nervous system where the most profound effects are exhibited. Mild intoxication occurs within minutes and can last as long as 30 minutes. Often, the drugs are inhaled repeatedly to maintain an intoxicated state for hours. Initially, the person experiences a sense of euphoria, but as the dose increases, confusion, perceptual distortions, and severe CNS depression occur. Inhalant users are also at risk for **sudden sniffing death**, which can occur when the inhaled fumes replace oxygen in the lungs and CNS, causing the user to suffocate. Inhalants can also cause death by disrupting the normal heart rhythm, which can lead to cardiac arrest (NIDA, 2017).

Long-Term Complications

Chronic neurologic syndromes can result from long-term use, which is linked to widespread brain damage and cognitive abnormalities that can range from mild impairment to severe dementia. In recent studies, considerably more inhalant users than cocaine users had brain abnormalities and their damage was more extensive. Inhalant users also performed significantly worse on tests of working memory with diminished ability to focus attention, plan, and solve problems. However, inhalants can change brain chemistry and may permanently damage the brain and CNS. Magnetic resonance imaging scans of users demonstrate severe changes in cerebral white matter (NIDA, 2017).

Steroids

Anabolic steroid is the name for synthetic substances related to the male sex hormones (androgens). Developed in the late 1930s to treat hypogonadism, they are also used to treat delayed puberty, some types of impotence, and wasting of the body caused by HIV infection or other diseases. They promote growth of skeletal muscle and the development of male sexual characteristics. More than 100 different types exist; to be used legally, all require a prescription. Some dietary supplements, such as dehydroepiandrosterone (DHEA) and androstenedione (Andro), can be purchased in commercial health stores. They are often used in the belief that large doses can convert into testosterone or a similar compound in the body that promote muscle growth. They can be taken orally or intramuscularly. Some are applied to the skin as a cream or gel. When abused, these preparations are taken at 10 to 100 times higher doses than are used for medical disorders. Although use among men is higher than among women, use among women is growing (NIDA, 2018k).

Case reports and small studies indicate that in high doses, anabolic steroids increase irritability and aggression. Some steroid users report that they have committed aggressive acts, such as physical fighting, armed robbery, using force to obtain something, committing property damage, stealing from stores, or breaking into a house or building. Users engage in these behaviors more often when they take steroids than when they are drug free. Other behavioral effects include euphoria, increased energy, sexual arousal, mood swings, distractibility, forgetfulness, and confusion (Ganson & Cadet, 2018.)

Anabolic steroids do not trigger a rapid increase in dopamine or cause the "high" associated with other drugs of abuse. However, long-term use can affect neurotransmitter pathways that regulate mood and behavior. With time, anabolic steroid use is associated with an increased risk for heart attacks and strokes, blood clotting, cholesterol changes, hypertension, depressed mood, fatigue, restlessness, loss of appetite, insomnia, reduced libido, muscle and joint pain, and severe liver problems (including hepatic cancer). Males can have reduced sperm production, shrinking of the testes, and difficulty or pain in urinating. Other undesirable body changes include breast enlargement in men and masculinization of women's bodies. Both sexes may experience hair loss and acne. Intravenous or intramuscular use of the drug and needle sharing put users at risk for HIV, hepatitis B and C, and infective endocarditis, as well as bacterial infections at injection sites (NIDA, 2018k).

EMERGING DRUGS AND TRENDS

New drugs and drug-use trends rapidly enter our communities. The National Institute of Drug Abuse continuously reports on these drugs. Some of the newer drugs include synthetic cathinones (bath salts, Flakka), Krokodil (toxic homemade opioid), and synthetic hallucinogens (N-bomb).

Bath salts contain cathinone, an amphetamine-like stimulant naturally found in the Khat plant (*Catha edulis*). Severe intoxication and dangerous health effects are associated with these drugs. These drugs, which are chemically similar to methamphetamines and MDMA, produce euphoria, increased sociability, and increased sex drive, as well as paranoia, agitation, and hallucinatory delirium. Indication is that they are strongly linked to abuse (NIDA, 2014).

Synthetic hallucinogens (e.g., the N-bomb) are being sold as substitutes for LSD or mescaline. These chemicals, considered more powerful than LSD, act on serotonin receptors and can cause seizures, heart attack, or respiratory arrest and death (NIDA, 2018l).

Recently, there has been a sharp increase in synthetic opioid deaths attributed to fentanyl. While the prescription rates have remained relatively stable, there have been unprecedented increases in the global supply, processing, and distribution of fentanyl by criminal elements beginning in 2013. An urgent, collaborative public health and law enforcement response is recommended by the CDC (NIDA, 2019c; Gladden, Martinez, & Seth, 2016).

GAMBLING: A NON–SUBSTANCE-RELATED DISORDER

Social gambling becomes a gambling disorder (also referred to as pathologic gambling) when it is persistent and recurrent leading to clinically significant impairment or distress. In the *DSM-5*, this disorder is classified as an addiction and a non–substance-related disorder (APA, 2013). Individuals with this disorder are preoccupied with gambling and experience an aroused, euphoric state during the actual betting. The action of seeking an aroused state is often more important to the pathologic gambler than the desire for money itself. They are drawn to the games and begin making bigger and bigger bets. Characteristically, they relentlessly chase their losses in an attempt to win them back. They are unable to control their gaming and may lie to family, friends, and employers to hide their gambling habit. They have an intense need to gamble and often turn to gambling when feeling distressed. These individuals are highly competitive, energetic, restless, and easily bored. Some evidence shows that changes in the serotonin system are associated with addiction behavior, similar to results reported for nicotine and alcohol dependence (van Timmeren, Daams, van Holst, & Goudriaan, 2018).

One study found a 1% to 3% lifetime prevalence (Grant, Schreiber, Odlaug, & Kim, 2010). According to the *DSM-5*, the lifetime prevalence rate is about 0.4% to 1% (APA, 2013). Individuals with gambling problems are more likely to commit suicide than those who do not have a gambling problem and are less likely to seek mental health treatment (Karlsson & Håkansson, 2018).

This disorder is conceptualized as similar to alcohol and other substances of dependence. When substances are used in conjunction with gambling, they cause a deterioration in play and accelerate the progression of the gambling disorder. Other comorbid disorders include depression, ADHD, Tourette syndrome, and personality disorders

(Karlsson & Håkansson, 2018). The disorder has four phases: winning, losing, desperation, and hopelessness. Pathologic gambling can be treated by psychotherapists experienced in this disorder; for many of these addicts, Gamblers Anonymous is sufficient to curb the disorder.

Compulsive gamblers feel omnipotent in their ability to win back what was lost. This omnipotence serves as self-deception that leads to denial. Care of these patients involves confronting such omnipotent beliefs. These individuals quickly irritate staff with their self-assurance and overbearing attitude. Staff education about the disorder is important. Family involvement is also crucial. Families often have been dealing with the patient in a dysfunctional manner. Relapse prevention involves learning about specific cues that trigger the gambling behavior.

EVIDENCE-BASED NURSING CARE FOR PERSONS WITH SUBSTANCE-RELATED DISORDERS

The assessment process is, in part, a treatment intervention. Patients are often in denial about the severity of the problem and about its emotional, social, legal, vocational, or other consequences.

Nursing Assessment

Assessment is crucial to understanding level of use, abuse, or dependence and to determining the patient's denial or acceptance of treatment. Assessment is often detailed and may involve family members and other loved ones. Along with the psychiatric nursing interview (see Chapter 9), specific items should be assessed. Box 25.6 gives examples of typical behaviors exhibited by individuals that are associated with each level of use, abuse, and addiction. The nurse can use the Substance Abuse Assessment as a guide in eliciting a substance use history in the assessment process (Box 25.7).

Usually, nurses encounter individuals during crisis when they are seeking professional help. These situations offer an opportunity to explore the denial that keeps their addiction thriving. The nurse's approach should be caring, matter-of-fact, gentle, and direct. Approaches that are punitive or attempt to elicit feelings of guilt or shame are destructive to the therapeutic relationship. Nursing Care Plan 25.1—which sets forth a plan of care for Gladys, the case study patient in this chapter—is available at http://thepoint.lww.com/BoydEssentials2e.

Denial of a Problem

Denial can be expressed in diverse behaviors and attitudes and may not be expressed as an overt denial of the problem. For example, patients may admit to a problem and even thank you for helping them to realize they have a problem but insist they can overcome the problem on their own and do not need outside help.

> **KEYCONCEPT Denial** is the patient's inability to accept his or her loss of control over substance use or the severity of the consequences associated with the substance abuse or addiction

---

BOX 25.6
Behaviors in Substance Use, Abuse, and Addiction

SUBSTANCE USE
- Does not have possible danger or potential legal problems
- Engages in use to enhance social situations and interaction
- Is not intended to result in intoxication
- Has control of the amount and frequency of use
- Exhibits socially acceptable behavior while using

PRESCRIPTION MEDICATION USE
- Use is for the dose, frequency, and indications prescribed.
- Use is for the particular episode of the condition for which it was prescribed.
- Use is coordinated among prescribing physicians.

SUBSTANCE ABUSE
- Use for intoxication or feeling of being "high"
- Use that interferes with normal life functions (e.g., producing sleep when inappropriate, excitability, or irritability interfering with social interaction)
- Potential harm to self or others (e.g., driving while intoxicated, use of injection drug equipment)
- Use that has legal consequences (e.g., all uses of illicit drugs)
- Use resulting in socially unacceptable behavior (e.g., public drunkenness, verbal or physical abuse)
- Use to alter normal feeling states such as sadness or anxiety

PRESCRIPTION MEDICATION ABUSE
- Use is at a higher dose and greater frequency than prescribed.
- Use is for indications other than prescribed or for self-diagnosed condition.
- Use results in feeling tired, having a clouded mental state, or feeling "hyperactive" or nervous.
- Supplementing medication with alcohol or drugs
- Soliciting more than one physician for the same medication
- Inability to control the amount and frequency of use
- Tolerance to larger amounts of the substance
- Withdrawal symptoms when stopping use
- Severe consequences from alcohol or drug use

SUBSTANCE ADDICTION
- Drug craving
- Compulsive use
- Presence of aberrant drug-related behaviors
- Repeated relapse into drug use after withdrawal

BOX 25.7
Substance Abuse Assessment

DRUG/LAST USE	PATTERN OF USE (AMOUNT, ROUTE, FIRST USE, FREQUENCY, AND LENGTH OF USE)
Alcohol/	
Stimulants/	
Opioids/	
Sedative–hypnotics and anxiolytic agents/	
Hallucinogens/	
Marijuana/	
Inhalants/	
Nicotine/	
Caffeine/	

ABUSE INDICATORS

1. Tolerance (increasing use of drug or alcohol with the same level of intoxication): _____
2. Withdrawal symptoms: a. Shakes? _____ b. Tremors? _____ c. Cramps, diarrhea, or rapid pulse? _____ d. Feeling paranoid, fearful? _____ e. Difficulty sleeping? _____
3. Consequences of use (e.g., presenting problems, persistent or recurrent emotional, social, legal, or other problems): _____
4. Loss of control of amount, frequency, or duration of use: _____
5. Desire or efforts to decrease use or control use: _____
6. Preoccupation (increasing focus or time spent on use and obtaining substances): _____
7. Social, vocational, recreational activities affected by use: _____
8. Previous alcohol or drug abuse treatment: _____

The following characteristics are typical of a person who has alcoholism and who is in denial:

- Confusion about severity of drinking history: "I went out drinking with friends last week and didn't have any problems; I don't get drunk all the time."
- Difficulty reconciling early positive experiences of alcohol use with current problems: "I used to drink with my buddies after work to unwind. We had a great time. Those were some good times. …"
- Confusion regarding the definition of *alcoholic*: "Well, I don't have withdrawal symptoms, so I can't be an alcoholic."
- Relief when they compare themselves with others and find the others in worse condition: "They are the alcoholics, not me!"
- A delusion that drinking can be self-controlled: "If I search hard enough or long enough, I will find a way to control and enjoy drinking."
- Confusion or trouble accepting that behavior is different when intoxicated: "I couldn't have done that; that's just not like me."

This quandary about the nature of the problem has often been met with confrontation by nurses and other professionals in the past. But argumentation, presenting evidence of addiction, and lecturing often fail to elicit admission of a problem or induce behavior change.

Gladys and Denial

Gladys continues to deny that she has a drinking problem. She is angry with her son for suggesting that she has a problem and refuses to sign a release of information for him.

Motivation for Change

Motivation is a key predictor of whether individuals will change their substance use behavior (Collins, Malone, & Larimer, 2012).

KEYCONCEPT Motivation is a goal-oriented attitude that propels action for change and can help sustain the development of new activities and behaviors.

Ambivalence about substance use is normal and can be dealt with by working with the patients' own concerns about their use of alcohol and other drugs. Motivation is fluid and can be modified. Experiences such as increased distress levels, critical life events, a period of evaluation or appraisal of one's life, recognizing negative consequences of use, and positive and negative external incentives for change can all influence a patient's commitment to change.

Techniques that enhance motivation are associated with increased success in treatment, higher rates of

> **BOX 25.8**
>
> ### FRAMES—Effective Elements of Brief Intervention
>
> **FEEDBACK**
> Provide patients with personal feedback regarding their individual status, such as personal alcohol and other drug consumption relative to norms, information about elevated liver enzyme values, and other factors.
>
> **RESPONSIBILITY**
> Emphasize the individual's freedom of choice and personal responsibility for change. General themes are as follows:
>
> 1. It's up to you; you're free to decide to change or not.
> 2. No one else can decide for you or force you to change.
> 3. You're the one who has to do it if it's going to happen.
>
> **ADVICE**
> Include a clear recommendation or advice on the need for change, typically in a supportive and concerned, rather than in a judgmental, manner.
>
> **MENU**
> Provide a menu of treatment options from which patients may pick those that seem more suitable or appealing.
>
> **EMPATHIC COUNSELING**
> Show warmth, support, respect, and understanding in communication with patients.
>
> **SELF-EFFICACY**
> Reinforce self-efficacy or an optimistic feeling that he or she can change.

abstinence, and successful follow-up treatment (Teeters, Lancaster, Brown, & Back, 2017). **Motivational interviewing** is a method of therapeutic intervention that seeks to elicit self-motivational statements from patients, supports behavioral change, and creates a disconnect between the patient's goals and their continued alcohol and other drug use. The acronym FRAMES (which is short form for feedback, responsibility, advice, menu of strategies, empathy, and self-efficacy) summarizes elements of brief interventions with patients using motivational interviewing (Box 25.8).

> **NCLEXNOTE** Motivational approaches are priority interventions for patients with substance-related disorders. They help patients recognize a problem and develop change strategies.

Countertransference

Countertransference is the total emotional reaction of the treatment provider to the patient (see Chapter 5). Patients with substance-related disorders can generate strong feelings and reactions in nurses and other health care providers (Table 25.5). These feelings can be generated by overtly unpleasant behaviors of the substance-dependent persons, such as lying, deceit, manipulation, or hostility, or these feelings may be more subconscious and stem from past experiences with people with alcoholism or addicts or even from dealing with situations in the health care provider's own family.

Codependence

The concept of **codependence** emerged out of studies of women's relationships with husbands who abused alcohol. Today, the scope of codependency includes both men and women who grew up in any type of dysfunctional family system in which substance abuse may or may not have been a problem. Codependence has also been described as "enabling," in which an individual in a relationship with a person who abuses alcohol inadvertently reinforces the

TABLE 25.5 PATIENT BEHAVIORS AND COUNTERTRANSFERENCE REACTIONS

Patient Behavior	Common Nursing Reaction
Behaves as a victim	Feels a sense of helplessness, increased need to give advice and "fix" the situation and the patient; shows anger toward the patient for not being able to take care of the situation him- or herself
Is intrusive, hostile, belittling	Can be frightened, withdraw from patient, express anger overtly, or be passive-aggressive (i.e., suggesting discharge to the team or ignoring legitimate requests from patient)
Does everything right, is insightful, pleasant, and so forth	Congratulates self on therapeutic interventions; can become bored or complacent
Relapses into drug or alcohol use	Feels angry, personally betrayed; withdraws from other patients; doubts own abilities
Asks personal questions about staff qualifications or prior drug or alcohol abuse	Reveals personal information, resents the intrusion, and may regret divulging information
Is silent or divulges minimal information	Tries harder, doubts own therapeutic ability, is angered by patient's resistance
Tries to "bend" or ignore rules of milieu and group rules	May permit program rule infractions; may feel pressured, angry, or passive-aggressive
Insists that no one can help him or her	Feels pressure to be the one who can help; may feel angry and inept or helpless

Adapted from Imhoff, J. E. (1991). Countertransference issues in alcoholism and drug addiction. *Psychiatric Annals*, 21(5), 292–306.

BOX 25.9 • THERAPEUTIC DIALOGUE • The Patient With Alcoholism

INEFFECTIVE APPROACH

Nurse: I would like to talk with you about your problem with alcoholism.

Gladys: Alcoholism! It's not that bad. Everyone gets loaded!

Nurse: You tell me why you were drinking. Your wife left you. You drink a quart of vodka a day. Your BAL was 0.15% when you were admitted.

Gladys: So what! I do have some problems or I wouldn't be here. But, I'm not an alcoholic. (Denial)

Nurse: Do you know what an alcoholic is?

Gladys: Sure I do. My father was one. He was a useless bum. I'm not anything like him.

Nurse: It sounds like you are a lot like him.

Gladys: I think I need to rest now. My back is killing me (avoidance).

EFFECTIVE APPROACH

Nurse: I would like to talk with you about what happens when you drink.

Gladys: It's not that bad. Everyone gets loaded!

Nurse: What concerns do you have about your drinking?

Gladys: I'm not really concerned. My son is. He thinks I drink too much.

Nurse: What does he tell you about that?

Gladys: Well, complains about it, but I just have a glass of wine at night.

Nurse: It sounds as if he is concerned about this, but you have your doubts about how serious it is. Your son is invited to our family education group, so he can learn about alcohol abuse.

Gladys: I have a lot of problems besides alcohol. I never use drugs. I only drink because it relaxes me and makes it easier to deal with stress.

Nurse: Many people drink to help them cope with stress. Sometimes the drinking itself can cause stress. While you are here, do you think it would be useful to look at the stress in your life and how it relates to your drinking?

Gladys: Yes. But I only drink when things get too out of hand. My health is pretty good.

Nurse: We can provide information about your health and alcohol use. To evaluate what information may be helpful, I would like to get a little more information about your drinking.

CRITICAL THINKING CHALLENGE

- What effect did the nurse have on the patient in using the word *alcoholism* in the first interaction?
- Discuss what communication approaches the nurse used in the second scenario to engage the patient in disclosing problems with alcohol and her relationship with her son. How does this nurse's approach vary from the one in the first interaction?

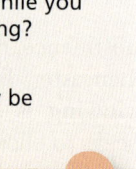

drinking behavior of the other person. The codependency label remains controversial and is viewed by some as an oversimplification of complex emotions and behaviors of family members. Mental health professionals should be careful not to use it as a catch-all diagnosis and to take special care to assess and plan interventions that address each person's particular situation, problems, and needs (Mental Health America, 2019).

Priority of Care

For a hospitalized patient, the first priority is to determine whether the person will be withdrawing. After the person is no longer in danger of withdrawal symptoms, the nurse can discuss the use of substance and encourage the individual to seek help for the addiction. A patient's denial of a problem with substances is common and often a priority.

Therapeutic Relationship

It is critical that the nurse establish a therapeutic relationship with these patients (Box 25.9). Several general guidelines are available for establishing therapeutic interactions with patients in substance abuse treatment programs:

- Encourage honest expression of feelings.
- Listen to what the individual is really saying.
- Express caring for the individual.
- Hold the individual responsible for his or her behavior.
- Provide fair and consistent consequences for negative behavior.
- Talk about specific objectionable actions.
- Do not compromise your own values or nursing practice.
- Communicate the treatment plan to the patient and to others on the treatment team.
- Monitor your own reactions to the patient.

Confrontation, or pointing out the inconsistencies in thoughts, feelings, and actions, can promote the person's experience of the natural consequences of one's behavior. Learning from previous behavior and its consequences is how change occurs. Confrontation can be very threatening to patients and should only occur within the context of a trusting relationship.

Mental Health Nursing Interventions

Several treatment modalities are used in most addiction treatment (pharmacologic modalities were discussed earlier in this chapter), including 12-step program-focused, cognitive or psychoeducation, behavioral, group psychotherapy, and individual and family therapy. Discharge planning and relapse prevention are also essential components of successful treatment and so are incorporated into most programs. See Table 25.6 for different treatment approaches to chemical addiction and Box 25.10.

Because patients with substance-related disorders differ greatly, no single type of treatment program will work for every individual. Often, several approaches can work together, but others may be inappropriate. Treatment programs usually combine many different interventions to provide a comprehensive approach based on the individual's needs. Nursing interventions vary depending on the nature of the current problems and their severity. For a patient who is being detoxified, physical interventions (e.g., monitoring vital signs and neurologic functioning) are necessary. When the substance use disorder is secondary to other physical or psychiatric problems, education of patient and family may be a priority.

Assessment and interventions should include culturally relevant data such as unique physiologic responses to substances, behavioral responses to dependence, and social expectations and sanctions. Staff who are knowledgeable about cultural differences and issues are integral to successful treatment.

Brief Intervention

A growing body of evidence indicates that brief interventions are more effective than no treatment, and indications suggest that they are as effective as more intensive interventions. Screening, brief intervention, and referral to treatment (SBIRT) has been shown to be an effective in helping individuals with high-risk alcohol use to seek help (Biroscak, Pantalon, Dziura, Hersey, & Vaca, 2019). Within the alcohol and other drugs field, brief intervention is a highly developed, researched, and widely accepted approach.

Screening and brief intervention are two separate skills that can be used together to reduce risky substance use. Screening involves asking questions about alcohol or drug use. A **brief intervention** is a negotiated conversation between the professional and patient designed to reduce or eliminate alcohol and drug use.

Not everyone who is screened will need a brief intervention and not everyone who needs a brief intervention will require treatment. In fact, the goals of screening and brief intervention are to reduce risky substance use before people become dependent or addicted.

Brief intervention is effective for several reasons. Research indicates that brief interventions are an appropriate response to patients presenting in a general health or community setting and who are unlikely to need, seek, or attend specialist treatment. Brief intervention—to be given clear concise information by a professional—may be all the patients may want. It is also an important part of the overall approach of harm reduction (discussed later in this chapter).

BOX 25.10

Principles of Effective Treatment for Addiction

1. Addiction is a complex but treatable disease that affects brain function and behavior.
2. No single treatment is appropriate for everyone.
3. Treatment needs to be readily available.
4. Effective treatment attends to multiple needs of the individual, not just his or her drug use.
5. Remaining in treatment for an adequate period of time is critical.
6. Behavioral therapies—including individual, family, or group counseling—are the most commonly used forms of drug abuse treatment.
7. Medications are an important element of treatment for many patients, especially when combined with counseling and other behavioral therapies.
8. An individual's treatment and service plan must be assessed continually and modified as necessary to ensure that it meets his or her changing needs.
9. Many drug-addicted individuals also have concurrent mental disorders.
10. Medically assisted detoxification is only the first stage of addiction treatment and by itself does little to change long-term drug abuse.
11. Treatment does not need to be voluntary to be effective.
12. Drug use during treatment must be monitored continuously because lapses during treatment do occur.
13. Treatment programs should provide assessment for HIV/AIDS, hepatitis B and C, tuberculosis, and other infectious diseases, as well as provide targeted risk-reduction counseling, linking patients to treatment as necessary.

National Institute on Drug Abuse. (2018). *Principles of drug addiction treatment: A research-based guide* (3rd ed., pp. 3–4). Bethesda, MD. Retrieved March 24, 2019, from https://www.drugabuse.gov/publications/principles-drug-addiction-treatment-research-based-guide-third-edition/principles-effective-treatment

TABLE 25.6 TREATMENT APPROACHES TO CHEMICAL DEPENDENCE

Approach	Conception of Etiology	Conception of Patient	Conception of Treatment Outcome	Conception of Treatment Process	Advantages of Approach	Disadvantages of Approach
Psychiatric	Symptom of underlying emotional problem	Emotionally disturbed	Emotional conflicts are resolved; emotional health improves	Psychotherapy, medication to treat cause of substance abuse	Not punitive, treats comorbidity	Focus is only on treatment of mental disorder
Social	Society and environment cause dependence	Victim of circumstance	Improved social functioning or improved environment	Removal of environmental influences and increasing coping responses to it	Stresses social supports and coping skills	Blames "ills of society"—the person not responsible for addiction
Moral	Person is morally weak—can't say "no"	"Hustler," morally deficient	Moral recovery, increased willpower, self-control, and responsible behavior	"Street addict" behavior and manipulation confronted	Holds person responsible for actions and making amends	Punitive, increases low self-esteem and sense of failure
Learning	Abuse is a learned, reinforced behavior	Has distorted thinking, poor coping skills	Patient learns new ways of thinking and new coping skills	Cognitive therapy techniques and coping skills taught	Not punitive; teaches new coping skills	Places emphasis on control of use
Disease	Probably caused by genetic or biologic factors	Has a chronically progressive disease	Abstinence, arresting disease progression, and beginning of recovery process	Is treated as a primary disease, reinforces patient is an addict and is sick	Not punitive, stresses social support and education	Minimizes mental health disorders; discounts return to social use
12-Step	Combination of disease concept and "spiritual bankruptcy"	Has an addiction and is powerless over substances	Abstinence, ongoing spiritual recovery	Use 12 steps, seeking spiritual support, making amends, serving others in need	Widespread success, emphasis is on quality of life and spiritual growth	Self-help group, not a treatment program
Dual diagnosis	Both a primary substance dependency and a mental health disorder	Has both mental and substance abuse disorder	Improvement in both mental health and substance abuse disorders	Concurrent treatment of both disorders	Treats both mental health disorder and dependency, minimizing relapse potential	Not inclusive enough; does not include social or other issues
Biopsychosocial	Biologic basis, with social and psychological influences	Has deficiencies in all three interacting areas	Improvement in mental and physical health, utilization of social supports	Concurrent treatment of all issues	Uses different modalities; is more inclusive	Does not match patient and specific interventions
Multivariant	Many different causes; may be different for each individual	Has multiple issues to be assessed and addressed	Particular issues for individual addressed, so improvement occurs	Treatment strategies are matched with individual patient needs	Treatment matched to individual's needs	Logistical problems can occur during its implementation

Brief intervention is most successful when working with people who:

- Are experiencing few problems with their drug use
- Have low levels of dependence
- Have a short history of drug use
- Have stable backgrounds
- Are unsure or ambivalent about changing or ending their drug use

It is recommended that brief intervention at a minimum include:

- Advising how to reduce patient's drug use
- Providing harm reduction information or self-help manuals relevant to the patient
- Giving the patient relevant information about
  - The consequences of a drug conviction in terms of international travel and employment
  - Consequences of further or heavier drug charges

Discussing harm reduction strategies, especially those relating to:

- Overdose
- Violence
- Driving under the influence
- Safe practices (e.g., safe injecting, safe sex)
- Offering and arranging a follow-up visit

Cognitive and Cognitive Behavioral Interventions and Psychoeducation

Cognitive approaches to addiction hypothesize that if a patient can change the way he or she thinks about a situation, both the emotional reaction to it and the behavioral response will change. Psychoeducational materials, groups, and one-on-one interactions with nurses also impart information to reduce knowledge deficits related to alcohol and drug dependence (Box 25.11). CBT is a brief structured treatment that focuses on immediate problems. It enables patients to examine the thinking process that leads to decisions to use substances, analyze distortions in thinking, and develop rational responses to these distortions. See Box 25.12.

BOX 25.11

Substance Abuse

When caring for the patient and family with substance abuse, be sure to include the following topic areas in the family's teaching plan:

- Psychopharmacologic agents, if used, including drug action, dosage, frequency, and possible side effects
- Manifestations of intoxication, overdose, and withdrawal
- Emergency medical system activation
- Nutrition
- Coping strategies
- Structured planning
- Safety measures
- Available treatment programs
- Family therapy referral
- Self-help groups and other community resources
- Follow-up laboratory testing, if indicated

BOX 25.12

Research for Best Practice. Behavioral Interventions and Substance Use Disorder in Primary Care

Barrett, K., & Chang, Y. (2016). Behavioral interventions targeting chronic pain, depression, and substance use disorder in primary care. *Journal of Nursing Scholarship, 48*(4), 345–353.

QUESTION: Which behavioral interventions target chronic pain, depression, and substance use disorder in primary care settings?

METHODS: Major health care databases were searched to identify randomized controlled trials using a behavioral intervention involving adults with at least two of the three conditions. There were over 1,800 relevant records found with only 6 articles meeting the final selection criteria. A total of 696 participants were studied.

FINDINGS: Behavioral interventions varied in content, format, and duration. Mindfulness-oriented therapy, interpersonal psychotherapy adapted for pain, and cognitive behavioral therapy showed promising improvements across all studies with small to moderate effects.

IMPLICATIONS FOR NURSING: Evidence is increasing that behavioral interventions are effective strategies for managing patients with comorbidities of chronic pain, depression and substance use disorder in primary care. Integrated delivery of behavioral interventions through group sessions, computers, and smart phones may increase patients' access to treatment.

Enhancing Coping Skills

Improving coping skills is thought to be one component of preventing relapse into alcohol and drug use. Coping skills include the ability to use thought, emotion, and action effectively to solve interpersonal and intrapersonal problems and to achieve personal goals. Groups in addiction treatment programs that also have a relapse prevention component look at coping. The skills listed in Box 25.13 are often taught as coping strategies for dealing with alcohol and drug cravings. Patients role-play new behaviors and learn from the feedback they receive from other group members. They also increase their sense of competency to use these skills in real-life situations.

Group Interventions and Early Recovery

Isolation and alienation from friends and family are common themes in patients with substance-related disorders. In addition, thinking that has become distorted is left unchallenged without contact with others; thus, change is difficult. When a patient enters a group that is working

> **BOX 25.13**
> **Skills Training Group Topics**
>
> **INTERPERSONAL**
> Starting conversations
> Giving and receiving compliments
> Nonverbal communication
> Receiving criticism
> Receiving criticism about drinking
> Drink and drug refusal skills
> Refusing requests
> Close and intimate relationships
> Enhancing social support networks
>
> **INTRAPERSONAL**
> Managing thoughts about alcohol
> Problem solving
> Increasing pleasant activities
> Relaxation training
> Awareness and management of anger
> Awareness and management of negative thinking
> Planning for emergencies
> Coping with persistent problems

with the goals of continuing recovery, numerous healing advantages can occur.

Groups in treatment settings focus on immediate goals of maintaining sobriety and not on childhood issues. The emphasis is on using problem solving and other skills to deal with stressful events that threaten abstinence. This type of support group is also extremely effective in outpatient treatment settings. After a period of successful abstinence, group therapy can focus more on traditional psychotherapy work.

Individual Therapy

Often, individual therapy is helpful, particularly in conjunction with group therapy or family therapy. In addiction treatment settings, counselors meet with individuals to maintain focus on the goals and objectives of their treatment, to review the fears and anxieties that often arise in early recovery, and to devise new and healthy responses and solutions to stressful and difficult situations.

Family Interventions

Family therapy, a vital part of addiction treatment, can be used in several beneficial ways to initiate change and help the family when the substance-abusing person is unwilling to seek treatment. Behavioral couples therapy for people with alcoholism can improve family functioning, reduce stressors, smooth marital adjustment, and lessen domestic violence and verbal conflict. When the substance-abusing person seeks help, family therapy can help stabilize abstinence and relationships. Often, inpatient substance abuse treatment programs have family education and group therapy components that help meet these goals. Family therapy can also help to maintain long-term recovery and prevent relapse. Goals of family therapy should be realistic and obtainable. Action plans must be specific and organized into manageable increments. Target dates should be realistic, so pressure is minimal, yet there is motivation to act in a timely manner. Planning for the future is very difficult as long as alcohol or drug abuse continues.

Harm-Reduction Strategies

Harm reduction, a community health intervention designed to reduce the harm of substance use to the individual, the family, and society, has replaced a moral or criminal approach to drug use and addiction. It recognizes that the ideal is abstinence but works with the individual regardless of his or her commitment to reduce use. The goal is to reduce the potential harm of the associated behavior. Harm reduction initiatives range from widely accepted designated driver campaigns to controversial initiatives such as provision of condoms in schools, safe injection rooms, needle exchange programs, and heroin maintenance programs.

Peer Support Self-Help Group

Alcoholics Anonymous (AA) was the first 12-step, self-help program (see Box 25.14 for a list of these steps).

> **BOX 25.14**
> **The 12 Steps of Alcoholics Anonymous**
>
> 1. We admitted we were powerless over alcohol—that our lives had become unmanageable.
> 2. Came to believe that a Power greater than ourselves could restore us to sanity.
> 3. Made a decision to turn our will and our lives over to the care of God *as we understood Him.*
> 4. Made a searching and fearless moral inventory of ourselves.
> 5. Admitted to God, to ourselves, and to another human being the exact nature of our wrongs.
> 6. Were entirely ready to have God remove all these defects of character.
> 7. Humbly asked Him to remove our shortcomings.
> 8. Made a list of all persons we had harmed, and became willing to make amends to them all.
> 9. Made direct amends to such people wherever possible, except when to do so would injure them or others.
> 10. Continued to take personal inventory and, when we were wrong, promptly admitted it.
> 11. Sought through prayer and meditation to improve our conscious contact with God, as we understood Him, praying only for knowledge of His will for us and the power to carry that out.
> 12. Having had a spiritual awakening as a result of these steps, we tried to carry this message to alcoholics and to practice these principles in all our affairs.
>
> The Twelve Steps are reprinted with permission of Alcoholics Anonymous World Services, Inc. Permission to reprint the Twelve Steps does not mean that A.A. has reviewed or approved the contents of this publication, nor that A.A. agrees with the views expressed herein. A.A. is a program of recovery from alcoholism only—use of the Twelve Steps in connection with programs and activities which are patterned after A.A., but which address other problems, or in any other non-A.A. context, does not imply otherwise.

AA is a worldwide fellowship of people with alcoholism who provide support, individually and at meetings, to others who seek help. The program steps include spiritual, cognitive, and behavioral components. Many treatment programs discuss concepts from AA, hold meetings at the treatment facilities, and encourage patients to attend community meetings when appropriate. They also encourage continuing use of AA and other self-help groups as part of an ongoing plan for continued abstinence. Twelve-step programs do not solicit members; engage in political or religious activities; make medical or psychiatric diagnoses; engage in education about addiction to the general population; or provide mental health, vocational, or legal counseling (Alcoholics Anonymous, 2019).

Alternative peer support groups differ from these programs in their approach. Four such groups in the United States are Women for Sobriety, Moderation Management, Men for Sobriety, and SMART Recovery. These groups are based on harm reduction philosophies and missions.

Evaluation and Treatment Outcomes

Recovery from alcoholism is a journey, often lasting a lifetime. Recovery involves a change in lifestyle and, often, new relationships. Short-term outcomes can be evaluated within the treatment setting. Long-term outcomes are established and evaluated by the patient who often continues to use professional and nonprofessional support as needed.

CHEMICAL DEPENDENCY AND PROFESSIONAL NURSES

Although accurate epidemiologic data specific to nursing are scarce, evidence suggests that the prevalence of substance use disorders among nurses is similar to that of the general public (Kunyk, 2015). A nurse is just as susceptible to addiction as any other individual, but additional risk factors exist such as access and availability of drugs, training in the administration and injection of drugs, and a familiarity with and a frequency of administering drugs. Working conditions may be difficult and involve staffing shortages, acutely ill patients, inadequate patient to nurse ratios, shift rotation, shifts lasting longer than 8 hours, and increased overtime all add additional stress to the nurse which increases the risk of substance abuse. Because of the risk of losing a license to practice, nurses are very reluctant to seek help. To protect patients' safety and maintain the standards of the profession, many states have mandatory reporting laws. According to the nurse practice acts, any nurse who knows of any health care provider's incompetent, unethical, or illegal practice must report that information through proper channels.

In 1982, the American Nurses Association House of Delegates adopted a national resolution to provide assistance to impaired nurses. The peer assistance programs strive to intervene early, reduce hazards to patients, and increase prospects for the nurse's recovery. The program offers consultation, referral, and monitoring for nurses whose practice is impaired, or potentially impaired, because of the use of illicit drugs or alcohol or a psychological or physiologic condition.

A referral can be made confidentially by the employer, Employee Assistance Program, coworker, family member, friend, or the nurse herself or himself. If the nurse is willing to undergo a thorough evaluation to determine the extent of the problem and any treatment needed, all information is kept confidential from the Board of Nursing, so that the nurse does not face disciplinary action against his or her nursing license.

Some signs of substance abuse in nurses include mood swings; inappropriate behavior at work; frequent days off for implausible reasons; noncompliance with acceptable policies and procedures; deteriorating appearance; deteriorating job performance; sloppy illegible charting; errors in charting; alcohol on the breath; forgetfulness; poor judgment and concentration; lying; and volunteering to act as the medications nurse.

Other characteristics of nurses with substance abuse include high achievement, both as a student and a nurse; volunteering for overtime and extra duties; no drug use unless prescribed after surgery or for a chronic illness; and family history of alcoholism or addiction.

SUMMARY OF KEY POINTS

- Substance use disorders are categorized according to the following substances: alcohol, caffeine, cannabis (marijuana), hallucinogens, inhalants, opioids, sedative–hypnotics, stimulants, tobacco, and others.

- Addiction is a condition of continued use of substances despite adverse consequences. Abuse occurs when a person uses alcohol or drugs for the purpose of intoxication or, in the case of prescription drugs, for purposes beyond their use.

- Accurate and comprehensive assessment is crucial in planning addiction treatment interventions. This assessment should consider all substances for pattern of use, including factors of tolerance; withdrawal symptoms; consequences of use; loss of control over amount, frequency, or duration of use; desire or efforts to cease or control use; and social, vocational, and recreational activities affected by use, history of previous addiction treatment, and family and social support systems.

- Denial of a substance use disorder is the individual's attempt to avoid accepting its diagnosis; it can be manifest in attempts to rationalize the substance use, minimize the harmful results, deflect attention from one's own problem to society's or someone else's, or blame childhood trauma.

- Nurses should use a nonconfrontational approach when dealing with patients in denial of their problem. Motivational interviewing approaches are most effective, using empathy and a nonjudgmental approach and to help the patient to realize the discrepancy between life goals and engaging in substance use, thus, motivating patients to change their self-destructive behaviors and make personal choices regarding treatment goals.

- Several effective modalities are used in addiction treatment, and many programs combine them, which may include 12-step programs, social skills groups, psychoeducational groups, group therapy, and individual and family therapies. No one best treatment method exists for all people.

- Substance use disorders have many social and political ramifications. Even the profession of nursing is not immune to substance use disorders among its members.

CRITICAL THINKING CHALLENGES

1. Jeff H, a 35-year-old patient who abuses cocaine, has entered a rehabilitation program. What goals do you believe would be realistic to achieve by the end of his projected 30-day inpatient stay?
2. You are working in an orthopedic unit, and Mary L has been admitted for treatment for a fractured femur. She has been drinking recently and has a BAL of 0.08%. What further information in the following areas would you need to plan her care?
    a. Medical
    b. Alcohol and drug use related
    c. Other psychosocial issues
3. Normal adolescent behavior is often similar to that associated with substance abuse. How would you differentiate this normal behavior from possible substance abuse or addiction?
4. John M has sought treatment for depression and job stress. He came to your psychiatric assessment unit smelling of alcohol. He believes that he does not have a drinking problem but a job problem. What interventions would you use for possible alcohol abuse or addiction?
5. Sylvia G has been abusing heroin intravenously heavily for 2 years. She has come into the hospital with an abscess on her leg. What symptoms would you expect to observe as she experiences withdrawal? What medications would likely be used to ease these symptoms?
6. After Sylvia G is free from withdrawal symptoms, she expresses interest in obtaining drug treatment. What are her options? How would you describe them to her?
7. Raymond L has been treated for hypertension at your clinic. You notice that he complains of peripheral neuropathy and has an unsteady gait. What other medical signs would corroborate alcoholism?
8. What laboratory test results would help confirm a diagnosis of alcoholism?

2004: *Ray*
This award-winning film is based on the life of Ray Charles (played by Jamie Foxx), the musical genius of rhythm and blues. His early childhood experiences included racial discrimination, extreme poverty, an absent father, the traumatic drowning of his younger brother, and the loss of his sight. The film depicts Ray Charles' struggle with his heroin addiction.
Viewing Points: Identify the role of heroin in the development of Ray Charles as a performer, adult, husband, and father. How did denial shape his use of heroin? What was his primary reason for entering treatment? What motivated him to stay clean for the rest of his life?

 Related Psychiatric–Mental Health Nursing videos on the topics of Addiction and Alcohol Withdrawal are available at http://thepoint.lww.com/BoydEssentials2e.

 Psychiatric–Mental Health Nursing Practice and Learn Interactive Case Studies related to the videos on the topics of Addiction and Alcohol Withdrawal are available at http://thepoint.lww.com/BoydEssentials2e.

REFERENCES

Alcoholics Anonymous. (2019). Alcoholics anonymous information on AA [Online]. Retrieved March 24, 2019, from http://www.aa.org

American Psychiatric Association. (2013). *Diagnostic and statistical manual of mental disorders* (5th ed.). Arlington, VA: Author.

Biroscak, B. J., Pantalon, M. V., Dziura, J. D., Hersey, D. P., & Vaca, F. E. (2019). Use of non-face-to-face modalities for emergency department screening, brief intervention, and referral to treatment (ED-SBIRT) for high-risk alcohol use: A scoping review. *Substance Abuse, 4*, 1–13.

Brosen, K. (2015). Pharmacogenetics of drug oxidation via cytochrome P450 (CPY) in the populations of Denmark, Faroe Islands and Greenland. *Drug Metabolism and Personalized Therapy, 30*(3), 147–163.

Centers for Disease control and Prevention. (2018\9). Prescription opioid data. Retrieved March 21, 2019, from https://www.cdc.gov/drugoverdose/data/prescribing.html

Chrysant, S. G., & Chrysant, G. S. (2015). Cardiovascular complications from consumption of high energy drinks: Recent evidence. *Journal of Human Hypertension, 29*(2), 71–76.

Collins, S. E., Malone, D. K., & Larimer, M. E. (2012). Motivation to change and treatment attendance as predictors of alcohol-use outcomes among project-based Housing First residents. *Addictive Behaviors, 37*(8), 931–939.

Cruz, S. L., Torres-Flores, M., Galván, E. J. (2019). Repeated toluene exposure alters the synaptic transmission of layer 5 medial prefrontal cortex. *Neurotoxicology and Teratology, 28*(73), 9–14.

Donoghue, K., Elzerbi, C., Saunders, R., Whittington, C., Pilling, S., & Drummond, C. (2015). The efficacy of acamprosate and naltrexone in the treatment of alcohol dependence, Europe versus the rest of the world; a meta-analysis. *Addiction*, *110*(6):920–930.

Ewing, J. A. (1984). Detecting alcoholism. The CAGE questionnaire. *Journal of the American Medical Association*, *252*(14), 1905–1907.

Ganson, K. T., & Cadet, T. J. (2018). Exploring anabolic-androgenic steroid use and teen dating violence among adolescent males. *Substance Use & Misuse*. *54*(5), 779–786. doi: 10.1080/10826084.2018.1536723.

Gladden, R. M., Martinez, P., & Seth, P. (2016). Fentanyl law enforcement submissions and increases in synthetic opioid-involved overdose deaths – 27 states, 2013–2014. *MMWR Morbidity Mortality Weekly Reports*, *65*(33), 837–843.

Grant, J. E., Schreiber, L., Odlaug, B. L., & Kim, S. W. (2010). Pathologic gambling and bankruptcy. *Comprehensive Psychiatry*, *51*(2), 115–120.

Karlsson, A., & Håkansson, A. (2018). Gambling disorder, increased mortality, suicidality, and associated comorbidity: A longitudinal nationwide register study. *Journal of Behavioral Addictions*, *7*(4), 1091–1099.

Kunyk, D. (2015). Substance use disorders among registered nurses: prevalence, risks and perceptions in a disciplinary jurisdiction. *Journal of Nursing Management*, *23*(1):54–64.

Mental Health America. (2019). Co-dependency [Online]. Retrieved March 24, 2019, from http://www.mentalhealthamerica.net/go/codependency

National Institute on Drug Abuse. (2014) Synthetic Cathinones (Bath Salts). National Institute on Drug Abuse; National Institutes of Health; U.S. Department of Health and Human Services. Retrieved March 22, 2019, from https://www.drugabuse.gov/drugs-abuse/synthetic-cathinones-bath-salts

National Institute on Drug Abuse. (2017). Inhalants. Drug facts. National Institute on Drug Abuse; National Institutes of Health; U.S. Department of Health and Human Services. Retrieved March 22, 2019, from https://www.drugabuse.gov/publications/drugfacts/inhalants

National Institute on Drug Abuse. (2018a). Cocaine. National Institute on Drug Abuse; National Institutes of Health; U.S. Department of Health and Human Services. Retrieved March 21, 2019, from https://www.drugabuse.gov/publications/drugfacts/cocaine

National Institute on Drug Abuse. (2018b). Methamphetamine. *Research Report Series. NIH Publication Number 13–4210*. National Institutes of Health. Bethesda, MD: U.S. Department of Health and Human. Retrieved March 21, 2019, from https://www.drugabuse.gov/publications/drugfacts/methamphetamine

National Institute on Drug Abuse. (2018c). MDMA ("ecstasy" or "Molly"). National Institute on Drug Abuse; National Institutes of Health; U.S. Department of Health and Human Services. Retrieved March 21, 2019, from https://www.drugabuse.gov/publications/drugfacts/mdma-ecstasymolly

National Institute on Drug Abuse. (2018d). Commonly abused drug. National Institute on Drug Abuse; National Institutes of Health; U.S. Department of Health and Human Services. Retrieved March 21, 2019, from https://www.drugabuse.gov/drugs-abuse/commonly-abused-drugs-charts#lsd

National Institute on Drug Abuse. (2018e). Tobacco, nicotine, and e-cigarettes. *Research Report Series*. National Institute on Drug Abuse; National Institutes of Health; U.S. Department of Health and Human Services. Retrieved March 21, 2019, from https://www.drugabuse.gov/publications/research-reports/tobacco-nicotine-e-cigarettes/what-scope-tobacco-use-its-cost-to-society

National Institute on Drug Abuse. (2018f). Marijuana as medicine. Drug facts. National Institute on Drug Abuse; National Institutes of Health; U.S. Department of Health and Human Services. Retrieved March 21, 2019, from https://www.drugabuse.gov/publications/drugfacts/marijuana-medicine

National Institute on Drug Abuse. (2018g). Synthetic Cannabinoids (K2/Spice). Drug facts. National Institute on Drug Abuse; National Institutes of Health; U.S. Department of Health and Human Services. Retrieved March 21, 2019, from https://www.drugabuse.gov/publications/drugfacts/synthetic-cannabinoids-k2spice

National Institute on Drug Abuse. (2018h). Hallucinogens and dissociative drugs. Research Reports. National Institute on Drug Abuse; National Institutes of Health; U.S. Department of Health and Human Services. Retrieved March 21, 2019, from https://www.drugabuse.gov/publications/research-reports/hallucinogens-dissociative-drugs/what-are-dissociative-drugs

National Institute on Drug Abuse. (2018i) Misuse of prescription drugs. National Institute on Drug Abuse; National Institutes of Health; U.S. Department of Health and Human Services. Retrieved March 21, 2019, from https://www.drugabuse.gov/publications/misuse-prescription-drugs/overview

National Institute on Drug Abuse. (2018j). Heroin. Drug facts. National Institute on Drug Abuse; National Institutes of Health; U.S. Department of Health and Human Services. Retrieved March 21, 2019, from https://www.drugabuse.gov/publications/drugfacts/heroin.

National Institute on Drug Abuse. (2018k). Inhalants. Drug facts. National Institute on Drug Abuse; National Institutes of Health; U.S. Department of Health and Human Services. Retrieved March 22, 2019, from https://www.drugabuse.gov/publications/drugfacts/anabolic-steroids

National Institute on Drug Abuse. (2018l). Other drugs. National Institute on Drug Abuse; National Institutes of Health; U.S. Department of Health and Human Services. Retrieved March 22, 2019, from https://www.drugabuse.gov/drugs-abuse/other-drugs

National Institute on Drug Abuse. (2019a). Alcohol. Drugs of abuse. National Institute on Drug Abuse; National Institutes of Health; U.S. Department of Health and Human Services. Retrieved March 20, 2019, from https://www.drugabuse.gov/drugs-abuse/alcohol

National Institute on Drug Abuse. (2019b). Tobacco/Nicotine and E-Cigs. National Institute on Drug Abuse; National Institutes of Health; U.S. Department of Health and Human Services. Retrieved March 20, 2019, from https://www.drugabuse.gov/drugs-abuse/tobacconicotine-e-cigs

National Institute on Drug Abuse. (2019c). Overdose Death Rates. National Institute on Drug Abuse; National Institutes of Health; U.S. Department of Health and Human Services. Retrieved March 22, 2019, from https://www.drugabuse.gov/related-topics/trends-statistics/overdose-death-rates

Piper, M. E., Cook, J. W., Schlam, T. R., Smith, S. S., Bolt, D. M., Collins, L. M., et al. (2017). Toward precision smoking cessation treatment II: Proximal effects of smoking cessation intervention components on putative mechanisms of action. *Drug and Alcohol Dependence*, *171*:50–58.

Prochaska, J. J., Das, S., & Young-Wolff, K. C. (2017). Smoking, mental illness, and public health. *Annual Review of Public Health*, *38*, 165–185.

Singh, A. K. (2019). Alcohol Interaction with cocaine, methamphetamine, opioids, nicotine, cannabis, and γ-hydroxybutyric acid. *Biomedicines*, *7*(1), E16.

Srivastava, A. B., & Gold, M. S. (2018). Naltrexone: A History and Future Directions. *Cerebrum*. pii: cer-13-18. eCollection 2018 Sep-Oct. Retrieved March 21, 2019.

Substance Abuse and Mental Health Services Administration (SAMHSA). (2014). Results from the 2013 National Survey on Drug Use and Health: Summary of national findings. NSDUH Series H-48, HHS Publication No. (SMA) 14–4863. Rockville, MD: Substance Abuse and Mental Health Services Administration. Retrieved March 21, 2019, from http://www.samhsa.gov/data/sitesdefault/files/NSDUHresultsPDFWHTML2013/Web/NSDUHresults2013.pdf

Substance Abuse and Mental Health Services Administration (SAMHSA). (2018). *Key substance use and mental health indicators in the United States: Results from the 2017 National Survey on Drug Use and Health* (HHS Publication No. SMA 18–5068, NSDUH Series H-53). Rockville, MD: Center for Behavioral Health Statistics and Quality, Substance Abuse and Mental Health Services Administration.

Teeters, J. B., Lancaster, C. L., Brown, D. G., & Back, S. E. (2017). Substance use disorders in military veterans: prevalence and treatment challenges. *Substance Abuse and Rehabilitation*, *8*, 69–77.

U.S. Department of Health and Human Services. (2010). *Healthy People 2020*. Washington, DC: U.S. Government Printing Office. Retrieved March 20, 2019, from http://www.healthypeople.gov.

van Timmeren, T., Daams, J. G., van Holst, R. J., & Goudriaan, A. E. (2018). Compulsivity-related neurocognitive performance deficits in gambling disorder: A systematic review and meta-analysis. *Neuroscience Biobehavioral Review*, *84*, 204–217.

Vieira, A., Reis, A. M., Matos, L. C., Machado, J., & Moreira, A. (2018). Does auriculotherapy have therapeutic effectiveness? An overview of systematic reviews. *Complementary Therapies in Clinical Practice*, *33*, 61–70.

Winhusen, T., Theobald, J., Kaelber, D. C., & Lewis, D. (2019). Medical complications associated with substance use disorders in patients with type 2 diabetes and hypertension: Electronic health record findings. *Addiction*, doi: 10.1111/add.14607

Yoon, C., Gedzior, J., & DePry, D. (2019). Wernicke-Korsakoff syndrome: Focus on low-threshold diagnosis and prompt treatment in the primary care setting. *International Journal of Psychiatry in Medicine*, *54*(3):172–180.

Zhang, B., Chaiton, M. O., Diemert, L. M., Bondy, S. J., Brown, K. S., & Ferrence, R. (2016). Health professional advice, use of medications and smoking cessation: A population-based prospective cohort study. *Preventive Medicine*, *91*, 117–122.

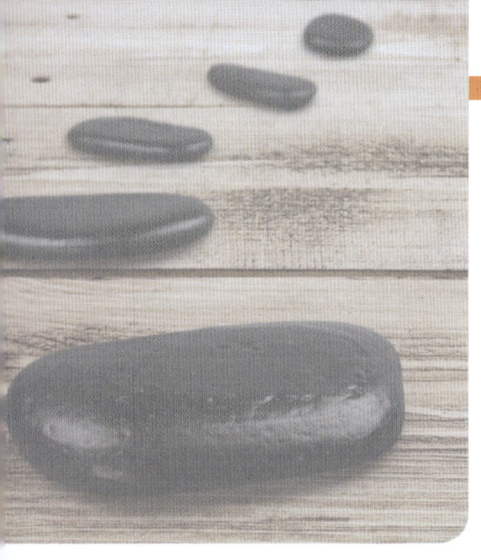

26
Eating Disorders

Nursing Care of Persons With Eating and Weight-Related Disorders

Jane H. White

KEY CONCEPTS

- body dissatisfaction
- body image distortion
- dietary restraint
- drive for thinness
- emotional dysregulation
- perfectionism

LEARNING OBJECTIVES

After studying this chapter, you will be able to:

1. Distinguish the signs and symptoms of anorexia nervosa (AN) from those of bulimia nervosa (BN).
2. Describe theories explaining anorexia nervosa and bulimia nervosa.
3. Differentiate binge-eating disorder (BED) from anorexia nervosa and bulimia nervosa.
4. Describe the risk factors and protective factors associated with the development of eating disorders.
5. Explain the importance of body image, body dissatisfaction, and gender identity in developmental theories that explain etiology of eating disorders.
6. Explain the impact of sociocultural norms on the development of eating disorders.
7. Implement nursing process for persons with eating and weight-related disorders.
8. Analyze special concerns within the therapeutic relationship for the nursing care of individuals with eating disorders.
9. Identify strategies for prevention and early detection of eating disorders.
10. Develop wellness strategies for persons with eating disorders.
11. Discuss the importance of integrated health care for persons with eating disorders.

KEY TERMS

• anorexia nervosa • binge eating • binge-eating disorder (BED) • bulimia nervosa • enmeshment • night eating syndrome • refeeding • self-monitoring • purging disorder

Case Study: Ellen

Ellen is a 20-year-old college sophomore admitted to an inpatient mental health unit after treatment on a medical unit where she was admitted for dehydration and electrolyte imbalance. Ellen has been binging and purging while in school to maintain a normal body weight.

Only since the 1970s have eating disorders received national attention, primarily because several high-profile personalities and athletes with these disorders have received front-page news coverage. Since the 1960s, the increased incidence of anorexia nervosa and bulimia nervosa has prompted mental health professionals to address their causes and devise effective treatments.

This chapter focuses on anorexia nervosa and bulimia nervosa and briefly discusses **binge-eating disorder (BED)**. Eating disorders differ in definition, clinical course, etiologies, and interventions and are presented separately in this chapter. However, symptoms of these

FIGURE 26.1 Progression of symptoms leading to an eating disorder.

> **BOX 26.1**
> ### Psychological Characteristics Related to Eating Disorders
>
> **ANOREXIA NERVOSA**
> Sexuality conflict or fears
> Maturity fears
> Ritualistic behaviors
> Perfectionism
> Emotional Dysregulation
>
> **BULIMIA NERVOSA**
> Impulsivity
> Boundary problems
> Limit-setting difficulties
>
> **ANOREXIA NERVOSA AND BULIMIA NERVOSA**
> Difficulty expressing anger
> Low self-esteem
> Body dissatisfaction
> Powerlessness
> Ineffectiveness
> Perfectionism
> Dietary restraint
> Obsessiveness
> Compulsiveness
> Nonassertiveness
> Cognitive distortions

disorders, such as dieting, **binge eating**, and preoccupation with weight and shape overlap significantly. Viewing the symptoms along a continuum from less to more severe eating behaviors helps with this conceptualization, as shown in Figure 26.1. There are also common psychological characteristics of people with eating disorders (Box 26.1). Subclinical cases, in the past diagnosed as ED NOS are now classified in the *DSM-5* (American Psychiatric Association [APA], 2013) as Other Specified Feeding and Eating Disorders (OSFED) or Unspecified Feeding and Eating Disorders (UFED) also called partial syndromes. These individuals still need treatment despite not meeting criteria for anorexia nervosa or bulimia nervosa. In addition, disordered eating behaviors are often classified as subclinical or subthreshold cases of true eating disorders such as anorexia nervosa and bulimia nervosa which are psychiatric diagnoses.

ANOREXIA NERVOSA

Anorexia nervosa is a mixture of symptoms that include significantly low body weight, intense fear of gaining weight or becoming fat, and a disturbance in experiencing body weight or shape (undue influence or distorted self-evaluation of body weight or shape or lack of recognition of the seriousness of low body weight).

Anorexia nervosa is further categorized into two major types: *restricting* (dieting and exercising with no binge eating or misuse of laxatives, diuretics, or enemas) and *binge eating and purging* (binge eating and misuse of laxatives, diuretics, or enemas). Malnutrition and semistarvation result in a preoccupation with food, binge eating, depression, obsession, and apathy, as well as compromising several body systems, leading to medical complications and, in some instances, death (APA, 2013).

Clinical Course

The onset of anorexia nervosa usually occurs in early adolescence. The onset can be slow with serious dieting occurring before an emaciated body—the result of starvation—is noticed. This discovery often prompts diagnosis. Because the incidence of subclinical or partial-syndrome cases, in which the symptoms are not severe enough to use an anorexia nervosa diagnosis, is higher than that of anorexia nervosa, many young women may not receive early treatment for their symptoms, or in some cases, they receive no treatment. The individual's refusal to maintain a normal weight because of a distorted body image and an intense fear of becoming fat make individuals with this disorder difficult to identify and treat.

It can be a chronic condition with relapses that are usually characterized by significant weight loss. Reporting conclusive outcomes for anorexia nervosa is difficult because of the variety of definitions used to determine recovery. Although patients considered to have recovered have restored normal weight, menses, and eating behaviors, some continue to have distorted body images and be preoccupied with weight and food; many develop bulimia nervosa; and many continue to have symptoms of other psychiatric illnesses, especially of the anxiety disorders.

Body Distortion

For most individuals, body image (a mental picture of one's own body) is consistent with how others view them. However, individuals with anorexia nervosa have a body image that is severely distorted from reality. Because of this distortion, they see themselves as obese and undesirable even when they are emaciated. They are unable to accept objective reality and the perceptions of the outside world.

> **KEYCONCEPT** **Body image distortion** occurs when the individual perceives his or her body disparately from how the world or society views it.

Concept Mastery Alert

People with anorexia nervosa have a distorted image of the appearance of their bodies. They can be very thin and still perceive that they are heavy and need to lose weight.

Drive for Thinness

Because of body distortion, individuals with anorexia nervosa have an intense drive for thinness. They see themselves as fat, fear becoming fatter, and are "driven" to work toward "undoing" this fear.

> **KEYCONCEPT** **Drive for thinness** is an intense physical and emotional process that overrides all physiologic body cues.

The individual with anorexia nervosa ignores body cues, such as hunger and weakness, and concentrates all efforts on controlling food intake. The entire mental focus of the young patient with anorexia nervosa narrows to only one goal: weight loss. Typical thought patterns are: "If I gain a pound, I'll keep gaining." This all-or-nothing thinking keeps these patients on rigid regimens for weight loss.

The behavior of patients with anorexia nervosa becomes organized around food-related activities, such as preparing food, counting calories, and reading cookbooks. Much behavior concerning what, when, and how they eat is ritualistic. Food combinations and the order in which foods may be eaten, and under which circumstances, can seem bizarre. One patient, for example, would eat only cantaloupe, carrying it with her to all meals outside of her home and consuming it only if it were cut in smaller than bite-sized pieces and only if she could use chopsticks, which she also carried with her.

> **KEYCONCEPT** **Emotional dysregulation** is a difficulty regulating expression of feelings. Emotional dysregulation and increased sensory sensitivity are linked to anorexia nervosa. Emotion dysregulation comprises one's inability to accept one's emotional responses, to accomplish goals in the midst of distress, and to be aware of and acknowledge the significance of developing and implementing coping strategies to influence and manage emotions effectively (Rotella et al., 2018).

> **NCLEXNOTE** The emotional dysregulation model links deficits in emotional regulation with anorexia nervosa. That is, those with anorexia nervosa have deficits in the ability to understand and modulate emotions, which results in experiencing emotions as overwhelming and unmanageable. Consequently, those with anorexia nervosa use disordered eating to regulate their affective state by either reducing negative affect or increasing positive affect and thus disordered eating, through reinforcement, is maintained (Rotella et al., 2018). Treatment programs that address emotional regulation and focus on teaching skills to regulate emotions may therefore be effective especially with anorexia nervosa patients.

Guilt and Anger

Patients with anorexia nervosa tend to avoid conflict and have difficulty expressing negative emotions, especially anger (Duarte, Ferreira, & Pinto-Gouveia, 2016; Monell, Clinton, & Birgegård, 2018). They have an overwhelming sense of guilt and anger, which leads to conflict avoidance, which is common in families of those with anorexia nervosa. Because of the ritualistic behaviors, an all-encompassing focus on food and weight, and feelings of inadequacy, social contacts are gradually reduced, and the patient becomes isolated. More severe weight loss is associated with other symptoms, such as apathy, depression, and even mistrust of others.

Perfectionism

Emotional dysregulation is hypothesized to relate to perfectionism. Perfectionistic behavior, such as making sure that everything is symmetrical or that objects are placed the same distance from each other, or in performance-based tasks is a typical significant symptom of anorexia nervosa and bulimia nervosa and is hypothesized to develop long before eating symptoms occur. Findings from research demonstrate that perfectionism is a significant personality symptom risk factor in eating disorders (Wagner & Vitousek, 2019).

> **KEY CONCEPT** **Perfectionism** consists of personal standards (the extent to which the individual sets and tries to achieve high standards for oneself) and concern over mistakes and their consequences for their self-worth and others' opinions.

It is now accepted that perfectionism precedes the development of weight and shape concerns. The more severe the disorder, the more perfectionistic. As symptoms are resolved, perfectionism may decrease (Larsson, Lloyd, Westwood, & Tchanturia, 2018).

Outcomes

Short-term outcomes for individuals with anorexia nervosa after hospitalization are generally poor. Poor outcomes are related to lower body mass indices (BMI) at the beginning of treatment, the level of impulsivity, self-induced vomiting, and higher trait anxiety purging (vomiting and laxative use).

Long-term outcomes are more positive than short-term outcomes, but remission rates vary from 20% to 70%, depending on the criteria used in the studies. Many individuals do recover, but recovery often takes years and can be characterized by residual symptoms (Fichter, Quadflieg, Crosby, & Koch, 2017).

Diagnostic Criteria

The diagnosis of anorexia is made when there is a restriction of intake leading to significantly low body weight. The BMI is used as a measure of severity. Other criteria include an intense fear of gaining weight or becoming fat, and body image issues including an undue influence of body weight on self-concept and lack of recognition of seriousness of low body weight (APA, 2013). See Key Diagnostic Characteristics 26.1 for an overview of diagnostic criteria and associated findings.

Epidemiology

The 12-month prevalence of anorexia nervosa among young females is approximately 0.4%, but many researchers believe this figure does not reflect the true prevalence of this serious disorder (APA, 2013). Adjusted approximations estimate that eating disorders affect over 13% of adolescents and adult women, and 1% to 2% of men. The age

---

KEY DIAGNOSTIC CHARACTERISTICS 26.1 • ANOREXIA NERVOSA

A. Restriction of energy intake relative to requirements, leading to a significantly low body weight in the context of age, sex, developmental trajectory, and physical health. *Significantly low weight* is defined as a weight that is less than minimally normal or, for children and adolescents, less than that minimally expected.

B. Intense fear of gaining weight or of becoming fat, or persistent behavior that interferes with weight gain, even though at a significantly low weight.

C. Disturbance in the way in which one's body weight or shape is experienced, undue influence of body weight or shape on self-evaluation, or persistent lack of recognition of the seriousness of the current low body weight.

Specify whether:
- **Restricting type:** During the last 3 months, the individual has not engaged in recurrent episodes of binge eating or purging behavior (i.e., self-induced vomiting or the misuse of laxatives, diuretics, or enemas). This subtype describes presentations in which weight loss is accomplished primarily through dieting, fasting, and/or excessive exercise.
- **Binge-eating/purging type:** During the last 3 months, the individual has engaged in recurrent episodes of binge eating or purging behavior (i.e., self-induced vomiting or the misuse of laxatives, diuretics, or enemas).

Specify if:
- **In partial remission:** After full criteria for anorexia nervosa were previously met, Criterion A (low body weight) has not been met for a sustained period, but either Criterion B (intense fear of gaining weight or becoming fat or behavior that interferes with weight gain) or Criterion C (disturbances in self-perception of weight and shape) is still met.
- **In full remission:** After full criteria for anorexia nervosa were previously met, none of the criteria have been met for a sustained period of time.

Specify current severity:
The minimum level of severity is based, for adults, on current body mass index (BMI) (see below) or, for children and adolescents, on BMI percentile. The ranges below are derived from World Health Organization categories for thinness in adults; for children and adolescents, corresponding BMI percentiles should be used. The level of severity may be increased to reflect clinical symptoms, the degree of functional disability, and the need for supervision.

- **Mild:** BMI ≥17 kg/m^2
- **Moderate:** BMI 16–16.99 kg/m^2
- **Severe:** BMI 15–15.99 kg/m^2
- **Extreme:** BMI <15 kg/m^2

Reprinted with permission from the. American Psychiatric Association. (2013). *Diagnostic and statistical manual of mental disorders* (5th ed.). Arlington, VA: American Psychiatric Association. All Rights Reserved.

> **BOX 26.2**
>
> **Boys and Men With Eating Disorders**
>
> Eating disorders in boys and men are becoming more prevalent. Males present with eating disorders between the ages of 16 and 24. The stigma that eating disorders are a women's disease may inhibit identification in primary care. In a study comparing males and females on prevalence of eating disorders, Shu et al. (2015) found boys to have a lower prevalence of bulimia nervosa and self-induced vomiting but were similar to females on the prevalence of anorexia nervosa. Males also had an earlier onset of eating disorder, a mean of age 12. Men and women do not differ with regard to comorbid conditions, such as depression and substance abuse and men with an eating disorder are also more likely to be involved in an occupation or sport in which weight control influences performance, such as wrestling, or sports in which low body fat is advantageous. Because many of the assessment instruments and treatment protocols are geared toward females, males suffer from a lack of early identification of their disorders and early as well as successful treatment.

of onset is typically between 14 and 16 years but can occur much earlier. Adolescents are vulnerable because of stressors associated with their development, especially concerns about body image, autonomy, and peer pressure, and their susceptibility to such influences as the media, which extols an ideal body type (Cheng, Perko, Fuller-Marashi, Gau, & Stice, 2019; Mangweth-Matzek & Hoek, 2017).

Gender

Females are 10 times more likely than males to develop anorexia nervosa. This disparity has been attributed to society's influence on females to internalize a thin body as ideal highlights some of the findings about eating disorders in males. See Box 26.2.

Ethnicity and Culture

In the United States, eating disorders occur in all ethnic and racial groups, and recent studies show there are very few differences in prevalence among Whites, Hispanic Americans, Asian Americans, and African Americans (Cheng et al., 2019). However, research findings demonstrate that Asian Americans have a higher level of belief that the ideal body is thin than other groups (Cheng et al., 2019). In Asian countries, eating disorders have risen over the last 10 years, attributed to not only the influence of Western countries' media but also to economic development itself (Pike & Dunne, 2015).

Comorbidity

Depression is common in individuals with anorexia nervosa, and these individuals are at risk to attempt suicide (Thornton, Welch, Munn-Chernoff, Lichtenstein, & Bulik, 2016). However, anxiety disorders such as obsessive-compulsive disorder (OCD), phobias, and panic disorder are even more strongly associated with anorexia nervosa. In many individuals with anorexia nervosa, OCD symptoms predate the anorexia nervosa diagnosis by about 5 years, leading many researchers to consider OCD a causative or risk factor for anorexia nervosa (Udo & Gilo, 2019). In fact, perfectionism is an aspect of both OCD and anorexia nervosa and is considered a risk factor for anorexia nervosa (Wagner & Vitousek, 2019). These comorbid conditions may often resolve when anorexia nervosa has been treated successfully. However, in many cases, an anxiety disorder may continue even following successful treatment of anorexia nervosa.

Etiology

The etiology of anorexia nervosa is multidimensional. Some of the risk factors (discussed later) and the etiologic factors overlap. For example, dieting is a risk factor for the development of anorexia nervosa, but it is also an etiologic factor, and in its most serious form—starving—it is also a symptom.

Biologic Theories

There is evidence that the volume of gray and white matter in the brains of persons with anorexia nervosa are reduced but are normalized during weight restoration. These deficits may reflect malnourishment. Other studies suggest that there may structural alterations even after long-term recovery (King, Frank, Thompson, & Ehrlich, 2018). Research is ongoing.

Genetic Theories

First-degree relatives of people with anorexia nervosa have higher rates of this disorder. Rates of partial-syndrome or subthreshold cases among female family members of individuals with anorexia nervosa are even higher (Bulik, Blake, & Austin, 2019). Female relatives also have high rates of depression, leading researchers to hypothesize that a shared genetic factor may influence development of both disorders.

Genetic research shows that there is a genetic vulnerability to anorexia nervosa, especially in females. Genetic heritability accounts for an estimated 50% to 80% of the risk of developing an eating disorder. Separating genetic influences from environmental influences is difficult when twins share a similar family environment (Bulik et al., 2019).

Neuroendocrine and Neurotransmitter Changes

Several neurobiologic changes occur in an eating disorder. The most common findings are increased activation of the amygdala and changes in the activation of the cingulate cortex. An increase in endogenous opioids (through exercise) contributes to denial of hunger. Malnutrition leads to a decrease in thyroid function. Serotonergic functioning is also blunted in low-weight patients (Dwarkasing et al., 2016; Scharner & Stengel, 2019).

Psychological Theories

Historically, the most widely accepted explanation of anorexia nervosa was the psychoanalytic paradigm that focused on conflicts of separation—individuation and autonomy. Usually diagnosed between 14 and 18 years of age, anorexia nervosa was thought to occur as a result of a developmental arrest of normal adolescent struggles around identity and role, body image formation, and sexuality (Bruch, 1973). Dieting and weight control were viewed as a means to defend against these feelings of inadequacy and growing into adulthood.

The psychoanalytic paradigm explained the disparity in the prevalence of eating disorders between boys and girls as being related to the development of self-esteem in adolescent girls. It was believed that the normal adolescent increase in self-doubt was linked to naturally occurring pubertal weight gain, which in turn resulted in confusion about one's identity. Unfortunately, this psychoanalytic perspective tended to blame parents, especially mothers, for the development of their child's illness. Today, the psychoanalytic theory is used in some psychotherapies, but it is no longer a competing theory of causation.

Internalization of Peer Pressure

Some adolescents have reported that dieting, binge eating, and purging initially began as a result of peer pressure and a need to conform. Subsequently many factors then converge that influence the initials behaviors to develop into a full syndrome eating disorder. Peers and friends, as well as peers in the larger school system, influence unhealthy weight-control behaviors among preadolescent and adolescent girls (Haynos, Watts, Loth, Pearson, & Neumark-Stzainer, 2016).

Body Dissatisfaction

Once the body is considered all important, the individual begins to compare her body with others, such as those of celebrities. Images from television and fashion magazines are particularly powerful for young girls and adolescents struggling with the tasks of identity and body image formation. Body dissatisfaction resulting from this comparison, in which one's own body is perceived to fall short of an ideal, may be dissatisfaction about one's weight, shape, size, or even a certain body part. Even in the absence of overweight, most adolescents surveyed in numerous studies were dissatisfied with their bodies (Waszczuk, Waaktaar, Eley, & Torgersen, 2019). Because this factor is so prevalent in women and especially adolescents in this country, body dissatisfaction is considered less predictive for a diagnosis of anorexia nervosa (APA, 2013). Yet it remains as an important factor that follows the internalizing of an idea body weight.

> **KEYCONCEPT** **Body dissatisfaction** occurs when the body is viewed negatively and becomes overvalued as a way of determining one's worth.

Many adolescents attempt to overcome this dissatisfaction through dieting and overexercising.

Social Theories

More than with any other psychiatric condition, society plays a significant role in the development of eating disorders with conflicting messages that young women receive from society about their roles in life. Young girls may interpret expectations about how they should look, what roles they should perform, and what they should achieve in society. Exposure to social media sites idealizing excessively thin bodies and glorifying extreme caloric restriction is associated with disordered eating behaviors (Griffiths et al., 2018).

The media, the fashion industry, and peer pressure are significant social influences. Magazines, television, videos, and the Internet depict young girls and adolescents, with thin and often emaciated bodies, as glamorous, successful, popular, and powerful. Girls diet because they want to be similar to these models both in character and appearance.

Preoccupation with body image and weight is also influenced by the obesity epidemic. A study on body dissatisfaction demonstrated that high BMIs and body dissatisfaction were more likely to occur in adolescents who later developed eating disorder symptoms (Goldstein & Gvion, 2019).

Preadolescent children are extremely susceptible to the message to reduce intake and increase exercise as a way to lose weight and maintain health. Coupled with Internet videos that sanction self-starvation, emerging adolescents are already dissatisfied with their bodies and have the tools to lose weight through dieting and exercise.

Feminists have focused on the role of this pressure regarding the female body as one part of an explanation for the significant increase in eating disorders and for the greater prevalence in females. Box 26.3 outlines some feminist assumptions regarding role, feminism, and the development of eating disorders.

BOX 26.3
Feminist Ideology and Eating Disorders

Since the 1970s, proponents of the feminist cultural model of eating disorders have advanced a position to explain the higher prevalence of these disorders in women. Feminists believe there is a struggle women have today similar to ones they believe women have had in history. They believe that during the Victorian era, "hysteria," a well-known emotional illness, developed as a result of oppression when women were not allowed to express their feelings and opinions and were "silenced" by a male-dominated society. Feminist scholars today have advanced the feminist relational model to understand the development of eating disorders. They view a major issue in development that causes conflict for young girls as the need to be connected versus society's view of the importance of separation. This confusion can be a stress that may be converted into disordered eating. Often at the base of symptoms such as severe food restriction is the gaining of power lost possibly because of this confusion in one's development (Holmes, Drake, Odgers, & Wilson, 2017).

BOX 26.4
Research For Best Practice: Eating Disorders and Women Athletes

Joy, E., Kussman, A., & Nattiv, A. (2019). A 2016 update on eating disorders in athletes: A comprehensive narrative review with a focus on clinical assessment and management. *British Journal of Sports Medicine, 50*(3), 154–162.

THE QUESTION: Are there differences in eating disorder symptoms among undergraduate varsity athletes, club athletes, independent exercisers, and nonexercisers?

METHODS: In this comprehensive review, across published research studies, disordered eating findings from many studies were shown to be more prevalent in athletes' versus nonathletes.

FINDINGS: An eating disorder in one sample of over 400 elite athletes and nonathlete was found in 18% of the athletes and 5% of the nonathletes. Among female athletes, the rates of eating disorders vary by sport. There were higher prevalence rates for specific sports such as rowing and in sports in which a low body mass is advantageous such as in cycling. Male athletes had a lower prevalence of eating disorders than female athletes, but a higher prevalence than nonathletes. Males who participated in weight class sports (such as wrestling) were more likely to engage in pathologic eating and weight control behaviors and be symptomatic when they were compared to male athletes in endurance sports and ball games.

IMPLICATIONS FOR NURSING: Nurses should be aware that athletes have higher rates of disordered eating and should be assessed for eating disorders. Nurses can teach parents and adolescents about the value of healthy athletic competition and the need to maintain healthy eating habits. Coaches as well as parents should be involved in educational programs highlighting the risk factors for eating disorders and symptom identification. An accurate assessment of each young athlete, male or female, is important.

Risk Factors

Research demonstrates that genetic risks play an important role in the development of eating disorders in both men and women. Eating disorders are highly inheritable. Puberty is a risk period for the development of anorexia nervosa. Girls often begin to diet at an early age because of body dissatisfaction, and the need for control of prepubertal weight increases. Restricting food can lead to starvation, binge eating, and purging. Males are more likely to engage in physical activity than dieting. Females demonstrate a drive for thinness; males have increased concern with muscularity and shape (Timko, DeFilipp, & Dakanalis, 2019).

Psychiatric disorders increase the risks of eating disorders. Low self-esteem, body dissatisfaction, and feelings of ineffectiveness also put individuals at risk. Bullying and weight teasing are other risk factors for the development of an eating disorder (Lie, Rø, & Bang, 2019).

Elite athletes participating in lean sports such as running and gymnastics, and nonelite athletes taking part in nonlean sports such as soccer, experience a triad of symptoms (disordered eating, menstrual dysfunction, and osteoporosis). See Box 26.4. Athletes involved in lean sports are at higher risk than nonelite athletes and the general population (Joy, Kussman, & Nattiv, 2019).

Family Response to Disorder

Historically, the family of the patient with anorexia was labeled as overprotective, enmeshed, being unable to resolve conflicts, and being rigid regarding boundaries. Although an uninformed family can delay and complicate treatment, there is no evidence that family interactions are the cause of eating disorders but can contribute to its development (Kluck, Dallesasse, & English, 2017). Some family interactions can be problematic for the adolescent with an eating disorder. For example, when conflict erupts between two family members and direct communication is blocked, interaction patterns are changed that may result in a dysfunction relay of messages through other family members.

Enmeshment refers to an extreme form of intensity in family interactions and represents low individual autonomy in a family. In an enmeshed family, the individual gets lost in the family system. The boundaries that define individual autonomy are weak. This excessive togetherness intrudes on privacy (Minuchin, Rosman, & Baker, 1978).

Overprotectiveness is defined as a high degree of concern for one another and can be detrimental to children at high risk for anorexia nervosa. The parents' overprotectiveness retards the child's development of autonomy and competence (Minuchin et al., 1978). *Rigidity* refers to families that are heavily committed to maintaining the status quo and find change difficult. Conflict is avoided, and a strong ethical code or religious orientation is usually the rationale.

The family, often unwittingly, can transmit unrealistic attitudes about weight, shape, and size. Adolescents are particularly sensitive to comments about their bodies because this is the stage for body image formation. Parental attitudes about weight have been found to influence body dissatisfaction and dieting; parental comments about weight or shape or even parents' worrying about their own weight can influence adolescents in much the same way as the media does. See Box 26.5.

Hurtful weight–related comments by family members and significant others have been associated with disordered eating in both females and males. Adolescents' perceived family functioning and the quality of their relationship with each parent have been shown to positively influence body image dissatisfaction and disordered eating. Therefore, healthy family relationships are believed to be a protective factor for developing an eating disorder as well as support research findings linking parental-focused treatment programs to positive outcomes for those with eating disorders (Wallis et al. 2018).

Recovery-Oriented Care for Persons With Anorexia Nervosa

Teamwork and Collaboration: Working Toward Recovery

Treatment for the patient with anorexia nervosa focuses on initiating nutritional rehabilitation to restore the individual to a healthy weight, resolving psychological conflicts around body image disturbance, increasing effective coping, addressing the underlying conflicts related to maturity fears and role conflict, and assisting the family with healthy functioning and communication. Several methods are used to accomplish these goals during the stages of illness and recovery.

The medical complications presented in Table 26.1 influence the decision to hospitalize an individual with an eating disorder. Suicidality is another reason for hospitalization. The criteria for hospital admission vary, and there is a lack of evidence-based studies determining when adolescents with anorexia nervosa should be hospitalized. The APA criteria are outlined in Box 26.6.

After an acceptable weight (at least 85% of ideal) is established, the patient is discharged to a partial hospitalization program or an intensive outpatient program. The intensive therapies needed to help patients with their underlying issues (e.g., body distortion and maturity fears) and to help families with communication and enmeshment usually begin after refeeding because concentration is usually impaired in severely undernourished patients with anorexia.

Family therapy typically begins while the patient is still hospitalized. Recently family-based therapies and

---

BOX 26.5

Research For Best Practice: Mothers, Daughters, and Body Image

Handford, C. M., Rapee, R. M., & Fardouly, J. (2018). The influence of maternal modeling on body image concerns and eating disturbances in preadolescent girls. *Behaviour Research and Therapy, 100,* 17–23.

THE QUESTION: Do maternal attitudes and behavior about their daughter's weight and eating habits influence body esteem, body satisfaction, eating attitudes, and eating behaviors of young girls?

METHODS: Fifty mother–daughter pairs were recruited from the community and allocated to one of two conditions: maternal modeling (self-critical remarks about their own weight, shape, and diet) or no modeling. Daughters were then asked to complete body esteem, body satisfaction, and eating attitudes questionnaires (pre- and post-maternal modeling).

FINDINGS: Girls whose mothers made self-critical comments about their own appearance and diet reported lower body esteem, lower body satisfaction, more problematic eating attitudes, and ate significantly fewer sweets than girls whose mothers had not made self-critical comments.

IMPLICATIONS FOR NURSING: Families should be cautioned that self-critical statements can lead to daughters' lower esteem, body dissatisfaction, and more problematic eating attitudes.

BOX 26.6

Criteria for Hospitalization of Patients With Eating Disorders

MEDICAL
- Acute weight loss, <85% below ideal
- Heart rate near 40 beats/min
- Temperature, <36.1°C
- Blood pressure, <80/50 mm Hg
- Hypokalemia
- Hypophosphatemia
- Hypomagnesemia
- Poor motivation to recover

PSYCHIATRIC
- Risk for suicide
- Severe depression
- Failure to comply with treatment
- Inadequate response to treatment at another level of care (outpatient)

Adapted from American Psychiatric Association (2006). Treatment of patients with eating disorders, third edition. American Psychiatric Association. *American Journal of Psychiatry, 163*(7 suppl), 4–54.

TABLE 26.1	COMPLICATIONS OF EATING DISORDERS
Body System	Symptoms
From Starvation to Weight Loss	
Musculoskeletal	Loss of muscle mass, loss of fat (emaciation), osteoporosis
Metabolic	Hypothyroidism (symptoms include lack of energy, weakness, intolerance to cold, and bradycardia), hypoglycemia, decreased insulin sensitivity
Cardiac	Bradycardia; hypotension; loss of cardiac muscle; small heart; cardiac arrhythmias, including atrial and ventricular premature contractions, prolonged QT interval, ventricular tachycardia, sudden death
Gastrointestinal	Delayed gastric emptying, bloating, constipation, abdominal pain, gas, diarrhea
Reproductive	Amenorrhea, low levels of luteinizing hormone and follicle-stimulating hormone, irregular periods
Dermatologic	Dry, cracking skin and brittle nails caused by dehydration, lanugo (fine, baby-like hair over the body), edema, acrocyanosis (bluish hands and feet), thinning hair
Hematologic	Leukopenia, anemia, thrombocytopenia, hypercholesterolemia, hypercarotenemia
Neuropsychiatric	Abnormal taste sensation (possible zinc deficiency)
	Apathetic depression, mild organic mental symptoms, sleep disturbances, fatigue
Related to Purging (Vomiting and Laxative Abuse)	
Metabolic	Electrolyte abnormalities, particularly hypokalemia, hypochloremic alkalosis; hypomagnesemia; increased blood urea nitrogen
Gastrointestinal	Salivary gland and pancreatic inflammation and enlargement with increase in serum amylase, esophageal and gastric erosion (esophagitis) rupture, dysfunctional bowel with dilation, superior mesenteric artery syndrome
Dental	Erosion of dental enamel (perimylolysis), particularly of the frontal teeth, with decreased decay
Neuropsychiatric	Seizures (related to large fluid shifts and electrolyte disturbances), mild neuropathies, fatigue, weakness, mild organic mental symptoms
Cardiac	Ipecac cardiomyopathy arrhythmias

caregiver-based approaches have shown promise in the treatment of eating disorders. These assist in improving overall communication within the family and helps members understand the disorder (Wong, Goh, & Ramachandran, 2019).

Interpersonal therapy (IPT) is a type of treatment that focuses on uncovering and resolving the developmental and psychological issues underlying the disorder. Role transitions and negative social evaluations typically are the focus (Miniati, Callari, Maglio, & Calugi, 2018). IPT and family-based therapies are sometimes combined.

Dialectic behavioral therapy specifically designed for patients with anorexia nervosa has shown positive results. This skills training type of intervention focuses on emotional dysregulation viewed as a key symptom in anorexia nervosa (Accurso, Astrachan-Fletcher, O'Brien, McClanahan, & Le Grange, 2018).

Integration With Primary Care

Persons with eating disorders are frequently treated in primary care for medical issues related to their eating disorder. Care in the mental health and primary care services should be coordinated with the mental health service providing care focusing on mental health issues and primary care treating the medical issues. When there are few psychiatric services available, eating disorders are treated and monitored by the primary care provider. The patient should have access to a therapist and dietitian in any treatment setting. Due to the fast-paced nature of primary care, eating disorders are not as easily recognized in a general health care setting and are often missed.

Safety Issues

Mortality is high among patients with anorexia nervosa especially when compared with other mental illnesses and is reported to be 3% to 7% with a longer duration of the disorder predicting the higher range of the mortality rate (Chidiac, 2019).

Suicide and cardiopulmonary arrest are the leading cause of death for individuals with anorexia nervosa (Goldstein & Gvion, 2019). These individuals tend to commit suicide with highly lethal means in which rescue is unlikely. Nurses need to pay special attention to the risk of suicide with these individuals (see Chapter 21). A significant number of individuals with eating disorders also self-injure without suicide attempts (Cucchi et al., 2016).

Evidence-Based Nursing Care for Persons With Anorexia Nervosa Disorder

Mental Health Nursing Assessment

Physical Health Assessment

A thorough evaluation of body systems is important because many systems are compromised by starvation. A careful history from both the patient with anorexia nervosa and the family, including the length and duration of symptoms, such as fasting, avoiding meals, and overexercising, is necessary to assess altered nutrition. Nursing management involves various biopsychosocial assessment and interventions.

Patients with longer durations of these maladaptive behaviors typically have more difficult and prolonged recovery periods.

> **NCLEXNOTE** Eating disorders are serious psychiatric disorders that threaten life. Careful assessment and referral for treatment are important nursing interventions.

The patient's weight is determined using the BMI and a scale. Currently, criteria for discharge require patients to be at least 85% of ideal weight according to height and weight tables. BMI, thought to reflect weight most accurately because exact height is used, is calculated by dividing weight in kilograms by height in meters squared. An acceptable BMI is between about 19 and 25.

Menses history also must be explored in that it provides information about possible estrogen depletion. However, it is often difficult to conclude that amenorrhea is present due to starvation because females in this age group often have irregular periods and some are on oral contraceptives. However, if menses was regular prior to anorexia nervosa, a return to regular menses after treatment can signify substantial body fat restoration. Fat and weight restoration have been hypothesized aid in the loss of bone mineral density (Misra, Golden, & Katzman, 2016).

Behavioral Responses

The psychological symptoms that patients with anorexia experience are listed in Box 26.1. The classic symptoms of body distortion—fear of weight gain, unrealistic expectations and thinking, and ritualistic behaviors—are easily noted during a clinical interview. Often, people with anorexia nervosa avoid conflict and have difficulty expressing negative emotions, such as anger. Other conflicts, such as sexuality fears and feelings of ineffectiveness, may underlie this disorder. These symptoms may not be apparent during a clinical interview; however, a variety of instruments is available to clinicians and researchers for determining their presence and severity.

There is a high rate of nonsuicidal self-injury in patients with eating disorders and the type and frequency of these behaviors should be assessed (Cucchi et al., 2016).

The Eating Attitudes Test is frequently used in community samples (Garner, Olmsted, Bohr, & Garfinkel, 1982). There is also a child version of this test, the CHEAT. The results of these paper-and-pencil tests can help identify the most significant symptoms for an individual patient and indicate a focus for interventions, especially therapy. In clinical settings, the Eating Disorder Examination Questionnaire (EDEQ) is most often used (Hilbert, de Zwaan, & Braehler, 2012).

Self-Concept

Individuals with eating disorders are usually struggling with their self-concept. It is important to determine their self-concept and self-esteem. In many instances, these individuals appear to be very competent, but when queried about their views, they often feel that they are not good enough and will describe their perceived faults in great detail.

Stress and Coping Patterns

Individuals with an eating disorder are often coping with stress and anxiety through controlling eating. In times of perceived stressful events, the dysfunctional eating pattern often becomes worse. An assessment of the stress the person is experiencing and coping patterns is important because a part of successful treatment is developing healthy coping skills.

Social Assessment

The assessment should also focus on the family interaction, influence, and peer relationships. The role of the patient in the family and community should be considered, as well as the person's ability to cope in social situations. For adolescents who are attending school, a conference with the teacher or counselor provides information regarding the amount and frequency of social contacts.

Strengths Assessment

Strengths such as motivation to eat differently and have a more normal life may emerge during the interview. The following questions that could be asked to elicit personal strengths:

- Do you remember a time when you did not have to worry about what you ate? If so, how old were you and what did you like to do?
- Have you found any strategy that prevented you from worrying about what you hate?

- Are you ready to change your eating patterns? What do you think will help you change your eating patterns?
- When you are successful in other areas (school, athletics), how do you reward yourself?

Priority of Nursing Care

Medical complications and suicide ideation are the two top priorities. Bradycardia and hypotension are well-established responses to starvation. Cardiac issues should be treated before the psychological issues can be meaningfully addressed. Normal electrolyte balance should be restored. Suicidality is also a high priority of nursing care and should be carefully assessed.

Therapeutic Relationships

Establishing a therapeutic relationship with individuals with anorexia nervosa may be difficult initially because they tend to be suspicious and mistrustful especially of authority figures and health personnel whom they believe will intervene to disrupt their restricting and starvation behaviors placing them in a position of extreme fear of becoming fat. At the time they are hospitalized, mistrust can almost reach a state of paranoia. Because of their low body weight and starvation, they are often impatient and irritable. A firm, accepting, and patient approach is important in working with these individuals. Providing a rationale for all interventions helps build trust, as does a consistent, nonreactive approach. Power struggles over eating are common and remaining nonreactive is a challenge. During such power struggles, the nurse should always think about his or her own feelings of frustration and need for control.

Mental Health Nursing Interventions

Establishing Mental Health and Wellness Goals

The mental health and wellness goals are very closely aligned for people with eating disorders. Successful recovery from an eating disorder involves establishing positive wellness habits of nutrition, physical activity, sleep, coping with stress, and developing a support system. The nurse and patient should prioritize long- and short-term goals. For example, a long-term goal is to maintain a normal weight through healthy eating and exercise. A short-term goal is to increase food intake by 300 calories per day.

> **NCLEXNOTE** Setting realistic eating goals is one of the most helpful interventions for patients with eating disorders. Because individuals with anorexia nervosa are often perfectionistic, they often set unrealistic goals.

One of the most helpful skills the nurse can teach is to set realistic goals around food and around other activities or tasks. Because of perfectionism, patients with anorexia often set unrealistic goals and end up frustrated. The nurse can help them establish smaller, more realistic, and attainable goals.

Physical Health Interventions

The person with anorexia can usually perform self-care activities. They may actually be overly perfectionistic regarding daily self-care activities. If symptoms become severe, hospitalization may be necessary to re-establish a healthy body weight.

Refeeding. Refeeding, the most important intervention during the hospital or initial stage of treatment, is also the most challenging. The nurse will encounter resistance to weight gain and refusal to eat and must monitor and record all intake carefully as part of the weight gain protocol.

The refeeding protocol typically starts with 1,500 calories a day and is increased slowly until the patient is consuming at least 3,500 calories a day in several meals. The higher the initial number of calories prescribed has been demonstrated to influence a shorter length of hospital stay and recovery (Garber et al., 2016). The usual plan for patients with very low weights is a weight gain of between 1 and 2 lb a week. In severe malnourished adolescents and especially those resisting refeeding, nasogastric tube feeding of supplements alone, or combined with meals, may be instituted (Garber et al., 2016).

Weight-increasing protocols usually take the form of a behavioral plan using positive reinforcements (i.e., excursion passes) and negative reinforcements (i.e., returning to bed rest) to encourage weight gain. The nurse should help patients to understand that these actions are not punitive. When all staff members agree on a clear protocol for behaviors related to eating and weight gain, reactivity of the staff to the patient is greatly reduced. These protocols provide ready-made, consistent responses to food-refusal behaviors and should be carried out in a caring and supportive context. On rare occasions when the patient is unable to recognize or accept her illness (denial), nasogastric tube feedings may be necessary.

Electrolytes may be completely depleted in anorexia nervosa, so nursing care involves stabilizing electrolyte balance. Potassium depletion usually results from use of diuretics, diarrhea, and vomiting. Calcium depletion is related to large intake of dietary fiber, which decreases calcium absorption. Many individuals also need phosphorus replacement (Peebles et al., 2017). During hospitalization, these electrolytes if warranted are replaced through oral or intravenous therapy.

Promotion of Sleep. Sleep disturbance is also common, and these individuals are viewed as hyperkinetic. They sleep little, but they usually awaken in an energized state. A structured, healthy sleep routine must be established immediately to conserve energy and calorie expenditure because of low weight. To further conserve energy, patients are often relegated to bed rest until a certain amount of weight is regained. Exercise is generally not permitted during refeeding and only with caution after this phase. Inpatients must be closely supervised because they are often found exercising in their rooms, running in place, and doing calisthenics.

Medication Interventions. Selective serotonin reuptake inhibitors (SSRIs) are useful in the treatment of AN especially regarding comorbid influences and symptoms such as OCD. The SSRI fluoxetine (Prozac) is approved by the Food and Drug Administration for the treatment of anorexia nervosa. Of course, comorbid conditions such as depression or OCD should be treated with appropriate medication. The nurse may be responsible for administering medications or providing patient and family teaching. See Box 26.7.

Psychosocial Interventions

Helping Patients Understand Feelings

Identifying feelings, such as anxiety and fear, and especially negative emotions, such as anger, is the first step in helping patients to decrease conflict avoidance and develop effective strategies for coping with these feelings.

Do not attempt to change distorted body image by merely pointing out that the patient is actually too thin. This symptom is often the last to resolve itself, and some individuals may take years to see their bodies realistically. However, although this symptom is difficult to abate, patients can continue to fear becoming fat but not be driven to act on the distortion by starving. The fear of becoming fat eventually lessens with time.

Cognitive Interventions

The nurse can help individuals with cognitive distortions and unrealistic assumptions to restructure the way they view the world, especially relative to food, eating, weight, and shape. Faulty ways of viewing these situations result in ineffective coping. Table 26.2 lists some distortions commonly experienced by individuals with eating disorders and some typical restructuring responses or statements that challenge the distortion, which the nurse can present as more realistic ways of perceiving situations. Imagery and relaxation are often used to overcome distortions and to decrease anxiety stemming from a distorted body image.

BOX 26.7

Drug Profile: Fluoxetine Hydrochloride (Prozac)

DRUG CLASS: Selective serotonin reuptake inhibitor

RECEPTOR AFFINITY: Inhibits central nervous system neuronal uptake of serotonin with little effect on norepinephrine; thought to antagonize muscarinic, histaminergic, and α-adrenergic receptors

INDICATIONS: Treatment of depressive disorders, obsessive-compulsive disorder, bulimia nervosa, and panic disorder

ROUTES AND DOSAGE: Available in 10- and 20-mg capsules and 20-mg/5-mL oral solution

Adults: 20 mg/d in the morning, not to exceed 80 mg/d. Full antidepressant effect may not be seen for up to 4 weeks. If no improvement, dosage is increased after several weeks. Dosages greater than 20 mg/d are administered twice daily. For eating disorders: typically, 60 mg/d is recommended.

Geriatric: Administer at lower or less frequent doses; monitor responses to guide dosage.

Children: Safety and efficacy have not been established.

HALF-LIFE (PEAK EFFECT): 2 to 3 days (6 to 8 hours)

SELECTED ADVERSE REACTIONS: Headache, nervousness, insomnia, drowsiness, anxiety, tremors, dizziness, lightheadedness, nausea, vomiting, diarrhea, dry mouth, anorexia, dyspepsia, constipation, taste changes, upper respiratory infections, pharyngitis, painful menstruation, sexual dysfunction, urinary frequency, sweating, rash, pruritus, weight loss, asthenia, and fever

BOXED WARNING: Increased risk of suicidal thoughts and behaviors in children, adolescents, and young adults.

WARNINGS: Avoid use in pregnancy and while breastfeeding. Use with caution in patients with impaired hepatic or renal function and diabetes mellitus. Possible risk for toxicity if taken with tricyclic antidepressants.

SPECIAL PATIENT AND FAMILY EDUCATION

- Be aware that the drug may take up to 4 weeks to get a full antidepressant effect.
- Take the drug in the morning or in divided doses, if necessary.
- Families and caregivers of pediatric patients being treated with antidepressants should monitor patient for agitation, irritation, and unusual changes in behavior.
- Report any adverse reactions.
- Avoid driving a car or performing hazardous activities because the drug may cause drowsiness or dizziness.
- Eat small, frequent meals to help with complaints of nausea and vomiting.

Psychoeducation

When weight is restored and concentration is improved, patients with anorexia nervosa can benefit from psychoeducation. Although these individuals have a wealth of knowledge about food and calories, they also have misinformation that needs clarifying. For example, they are often unclear about the role of "fats" in a healthy diet and try to be as "fat free" as possible. A thorough assessment of their knowledge is important because they seem to be "walking calorie books" with little information on the role of all of the nutrients and the importance of including

TABLE 26.2   COGNITIVE DISTORTIONS TYPICAL OF PATIENTS WITH EATING DISORDERS, WITH RESTRUCTURING STATEMENTS

Distortion	Clarification or Restructuring
Dichotomous or All-or-Nothing Thinking "I've gained 2 lb, so I'll be up to 100 lb soon."	"You have never gained 100 lb, but I understand that gaining 2 lb is scary."
Magnification "I binged last night, so I can't go out with anyone."	"Feeling bad and guilty about a binge are difficult feelings, but you are in treatment, and you have been monitoring and changing your eating."
Selective Abstraction "I can only be happy 10 lb lighter."	"When you were 10 lb lighter, you were hospitalized. You can choose to be happy about many things in your life."
Overgeneralization "I didn't eat anything yesterday and did okay, so I don't think not eating for a week or 2 will harm me."	"Any starvation harms the body, whether or not outward signs were apparent to you. The more you starve the more problems your body will encounter."
Catastrophizing "I purged last night for the first time in 4 months—I'll never recover."	"Recovery includes up and downs, and it is expected you will still have some mild but infrequent symptoms."

them in a healthy diet. There are several topic areas that should be included in a teaching plan. See Box 26.8.

Wellness Strategies

Individuals with anorexia focus on body weight, nutrition, and exercise. They often ignore the other wellness dimensions such as developing positive coping skills for stress management, developing a sense of connection with others, and searching for meaning or a purpose in life. See Box 26.9.

Evaluation and Treatment Outcomes

Several factors influence the outcome of treatment for individuals with anorexia nervosa. Particularly long duration of symptoms and low weight when treatment begins predict poor outcomes, but family support and involvement generally improve outcomes. Comorbid conditions and their severity also influence recovery especially anxiety disorders. Although patients are discharged from the hospital when their weight has reached 85% of what is considered ideal, restoration of healthy eating and changes in maladaptive thinking may not have yet occurred. Individuals often continue to restrict foods. Therefore, without intensive outpatient treatment, including nutritional counseling and support, they are unlikely to recover fully. Distorted thinking and eating patterns can set the stage for a relapse and later for the possible development of bulimia nervosa.

BOX 26.8

Anorexia Nervosa

When caring for a patient with anorexia nervosa, be sure to include the following topic areas in the teaching plan:

- Psychopharmacologic agents, if used, including drug, action, dosage, frequency, and possible adverse effects
- Nutrition and eating patterns
- Effect of restrictive eating or dieting
- Weight monitoring
- Safety and comfort measures
- Avoidance of triggers
- Self-monitoring techniques
- Trust
- Realistic goal setting
- Resources

BOX 26.9

Wellness Challenges

- Recognizing the need for moderate physical activity, healthy foods, and sleep
  - Strategies: Limit physical activity to a reasonable schedule
  - Practice increasing amounts of healthy food
  - Track sleep and increase amount of sleep (if needed) and engage sleep hygiene techniques
- Coping effectively with drive for thinness.
  - Strategies: Identify times when the need to restrict diet occurs; examine other strategies in dealing with the situation
- Stress management
  - Strategies: Practice meditation, use cognitive strategies to examine beliefs and thoughts
- Increase self-concept
  - Strategies: Keep a list of accomplishments, help others; keep busy; counseling or therapy
- Developing a sense of connection, belong, and a support system
  - Strategies: Develop a plan to increase social contact
- Expanding a sense of purpose and meaning in life
  - Strategies: Pray, meditate, help others, volunteer

Continuum of Care

Inpatient

Hospitalization is required based on criteria noted in Box 26.6. Because of its life-threatening nature, anorexia nervosa in its very acute stage is unlikely to be manageable in outpatient settings.

The patient's systems are monitored closely because at the time of admission, most patients are severely malnourished (see Table 26.1). Patients usually are placed on a privilege-earning program in which privileges, such as having visitors and receiving passes to go outside the hospital, are earned based on weight gain. See Chapter 10.

Emergency Care

Emergency care is not usually needed for individuals with anorexia nervosa. Family members and peers usually notice the weight loss and emaciation before patients' systems are compromised to the degree that they require emergency treatment. If systems are compromised enough to warrant emergency treatment, patients usually are admitted immediately for medical-surgical inpatient care.

Outpatient Treatment

After refeeding, treatment of anorexia nervosa takes place on an outpatient basis and involves individual and family therapy, nutrition counseling to reinforce healthy eating patterns and attitudes, and physician visits to monitor weight and evaluate somatic recovery. Support groups, which are often suggested, should not be substituted for therapy. Following an inpatient treatment program, many anorexia nervosa patients are referred for intensive outpatient therapy or day treatment programs prior to the usual outpatient therapy of one or two hourly sessions a week. In intensive outpatient therapy, patients may return to school but participate four to five evenings a week in a 4- to 5-hour structured program that includes group therapy, meeting with a dietician, and individual therapy. After full recovery, support groups are useful in maintaining recovery.

Family Interventions. Denial, guilt, and subsequent greater overprotectiveness are common reactions of the family, especially when hospitalization has been necessary. In addition to family therapy with a skilled therapist, the nurse can help family members express their feelings, increase effective communication, decrease protectiveness, and resolve guilt. Often, siblings become resentful of the patient with an eating disorder because of the significant amount of attention they get from their parents. Having siblings discuss these feelings and the effect the illness has had on them is helpful. Families and friends are eager to help the patient with anorexia but often need direction. Box 26.10 provides a list of strategies that may assist them.

School Interventions. Younger patients with anorexia nervosa may have lost some school time because of hospitalization. Integrating back into a school and classroom setting is difficult for most. Shame and guilt about having an eating disorder and being hospitalized must be addressed. Because these patients typically have isolated themselves before hospitalization and treatment, renewing friendships and relationships with peers may provoke anxiety. Involving school nurses and teachers in the reentry process may help.

Prevention and early detection strategies for parents and schoolteachers are often the focus of school nurses and mental health nurses who work in the community. Some of these strategies appear in Box 26.11 and are based on the research on risk factors and protective factors.

National eating disorder awareness and advocacy groups work toward educating the general public; those at risk; and those who work with groups at risk, such as teachers and coaches. They also monitor the media and work to remove unhealthy advertisements and articles that appear in magazines appealing to young girls. Policies, both health and social, can decrease the prevalence of eating disorders. Strategies include improving school-based curriculum to include content on prevention of EDs; implementing school-based anti-bullying policies that protect students from being bullied about their weight;

BOX 26.10

What Family and Friends Can Do to Help Those With Eating Disorders

- Tell the person you are concerned, you care, and you would like to help. Suggest that the person seek professional help from a physician or therapist.
- If the person refuses to seek professional help, encourage reaching out to an adult, such as a teacher, school nurse, or counselor.
- Do not discuss weight, the number of calories being consumed, or particular eating habits.
- Do try to talk about things other than food, weight, counting calories, and exercise.
- Avoid making comments about a person's appearance. Concern about weight loss may be interpreted as a compliment; comments regarding weight gain may be felt as criticism.
- It will not help to become involved in a power struggle. You cannot force the person to eat.
- You can offer support. Ultimately, however, the responsibility and the decision to accept help and to change rest with the person.
- Read and educate yourself regarding these disorders.

> **BOX 26.11**
>
> **Eating Disorder Prevention Strategies for Parents and Children**
>
> **EDUCATION FOR PARENTS**
> - Real versus ideal weight
> - Influence of attitudes, behaviors, teasing
> - Ways to increase self-esteem
> - Role of media: TV, magazines
> - Signs and symptoms
> - Interventions for obesity
> - Boys at risk also
> - Observe for rituals
> - Supervision of eating and exercise
>
> **STRATEGIES FOR CHILDREN**
> *Education*
> - Peer pressure regarding eating, weight
> - Menses, puberty, normal weight gain
> - Strategies for obesity
> - Ways to develop or improve self-esteem
> - Body image traps: media, retail clothing
> - Adapting and coping with problems
> - Reporting friends with signs of eating disorders
>
> **Screening:** Screen for risk factors
> **Assessment:** Assess for treatment
> **Follow-up:** Monitor for relapse

and training educators including coaches and health providers on prevention and early identification.

BULIMIA NERVOSA

Bulimia nervosa was once thought to be a type of anorexia nervosa. However, findings from extensive investigations have identified its characteristics as a separate entity. It is more prevalent than anorexia nervosa. Individuals with bulimia nervosa are usually older at onset than are those with anorexia nervosa. The disorder generally is not as life threatening as anorexia nervosa. The usual treatment is outpatient therapy. Outcomes are better for bulimia nervosa than for anorexia nervosa, and mortality rates are lower.

Clinical Course

Few outward signs are associated with bulimia nervosa. Individuals binge (eating an excessive amount, usually at one sitting) and purge (purposeful initiation of stomach or bowel evacuation through artificial means such as vomiting or laxatives) in secret and are typically of normal weight; therefore, it does not come to the attention of parents and peers as readily as does anorexia nervosa. Treatment consequently can be delayed for years as individuals attempt on their own to get their eating under control. Patients usually initiate their own treatment when control of their eating becomes impossible. When treatment is undertaken and completed, patients typically recover completely, except in cases in which personality disorders and comorbid serious depression are also present.

Patients with bulimia nervosa present as overwhelmed and overly committed individuals, "social butterflies" who have difficulty with setting limits and establishing appropriate boundaries. They have an enormous number of rules regarding food and food restriction, and they feel shame, guilt, and disgust about their binge eating and purging. They may also be impulsive in other areas of their lives, such as spending.

Diagnostic Criteria

Bulimia nervosa involves eating a large amount of food within a discrete period of time (e.g., 2 hours) and engaging in recurrent episodes of binge eating and compensatory purging in various forms such as vomiting or using laxatives, diuretics, or emetics or in nonpurging compensatory behaviors, such as fasting or overexercising in order to avoid weight gain. These episodes must occur at least once a week for a period of at least 3 months to meet the *DSM-5* criteria. Self-evaluation is excessively and inappropriately influenced by body weight and shape. Unlike anorexia nervosa, there is little or no weight loss. See Box 26.1 for characteristics related to bulimia nervosa.

>
> **Remember Ellen?**
> She is normal weight but has been vomiting one to two times a week for several months after binging. She has callouses on her hands from her teeth when she gagged herself. She sees herself as very overweight. Does Ellen have characteristics of bulimia nervosa? If she did not know that these behaviors were symptoms of bulimia, how would you explain to her what her symptoms might mean?

Binge eating is defined as rapid, episodic, impulsive, and uncontrollable ingestion of a large amount of food during a short period of time, usually 1 to 2 hours. Eating is followed by feelings of guilt, remorse, and often self-contempt, leading to purging. To assuage the out-of-control feeling, severe dieting is instituted, and these restrictions, referred to as *dietary restraint*, precipitate the next binge. The restrictions are viewed as "rules," such as no sweets, no fats, and so forth. The rules may be about what one can and cannot eat. Each binge sets up an out of control feeling and thus the individual then sees the need for even stricter rules about what can and cannot be consumed, leading to more frequent binge eating. This cycle has prompted clinicians to focus treatment primarily on interventions related to dietary restraint. When dietary restraint is resolved, binge eating is decreased, and generally the purging that follows binge eating also is decreased. Feeling out of control with food is often the major complaint when individuals seek treatment for bulimia nervosa.

> **KEYCONCEPT** **Dietary restraint** has been described by researchers in the field of eating disorders as a way to explain the relationship between dieting and binge eating.

Dieters' deprivation, or restraint, whether real or imagined, contributes to overeating and binging. Genetic predisposition for binge eating and deprivation may make dieters more prone to feel distress over their dietary "failures," especially if dieting has become a way to overcome body dissatisfaction and to compensate for distress through dietary restraint that leads to overeating (Castillo & Weiselberg, 2017). Whether the eating is influenced by the attraction of forbidden foods or by internal needs to assuage failure, there is significant evidence that restraining one's intake is a precondition for bouts of overeating.

Bulimia Nervosa Across the Life Span

Bulimia nervosa occurs in all age groups. It is not as common in children as in adolescents and adults; children appear more likely to have BED, discussed later. This finding has only recently been reported, and more data are needed to substantiate this finding.

Epidemiology

Recent epidemiologic data report the lifetime prevalence of bulimia nervosa to be as high as 2.3% depending on whether clinical or community populations are sampled, but it is estimated that less than one third of the cases have been detected. Strict criteria are used when clinical groups are studied as opposed to self-reported symptoms in community surveys, making the community sample prevalence rates higher (Wade, 2019).

Age of Onset

Typically, the age of onset is between 15 and 24 years, which is later than the typical onset of anorexia nervosa. Some women older than the typical age of onset have developed bulimia nervosa and symptom cases have been identified as subsequent to life stressors such as a loss (Volpe et al., 2016).

Gender

As with anorexia nervosa, females are 10 times more likely than males to experience bulimia nervosa. Box 26.2 highlights boys and men with eating disorders.

Ethnicity and Culture

Bulimia nervosa is related to culture in the same way as anorexia nervosa. In western cultures and those becoming westernized in their norms, the focus on achieving a thin body ideal underlies the dieting and dietary restraint that set up the trajectory toward a diagnosable eating disorder. Any ethnic differences have to do with the degree to which individuals from specific cultural backgrounds internalize the thin ideal.

Comorbidity

The most common comorbid conditions are anxiety disorders, mood disorders, self-harm, and substance use. If a comorbid condition occurs before the eating disorder develops, it may actually have a role in precipitating the disorder (Wade, 2019). The suicide rate for bulimia is around 7.5%, with suicide attempts and ideation ranging from 15% to 40%.

There are several medical complications affecting those with bulimia. Electrolyte imbalance can lead to cardiac arrhythmia, seizure, and death. Self-induced vomiting with loss of stomach acid can result in hyperchloremic alkalosis and hypokalemia. Chronic vomiting can result in subconjunctival hemorrhages, esophageal damage, acid reflux, and dental lesions (Castillo & Weiselberg, 2017).

Etiology

As with anorexia nervosa, theories do not individually explain the development of bulimia nervosa. Rather, the convergence of many of these factors at a vulnerable stage of individual development best explains causality.

Some of the predisposing or risk factors for anorexia nervosa and bulimia nervosa overlap with theories of causality. For example, dieting puts an individual at risk for the development of bulimia nervosa. The dieting can turn into dietary restraint, a symptom that leads to binge eating and purging. However, not all individuals who diet experience bulimia nervosa. The interplay of other risk factors (e.g., body dissatisfaction and separation individuation issues) most likely explains the development of this disorder.

Biologic Theories

Some progress has been made in understanding the biologic changes in bulimia nervosa. Dieting and binging can affect brain function. Dieting is believed to affect serotonergic regulation and binging affects the dopamine (DA), acetylcholine (ACh), and opioid reward–related systems. The changes are the result of eating dysregulation rather than the cause. As with anorexia nervosa, these changes often disappear when symptoms such as dietary restraint, binge eating, and purging remit (Wade, 2019).

Genetic and Familial Predispositions

Bulimia nervosa runs in families, with an increased risk for individuals if family members are diagnosed with this disorder. Although anorexia and bulimia are both strongly related to genetics, it is believed that only bulimia has genetic specificity—that is, if one twin has bulimia nervosa, the other twin is at higher risk for developing that disorder (Bulik et al., 2019).

Psychosocial Theories

Symptoms of bulimia nervosa develop when psychological, sociocultural, or environmental events occur. Because the age of onset for bulimia nervosa is late adolescence—going away to college, for example—may represent the first physical separation for some adolescents, who are unprepared for the emotional separation. In addition, an inability to set limits and develop healthy boundaries leads to a sense of being overwhelmed and "drained." Overwhelming feelings often lead to binge eating, either to avoid or to distract oneself from feelings such as resentment, or binge eating can serve to assuage emptiness or to fill up a "drained" self with food.

Cognitive Theory

Many experts view bulimia nervosa as a disorder of thinking in that distortions are the basis for behaviors such as binge eating and purging. Psychological triggering mechanism models explain that cues such as stress, negative emotions, and even environmental cues (e.g., the presence of attractive food) play a role in etiology. However, today these cognitive and triggering theories are viewed as an explanation for maintaining the binge eating after it has been established rather than an explanation of causality.

The same sociocultural factors that underlie anorexia nervosa play a significant role in the development of bulimia nervosa.

Ellen's Triggers
Some of Ellen's triggers are anxiety, boredom, alcohol use, exhaustion, anger, and social situations where food is readily available. What are the theoretical explanations that relate her triggers to the bulimia behavior? What interventions would you suggest for these triggers?

Family Factors

Dysfunctional family relationships of persons with eating disorders have been implicated for years. Current research indicates that perceived lack of cohesion in a family relates to depressive and bulimic behaviors. That is, if a person is depressed and views family members as less cohesive, close, or supportive, the individual would be more likely to have depression and/or bulimia (Kluck, Dallesasse, & English, 2017).

Risk Factors

There are numerous risk factors associated with bulimia nervosa including genetic risk, female gender, obstetric complication and perinatal factors, higher body mass index, frequent dieting, overexercising, and concern about body weight. Childhood sexual abuse and/or neglect has often been suggested as a risk factor for eating disorders. The beginning of puberty and the start of early adulthood are high-risk periods when adverse life events or peer teasing about appearance may trigger bulimic behavior, particularly if there is genetic susceptibility (Wade, 2019).

Teamwork and Collaboration: Working Toward Recovery

Individuals with bulimia nervosa benefit from a comprehensive multimodal treatment approach. The goals for treatment for individuals with bulimia nervosa focus on stabilizing and then normalizing eating, which means stopping the binge–purge cycles; restructuring dysfunctional thought patterns and attitudes, especially about eating, weight, and shape; teaching healthy boundary setting; and resolving conflicts about separation–individuation. Treatment usually takes place in an outpatient setting except when the patient is suicidal or when past outpatient treatment has failed (see Box 26.6).

Pharmacologic interventions paired with cognitive-behavioral therapy (CBT) or interpersonal psychotherapy is also effective. Antidepressants demonstrate effectiveness in treating binge eating and purging even without comorbid depression. Nutrition counseling is an important part of outpatient treatment to stabilize and normalize eating. Some mental health professionals, psychologists, advanced practice psychiatric nurses, and social workers specialize in treating eating disorders, often working with nutritionists who also have expertise with this population. Group psychotherapy and support groups are also used. Family therapy is not usually a part of the treatment because many people with bulimia nervosa live on college campuses away from home or are older and live on their own. Usually, treatment becomes less intensive as symptoms remit. Therapy focuses on psychological issues, such as boundary setting and separation—individuation conflicts and on changing problematic behaviors and dysfunctional thinking using CBT.

Safety Issues

Bulimia nervosa is associated with a high risk of suicide independent of other comorbid disorders. Individuals with bulimia nervosa are also often at risk for self-harm. Because they display high levels of impulsivity, shoplifting, and overspending, financial and legal difficulties have been associated with this disorder (Wade, 2019).

Evidence-Based Nursing Care for Persons With Bulimia Nervosa Disorder

Mental Health Nursing Assessment

Physical Health Assessment

Even though most individuals with bulimia nervosa maintain normal weights, the physical ramifications of this disorder may be similar to those of anorexia nervosa. Hypokalemia can contribute to muscle weakness and fatigability, as well as to the development of cardiac arrhythmias, palpitations, and cardiac conduction defects. Patients who purge as well as abuse laxatives risk fluid and electrolyte abnormalities that can further compromise cardiac status. Tooth enamel erosion because of frequent purging is also a consequence of bulimia nervosa. Neuropsychiatric disturbances, such as poor concentration and attention, and sleep disturbances are common.

The nurse should assess current eating patterns, determine the number of times a day the individual binges and purges, and note dietary restraint practices. Sleep patterns and exercise habits are also important.

Psychosocial Assessment

For the individual with bulimia nervosa, psychological assessment focuses on cognitive distortions—cues or stimuli that lead to dysfunctional behavior affecting symptom development—and knowledge deficits. The psychological characteristics typical of patients with bulimia nervosa are presented in Box 26.1.

Individuals with bulimia nervosa display a significant number of cognitive distortions, examples of which are found in Table 26.2. These thought patterns form the basis for "rules" and lead the way to destructive eating patterns. During routine history taking, patients relate many of these erroneous assumptions. Situations that produce feelings of being overwhelmed and powerless need to be explored, as does the patient's ability to set boundaries, control impulsivity, and maintain quality relationships. These underlying issues precipitate binge eating. Body dissatisfaction should be openly explored. Mood is an important area for evaluation because many people with bulimia nervosa also have depression.

Symptoms of depression should be thoroughly explored (see Chapter 23). See Nursing Care Plan 26.1—which sets forth a plan of care for Ellen, the case study patient in this chapter—is available at http://thepoint.lww.com/BoydEssentials2e.

Strengths Assessment

Persons with bulimia can usually identify periods of time when they were able to resist binging and purging. They are usually motivated to reduce or eliminate the binging and purging. The following questions can be used if the strengths do not emerge during the assessment interview.

- How have you curtailed the binging and purging behavior in the past?
- What do you do to reduce your anxiety (instead of binging)?
- Is there anyone in your life that you feel understands your situation?
- How motivated are you to change your eating behaviors and work on body image issues?

Priority of Nursing Care

The first priority is to address emerging medical problems such as electrolyte imbalances. Suicide or self-harm behaviors should also be addressed.

Establishing a Therapeutic Relationship

Individuals with bulimia nervosa experience a great deal of shame and guilt. They also often have an intense need to please and be liked and may approach the nurse–patient relationship in a superficial manner. They are too ashamed to discuss their symptoms but do not want to disappoint others, so they may discuss more social or unrelated issues in an attempt to engage the nurse (Box 26.12). A nonjudgmental, accepting approach, stressing the importance of the relationship and outlining its purpose, is important at the outset. Explaining the nature of the relationship and the goals of therapy will help clarify the boundaries.

> **Consider This:**
>
> Ellen feels shame and guilt over her binging and purging. She does not like to talk about it and is very reluctant to talk to the nurse about the behavior. Which interventions would be helpful to help Ellen deal with her guilt? Would she be a candidate for a support group?

BOX 26.12 • THERAPEUTIC DIALOGUE • The Patient With an Eating Disorder

INEFFECTIVE APPROACH

Nurse: Ellen, I am glad to see that you ate your lunch.
Ellen: Thanks, I feel so fat after I eat.
Nurse: I will lock the bathroom so you are not tempted to purge.
Ellen: What, don't you trust me?
Nurse: It is not about trust, but I don't feel comfortable leaving you alone with bathroom access.
Ellen: Really? You have your nerve.
Nurse: We are just trying to help.
Ellen: Some help you are. I know you don't trust me.
Nurse: Now, Ellen that is not what I said.
Ellen: No, but that is what you meant.

EFFECTIVE APPROACH

Nurse: Ellen, how was your lunch.
Ellen: I was ok. I always feel so fat after I eat.
Nurse: That is understandable. How long does that feeling last.
Ellen: Well, it depends on how much I have eaten. Since I didn't eat much, it will last for about an hour?
Nurse: Oh, I see. For many people with bulimia, the urges to purge are strongest after a meal? Is this a hard time for you?
Ellen: Sometimes it is.
Nurse: How can I help you resist the urges? Would you like me to stay with you until group time?
Ellen: That would be great.

CRITICAL THINKING CHALLENGE

- What effect did the first interaction have on the Ellen's behavior? Why?
- In the second interaction, what theories and interventions regarding eating disorders did the nurse use in her approach to the Ellen?

Mental Health Nursing Interventions

Physical Health Interventions

If the patient is admitted to the hospital, meals and all food intake are strictly monitored to normalize eating. Bathroom visits may also be supervised to prevent purging. Outpatients are asked to record their intake, binges, and purges. Because individuals with bulimia nervosa have chaotic lifestyles and are often overcommitted, sleep may be a low priority. Sleep-deprived individuals may assume that food would be helpful, and they begin to eat, triggering a binge. To encourage regular sleep patterns, sleep hygiene strategies are implemented.

Medication Interventions

Fluoxetine is approved by the FDA for treating bulimia nervosa. This SSRI has been shown to reduce vomiting and binging episodes (Bello & Yeomans, 2018).

Teaching Points

Patients should be instructed to take medication as prescribed. SSRIs must be taken in the morning because they can cause insomnia. Patients should be informed that any weight loss they initially experience is temporary and is usually regained after a few weeks when the medication dosage has stabilized.

Psychosocial Interventions

Behavioral Strategies

The behavioral techniques, such as cue elimination and response prevention, require self-monitoring to individualize the therapy. **Self-monitoring** is accomplished using a diary in which the patient records binges and purges and precipitating emotions and environmental cues. Emotional and environmental cues are identified, and alternative responses are suggested, tried, and reinforced. When a cue or stimulus leads to a dysfunctional or unhealthy response, the response can be eliminated or an alternate, healthier response to the cue can be substituted, tried, and then reinforced. Figure 26.2 gives two examples of behavioral interventions. In Example 1, for the patient with anorexia nervosa, the response is modified or altered to a healthier one; In Example 2, for the patient with bulimia nervosa, the cue is changed to

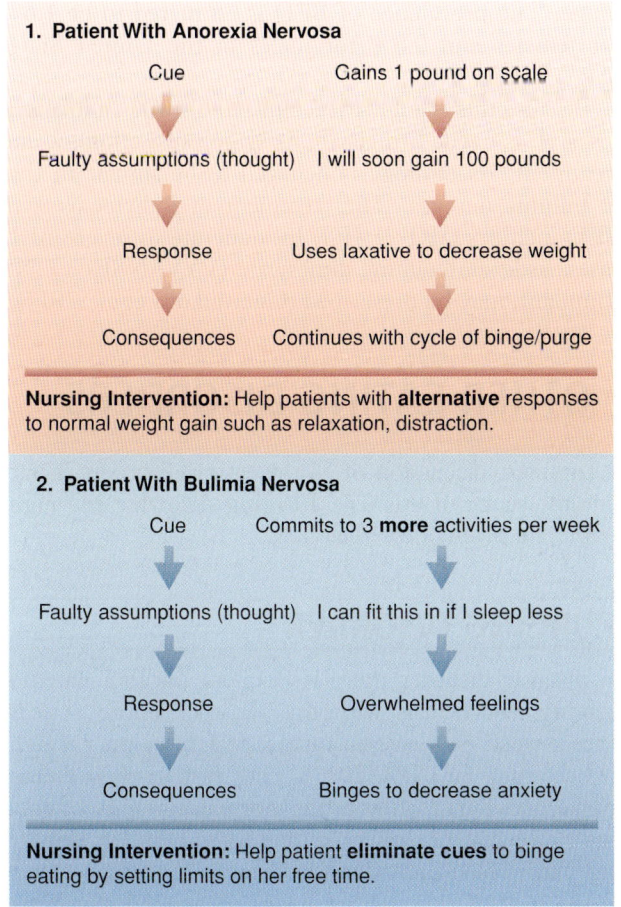

FIGURE 26.2 Examples of the relationship of cues, thoughts, responses, and behavioral interventions.

produce a different, healthier response. Other techniques, such as postponing binges and purges through distraction, a technique to interrupt the cycle, are also effective.

> **NCLEXNOTE** Cognitive interventions within the context of a therapeutic relationship are a priority in the nursing care of patients with eating disorders.

Group Interventions

Group interventions are cost effective and increase learning more effectively than does individual treatment because patients learn from each other as well as from the nurse, therapist, or leader. Some experts have recommended 12-step programs for treating bulimia nervosa. However, many clinicians who work in this specialty have noted that these programs, with their strict rules, can be counterproductive for patients with bulimia nervosa, who already have rigid rules and are "abstinent" in many ways that lead to binge eating. Broad parameters regarding food choices (e.g., all foods allowed in moderation) in combination with knowledge about healthy eating should be encouraged instead.

After symptoms subside, patients can concentrate on interpersonal issues in therapy, such as a fused relationship with their mothers or feelings of inadequacy and low self-esteem, which often underlie their lack of assertiveness.

Psychoeducation

In addition to cognitive and behavioral techniques, educational strategies are also incorporated into treatment. For individuals with bulimia nervosa, psychoeducation focuses on setting boundaries and healthy limits, developing assertiveness, learning nutritional concepts related to healthy eating, and clarifying the many misconceptions they have about food and its influence on weight. Rules that result from dichotomous thinking also must be addressed because of their role in dietary restraint and resulting binge eating.

The nurse can assist patients to understand the binge–purge cycle and the role of rigid rules in contributing to this cycle. The value of eating meals regularly to ward off hunger and reduce the possibility of a binge is also important. Patients who abuse laxatives must be taught that although these drugs produce water-weight loss, they are ineffective for true, lasting weight loss because they work on the colon and not the small intestine or stomach where food is absorbed. Patients also need information about potassium depletion, electrolyte imbalances, dehydration, and the medical consequences of binge eating and purging. Other topics for psychoeducation are included in Box 26.13.

Evaluation and Treatment Outcomes

Most people recover from bulimia nervosa over time. Rates of recovery from bulimia peak within the first 10 years. Patients with bulimia nervosa have better and

---

BOX 26.13

Bulimia Nervosa

When caring for the patient with bulimia nervosa, be sure to include the following topic areas in the teaching plan:
- Psychopharmacologic agents, if used, including drug, action, dosage, frequency, and possible adverse effects
- Binge–purge cycle and effects on the body
- Nutrition and eating patterns
- Hydration
- Avoidance of cues
- Cognitive distortions
- Limit setting
- Appropriate boundary setting
- Assertiveness
- Resources
- Self-monitoring and behavioral interventions
- Realistic goal setting

quicker recovery than do those with anorexia nervosa (Eddy et al., 2017).

Continuum of Care

Although patients with bulimia nervosa are less likely than those with anorexia nervosa to require hospitalization, those with extreme dehydration and electrolyte imbalance, depression and suicidality, or symptoms that have not remitted with outpatient treatment need hospitalization.

However, most treatment takes place in outpatient settings. After treatment, referrals to recovery groups and support groups are important to prevent relapse. Rarely do patients with bulimia nervosa require emergency care.

Community Interventions

As with anorexia nervosa, preventing bulimia nervosa requires effort on the part of teachers, school nurses, parents, and society as a whole. Because many of the risk factors are seen early in children attending elementary school, educating school nurses and teachers is an important focus for psychiatric–mental health nurses working in the community. Protective factors that mediate between risk factors and the development of an eating disorder must be emphasized and developed. Box 26.11 covers important prevention strategies for parents and their children or adolescents.

Society has begun to engage in an effort to help young girls. The federal government has developed a website called *girlshealth* that is devoted to areas such as body changes, body image, relationships, and self-confidence.

BINGE-EATING DISORDER

BED is the most common eating disorder, with a worldwide prevalence of 1.4%. In the United States, the prevalence of BED is estimated to be 2.8%. Several studies have uncovered a group of individuals who binge in the same way as those with bulimia nervosa do, but these individuals do not purge or compensate for binges through other behaviors. BED differs from other eating disorders in that it is associated with obesity and the development of obesity (Guerdjikova, Mori, Casuto, & McElroy, 2017).

The diagnostic criteria for BED consist of binge eating, which includes both the ingestion of a large amount of food in a short period of time and a sense of loss of control during the binge, distress regarding the binge; eating until uncomfortably full, and feelings of guilt or depression after the binge. As mentioned, purging or other compensatory behavior does not follow the binge. The prevalence of BED is estimated to be 1.6% for females and 0.8% for males in the United States (APA, 2013).

Because this is a newly recognized disorder, additional research is needed to clarify its symptoms, etiology, and treatment. Its etiology is believed to be similar to that of bulimia nervosa. The treatment of individuals with BED includes CPT or IPT. In moderate to severe BED cases, lisdexamfetamine dimesylate (VYVANSE) a CNS stimulant, may be prescribed (Guerdjikova et al., 2017).

OTHER EATING DISORDERS

A complete discussion of all the eating disorders is outside the scope of this text. **Purging disorder** and night eating are briefly described here.

PURGING DISORDER

In purging disorder there is frequent purging, but not binging. Individuals with this disorder purge at least once a week and have an intense fear of gaining weight or becoming fat (APA, 2013). They restrict their dietary intake and purge after eating normal amounts of food due to the fear of eating, gaining weight, and/or appearing "fat." These individuals have increased levels of body image disturbance, higher levels of general psychopathology, distress, eating pathology, and personality disorders when compared to a comparable group of persons without purging disorder. While individuals with this disorder do not overeat as those with bulimia nervosa, they do report more dietary restraint, greater fear of losing control, and greater guild over eating than control groups. On a continuum of bulimic symptomatology, purging disorder may be the midpoint with bulimia nervosa the more severe (Smith, Crowther, & Lavender, 2017).

NIGHT EATING SYNDROME

In **night eating syndrome**, the individual eats after awakening from sleep or consumes an excessive amount of food after the evening meal (APA, 2013). The person is aware of the overeating, which causes significant distress or impairment to the individual. There is a feeling of loss of control over consumption, sleep fragmentation, and morning anorexia. Night eating syndrome is conceptualized as a disorder of circadian modulation of food intake and sleep. It is mainly attributed to an endocrine metabolic or psychological trigger factor. These individuals typically experience insomnia and nighttime awakenings (Haraguchi, Komada, Inoue, & Shibata, 2019).

SUMMARY OF KEY POINTS

- Anorexia nervosa and bulimia nervosa have some common symptoms but are classified as discrete disorders.
- Eating disorders are best viewed along a continuum that includes subclinical or partial-syndrome disorders; because these disorders occur more frequently than full syndromes, they are often overlooked but, after they are identified, they can be prevented from worsening.
- Similar factors predispose individuals to the development of anorexia nervosa and bulimia nervosa, and these factors represent a biopsychosocial model of risk. These disorders are preventable, and identifying risk factors assists with prevention strategies.
- Etiologic factors contribute in combination to the development of eating disorders; no one factor provides an explanation.
- Treatment of anorexia nervosa frequently includes hospitalization for refeeding; bulimia nervosa is treated primarily on an outpatient basis.
- Cognitive-behavioral therapy and medications improve the symptoms. Individual and group interpersonal psychotherapy are also effective in self-evaluation and communication.
- The outcomes for bulimia nervosa are better than those for anorexia nervosa. The type and severity of comorbid conditions and the length of the illness influence outcomes.
- BED is characterized by periods of binge eating not followed by purging or any other compensating behaviors.

CRITICAL THINKING CHALLENGES

1. Discuss the potential difficulties and risks in attempting to treat a patient with anorexia nervosa in an outpatient setting.
2. Parents are often in need of support and suggestions for how to help prevent eating disorders. Develop a teaching program and include the topics and rationale for suggestions chosen.
3. Identify the important nursing management components of a refeeding program for a hospitalized patient with anorexia nervosa.
4. Bulimia nervosa is often described as a closet disorder with secretive binge eating and purging. Identify the signs and symptoms of each system involved for someone with this disorder.
5. Positive outcomes for the recovery of bulimia nervosa and anorexia nervosa depend on many factors. Identify the factors that promote positive outcomes and those related to poorer outcomes and prognosis.

 A related Psychiatric–Mental Health Nursing video on the topic of Eating Disorder is also available at http://thePoint.lww.com/BoydEssentials2e.

 A Psychiatric–Mental Health Nursing Practice and Learn Interactive Case Study related to the video on the topic of Eating Disorder is also available at http://thePoint.lww.com/BoydEssentials2e.

REFERENCES

Accurso, E. C., Astrachan-Fletcher, E., O'Brien, S., McClanahan, S. F., & Le Grange, D. (2018). Adaptation and implementation of family-based treatment enhanced with dialectical behavior therapy skills for anorexia nervosa in community-based specialist clinics. *Eating Disorders*, 26(2), 149–163.

American Psychiatric Association. (2013). *Diagnostic and statistical manual of mental disorders* (5th ed.). Arlington, VA: American Psychiatric Association.

Bello, N. T., & Yeomans, B. L. (2018). Safety of pharmacotherapy options for bulimia nervosa and binge eating disorder. *Expert Opinion on Drug Safety*, 17(1), 17–23. doi: 10.1080/14740338.2018.1395854.

Bruch, H. (1973). *Eating disorders: Obesity, anorexia nervosa and the person within*. New York: Basic Books.

Bulik, C. M., Blake, L., & Austin, J. (2019). Genetics of eating disorders: What the clinician needs to know. *Psychiatric Clinics of North America*, 42, 59–73.

Castillo, M., & Weiselberg, E. (2017). Bulimia nervosa/purging disorder. *Current Problems in Pediatric & Adolescent Health Care*, 47(4), 85–94.

Cheng, Z. H., Perko, V. L., Fuller-Marashi, L., Gau, J. M., & Stice, E. (2019). Ethnic differences in eating disorder prevalence, risk factors, and predictive effects of risk factors among young women. *Eating Behaviors*, 32, 23–30.

Chidiac, C. W. (2019). An update on the medical consequences of anorexia nervosa. *Current Opinion in Pediatrics*.

Cucchi, A., Ryan, D., Konstantakopoulos, G., Stroumpa, S., Kaçar, A. S., Renshaw, S., et al. (2016). Lifetime prevalence of non-suicidal self-injury in patients with eating disorders: A systematic review and meta-analysis. *Psychological Medicine*, 46, 1345–1358.

Duarte, C., Ferreira, C., & Pinto-Gouveia, J. (2016). At the core of eating disorders: Overvaluation, social rank, self-criticism and shame in anorexia, bulimia and binge eating disorder. *Comprehensive Psychiatry*, 66, 123–131.

Dwarkasing, J. T., Witkamp, R. F., Boekschoten, M. V., Ter Laak, M. C., Heins, M. S., & van Norren, K. (2016). Increased hypothalamic serotonin turnover in inflammation-induced anorexia. *BMC Neuroscience*, 17(1), 26.

Eddy, K. T., Tabri, N., Thomas, J. J., Murray, H. B., Keshaviah, A., Hastings, E., et al. (2017). Recovery from anorexia nervosa and bulimia nervosa at 22-year follow-up. *The Journal of Clinical Psychiatry*, 28(2), 184–189.

Fichter, M. M., Quadflieg, N., Crosby, R. D., & Koch, S. (2017). Long-term outcome of anorexia nervosa: Results from a large clinical longitudinal study. *International Journal of Eating Disorders*, 50(9), 1018–1030.

Garber, A. K., Sawyer, S. M., Golden, N. H., Guarda, A. S., Katzman, D. K., Kohn, M. R., et al. (2016). A systematic review of approaches to refeeding in patients with anorexia nervosa. *International Journal of Eating Disorders*, 49(3), 293–310.

Garner, D. M., Olmsted, M. P., Bohr, Y., & Garfinkel, P. E. (1982). The eating attitudes test: Psychometric features and clinical correlates. *Psychological Medicine*, 12(4), 871–878.

Goldstein, A., & Gvion, Y. (2019). Socio-demographic and psychological risk factors for suicidal behavior among individuals with anorexia and bulimia nervosa: A systematic review. *Journal of Affective Disorders*, 245, 1149–1167.

Griffiths, S., Castle, D., Cunningham, M., Murray, S. B., Bastian, B., & Barlow, F. K. (2018). How does exposure to thinspiration and fitspiration relate to symptom severity among individuals with eating disorders? Evaluation of a proposed model. *Body Image, 27*, 187–195.

Guerdjikova, A. I., Mori, N., Casuto, L. S., & McElroy, S. L. (2017). Binge eating disorder. *Psychiatric Clinics of North America, 40*(2), 255–266.

Haraguchi, A., Komada, Y., Inoue, Y., & Shibata, S. (2019). Correlation among clock gene expression rhythms, sleep quality, and meal conditions in delayed sleep-wake phase disorder and night eating syndrome. *Chronobiology International, 28*, 1–14.

Haynos, A. F., Watts, A. W., Loth, K. A., Pearson, C. M., & Neumark-Stzainer, D. (2016). Factors predicting an escalation of restrictive eating during adolescence. *Journal of Adolescent Health, 59*(4), 391–396.

Hilbert, A., de Zwaan, M., & Braehler, E. (2012). How frequent are eating disorders in the population? Norms of the eating disorder examination questionnaire. *PLoS One, 7*(1), e29125.

Holmes, S., Drake, S., Odgers, K., & Wilson, J. (2017). Feminist approaches to Anorexia Nervosa: A qualitative study of a treatment group. *Journal of Eating Disorders, 5*, 36.

Joy, E., Kussman, A., & Nattiv, A. (2019). 2016 update on eating disorders in athletes: A comprehensive narrative review with a focus on clinical assessment and management. *British Journal of Sports Medicine, 50*(3), 154–162.

King, J. A., Frank, G. K. W., Thompson, P. M., & Ehrlich, S. (2018). Structural neuroimaging of anorexia nervosa: Future directions in the quest for mechanisms underlying dynamic alterations. *Biological Psychiatry, 83*(3), 224–234. doi: 10.1016/j.biopsych.2017.08.011.

Kluck, A. S., Dallesasse, S., & English, E. M. (2017). Family relations and psychopathology: Examining depressive and bulimic symptomatology. *Child Psychiatry and Human Development, 48*(5), 818–827.

Larsson, E., Lloyd, S., Westwood, H., & Tchanturia, K. (2018). Patients' perspective of a group intervention for perfectionism in anorexia nervosa: A qualitative study. *Journal of Health Psychology, 23*(12), 1521–1532.

Lie, S. Ø., Rø, Ø., & Bang, L. (2019). Is bullying and teasing associated with eating disorders? A systematic review and meta-analysis. *International Journal of Eating Disorders, 52*(5), 497–514.

Mangweth-Matzek, B., & Hoek, H. W. (2017). Epidemiology and treatment of eating disorders in men and women of middle and older age. *Current Opinion in Psychiatry, 30*(6), 446–451.

Miniati, M., Callari, A., Maglio, A., & Calugi, S. (2018). Interpersonal psychotherapy for eating disorders: Current perspectives. *Psychology Research & Behavior Management, 11*, 353–369.

Minuchin, S., Rosman, B., & Baker, L. (1978). *Psychosomatic families.* Cambridge, MA: Harvard University Press.

Misra, M., Golden, N. H., & Katzman, D. K. (2016). State of the art systematic review of bone disease in anorexia nervosa. *International Journal of Eating Disorders, 49*(3), 276–292.

Monell, E., Clinton, D., & Birgegård, A. (2018). Emotion dysregulation and eating disorders-Associations with diagnostic presentation and key symptoms. *International Journal of Eating Disorders, 51*(8), 921–930.

Peebles, R., Lesser, A., Park, C. C., Heckert, K., Timko, C. A., Lantzouni, E., et al. (2017). Outcomes of an inpatient medical nutritional rehabilitation protocol in children and adolescents with eating disorders. *Journal of Eating Disorders, 5*, 7.

Pike, K., & Dunne, P. E. (2015). The rise of eating disorders in Asia: A review. *Journal of Eating Disorders, 3*, 33.

Plana, M. T., Torres, T., Rodríguez, N., Boloc, D., Gassó, P., Moreno, E., et al. (2019). Genetic variability in the serotoninergic system and age of onset in anorexia nervosa and obsessive-compulsive disorder. *Psychiatry Research, 271*, 554–558.

Rotella, F., Mannucci, E., Gemignani, S., Lazzeretti, L., Fioravanti, G., & Ricca, V. (2018) Emotional eating and temperamental traits in Eating Disorders: A dimensional approach. *Psychiatry Research, 264*, 1–8.

Scharner, S., & Stengel, A. (2019). Alterations of brain structure and functions in anorexia nervosa. *Clinical Nutrition Experimental.*

Shu, C. Y., Limburg, K., Harris, C., McCormack, J., Hoiles, K. J., Hamilton, M. J., et al. (2015). Clinical presentation of eating disorders in young males in a tertiary setting. *Journal of Eating Disorders, 3*, 39.

Sjögren, M., Nielsen, A. S., Hasselbalch, K. C., Wøllo, M., & Hansen, J. S. (2018). A systematic review of blood-based serotonergic biomarkers in Bulimia Nervosa. *Psychiatry Research*, pii: S0165-1781(18)31579-8.

Smith, K. E., Crowther, J. H., & Lavender, J. M. (2017). A review of purging disorder through meta-analysis. *Journal of Abnormal Psychology, 126*(5), 565–592.

Thornton, L. M., Welch, E., Munn-Chernoff, M. A., Lichtenstein, P., & Bulik, C. M. (2016). Anorexia nervosa, major depression, and suicide attempts: Shared genetic factors. *Suicide & Life Threatening Behavior, 46*(5), 525–534.

Timko, C., DeFilipp, L., & Dakanalis, A. (2019). Sex differences in adolescent anorexia and bulimia nervosa: Beyond the signs and symptoms. *Current Psychiatry Reports, 21*(1), 1.

Udo, T., & Grilo, C. M. (2019). Psychiatric and medical correlates of DSM-5 eating disorders in a nationally representative sample of adults in the United States. *International Journal of Eating Disorders, 52*(1), 42–50.

Volpe, U., Tortorella, A., Manchia, M., Monteleone, A. M., Albert, U., & Monteleone, P. (2016). Eating disorders: What age at onset?. *Psychiatry Research, 238*, 225–227.

Wade, T. D. (2019). Recent research on bulimia nervosa. *Psychiatric Clinics of North America, 42*, 21–32.

Wagner, A. F., & Vitousek, K. M. (2019). Personality variables and eating pathology. *Psychiatric Clinics of North America, 42*(1), 105–119.

Wallis, A., Miskovic-Wheatley, J., Madden, S., Rhodes, P., Crosby, R. D., Cao, L., et al. (2018). Family functioning and relationship quality for adolescents in family-based treatment with severe anorexia nervosa compared with non-clinical adolescents. *European Eating Disorders Review, 6*(1), 29–37.

Waszczuk, M. A., Waaktaar, T., Eley, T. C., & Torgersen, S. (2019). Etiological influences on continuity and co-occurrence of eating disorders symptoms across adolescence and emerging adulthood. *International Journal of Eating Disorders.*

Wong, L., Goh, L. G., & Ramachandran, R. (2019). Family-based therapy for anorexia nervosa: results from a 7-year longitudinal Singapore study. *Eating & Weight Disorders.* doi: 10.1007/s40519-019-00654-3

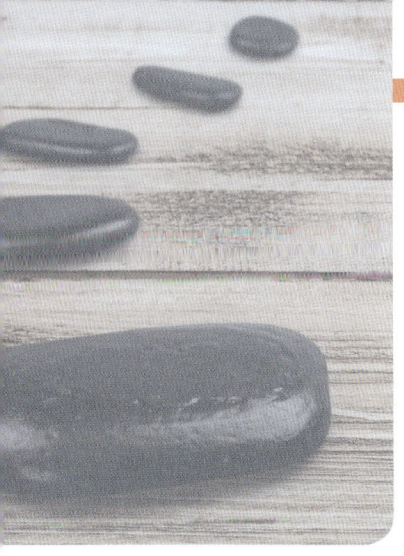

27

Somatic Symptom and Related Disorders

Management of Somatic Problems

Victoria Soltis-Jarrett

KEY CONCEPT
- somatization

LEARNING OBJECTIVES

After studying this chapter, you will be able to:

1. Explain the concept of somatization and the occurrence of somatic symptom and related disorders in people with mental health problems.
2. Discuss the prevailing theories related to somatic symptom and related disorders.
3. Identify evidence-based nursing assessment and outcomes for persons with somatization and cognitive distortions.
4. Develop recovery-oriented nursing interventions for patients with somatic symptoms and related disorders.
5. Discuss special concerns within the therapeutic relationship common for those with somatic symptom and related disorders.
6. Define the relationship between mental health care and primary care.
7. Develop wellness strategies for persons with somatic disorders.

KEY TERMS

- alexithymia • somatic symptom disorder (SSD) • conversion disorder • factitious disorder • factitious disorder imposed on another • illness anxiety disorder • pseudologia fantastica • psychosomatic

Case Study: Carol

Carol is a 48-year-old woman with obesity who is very angry at being forced to see a mental health care provider. She has had multiple surgeries including hysterectomy, gastric bypass, carpal tunnel release. She suffers from shoulder and neck pain and from vertigo. She takes multiple medications.

The connection between the "mind" and "body" has been hypothesized and described for centuries. The term **psychosomatic** has been traditionally used to describe, explain, and predict the psychological origins of illness and disease. Unfortunately, this notion perpetuates the stigma that certain disorders are purely "psychological" in nature and thus that they are not real or valid. For example, it was formerly believed that people with asthma were behaviorally "acting out" their anger, fear, or emotional pain and were seeking attention rather than experiencing an alteration in their respiratory status.

In contrast, the concept of *somatization* acknowledges and respects that bodily sensations and functional changes are expressions of health and illness, and, even though they may be unexplained, they are not imaginary or "all in the head" (Boutros & Peters, 2012).

KEYCONCEPT Somatization (from *soma,* meaning body) is the manifestation of psychological distress as physical symptoms that may result in functional changes, somatic descriptions, or both.

Whereas some evidence suggests that somatization is a result of abnormally high levels of physiologic response

(Guo, Kleinstäuber, Johnson, & Sundram, 2019), other evidence supports the idea that somatization is the physical expression of personal problems or the internalization and expression of stress through physical symptoms (Kounou et al., 2017). For example, a woman quits her job complaining of chronic fatigue syndrome rather than recognizing that she is emotionally stressed from the constant harassment of a coworker.

Historically, the concept of somatization was linked to women and was related to a woman's body, mind, or even her soul. For example, the term *hysteria*, frequently associated with somatization, actually comes from ancient times when it was believed that a woman's unfounded physical symptoms were related to her "wandering or discontented uterus." Because *hystera* is the Greek word for uterus, the terms *hysteria* and *hysterical* were used to describe a woman whose physical or emotional symptoms could not be substantiated by physicians at that time.

Today, we understand that somatization is not linked to the uterus; both men and women can be affected by somatization. Much research is still needed in this area to be able to make any valid and reliable conclusions about gender and somatization (Soltis-Jarrett, 2004). Somatization also crosses all cultures and is recognized in almost every society (Wong, Tiwari, Fong, & Bullock, 2016). In many cultures, the expression of physical discomfort is more acceptable than acknowledging psychological distress. The disruption of routine body cycles, such as digestion, menstruation, or sleep, is more socially acceptable than having emotional responses related to interpersonal relationships, economic crises, adjustment to marriage, infertility, or the death of a spouse.

This chapter explores the holistic evidence-based nursing care for people experiencing the *DSM-5* group of disorders with the prominent symptom of somatization (American Psychiatric Association [APA], 2013). Somatic symptom disorder (SSD) is highlighted and illness anxiety disorder, conversion disorder, and factitious disorders are discussed.

SOMATIC SYMPTOM DISORDER

Nurses in primary care and medical–surgical settings are more likely than mental health nurses to encounter persons with these problems. Note: the term *somatoform* is no longer used in the *DSM-5* to describe these disorders (APA, 2013).

Clinical Course

Somatic symptom disorder (SSD) is one of the most difficult disorders to manage because its symptoms tend to change, are diffuse and complex, and vary and move from one body system to another. For example, initially gastrointestinal (e.g., nausea, vomiting, diarrhea) and neurologic (e.g., headache, backache) symptoms may be present that change to musculoskeletal (e.g., aching legs) and sexual issues (e.g., pain in the abdomen, pain during intercourse). Physical symptoms may last for 6 to 9 months (Kurlansik & Maffei, 2016).

Individuals with SSD perceive themselves as being "sicker than the sick" and report all aspects of their health as poor. Many eventually become disabled and unable to work. They typically visit health care providers many times each month and quickly become frustrated because their primary health care providers do not appreciate their level of suffering and are unable to validate that a particular problem accounts for their extreme discomfort. Consequently, individuals with SSD tend to "provider shop," moving from one to another until they find one who will give them new medication, hospitalize them, or perform surgery. Because the source of worrisome physical symptoms cannot be determined through medical or laboratory tests, medical or psychiatric interviews, or medical imaging, they repeatedly seek a medical reason for their discomfort and ask for relief from suffering. Depending on the severity, these individuals undergo multiple surgeries and even develop iatrogenic illnesses. People with SSD often evoke negative subjective responses in health care providers, who usually wish that the patient would go to someone else.

The most common characteristics are:

- Reporting the same symptoms repeatedly
- Receiving support from the environment that otherwise might not be forthcoming (e.g., gaining a spouse's attention because of severe back pain)
- Expressing concern about the physical problems inconsistent with the severity of the illness (being "sicker than the sick")

NCLEXNOTE Patients with SSD seek health care from multiple providers but often avoid mental health specialists.

Diagnostic Criteria

The diagnostic criteria of SSD include one or more symptoms that cause persistent distress or significant disruption in daily lives for at least 6 months and excessive thoughts about the seriousness of the symptoms, feelings (such as anxiety about the symptoms or overall health), or behaviors related to the symptoms or health concerns (e.g., spending excessive time and energy focusing on these symptoms or health) (APA, 2013). These symptoms may or may not be explained by medical evidence. The expression of the symptoms varies from population to population.

Somatic Symptom Disorder Across the Life Span

SSD is found in most populations and cultures even though its expression may vary from population to population. In cultures that highly stigmatize mental illness, somatic symptoms are more likely to appear (Lau et al., 2016).

Children and Adolescents

Although many children have somatic symptoms, SSD is not usually diagnosed until adolescence. However, when children have medical symptoms, further evaluation is needed so they are often referred to specialists to rule out physical, sexual, or emotional abuse or a comorbid psychiatric illness, such as depression or anxiety. In children, the most common symptoms are frequent abdominal pain, headache, fatigue, and nausea. Expression of somatic symptom in children tends to be overlooked or minimized when it needs to be identified as a risk factor for follow-up (Cerutti et al., 2017). In adolescents, initial symptoms are typically menstrual difficulties, and pelvic or abdominal pain. Risk factors for both children and adolescents need to be taken seriously. Research has shown a link between childhood sexual abuse and somatization, substance use, and depression in adults (Kealy, Rice, Ogrodniczuk, & Spidel, 2018; López & Yeater, 2018).

Older Adults

SSD can involve a lifelong pattern of symptoms that persist into old age. The symptoms of SSD, however, are often unrecognized by health care providers who tend to accept and minimize them as a part of the natural aging process after no medical cause is found.

Epidemiology

The estimated prevalence of SSD ranges from 5% to 7% (APA, 2013). Millions of dollars of lost revenue and the increased use of short- and long-term disability have prompted employers to study this unique population of employees. This disorder in believed to be higher than reported. In persons with fibromyalgia syndrome, nearly 25% meet the criteria for SSD (Hennignsen, 2018.)

Age of Onset

SSD usually begins before the age of 30 years with the first symptom often appearing during adolescence. Rarely diagnosed until several years later, seeking help can last for many years with the individual frequently going from one health care provider to another to no avail. The use of specific assessment instruments is increasing the likelihood of earlier diagnosis and treatment (Toussaint, Husing, Kohlmann, & Lowe, 2019).

Gender, Ethnic, and Cultural Differences

Epidemiologic studies have reported that SSD occurs primarily in nonwhite, less educated women, particularly those with a lower socioeconomic status and high emotional distress (Granot et al., 2018). Men are less likely to be diagnosed with SSD, partly because of stereotypic male traits, such as a disinclination to admit discomfort or seek help for their symptoms (APA, 2013).

Risk Factors

SSD tends to run in families, and children of parents with multiple unexplained somatic complaints are more likely to have somatic problems. Individuals with a tendency toward heightened physiologic arousal and a tendency to amplify somatosensory information have a greater risk of developing this disorder. Data have also confirmed a strong association between sexual trauma exposure and somatic symptoms, illness attitudes, and health care utilization in women (Granot et al., 2018; Henningsen, 2018).

Comorbidity

SSD frequently coexists with other psychiatric disorders, most commonly depression and anxiety. Others include posttraumatic stress disorder, panic disorder, social phobia, obsessive-compulsive disorder (OCD), psychotic disorders, and personality disorders (Newby, Hobbs, Mahoney, Wong, & Andrews, 2017). Older adults are at particularly high risk for comorbid depression (Johnson et al., 2017).

Ultimately, numerous unexplained medical problems also coexist with this disorder because many patients have received medical and surgical treatments, often unnecessarily, and are plagued with side effects. A disproportionately high number of women who eventually receive diagnoses of SSD have been treated for irritable bowel syndrome, polycystic ovary disease, and chronic pain.

Etiology

Biologic Theories

The cause of SSD is unknown. General agreement exists that somatization has a biopsychosocial basis with the possibility of biologic dysfunction common in depression and chronic fatigue syndrome. There are data to support the presence of anatomical and functional deficits in the cortico-limbic-cerebellar circuit (Li et al., 2018).

Although SSD has been shown to run in families, the exact transmission mechanism is unclear. Strong evidence suggests an increased risk for SSD in first-degree relatives, indicating a familial or genetic effect. Because many individuals with SSD live in chaotic families, the high prevalence in first-degree relatives could be explained by environmental influence.

Psychological Theories

Somatization has been explained as a form of social or emotional communication, meaning that the bodily symptoms express an emotion that cannot be verbalized by the individual. An adolescent who experiences severe abdominal pain after her parents argue or a wife who receives nurturing from her husband only when she has back pain are two examples. From this perspective, somatization may be a way of communicating and maintaining relationships. Following this line of reasoning, an individual's physical problems may also become a way of controlling relationships, so somatization becomes a learned behavior pattern. With time, physical symptoms develop automatically in response to perceived threats. Finally, SSD develops when somatizing becomes a way of life (Davoodi et al., 2018).

Consistent with a communication explanation, cognitive behaviorists explain somatization symptoms as an interaction of negative views of the world with physical factors (e.g., pain, discomfort). In this model, individuals have a heightened response based on their experiences with a stressor, especially if the stressor is uncontrollable and unpredictable. Over time, their exaggerated responses become an automatic pattern, resulting in "sick role" behavior, which in turn provokes either a negative or positive response in others (Dumont & Olson, 2012; Mik-Meyer & Obling, 2012).

Another theoretical explanation for somatization is the personality trait **alexithymia**, which is associated with SSD. Individuals with alexithymia have difficulty identifying and expressing their emotions. They have a preoccupation with external events and are described as concrete externally oriented thinkers (Taycan, Özdemir, & Erdoğan Taycan, 2017).

Credible evidence suggests a link between a history of childhood sexual abuse, rape, and domestic violence, and subsequent lifetime sequelae of somatic symptoms and somatic disorders (Granot et al., 2018).

Social Theories

SSD has been reported globally even though its conceptualization is primarily Western. The symptoms may vary from culture to culture. For example, studies in China have identified and discussed the notion of somatization as a moral issue rather than a medical problem. Somatization is a more socially acceptable way to express behavior in lieu of being diagnosed as depressed because in China, where mental illness is perceived as a character flaw. In many non-Western societies, where the mind–body distinction is not made and symptoms have different meanings and explanations, these physical manifestations are not labeled as a psychiatric disorder (Zhou et al., 2016) (Box 27.1). In Latin-American countries, depression is more likely described in somatic symptoms, such as headaches, gastrointestinal disturbances, or complaints of "nerves," rather than sadness or guilt (Yusim et al., 2010).

> **BOX 27.1**
>
> **Somatization in Chinese Culture**
>
> In Chinese tradition, the health of the individual reflects a balance between positive and negative forces within the body. Five elements at work in nature and in the body control health conditions (e.g., fire, water, wood, earth, metal), five viscera (e.g., liver, heart, spleen, kidneys, lungs), five emotions (anger, joy, worry, sorrow, fear), and five climatic conditions (e.g., wind, heat, humidity, dryness, cold). All illness is explained by imbalances among these elements. Because emotion is related to the circulation of vital air within the body, anger is believed to result from an adverse current of vital air to the liver. Emotional outbursts are seen as results of imbalances among the natural elements rather than the results of behavior of the person.
>
> The stigma of mental illness in the Chinese culture is so great that it can have an adverse effect on a family for many generations. If problems can be attributed to natural causes, the individual and family are less responsible, so that stigma is minimized. The Chinese have a culturally acceptable term for symptoms of mental distress—the closest translation of which would be *neurasthenia*—which comprises somatic complaints of headaches, insomnia, dizziness, aches and pains, poor memory, anxiety, weakness, and loss of energy.

Family Response to Disorder

Family dynamics are shaped by all members, including the person with SSD. When one member has several ongoing chronic health issues, family members' activities and interactions are affected. The physical symptoms of the individual become the focus of family life, so activities are planned around that person. Because so much time and so many resources are used trying to discover an underlying illness, resources to other family member are reduced. Because the person is always sick, expressing anger about the situation is difficult. The family members need support as they learn to understand the seriousness and difficulty of experiencing an SSD.

Recovery-Oriented Care for Persons With Somatic Symptom Disorder

Teamwork and Collaboration: Working Toward Recovery

The care of patients with SSD involves three approaches:

- Providing long-term supportive general management of the chronic condition

- Treating symptoms of comorbid psychiatric and physical problems (Soltis-Jarrett, 2011)
- Providing care in special settings, including individual and group treatment and the use of complementary and alternative medicine (Henningsen, 2018)
- The cornerstones of management are trust and believing. Ideally, the patient should see only one health care provider at regularly scheduled visits. During each primary care visit, the provider should conduct a holistic assessment including a partial physical examination of the organ system, focusing on the areas where the patient has complaints. Physical symptoms are treated conservatively using the least intrusive approach. The provider should also assess for any stressors, life changes, and/or a history of trauma that has been linked to the excessive expression of somatic symptoms. In the mental health setting, the use of cognitive behavioral therapy (CBT) can be effective (Liu, Gill, Teodorczuk, Li, & Sun, 2019).

Evidence-Based Mental Health Nursing Care of the Person With Somatic Symptom Disorder

Mental Health Nursing Assessment

During the assessment interview, the nurse should allow enough time for the patient to explain all medical problems; a hurried assessment interview blocks communication. Nursing Care Plan 27.1—which sets forth a plan of care for Carol, the case study patient in this chapter—is available at http://thepoint.lww.com/BoydEssentials2e.

> **NCLEXNOTE** Encourage and allow patients with SSD to discuss their physical problems before focusing on psychosocial issues.

Physical Health Assessment

Psychiatric–mental health nurses typically see these patients for problems related to a coexisting psychiatric disorder, such as depression, not because of the SSD. While taking the patient's history, the nurse may discover that the individual has had multiple surgeries or medical problems, making SSD a strong possibility. If the patient has not already received a diagnosis of SSD, the nurse should screen for it by determining the presence of the most commonly reported problems associated with this disorder, which include dysmenorrhea, a lump in the throat, vomiting, shortness of breath, burning sensation in the sex organs, painful limbs, and amnesia. If the patient has these symptoms, he or she should be seen by a mental health provider qualified to make the diagnosis. Box 27.2 presents the Health Attitude Survey, which can be used as a screening test for somatization.

BOX 27.2

Health Attitude Survey

On a scale of 1 to 5, please indicate the extent to which you agree (5) or disagree (1).

DISSATISFACTION WITH CARE
1. I have been satisfied with the medical care I have received. (R)
2. Doctors have done the best they could to diagnose and treat my health problems. (R)
3. Doctors have taken my health problems seriously.
4. My health problems have been thoroughly evaluated. (R)
5. Doctors do not seem to know much about the health problems I have had.
6. My health problems have been completely explained. (R)
7. Doctors seem to think I am exaggerating my health problems.
8. My response to treatment has not been satisfactory.
9. My response to treatment is usually excellent. (R)

FRUSTRATION WITH ILL HEALTH
10. I am tired of feeling sick and would like to get to the bottom of my health problems.
11. I have felt ill for quite a while now.
12. I am going to keep searching for an answer to my health problems.
13. I do not think there is anything seriously wrong with my body. (R)

HIGH UTILIZATION OF CARE
14. I have seen many different doctors over the years.
15. I have taken a lot of medicines recently.
16. I do not go to the doctor often. (R)
17. I have had relatively good health over the years.

EXCESSIVE HEALTH WORRY
18. I sometimes worry too much about my health.
19. I often fear the worst when I develop symptoms.
20. I have trouble getting my mind off my health.

PSYCHOLOGICAL DISTRESS
21. Sometimes I feel depressed and cannot seem to shake it off.
22. I have sought help for emotional or stress-related problems.
23. It is easy to relax and stay calm. (R)
24. I believe the stress I am under may be affecting my health.

DISCORDANT COMMUNICATION OF DISTRESS
25. Some people think that I am capable of more work than I feel able to do.
26. Some people think that I have been sick just to gain attention.
27. It is difficult for me to find the right words for my feelings.

(R) indicates items reversed for scoring purposes. Scoring—The higher the score, the more likely somatization is a problem.

From Noyes, R. Jr., Langbehn, D., Happel, R., Sieren, L., & Muller, B. (1999). Health Attitude Survey: A scale for assessing somatizing patients. *Psychosomatics, 40*(6), 470–478.

Review of Systems. Although these patients' symptoms have usually received considerable attention from the medical community, a careful review of systems is important because the appearance of physical problems is usually related to psychosocial problems. Even as the patient continues to be seen for mental health problems, an ongoing awareness of biologic symptoms is important, particularly because these symptoms are de-emphasized in the overall case management.

Pain is the most common finding in people with this disorder. Because the pain is usually related to symptoms of all the major body systems, it is unlikely that a somatic intervention such as an analgesic will be effective on a long-term basis. Remember that although no medical explanation exists for the pain, the patient's pain is real and has serious psychosocial implications. A careful assessment should include the following questions:

- What is the pain like?
- What is the extent of the pain?
- What helps the pain get better?
- When is the pain at its worst?
- What has worked in the past to relieve the pain?

Physical Functioning. The actual physical functioning of these individuals is often marginal. They usually have problems with sleep, fatigue, activity, and sexual functioning. Assessment of these areas generates data to be used in planning interventions. The amount and quality of sleep are important, as are the hours when the individual sleeps. For example, an individual may sleep a total of 6 hours each diurnal cycle but only from 2:00 to 6:00 am plus an afternoon nap.

Fatigue is a constant problem for many people with SSD, and because various physical problems interfere with normal activity. These patients report an overwhelming lack of energy, which makes maintaining usual routines or accomplishing daily tasks impossible. Fatigue is accompanied by the inability to concentrate on simple functions, leading to decreased performance and disinterest in surroundings. Patients tend to be lethargic and listless and often have little energy (Box 27.3).

Female patients with this disorder usually have had multiple gynecologic problems, so that the physical manifestations of SSD often lead to altered sexual behavior. Symptoms of dysmenorrhea and painful intercourse may indicate a history of sexual abuse and sexual trauma. Physiologic indicators, such as those produced by laboratory tests, are not available. However, a careful assessment of the patient's menstrual history, gynecologic problems, and sexual functioning is important. It is also important to assess whether abuse or trauma has occurred in the past or continues in the present, and whether such abuse is sexual, physical, or emotional.

Medication Assessment. A medication assessment of these patients can be challenging. Patients with SSD frequently seek help from numerous providers because they do not feel that they are believed, or they think that providers don't care about their suffering. Because they often receive medications from each provider, they are usually taking a large number of drugs. A medication assessment is needed not only because of the number of medications but also because these individuals frequently experience

BOX 27.3 CLINICAL VIGNETTE

Somatic Symptom Disorder and Stress

Ms. J, age 42 years, has been coming to the mental health clinic for 2 years for her nerves. She has seen only the physician for medication but now has been referred to the nurse's new stress management group because she is experiencing side effects to all the medications that have been tried. The psychiatrist has diagnosed SSD and wants her to learn to manage her "nerves" without medication.

At the first meeting with the nurse, Ms. J was preoccupied with chest pain and bloating that had lasted for the past 6 months. Her chest pain is constant and sharp at times. The pain does not prevent her from going to her job as a waitress but does interfere with meal preparation at night for her family and her ability to have sexual intercourse. She has numerous other physical problems, including allergies to certain perfumes, dysmenorrhea, ovarian polycystic disease (ovarian cysts), chronic urinary tract infections, and rashes. She is constantly fatigued and has frequent leg cramps. She states that she is too tired to fix dinner for her family. On days off from work, she takes a nap in the afternoon, sleeping until evening. She is unable to fall asleep at night.

She believes that she will soon have to have her gallbladder removed because of occasional referred pain to her back and nausea that occurs a couple hours after eating. She is not enthusiastic about a stress management group and does not believe it will help her problems. However, she has agreed to consider it for as long as the psychiatrist will continue prescribing diazepam (Valium).

What Do You Think?
- How would you prioritize Ms. J's physical symptoms?
- What are some possible explanations for Ms. J's fatigue?

unusual side effects, or they report that they are "sensitive" to medications. Because of their somatic sensitivity, they often overreact to medication. Developing a therapeutic relationship promotes trust and can minimize these patients' search for a health care professional who believes their symptoms and suffering.

These patients spend much of their lives trying to find out what is wrong with them. When one health care provider after another can find little if any explanation for their symptoms, many patients become anxious and/or depressed. To alleviate their symptoms of anxiety, they sometimes self-medicate with over-the-counter (OTC) medications and/or substances of abuse (e.g., alcohol, marijuana), or they seek a health care provider who prescribes a benzodiazepine such as alprazolam. Because symptoms associated with their disorder cannot be treated within a few weeks with a benzodiazepine, they can become dependent on medication that should not have been prescribed in the first place.

Although benzodiazepines have a place in therapeutics, they are not recommended for long-term use and only complicate the treatment of individuals with SSD. These medications should also be avoided because of their addictive qualities, which place patients at risk of addiction. Unfortunately, by the time patients with SSD see a mental health provider, they often have already begun taking the medications for anxiety. Many times, they only agree to see a mental health provider because the last provider would no longer prescribe an anxiolytic without a psychiatric evaluation.

Remember Carol?
Carol has been taking alprazolam for stress for years. Her primary health care provider is refusing to prescribe it again until she has a complete mental health examination. No other health care providers will prescribe alprazolam for her.

Psychosocial Assessment

The mental status of individuals with SSD can be within normal limits, although most patients report frustration, depression, and hopelessness about their situation. What is most noticeable is their intense focus on their bodies and the physical symptoms that are causing them distress and disability.

Generally, cognition is not impaired in people with SSD, but it may be distorted, such as believing the pain means a life-threatening condition. These individuals seem preoccupied with the signs and symptoms of their illnesses and may even keep a record of their experiences. Living with illness, diseases, and suffering truly becomes a way of life.

Some individuals with SSD have intense emotional reactions to life stressors and have led or are leading traumatic or chaotic lives. These patients usually have had a series of personal crises beginning at an early age. Examples include severe sexual and physical abuse and psychological trauma. Typically, a new symptom or medical problem develops during times of emotional stress as well as during anniversaries of losses or traumas that have occurred in the patient's lifetime. It is critical that the link between the physical assessment data and the patient's psychological and social history are considered. A thorough history of major psychological events should be compared with the chronology of physical problems. Special attention should be paid to any history of sexual abuse or trauma in the patient's younger years. Early sexual abuse also may prevent the individual from being able to perform sexually or to have to endure chronic abdominal pain or discomfort during sexual relations.

The individual's mood is usually labile, often shifting from extremely excited or anxious to being depressed and hopeless. Response to physical symptoms is usually magnified, such as interpreting a simple cold as pneumonia or a brief chest pain as a heart attack. Family members may not believe the physical symptoms are real and may view them as attention-getting behavior because symptoms often improve when the patient receives attention. For example, a woman who has been in bed for 3 weeks with severe back pain may suddenly feel much better when her children visit her.

Social Network. People with this disorder spend excessive time seeking medical care and treating their multiple illnesses. Because they believe themselves to be very sick, they also believe that they are disabled and cannot work. Many are unemployed, so frequently these individuals have changed jobs, had multiple positions over their lifetimes or careers, or have had absences or gaps in employment (Sharma & Manjula, 2013).

Because their symptoms are often inconsistent with any identifiable medical diagnosis, these individuals are rarely satisfied with their health care providers who can find nothing wrong. However, their social network often consists of a series of health care providers, rather than peers or family members, who can also become weary of the individual's constant complaints of physical problems. Identifying a support network requires sorting out the health care providers from family and friends.

Consider Carol's Limited Social Network
Carol has no friends and spends her time going from provider to provider. Her anxiety about her symptoms have impacted her ability to maintain friendships and other close relationships.

Family Issues. Individuals with SSD sometimes live in chaotic families with multiple problems. In assessing the family structure, other members with psychiatric disorders must be identified. Women may be married to abusive men who have antisocial personality disorders; substance use disorders are common. Identifying the positive and negative relationships within the family is important.

SSD is particularly problematic because it disrupts the family's social life. Changes in routine or major life events often precipitate the appearance of a symptom. For example, a person may be planning a vacation with the family but at the last minute decides she cannot go because her back pain has returned, and she will not be able to sit in the car. These family disruptions are common. In addition, as already noted, employment history for the person with SSD may be erratic.

Strengths Assessment

A person with SSD may have difficulty identifying *any* personal strengths. The nurse should help the person focus on daily activities and suggest strengths that emerge. For example, some strengths might be that the person has a place to live, has a caring family, or some educational attainment. The nurse also elicits motivation to feel better.

Priority of Nursing Care

The physical issues dominate the individual's concern and should not be dismissed. They may have a variety of health issues to discuss including fatigue, pain, and insomnia. Psychologically, depression and suicidal behavior should always be considered. Social isolation may be an outward expression of depression.

Development of a Therapeutic Relationship

The most difficult aspect of nursing care is developing a sound, positive, nonjudgmental nurse–patient relationship, yet this relationship is crucial. Without it, the nurse is just one more provider who fails to meet the patient's expectations. Developing this relationship requires time and patience. Therapeutic communication techniques should be used to refocus the patient on psychosocial problems related to the physical manifestations (Box 27.4).

During periods when symptoms of other psychiatric disorders surface, additional interventions are needed. For example, if depression occurs, additional supportive or cognitive approaches may be needed.

Carol's Behavior on the Mental Health Unit
Carol felt she was tricked into agreeing to be admitted to a mental health unit for medication evaluation. She believes she should be on a medical unit for her constant pain.

Mental Health Nursing Interventions

Establishing Recovery and Wellness Goals

Establishing recovery and wellness goals may seem to be out of the question with individuals who defines themselves as "ill," "sick," and/or in "chronic pain." However, helping such individuals define their symptoms and validate them is a start to recovery. Nurses are poised to educate individuals with multiple somatic problems to better understand their symptoms (e.g., what triggers them) and to define short-term goals for recovery. The notion of recovery itself is patient-centered and focused on what the patient believes is realistic and possible. For example, some patients with this disorder may choose to learn to live with their symptoms (e.g., pain) and find alternative ways of coping. Nursing interventions can focus on individuals learning the triggers in their lives that worsen their symptoms as well as those activities that lessen them. Even though a patient may suffer from multiple somatic symptoms and/or this chronic illness, together the nurse and the patient can work toward setting short- and long-term goals that promote health and wellness.

Physical Health Interventions

Nursing interventions that focus on physical health become especially important because medical treatment must be conservative; aggressive pharmacologic treatment must be avoided. Each time a nurse sees the patient, some of that time should be spent respectfully discussing physical complaints and validating the patient's distress. During the discussion, it is important that the nurse project the belief that the patient is truly experiencing the symptoms. Several physically focused interventions, including pain management, activity enhancement, nutrition regulation, relaxation, and pharmacologic interventions, may be useful in caring for patients with SSD.

Pain Management

In pain management, a single approach rarely works. Pain is a primary issue and was previously considered a separate disorder. Nursing care focuses on helping patients identify strategies to relieve pain and to examine stressors in their lives. After a careful assessment of the pain, nonpharmacologic strategies should be developed to reduce it. If gastrointestinal pain is frequent, eating and bowel habits should be explored and modified as needed. For back pain, exercises and consultation from a physical therapist may be useful. Headaches are a challenge. Self-monitoring and tracking them engages the patient in the therapeutic process and helps to identify psychosocial triggers. In addition, suggesting or referring the individual for complementary and alternative treatments may be useful (Henningsen, 2018). Relaxation techniques, identifying thoughts and feelings about pain or discomfort, and including family members in the intervention have also been shown to be useful.

Activity Enhancement

Helping the patient establish a daily routine may alleviate some of the difficulty with sleep, but doing so may be difficult because most of these patients are not employed. Encouraging the patient to get up in the morning and go to bed at night at specific times can help the patient to establish a routine. These patients should engage in regular exercise to improve their overall physical state, although they often have numerous reasons why they cannot. This is where the nurse's patience is tested; the nurse ultimately needs to remember that the patient's symptoms are an expression of suffering. Agreeing that daily exercise is difficult but continuing to emphasize the

BOX 27.4 • THERAPEUTIC DIALOGUE • Establishing a Relationship

INEFFECTIVE APPROACH

Nurse: Good morning, Carol.
Carol: I'm in so much pain. Take that breakfast away.
Nurse: You don't want your breakfast?
Carol: Can't you see? I hurt! When I hurt, I can't eat!
Nurse: If you don't eat now, you probably won't be able to have anything until lunch.
Carol: Who cares? I have no intention of being here at lunchtime. I don't belong here.
Nurse: Carol, I don't think that your doctor would have admitted you unless there were a problem. I would like to talk to you about why you are here.
Carol: Nurse, I'm just here. It's none of your business.
Nurse: Oh.
Carol: Please leave me alone.
Nurse: Sure, I will see you later.

EFFECTIVE APPROACH

Nurse: Good morning, Carol.
Carol: I'm in so much pain. Take that breakfast away.
Nurse: (Silently removes tray. Pulls up chair and sits down.)
Carol: My back hurts.
Nurse: Oh, when did the back pain start?
Carol: Last night. It's this bed. I couldn't get comfortable.
Nurse: These beds can be pretty uncomfortable.
Carol: My back pain is shooting down my leg.
Nurse: Does anything help it?
Carol: Sometimes if I straighten out my leg it helps.
Nurse: Can I help you straighten out your leg?
Carol: Oh, it's OK. The pain is going away. What did you say your name is?
Nurse: I'm Susan Miller, your nurse while you are here.
Carol: I won't be here long. I don't belong in a psychiatric unit.
Nurse: While you are here, I would like to spend time with you.
Carol: OK, but you understand, I do not have any psychiatric problems.
Nurse: We can talk about whatever you want. But because you want to get out of here, we might want to focus on what it will take to get you ready for discharge.

CRITICAL THINKING CHALLENGE

- What communication mistakes did the nurse in the first scenario make?
- What communication strategies helped the patient feel comfortable with the nurse in the second scenario?
- How is the first scenario different from the second?

---

importance of exercise can counter some of the reluctance to exercise.

Nutrition Regulation

Patients with SSD often have gastrointestinal problems and may have special nutritional needs. The nurse should discuss the nutritional value of foods with the patient. Discussing the use of whole healthy food sources rather than processed or "junk" food is a strategy nurses can use to assist the patient with gastrointestinal distress to consider dietary changes. The act of talking with patients about ways that they can exert some control of their bodies can have a positive effect and assist them with managing some of their symptoms. If patients are being prescribed medications that promote weight gain, weight control strategies may be discussed, including exercise or increasing movement with physical therapy.

Relaxation

Patients taking anxiety-relieving medication can be taught relaxation techniques to alleviate stress. It is a challenge to help these patients really use these strategies. The nurse should consider various techniques, including simple relaxation techniques, distraction, and guided imagery (see Chapter 9).

Medications Interventions

No medication is specifically recommended for patients with SSD; however, psychiatric symptoms of comorbid disorders, such as depression and anxiety, should be treated pharmacologically as appropriate (Soltis-Jarrett, 2011). Usually, the patients who are depressed or anxious are taking an antidepressant to treat their symptoms (see Chapter 21).

Multiple antidepressants have been shown to be effective for treating pain and the symptoms of depression. Duloxetine—a serotonin and norepinephrine reuptake inhibitor that is indicated for neuropathy, depression, and anxiety—is also used to manage pain (Brammer, 2018). See Box 27.5.

Patients who report symptoms of anxiety are treated pharmacologically, similar to those with depression. The first line of treatment for all anxiety disorders is with a selective serotonin reuptake inhibitor (SSRI). Doses for SSD are usually higher than those prescribed for depression to relieve and manage the symptoms of the anxiety disorders, including panic, social phobia, generalized anxiety, OCD, and posttraumatic stress disorder.

Nonpharmacologic approaches such as biofeedback and relaxation are also quite useful in conjunction with pharmacologic treatment. Benzodiazepines may be used initially in the treatment of those with anxiety but should be slowly decreased and discontinued because of the psychological and physiologic dependence associated with these medications. Buspirone (Buspar), a nonbenzodiazepine, does not lead to tolerance or withdrawal and may be useful for relief of acute anxiety. Buspar should be used cautiously with other serotonin-related medications (such as SSRIs) because of its high affinity for serotonin receptors. If panic disorder is present, it should be treated aggressively with SSRIs and frequently at higher doses.

Pain medication should be prescribed conservatively. If mood disorders are also present, some mood stabilizers not only treat the depression but also may treat the pain.

BOX 27.5

Drug Profile: Duloxetine

DRUG CLASS: Serotonin and norepinephrine reuptake inhibitor (SNRI)

RECEPTOR AFFINITY: Binds selectively and has a high affinity to both norepinephrine (NE) and serotonin (5-HT) transporters yet lacks affinity for monoamine receptors within the central nervous system.

INDICATIONS: Treatment of depression, generalized anxiety disorder, chronic musculoskeletal pain, diabetic peripheral neuropathic pain, fibromyalgia

ROUTE AND DOSAGE: Available as capsules: 30 mg, 60 mg

Adults: Initially, 60 mg daily and increasing to 90 mg/d consistent with patient tolerance. Therapy at 120 mg/d may be necessary before response occurs. Can be given in divided doses for individuals who are used to taking pain medication twice a day.

Geriatric: Adjust dosage as needed because older patients—particularly those on other medications—are more prone to develop side effects. May initiate dose of 30 mg daily for 2 weeks.

Pediatric: Not recommended for children younger than 18 years of age

HALF-LIFE (PEAK EFFECTS): Duloxetine has an elimination half-life of about 12 hours (the range is 8 to 17 hours). Steady state is usually achieved after 3 days.

SELECTED SIDE EFFECTS: Nausea, dry mouth, constipation, diarrhea, fatigue, difficulty sleeping, and dizziness. Increased blood pressure can occur and should be monitored. Seizures have been reported. Sexual dysfunction (decreased sex drive and delayed orgasm and ejaculation) has been associated with duloxetine.

BOXED WARNING: Suicidal thoughts and behaviors

WARNINGS: Screen for bipolar disorder, monitor for serotonin syndrome; monitor blood pressure before and after dosage is initiated (e.g., weekly for 1 month), screen for medication-to-medication interactions.

SPECIFIC PATIENT/FAMILY EDUCATION

- Take drug exactly as prescribed; do not stop taking it abruptly or without consulting your health care provider.
- If patients wish to stop the medication, they need to consult with their provider about tapering the dose due to discontinuation syndrome, a cluster of physical and emotional symptoms that are associated with decreasing SNRIs and SSRIs too quickly. Symptoms of abrupt discontinuation can include: dizziness, anxiety, nausea, vomiting, nervousness, and diarrhea.
- Families and caregivers of patients should be advised to observe for the emergence of anxiety, agitation, panic attacks, insomnia, irritability, hostility, aggressiveness, impulsivity, hypomania, mania, other unusual changes in behavior, worsening of depression, and suicidal ideation. Such symptoms should be reported to the patient's prescriber or health professional, especially if side effects are severe, abrupt in onset, or were not part of the patient's presenting symptoms.
- Report any signs and symptoms of side effects.
- Combining duloxetine with aspirin, nonsteroidal anti-inflammatory drugs (NSAIDs), warfarin (Coumadin), or other drugs that are associated with bleeding may increase the risk of bleeding.

An example is gabapentin, another frequently prescribed medication for neuropathic pain experienced during and after herpes zoster (also commonly known as shingles).

Administering and Monitoring Medications. In SSD, patients are usually treated in the community, where they commonly self-medicate. Carefully question patients about self-administered medicine and determine which medicines or substances they are currently using to relieve their pain and/or discomfort (including OTC, herbal supplements, and/or illicit substances). Also listen carefully to determine any side effects the patient attributes to the medication. This information should be documented and reported to the rest of the team. The patient should be encouraged to continue taking only prescribed medication and to seek approval before taking any additional OTC or other prescribed medications. SSD patients are at high risk for prescription drug misuse and abuse as well as for purchasing substances illicitly. The recent trends of prescription drug misuse have been linked to opioid use disorder and overdose (SAMHSA, 2018).

Managing Side Effects. These individuals often have atypical reactions to their medications. Side effects should be assessed, but the patient should be encouraged to compare the benefits of the medication with any problems related to side effects. Patients should also be encouraged to give the medications enough time to be effective because many medications require up to 6 weeks before the patient has a response or experiences a relief of symptoms. This is especially true for patients who are prescribed some of the antidepressants that have been in use the longest, such as fluoxetine.

Monitoring for Drug Interactions. In working with patients with SSD, always be on the lookout for drug–drug interactions. Medications these patients take for physical problems could interact with psychiatric medications. Patients may be taking alternative medicines, such as herbal supplements, but they usually willingly disclose doing so. The patient should be encouraged to use the same pharmacy for filling all prescriptions so possible interactions can be checked and monitored.

Psychosocial Interventions

The choice of psychosocial intervention depends on the specific problem the patient is experiencing. The most important and ongoing intervention is the maintenance of a therapeutic relationship.

Reduction of Patient Anxiety About Illness

Several interventions are effective in reducing patients' fears of experiencing serious illnesses. CBT, stress management, and group interventions may lead to a decrease in intensity and increase in control of symptoms (Wortman et al., 2018). Whether the positive outcomes result from the intervention itself or from the symptom validation and increased attention given to the patient remains unknown. Other interventions include the use of antidepressants in reducing depressive and anxiety-related symptoms. Nursing care should include listening to the patient's report of symptoms and fears, validating it by acknowledging that the fears may be real, asking the patient to monitor symptoms in a journal, and encouraging the patient to bring the journal to the next visit. By reviewing the symptom pattern, it is possible to continue to educate the patient and assess for significant symptoms. The outcome of this approach should be a decrease in fears and better control of the symptoms.

Counseling

Counseling with a focus on problem-solving is needed from time to time. These patients often have chaotic lives and need support through the multitude of crises. Although they may appear fascinating and at times self-assured, they can easily irritate others because of their constant complaints. The consequences of their impaired social interaction with others must be examined within a counseling framework. It will become evident that the patient's problem-solving and decision-making skills could be improved. Identifying stresses and strengthening positive coping responses helps the patient deal with a chaotic lifestyle.

Psychoeducation

Health teaching is useful throughout the nurse–patient relationship. These patients have many questions about illnesses, symptoms, and treatments. Emphasize positive health care practices and minimize the effects of serious illness. Because of problems in managing medications and treatment, the therapeutic regimen needs constant monitoring, resulting in ample opportunities for teaching. Patients with SSD should focus on "staying healthy" instead of focusing on their illnesses. For these individuals, approaching the topic of health promotion usually has to be within the context of preventing further problems. Setting aside time for themselves and identifying activities that meet their psychological and spiritual needs, such as going to church or synagogue, are important in maintaining a healthy balance (Box 27.6).

Social Relationships. Patients with SSD are usually isolated from their families and communities. Strengthening social relationships and activities often becomes the focus of the nursing care. The nurse should help the patient identify individuals with whom contact is desired, ask

BOX 27.6

Psychoeducation Checklist: Somatic Symptom Disorder

When caring for a patient with SSD, be sure to include the following topic areas in the teaching plan:
- Psychopharmacologic agents (anxiolytics) if ordered, including drug, action, dosage, frequency, and possible side effects
- Nonpharmacologic pain relief measures
- Exercise
- Nutrition
- Social interaction
- Appropriate health care practices
- Problem-solving
- Relaxation and anxiety-reduction techniques
- Sexual functioning

for a commitment to contact them, and encourage them to reinitiate the relationship. The nurse should counsel patients about talking too much about their symptoms with these individuals and emphasize that medical information should be shared with the nurse instead. The nurse must also ensure that patients know when their next appointments are scheduled.

Group Interventions. Although these patients may not be candidates for insight group psychotherapy, they do benefit from cognitive behavioral groups that focus on developing coping skills for everyday life (Liu et al., 2019). Because most are women, participation in groups that address feminist issues should be encouraged to strengthen their assertiveness skills and improve their generally low self-esteem.

When leading a group that has members with this disorder, redirection can keep the group from giving too much attention to a person's illness. However, these individuals need reassurance and support while in a group. They may say that they do not fit in or belong in the group. In reality, they are feeling insecure and threatened by the situation. The group leader needs to show patience and understanding to engage the individual effectively in meaningful group interaction.

Family Interventions

The results of a family assessment often reveal that families of these individuals need education about the disorder, helpful strategies for dealing with the multiple complaints of the patient, and usually help in developing more effective communication patterns. Because of the chaotic nature of some of the families and the lack of healthy problem-solving, physical, sexual, and psychological abuse may be evident. It is important to be particularly sensitive to any evidence of current physical or sexual abuse because this may lead to a need for additional interventions.

Wellness Strategies

Wellness strategies should be included in the discussion of the interventions. The same interventions that were discussed in reducing the symptoms of SSD are also used as wellness strategies.

Evaluation and Treatment Outcomes

Recovery outcomes for patients with SSD should be realistic. Because this is a lifelong disorder, small successes should be expected. Specific outcomes should be identified, such as gradually increasing social contact. Over time, a gradual reduction in the number of health care providers the individual contacts should occur and a slight improvement in the ability to cope with stresses should follow.

Continuum of Care

Inpatient Care

Ideally, individuals with SSD spend minimal time in the hospital for treatment of their medical or comorbid mental disorders. While an inpatient, the patient should have consistency in providers who care or oversee all nursing care. Therapeutic interactions and relationships are very important and can help move the individual toward recovery.

Emergency Care

The emergencies these individuals experience may be physical (e.g., chest pain, back pain, gastrointestinal symptoms) or stress responses related to a psychosocial crisis. Occasionally, these individuals become suicidal and require an intensive level of care. Generally speaking, nonpharmacologic interventions should be tried first, with very conservative use of antianxiety medications. All attempts should be made to retrieve records from other facilities.

Community Treatment

These patients can spend a lifetime in the health care system and still have little continuity of care. Switching from one health care provider to others is detrimental to their long-term care. Most are outpatients. When they are hospitalized, it is usually for evaluation of medical problems or to receive care for comorbid disorders.

ILLNESS ANXIETY DISORDER

Illness anxiety disorder is a new classification in the *DSM-5*. Previously, the term *hypochondriasis* (or hypochondria) was used to designate this disorder. Most of the persons with hypochondriasis were also diagnosed with SSD. However, there are some individuals who either do not have somatic symptoms or have only very mild symptoms, but who remain preoccupied with having or developing a medical illness (APA, 2013). These individuals would receive the diagnosis of illness anxiety disorder and would be encouraged to seek mental health treatment for their anxiety and preoccupation.

Individuals with illness anxiety disorder are fearful about developing a serious illness based on their misinterpretation of body sensations. The fear of having an illness continues despite medical reassurance and interferes with psychosocial functioning. They spend time and money on repeated examinations looking for feared illnesses. For example, an occasional cough or the appearance of a small sore results in the person's making an appointment with an oncologist. An illness anxiety disorder sometimes appears if the person had had a serious childhood illness or if a family member has a serious illness.

CONVERSION DISORDER (FUNCTIONAL NEUROLOGIC SYMPTOM DISORDER)

Conversion disorder is a psychiatric condition in which severe emotional distress or unconscious conflict is expressed through physical symptoms (APA, 2013). Patients with conversion disorder have neurologic symptoms that include impaired coordination or balance, paralysis, aphonia (i.e., inability to produce sound), difficulty swallowing or a sensation of a lump in the throat, and urinary retention. They may also have loss of touch, vision problems, blindness, deafness, and hallucinations. In some instances, they may have seizures (Galli, Tatu, Bogousslavsky, & Aybek, 2018). However, laboratory, electroencephalographic, and neurologic test results are typically negative. The symptoms, different from those with an organic basis, do not follow a neurologic course but rather follow the person's own perceived conceptualization of the problem. For example, if the arm is paralyzed and will not move, reflexes and muscle tone may still be present.

Some evidence suggests that there are neurobiologic changes in the brains of people with this disorder that may be responsible for the loss of sensation or control of movement. Stress may also be a contributing factor. Published reports state that childhood trauma (e.g., sexual abuse) is associated with the later development of conversion disorder (Conejero et al., 2018).

It is important to understand that the lack of physical sensation and movement is real for the patient. In approaching the patient, the nurse treats conversion symptoms as real symptoms that may have distressing psychological aspects. Acknowledging the symptoms helps the patient deal with them. As trust develops within the nurse–patient relationship, the nurse can help the patient develop problem-solving approaches to everyday problems.

FACTITIOUS DISORDERS

Factitious disorders are very different from SSDs. Persons with **factitious disorders** intentionally cause an illness or injury to receive the attention of health care workers. These individuals are motivated solely by the desire to become a patient and develop a dependent relationship with a health care provider. There are two types of factitious disorders: factitious disorder and factitious disorder imposed on another.

FACTITIOUS DISORDER

Although feigned illnesses have been described for centuries, it was not until 1951 that the term *Münchausen's* [sic] *syndrome* was used to describe the most severe form of this disorder, which was characterized by fabricating a physical illness, having recurrent hospitalizations, and going from one health care provider to another (Asher, 1951). Today, this disorder is called *factitious disorder* and is differentiated from malingering, in which the individual who intentionally produces symptoms of illness and is motivated by another specific self-serving goal, such as being classified as disabled or avoiding work.

Clinical Course and Diagnostic Criteria

Unlike people with borderline personality disorder, who typically injure themselves overtly and readily admit to self-harm, patients with factitious disorder injure themselves covertly. The illnesses are produced in such a manner that the health care provider is tricked into believing that a true physical or psychiatric disorder is present (Tatu, Aybek, & Bogousslavsky, 2018).

The self-produced physical symptoms appear as medical illnesses and involve all body systems. They include seizure disorders, wound-healing disorders, the abscess processes (i.e., introduction of infectious material below the skin surface), and feigned fever (rubbing the thermometer). These patients are extremely creative in simulating illnesses. They tell fascinating but false stories of personal triumph. These tales are referred to as pseudologia fantastica and are a core symptom of the disorder. **Pseudologia fantastica** are stories that are not entirely improbable and often contain a mixture of truth and falsehood. These patients falsify blood, urine, and other samples by contaminating them with protein or fecal matter. They self-inject anticoagulants to receive diagnoses of "bleeding of undetermined origin" or ingest thyroid hormones to produce thyrotoxicosis. They also inflict injury on themselves by inserting objects or feces into body orifices, such as the urinary tract, open wounds, or even intravenous tubing. They produce their own surgical scars, especially abdominal, and when treated surgically, they delay wound healing through scratching, rubbing, or manipulating the wound and introducing bacteria into the wound. These patients put themselves in life-threatening situations through actions such as ingesting allergens known to produce an anaphylactic reaction.

Patients who manifest primarily psychological symptoms produce psychotic symptoms such as hallucinations and delusions, cognitive deficits such as memory loss, dissociative symptoms such as amnesia, and conversion symptoms such as pseudoblindness or pseudoparalysis. These individuals often become psychotic, depressed, or suicidal after an unconfirmed tragedy. When questioned about details, they become defensive and uncooperative. Sometimes these individuals have a combination of both physical and psychiatric symptoms.

Epidemiology and Risk Factors

The prevalence of factitious disorder is unknown because diagnosing it and obtaining reliable data are difficult. The prevalence was reported to be high when researchers were actually looking for the disorder in specific populations. Within large general hospitals, factitious disorders are diagnosed in about 1% of patients with whom mental health professionals consult. The age range of patients with the disorder is between 19 and 64 years. The median age of onset is the early 20s. Formerly thought to occur predominantly in men, this disorder is now reported predominantly in women. No genetic pattern has been identified, but it does seem to run in families. The presence of comorbid psychiatric disorders, such as mood disorders, personality disorders, and substance-related disorders, is common. Health care professionals, nurses, pharmacists, and physicians are over-represented in the occurrence of this disorder (Jimenez, Nkanginieme, Dhand, Karafa, & Salerno, 2019).

Etiology

Many people with factitious disorder have experienced severe sexual abuse, trauma, and/or distress before the development of the disorder. The psychodynamic explanation is that these individuals, who were often abused as children, received nurturance only during times of illness; thus, they try to recreate illness or injury in a desperate attempt to receive love and attention. During the actual self-injury, the individual is reported to be in a trancelike, dissociative state. Many patients report having an intimate relationship with a health care provider, either as a child or as an adult, and then experiencing rejection when the relationship ended. The self-injury and subsequent attention is an attempt by the individual to re-enact those experiences and gain control over the situation and the other person (Jimenez et al., 2019).

These patients are usually discovered in medical–surgical settings. They are hostile and distance themselves from others. Their network is void of friends and family and usually consists only of health care providers, who change at regular intervals. In factitious disorder, the patient fabricates a detailed and exaggerated medical history. When the interventions do not work and the fabrication is discovered, the health care team feels manipulated and angry. When the patient is confronted with the evidence, he or she becomes enraged and often leaves that health care system, only to enter another. Eventually, the person is referred for mental health treatment. The course of the disorder usually consists of intermittent episodes.

Evidence-Based Nursing Care for Persons With Factitious Disorder

The overall goal of treatment for a patient with factitious disorder is to replace the dysfunctional attention-seeking behaviors with positive behaviors. To begin treatment, the patient must acknowledge the deception. Because the pattern of self-injury is well established and meets overwhelming psychological needs, giving up the behaviors is difficult. The treatment is long-term psychotherapy. The psychiatric–mental health nurse will most likely care for the patient during or after periods of feigned illnesses.

Mental Health Nursing Assessment

A nursing assessment should focus on obtaining a history of medical and psychological illnesses. Physical disabilities should be identified. Early childhood experiences, particularly instances of abuse, neglect, or abandonment, should be identified to understand the underlying psychological dynamics of the individual and the role of self-injury. Family assessment is important because family relationships become strained as the members become aware of the self-inflicted nature of this disorder.

Priority of Care

The consequences of self-injury are the first priority. Medical treatment may be needed. The patient is at high risk for self abuse as discovery unfolds.

Desired outcomes include decreased self-injurious behavior and increased positive coping behaviors. Any nursing intervention must be implemented within the context of a strong nurse–patient relationship. A nonjudgmental attitude is imperative.

Nursing Interventions

The fabrications and deceits of patients with factitious disorder provoke anger and a sense of betrayal in many nurses. To be effective with these patients, it is important to be aware of these feelings and resolve them by developing a better understanding of the underlying psychodynamic issues. Confronting the patient has been reported to be effective only if the patient feels supported and accepted and if there is clear communication among the patient, the mental health care team, and family members. All care should be centralized within one facility. The patient should see health care providers regularly even when not in active crisis. Offering the patient a tactful way of giving up the behaviors is often crucial. Behavioral techniques that shape new behaviors help the patient move forward toward a new life.

The health care team that knows the patient, agrees on a treatment approach, and follows through is crucial to the patient's eventual recovery. For this to happen, the medical, psychiatric, inpatient, and outpatient teams need to communicate with each other on a regular basis. Family members must also be aware of the need for consistent treatment.

FACTITIOUS DISORDER IMPOSED ON ANOTHER

A rare but dramatic disorder, **factitious disorder imposed on another** (previously *factitious disorder by proxy* or *Münchausen's* [sic] *by proxy*), involves a person who inflicts injury on another person. It is commonly a mother, who inflicts injuries on her child to gain the attention of the health care provider through her child's injuries. These actions include inducing seizures, poisoning, or smothering. This most severe form of child abuse is usually identified in the emergency department. The mother rarely admits injuring the child and thus is not amenable to treatment; the child is frequently removed from the mother's care. This form of child abuse is distinguished from other forms by the routine unwitting involvement of health care workers, who subject the child to physical harm and emotional distress through tests, procedures, and medication trials. Some researchers suspect that children who are abused in this way may later experience factitious disorder themselves (Abeln & Love, 2018).

SUMMARY OF KEY POINTS

- Somatization is affected by sociocultural and gender factors. It occurs more frequently in women than men and in those who are less educated. It also has been strongly associated with individuals who have been sexually abused as children.

- SSD is a chronic relapsing condition characterized by multiple physical symptoms of unknown origin that develop during times of emotional distress.

- Conversion disorder is a condition of neurologic symptoms (e.g., impaired voluntary muscles or sensory stimulation) that is associated with severe emotional distress.

- Factitious disorders include two types, factitious disorder and factitious disorder imposed on another. In factitious disorder, physical or psychological symptoms (or both) are fabricated to assume the sick role. In factitious disorder imposed on another, the intentional production of symptoms is in others, usually children.

- Identifying somatic symptom disorders is very complex because patients with these disorders refuse to accept any psychiatric basis to their health problems and often go for years moving from one health care provider to another to receive medical attention and avoid psychiatric assessment.

- These patients are often seen on the medical–surgical units of hospitals and go years without receiving a correct diagnosis. In most cases, they finally receive mental health treatment for comorbid conditions, such as depression, anxiety, and panic disorder.

- The development of the nurse–patient relationship is crucial to assessing these patients and identifying appropriate interventions. Because these patients deny any psychiatric basis to their problem and continue to focus on their symptoms as being medically based, the nurse must take a flexible, relaxed, and nonjudgmental approach that acknowledges the symptoms but focuses on new ways of coping with stress and avoiding recurrence of symptoms.

- Health teaching is important to help the individual develop positive lifestyle changes in place of somatization responses. Identifying personal strengths and supporting the development of positive skills improve self-esteem and personal confidence. Teaching the use of stress management provides the patient with positive coping skills.

CRITICAL THINKING CHALLENGES

1. A depressed young woman is admitted to a psychiatric unit in a state of agitation. She reports extreme abdominal pain. Her admitting provider tells you that she has a classic case of somatization disorder and to de-emphasize her physical symptoms. Under no circumstances can she have any more pain medication. Conceptualize the assessment process and how you would approach this patient.
2. Develop a continuum of "self-injury" for patients with borderline personality disorder, SSD, factitious disorder, and factitious disorder imposed on another.
3. Develop a teaching plan for an individual who has a long history of somatization but who recently received a diagnosis of breast cancer. How will the patient be able to differentiate the physical symptoms of somatization from those associated with the treatment of her breast cancer?
4. A Chinese American patient was admitted for panic attacks and numerous somatic problems, ranging from dysmenorrhea to painful joints. The results of all medical examinations have been negative. She truly believes that her panic attacks are caused by a weak heart. What approaches should the nurse use in providing culturally sensitive nursing care?
5. A person with depression is started on a regimen of phenelzine, 15 mg three times a day. She believes that she is allergic to most foods but insists on having wine in the evenings because it helps digest her food. Develop a teaching plan that provides the knowledge that she needs to prevent a hypertensive crisis caused by excessive tyramine but that is sensitive to the patient's food preferences.

1995: *Safe*

This is a story of Carol White (Julianne Moore), a married stay-at-home mother who appears to have everything. She begins having headaches that lead to a grand mal seizure. As the movie unfolds, she becomes sicker and sicker as she reports she is allergic to environmental toxins. She seeks help from an allergist and psychiatrists. She eventually leaves her husband for a retreat that is actually a scam.

Significance: The film depicts the pain and suffering that is characteristic of somatization and its impact on the family. It also shows how desperate a person can be to seek out relief of symptoms.

Viewing Points: Identify the mistakes in recognizing and treating the somatic disorder.

REFERENCES

Abeln, B., & Love, R. (2018). An overview of Munchausen Syndrome and Munchausen Syndrome by Proxy. *Nursing Clinics of North America, 53*(3), 375–384. doi: 10.1016/j.cnur.2018.04.005.

American Psychiatric Association (APA). (2013). *Diagnostic and statistical manual of mental disorders* (5th ed). Arlington, VA: American Psychiatric Association.

Asher, R. (1951). Münchausen's syndrome. *Lancet, 1,* 339–341.

Boutros, N. N., & Peters, R. (2012). Internal gating and somatization disorders: Proposing a yet un-described neural system. *Medical Hypotheses, 78*(1), 174–178.

Brammer, S. V. (2018). What interventions improve outcomes for the patient who is depressed and in pain? *Pain Management Nursing, 19*(6), 580–584. doi: 10.1016/j.pmn.2018.06.006.

Cerutti, R., Spensieri, V., Valastro, C., Presaghi, F., Canitano, R., & Guidetti, V. (2017). A comprehensive approach to understand somatic symptoms and their impact on emotional and psychosocial functioning in children. *PLoS One, 12*(2), e0171867.

Conejero, I., Thouvenot, E., Abbar, M., Mouchabac, S., Courtet, P., & Olié, E. (2018). Neuroanatomy of conversion disorder: Towards a network approach. *Reviews in the Neurosciences, 29*(4), 355–368.

Davoodi, E., Wen, A., Dobson, K. S., Noorbala, A. A., Mohammadi, A., & Farahmand, Z. (2018). Early maladaptive schemas in depression and somatization disorder. *Journal of Affective Disorders, 35,* 82–89.

Dumont, I. P., & Olson, A. L. (2012). Primary care, expression, and anxiety: Exploring somatic and emotional predictors of mental health status in adolescents. *Journal of the American Board of Family Medicine, 25*(3), 291–299.

Galli, S., Tatu, L., Bogousslavsky, J., & Aybek, S. (2018). Conversion, factitious disorder and malingering: A distinct pattern or a continuum? *Frontiers of Neurology and Neuroscience, 42,* 72–80.

Granot, M., Yovell, Y., Somer, E., Beny, A., Sadger, R., Uliel-Mirkin, R., et al. (2018). Trauma, attachment style, and somatization: a study of women with dyspareunia and women survivors of sexual abuse. *BMC Women's Health, 18*(1), 29.

Guo, D., Kleinstäuber, M., Johnson, M. H., & Sundram, F. (2019). Evaluating commonalities across medically unexplained symptoms. *International Journal of Environmental Research and Public Health, 16*(5), pii: E818.

Henningsen, P. (2018). Management of somatic symptom disorder. *Dialogues in Clinical Neuroscience, 20*(1), 23–31.

Jimenez, X. F., Nkanginieme, N., Dhand, N., Karafa, M., & Salerno, K. (2019). Clinical, demographic, psychological, and behavioral features of factitious disorder: A retrospective analysis. *General Hospital Psychiatry, 31,* pii: S0163-8343(19)30005-2.

Johnson, K., Politis, M. D., Hansen, A. R., McKenzie, L. E., Duncan, D. T., & Zhang, J. (2017). It is a painful somatic symptom, not the history of cancer/malignancy that is associated with depression: Findings from multiple national surveys. *Pain, 158*(4), 740–746.

Kealy, D., Rice, S. M., Ogrodniczuk, J. S., & Spidel, A. (2018). Childhood trauma and somatic symptoms among psychiatric outpatients: Investigating the role of shame and guilt. *Psychiatry Research, 268,* 169–174.

Kounou, K. B., Brodard, F., Gnassingbe, A., Dogbe Foli, A. A., Sager, J. C., Schmitt, L., et al. (2017). Posttraumatic stress, somatization, and quality of life among Ivorian refugees. *Journal of Traumatic Stress, 30*(6):682–689.

Kurlansik, S. L., & Maffei, M. S. (2016). Somatic symptom disorder. *American Family Physician, 93*(1), 49–54.

Lau, A. S., Guo, S., Tsai, W., Nguyen, D. J., Nguyen, H. T., Ngo, V., et al. (2016). Adolescents' stigma attitudes toward internalizing and externalizing disorders: Cultural influences and implications for distress manifestations. *Clinical Psychological Science, 4*(4), 704–717.

Li, R., Liu, F., Su, Q., Zhang, Z., Zhao, J., Wang, Y., et al. (2018). Bidirectional causal connectivity in the cortico-limbic-cerebellar circuit related to structural alterations in first-episode, drug-naive somatization disorder. *Frontiers in Psychiatry, 9,* 162.

Liu, J., Gill, N. S., Teodorczuk, A., Li, Z. J., & Sun, J. (2019). The efficacy of cognitive behavioural therapy in somatoform disorders and medically unexplained physical symptoms: A meta-analysis of randomized controlled trials. *Journal of Affective Disorders, 245,* 98–112.

López, G., & Yeater, E. A. (2018). Comparisons of sexual victimization experiences among sexual minority and heterosexual women. *Journal of Interpersonal Violence,* 886260518787202. doi: 10.1177/0886260518787202.

Mik-Meyer, N., & Obling, A. R. (2012). The negotiation of the sick role: General practitioners; classification of patients with medically unexplained symptoms. *Sociology of Health & Illness, 34*(7), 1025–1038.

Newby, J. M., Hobbs, M. J., Mahoney, A. E., Wong, S. K., & Andrews, G. (2017). DSM-5 illness anxiety disorder and somatic symptom disorder: Comorbidity, correlates, and overlap with DSM-IV hypochondriasis. *Journal of Psychosomatic Research, 101*, 31–37.

Noyes, R. Jr., Langbehn, D., Happel, R., Sieren, L., & Muller, B. (1999). Health Attitude Survey: A scale for assessing somatizing patients. *Psychosomatics, 40*(6), 470–478.

Sharma, M. P., & Manjula, M. (2013). Behavioural and psychological management of somatic symptom disorders: An overview. *International Review of Psychiatry, 25*(1), 116–124

Soltis-Jarrett, V. (2004). Interactionality: Willfully extending the boundaries of participatory research in psychiatric-mental health nursing. *Advances in Nursing Science, 27*(4), 316–329.

Soltis-Jarrett, V. (2011). His-story or Her-story: Deconstruction of the concepts of somatization towards a new approach in advanced nursing practice care. *Perspectives in Psychiatric Care, 47*(4), 183–193.

Substance Abuse and Mental Health Services Administration (SAMHSA). (2018). 2017 National Survey on Drug Use and Health: Detailed Tables. Center for Behavioral Health Statistics and Quality. Rockville, Maryland. https://www.samhsa.gov/data/sites/default/files/cbhsq-reports/NSDUHDetailedTabs2017/NSDUHDetailedTabs2017.pdf. Retrieved April 19, 2019.

Tatu, L., Aybek, S., & Bogousslavsky, J. (2018). Munchausen syndrome and the wide spectrum of factitious disorders. *Frontiers of Neurology and Neuroscience, 42*, 81–86

Taycan, O., Ozdemir, A., & Erdogan Taycan, O. (2017). Alexithymia and somatization in depressed patients: The role of the type of somatic symptom attribution. *Noro Psikiyatri Arsivi, 54*(2), 99–104.

Toussaint, A., Hüsing P., Kohlmann, S., & Löwe, B. (2019). Detecting DSM-5 somatic symptom disorder: Criterion validity of the Patient Health Questionnaire-15 (PHQ-15) and the Somatic Symptom Scale-8 (SSS-8) in combination with the Somatic Symptom Disorder – B Criteria Scale (SSD-12). *Psychological Medicine, 7*, 1–10.

Wong, J. Y., Tiwari, A., Fong, D. Y., & Bullock, L. (2016). A cross-cultural understanding of depression among abused women. *Violence Against Women, 2*(11), 1371–1396.

Wortman, M.S.H., Lokkerbol, J., van der Wouden, J. C., Visser, B., van der Horst, H, E., & Hartman, T. C. O. (2018). Cost-effectiveness of interventions for medically unexplained symptoms: A systematic review. *PLoS One. 13*(10):e0205278. doi: 10.1371/journal.pone.0205278.

Yusim, A., Anbarasan, D., Hall, B., Goetz, R., Neugebauer, R., Stewart, T., et al. (2010). Sociocultural domains of depression among indigenous populations in Latin America. *International Review of Psychiatry, 22*(4), 370–377.

Zhou, X., Peng, Y., Zhu, X., Yao, S., Dere, J., Chentsova-Dutton, Y. E., et al. (2016). From culture to symptom: Testing a structural model of "Chinese somatization." *Transcultural Psychiatry, 53*(1), 3–23.

28
Sleep–Wake Disorders

Nursing Care of Persons With Insomnia and Sleep Problems

Sheri Compton-McBride

This chapter is available at http://thepoint.lww.com/BoydEssentials2e and in the CoursePoint ebook.

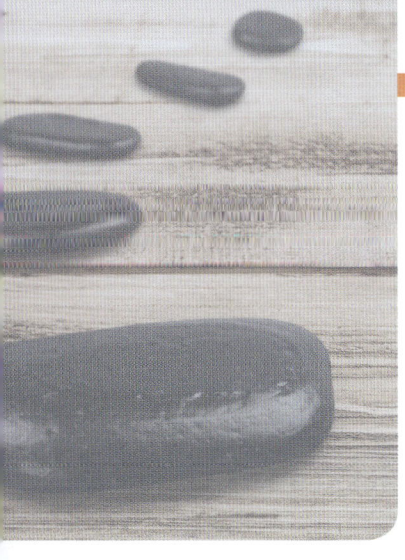

29

Sexual Disorders

Nursing Care of Persons With Sexual Dysfunction and Paraphilias

Mary Ann Boyd

KEY CONCEPTS
- sexual arousal
- sexual disorders
- sexuality
- sexual health

LEARNING OBJECTIVES

After studying this chapter, you will be able to:

1. Discuss the development of sexual behavior.
2. Compare male and female sexual response and theoretical models.
3. Discuss sexuality and wellness.
4. Identify common sexual disorders that co-occur with other mental disorders.
5. Develop a nursing care plan for a person with a sexual disorder.
6. Identify nursing intervention strategies common to treating those with sexual disorders.
7. Discuss the integration of primary care for persons with sexual disorders.

KEY TERMS

- anorgasmia • biosexual identity • dyspareunia • erectile dysfunction • excitement phase • gender dysphoria • gender identity • human sexual response cycle • orgasmic disorder • orgasmic phase • paraphilias • plateau phase • premature ejaculation • resolution • sensate focus • sex role identity • sex therapist • sexual desire • sexual maturation • sexual orientation • vaginismus

Case Study: Alice

Alice is a 35-year-old woman diagnosed with multiple sclerosis 3 years ago. She experiences transitory visual blurring, weakness of the lower limbs, and mood swings. She also has problems with urinary leakage and occasional bowel incontinence.

Sexuality is associated with sensuality, pleasure and pleasuring, intimacy, trust, communication, love and affection, attractiveness, affirmation of one's masculinity and femininity, and reverence for life. Sexuality influences how we view ourselves (self-concept) and consequently how we relate to others.

Sexuality is influenced by a person's emotional and physiologic status, beliefs and values, and morals and laws of society. Barriers to sexual fulfillment can arise from medical problems (e.g., neurologic, musculoskeletal, cardiovascular, respiratory, renal, hepatic, and cognitive impairments); from pain, weakness, and fatigue; and from sequelae of surgical procedures and drugs. More often, sexual problems are a result of the interplay of multiple causes that can include intrapsychic, interpersonal, and sociocultural factors. This chapter focuses on sexuality and sexual functioning and discusses nursing care for persons experiencing sexual dysfunction.

> **KEYCONCEPT Sexuality** is a life force that encompasses all that is male or female and how these characteristics relate to all that is human.

SEXUAL DEVELOPMENT

All of us are sexual beings, whether we are or are not sexually active. Sex is what we are, not what we do—the sum total of all of our biologic and experiential influences. **Sexual maturation** encompasses four areas: biosexual identity, gender identity, sex role identity, and sexual orientation. Although **biosexual identity** refers to the anatomic and physiologic states of being male or female, **gender identity** is the conviction of belonging to a male or female gender. Both biosexual and gender identities result from genetic and intrauterine hormonal influences, not learned behavior. **Sex role identity** (or gender role) is the outward expression of gender, including behaviors, feelings, and attitudes. **Sexual orientation** refers to a person's sexual attraction to those of the opposite sex (heterosexual), same sex (homosexual), or both sexes (bisexual). Sexual orientation is determined early in development as a result of the influence of genetic factors and the interactions between sex hormones and the developing brain and should not be considered a lifestyle choice. There is no evidence that interventions can change sexual orientation (Grabowska, 2017; Substance Abuse and Mental Health Services Administration [SAMHSA], 2015).

Genes and Determination of Sex

As a result of the sex-determining genes on the Y chromosome, testosterone is present in male fetuses and, by weeks 6 to 12, is responsible for the formation of the penis, prostate, and scrotum. The formation of ovaries in female fetuses depends on the absence of this male hormone. After the male sex organs are formed, testosterone levels temporarily rise, causing a permanent sexual organization of the brain that is different than that of females. Testosterone is also elevated during the first 3 months after birth, causing the brain's structures and circuits to be fixed for the rest of a boy's life.

These structural differences are thought to be the basis of sex differences that are reflected in behavior from birth. For example, female newborns are more likely to watch human faces; male infants look more at mobiles. Toy preference (i.e., choosing dolls vs. cars) is obvious at 3 to 8 months. During puberty, rising hormones stimulate these structures and circuits that were set up many years earlier to further respond in feminine or masculine directions. Since the sexual differentiation of the genitals takes place earlier (during the first 2 months of pregnancy) than the sexual differentiation of the brain (second half of pregnancy), these two processes may be influenced differently. In rare cases, transsexuality may occur. For example, people with male sexual organs may experience their identity as female (Eid & Biason-Lauber, 2016).

Sexual Behaviors in Children and Adolescents

In infants, sexual behaviors are rare with the exception of hand-to-genital contact. As children become more aware of their body parts and the physical sensations deriving from their genitals, they become more interested in gender differences. For 2- to 5-year-old children, sexual behaviors are varied and more common than in older children, who are more aware of the social norms of concealing sexual behaviors. For example, young children observe and comment on body differences, demonstrate interest in bathroom habits and urination, and handle their genitals for pleasure and comfort. Their curiosity leads them to want to look at and touch adult bodies and breasts. Mutual genital exploration or urination among children may be seen at this time along with questions about where babies come from.

Age-appropriate solitary sexual behaviors (i.e., touching one's own genitals) are also common. At this early age, these behaviors do not have the sexualized meaning they do in adults. However, if young children are exposed to sexually explicit material (Internet, movies, observation of parental sexual activities) or if their parents overreact to age-appropriate behaviors, these activities can take on additional, more adult-like, meanings. If preoccupation with the sexual behaviors interferes with the child's ability to grow and function, then the behaviors are problematic. For example, an 8-year-old boy sneaking to the bathroom several times a day to touch his genitals needs help in addressing this behavior.

Sexual behaviors are common and occur in 42% to 73% of children by the time they reach 13 years of age. Generally, the frequency of overt sexual behaviors decrease with age. These behaviors may not be as obvious because as children mature, they become increasingly more covert in their sexual behavior. For example, whereas 6- to 9-year-old boys and girls often touch their genitals at home, stand too close to others, and try to look at persons when they are nude, 10- to 12-year-old children, who are actually more interested in and know more about sex, limit their behavior to looking at nudity in magazines, television, and the internet (Lussier, McCuish, Mathesius, Corrado, & Nadeau, 2018; Miragoli, Camisasca, & Di Blasio, 2017).

Sexual contact with others occurs at a relatively early age in the United States. In a nationwide survey of 9th through 12th grade students in 50 states, 34.2% were currently sexually active, 46% had had sexual intercourse, and 5.9% of students had sexual intercourse for the first time before age 13 years (Kann et al., 2016). A variety of circumstances lead to this sexual activity. Sex may be engaged in because of peer pressure or because friends or social groups condone sex. The need to be convinced of being in love, wanting to feel loved, and fear of rejection all precipitate risk-taking behavior. Depending on the family environment, stresses, and observation of adult sexual activities, children may exhibit more adult sexual behaviors, which may be considered normal for the environment in which they live. For children and adolescents, sexual behavior (usually involving other people) is considered abnormal when it occurs at a greater frequency or at a much earlier age than would be developmentally or culturally expected.

Sexual Behaviors in Adulthood

Sexual activities occur throughout young adulthood and continue through middle and late adulthood into the 1980s and 1990s. Although the frequency and types of sexual encounters may change, the quality need not change. During the fourth to fifth decades of life, physical changes become more obvious, and so various chronic illnesses, such as hypertension or arthritis, may also develop. As a result of decreased endocrine production, gradual changes to body tissues occur over a 15- to 20-year span. Most physical symptoms arise from vasomotor instability, which can include morning fatigue, vague pains, hot flashes, dizziness, chills, sweating, nervousness, crying spells, decreased sexual potency, and palpitations.

In women, estrogen deficiency during menopause affects the sexual system by causing a gradual thinning of the vaginal mucosa, decreasing the elasticity of muscles and orgasmic force, and increasing breast involution (sagging of breast tissue). Vaginal lubrication decreases, which may cause dyspareunia (i.e., pain during intercourse), often requiring the use of a water-soluble lubricant or saliva. Although many women experience little or no change in sexual function, both decreased and increased sexual activity and interest are possible. In some women, more time is required to lubricate the vulvovaginal areas and to strengthen clitoral response. Orgasmic capacity and breast response remain fairly constant in appropriately stimulated women.

In men, decreasing testosterone production is responsible for sexual changes. The amount and viability of sperm decrease, erections become less firm, and more direct sexual stimulation is needed. The testicles begin to decrease in elasticity and size, ejaculation time increases, and the force of ejaculation decreases. Spermatogenesis decreases, although viable sperm, capable of impregnation, continue to be produced. Seminal fluid is less voluminous and viscous, and ejaculatory force is decreased. Older men, however, are capable of sustaining erection much longer with decreased ejaculatory demand, potentially benefiting older women, who require increased time to reach orgasm. Coupled with women's increased sexual enjoyment in the later years, sexual activity is often perceived as more satisfactory than previously experienced.

Sexual continuity depends to a great extent on good physical health, activity, and regular opportunities for sexual expression and sexual activity in all forms, including masturbation and same-gender behavior. An important influence on sexuality is the attitudes of others, especially attitudes that define specific behaviors as acceptable or unacceptable. This is especially true in later life (Miragoli et al., 2017; Syme & Cohn, 2016). In healthy adults, sexual function, although modified by the aging process, should remain satisfying despite a differently timed sequence. Frequent sexual activity, whether by coitus, masturbation, or other practices, usually preserves sexual potency.

SEXUAL RESPONSES

Understanding normal sexual responses helps when discussing this very personal but important aspect of being human with patients. The following section provides an overview of major concepts and theories related to sexual responses.

Sexual Desire and Arousal

Sexual desire is the ability, interest, or willingness to receive or a motivational state to seek sexual stimulation. In healthy adults, the sex drive is integrated through the central nervous system (CNS) with the autonomic nervous system governing extragenital changes (increased respiration and heart rate). The parasympathetic nervous system largely controls arousal; the sympathetic nervous system largely controls orgasmic discharge. Sexual stimulation brings about a total-body response with dramatic changes seen in the genitals and breasts. Sex hormones, particularly androgen, influence desire in both genders, but less is known about hormonal influence in women. That the higher centers of the brain apparently mediate the lower reflex response centers supports the relationship between cognitive and affective states and sexual function.

During sexual arousal, both men and women experience an increased heart rate, blood pressure, respiration, and myotonia.

> **KEYCONCEPT** **Sexual arousal** is state of mounting sexual tension characterized by vasoconstriction and myotonia.

In men, visual stimulation (i.e., seeing a naked person), fantasies, memories, or physical stimulation of the genitals or other regions (e.g., nipples) causes the parasympathetic system to involuntarily release chemicals that dilate penile arteries. A rapid inflow of arterial blood to the cavernous spaces of corpora cavernosa, facilitated by high levels of intrapenile nitric oxide, causes stiffening and elongation of the penis. With continued stimulation, an emission of semen and an ejaculation occurs. Dopaminergic activity in the CNS facilitates arousal and ejaculation; serotonergic systems inhibit them (Will, Hull, & Dominguez, 2014).

Fantasies, visual stimuli, and physical stimulation are also important for sexual arousal in women, but physical stimulation seems more important for women and visual stimuli for men. Similar to the case in men, the parasympathetic nervous system increases blood flow to the female genitalia, lubricating the vagina and enlarging the breast and clitoris. Estrogens and progestins are involved in female sexual functioning, but androgens are needed by people of both genders to maintain arousal.

Theoretical Models of Sexual Response

In 1966, Masters and Johnson described the classic **human sexual response cycle** as consisting of four phases: excitement, plateau, orgasm, and resolution. In the **excitement phase**, erotic feelings of both genders lead to a penile erection in men and vaginal lubrication in women. Heart rate and respirations also increase. The **plateau phase** is represented by sexual pleasure and increased muscle tension, heart rate, and blood flow to the genitals. For men, the **orgasmic phase** is ejaculation of semen, and for women, it consists of rhythmic contractions of the vaginal muscles. For most men, immediately after orgasm and before resolution, a refractory period occurs when no response is possible. **Resolution** is the gradual return of the organs and body systems to the nonaroused state. Muscle tension and vasocongestion subside. Breathing and heart rate gradually return to normal rates. Usually, the person feels a sense of relaxation, relief of tension, and satisfaction (Masters & Johnson, 1966, 1970).

After publication of Masters and Johnson's works, Kaplan (1979) proposed a three-phase model of sexual response—desire, excitement, and orgasm—and identified low-desire states as a frequent cause of sexual dysfunction.

This linear approach is criticized as being primarily a biologic model and does not account for nonbiologic experiences such as pleasure, satisfaction, and the context of the relationship. To account for emotional and psychological aspects of sexual response, a circular model focusing on women's sexual responses was developed by Basson (2001). This model proposes that nonsexual interpersonal factors, such as a desire for physical connection and intimacy needs, also motivate women to engage in sexual relations, not only sexual release. Arousal and desire appear to be interchangeable and inseparable from one another, with one reinforcing the other. Subjective feelings of interest may follow the sensation of arousal, and sexual satisfaction may be experienced without orgasm.

These two models—linear and circular—have been debated for years. Both models are supported empirically as being relevant to sexual responses in women. Women report that sexual experiences are at times consistent with the linear and circular models at other times (Ferenidou, Kirana, Fokas, Hatzichristou, & Athanasiadis, 2016). There is emerging evidence that the circular model is a better fit for men than the linear model (Connaughton, McCabe, & Karantzas, 2016).

Dual-Control Model

Another conceptualization, the dual-control model focuses on individual variability and proposes that sexual responses involve an interaction between sexual excitement and sexual inhibition (Bancroft, Graham, Janssen, & Sanders, 2009). This model assumes that (1) neurobiologic inhibition of sexual response is adaptive and occurs in situations when sexual activity would be a disadvantage, dangerous, or distracting; (2) individuals vary in their propensity for sexual excitation and inhibition; and (3) the context and cultural meaning attributed to the interaction of the individuals are important stimuli for both excitatory and inhibitory processes. Emerging research is showing that the dual-control model is an important framework in understanding how mood influences both subjective and genital sexuality in both males and females (Hodgson, Kukkonen, Binik, & Carrier, 2016; Turner et al., 2019; Velten, Zahler, Scholten, & Margraf, 2019).

SEXUAL HEALTH AND WELLNESS

Sexual health is an important aspect of wellness. Sexual health is viewed holistically and positively and is relevant throughout the individual's life span from the young to the old. Influenced by gender norms, expectations, and power dynamics, sexual health is understood within specific social, economic, and political contexts (WHO, 2019). Major health threats related to sexuality are HIV/AIDS, hepatitis, and sexually transmitted diseases.

> **KEYCONCEPT** According to the working definition of the World Health Organization (WHO), **sexual health** is "a state of physical, emotional, mental and social well-being in relation to sexuality; it is not merely the absence of disease, dysfunction or infirmity. Sexual health requires a positive and respectful approach to sexuality and sexual relationships, as well as the possibility of having pleasurable and safe sexual experiences, free of coercion, discrimination and violence. For sexual health to be attained and maintained, the sexual rights of all persons must be respected, protected and fulfilled" (WHO, 2019).

The mental health of members of the LGBTQ (lesbian, gay, bisexual, transgender, questioning) community is at risk due to discrimination in environments where they live, learn, and work (Cicero & Wesp, 2017). Sexual orientation discrimination is most prevalent in early young adulthood, but it occurs in all ages. Higher risks for alcohol, tobacco, and drug use disorders are associated with discrimination at the older ages (Evans-Polce, Veliz, Boyd, Hughes, & McCabe, 2019). LGBT youth are two to three times more likely to attempt suicide, more likely to be homeless. Lesbians are less likely to get preventive cancer services. Gay men are at higher risk of HIV and other STIs. Transgender individuals are highly stigmatized and are most likely to be victimized than heterosexual or LGB. LGBT populations have the highest rates of tobacco, alcohol, and other drug use. One of the goals of *Healthy People 2020* is to improve the health, safety, and well-being of LGBT individuals (Healthy People 2020, 2017). Nurses are in a unique position to provide gender-affirming care in order to improve the safety and well-being of the LGBTQ communities.

SEXUAL DYSFUNCTIONS AND PROBLEMATIC BEHAVIORS

Sexual dysfunctions are a group of disorders that are characterized by clinically significant disturbances in the person's ability to respond sexually or to experience sexual pleasure (American Psychiatric Association [APA], 2013). The *DSM-5* identifies the following as sexual disorders: delayed ejaculation (DE), erectile disorder, female orgasmic disorder, female sexual interest/arousal disorder, genitopelvic pain/penetration disorder, male hypoactive sexual desire disorder, and premature ejaculation (PE). These dysfunctions can be lifelong or acquired and are categorized as mild, moderate, or severe. An occasional episode is not considered dysfunctional (APA, 2013). In this chapter, female orgasmic disorder is highlighted because it is among the most commonly occurring sexual disorders in women, and **anorgasmia** (the inability to achieve an orgasm) is a frequent medication side effect.

> **KEYCONCEPT** **Sexual disorders** are clinical disturbances caused by the inability to respond sexually or to experience sexual pleasure.

FEMALE ORGASMIC DISORDER

A female orgasm is the least understood of all sexual responses; no universal definition exists (Bancroft & Graham, 2011). Women's descriptions of the orgasmic experience vary from altered consciousness to focused sensation. Many women require clitoral stimulation to reach orgasm and only a minority of women report that they always experience orgasm during intercourse.

According to *DSM-5*, an **orgasmic disorder** is the inability to reach orgasm by any means, either alone or with a partner and/or markedly reduced intensity of orgasmic sensations for at least 6 months. The inability to experience an orgasm causes clinically significant distress (APA, 2013).

Diagnostic Criteria

Female orgasmic disorder is characterized by the inability of a woman to experience orgasm or the intensity of the orgasm is markedly reduced at least 75% of the time. If other explanations for the anorgasmia exist, such as substance use, medications, or interpersonal issues, the diagnosis is not used.

Epidemiology and Risk Factors

Debate about the issue of female orgasms is considerable. Estimated prevalence of women's inability to reach orgasm ranges from 9% (in the United States) to 41.2% in Southeast Asia (Bancroft & Graham, 2011).

Poor physical health, mental health, and relationship issues, especially partner difficulties, are the primary risk factors. Age, arousal difficulty, and lubrication difficulty are related to difficulty reaching orgasm (Rowland, Cempel, & Tempel, 2018).

Etiology

In general, any local genital or pelvic pathology, trauma, or surgery that causes pain on intercourse can produce impaired response to sexual stimulation. Spinal cord damage, endocrine disorders, systemic diseases, chronic pain, and general debility can interfere with sexual responses. CNS depressants (e.g., alcohol, barbiturates, narcotics), psychiatric disorders, infections, inflammatory disorders, and pregnancy have all been associated with female orgasmic disorder. Additionally, many medications such as antidepressants, antihypertensives, and substances (e.g., alcohol) can also affect the sexual response (Thomas, Neal-Perry, & Hess, 2018).

> **Consider Alice**
>
> Alice admits that her sexual activity is far less frequent than before her illness. She feels she is no longer attractive or able to fulfill her functions as a wife.
> How would you discuss her feelings? What information would you give her to help her look at her situation realistically?

Sexual responses can be inhibited by many different emotions and cognitions, including sexual anxiety and guilt, anger or hostility toward one's partner, indifference toward one's partner, depression, or excessive and intrusive thoughts. Misinformation or lack of information contributes to the inhibition. Cultural expectations also play an important role in the sexual experience. Religious prohibitions and cultural taboos often contribute to a woman's view of her sexuality. If a woman believes that sexual relationships are sinful or "a woman's duty," she is not as likely to explore her own sexual potential.

Recovery-Oriented Care for Persons With Female Orgasmic Disorder

Teamwork and Collaboration: Working Toward Recovery

The treatment of the woman with an orgasmic disorder is best left to clinicians who specialize in this area, but other health care providers can first treat underlying health, mental health, and relationship issues. If the orgasmic problem is not related to any of these areas, she should be referred to a qualified **sex therapist**, who blends education and counseling with psychotherapy and specific sexual exercises. For example, **sensate focus** is a method for partners to learn what each finds arousing and to learn to communicate those preferences. It begins with nongenital contact and gradually includes genital touch and sexual intercourse.

Integration With Primary Care

Sexual disorders are treated by specialists, but often the patient's initial concern is shared with a nurse. It is important that mental and health problems are treated from a holistic perspective. Mental health and primary health clinicians should be monitoring the sexual health of the patient and provide appropriate, evidence-based interventions.

Evidence-Based Nursing Care for the Woman With Female Orgasmic Disorder

The psychiatric–mental health nurse has a responsibility to conduct an assessment to determine the presence of any sexual issues or problems. The scope of practice dictates the level of assessment and interventions. The nurse will most likely be seeing the patient for a different problem (e.g., psychiatric problem, acute or chronic physical health problem) and will discover a sexual problem during a health assessment. Patients are sometimes reluctant to discuss sexual problems, especially those who are socially stigmatized (same-sex couples, developmentally disabled people, and old people).

Attention should be paid to special populations' high risk for sexual problems, such as those with mental illnesses or chronic health problems. For older adults, poor physical health and lack of a partner are common barriers to sexual continuity. Other barriers include a lack of privacy or institutionalization. Lack of knowledge about the impacts of aging or health conditions on sexuality, the normality of continued sexual desire and interest, and the alternatives for sexual gratification may also inhibit sexual activity.

Remember Alice?
Alice believed that she could not have sexual relations with her husband because of her physical problems. Her nurse practitioner provided education and hope.
What information would you reinforce through discussion? What would you say to reinforce her self-esteem and hope for sexual relations?

If sexual dysfunction exists, one of the most important questions is does the individual want to change sexual functioning? Many women may not see a need to pursue therapy even if a sexual problem exits. See Box 29.1.

Mental Health Nursing Assessment

Current sexual functioning, age, physical health, and the presence of any medical or psychiatric and substance use problems as well as factors that contribute to sexual functioning (e.g., rest, nutrition, personal hygiene) are considered in the sexual assessment (Box 29.2). A careful medication history is important because so many medications have a negative effect on sexual performance (see Chapter 11).

Adults with chronic medical illnesses and disabilities who have problems with sensation, movement, body structure, fertility, or energy should be asked about the impact of the medical problems on their sexual function. Diabetes mellitus, heart disease, hormonal imbalances, menopause, and chronic illness such as kidney disease or liver failure are associated with sexual dysfunction in women (Phillips & Phillips, 2015). Sexual activity often changes after a cardiac event because of fear about causing another attack (Steinke, Mosack, & Hill, 2015). Obesity and pregnancy can both compromise sexual responses (Sarwer, Hanson, Voeller, & Steffen, 2018).

The woman's sexual knowledge should also be determined. Does she understand the sexual responses, effects of medications, hormonal changes that occur during the woman's life cycle (e.g., adolescence, menstruation, pregnancy, menopause, aging), and the importance of adequate rest and nutrition?

The assessment also includes the woman's self-concept and body image and her relationship with her partner. A poor self-concept can prevent a woman from engaging in sexual relationships. Mood states, such as chronic depression and grief, also seriously affect the woman's ability to have an orgasm. The amount of stress and the ability to relax and focus on her sexuality are important assessment data. An unsatisfactory partner relationship may be at the

BOX 29.1 • THERAPEUTIC DIALOGUE • Assessing Interest in Sexual Activity

INEFFECTIVE APPROACH

Nurse: Alice, are you currently sexually active?
Alice: Once in a while.
Nurse: How would you describe your sexual activity?
Alice: How would you feel if you were in my condition?
Nurse: Well, you could still have sexual relations.
Alice: Sure thing. (Getting irritated)
Nurse: Is there a problem?
Alice: Look, I just don't want to talk about it.

EFFECTIVE APPROACH

Nurse: Alice are you currently sexually active?
Alice: Once in a while.
Nurse: Once in a while?
Alice: Yeah, I really don't feel like it any more.
Nurse: Oh (Silence)
Alice: My illness is messing up things in the bedroom.
Nurse: How so?
Alice: Well, I just feel so ugly—I have to urinate, my legs are weak.
Nurse: Are you feeling that you want to have sex?
Alice: Sometimes I think about it, but then I remember my illness. My poor husband. He should find someone else.
Nurse: Have you talked with him about your feelings?
Alice: Well, no. He is so patient.
Nurse: There are many women who have similar feelings but are able to begin to enjoy sex again. Is that something that you would like to consider?
Alice: Well, maybe.
Nurse: We can talk more about this. There are resources that can help you and your husband.
Alice: OK, sounds good.

CRITICAL THINKING CHALLENGE

- Compare the course of the first dialogue with the second one. What did the second nurse do differently to elicit information about Alice's feelings and concerns?
- What is problematic about the first dialogue?

BOX 29.2

Medical Conditions and Substances Affecting Sexual Function

- Cardiovascular conditions and vascular conditions
- Endocrine conditions, particularly diabetes mellitus, which cause gradual impotence in half of men and orgasmic dysfunction in one third of women
- Cancer or cancer treatments, such as radiation
- Surgery, particularly hysterectomy, mastectomy, prostatectomy, and bowel surgery
- Arthritis and neuromuscular disorders
- Spinal cord injury
- Head injury
- Cerebrovascular accident (stroke)
- Organic brain syndrome (senile dementia, Alzheimer disease)
- Cerebral palsy
- Asthma, emphysema, and chronic obstructive pulmonary disease
- Chronic renal failure
- Obesity
- Localized genital conditions, such as Sjögren syndrome, balanitis, vulvar ulcers, and psoriasis
- Prescription medications (e.g., antihypertensive drugs, anticholinergic drugs, some antidepressants)
- Chronic use of most recreational drugs
- Chronic alcohol abuse

core of the sexual problem. Cultural and family values play an important role in understanding a patient's response to orgasmic dysfunction and should be considered. Lifestyle disruptions, a birth of a child, a move to another city, or a change in financial or social status may coincide with sexual dysfunction. Nursing Care Plan 29.1—which sets forth a plan of care for Alice, the case study patient in this chapter—is available at http://thepoint.lww.com/BoydEssentials2e.

Priority of Nursing Care

Low self-esteem and depression are nursing care priorities for a woman with a sexual disorder. The nurse should determine the significance of this disorder to the person. For some women, this problem may not be a major concern; for others, it may represent loss of femininity.

Nursing Interventions

Establishing Mental Health and Wellness Goals

Sexual problems impact all aspects of health and wellness. The nurse should help a person examine current sexual needs. The nurse can help the person identify ways to enhance sexual health. If there is a sexual problem, the nurse and the patient can collaborate on establishing realistic goals. For example, encouraging patient to discuss sexual needs with partner is a beginning step.

Self-Care and Wellness Challenges

Wellness activities are especially challenging because of the importance of sexual health to a person's well-being. Co-occurring illnesses may interfere with sexual functioning. Feeling unattractive or stigmatized can compromise the willingness to discuss sexual needs. Wellness strategies can support sexual health (see Box 29.3).

BOX 29.3

Wellness Challenges

- Feeling positive about sexuality and sexual health
  - Strategies: Discuss the importance of sexual health to wellness
- Seeking pleasant environments that support sexual activities
  - Strategies: Discuss realistic environmental changes that are conducive to sexual activity
- Recognizing the need for physical activity, healthy foods, and sleep
  - Strategies: Encourage regular physical activity, discuss healthy diets, encourage establishing healthy sleep hygiene routines
- Developing a sense of connection, belonging, and a support system
  - Strategies: Seek positive relationships and reduce number of unpleasant interactions

---

BOX 29.4

Psychoeducation Checklist: Female Orgasmic Disorder

When caring for the patient with female orgasmic disorder, be sure to include the following topics in your teaching plan for the patient and partner:
- Possible etiologic factors
- Anxiety reduction techniques
- Communication skills
- Impact of medication on orgasm

Nursing interventions include providing counseling, sex education, problem-solving opportunities, or referrals. Several health care practices are also known to promote sexual health such as getting adequate rest, maintaining optimal nutrition, and exercising regularly. Explaining the dynamics of sexual responses is another important nursing action. Individuals who report difficulties with sexual response often benefit from factual information and helpful suggestions and do not need sex therapy. However, when long-standing or highly complex problems emerge in the assessment, it is better to refer the individual or couple to a formally trained, certified, sex therapist. Nurses should be aware that certain processes, techniques, and adaptive devices can improve sexual functioning.

Unless the nurse has had additional preparation in sexual counseling, simply providing factual information and helping patients identify issues related to sexual problems and develop problem-solving skills are the primary psychosocial interventions. Patients often benefit from learning how to communicate their sexual needs better in such areas as type of stimulation desired, positioning, and the amount of time required for maximum sexual pleasure. Resource materials and referral sources can be recommended. Box 29.4 outlines topics for patient education.

Women with orgasmic dysfunction can also benefit from a support group that includes women with similar problems. Group modalities, such as psychoeducation groups, are useful in helping patients decrease their embarrassment and uneasiness about sexual topics and increase their knowledge. Partner support is critical and should be encouraged throughout treatment.

Evaluation and Treatment Outcomes

Outcomes related to improved sexual functioning are developed with the patient and may vary from acquiring knowledge to increasing communication with her partner and to deciding about a referral for specialized treatment.

EJACULATORY DYSFUNCTION

Ejaculatory dysfunction is one of the most common male sexual disorders and ranges from **premature ejaculation** (PE), inability to control ejaculation before or shortly after penetration to DE, delay or absence of ejaculation. These types of dysfunction cause negative personal consequences, clinical distress, frustration, and the avoidance of sexual intimacy (Stephenson, Truong, & Shimazu, 2018). The dysfunction needs to be present for 6 months to be diagnosed as a sexual dysfunction and is not diagnosed in a man whose difficulty is caused by drug or alcohol abuse. In those cases, a substance abuse diagnosis is made, with the sexual disorder generally resolving when the substance abuse is treated (APA, 2013).

Epidemiology

Based on patient self-report, PE is viewed as the most common male sexual dysfunction, with prevalence rates of up to 30% of men with an erectile dysfunction (ED). It is estimated that about 27% of men seeking treatment report PE as a problem. Most men with PE, however, do not seek treatment (Rastrelli, Cipriani, Corona, Vignozzi, & Maggi, 2019).

Etiology

The etiology of PE is unknown with few data to support suggested biologic or psychological theories such as anxiety, penile hypersensitivity, and serotonin receptor dysfunction. Age does not seem to be an etiologic factor or a risk (El-Hamd, Saleh, & Majzoub, 2019).

Recovery-Oriented Care for Persons With Premature Ejaculation

Teamwork and Collaboration: Working Toward Recovery

The treatment of PE involves medication and behavioral strategies. Men with PE are usually treated by specialists. Nurses are instrumental in teaching patients about the disorder and potential treatments and facilitating decision-making about seeking treatment.

Integration With Primary Care

Treatment of PE should be coordinated within the context of primary care. Since medications and medical illness can impact sexual functioning, it is important that one provider coordinates care. There is emerging evidence that alternative treatments, such as acupuncture, may be helpful (Cooper et al., 2017).

Evidence-Based Nursing Care for Men With Premature Ejaculation

The problem of PE may become apparent during a health history that includes specific sexual data. Patients

BOX 29.5

Psychoeducation Checklist: Premature Ejaculation

When caring for the patient with premature ejaculation, be sure to include the following topics in your teaching plan for the patient and partner:
- Possible etiologic factors
- Pharmacologic agents, if indicated, including drug, dosage, action, frequency, and possible side effects
- Measures to decrease anxiety performance
- Communication skills
- Sexual counseling
- Sensate focus
- Sex therapy

need assurance that many men have similar problems and that treatment is possible (Box 29.5). Patients can be referred to specialists for behavioral strategies. Younger men may find that masturbation before anticipation of sexual intercourse may help.

ERECTILE DYSFUNCTION

Erectile dysfunction (ED) refers to the inability of a man to achieve or maintain an erection sufficient for satisfactory completion of the sexual activity.

Diagnostic Criteria

Although most men experience an occasional lack of erection, intervention is required when there is consistent (more than 6 months) erectile inefficiency during masturbation, intercourse, or on awakening (APA, 2013).

Epidemiology

Estimates of ED vary in 5% to 20% of men. ED may occur at any age although incidence increases with aging. Men with diabetes mellitus, cardiovascular disease, or chronic renal failure also have a higher incidence of ED. For those undergoing treatment for prostate cancer, there is a high probability of ED (Donovan et al., 2016). Approximately, 10% to 52% of men aged 40 to 70 have ED (Colson, et al., 2018). Although less common in younger men, ED still affects 5% to 10% of men below the age of 40. Findings from these studies show that ED impacts significantly on mood state, interpersonal functioning, and overall quality of life (Nguyen, Gabrielson, & Hellstrom, 2017).

Etiology

Biologic Theories

Common biologic causes of ED include genital trauma, vascular insufficiency, renal disease, hormonal deficiencies, Parkinson disease, diabetes mellitus, multiple sclerosis, surgical procedures, use of antihypertensive and antidepressant drugs, and heavy cigarette smoking. Long-term alcohol or cocaine consumption can affect the erectile response. It is also more common with the aging process (Eisenberg & Meldrum, 2017).

Many men with mental disorders attribute their ED to their psychiatric medication. Consequently, these individuals stop taking their medications. Within a few weeks to months, they have a psychiatric relapse.

Psychological Theories

ED may also have a psychogenic basis. Numerous psychosocial etiologies have been identified. Fear of failure, relationship stress, poor body image, fear of rejection, partner hostility, guilt, cultural taboos, religious proscriptions, lack of knowledge, and negative attitudes are some of the identified related factors (Balon, 2017; Chen et al., 2018).

Recovery-Oriented Care for Persons With Erectile Dysfunction

Teamwork and Collaboration: Working Toward Recovery

The treatment of men with ED is usually managed in primary care setting except for those with mental disorders, who may seek treatment within the mental health system. Since the introduction of the phosphodiesterase 5 (PDE5) inhibitors, pharmacologic agents such as sildenafil citrate, tadalafil, and vardenafil, many men choose the convenience of medication. For persons with psychiatric disorders, monitoring medications and their potential interaction is important. However, behavioral interventions have also been shown to be useful.

Evidence-Based Nursing Care for the Person With Erectile Dysfunction

Mental Health Nursing Assessment

Some men are not comfortable discussing sexuality and sexual problems. The assessment should be conducted in an atmosphere of trust and understanding. In many cultures, male self-esteem is related to the ability to perform sexually. When a man has problems maintaining an erection, it is embarrassing and demeaning to him. Sensitivity to the patient's feelings should be reflected throughout the assessment.

Many medical problems are reported that compromise male sexual activity and responses. Obesity, smoking, diabetes mellitus, hypertension, hyperlipidemia, cardiovascular disease, and obstructive sleep disorder are a few.

In addition, low testosterone, chronic kidney disease, and some neurologic disorders also associated with male sexual dysfunction (Costa, Ponciano, Costa, Gomes, & Oliveira, 2018; Huang et al., 2019; Zamorano-Leon et al., 2018.).

Assessment should include a discussion about the impact of sexual dysfunction on the quality of the relationship with the partner. If a mental disorder, such as depression or posttraumatic stress disorder, is present, comparing the timing of the dysfunction with the onset of symptoms and prescribed medication can determine whether the ED is related to the disorder and medication.

Priority of Nursing Care

ED affects men differently, and the priorities of care will depend on its meaning to the patient. Low self-esteem and self-identity are two priorities that should be considered. ED may indicate an undiagnosed medical disorder such as diabetes or a medication side effect. There may be wellness priorities such as diet and exercise modifications that emerge.

Nursing Interventions

Wellness Strategies

Promotion of positive health practices that focus on adequate nutrition, rest, and exercise is important in promoting erectile functioning. Weight loss may improve overall health and enhance the strength of the erection. Regular exercise is also related to sexual health. Helping the patient develop a better lifestyle is important in promoting sexual functioning. Reducing alcohol consumption can also improve sexual performance.

Pharmacologic Interventions

PDE5 inhibitors are the treatment of choice. With sexual stimulation, nitric oxide is released into the nerve terminations and endothelial cell, stimulating the production of cyclic guanosine monophosphate (cGMP), a substance that enables the smooth muscle cells of the corpora cavernosa to relax. The PDE enzymes are involved in the breakdown of cGMP. The PDE inhibitors inactivate PDE5, thereby enabling the buildup of cGMP, sustaining relaxation of the corpora cavernosa.

Approved PDE5 inhibitors include sildenafil citrate (Viagra), vardenafil HCl (Levitra), tadalafil (Cialis), and avanafil (Stendra). These medications enhance the effect of nitric oxide, which is released in the corpora cavernosa during sexual stimulation. These medications are rapidly absorbed, with maximum observed plasma concentrations reached within 30 to 120 minutes of oral dosing in the fasted state. Cialis acts for up to 36 hours. Although these medications are approved for the treatment of ED in men, they have not been shown to be efficacious in sexual arousal disorders in women.

Before the introduction of PDE5 inhibitors, intracavernosal pharmacotherapy was the treatment of choice for ED. A vascular smooth muscle relaxant such as papaverine hydrochloride, phentolamine mesylate, or prostaglandin is directly injected into the corpora cavernosa by the patient or partner. This increases arterial flow of blood into the corpora cavernosa and decreases venous outflow. Neurogenic rather than vascular ED appears to respond better. Complications can include excessive bleeding, scarring and priapism, and potential hepatic involvement. Counseling, strict monitoring, and specific teaching are required (Rew & Heidelbaugh, 2016).

Another treatment is the use of alprostadil (prostaglandin) in microsuppository form inserted into the urethra using a special applicator. The system called MUSE causes a rapid absorption of the medication through the urethral mucosa into the corpus spongiosum. It is particularly useful for men who are unable to inject themselves (Rew & Heidelbaugh, 2016).

Other Treatments

When erection is determined to be permanently impaired, several options may be considered to facilitate intercourse. An external penile prosthesis can be placed over the flaccid penis although some find this esthetically displeasing. A pumping device that creates a vacuum can be used for blood entrapment followed by placement of a rubber band at the base of the penis. Surgical techniques for improving vascular sufficiency are also showing promising results.

Psychoeducation

Education is important for the patient with ED. Teaching the patient about positive health practices and treatment options (i.e., mechanical devices, medications, surgical procedures) is usually needed (Box 29.6). The patient's concern about his partner's satisfaction needs to be explored. Many times, men believe that partner satisfaction is related only to penile penetration and their ability to sustain an erection. Encouraging the patient to talk with his partner about her (or his) sexual needs and other aspects of their sexual experience (physical closeness, kissing, hugging, mutual exploration of their bodies) helps him broaden his understanding of the sexual experience.

> **BOX 29.6**
> **Psychoeducation Checklist: Male Erectile Dysfunction**
>
> When caring for the patient with male erectile disorder, be sure to include the following topics in your teaching plan for the patient and partner:
> - Possible etiologic factors
> - Psychopharmacologic agents (e.g., intracavernosal therapy, yohimbine), including drug, action, frequency, administration technique, and possible side effects
> - Alternative methods of sexual expression
> - Prosthesis use
> - Sexual education and counseling
> - Communication skills
> - Sex therapy

Evaluation and Treatment Outcomes

The primary outcome for ED is improved sexual functioning. Acceptance of change of physical status is an outcome that is difficult to obtain. Improvement in sexual satisfaction may include increasing the ability for erectile functioning. If ED is permanent, exploration of other avenues of sexual expression may indicate a successful outcome. In this disorder, partner satisfaction is usually of prime concern. Improved communication with the man's partner may also be a positive outcome.

FEMALE SEXUAL INTEREST/AROUSAL DISORDER

A female sexual interest/arousal disorder may occur at any age and may cause relationship difficulties and personal stress along with avoidance of sexual activity and impaired communication. Other etiologic factors, such as anxiety, guilt, and history of sexual abuse, and changes in androgen levels during the menstrual cycle have been shown to affect arousal. Aging also affects sexual arousal because vasocongestion develops more slowly in older women, so vaginal lubrication decreases after menopause; lower estrogen levels at this life stage may affect sexual arousal.

Intervention focuses on treating factors that contribute to the lack of arousal. Flibanserin, a medication designed and studied for premenopausal women with sexual desire disorder, is approved by the FDA for generalized hypoactive sexual desire disorder. The primary side effects of the daily pill are dizziness, sleepiness, and fatigue (Sprout

Pharmaceuticals, 2015). Cognitive behavioral therapy is recommended for psychosocial issues. For hormonal changes, a referral to a women's health provider is useful (Balon & Segraves, 2014).

MALE HYPOACTIVE SEXUAL DESIRE DISORDER

Male hypoactive sexual desire disorder is a recurrent deficiency or absence of sexual fantasies and desire for sexual activity. Individuals with this disorder are not interested in sex, do not or cannot get "turned on," and require no sexual gratification. Active avoidance of potential sexual relationships may exist. The prevalence is unknown, but it is believed to affect only a small proportion of men. Often, the disorder develops in adulthood after a period of adequate sexual interest and is associated with psychological distress, stressful life events (e.g., childbirth), or relationship difficulties (Balon & Segraves, 2014; Parish & Hahn, 2016).

Therapy for psychological issues related to hypoactive sexual desire aims at helping the patient understand the problem and develop strategies to enhance sexual arousal. Treatment approaches may include individual and couples therapy, sex-therapy techniques, clinical hypnosis, cognitive behavioral therapy, guided fantasy exercises, and sexual assertiveness training. If the problem is related to medication, changing to another classification of medication, giving drug holidays, or lowering the dose may help.

GENITOPELVIC PAIN/PENETRATION DISORDER

Genitopelvic pain/penetration disorder is characterized by persistent or recurrent difficulties with vaginal penetration during intercourse, marked vulvovaginal or pelvic pain during vaginal intercourse or penetration attempts, or significant fear or anxiety about the vulvovaginal or pelvic pain in anticipation of, during, or as a result of vaginal penetration (APA, 2013).

Dyspareunia is a term used to describe the genital pain associated with sexual intercourse that may be caused by **vaginismus**, which is spastic involuntary constriction of the perineal and outer vaginal muscles fostered by imagined, anticipated, or real attempts at vaginal penetration. This disorder may be related to interpersonal or emotional factors such as sexual dissatisfaction or poor technique leading to inadequate relaxation and lubrication. Biologic etiologies include intact or biperforate hymen, postmenopausal atrophic changes, trauma, malignancy, intestinal disease, or other pelvic disorders (Balon & Segraves, 2014).

PARAPHILIAS

Paraphilias are described as "intense and persistent sexual interest other than sexual interest in genital stimulation or preparatory fondling with phenotypically normal, physically mature, consenting human partners characterized by recurrent, intense sexual urges, fantasies, or behaviors involving unusual objects, activities, or situations" (APA, 2013, p. 685). These interests cause significant distress to the individual or impair social or occupational functioning. The paraphilias include voyeurism, exhibitionism, frotteurism, sexual masochism, sexual sadism, pedophilia, fetishism, and the transvestism disorders (APA, 2013).

Paraphilias are rarely diagnosed; the situation is complicated across cultures because acceptability of sexual practices varies across cultures. Although very few studies exist, some assert that comorbid mood disorders are often associated with paraphilia disorders (Becker & Johnson, 2014). These disorders often come to the attention of mental health professionals within the context of illegal sexual activity or sexually violent predators. Treatment of paraphilias is rarely sought by the individual; rather, it is a result of the psychosocial or criminal ramifications.

Certain behaviors and fantasies associated with paraphilias are said to begin in childhood and become more elaborate and better defined during adolescence and early adulthood. The disorders are often found to be chronic and lifelong, with the fantasies and behavior finally diminishing with old age. Table 29.1 includes the different categories of paraphilias along with their descriptions.

GENDER DYSPHORIA

Gender dysphoria is the term used to describe an incongruence between an individual's experienced/expressed gender and assigned gender (APA, 2013). Gender dysphoria is not classified as a sexual dysfunction. These individuals have a strong desire to be of the other gender. In boys (assigned gender), a strong preference for is shown for cross-dressing or simulating female attire. In girls (assigned gender), a strong preference is shown for wearing typically masculine clothing and a strong resistance to the wearing of typical female clothing (APA, 2013).

In child clinical samples, about four boys for each girl are referred with this disorder, but these differences disappear in adolescence (Becker & Perkins, 2014). Gender dysphoria does not necessarily persist into adulthood. Treatment focuses on acceptance, support, and self-esteem enhancement for both children and parents. Treatment goals should be made by the patient and family with the clinician providing the research literature.

TABLE 29.1 PARAPHILIAS

Paraphilia	Description
Exhibitionism	The behavior involves exposing one's genitals to strangers, with occasional masturbation. There may be an awareness of the desire to shock the individual or the fantasy that the individual will become sexually aroused on observation of the exposure.
Fetishism	An object such as women's undergarments or foot apparel is used for sexual arousal. The individual usually masturbates while holding, rubbing, or smelling the item or it is worn by a partner during sexual activity. Fetishism usually begins in adolescence and continues throughout life.
Frotteurism	Sexually arousing urges, fantasies, and behaviors occur when touching or rubbing one's genitals against the breasts, genitals, or thighs of a nonconsenting person. This paraphilia usually begins in early adolescence or young adulthood and diminishes with age.
Pedophilia	Sexual activity occurs with a child usually 13 yrs of age or younger by an individual at least 16 yrs of age or 5 yrs older than the child. Pedophilic acts include fondling, oral sex, and anal or vaginal intercourse with the penis, fingers, or objects, with varying amounts of force.
Sexual masochism	This behavior involves the act of being humiliated, beaten, bound, or made to suffer. Self-induced masochistic acts include use of electric shock, pin sticking, restraints, and mutilation; partner-induced acts may include bondage, whipping, being urinated or defecated on; and being forced to crawl, bark, or wear diapers. One dangerous form of sexual masochism that may be practiced alone or with a partner is "hypoxyphilia." Oxygen deprivation by means of a noose, plastic bag, chest compression, or drug effect is used during sexual activity to heighten orgasmic sensation. Deaths have occurred as a result of these techniques.
Sexual sadism	Sexual excitement occurs when causing physical or psychological suffering to another individual. Commonly, the individual with sadistic behavior interacts with a masochistic partner. Sadistic behavior includes various forms of physical punishment, use of restraints, rape, burning, stabbing, strangulation, torture, and murder. This is usually a chronic paraphilia that begins as early sexual fantasies and increases in severity over time.
Transvestic fetishism	This behavior applies generally to the heterosexual man who cross-dresses for the purpose of sexual excitement. The fantasies, sexual urges, or behaviors associated with the cross-dressing are recurrent and cause clinically significant distress or impairment in social, occupational, or other important areas of functioning.
Voyeurism	This behavior involves "peeping," for the purpose of sexual excitement, at unsuspecting people who are nude, undressing, or engaged in sexual activity.
Other paraphilias	Sexual fantasies, urges, and activities involving animals (zoophilia), corpses (necrophilia), feces (coprophilia), urine (urophilia), body parts (partialism), and obscene telephone calls (telephone scatalogia).

SUMMARY OF KEY POINTS

- Female orgasmic disorder is a common disorder affecting women; ED and PE are the most common disorders affecting men.
- Nursing interventions for people experiencing sexual dysfunction include (but are not limited to) counseling, education, and referral to sex therapists.
- Various medical conditions, psychological states, and medications negatively affect the sexual response cycle. Education about medication side effects and sexual experiences is important in maintaining health.
- Paraphilias are rarely diagnosed, but the prevalence may be higher than usually presented.
- Gender dysphoria occurs when the individual is uncomfortable with assigned sex or gender role.

CRITICAL THINKING CHALLENGES

1. A 36-year-old woman was recently diagnosed with depression and treated with a selective serotonin reuptake inhibitor (an antidepressant). Her depression is improving, but she has not been interested in sexual relations with her husband. Her lack of sexual interest is beginning to cause problems in her marriage. What could account for the changes in sexual interest?

2. A 52-year-old married man who is being successfully treated with lithium carbonate for his bipolar disorder was recently diagnosed with diabetes mellitus. He was told that his diabetes mellitus could be controlled by weight loss and diet. His major worry is that the disease and lithium are causing his impotence. He casually mentions that he is considering stopping the lithium. What issues should the nurse explore with the patient? What actions could the patient begin that would improve his sexual health?

3. During a nursing assessment, a young adult woman reveals that she is a lesbian and that she is currently living with her partner. She has not yet told her parents about her sexual orientation and is experiencing some anxiety about sharing this part of her life with her family. Her partner is supportive and encourages the young woman to take her time in telling her family members. Is this patient experiencing symptoms of a gender dysphoria? Explain.

2004: *Kinsey*

This critically acclaimed, American biographical drama describes the life of Alfred Charles Kinsey, a pioneer in the area of sexology. Professor Kinsey is being interviewed about his sexual history. During the interview, he has flashbacks to his childhood and young adulthood. His father, a minister, denounces modern inventions as leading to sexual sin and is shown as humiliating his young son. Kinsey, a biologist at Indiana University, marries a student in his class. He comes to terms with his own sexual needs and realizes that sexuality is more varied than originally thought. He publishes books on sexual habits and debunks many 1950s-era myths.

Viewing Points: How did Dr. Kinsey's work contribute to normalizing same-sex relationships and premarital sex? Identify the sexual myths that Dr. Kinsey was able to challenge.

REFERENCES

Akdemir, A. O., Karabakan, M., Aktas, B. K., Bozkurt, A., Ozgur, E. G., Akdogan, N., et al. (2019). Visceral adiposity index is useful for evaluating obesity effect on erectile dysfunction. *Andrologia, 2*, e13282.

American Psychiatric Association. (2013). *Diagnostic and statistical manual of mental disorders* (5th ed.). Arlington, VA: Author.

Balon, R. (2017). Burden of sexual dysfunction. *Journal of Sex and Marital Therapy, 43*(1), 49–55.

Balon, R., & Segraves, R. (2014). Sexual dysfunctions. In R. E. Hales, S. C. Yudofsy, & L. W. Roberts (Eds.). *The American psychiatric publishing textbook of psychiatry* (6th ed.). Arlington, VA: American Psychiatric Association.

Bancroft, J., & Graham, C. A. (2011). The varied nature of women's sexuality: Unresolved issues and a theoretical approach. *Hormones and Behavior, 59*(5), 717–729.

Bancroft, J., Graham, C. A., Janssen, E., & Sanders, S. A. (2009). The dual control model: Current status and future directions. *Journal of Sex Research, 46*(2–3), 121–142.

Basson, R. (2001). Female sexual response: The role of drugs in the management of sexual dysfunction. *Obstetrics and Gynecology, 98*(2), 350–353.

Becker, J., & Johnson, B. (2014). Paraphilic disorders. In R. E. Hales, S. C. Yudofsy, & L. W. Roberts (Eds.). *The American psychiatric publishing textbook of psychiatry* (6th ed.). Arlington, VA: American Psychiatric Association.

Becker, J., & Perkins, A. (2014). Gender dysphoria. In R. E. Hales, S. C. Yudofsy, & L. W. Roberts (Eds.). *The American psychiatric publishing textbook of psychiatry* (6th ed.). Arlington, VA: American Psychiatric Association.

Chen, J., Chen, Y., Gao, Q., Chen, G., Dai, Y., Yao, Z., et al. (2018). Impaired prefrontal-amygdala pathway, self-reported emotion, and erection in psychogenic erectile dysfunction patients with normal nocturnal erection. *Frontiers in Human Neuroscience, 2*, 157.

Cicero, E. C., & Wesp, L. M. (2017). Supporting the health and well-being of transgender students. *The Journal of School Nursing, 33*(2), 95–108.

Colson, M. H., Cuzin, B., Faix, A., Grellet, L., & Huyghes, E. (2018). Current epidemiology of erectile dysfunction, an update. *Sexologies, 27*(1), e7–e13.

Connaughton, C., McCabe, M., & Karantzas, G. (2016). Conceptualization of the sexual response models in men: Are there differences between sexually functional and dysfunctional men? *The Journal of Sexual Medicine, 13*(3), 453–463.

Cooper, K., Martyn-St James, M., Kaltenthaler, E., Dickinson, K., Cantrell, A., Ren, S., et al. (2017). Complementary and alternative medicine for management of premature ejaculation: A systematic review. *Sexual Medicine, 5*(1), e1–e18.

Costa, M. R., Ponciano, V. C., Costa, T. R., Gomes, C. P., & Oliveira, E. C. (2018). Stage effect of chronic kidney disease in erectile function. *International Brazilian Journal of Urology, 44*(1), 132–140.

Donovan, J. L., Hamdy, F. C., Lane, J. A., Mason, M., Metcalfe, C., Walsh, E., et al. (2016). Patient-reported outcomes after monitoring, surgery, or radiotherapy for prostate cancer. *New England Journal of Medicine, 375*(15), 1425–1437.

Eid, W., & Biason-Lauber, A. (2016). Why boys will be boys and girls will be girls: Human sex development and its defects. *Birth Defects Research (Part C), 108*, 365–379.

Eisenberg, M. L., & Meldrum, D. (2017). Effects of age on fertility and sexual function. *Fertility and Sterility, 107*(2), 301–304.

El-Hamd, M. A., Saleh, R., & Majzoub, A. (2019). Premature ejaculation: An update on definition and pathophysiology. *Asian Journal of Andrology*. doi: 10.4103/aja.aja_122_18.

Evans-Polce, R. J., Veliz, P. T., Boyd, C. J., Hughes, T. L., & McCabe, S. E. (2019). Associations between sexual orientation discrimination and substance use disorders: differences by age in US adults. *Social Psychiatry and Psychiatric Epidemiology*, 1–10. doi: 10.1007/s00127-019-01694-x

Ferenidou, F., Kirana, P. S., Fokas, K., Hatzichristou, D., & Athanasiadis, L. (2016). Sexual response models: Toward a more flexible patter of women's sexuality. *The Journal of Sexual Medicine, 13*(9), 1369–1376.

Grabowska, A. (2017). Sex on the brain: Are gender-dependent structural and functional differences associated with behavior? *Journal of Neuroscience Research, 95*, 200–212.

Healthy People 2020. (2017). *Lesbian, gay, bisexual, and transgender health*. Washington, DC: U.S. Department of Health and Human Services, Office of Disease Prevention and Health Promotion. Retrieved April 2017, from https://www.healthypeople.gov/2020/topics-objectives/topic/lesbian-gay-bisexual-and-transgender-health

Hodgson, B., Kukkonen, T. M., Binik, Y. M., & Carrier, S. (2016). Using the dual control model to investigate the relationship between mood, genital, and self-reported sexual arousal in men and women. *The Journal of Sex Research, 4*(8), 1–15.

Huang, Y. P., Liu, W., Chen, S. F., Liu, Y. D., Chen, B., Deng, C. H., et al. (2019). Free testosterone correlated with erectile dysfunction severity among young men with normal total testosterone. *International Journal of Impotence Research, 31*(2), 132–138.

Kann, L., McManus, T., Harris, W. A., Shanklin, S. L., Flint, K. H., Hawkins, J., et al. (2016). Youth risk behavior surveillance—United States, 2015. *Morbidity and Mortality Weekly Report. Surveillance Summaries, 65*(6), 1–174.

Kaplan, H. S. (1979). *Disorders of sexual desire and other concepts and techniques in sex therapy*. New York: Simon & Schuster.

Lussier P., McCuish, E., Mathesius, J., Corrado, R., & Nadeau, D. (2018). Developmental trajectories of child sexual behaviors on the path of sexual behavioral problems: Evidence from a prospective longitudinal study. *Sexual Abuse, 30*(6), 622–658.

Masters, W. H., & Johnson, V. E. (1966). *Human sexual response*. Boston, MA: Little, Brown.

Masters, W. H., & Johnson, V. E. (1970). *Human sexual inadequacy*. Boston, MA: Little, Brown and Co.

Miragoli, S., Camisasca, E., & Di Blasio, P. (2017). Child sexual behaviors in school context: Age and gender differences. *Journal of Child Sexual Abuse, 26*(2), 213–231.

Nguyen, H. M. T., Gabrielson, A. T., & Hellstrom, W. J. G. (2017). Erectile dysfunction in young men—A review of the prevalence and risk factors. *Sexual Medicine Reviews, 5*(4), 508–520.

Parish, S. J., & Hahn, S. R. (2016). Hypoactive sexual desire disorder: A review of epidemiology, biopsychology, diagnosis, and treatment. *Sexual Medicine Reviews, 4*(2), 103–120.

Phillips, A., & Phillips, S. (2015). Recognising female sexual dysfunction as an essential aspect of effective diabetes care. *Applied Nursing Research, 28*, 235–238.

Rastrelli, G., Cipriani, S., Corona, G., Vignozzi, L., & Maggi, M. (2019). Clinical characteristics of men complaining of premature ejaculation together with erectile dysfunction: a cross-sectional study. *Andrology, 7*(2), 163–171.

Rew, K. T., & Heidelbaugh, J. J. (2016). Erectile dysfunction. *American Family Physician, 94*(10), 820–827.

Rowland, D. L., Cempel, L. M., & Tempel, A. R. (2018). Women's attributions regarding why they have difficulty reaching orgasm. *Journal of Sex and Marital Therapy, 44*(5), 475–484.

Sarwer, D. B., Hanson, A. J., Voeller, J., & Steffen, K. (2018). Obesity and sexual functioning, *Current Obesity Reports, 7*(4), 301–307.

Sprout Pharmaceuticals. (2015). FDA Advisory Committee recommends approval for sprout Pharmaceuticals' ADDYI™ (flibanserin) to treat hypoactive sexual desire disorder in premenopausal women. Retrieved April 11, 2019, from www.sproutpharma.com.

Steinke, E. E., Mosack, V., & Hill, T. J. (2015). Change in sexual activity after cardiac event: The role of medications, comorbidity, and psychosocial factors. *Applied Nursing Research, 28*(3), 244–250.

Stephenson, K. R., Truong, L., & Shimazu, L. (2018). Why is impaired sexual function distressing to men? Consequences of impaired male sexual function and their associations with sexual well-being. *Journal of Sexual Medicine, 15*(9), 1336–1349.

Substance Abuse and Mental Health Services Administration. (2015). *Ending conversion therapy: Supporting and affirming LGBTQ youth (HHS Publication No. (SMA) 15-4928)*. Rockville, MD: Substance Abuse and Mental Health Services Administration.

Syme, M. L., & Cohn, T. J. (2016). Examining aging sexual stigma attitudes among adults by gender, age, and generational status. *Aging and Mental Health, 20*(1), 36–45.

Thomas, H. N., Neal-Perry, G. S., & Hess, R. (2018). Female sexual function at midlife and beyond. *Obstetrics and Gynecology Clinics of North America, 45*(4), 709–722.

Turner, D., Wittekind, C. E., Briken, P., Fromberger, P., Moritz, S., & Rettenberger, M. (2019). Approach and avoidance biases toward sexual stimuli and their association with the Dual Control Model of Sexual Response in heterosexual men. *Archives Sexual Behavior, 48*(3), 867–880.

Velten, J., Zahler, L., Scholten, S., & Margraf, J. (2019). Temporal stability of sexual excitation and sexual inhibition in women. *Archives of Sexual Behavior, 48*(3), 881–889.

Will, R. G., Hull, E. M., & Dominguez, J. M. (2014). Influences of dopamine and glutamate in the medial preoptic area on male sexual behavior. *Pharmacology Biochemistry, and Behavior, 121*, 115–123.

World Health Organization. (2019). Sexual and reproductive health. *The World Health Organization's department of reproductive health and research, Geneva*. Retrieved April 8, 2019, from http://www.who.int/reproductive-health/topics/sexual_health/sh_definitions/en/

Zamorano-Leon, J. J., Segura, A., Lahera, V., Rodriguez-Pardo, J. M., Prieto, R., Puigvert, A., et al. (2018). Relationship between erectile dysfunction, diabetes and dyslipidemia in hypertensive-treated Men. *Urology Journal, 15*(6), 370–375.

UNIT VI
CARE OF SPECIAL POPULATIONS

30
Mental Health Disorders of Childhood and Adolescence

Rebecca Luebbert

KEY CONCEPTS
- attention
- neurodevelopmental delay
- hyperactivity
- impulsiveness
- tics

LEARNING OBJECTIVES

After studying this chapter, you will be able to:

1. Describe mental disorders usually diagnosed in childhood or adolescence.
2. Discuss prevailing theories relevant to the mental health disorders in childhood and adolescence.
3. Discuss the nursing care of children with neurodevelopmental disorders.
4. Analyze the nursing assessment, diagnosis, intervention, and evaluation processes in caring for a child or adolescent with attention-deficit hyperactivity disorder.
5. Discuss the epidemiology, etiology, medications, and nursing care of children with tic disorders.
6. Discuss the nursing care of children and adolescents with separation anxiety and obsessive-compulsive disorders.
7. Compare the nursing care of children and adolescents with mood disorders and schizophrenia with that for adults with similar disorders.
8. Discuss the significance of behavioral intervention strategies for children who have elimination disorders.

KEY TERMS

- adaptive behavior • attention-deficit hyperactivity disorder (ADHD) • autism spectrum disorder (ASD) • communication disorders • dyslexia • encopresis • enuresis • intellectual disability • learning disorder • motor tics • phonic tics • phonologic processing • separation anxiety disorder • Tourette disorder

Psychiatric problems are less easily recognized in children than in adults. Normal growth and development behaviors of one age group may be a symptom of a disorder in another age group. For example, an imaginary friend is age appropriate for a 4-year-old child but not for an adolescent. Despite the difficulty in diagnosis, about 20% of U.S. youth in their lifetimes are affected by a mental disorder that impairs their ability to function (NAMI, 2019). Unfortunately, although depression, anxiety, and behavioral and disorders are prevalent among children and adolescents, significant gaps in treatment exist (Ghandour et al., 2019).

This chapter presents an overview of selected childhood disorders and discusses nursing care for children and their families with these problems. Because it is beyond the scope of this text to present all child psychiatric disorders, this chapter discusses selected ones, including neurodevelopment disorders (intellectual disability, autism spectrum disorder, attention-deficit hyperactivity disorder, and tic disorders), separation anxiety disorder, obsessive-compulsive disorder (OCD), mood disorders, childhood schizophrenia, and elimination disorders (enuresis and encopresis). Oppositional defiant and conduct disorders are discussed in Chapter 24.

> **NCLEXNOTE** All the psychiatric disorders of childhood and adolescence should be viewed within the context of growth and development models. Safety and self-esteem are priority considerations.

NEURODEVELOPMENTAL DISORDERS OF CHILDHOOD

The neurodevelopmental disorders occur early in a child's development, often before grade school. These disorders include developmental deficits that range from very specific limitations of learning to global impairments of social skills. They impact personal, social, academic, or occupational functioning. Under the primary influences of genes and environment, neurodevelopment of attention, cognition, language, affect, and social and moral behavior proceeds along several pathways. Developmental pathways and developmental delays are closely interwoven. For example, a language delay can interfere with a child's social development and contribute to behavior problems (Yew & O'Kearney, 2017). This section discusses neurodevelopmental disorders of childhood that include several conditions that are etiologically unrelated; however, their common feature is a significant delay in one or more lines of development.

> **KEYCONCEPT** **Neurodevelopmental delay** means that the child's development in attention, cognition, language, affect, and social or moral behavior is outside the norm and is manifested by delayed socialization, communication, peculiar mannerisms, and idiosyncratic interests.

INTELLECTUAL DISABILITY

Intellectual disability is defined as a disability characterized by significant limitations in both intellectual function and in adaptive behavior that covers many everyday social and practical skills (American Association on Intellectual and Developmental Disabilities [AAIDD], 2019). The disability begins before the age of 18 years.

Diagnostic Criteria and Clinical Course

The diagnosis of intellectual disability involves an assessment of intellectual function such as reasoning, problem solving, and adaptive function in personal independence and social responsibility (American Psychiatric Association [APA], 2013). A diagnosis is made through clinical assessment of behavioral features; historical accounts from parents and teachers; and performance on standardized tests such as the Stanford-Binet or the Wechsler Intelligence Scales for Children. The usual threshold for intellectual disability is an intelligence quotient (IQ) of 70 or less (i.e., two standard deviations below the population mean).

Adaptive behavior is composed of three skill types: *conceptual skills* (e.g., language and literacy, money, time, number concepts, and self-direction); *social skills* (e.g., interpersonal skills, social responsibility, self-esteem, gullibility, social problem-solving, and the ability to follow rules and obey laws and to avoid being victimized); and *practical skills* (e.g., activities of daily living [ADLs], occupational skills, health care, travel and transportation, schedules and routines, safety, use of money, use of telephone) (AAIDD, 2019). Impaired adaptive functioning is primarily a clinical judgment based on the child's capacity to manage age-appropriate ADLs. However, standardized assessment instruments are available to assist with determination of the child's capabilities (Lyons, Huber, Carter, Chen, & Asmus, 2016).

An intellectual disability is not necessarily lifelong. Some children may be diagnosed at school age as having an intellectual disability, but with guidance and education, they may no longer meet the criteria as adults.

Epidemiology and Etiology

A large meta-analysis estimated the prevalence of intellectual disabilities to be about 1% in the United States and worldwide (McKenzie, Milton, Smith, & Ouellette-Kuntz, 2016). A considerable variability worldwide exists, with low- and middle-income countries reporting significantly higher rates of disability than high-income countries (Global Research on Developmental Disabilities Collaborators, 2018). Children and adolescents with intellectual disabilities are at significantly higher risk for other mental disorders than those without an intellectual disability. In a national study of adolescents with intellectual disability, 65% met lifetime criteria for a mental disorder (Platt, Keyes, McLaughlin, & Kaufman, 2019).

Intellectual disabilities result from a variety of causes with the most common etiology related to genetic syndromes. Chromosomal changes or defects (e.g., Down syndrome) and exposure to toxins during prenatal development (e.g., fetal alcohol syndrome), heredity, pregnancy and perinatal complications, medication conditions, and environmental influences are all associated with intellectual disabilities. The cause is unknown in many of the cases (Batshaw, Roizen, & Lotrecchiano, 2013).

> **BOX 30.1**
>
> **History and Hallmarks of Childhood and Adolescent Disorders**
>
> - Maternal age and health status during pregnancy
> - Exposure to medication, alcohol, or other substances during pregnancy
> - Course of pregnancy, labor, and delivery
> - Infant's health at birth
> - Eating, sleeping, and growth in first year
> - Health status in first year
> - Interest in others in first 2 years
> - Motor development
> - Mastery of bowel and bladder control
> - Speech and language development
> - Activity level
> - Response to separation (e.g., school entry)
> - Regulation of mood and anxiety
> - Medical history in early childhood
> - Social development
> - Interests

Nursing Care of Children With Intellectual Disability

Assessment of a child with an intellectual disability focuses on current adaptive skills, intellectual status, and social functioning. A developmental history is a useful way to gather information about past and current capacities (Box 30.1). The nurse compares these data with normal growth and development. Developmentally delayed children who have not had a psychological evaluation should be considered for referral. These children also require evaluation for other comorbid psychiatric disorders, which may be a challenge because of the child's cognitive limitations. Discussions about feelings and behavior may be too complex for these children. If children or adolescents with intellectual disabilities have a comorbid mental disorder or serious behavioral problems, a carefully constructed interdisciplinary behavioral plan will guide care and treatment.

The nurse also assesses the child's support systems (family, school, rehabilitative, and psychiatric) to ensure that the child's special needs have been identified and are being addressed. For example, occupational therapy may be recommended to improve motor coordination, but the family may not have transportation to these services available, so availability to alternative services should be explored.

The child and family's response to intellectual disability and other comorbid conditions will determine the nursing diagnoses, planning, and implementation of nursing interventions. Associated nursing diagnoses include Ineffective Coping, Delayed Growth and Development, and Interrupted Family Processes. Nursing interventions include promoting coping skills (i.e., interventions directed at building strengths, adapting to change, and maintaining or achieving a higher level of functioning), patient education, and parent education.

The overall goals of treatment and nursing care are an optimal level of functioning for the family and eventual independent functioning within a normal social environment for the child. For many children with intellectual disability, achieving independence in adulthood will be delayed but not impossible.

Continuum of Care

Children and families may require varying levels of interventions at different times throughout the life cycle. When a child is young, the family requires special educational support and, for some, residential services. The need for psychiatric intervention varies according to the severity of disability, family functioning, and the coexistence of other disorders. Feelings of grief and loss in family members (especially parents) related to having a child with a disability may be relieved through family therapy. More specific parent training may be needed to deal with emerging maladaptive behaviors.

AUTISM SPECTRUM DISORDER

Autism spectrum disorder (ASD) is characterized by persistent impairment in social communication and social interaction with others (APA, 2013). Children with ASD may or may not have an intellectual disability, but they commonly show an uneven pattern of intellectual strengths and weaknesses. This condition may be a lifelong pattern of being rigid in manner, intolerant of change, and prone to behavioral outbursts in response to environmental demands or changes in routine. Two conditions, autism disorder and Asperger syndrome, were previously diagnosed as separate disorders. However, because they have many overlapping symptoms and are difficult to differentiate from each other, the *DSM-5* no longer considers autism and Asperger syndrome as separate disorders, but considers both as an ASD differentiated by language or intellectual impairment (APA, 2013).

ASD with restricted repetitive patterns of behavior such as stereotypic or repetitive motor movement, use of objects, inflexible adherence to routine or ritualized patterns, and fascination with lights or movement has been a subject of considerable interest and research effort since its original description more than 70 years ago. Leo Kanner (1943) described the profound isolation of these children and their extreme desire for sameness. These children appear aloof and indifferent to others and often seem to prefer inanimate objects.

Impairment in communication is severe and affects both verbal and nonverbal communication. Children with ASD may manifest delayed and deviant language development, as evidenced by echolalia (repetition of words or phrases spoken by others) and a tendency to be extremely literal in interpretation of language. Pronoun reversals and abnormal intonation are also common. Other common features of ASD are stereotypic behavior, self-stimulating, nonfunctional repetitive behaviors, such as repetitive rocking, hand flapping, and an extraordinary insistence on sameness. These children may also engage in self-injurious behavior, such as hitting, head banging, or biting. In some children, their unusual interests may evolve into fascination with specific objects, such as fans or air conditioners, or a particular topic, such as U.S. Civil War generals.

A child with ASD may have age-appropriate language and intelligence but also have severe and sustained impairment in social interaction and restricted, repetitive patterns of behavior, interests, and activities. This type of ASD was previously known as Asperger syndrome and appears to be a milder form of ASD. These children have social deficits marked by inappropriate initiation of social interactions, an inability to respond to normal social cues, and a tendency to be literal in their interpretation of language (APA, 2013). They may also display stereotypic behaviors, such as rocking and hand flapping, and have highly restricted areas of interest, such as train schedules, fans, air conditioners, or dogs. Signs of developmental delay may not be apparent until preschool or school age, when social deficits become evident (Box 30.2).

Epidemiology and Etiology

Recent studies by the CDC find that approximately 1 in 59 children has been identified with ASD. It is found approximately four times more often in boys than in girls and is found in all racial, ethnic, and socioeconomic groups (Baio et al., 2018). Intellectual disability and seizures often occur in ASD (Strasser, Downes, Kung, Cross, & De Haan, 2018). Published claims that the prevalence of autism is increasing are confounded by improved methods of diagnosis (El Achkar & Spence, 2015).

Research is accelerating in understanding the etiology of ASD because structural and functional imaging studies provide intriguing leads for future inquiry (Fig. 30.1). Multiple etiologic hypotheses are related to this disorder. Recent studies support a shared genetic etiology between ASD and schizophrenia (McCarthy, Gillis, Kramer, Lihm, Yoon, Berstein, et al., 2014). Expression of multiple genes related to the regulation of neurogenesis, brain, and differentiation process are implicated in ASD (Vaishnavi, Manikandan, & Munirajan, 2014). One line of research is determining defects in the metabolism of cellular antioxidants (Raymond, Deth, & Ralston, 2014). Studies show that higher levels of lead and mercury and lower levels of antioxidants are found in inpatients with ASD when compared to control groups (Alabdali, Al-Ayadhi, & El-Ansary, 2014). Symptoms of gastrointestinal disturbance have focused other research on the

BOX 30.2 CLINICAL VIGNETTE

Frank (Autism Spectrum Disorder Asperger Syndrome)

A pediatrician refers Frank, age 5 years, 6 months, for an evaluation because of Frank's unusual preoccupation with ceiling fans and lawn sprinklers. According to his mother, Frank became interested in ceiling fans at age 3 years when he began drawing them, tearing pictures of them out of magazines, and engaging others in discussions about them. In the months before the evaluation, Frank also became fascinated by lawn sprinklers. These preoccupations dominated Frank's interactions with others so much that he was practically incapable of discussing any other topics. He remained on the periphery of his kindergarten class and had few friends. Although he tried to make friends, his approaches were inept, and he had trouble reading others.

Frank was the product of a full-term uncomplicated pregnancy, labor, and delivery to his then 25-year-old mother. It was her first pregnancy, and both parents eagerly anticipated Frank's birth. As an infant, Frank was healthy but seemed to cry a lot and was difficult to comfort, causing his mother to feel inadequate and depleted. His motor development was also delayed, and at age 3 years, nonfamily members had difficulty understanding his speech. His articulation, however, was within normal limits at the time of consultation. Frank received regular pediatric care and had no history of serious illness or injury. There was no family history of intellectual disability or psychiatric illness; results of genetic testing for chromosomal abnormality were negative.

In addition to his unusual preoccupations and social deficits, Frank resisted any change in his routine, was easily frustrated, and was prone to temper tantrums. His parents sharply disagreed about the nature of and appropriate response to his problems.

What Do You Think?
- What effect do you think Frank's preoccupation may have on his family and their relationships?
- What kind of teaching program would you develop if you were the nurse assigned to this family?

FIGURE 30.1 Patients with autism (*right*) may have decreased metabolic rates in the cingulate gyrus and other associated areas; however, wide heterogeneity in brain metabolic patterns is seen in patients with autism. (Courtesy of Monte S. Buchsbaum, MD, The Mount Sinai Medical Center and School of Medicine, New York.)

role of the GI microbiota and their fermentation products (Wang, Conlon, Christophersen, Sorich, & Angley, 2011). Other researchers suggest a role for maternal autoantibodies in the fetal brain in some cases (Elamin & Al-Ayadhi, 2014).

Recovery-Oriented Care for Children With Autism Spectrum Disorder

Teamwork and Collaboration: Working Toward Recovery

ASDs require long-term care at various levels of intensity. Treatment consists of designing academic, interpersonal, and social experiences that support the child's development. Children with autism, even those who are severely affected, may be able to live at home and attend special schools that use behavioral techniques. Other outpatient services may include family counseling, home care, and medication. As the child moves toward adulthood, living at home may become more difficult given the appropriate need for greater independence. The level of structure required depends primarily on IQ and adaptive functioning.

Planning interventions for children with an ASD considers the child; family; and community supports, such as schools, rehabilitation centers, or group homes. First and foremost, the clinicians involved in the child's treatment should collaborate with the family toward the same general goals. As the number of clinicians and educators involved increases, the chance of fragmentation in treatment planning also increases. The nurse can serve as a case coordinator.

Residential care may be necessary in some cases. After making the decision to place a child into a residential facility, family members may experience guilt, loss, and a sense of failure concerning their inability to care for the child at home.

Evidence-Based Nursing Care for Children With Autism Spectrum Disorder

Mental Health Nursing Assessment

Physical Health Assessment

Physical health assessment should include a review of physical health and neurologic status, giving particular attention to coordination, childhood illnesses, injuries, and hospitalizations. The nurse should assess sleep, appetite, and activity patterns because they may be disturbed in affected children. Lack of adequate sleep can increase irritability. Comorbid seizure disorders are common in those with autism; depression is often seen concurrently even when no intellectual or language impairment is evident. Thus, the nurse should consider these conditions in the assessment.

Children with additional psychiatric disorders or seizures may be receiving multiple medications and require the care of several clinicians. Therefore, assessment should include a careful review of current medications and treating clinicians.

Psychosocial Assessment

Communication, behaviors, and flexibility are critical assessment areas. Direct behavioral observation is important to evaluate the child's ability to relate to others, to verify the selection of age-appropriate activities, and to watch for stereotypic behaviors. Assessment of the child with ASD can be based on the following categories:

- Communication
  - Verbal and nonverbal
  - Use of picture cards, writing, or drawing
  - Comfortable with eye contact
  - Understand emotional cues
  - Presence of pain
  - Preoccupation with restricted interests
- Behaviors
  - Items of fixation (how does family manage?)
  - Triggers for agitation
  - Early signs that indicate beginning of agitation
  - Interventions that work when child is overstimulated or agitated
  - Repetitive behaviors
- Flexibility or adherence to routine
  - Home schedule
  - What aggravates or irritates the person
  - Early warning signs of agitation
  - When overagitated, what interventions work best

The child's behavior, need for structure, and communication style can affect family functioning. Having a child with ASD is bound to influence family interaction; responding to the child's needs may adversely affect family functioning. For example, sleep disruption in family members who care for these children may increase family stress.

Priority of Nursing Care

Treatment outcomes need to be individualized to the child, family, and social environment and may change with time. Ensuring physical safety is a priority for the nurse. The nurse will need to develop a plan of care that takes into consideration the child's ability to communicate effectively with others. The child may also have difficulty completing ADLs and may demonstrate poor coping and impaired social skills. Determining the need for predictability and stability in routine for the child is also important.

Mental Health Nursing Interventions

Physical Health Interventions

In teaching self-care skills, the nurse needs to consider the child's current adaptive skills and language limitations. Developing a list of activities for the child to post in his or her bedroom may be effective for some children. Drawings or symbols may be useful for nonverbal children. Physical safety is an important concern for children who are cognitively delayed and may have impaired judgment.

No medication has proved effective at changing the core social and language deficits of autism. However, some atypical antipsychotics (i.e., risperidone, aripiprazole) are approved for the treatment of irritability associated with autism. Weight gain and metabolic syndrome are concerns with these agents. Evidence is minimal that anticonvulsants and traditional mood stabilizers are useful in managing mood lability and aggression (Bertelli, Rossi, Keller, & Lassi, 2016).

Psychosocial Interventions

When working with children with neurodevelopmental disorders, building on their strengths and using positive reinforcement are very important. If these children feel that they are constantly criticized or need "fixing," their self-esteem will be eroded and they will be unlikely to cooperate and learn.

Promoting Interaction

Structuring interventions for social isolation should fit the child's cognitive, linguistic, and developmental levels. Interventions fostering nonverbal social interactions may be more useful than those based on speech. For higher functioning children, activities such as getting the mail, passing out snacks, or taking turns in the context of simple games can engage them in social activities without requiring the use of their limited language skills. Structuring social interactions so that the child shares a task with another, such as carrying a load of books, may help boost confidence in relating to others.

ASDs call for extraordinary patience and determination. With help, these children can learn social and communication skills, such as taking turns in conversation and warning the listener before changing the subject in the context of milieu.

Ensuring Predictability and Safety

When children with ASDs are hospitalized, milieu management—a consistent, structured environment with predictable routines for activities, mealtimes, and bedtimes—is necessary for successful treatment. Changes in routine may provoke disorganization in the child, leading to emotional disequilibrium and explosive behavior. The safety of the inpatient unit offers an opportunity to try behavioral strategies, such as rewards for managing transitions. Health care professionals can pass on successful strategies to parents or primary caretakers (Anderson & Byrne-Barta, 2015).

A structured physical environment will most likely be important to a child with a development disorder. Keeping furniture, dishes, and toys in the same place helps ease anxiety and fosters secure feelings. The nurse should identify the child's individually specific needs for structure.

Behavioral Interventions

Children with ASDs often need specific behavioral interventions to reduce the frequency of inappropriate or aggressive behavior (Anderson & Byrne-Barta, 2015). For example, a child may have angry outbursts in response to routine transitions. If the tantrum is dramatic, the consequence may be that the transition does not take place. By structuring the environment and using visual cues to signal the end of one activity and the start of another, it may be possible to reduce the number and intensity of responses to transitions. Safety is always a concern. Self-injury and aggression are sometimes present, so children may need to be protected from hurting themselves and others. If aggressive or assaultive behavior is a problem, a brief "time out" followed by prompt reentry into activities is usually effective.

Managing the repetitive behaviors of these children depends on the specific behavior and its effects on others or the environment. If the behavior, such as rocking, has no negative effects, ignoring it may be the best approach. If the behavior, such as head banging, however, is unacceptable, redirecting the child and using positive reinforcement are recommended. In some cases, especially in severely delayed children, these strategies may not work, and environmental alterations and perhaps protective headgear will be needed.

Supporting Family

Unfortunately, lack of integration of medical, psychiatric, social, and educational services can add to the family's burden. Parents may manifest denial, grief, guilt, and anger at various points as they adjust to their child's disability. The nurse can offer parents the opportunity to express their frustrations and disappointments and can be alert for indications that parents are in need of additional assistance, such as parent support groups or respite care.

Family interventions include support, education, counseling, and referral to self-help groups. Whenever possible, the nurse provides education to help parents determine appropriate expectations for their child and to meet the child's special needs. The following are examples of potentially useful nursing interventions focusing on the family:

- Interpreting the treatment plan for parents and child
- Modeling appropriate behavior modification techniques

- Including the parents as co-therapists for the implementation of the care plan
- Assisting the family in identifying and resolving their sense of loss related to the diagnosis
- Coordinating support systems for parents, siblings, and family members
- Maintaining interdisciplinary collaboration

Evaluation and Treatment Outcomes

Evaluation of patient and family outcomes is an ongoing process. Short-term outcomes might consist of discrete behavioral improvements, such as reducing self-injurious behavior by 50%. The long-term goal is for the patient to achieve the highest level of functioning.

ATTENTION-DEFICIT HYPERACTIVITY DISORDER

Attention-deficit hyperactivity disorder (ADHD) is one of the most commonly diagnosed disorders in school-aged children (Centers for Disease Control and Prevention [CDC], 2019a). It is almost certainly a heterogeneous disorder with multiple etiologies. The relatively high frequency of ADHD and associated behavior problems virtually guarantees that nurses will meet affected children in all pediatric treatment settings. ADHD is also diagnosed in adults, but it is less common than in children (Torgersen, Gjervan, Lensing, & Rasmussen, 2016).

Clinical Course and Diagnostic Criteria

A persistent pattern of inattention, hyperactivity, and impulsiveness that interferes with functioning characterizes ADHD (APA, 2013). A diagnosis is made based on school behavior, parents' reports, and direct observation of inattention and hyperactivity–impulsivity that are inconsistent with developmental level. Parents and teachers describe children with ADHD as restless, always on the go, highly distractible, unable to wait their turn, heedless, and frequently disruptive. Indeed, it is often disruptive behavior that brings these children into treatment.

> **KEYCONCEPT Attention** involves concentrating on one activity to the exclusion of others, as well as the ability to sustain focus.

In ADHD, the person finds it difficult to attend to one task at a time and is easily distracted. For some, the lack of attention is related to being unable to filter incoming information, which leads to being unable to screen and select the important information. That is, all incoming stimuli are treated the same (e.g., directions from a teacher elicits the same importance as noise in the hallway). For others, the distractibility may be related to stimuli seeking behavior. Given the heterogeneity of ADHD, either of these models may explain problems of attention for subgroups of affected children.

Children with ADHD are prone to impulsive, risk-taking behavior and often fail to consider the consequences of their actions (CDC, 2019a). They tend to exercise poor judgment and seem to have more than the usual lumps, bumps, and bruises because of their risk-taking behavior. They often require a high degree of structure and supervision (Daley et al., 2018).

> **KEYCONCEPT Impulsiveness** is the tendency to act on urges, notions, or desires without adequately considering the consequences.

Although hyperactivity is a characteristic often associated with ADHD, controversy is long-standing about whether attention-deficit disorder can occur without overactivity. In many cases, the hyperactivity prompts the search for treatment. Parents typically report that a child's hyperactivity was manifested early in life and is evident in most situations (APA, 2013). Hyperactivity and impulsivity in childhood are associated with conduct disorder (Chapter 24) and intimate partner violence perpetration in adults (Guendelman, Ahmad, Meza, Owens, & Hinshaw, 2016).

> **KEYCONCEPT Hyperactivity** is excessive motor activity, as evidenced by restlessness, an inability to remain seated, and high levels of physical motion and verbal output.

ADHD Across the Life Span

ADHD is usually diagnosed in childhood and was traditionally viewed as a problem of children. We now understand that ADHD persists into adulthood and it is sometimes first diagnosed later than in childhood. In adults, symptoms of hyperactivity and impulsivity tend to decline with age and deficit of attention persist and become more varied (Torgersen et al., 2016). However, the majority of the adults with ADHD are undiagnosed and untreated (Ginsberg, Quintero, Anand, Casillas, & Upadhyaya, 2014). Many of the adults with ADHD become the parents of children with the same disorder (Deater-Deckard, 2017).

Epidemiology and Risk Factors

Although prevalence estimates vary depending on the diagnostic criteria used, the sources of data, and the sampling procedure, ADHD has been diagnosed in as many as 9.4% of children aged 2 to 17 (Danielson, Ghandour, Holbrook, Kogan, & Blumberg, 2018). Boys are twice as likely as girls to be diagnosed with ADHD (CDC, 2019a). A familial history of ADHD, bipolar disorder, or substance use (Sanchez-Gistau et al., 2015), early exposure to pesticides and lead (Rauh, 2016), and prenatal tobacco exposure (Joelsson et al., 2016) are associated with an increased risk for ADHD.

Etiology

No single explanation for the occurrence of ADHD exists; instead, this disorder is viewed as having multiple causes. Genetic factors are implicated in the etiology of ADHD. They clearly play a fundamental role in the manifestation of the ADHD behavior (Scibberas, Mulraney, Silva, & Coghill, 2017). In some children, ADHD may have developed because of being hypersensitive to environmental stimuli such as foods. This hypersensitivity to foods may be allergies to specific foods (e.g., wheat, milk, peanuts, eggs, soy) or to other substances such as artificial dyes and flavors or salicylates (Stevenson et al., 2014).

Biologic Theories

Although the etiology of ADHD is uncertain, evidence about neurobiologic dysfunction is pervasive. Several lines of research have shown that the frontal lobe and functional connections are impacted with specific subcortical structures also dysregulated. One clearly dysfunctional area is the dorsolateral prefrontal cortex, the center of directed attention and the ability to manage emotions or delay emotional reactions. Several neurotransmitters (e.g., dopamine, serotonin) are dysregulated (Zhu et al., 2016). Clinically, the hyperactive–impulsive behavior characteristic of ADHD has been shown to be predominantly related to biologic factors, not psychosocial factors (Freitag et al., 2012).

Psychosocial Theories

Although genetic endowment is clearly a fundamental element in the etiology of ADHD, psychosocial factors are also important risk factors, particularly those related to inattention (Freitag et al., 2012). Family stress, marital discord, and parental substance use are also associated with exacerbation of ADHD behaviors (Sigfusdottir et al., 2017). Other implicated psychosocial factors are poverty, overcrowded living conditions, and family dysfunction.

Family Response to ADHD

Living with a child who has ADHD is a challenge for all family members, particularly those members who also have issues similar to those of the affected child. The family will not only be raising a child who needs a structured environment that helps support focus and attention, but the parents have to partner with their children's school system. For some families, the relationship with the school is positive and supportive. For others, the relationship with the school can be strained and lead to additional stress. It is important that the teachers and parents work together and provide consistent directions to the child.

If parents also have problems related to attention, impulse, and hyperactivity, home chaos, and ineffective parenting practices can occur (Deater-Deckard, 2017). If the parents also have ADHD, they might not be able to provide a calm structured environment for the child. Effective parenting requires the ability to resist overreacting emotionally, to focus on the child, to keep track of activities, and to provide consistency in discipline.

Recovery-Oriented Care for Persons With ADHD

Teamwork and Collaboration: Working Toward Recovery

Children with ADHD and their families benefit from symptom management, education, and support from various disciplines to have a high-quality life. Successful recovery efforts involve early recognition and treatment. By recognizing the problem early, family members and teachers can structure the child's interactions, develop meaningful discipline strategies, and modify the physical environment so the child can learn coping skills to deal with impulsivity, distractibility, and hyperactivity. Evidence has accumulated over the years that medication is helpful, especially in the early years, but for long-term effects, a combination of medication management and behavioral approaches results in the best outcomes for the children and their families (CDC, 2019a).

ADHD is not an easy disorder to treat or manage. Comorbidity complicates successful recovery. Children with ADHD have more conduct problems (e.g., run-ins with police), depression, and anxiety (CDC, 2019a). Many other problems interfere with recovery efforts, such as family disruptions and economic problems, as well as naturally occurring changes such as maturational issues during their adolescent years. Additionally, children from disadvantaged backgrounds fare worse than those children who have socioeconomic and educational support (Huang, Xu, Au, Xu, & Wu, 2018).

Safety Issues

Due to increased impulsivity and inattention, children and adolescents with ADHD are at greater risk for injury than those without ADHD. Research finds that children with ADHD are significantly more likely to experience injury while riding a bike, have more head injuries and injuries to multiple body parts, and are more likely to be hospitalized for unintentional poisoning. Teenagers with ADHD are more likely to break traffic rules and are more likely to be involved in a car accident than those without ADHD (CDC, 2019a).

Individuals of all ages with ADHD are at high risk for moodiness that could lead to risk-taking behavior and suicide ideation or attempts (Balazs, Miklósi, Keresztény, Dallos, & Gádoros, 2014). Mood lability, the presence of depression, and potential for self-harm should be carefully assessed in these individuals. These children are also at risk for depression and suicidal ideation, especially in adolescence.

Evidence-Based Nursing Care for Children with ADHD

The planning of nursing interventions must be done within the context of the family, treatment setting, and school environment. With the parents, clinical team members, and school personnel, the nurse participates in designing a plan of care that fits the child's and family's needs. Persons with ADHD and their families will benefit from nursing care at many different times in the course of the disorder. Unless hospitalized for a comorbid mental health problem, most treatment will occur outside the mental health system. School nurses often provide most of the nursing care and family education.

Mental Health Nursing Assessment

In the school setting, the primary focus of the assessment is the impact of ADHD on classroom behavior and school performance. In the hospital, the nurse tries to determine the contribution of ADHD to the acute psychiatric problem. In both cases, the nurse collects assessment data through direct interview, observation of the child and parent, and teacher ratings. Because children with ADHD may have difficulty sitting through long sessions, interviews are typically brief. Parents and teachers are extremely important sources for assessment data. To this end, the nurse can make use of several standardized instruments (Box 30.3). See Nursing Care Plan 30.1 at http://thepoint.lww.com/BoydEssentials2e.

Physical Health Assessment

As with other psychiatric disorders with onset in childhood, the nursing assessment of children with ADHD begins with identification and exploration of the presenting problems, usually hyperactivity, impulsivity, and inattention. This typically entails a review of the child's developmental course, the onset and pattern of the current symptoms, factors that have worsened or improved the child's problems, and prior treatment or self-initiated efforts to remedy the situation. Medical history is also essential, consisting of perinatal course, childhood illnesses, hospital admissions, injuries, seizures, tics, physical growth, general health status, and date of the child's last physical examination.

The behavior of these children is characteristically very active and can often be observed in the office. They cannot sit still. They fidget. Even in sleep, they may be more active than normal children. Thus, a careful assessment of eating, sleeping, and activity patterns is essential. Assessing daily food intake, typical diet, and frequency of eating will help identify any nutritional problems. Caffeinated products can contribute to hyperactivity in some children. Sleep is often disturbed for children with ADHD and consequently also the family. A detailed sleep assessment can provide points for interventions and help the interpretation of drug effects.

Psychosocial Assessment

Data regarding school performance, behavior at home, and comorbid psychiatric disorders are essential for developing school interventions and behavior plans and establishing the baseline severity for medication. Children with ADHD are more likely to have problems with their cognitive process during changing demands of teachers and parents (cognitive processing, attention, language, and memory) (Korrel, Mueller, Silk, Anderson, & Sciberras, 2017; Yang, Allen, Holmes, & Chan, 2017). Consequently, they may have more difficulty in school with decision-making. These children are often behind

---

BOX 30.3

Standardized Tools for ADHD Diagnosis[a]

CONNERS QUESTIONNAIRES
The Conners Parent Questionnaire is a 48-item scale that a parent completes about his or her child. Each item is a statement that the parent rates on a 4-point scale from 0 (not at all) to 3 (very much). The Conners Teacher Questionnaire is a 28-item questionnaire that the child's teacher completes according to the same 4-point scale as the Parent Questionnaire. Both questionnaires have been standardized by age and gender for a mean of 50 and a standard deviation of 10 (Conners, 1989; Goyette, Connors, & Ulrich, 1978).

CHILD BEHAVIOR CHECKLIST
The Child Behavior Checklist (CBCL) is a 118-item questionnaire that a parent completes. In addition to the 118 questions about specific behaviors and psychiatric symptoms, the CBCL also includes questions concerning the child's competence in social and academic spheres as well as age-appropriate activities. Normative data are available, allowing the conversion of raw scores to standard scores for age and gender. A teacher version of this scale is also available.

[a]Note that the diagnosis of ADHD is not made on the basis of questionnaires alone. Data from these rating scales augment the information gathered through interview and observation. These questionnaires can be especially useful before and after initiating a treatment plan to measure change.

in their work at school because of poor organization, off-task behavior, and impulsive responses.

Dysfunctional interactions can develop within the family. Discipline is frequently an issue because parents may have difficulty controlling their child's behavior, which is disruptive and occasionally destructive. They can exhaust their parents, aggravate teachers, and annoy siblings with their intrusive and disruptive actions. Reviewing the problem behaviors and the situations in which they occur is a way to identify negative interaction patterns.

Because ADHD often occurs in the context of psychosocial adversity, it is important to review the family situation, including parenting style, stability of household membership, consistency of rules and routines, and life events (e.g., divorce, moves, deaths, job loss). Identification of these factors can be useful in shaping a care plan that builds on potential strengths and mitigates the effects of environmental factors that may perpetuate the child's disruptive behavior.

Priority of Nursing Care

Priorities of nursing care will depend on the severity of the responses, family situation, and school environment. Increased impulsivity and intention puts the child or adolescent at greater risk for injury. Comorbid disorders, such as mood or conduct disorders, may also be present. Sleep deprivation, inadequate nutrition, and the inability to carry out daily routines may require intervention. The child may demonstrate poor coping skills and may not function well in social settings or in structured activities (such as in the school environment). Outcomes should be individualized to the child. Short-term outcomes, such as decreasing the number of classroom ejections within a 2-week period, may be useful for one child, but reducing the frequency and amplitude of angry outbursts at home may be relevant to another child.

Nursing Interventions

Physical Health Interventions

Modifying Nutrition. A link between adverse reaction to food (e.g., dietary salicylates and artificially added food colors, flavors, preservatives) and ADHD was suggested many years ago when the Feingold diet was introduced (Feingold, 1975). Over the years, interest in the link between food and behavior continues to spark interest in ADHD as a problem related to food. Study outcomes are mixed. Agreement exists that in some children the behaviors associated with ADHD can be decreased with diet changes (Pelsser, Frankena, Toorman, & Pereira, 2017). Study outcomes are mixed. A review of the artificial food color elimination diet (restricted elimination diet), a few foods diet, and polyunsaturated fatty acid supplementation diet indicates that the free foods diet provides a contribution to ADHD treatment (Pelsser et al., 2017). The others did not have the research to support their efficacy.

The *few foods diet* includes basic foods that are not likely to produce adverse effects, such as lamb, chicken, potatoes, bananas, and apples. Grains, dairy products, and processed foods are avoided in the few foods diet. The *restricted elimination diet* includes all-natural, chemical-free foods. Fruits, vegetables, nuts, nut butters, beans, seeds, gluten-free grains such as rice and quinoa, fish, lamb, wild game meats, organic turkey, and large amounts of water are consumed. This diet is very restricted and consequently difficult to follow all of the time. The polyunsaturated diet suggests that children with ADHD have low levels of omega-3 polyunsaturated fatty acids. Supplements are encouraged for these individuals (Pelsser et al., 2017).

Supplementation with free fatty acids has been shown to be helpful for children who have deficiencies in free fatty acid such as omega-3 free fatty acid, omega-6 free fatty acid, and linolenic acid. This supplementation is usually achieved with capsule-containing oils or diets rich in fish products.

If patients adhere to any of these diets, the nurse should support the patient and family in providing the nutritional information needed for the diet. Additionally, the patient and family will need education regarding those foods that are chemical free. A referral to a dietician will benefit both patient and family.

Children with ADHD seem to be more susceptible to being overweight and developing obesity (Cortese & Tessari, 2017). Because of the impulsivity and inattention characteristic of ADHD, these children may be unable to resist external cues for high-fat foods. The nurse can help the family and patient structure the external environment so the child has healthy choices available.

Promoting Sleep. Sleep can be a problem for children with ADHD for many reasons. The overactivity of the disorder itself and the side effects of the psychostimulants contribute to sleep problems. A sleep history should be taken before medications are prescribed. If problems exist, atomoxetine (Strattera) should be considered before the psychostimulants (see next section). If sleep problems arise while taking medications, sleep diaries should be kept. Sleep hygiene and behavior therapy techniques should be implemented (Um, Hong, & Jeong, 2017). See Chapter 28.

Using Pharmacologic Interventions. The first-line recommended medications for ADHD symptoms are the psychostimulants and atomoxetine (Strattera). Alpha$_{2A}$ agonists, guanfacine extended release (Intuniv) is also approved for the treatment of ADHD alone or adjunctive to stimulants (Jain & Katic, 2016; Hirota, Schwartz, & Correll, 2014).

Psychostimulants. Psychostimulants (see Chapter 11) are by far the most commonly used medications for the treatment of ADHD. These medications enhance dopamine and norepinephrine activity and thereby improve attention and focus, increase inhibition of impulsive actions, and quiet the "noise" associated with distractibility and shifting attention (Jain & Katic, 2016).

Methylphenidate (Ritalin) has a total duration of action of about 4 hours (Box 30.4). Thus, parents or teachers often describe a return of overactivity and distractibility as the first dose of medication wears off. This "rebound effect" can often be managed by moving the second dose of the day slightly closer to the first dose. Longer-acting preparations of methylphenidate, such as Concerta, Ritalin LA, and Metadate or amphetamine–dextroamphetamine (Adderall XR), do not require such frequent dosing and may be a better fit with a school day schedule.

One major concern with the psychostimulants is the potential for abuse. With the increase in recognition of ADHD, psychostimulant prescriptions have increased, as well as an increase in teen and preteen abuse of amphetamine products. These abused prescription medications most often belong to the adolescents or a friend. Nurses should caution parents about the potential for abuse and prevent their child's medication from being a source of recreational use.

Atomoxetine. Atomoxetine (Strattera), a noradrenergic reuptake inhibitor, is not classified as a stimulant and is effective in the treatment of ADHD, especially when it is used in combination with the psychostimulants. Because it has little risk of abuse or misuse, it is often used for those who have comorbid substance abuse issues. This medication is generally well tolerated in children and adults. Common side effects include headache, abdominal pain, decreased appetite, vomiting, somnolence, and nausea (Briars & Todd, 2016).

Teaching Points. Medication can help the child's hyperactivity, impulsiveness, and inattention; therefore, teaching the parent, child, and school personnel about the importance of the medication in ADHD and the potential side effects is a place to begin. Explaining to the child that the medication improves concentration and the ability to sit still can help strengthen patient motivation.

Many times parents are reluctant to initiate treatment with psychostimulants because of the fear that their use in childhood will increase the risk of using substances in adulthood. Studies show that treatment of ADHD is not associated with a risk of substance use disorders (Humphreys, Eng, & Lee, 2013). Teaching patients and families about the biologic basis of ADHD helps parents understand that these children are not "bad" kids but that they have problems with impulse control and attention. It may be helpful to review the purposes of the medications and assure parents that evidence shows medications help most affected children.

BOX 30.4

Drug Profile: Methylphenidate (Ritalin)

DRUG CLASS: Central Nervous System Stimulant

RECEPTOR AFFINITY: The mechanisms of pharmacologic effect are not completely clear. At low doses, it provides mild cortical stimulation similar to that of amphetamines. This stimulation results from methylphenidate's ability to promote release and interfere with the reuptake of dopamine in the synaptic cleft. Main sites appear to be the brain stem arousal system and cortex to produce its stimulant effect.

INDICATIONS: Treatment of narcolepsy, attention-deficit disorders, and hyperkinetic syndrome.

ROUTES AND DOSAGE: Available in 5- to 10-mg immediate-release tablets and 20-mg sustained-release tablets (Ritalin-SR). Newer long-acting preparations such as Concerta and Metadate, in various dose strengths, are also available.

Adult dosage: Must be individualized; range from 10 to 60 mg/d orally in divided doses bid (twice a day) to tid (three times a day), preferably 15 to 30 minutes before meals. If insomnia is a problem, drug should be administered before 6 PM.

Child dosage: The immediate-release formulation can be started at 5 mg twice or three times daily on a 4-hour schedule with weekly increases depending on response. Starting doses of the long-acting preparations are equivalent to the total tid dose (e.g., 5 tid of short-acting would translate into 18 mg of Concerta). Usually given on a tid schedule, with the last dose being roughly half that of the first and second dose. Daily dosage of more than 60 mg is not recommended. Discontinue after 1 month if no improvement is seen.

PEAK EFFECT: 1 hour; half-life: 3 to 4 hours for the immediate-release preparations

SELECT SIDE EFFECTS: Nervousness, insomnia, dizziness, headache, dyskinesias (including tics), toxic psychosis, anorexia, nausea, abdominal pain, increased pulse and blood pressure, palpitations, tolerance, psychological dependence

WARNING: The drug is discontinued periodically to assess the patient's condition. Contraindications include marked anxiety, tension and agitation, glaucoma, severe depression, and obsessive-compulsive symptoms. Use cautiously in patients with a personal or family history of tic disorders, seizure disorders, hypertension, drug dependence, alcoholism, or emotional instability.

SPECIFIC PATIENT AND FAMILY EDUCATION

- Do not chew or crush sustained-release tablets; they must be swallowed whole.
- Take the drug exactly as prescribed; if insomnia is a problem, the time and dose may need adjustment. The drug is rarely taken after 5 pm.
- Avoid alcohol and over-the-counter products, including decongestants, cold remedies, and cough syrups; these could accentuate side effects of the stimulant.
- Keep appointments for follow-up, including evaluations for monitoring the child's growth and use of parent and teacher ratings to monitor benefit.
- Note that the prescriber may discontinue the drug periodically to confirm effectiveness of therapy.

Psychosocial Interventions

Behavioral programs based on rewards for positive behavior, such as waiting turns and following directions, can foster new social skills. Behavioral parent training, behavioral classroom management, and behavioral peer interventions are well-established treatments. Specific cognitive behavioral techniques are helpful in which the child learns to "stop, look, and listen" before doing. These approaches have been refined and several useful treatment manuals are available (Evans, Owens, & Bunford, 2014). In general, interactions with children can be guided by the following:

- Set clear limits with clear consequences. Use few words and simplify instructions.
- Establish and maintain a predictable environment with clear rules and regular routines for eating, sleeping, and playing.
- Promote attention by maintaining a calm environment with few stimuli. These children cannot filter out extraneous stimuli and react to all stimuli equally.
- Establish eye contact before giving directions; ask the child to repeat what was heard.
- Encourage the child to do homework in a quiet place.
- Help the child work on one assignment at a time (reward with a break after each completion).

Family treatment is nearly always a component of cognitive behavioral treatment approaches with the child. This may involve parent training that focuses on principles of behavior management, such as appropriate limit setting and use of reward systems, as well as revising expectations about the child's behavior. School programming often involves increasing structure in the child's school day to offset the child's tendency to act without forethought and to be easily distracted by extraneous stimuli. Specific remediation is required for the child with comorbid deficits in learning or language. Some children may require small self-contained classrooms.

Evaluation and Treatment Outcomes

Children may not notice any effects after taking medication, but people in their environment do. Often, within 1 to 2 weeks of initiating therapy, children with ADHD become more attentive, less impulsive, and less active. Parents and teachers are often the first to notice improvement. With time, academic achievement also may improve (Fig. 30.2).

Continuum of Care

Treatment of ADHD typically is conducted in outpatient settings. Optimal treatment is multimodal (i.e., includes several types of interventions), encompassing four main areas: individual treatment for the child, family treatment, school accommodations, and medication. Parent training and social skills training also help diminish disruptive and defiant behavior.

FIGURE 30.2 Long-term outcomes of optimal treatment for patients with attention-deficit hyperactivity disorder.

TIC DISORDERS AND TOURETTE DISORDER

Tics are a part of several mental health problems. **Motor tics** are usually quick jerky movements of the eyes, face, neck, and shoulders, although they may involve other muscle groups as well. Occasionally, tics involve slower, more purposeful, or dystonic movements. **Phonic tics** typically include repetitive throat clearing, grunting, or other noises but may also include more complex sounds, such as words; parts of words; and in a minority of patients, obscenities. Transient tics by definition do not endure over time and appear to be fairly common in school-aged children. *Tic disorder* is a general term encompassing several syndromes that are chiefly characterized by motor tics, phonic tics, or both.

> **KEYCONCEPT** Tics are sudden, rapid, repetitive, stereotyped motor movements or vocalizations.

Tourette disorder, the most severe tic disorder, is defined by multiple motor and phonic tics for at least 1 year. Because no diagnostic tests are used to confirm this disorder, the diagnosis is based on the type and duration of tics present (Hirschtritt, Dy, Yang, & Schart, 2016). The typical age of onset for tics is about 7 years; motor tics generally precede phonic tics. Parents often describe the seeming replacement of one tic with another. In addition to this changing repertoire of motor and phonic tics, Tourette disorder exhibits a waxing and waning course. The child can suppress the tics for brief periods. Thus, it is not uncommon to hear from parents that their child has more frequent tics at home than at school. Older children and adults may describe an urge or a physical sensation before having a tic. The general trend is for tic symptoms to decline by early adulthood.

Epidemiology and Etiology

The prevalence of Tourette disorder is estimated to be 0.6% in children, with boys being affected three to five times more often than girls (CDC, 2019c). OCD frequently occurs in association with Tourette disorder (Hirschtritt et al., 2016).

The precise nature of the underlying pathophysiology in this primarily inherited disorder is unclear, but the basal ganglia and functionally related cortical areas are presumed to play a central role. Findings from neuroimaging studies are consistent with the presumption that a dysregulation of the corticostriatal–thalamic circuitry of the brain underlies Tourette disorder. Additionally, multiple genes on different chromosomes interacting with environmental factors are involved. Several neurochemical systems have been implicated in the etiology of Tourette disorder (Kanaan et al., 2017).

Family Response to Disorder

Before evaluation and diagnosis of Tourette disorder, most families struggle with various explanations for the child's tics. Because tics fluctuate in severity with time and may be more prominent in some settings than in others, family members may have difficulty understanding their involuntary nature. Some parents may be convinced that the tics are deliberate and done to secure attention; others may judge that the tics are "nervous habits" indicative of underlying trouble. Such views require reconciliation with the currently accepted view that tics are involuntary. Some parents may conclude that the child is incapable of controlling any behavior because of Tourette disorder. They may subsequently feel uncertain about setting limits. In these families, delineating the boundaries of Tourette disorder can be helpful (CDC, 2019c).

On learning that this disorder is probably genetic, some parents may harbor guilt for having passed it on to their child. The nurse can assist such families by listening to these concerns and providing information about the natural history of Tourette disorder—it is not a progressive condition, tics often diminish in adulthood, and it need not restrict what the child can achieve in life.

Evidence-Based Nursing Care for Children With Tourette Disorder

Mental Health Nursing Assessment

Nursing assessment of a child with tics includes a review of the onset, course, and current level of the symptoms. Goals of the assessment are to identify the frequency, intensity, complexity, and interference of the tics and their effects on functioning; determine the child's level of adaptive functioning; identify the child's areas of strength and weakness in general and in school; and identify social supports for the child and family.

Another important aspect of the assessment is to determine the effects of the tic symptoms on the child and family. Some children and families adjust well; however, others are embarrassed or devastated and tend to withdraw socially. Some children with Tourette disorder have ADHD, and a substantial percentage have symptoms of OCD (Hirschtritt et al., 2016). Therefore, in addition to inquiring about tics, the nurse should assess the child's overall development, activity level, and capacity to concentrate and persist with a single task, as well as explore repetitive habits and recurring worries.

Priority of Nursing Care

Children with Tourette disorder typically have normal intelligence, but their tics can interfere with their ability to relate to others and perform in school. The nurse should determine the degree of anxiety experienced by the child, the impact of the tics on the child's ability to cope, and whether the tics contribute to interference with social relationships and interactions.

Mental Health Nursing Interventions

The approach to planning nursing interventions depends on the primary source of impairment: tics themselves; OCD symptoms; or the triad of hyperactivity, inattention, and poor impulse control. The nurse can provide counseling and education for the patient, education for the parents, and consultation for the school. Most children and their families need some education about Tourette disorder. Individual psychotherapy with a mental health specialist (e.g., a psychologist or an advanced practice nurse) may be indicated for some children and adolescents with Tourette disorder to deal with maladaptive responses to the chronic condition. There is evidence that comprehensive behavior therapy is effective in reducing the tics (Sukhodolsky et al., 2017).

Medications

Two classes of drugs are commonly used in the treatment of tics: antipsychotics and α-adrenergic receptor agonists. Aripiprazole is replacing the use of older antipsychotics, such as haloperidol and pimozide (Zheng et al., 2016). These potent dopamine blockers are often effective at low doses. Attempts to eradicate all tics by increasing the dosages of these antipsychotics almost certainly will result in diminishing therapeutic returns and additional side effects. The most frequently encountered side effects include drowsiness, dulled thinking, muscle stiffness, akathisia, increased appetite and weight gain, and acute dystonic reactions. Long-term use carries a small risk for tardive dyskinesia.

Psychoeducation

Teachers, guidance counselors, and school nurses may need current information about Tourette disorder and its related problems. Discussions with school personnel often include issues such as how to deal with tic behaviors that are disruptive in the classroom, how to manage teasing from other children, and how to handle medication side effects. A careful discussion of the boundaries of Tourette disorder and tic symptomatology usually can resolve these matters. Teachers who understand the involuntary nature of tics can often generate creative solutions, such as excusing the child to do errands. This strategy allows the child to step out of the classroom briefly to release a bout of tics, thereby reducing stress. In some situations, a brief presentation about Tourette disorder to the class will reduce teasing and help both teachers and classmates tolerate the tic symptoms (Box 30.5).

Before initiating these interventions with the school personnel, it is essential to identify the child's needs and to pursue these strategies in collaboration with the family and other clinical team members. The Education for the Handicapped Act (Public Law 94–142) ensures that children with conditions such as Tourette disorder are eligible for special education services even if they do not meet full criteria for having a learning disability. Thus, if evidence shows that Tourette disorder is hindering academic progress, parents can demand special education services for their child. Nurses can help families negotiate with the school to obtain appropriate services.

Evaluation and Treatment Outcomes

Treatment outcomes will vary over the years and will be influenced by growth and development changes, family interaction and understanding of the disorder, and reduction or elimination of the frequency of the tics. Outcomes should include improvement of the child's quality of life and ability to learn to manage the symptoms of the disorder.

SEPARATION ANXIETY DISORDER

Separation anxiety is normal for very young children, but typically declines between 3 and 5 years of age. When

---

BOX 30.5 • THERAPEUTIC DIALOGUE • Tics and Disruptive Behaviors

INEFFECTIVE APPROACH

Teacher: I see the tics. He jerks his head, makes faces, and flicks his hands.
Nurse: What do you do about them?
Teacher: What can I do? If he isn't disrupting the class, I leave him alone. Even when he is throwing spitballs.
Nurse: Spitballs! He shouldn't be allowed to throw spitballs.
Teacher: Oh, I thought that was a part of his problem.
Nurse: Well, throwing spitballs has nothing to do with tics.

EFFECTIVE APPROACH

Teacher: I see the tics. He jerks his head, makes faces, and flicks his hands.
Nurse: He cannot help the tics that you are seeing. Tic disorders can exhibit a wide range of severity, from mild to severe and from simple to complex. Some complex tics may be difficult to distinguish from habits or rituals.
Teacher: What about things like throwing spitballs? When he does things like that, I try to ignore that behavior.
Nurse: Sounds like you give him the benefit of the doubt. (Validation) However, throwing a spitball is not a tic behavior.
Teacher: What should I do?
Nurse: How do you usually handle that type of behavior? (A modification of reflection)
Teacher: I'd ask him to stop and sometimes go into the hall.
Nurse: Disruptive behavior that is voluntary in a student with a tic disorder should be handled as you would handle any other child.

CRITICAL THINKING CHALLENGE

- Compare the responses of the nurse in these scenarios. What made the difference in the teacher's responsiveness to the nurse?

the child's fear and anxiety around separation become developmentally inappropriate, **separation anxiety disorder** is diagnosed. Separation anxiety disorder is the most common childhood anxiety disorder and occurs at a mean age of 7 years (Vaughan, Coddington, Ahmed, & Ertel, 2017). Although many children experience some discomfort on separation from their attachment figures, children with separation anxiety disorder suffer great worry or fear when faced with ordinary separations or being away from home, such as when going to school. When separation is about to occur, children often resist by crying or hiding from their parents (Milrod et al., 2014). When asked, most children with separation anxiety disorder will express worry about harm to or permanent loss of their major attachment figure. Other children may express worry about their own safety. For a discussion of other anxiety disorders, see Chapter 18.

A common manifestation of anxiety is school phobia, in which the child refuses to attend school, preferring to stay at home with the primary attachment figure. The term *school phobia* was coined to distinguish it from truancy; whether it is a phobia in the usual sense is a matter of some debate. However, school phobia is common in other disorders such as general anxiety disorder, social phobia, OCD, depression, and conduct disorder. When a comorbid disorder such as depression is identified, it becomes the focus of treatment. In some cases, school phobia may resolve when the primary disorder is successfully treated.

Epidemiology and Etiology

The prevalence of separation anxiety disorder is estimated at 1% to 4% of school-aged children, with an onset usually between 7 and 9 years of age; thus, it is relatively common (Vaughan et al., 2017). Insecure attachment, difficult temperaments, and genetic factors contribute to the development of separation anxiety disorder. Anxiety disorders are often familial, so it appears that both environmental and genetic factors affect the risk for separation anxiety disorder. For example, separation anxiety may emerge after a move, change to a new school, or death of a family member or pet.

No single etiologic factor, but instead several risk factors are associated with the onset of the disorder. For example, children of parents with at least one anxiety disorder have an increased risk of also having an anxiety disorder. The risk increases even more when two parents are affected. Parental depression is also associated the anxiety disorders and depression in children (Hammen, 2016).

Family Response to Disorder

There is no single family response to a child who is experiencing separation anxiety. Parenting style, life events, and environmental factors vary from family to family. The family dynamics related to the child's behavior have to be carefully assessed. In some instances, the family may be undergoing a separation of a significant family member through death, divorce, or military deployment. In other situations, the arrival of a new family member may precede the child's separation anxiety. A family assessment is important in determining the relationship of the child's fears and anxiety and the family dynamics.

Recovery-Oriented Care for Persons With Separation Anxiety Disorder

Teamwork and Collaboration: Working Toward Recovery

An interdisciplinary approach is needed for the treatment of separation anxiety disorder. Effective treatment includes child and parent psychoeducation, school consultation, cognitive behavioral therapy, and selective serotonin reuptake inhibitors (SSRIs) (Vaughan et al., 2017).

Evidence-Based Nursing Care for Children With Separation Anxiety Disorder

School refusal is often what prompts the family to seek consultation for the child. Because school refusal can be a behavioral manifestation of several different child psychiatric disorders, it requires careful assessment. Issues to consider are whether the parents have been aware that the child is avoiding school (separation anxiety versus truancy); what efforts the family has used to return the child to school; the presence of significant subjective distress in the child with anticipation of going to school; and whether the school refusal occurs in the context of other behavioral, social, or emotional problems. The nurse should also review the purpose and dose of current medications.

The child's developmental history and response to new situations and prior separations provide essential background information for understanding the child's current separation anxiety. The assessment should also include a review of recent life events and the methods the family has used to promote the child's return to school. Finally, the family history with respect to anxiety, panic attacks, or phobias is also informative.

Nursing priorities of care and interventions will depend on the role of the nurse (school nurse, acute care, or community practice) and the relationship with the child and family. In some instances, the nurse will be responsible for education of the child and family. If the child is receiving medication, nursing care related to administration of medications and education should be implemented. Nurses will also be involved in educating teachers and serving as a liaison between treating physicians, family and child, and school.

OBSESSIVE-COMPULSIVE DISORDER

OCD is characterized by intrusive thoughts that are difficult to dislodge (i.e., obsessions) or ritualized behaviors that the child feels driven to perform (i.e., compulsions) (see Chapter 20). Children tend to exhibit both multiple obsessions and compulsions that relate to fear of catastrophic family event, contamination, sexual or somatic obsessions, and overly moralistic thoughts. Washing, checking, repeating and ordering are the most commonly reported compulsions (Geller, 2016).

Epidemiology and Etiology

The prevalence rate of OCD is estimated at 1% to 2% with two peaks of incidence across the life span, one occurring in pre-adolescent children and later a peak in early adult life (Geller, 2016). More than half of the cases of OCD in youth involve a comorbid disorder such as a tic, mood, or anxiety disorder. The etiology of OCD in children is thought to be similar to that of adults (see Chapter 20). However, there is a subset of children whose OCD behavior that may be related to an immune response to group A beta-hemolytic streptococcal infections that led to inflammation of the basal ganglia (Geller, 2016).

Family Response to Disorder

Parents' responses to their child's obsessions and compulsions depend on their understanding of the thoughts and behaviors. Because OCD is highly familial, if the parents are recovering from their disorder, they may be able to support their child's ability to begin to deal with the symptoms. Conversely, the parents may find their child's thoughts and behaviors tiring so they become easily irritated with the multiple obsessions and compulsions. Parents need education and support to help their child.

Recovery-Oriented Care for Persons With OCD

Teamwork and Collaboration: Working Toward Recovery

Interdisciplinary treatment including school personnel is important for the child and family with OCD. Cognitive behavior therapy (CBT), including psychoeducation, cognitive training, exposure and response preventions, and relapse prevention is the treatment of choice.

Evidence-Based Nursing Care for Children With OCD

Recurrent worries and ritualistic behavior can occur normally in children at particular stages of development. The first step in the assessment of OCD in children is to distinguish between normal childhood rituals and worries and pathologic rituals and obsessional thoughts. Obsessional thoughts are recurrent, nagging, and bothersome. Although children may describe obsessions as occurring "out of the blue," external events may trigger obsessions. For example, a child may fear contamination whenever he or she is in contact with a certain person or object. Likewise, compulsions waste time, cause distress, and interfere with daily life (Box 30.6).

BOX 30.6 CLINICAL VIGNETTE

Kimberly and OCD

Kim, an 11-year-old fifth grader, comes for evaluation because her mother and teacher have become increasingly concerned about her repetitive behaviors. In retrospect, Kim's mother recalls first noticing repetitive rituals about 2 years before, but she did not become alarmed about these behaviors until recently when they began to interfere with daily living. At the time of referral, Kim exhibits complicated jumping rituals that involve a specific number of jumps and a particular manner of jumping. She also turns light switches off and on and performs complex movements, such as blinking in patterns and thrusting her arms back and forth a certain number of times. Her mother also reports Kim's near-constant request for reassurance about her own safety. In recent months, her incessant demands for reassurance have been more frequent and elaborate. For example, Kim's mother has to answer three times that everything is all right and then say, "I swear to it."

At the evaluation, Kim expresses fears that some ill fate, such as catastrophic illness or injury, will befall her. This fear is triggered by contact with any individual who seems sick, chance exposures to foul smells or dirt, and minor scrapes or bumps. When the fear is triggered, she becomes increasingly anxious and consumed with the fear that she will develop an illness and die. Sometimes her fears are specific, such as cancer or AIDS. Other times her fears are more ambiguous, as evidenced by statements such as, "Something bad will happen" if she doesn't complete the ritual. Kim acknowledges that the ritual is probably not related to the feared event, but she is reluctant to take a chance. If the ritual does not reduce her anxiety, she seeks reassurance from her mother.

Kim's medical history was negative for serious illness or injury. She was born after an uncomplicated pregnancy, labor, and delivery and achieved developmental milestones at appropriate times. Indeed, her mother could recall no unusual problems in the first few years of life except that Kim was typically anxious in unfamiliar situations. Kim's mother reports a prior history of panic attacks, but the family history is otherwise negative for anxiety disorders, including OCD.

What Do You Think?

- What assessment information would you want to elicit from Kim?
- What additional information should be considered from Kim's mother about her history of panic attacks?
- What nursing interventions should be considered if Kim were your patient?

The severity of the child's and family's response to OCD will determine the appropriate nursing diagnoses. When the obsessions and compulsions emerge, these children or adolescents are in distress because of the disturbing and relentless nature of the symptoms.

Nursing interventions will be guided by the needs of the family and the developmental needs of the child or adolescent. If medication is prescribed, it is important to emphasize safe management of medications. Because the antidepressants have a "black box" warning regarding suicide risk in adolescents, the nurse must discuss with the parents and child the importance of monitoring moods and keeping regularly scheduled mental health appointments.

OTHER NEURODEVELOPMENTAL DISORDERS

Other neurodevelopmental disorders are characterized by a narrower range of deficits. These include specific neurodevelopmental disorders generally classified as learning, communication, and motor skills disorders. This section focuses primarily on learning and communication disorders.

SPECIFIC LEARNING DISORDERS

Generally, a **learning disorder** (also called learning disability) is defined as a discrepancy between actual achievement and expected achievement based on the person's age and intellectual ability. The definition varies depending on the source and state statute. Learning disorders are typically classified as verbal (e.g., reading, spelling) or nonverbal (e.g., mathematics).

Reading disability, also called **dyslexia**, has been recognized for more than 100 years. It is defined as a significantly lower score for mental age on standardized tests in reading that is not the result of low intelligence or inadequate schooling. This relatively common problem affects about 5% of school-aged children, with some studies reporting higher prevalence. In clinical samples, dyslexia affects boys more often than girls. This discrepancy can be explained by slower and variable processing speed and less inhibitory control in males than females. Verbal reasoning in a strength in males (Arnett et al., 2017).

Although it is clear that no single cause will provide a sufficient explanation for reading disability, the underlying problem appears to be a deficit in **phonologic processing**, which involves the discrimination and interpretation of speech sounds. A disturbance in the development of the left hemisphere is believed to cause this deficit. Both genetic and environmental factors have been implicated in the etiology of reading disability. Data from family studies show that reading disability is familial and that shared environmental factors alone cannot explain the high rate of recurrence in affected families (Becker et al., 2017).

Less is known about the prevalence of nonverbal learning disorder (i.e., mathematics disorder), with estimates of occurrence ranging from 0.1% to 1.0% of school-aged children and no apparent difference between boys and girls. Mathematical ability is moderately inheritable and negatively associated with inattentiveness and hyperactivity–impulsivity symptoms of ADHD (Greven, Kovas, Willcutt, Petrill, & Plomin, 2014).

COMMUNICATION DISORDERS

Communication disorders involve speech or language impairments. *Speech* refers to the motor aspects of speaking; *language* consists of higher-order aspects of formulating and comprehending verbal communication. Communication disorders are fairly common and are yet more common in children with ASDs, ADHD, anxiety, and conduct disorders (Beitchman, Brownlie, & Bao, 2014). As with reading disability, undoubtedly multiple causes of speech or language deficit may be present.

A delay in speech or language development can adversely affect the child's socialization and education. For example, peers may rebuff or tease a child with an articulation defect or stutter, contributing to withdrawal and a negative self-image. The resulting isolation could limit opportunities to negotiate rules, take turns, and learn cooperation. These same tasks could also be difficult for children with language delay. Moreover, language appears to play a role in the regulation of behavior and impulses (Lyons et al., 2016).

Evidence-Based Nursing Care for Children With Communication Disorders

Nursing assessment of children with a known specific developmental disorder includes (1) evidence of interference in daily life, (2) determination of the child's ability (and limitations) to communicate during the interview, (3) assessment of the child's perception about his or her disability, (4) observation for impaired learning and communication, and (5) past and current interventions for the learning or communication deficit with data gathered through direct interview of the child and significant others such as parents.

For the child with learning disabilities, nurses can focus on building self-confidence and helping the family connect with guidance and educational resources that support the child's development into adulthood. For the child with communication disorders, the interventions focus on fostering social and communication skills and making referrals for specific speech or language therapy. Modeling appropriate communication in spontaneous situations with the child can be a useful intervention for some children. The following is an overview of nursing interventions for the child with specific developmental difficulties:

- Introduce strategies for increasing communication skills (e.g., initiating conversation, taking turns in conversation, facing the listener).
- Identify and develop specific intervention strategies for problems secondary to learning communication disorders, such as low self-esteem.
- Provide parental support for coping with the disorder.
- Maintain interdisciplinary medical, dental, and speech therapy, and also educational collaboration.
- Refer to learning or speech specialist for evaluation and assistance.

Continuum of Care

Children with learning disabilities obviously require careful psychoeducational and cognitive testing to identify their strengths and deficits. School or clinical psychologists usually perform this type of specialized testing. When a learning disability has been identified, the U.S. Education for All Handicapped Children Act (Public Law 94–142) mandates that public school systems provide remedial services in the least restrictive educational setting. Families occasionally need help in advocating for these services.

The same is true for children with communication disorders, although the services requested may be different. Speech pathologists conduct the diagnostic assessment of speech and language disorder. Nurses may be involved with formal screening for communication disorders. Services such as speech therapy (directed at the motor aspects of speaking) or social skills groups (directed at the social and interpersonal aspects of language) are often available in school districts and can be obtained if a speech or language disorder has been identified. For some children with communication disorders, the services offered by the school may be insufficient. In such cases, the nurse can help the family locate a facility that can provide these needed services.

OTHER MENTAL DISORDERS

MOOD DISORDERS

Mood disorders in children and adolescents are a major public health concern. The prevalence of diagnosed depression in children aged 3 to 17 is estimated to be 3.2%. Of these, nearly 75% have comorbid anxiety, and nearly 50% have additional behavior problems. An estimated 2.9% of adolescents are diagnosed with bipolar disorder, of which 2.6% are considered severely impaired. Girls are more likely to meet the diagnostic criteria for these disorders (Merikangas et al., 2010). (See Chapters 21 and 22 for a complete discussion of these disorders.)

Children with mood disorders may not spontaneously express feelings (e.g., sadness, irritability) and are more likely to show their suffering through their behavior. These children may act out their feelings rather than discuss them. Thus, behavior problems may accompany depression. Reports from parents are important sources of information about changes in sleep patterns, appetite, activity level and interests, and emotional stability.

Priorities of nursing care for children or adolescents who are depressed are similar to those for adults. Treatment goals include improving the mood and restoring sleep, appetite, and self-care. Interventions for responses to mood disorders in children and adolescents are also similar to those for adults. The psychiatric nurse develops a therapeutic relationship with the child and provides parent education and support. Developing sensitivity to the influence of environmental events on the child is important for the nurse, parents, and teachers (Box 30.7).

BOX 30.7

Questions, Choices, and Outcomes

Mrs. S has just returned with her son Jared to the child psychiatric inpatient services facility after an overnight pass. She reports that the visit did not go well because of Jared's anger and defiance. She remarked that this behavior was distressingly similar to his behavior before the hospitalization. She expressed additional concern because of the upcoming discharge from the hospital. After saying goodbye to Jared, she pulled the nurse aside and stated that she had decided to file for divorce.

Mrs. S indicated that she had not told her husband or the family therapist. When asked whether Jared knew about her decision, Mrs. S suddenly realized that he may have overheard her discussing the matter with her sister on the telephone during this home visit.

How should the nurse approach this situation?

CHOICE	POSSIBLE OUTCOMES
Discuss her hypothesis about Jared's behavior and his uncertainty.	Mother can see relationship between Jared's behavior and her plan for divorce. Mother ignores the nurse. Mother is interested but does not see the connection.
Ignore the statement	Child and family did not learn about the connection between Jared's behavior and the events at home.
Encourage Jared's mother to sort out her problems.	The focus is then on mother's problems.

ANALYSIS

The best response is focusing on the possible relationship between Jared's recent behavioral deterioration and his uncertainty about his family's future. If the nurse ignores the statement or focuses on the mother's interpretation of Jared's behavior, the mother is less likely to appreciate the connection between her pending divorce and Jared's behavior. The nurse should also emphasize the importance of discussing the matter in family therapy.

Children and adolescents may be treated with medication. Antidepressant medications are used for depression and mood antipsychotics for bipolar disorder. The controversy surrounding the use of SSRIs in children reminds us that all treatments involve a risk–benefit equation. Given the modest benefit of the SSRIs and the potential for side effects, these medications merit careful monitoring in children and adolescents. Patient monitoring should focus on evidence of benefit and side effects, including sleep problems, hyperactivity, sudden changes in mood or behavior, suicidal ideation, or self-injurious behavior.

CHILDHOOD SCHIZOPHRENIA

Childhood (early-onset) schizophrenia is diagnosed by the same criteria as those used in adults (see Chapter 23). Difficulty in diagnosing a psychiatric disorder in children has led to years of debate and controversy regarding whether childhood schizophrenia differs from the adult type or is merely an early manifestation of the same disorder. For many years, it was believed that autism represented the childhood form of schizophrenia. However, today autism and childhood schizophrenia are differentiated. As currently defined, childhood schizophrenia (onset before the age of 13 years) is very rare, but prevalence increases sharply during adolescence, especially in young men (Kodish & McClellan, 2016).

Childhood schizophrenia is usually characterized by poorer premorbid functioning than later-onset schizophrenia. Common premorbid difficulties include social, cognitive, linguistic, attentional, motor, and perceptual delays. Taken together, these findings suggest that early-onset schizophrenia is a more severe form of the disorder.

Nursing care for children with schizophrenia follows an approach similar to that for ASD. Antipsychotic medications are not generally approved for use in children, although the newer atypical antipsychotic medications appear to have a lower risk for neurologic effects; other side effects such as weight gain also warrant careful monitoring.

Development of an individualized care plan for children with schizophrenia begins with a nursing assessment to identify functional problems specific to the child. Similarly, the recognition that childhood schizophrenia is a chronic and severe condition should guide the identification of outcomes. Goals should be realistic; the nurse should pay special attention to the child's support systems. Parent education about the disorder, medications, and long-term management (including use of community resources) is an essential part of the treatment plan. Long-term management also requires monitoring of chronic antipsychotic therapy.

ELIMINATION DISORDERS

ENURESIS

Enuresis is the involuntary excretion of urine after the age at which the child should have attained bladder control. It usually involves involuntary bed-wetting at night, but repeated urination on clothing during waking hours can occur (diurnal enuresis). Enuresis is a self-limiting disorder, with most children experiencing a spontaneous remission.

Epidemiology and Etiology

The prevalence of nocturnal enuresis varies with age and gender, being most common in young boys—an estimated 5% to 10% of 5-year-old boys, and 3% to 5% in 10-year old boys have nocturnal enuresis (Mikkelsen, 2014). The frequency in girls is about half that of boys in each age group. The etiology of enuresis is unknown, with probably no single cause. Most children with nocturnal enuresis are urologically normal. Some evidence has shown that at least some children with nocturnal enuresis secrete decreased amounts of antidiuretic hormone during sleep, which may play a role in enuresis (Mikkelsen, 2014).

Nursing Care

Nursing assessment should include the child's developmental history, the onset and course of enuresis, prior treatment, presence of emotional problems, and medical history. The nurse should also explore the family's home environment, family attitudes about the child's enuresis, and the family's medical history. Routine laboratory tests such as urinalysis and a urine culture are used to identify the presence of infection. The nurse should obtain baseline data regarding toileting habits, including daytime incontinence, urinary frequency, and constipation. He or she should refer children with persistent daytime enuresis for consultation with a urologist.

In many cases, limiting fluid intake in the evening and treating constipation (if present) is sufficient to decrease the frequency of bed-wetting. One of the most effective methods is the bell and pad. In this approach, the child sleeps on a pad that has wires on it, and when the child voids, a bell sounds, waking up the child. With use, the child either wakes up to urinate or learns to sleep through the night without voiding. A more temporary solution is the use of desmopressin (DDAVP), a synthetic antidiuretic hormone that actually inhibits production of urine. After medication is withdrawn, the enuresis frequently returns (Mikkelsen, 2014).

ENCOPRESIS

Encopresis involves soiling clothing with feces or depositing feces in inappropriate places. Additional diagnostic criteria include that the child is older than 4 years; that the soiling occurs at least once per month; and that the soiling is not the result of a medical disorder, such as congenital aganglionic megacolon (Hirschsprung disease). The most common form of encopresis is fecal impaction accompanied by leakage around the hardened mass of stool. Because of the loss of muscle tone in the lower bowel, the child loses the usual urge to defecate and may not feel the leakage. Surprisingly, the child may not detect the smell of the stool because the olfactory apparatus becomes accustomed to the odor. If left untreated, this problem generally resolves independently by middle adolescence. Nonetheless, the social consequences may be substantial (Mikkelsen, 2014).

Epidemiology and Etiology

As with enuresis, encopresis is more common in boys, and the frequency of the condition declines with age. The current estimate of prevalence is 1.5% of school-aged children aged 7 to 8 years, with boys three times more likely to have encopresis than girls (Mikkelsen, 2014).

The reasons for withholding stool and starting the cycle of fecal impaction are unclear but are not usually the result of physical causes. However, as noted, when fecal impaction occurs, there is an accompanying loss of tone in the bowel and subsequent leakage.

Nursing Care

Assessment includes a detailed interview with the child and parent regarding the pattern of the encopresis. A calm matter-of-fact approach can help to reduce the child's embarrassment. Physical examination is also necessary; thus, collaboration with the child's primary care provider or consulting pediatric specialist is essential. The presence of encopresis does not necessarily signal severe emotional or behavioral disturbances, but the nurse should inquire about other psychiatric disorders. Diagnosis of encopresis is presumed given a history of intermittent constipation and soiling. Collaboration with primary care consultants is often helpful to rule out rare medical conditions, such as Hirschsprung disease.

Effective intervention begins with educating the parents and the child about normal bowel function and the self-perpetuating cycle of fecal impaction and leakage of stool around the hardened mass of feces. The short-term goal of this educational effort is to decrease the anger and recrimination that often complicate the picture in these families. Because encopresis often results in a loss of bowel tone, it may help to motivate children by emphasizing the need to strengthen their anal muscles.

In many cases, cleaning out the bowel is necessary before initiating behavioral treatment. The bowel catharsis is usually followed by administration of mineral oil, which is often continued during the bowel retraining program. A high-fiber diet is often recommended.

The behavioral treatment program involves daily sitting on the toilet after each meal for a predetermined period (e.g., 10 minutes). The child and parents can measure the time with an ordinary kitchen timer. The parents can encourage the child to read or look at picture books while sitting. They can give the child rewards in the form of stars, stickers, or points for complying with the retraining program and add bonuses for successful defecation. The family can tally stickers or points on a calendar, and the child can "cash in" collected points for small prizes.

Caring for children with encopresis on an inpatient unit is a challenge, because very little research provides direction for positive outcomes. Staff can become frustrated with the child's seemingly unwillingness to cooperate. Possible interventions include maintaining discretion, assisting children with the development of age-appropriate social skills and empathy, and providing positive peer pressure (Shepard, Poler, & Grabman, 2016).

SUMMARY OF KEY POINTS

- An estimated 20% of American youths are affected by a mental disorder that impairs their ability to function.

- In addressing intellectual disabilities, the emphasis is on determining adaptive behaviors (e.g., conceptual skills, concepts, self-direction), social skills, and practical skills. With guidance and education, many children will no longer have a disability as adults.

- Children with ASD benefit from structure and specific behavioral interventions.

- ADHD is defined by the presence of inattention; impulsiveness; and in most cases, hyperactivity. As currently defined, ADHD is the most common disorder of childhood. This heterogeneous disorder affects boys more often than girls. Nursing interventions involve family and child education and support. The family must partner with the school system to help the child receive the best educational experience. Effective treatment of ADHD often involves multiple approaches, including medication and parental education and support.

- Tourette disorder is a tic disorder characterized by motor and phonic tics. It is a frustrating disorder that requires patience and understanding. About half of the children with this disorder also have ADHD.

- Separation anxiety is relatively common in school-aged children. OCD becomes more common in adolescents. Treatment of separation anxiety and OCD may include medication, behavioral therapy, or a combination of these treatments.
- Elimination disorders include encopresis and enuresis. Behavioral therapy approaches are the most effective treatment for these disorders. Medication may also be used.
- Major depression in children is believed to be similar to major depression in adults.
- Childhood schizophrenia is a rare disorder, so other diagnoses should be carefully considered. Nursing care is similar to care of children with ASDs.

CRITICAL THINKING CHALLENGES

1. Interview parents of a child with an intellectual disability. Determine their approach to providing support in education and socialization.
2. Examine the differences and similarities between ASD with and without intellectual and language impairment. Determine whether differences exist in the nursing care according to the diagnoses. Develop a teaching plan for parents of children who have ASD and are trying to understand the underlying problems related to the disorder.
3. Compare and contrast nursing approaches for a child with ADHD with those used for a child with ASD. How are they different? How are they similar?
4. Learning disabilities and communication disorders are more common in children with psychiatric disorders than in the general population. How might a learning disability or a communication disorder complicate a psychiatric illness in a school-aged child?
5. How would you answer these questions from a parent: "What causes ADHD? Is it my fault?"
6. A child is threatening to kill himself. What information is needed in order to keep this child safe?

1988: *Rain Man*

This classic film stars Dustin Hoffman as Raymond Babbitt, a man who has autism (savant). Tom Cruise plays his brother Charlie, a self-centered hustler who believes that he has been cheated out of his inheritance. Discovering Raymond in an institution, Charlie abducts Raymond in a last-ditch effort to get his fair share of the family estate. The story revolves around the relationship that develops as the brothers drive across the country.

Dustin Hoffman brilliantly portrays the behaviors and symptoms of high-functioning autism, such as the monotone speech, insistence on sameness, and repetitive behavior.

Viewing Points: Identify and describe Raymond's ritualistic behaviors. Observe Raymond's language patterns and any distinct abnormalities. What happens when Raymond's rituals are interrupted?

UNFOLDING PATIENT STORIES FOR UNIT VI

Unfolding Patient Stories: Andrew Davis • Part 2

Think back to **Andrew Davis** in Unit V, who admitted himself to an alcohol rehabilitation facility. His alcohol abuse began in early adolescence. What factors can increase the risk for alcohol abuse and addiction as an adolescent? What are the psychosocial influences and consequences of alcohol abuse? What assessments can help the nurse identify the signs of alcohol abuse?

Care for Andrew and other patients in a realistic virtual environment: **vSim** *for Nursing* (thepoint.lww.com/vSimMental Health). Practice documenting these patients' care in DocuCare (thepoint.lww.com/DocuCareEHR).

Unfolding Patient Stories: George Palo • Part 2

Think back to 90-year-old **George Palo** in Unit IV, who was diagnosed with minor neurocognitive disorder, Alzheimer type, and who has been living independently in a retirement community since his wife died 3 years ago. His daughter has noticed some cognitive decline and social isolation after the recent loss of his dog. What assessments should the nurse perform during a home visit? How can the nurse determine if George is receptive to community resources for supporting his independent living and involvement in activities? Considering his neurocognitive disorder and response to recent loss, how would the nurse approach a discussion of his ability to maintain independence and when he should transfer to a higher level of care?

Care for George and other patients in a realistic virtual environment: **vSim** *for Nursing* (thepoint.lww.com/vSimMental Health). Practice documenting these patients' care in DocuCare (thepoint.lww.com/DocuCareEHR).

REFERENCES

Alabdali, A., Al-Ayadhi, L., & El-Ansary, A. (2014). A key role for an impaired detoxification mechanism in the etiology and severity of autism spectrum disorders. *Behavioral and Brain Functions, 10*(1), 14.

American Association on Intellectual and Developmental Disabilities. (2019). *Definition of intellectual disability*. Retrieved March 21, 2019, from http://aaidd.org/intellectual-disability/definition.

American Psychiatric Association. (2013). *Diagnostic and statistical manual of mental disorders* (5th ed). Arlington, VA: Author.

Anderson, D., & Byrne-Barta, D. (2015). Keeping the child with Autism Spectrum Disorder safe. *AAACN Viewpoint, 37*(1), 11–13.

Arnett, A. B., Pennington, B. F., Peterson, R. L., Willcutt, E. G., DeFries, J. C., & Olsen, R. K. (2017). Explaining the sex difference in dyslexia. *Journal of Child Psychology & Psychiatry, 58*(6), 719–727.

Baio, J., Wiggins, L., Christensen, D. L., Maenner, M. J., Daniels, J., Warren, Z., et al. (2018). Prevalence of Autism Spectrum Disorder among children aged 8 years—Autism and Developmental Disabilities Monitoring Network, 11 sites, United States, 2014. *Morbidity and Mortality Weekly Report (MMWR), 67*(6), 1–23.

Balazs, J., Miklósi, M., Keresztény, A., Dallos, G., & Gádoros, J. (2014). Attention-deficit hyperactivity disorder and suicidality in a treatment naïve sample of children and adolescents. *Journal of Affective Disorders, 152*, 282–287.

Batshaw, M. L., Roizen, N. J., & Lotrecchiano, G. R. (2013). *Children with disabilities* (7th ed.). Baltimore, MD: Paul H. Brookes Publishing Co.

Becker, N., Vasconcelos, M., Oliveira, V., Santos, F. C. D., Bizarro, L., Almeida, R., et al. (2017). Genetic and environmental risk factors for developmental dyslexia in children: A systematic review of the last decade. *Developmental Neuropsychology, 42*(7/8), 423–445.

Beitchman, J. H., Brownlie, E. B., & Bao, L. (2014). Age 31 mental health outcomes of childhood language and speech disorders. *Journal of the American Academy of Child & Adolescent Psychiatry, 53*(10), 1102–1110.

Bertelli, M. O., Rossi, M., Keller, R., & Lassi, S. (2016). Update on psychopharmacology for autism spectrum disorders. *Advances in Mental Health & Intellectual Disabilities, 10*(1), 6–26.

Briars, L., & Todd, T. (2016). A review of pharmacologic management of attention-deficit/ hyperactivity disorder. *Journal of Pediatric Pharmacology & Therapeutics, 21*(3), 192–206.

Centers for Disease Control and Prevention. (2019a). *Attention-deficit/hyperactivity disorder (ADHD)*. Retrieved March 23, 2019, from https://www.cdc.gov/ncbddd/adhd/index.html

Centers for Disease Control and Prevention. (2019b). *Children's mental health: Data and statistics on children's mental health*. Retrieved March 24, 2019, from https://www.cdc.gov/childrensmentalhealth/data.html

Centers for Disease Control and Prevention. (2019c). *Tourette syndrome (TS)*. Retrieved March 24, 2019, from https://www.cdc.gov/ncbddd/tourette/index.html

Conners, C. K. (1989). *Conners' rating scales manual*. North Tonawanda: Multi-Health Systems.

Cortese, S., & Tessari, L. (2017). Attention-deficit/hyperactivity disorder (ADHD) and obesity: Update 2016. *Current Psychiatry Reports, 19*(1), 4.

Daley, D., Van Der Oord, S., Ferrin, M., Cortese, S., Danckaerts, M., Doepfner, M., et al. (2018). Practitioner review: Current best practice in the use of parent training and other behavioural interventions in the treatment of children and adolescents with attention deficit hyperactivity disorder. *Journal of Child Psychology & Psychiatry, 59*(9), 932–947.

Danielson, M. L., Bitsko, R. H., Ghandour, R. M., Holbrook J. R., Kogan, M. D., & Blumberg, S. J. (2018). Prevalence of parent-reported ADHD diagnosis and associated treatment among U.S. children and adolescents, 2016. *Journal of Clinical Child & Adolescent Psychology, 47*(2), 199–212.

Deater-Deckard, K. (2017). Parents' and children's ADHD in a family system. *Journal of Abnormal Child Psychology, 45*(3), 519–525.

El Achkar, C. M., & Spence, S. J. (2015). Clinical characteristics of children and young adults with co-occuring autism spectrum disorder and epilepsy. *Epilepsy & Behavior, 47*, 183–190.

Elamin, N. E., & Al-Ayadhi, L. Y. (2014). Brain autoantibodies in autism spectrum disorders. *Biomarkers in Medicine, 8*(3), 345–352.

Evans, S. W., Owens, J. S., & Bunford, N. (2014). Evidence-based psychosocial treatments for children and adolescents with attention-deficit/ hyperactivity disorder. *Journal of Clinical Child and Adolescent Psychology, 43*(4), 527–551.

Feingold, B. F. (1975). Hyperkinesis and learning disabilities linked to artificial food flavors and colors. *American Journal of Nursing, 75*(5), 797–783.

Freitag, C. M., Hänig, S., Schneider, A., Seitz, C., Palmason, H., Retz, W., et al. (2012). Biological and psychosocial environmental risk factors influence symptom severity and psychiatric comorbidity in children with ADHD. *Journal of Neural Transmission, 119*(1), 81–94.

Geller, D. (2016). Obsessive-compulsive disorder. In M. K. Dulcan (Ed.). *Dulcan's textbook of child and adolescent psychiatry* (2nd ed.). Arlington, VA: American Psychiatric Publishing.

Ghandour, R. M., Sherman, L. J., Vladutiu, C. J., Ali, M. M., Lynch, S. E., Bitsko, R. H., et al. (2019) Prevalence and treatment of depression, anxiety, and conduct problems in US children. *Journal of Pediatrics, 206*, 256–267.

Ginsberg, Y., Quintero, J., Anand, E., Casillas, M., & Upadhyaya, H. P. (2014). Underdiagnosis of attention-deficit/ hyperactivity disorder in adult patients: A review of the literature. *Primary Care Companion CND Disorders, 16*(3), pii: PCC.13r01600.

Global Research on Developmental Collaborators. (2018). Developmental disabilities among children younger than 5 years in 195 countries and territories, 1990–2016: A systematic analysis for the Global Burden of Disease Study 2016. *Lancet Global Health, 6*(10), e1100–e1121.

Goyette, C. H., Connors, C. K., & Ulrich, R. F. (1978). Normative data on the Connors Parent and Teachers Rating Scales. *Journal of Abnormal Child Psychology, 6*(2), 221–236.

Greven, C. U., Kovas, Y., Willcutt, E., Petrill, S. A., & Plomin, R. (2014). Evidence for shared genetic risk between ADHD symptoms and reduced mathematics ability: A twin study. *Journal of Child Psychology and Psychiatry, 55*(1), 39–48.

Guendelman, M. D., Ahmad, S., Meza, J. I., Owens, E. B., & Hinshaw, S. P. (2016). Childhood attention-deficit/ hyperactivity disorder predicts intimate partner victimization in young women. *Journal of Abnormal Child Psychology, 44*(1), 155–166.

Hammen, C. (2016). Children of depressed parents: The long view. *American Journal of Psychiatry, 173*(10), 956–957.

Hirota, T., Schwartz, S., & Correll, C. U. (2014). Alpha-2 agonists for attention-deficit/hyperactivity disorder in youth: A systematic review and meta-analysis of monotherapy and add-on trials to stimulant therapy. *Journal of the American Academy of Child and Adolescent Psychiatry, 53*(2), 153–173.

Hirschtritt, M. E., Dy, M. E., Yang, K. G., & Scharf, J. M. (2016). Child neurology: Diagnosis and treatment of Tourette syndrome. *Neurology, 87*(7), e65–e67.

Huang, Y., Xu, H., Au, W., Xu, C., & Wu, K. (2018). Involvement of family environmental, behavioral, and social functional factors in children with attention-deficit/ hyperactivity disorder. *Psychology Research and Behavior Management, 9*(11), 447–457.

Humphreys, K. L., Eng, T., & Lee, S. S. (2013). Stimulant medication and substance use outcomes: A meta-analysis. *JAMA Psychiatry, 70*(7), 740–749.

Jain, R., & Katic, A. (2016). Current and investigational medication delivery systems for treating attention-deficit/ hyperactivity disorder. *Primary Care Companion CNS Disorders, 18*(4). doi: 10.4088/PCC.16r01979

Joelsson, P., Chudal, R., Talat, A., Suominen, A., Brown, A. S., & Sourander, A. (2016). Prenatal smoking exposure and neuropsychiatric comorbidity of ADHD: A Finnish nationwide population-based cohort study. *BMC Psychiatry, 16*, 306.

Kanaan, A. S., Gerasch, S., Garcia-Garcia, I., Lampe, L., Pampel, A., Anwander, A., et al. (2017). Pathological glutamatergic neurotransmission in Gilles de al Tourette syndrome. *Brain, 140*(Pt 1), 218–234.

Kanner, L. (1943). Autistic disturbances of affective contact. *Nervous Child, 2*, 217–250.

Kodish, I., & McClellan, J. M. (2016). Early-onset schizophrenia. In M. K. Dulcan (Ed.) *Dulcan's textbook of child and adolescent psychiatry* (2nd ed.). Arlington, VA: American Pscyhiatric Publishing.

Korrel, H., Mueller, K. L., Silk, T., Anderson, V., & Sciberras, E. (2017). Research review: Language problems in children with attention-deficit hyperactivity disorder: A systematic meta-analytic review. *Journal of Child Psychology and Psychiatry, and Allied Disciplines, 58*(6), 640–654.

Kuniyoshi, J. S., & McClellan, J. M. (2010). Early-onset schizophrenia. In M. K. Dulcan (Ed.). *Dulcan's textbook of child and adolescent psychiatry*. Arlington, VA: American Psychiatric Publishing.

Lomangino, K. (2011). Benefit for elimination diet in ADHD?. *Clinical Nutrition Insight, 37*(4), 8–9, 11.

Lyons, G. L., Huber, H. B., Carter, E. W., Chen, R., & Asmus, J. M. (2016). Assessing the social skills and problem behaviors of adolescents with severe disabilities enrolled in general education classes. *American Journal of Intellectual Developmental Disabilities, 121*(4), 327–345.

Matthews, C. A., & Grados, M. A. (2011). Familiarity of Tourette syndrome, obsessive-compulsive disorder, and attention-deficit/hyperactivity disorder: Heritability analysis in a large sib-pair sample. *Journal of the American Academy of Child & Adolescent Psychiatry, 50*(1), 46–54.

McCarthy, S. E., Gillis, J., Kramer, M., Lihm, J., Yoon, S., Berstein, Y., et al. (2014). De novo mutations in schizophrenia implicate chromatin remodeling and support a genetic overlap with autism and intellectual disability. *Molecular Psychiatry, 19*(6), 657–658.

McKenzie, K., Milton, M., Smith, G., & Ouellette Kuntz, H. (2016). Systematic review of the prevalence and incidence of intellectual disabilities: Current trends and issues. *Curriculum Developmental Disorders Reports, 3*(2), 104–115.

Merikangas, K. R., He, J., Burstein, M., Swanson, S. A., Avenevoli, S., Cui, L., et al. (2010). Lifetime prevalence of mental disorders in U.S. adolescents: Results from the National Comorbidity Survey Replication–Adolescent supplement (NCS-A). *Journal of the American Academy of Child & Adolescent Psychiatry, 49*(10), 980–989.

Mikkelsen, E. J. (2014). Elimination disorders. In R. E. Hales, S. C. Yudofsy, & L. W. Roberts (Eds.). *The American Psychiatric Publishing textbook of psychiatry* (6th ed.). Arlington, VA: American Psychiatric Publishing. Retrieved from www.psychiatryonline.org. http://dx.doi.org/10.1176/appi.books.9781585625031.rh01

Milrod, B., Markowitz, J. C., Gerber, A. J., Cyranowski, J., Altemus, M., Shapiro, T., et al. (2014). Childhood separation anxiety and the pathogenesis and treatment of adult anxiety. *American Journal of Psychiatry, 171*(1), 34–43.

Molina, B. S., Hinshaw, S. P., Swanson, J. M., Arnold, L. E., Vitiello, B., Jensen, P. S., et al. (2009). The MTA at 8 years: Prospective follow-up of children treated for combined-type ADHD in a multisite study. *Journal of the American Academy of Child & Adolescent Psychiatry, 48*(5), 484–500.

Murthy, P., & Chand, P. (2012). Treatment of dual diagnosis disorders. *Current Opinion in Psychiatry, 25*(3), 194–200.

NAMI. (2019). *Mental health facts: Children & teens*. Retrieved March 13, 2019, from https://www.nami.org/Learn-More/Mental-Health-By-the-Numbers.

Pelsser, L. M., Frankena, K., Toorman, J., & Pereira, R. R. (2017). Diet and ADHD, reviewing the evidence: A systematic review of meta-analyses of double-blind placebo-controlled trials evaluating the efficacy of diet interventions on the behavior of children with ADHD. *PLoS One, 12*(1), e0169277.

Platt, J. M., Keyes, K. M., McLaughlin, K. A., & Kaufman, A. S. (2019). Intellectual disability and mental disorders in a US population representative sample of adolescents. *Psychological Medicine, 49*(6), 952–961.

Rapp, A., Dodds, A., Walkup, J. T., & Runn, M. (2013). Treatment of pediatric anxiety disorders. *Annals of the New York Academy of Sciences, 1304*, 52–61.

Rauh, V. A., & Margolis, A. E. (2016). Research review: Environmental exposures, neurodevelopment, and child mental health—New paradigms for the study of brain and behavioral effects. *Journal of Child Psychology and Psychiatry and Allied Health, 57*(7), 775–793.

Raymond, L. J., Deth, R. C., & Ralston, N. V. (2014). Potential role of selenoenzymes and antioxidant metabolism in relation to autism etiology and pathology. *Autism Research and Treatment, 2014*, 164938.

Sanchez-Gistau, V., Romero, S., Moreno, D., de la Serna, E., Baeza, I., Sugranyes, G., et al. (2015). Psychiatric disorders in child and adolescent offspring of patients with schizophrenia and bipolar disorder: A controlled study. *Schizophrenia Research, 168*(1-2), 197–203.

Scibberas, E., Mulraney, M., Silva, D., & Coghill, D. (2017). Prenatal risk factors and the etiology of ADHD-Review of existing evidence. *Current Psychiatry Reports, 19*(1), 1.

Shepard, J. A., Poler, J. E., Jr., & Grabman, J. H. (2016). Evidence-based psychosocial treatments for pediatrician elimination disorders. *Journal of Clinical Child & Adolescent Psychology, 46*(6), 767–797.

Sigfusdottir, I. D., Asgeirsdottir, B. B., Hall, H. A., Sigurdsson, J. F., Young, S., & Gudjonsson, G. H. (2017). An epidemiological study of ADHD and conduct disorder: Does family conflict moderate the association?. *Social Psychiatry Psychiatric Epidemiology, 52*(4), 457–464.

Stevenson, J., Buitelaar, J., Cortese, S., Ferrin, M., Konofal, E., Lecendreux, M., et al. (2014). Research review: The role of diet in the treatment of attention-deficit/hyperactivity disorder—an appraisal of the evidence on efficacy and recommendations on the design of future studies. *Journal of Child Psychology and Psychiatry, 55*(5), 416–427.

Strasser, L., Downes, M., Kung, J., Cross, J. H., & De Haan, M. (2018). Prevalence and risk factors for autism spectrum disorder in epilepsy: A systematic review and meta-analysis. *Developmental Medicine & Child Neurology, 60*(1), 19–29.

Sukhodolsky, D. G., Woods, D. W., Piacentini, J., Wilhelm, S., Peterson, A. L., Katsovich, L., et al. (2017). Moderators and predictors of response to behavior therapy for tics in Tourette syndrome. *Neurology, 88*(11), 1029–1036.

The Foundation for Medical Practice Education. (2009). *ADHD rating scale*. Retrieved from http://www.fmpe.org/en/documents/appendix/Appendix%201%20-%20ADHD%20Rating%20Scale.pdf.

Torgersen, T., Gjervan, B., Lensing, M. B., & Rasmussen, K. (2016). Optimal management of ADHD in older adults. *Neuropsychiatric Disease and Treatment, 12*, 79–87.

Um, Y. H., Hong, S. C., & Jeong, J. H. (2017). Sleep problems and predictors in attention-deficit hyperactivity disorder: Causal mechanisms, consequences and treatment. *Clinical Psychopharmacology and Neuroscience, 15*(1), 9–18.

Vaishnavi, V., Manikandan, M., & Munirajan, A. K. (2014). Mining the 3'UTR of autism-implicated genes for SNPs perturbing microRNA regulation. *Genomics Proteomics Bioinformatics, 12*(2), 92–104.

Vaughan, J., Coddington, J. A., Ahmed, A. H., & Ertel, M. (2017). Separation anxiety disorder in school-age children: What health care providers should know. *Journal of Pediatric Health Care, 31*(4), 433-440.

Wagner, K. D., & Pliszka, S. R. (2011). Treatment of child and adolescent disorders. In A. F. Schatzberg & C. B. Nemeroff (Eds.). *The American Psychiatric Publishing Textbook of Psychopharmacology* (4th ed.). Arlington, VA: American Psychiatric Publishing.

Wang, L., Conlon, M. A., Christophersen, C. T., Sorich, M. J., & Angley, M. T. (2014). Gastrointestinal microbiota and metabolite biomarkers in children with autism spectrum disorders. *Biomarkers in Medicine, 8*(3), 331–334.

Yang, T. X., Allen, R. J., Holmes, J., & Chan, R. C. (2017). Impaired memory for instructions in children with attention-deficit hyperactivity disorder is improved by action at presentation and recall. *Frontiers in Psychology, 8*, 39.

Yew, S. G. K., & O'Kearney, R. (2017). Language difficulty at school entry and the trajectories of hyperactivity-inattention problems from ages 4 to 11: Evidence from a population-representative cohort study. *Journal of Abnormal Child Psychology, 45*(6), 1105–1118.

Zheng, W., Li, X. B., Xiang, Y. Q., Zhong, B. L., Chiu, H. F., Ungvari, G. S., et al. (2016). Aripiprazole for Tourette's syndrome: A systematic review and meta-analysis. *Human Psychopharmacology, 31*(1), 11–18.

Zhu, Y., Yang, D., Ji, W., Huang, T., Xue, L., Jiang, X., et al. (2016). The relationship between neurocircuitry dysfunctions and attention deficit hyperactivity disorder: A review. *BioMed Research International, 2016*(2016), 3821579.

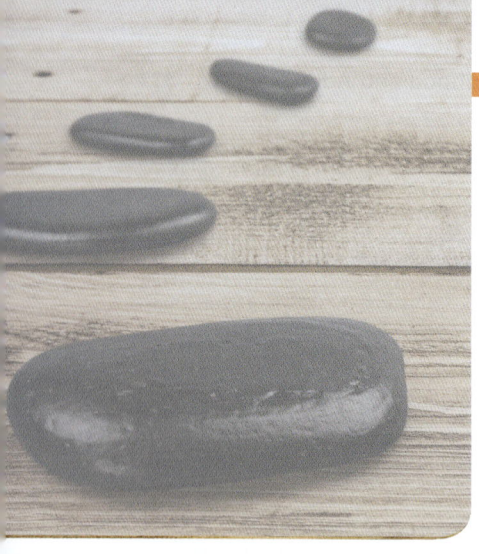

31
Mental Health Disorders of Older Adults

Mary Ann Boyd and Rebecca Luebbert

KEY CONCEPTS
- cognition
- delirium
- dementia
- memory

LEARNING OBJECTIVES

After studying this chapter, you will be able to:

1. Distinguish the clinical characteristics, onset, and course of delirium and dementia.
2. Integrate biologic, psychological, and social theories related to delirium and dementia.
3. Discuss the nursing care of persons with delirium and dementia.
4. Distinguish among other types of neurocognitive disorders.

KEY TERMS

- acetylcholine (ACh) • acetylcholinesterase (AChE) • acetylcholinesterase inhibitors (AChEIs) • agnosia • amyloid precursor protein (APP) • aphasia • apraxia • beta-amyloid plaques • catastrophic reactions • cortical dementia • disinhibition • disturbance of executive functioning • hypersexuality • hypervocalization • illusions • impaired consciousness • neurocognitive disorders • neurofibrillary tangles • oxidative stress • subcortical dementia

Most mental disorders occur in people of all ages and are not unique to the older adult. The first disorder discussed in this chapter, delirium, can occur at any time in a person's life, but frequently occurs in the older adult. The other disorders discussed in this chapter are unique to the older adult. This chapter focuses on changes in cognitive functioning and neurocognitive disorders that are associated with the older adult.

Cognition is an intellectual process of acquiring, using, or manipulating perceptions and information. It involves the perception of reality and an understanding of its representations. Cognitive functions to be noted include the acquisition and use of language, the orientation of time and space, and the ability to learn and solve problems. Cognition also is the basis of judgment, reasoning, attention, comprehension, concept formation, planning, and the use of symbols (e.g., numbers and letters used in mathematics and writing).

KEYCONCEPT Cognition is based on a system of interrelated abilities, such as perception, reasoning, judgment, intuition, and memory that allow one to be aware of oneself and one's surroundings. Impairments in these abilities can result in a failure of the afflicted person to recognize that he or she is ill and in need of treatment.

Memory, a facet of cognition, refers to the ability to recall or reproduce what has been learned or experienced. It is more than simple storage and retrieval; it is a complex cognitive mental function that includes most areas of the brain, especially the hippocampus, which is believed to be essential to the transfer of some memories from short- to long-term storage. Defects of memory are an essential feature of many cognitive disorders, particularly dementia.

> **KEYCONCEPT** **Memory** is a facet of cognition concerned with retaining and recalling past experiences, whether they occurred in the physical environment or internally as cognitive events.

Neurocognitive disorders are characterized by a decline in cognitive function from a previous level of functioning. These disorders are acquired and have not been present since early life. The diagnosis of a neurocognitive disorder is based on deficits in the following cognitive domains: *attention* (distractibility with multiple stimuli), *executive function* (planning, decision-making, working memory), *learning and memory* (recall and recognition), *language* (expressive, including naming, work finding, fluency, grammatical syntax, and receptive language), *perceptual-motor* (visual perception, visuoconstructional, perceptual-motor), and *social cognition deficits* (recognition of emotions, ability to consider another's mental state) (American Psychiatric Association [APA], 2013).

The neurocognitive disorders discussed in this chapter include delirium and dementia. Delirium is a disorder of acute cognitive impairment usually caused by a medical condition (e.g., infection), substance abuse, or multiple etiologies. Dementia is characterized by chronic cognitive impairments. Dementia is differentiated from delirium by underlying cause, not by symptom patterns, which are often similar.

> **KEYCONCEPT** **Delirium** is a disorder of acute cognitive impairment that is caused by a medical condition (e.g., infection), substance abuse, or multiple etiologies.

> **KEYCONCEPT** **Dementia** is characterized by chronic cognitive impairments and is differentiated by underlying cause, not by symptom patterns. Dementia can be further classified as cortical or subcortical to denote the location of the underlying pathology.

Cortical dementia results from a disease process that globally afflicts the cortex. **Subcortical dementia** is caused by dysfunction or deterioration of deep gray- or white-matter structures inside the brain and brain stem. Symptoms of subcortical dementia may be more localized and tend to disrupt arousal, attention, and motivation, but they can produce a variety of clinical behavioral manifestations. In this chapter, one type of cortical dementia, Alzheimer disease (AD), is highlighted because it is the most prevalent form of dementia.

DELIRIUM

Clinical Course

Delirium is a disturbance in consciousness and a change in cognition that develops over a short time. It is usually reversible if the underlying cause is identified and treated quickly. It is a serious disorder and should always be treated as a medical emergency.

> **EMERGENCY CARE ALERT !** Individuals with delirium are in a state of confusion and disorientation that develops during a period of a few hours or days. If delirium is not treated in a timely manner, irreversible neurologic damage can occur. Delirium is a common complication in patients admitted to intensive care units and inpatient psychiatric units (Slooter, Van De Leur, & Zaal, 2017).

Diagnostic Criteria

Impaired consciousness is the key diagnostic criterion for delirium. The patient becomes less aware of his or her environment and loses the ability to focus, sustain, and shift attention. Cognitive changes include problems with memory, orientation, and language. The patient may not know where he or she is, may not recognize familiar objects, or may be unable to carry on a conversation. This problem developed during a short period (compared with dementia, which develops gradually) (APA, 2013). Delirium is different than dementia, although the presenting symptoms are often similar. Impaired alertness, apathy, anxiety, disorientation, and hallucinations commonly occur. Table 31.1 highlights the differences between delirium and dementia.

> **NCLEXNOTE** Delirium and dementia have similar presentations. Because delirium can be life threatening, identifying the potential underlying cause for the symptoms is a priority.

Although delirium may occur in any age group, it is most common among older adults. In this age group, delirium is often mistaken for dementia, which in turn leads to inappropriate treatment. Patients with delirium have a reduced ability to focus, difficulty in sustaining or shifting attention, changes in cognition, or perceptual disturbances (Stelmokas et al., 2016).

Epidemiology and Risk Factors

Statistics concerning prevalence are based primarily on older adults in acute care settings. Estimated prevalence rates range from 10% to 50% of patients. Delirium is particularly common in older postoperative patients. In some groups, such as those with dementia, the prevalence may be higher (Stelmokas et al., 2016).

Pre-existing cognitive impairment is one of the greatest risk factors for delirium (Davis et al., 2017). See Boxes 31.1 and 31.2.

Etiology

Delirium in the older adult is associated with medications, infections, fluid and electrolyte imbalances,

TABLE 31.1	DIFFERENTIATING DELIRIUM FROM DEMENTIA	
Characteristics	Delirium	Dementia
Onset	Sudden	Insidious
24-h course	Fluctuating	Stable
Consciousness	Reduced	Clear
Attention	Globally disoriented	Usually normal
Cognition	Globally disoriented	Globally impaired
Hallucinations	Visual auditory	Possible
Orientation	Usually impaired	Often impaired
Psychomotor activity	Increased, reduced, or shifting	Often normal
Speech	Often incoherent; slow or rapid	Often normal
Involuntary movement	Often asterixis or coarse tremor	Rare
Physical illness or drug toxicity	One or both	Rare

Source: Lee, L., Weston, W. W., Heckman, G., Gagnon, M., Lee, F. J., & Stoke, S. (2013). Structured approach to patients with memory difficulties in family practice. *Canadian Family Physician, 59*(3), 249–254.

metabolic disturbances, hypoxia, or ischemia. The probability of the syndrome developing increases if some predisposing factors, such as advanced age, brain damage, or dementia, are also present. Sensory overload or underload, immobilization, sleep deprivation, and psychosocial stress also contribute to delirium (Todd & Teale, 2017).

Recovery-Oriented Care for Persons With Delirium

Teamwork and Collaboration: Working Toward Recovery

Although delirium may be recognized and diagnosed in any health care setting, appropriate intervention usually requires that the patient be admitted to an acute care setting for rigorous assessment and rapid treatment. Priority in care is identifying the underlying cause of the delirium. Interdisciplinary management of delirium includes two primary aspects: (1) elimination or correction of the underlying cause and (2) symptomatic and supportive measures (e.g., adequate rest, comfort, maintenance of fluid and electrolyte balance, and protection from injury).

Safety Issues

If possible, the use of all suspected medications should be stopped and vital signs should be monitored at least every 2 hours. Close observation of the patient with particular regard to changes in vital signs, behavior,

---

BOX 31.1

Risk Factors for Delirium

Advanced age
Pre-existing dementia
Functional dependence
Endocrine and metabolic disorders
Bone fracture
Infection (pneumonia, urinary tract)
Medications (anticholinergic side effects)
Changes in vital signs (including hypotension and hyper- or hypothermia)
Electrolyte or metabolic imbalance (dehydration, renal failure, hyponatremia)
Admission to a long-term care institution
Postcardiotomy
AIDS
Pain
Acute or chronic stress
Substance use and alcohol withdrawal

BOX 31.2 CLINICAL VIGNETTE

Delirium

Margaret, a widowed 72-year-old woman living in her own home, has been having trouble sleeping. Her daughter visits her and suggests that she try an over-the-counter (OTC) sleeping medication. Margaret also takes antihistamines for allergies and the antidepressant amitriptyline. Three nights later, a neighbor calls the daughter, concerned because Margaret is wandering the streets, unable to find her home. When the neighbor approached Margaret to help her home, she began to scream and strike out at the neighbor.

The daughter visits immediately and discovers that her mother does not know who she is, does not know what time it is, appears disheveled, and is suspicious that people have been in her home stealing the things she cannot find. Margaret does not recall taking any medication, but when her daughter investigates, she finds that 10 pills of the new sleeping aid have already been used.

What Do You Think?

- Identify risk factors that may have contributed to Margaret's experiencing delirium.
- How could the addition of an OTC sleeping medication interact with the antihistamine and antidepressant to be responsible for Margaret's delirium?

and mental status is required. Patients are monitored until the delirium subsides or until discharge. If the delirium still exists at discharge, it is critical that referrals for postdischarge follow-up assessment and care be implemented.

Evidence-Based Nursing Care for Persons With Delirium

The best management is prevention or early recognition of delirium. Special efforts should be made to include family members in the nursing process.

Mental Health Nursing Assessment

The onset of symptoms is typically signaled by a rapid or acute change in behavior. Assessing the symptoms first requires knowing what is normal for the individual. Caregivers, family members, or significant others should be interviewed because they can often provide valuable information. Family members may be the only resource for accurate information.

Physical Health Assessment

History should include a description of the onset, duration, range, and intensity of associated symptoms. Recent physical illness, dementia, depression, or other psychiatric illnesses should be identified. A physical examination should be conducted. Vital signs are crucial. Changes in activities of daily living (ADLs), use of sensory aids (eyeglasses and hearing aids), pain, and sleep should be documented.

Medication Assessment. Many medications are associated with delirium. See Table 31.2. Medications and recent changes in the type and number, including OTC medications should be documented. Combinations of medications can interact and cause delirium. Cold medications, taken in sufficient quantities may cause confusion, especially in older adults. A substance use history (including alcohol intake and smoking history) should be taken.

Psychosocial Assessment

Mental Status. Rapid onset of global cognitive impairment that affects multiple aspects of intellectual functioning is

TABLE 31.2 EXAMPLES OF DRUGS THAT CAN CAUSE DELIRIUM

Class	Specific Drugs	Class	Specific Drugs
Anticholinergic	Antihistamines	Cardiac	β-Blockers
	Chlorpheniramine		Propranolol (Inderal)
	Antiparkinsonian drugs (e.g., benztropine [Cogentin], biperiden [Akineton], or trihexyphenidyl)		Clonidine (Catapres)
			Digitalis (Digoxin, Lanoxin)
			Lidocaine (Xylocaine)
	Atropine		Methyldopa (Aldomet)
	Belladonna alkaloids		Quinidine
	Diphenhydramine		Procainamide (Pronestyl)
	Phenothiazines	Sedative–hypnotic	Barbiturates
	Scopolamine		Benzodiazepines
	Tricyclic antidepressants	Sympathomimetic	Amphetamines
Anticonvulsant	Phenobarbital		Phenylephrine
	Phenytoin (Dilantin)		Phenylpropanolamine
	Sodium valproate (Depakene, Depakote)	Over-the-counter medications	Compoz
			Excedrin PM
Anti-inflammatory	Corticosteroids		Sleep-Eze
	Ibuprofen (Motrin, Advil)		Sominex
	Indomethacin (Indocin)	Miscellaneous	Acyclovir (antiviral)
	Naproxen (Naprosyn)		Aminophylline
Antiparkinsonian	Amantadine		Amphotericin (antifungal)
	Carbidopa (Sinemet)		Bromides
	Levodopa (Larodopa)		Cephalexin (Keflex)
Antibiotics	Isoniazid		Chlorpropamide (Diabinese)
	Rifampin		Cimetidine (Tagamet)
Analgesic	Opioids		Disulfiram (Antabuse)
	Salicylates		Lithium
	Synthetic narcotics		Metronidazole (Flagyl)
			Theophylline
			Timolol ophthalmic

Source: Wynn, G. H., Oesterheid, J. R., Cozza, K. I., Armstrong, S. C. (2009). *Clinical Manual of Drug Interaction: Principles for Medical Practice.* Arlington, VA: American Psychiatric Publishing, Inc.

the hallmark of delirium. Mental status evaluation reveals several changes:

- Fluctuations in level of consciousness with reduced awareness of the environment
- Difficulty focusing and sustaining or shifting attention
- Severely impaired memory, especially immediate and recent memory

Patients may be disoriented to time and place but rarely to person. Environmental perceptions are often disturbed. The patient may believe shadows in the room are really people. Thought content is often illogical, speech may be incoherent or inappropriate to the context. Mental status tends to fluctuate over the course of the day.

Behavior. Persons with delirium exhibit a wide range of behaviors, complicating the process of making a diagnosis and planning interventions. At times, the individual may be restless or agitated and at other times lethargic and slow to respond.

Family Environment. An assessment of living arrangements may provide information about sensory stimulation or social isolation. Assessing family interactions, support for the patient, and family members' ability to understand delirium is also important. The behaviors exhibited by the person experiencing delirium may be frightening or at least confusing for family members. Some family members may actually contribute to the patient's increased agitation. At the same time, however, the family's presence may help to calm and reassure the patient.

Nursing Interventions

Determining the underlying cause for the delirium is priority. Important interventions include providing a safe and therapeutic environment; maintaining fluid and electrolyte balance and adequate nutrition and preventing aspiration and decubitus ulcers, which are common complications. Other interventions relate to individual symptoms and underlying causes.

Safety Interventions

Behaviors exhibited by the person with delirium, such as hallucinations, delusions, illusions, aggression, or agitation (restlessness or excitability), may pose safety problems. Because individuals with delirium are more likely to fall or injure themselves during a confused state, special precautions and safety measures should be considered. The patient must be protected from physical harm by using low beds, guardrails, and careful supervision. Delirium management and fall prevention may be implemented for any patient at risk for falls.

Complementary and Alternative Medication Interventions

There is strong evidence that complementary and alternative medicine interventions are effective in reducing agitation and delirium in older adults. Aromatherapy, massage, acupuncture, and therapeutic touch have been used successfully in reducing agitation and aggressive behavior (Levy, Attias, Ben-Arye, Bloch, & Schiff, 2017).

Medications

As the underlying medical problem is treated, the person may be given medication to treat the symptoms associated with delirium, such as agitation, inattention, combativeness, insomnia, and psychosis. Dosages are usually kept very low, especially with older adults and the medication is selected in light of the potential side effects (particularly anticholinergic effects, hypotension, and respiratory suppression) (Gray & Hanlon, 2016). Antipsychotics are often used for a targeted group of patients who experience hallucinations or delusions associated with delirium. Recent research suggests that supportive measures and treatment of precipitating factors are more effective than antipsychotics (Agar et al., 2017). Benzodiazepines are also used when the delirium is related to alcohol withdrawal. In some patients, benzodiazepines may further impair cognition because of the sedation.

Patients should be monitored for sedation, hypotension, or extrapyramidal symptoms. Although mental status often fluctuates during delirium, it may also be influenced by these medications, so any changes or worsening of mental status after administration of the medication should be reported immediately to the prescriber. Some side effects may also be confused with the symptoms of delirium. For example, akathisia (see Chapter 11), a side effect of antipsychotics, may appear as agitation or restlessness. Medications for treating symptoms related to delirium should be discontinued as soon as possible.

Teaching Points. To prevent future occurrences, provide education to the patient and family about the underlying cause of the delirium. If the delirium is not resolved before discharge, family members need to know how to care for the patient at home.

Psychosocial Interventions

Patients with delirium need frequent interaction and support if they are confused or hallucinating. Patients should be encouraged to express their fears and discomforts that result from frightening or disconcerting psychotic experiences. Adequate lighting, easy-to-read calendars and clocks, a reasonable noise level, and frequent verbal orientation may reduce this frightening experience. If the patient wears eyeglasses or uses a hearing aid, these devices should be used.

Including familiar personal possessions in the environment may also help. These interventions have been shown to reduce the need for antipsychotic medication and reduced length of hospitalization (Gorski et al., 2017).

A safe environment is important to protect the patient from injury. A predictable, orienting environment will help to reestablish order to the patient's life. That is, a calendar, clocks, and other items may be provided to help orient the patient to time, place, and person. If the patient is agitated, deescalation techniques should be used (see Chapter 14). Physical restraint should be avoided.

Families can also be encouraged to work with staff to reorient the patient and provide a supportive environment. Families need to understand that important decisions requiring the patient's input should be delayed if at all possible until the patient has recovered. Although patients may be able to participate in decision-making, they may not remember the decision later; therefore, it is important to have several witnesses present.

Evaluation and Treatment Outcomes

The primary treatment goal is prevention or resolution of the delirious episode with return to previous cognitive status. Outcome measures include:

- Correction of the underlying physiologic alteration
- Resolution of confusion
- Family member verbalization of understanding of confusion
- Prevention of injury

Resolution of confusion is the primary goal, however, the nursing care provided makes important contributions to all four of these outcomes. The end result of delirium may be full recovery, incomplete recovery, incomplete recovery with some residual cognitive impairment, or a downward course leading to death.

Continuum of Care

Patients with delirium may present in a number of treatment settings (e.g., home, nursing home, ambulatory care, day treatment, outpatient setting, hospital). Patients usually are admitted to an acute care setting for rapid evaluation and treatment of the underlying etiology. For more information on caring for patients with delirium, see Box 31.3.

> **BOX 31.3**
> **Psychoeducation Checklist: Delirium**
>
> When caring for the patient with delirium, be sure to include the caregivers, as appropriate, and address the following topic areas in the teaching plan:
>
> - Psychopharmacologic agents, if used, including drug action, dosage, frequency, and possible adverse effects
> - Underlying cause of delirium
> - Mental status changes
> - Safety measures
> - Hydration and nutrition
> - Avoidance of restraints
> - Decision-making guidelines

ALZHEIMER DISEASE

Clinical Course

AD is a degenerative, progressive, neuropsychiatric disorder that results in cognitive impairment, emotional and behavioral changes, physical and functional decline, and ultimately death. Gradually, the patient's ability to carry out ADLs declines, although physical status often remains intact until late in the disease. Although primarily a disorder of older adults, AD has been diagnosed in patients as young as age 35 years.

Two subtypes have been identified: early-onset AD (age 65 years and younger) and late-onset AD (age older than 65 years). Late-onset AD is much more common than early-onset AD, but early-onset AD has a more rapid progression. AD is also routinely conceptualized in terms of three stages: mild, moderate, and severe. Signs and symptoms of AD change as the patient passes from one phase of the illness to another (Fig. 31.1).

Dementia/Alzheimer

Stage	Mild	Moderate	Severe
Symptoms	Loss of memory Language difficulties Mood swings Personality changes Diminished judgment Apathy	Inability to retain new info Behavioral, personality changes Increasing long-term memory loss Wandering, agitation, aggression, confusion Requires assistance w/ADL	Gait and motor disturbances Bedridden Unable to perform ADL Incontinence Requires long-term care placement

FIGURE 31.1 Alzheimer disease progression.

Diagnostic Criteria

The diagnosis of AD is made on clinical grounds, but verification is only confirmed during autopsy. The essential feature of AD is cognitive decline from a previous level of functioning in one or more cognitive domains (attention, executive function, learning and memory, language, perceptual-motor or social cognition) (APA, 2013). These deficits interfere with independence in ADLs. Typical deficits include **aphasia** (i.e., alterations in language ability), **apraxia** (i.e., impaired ability to execute motor activities despite intact motor functioning), **agnosia** (i.e., failure to recognize or identify objects despite intact sensory function), or a **disturbance of executive functioning** (i.e., ability to think abstractly, plan, initiate, sequence, monitor, and stop complex behavior).

Mild neurocognitive impairment (*MCI*) is diagnosed if a modest cognitive decline from a previous level of function is found in one or more of the cognitive domains, but the cognitive deficits do not interfere with independence in daily activities (APA, 2013). MCI is thought to be related to multiple causes and some, but not all, progress to AD. MCI is categorized according to type of memory loss. In *amnestic MCI*, an individual may start to forget important information such as appointments, conversations, or events. In *nonamnestic MCI*, impairment in visual perception, the ability to make sound decisions, or the capacity to judge the time or sequence of steps needed to complete a complex task occurs (Csulky et al., 2016).

Epidemiology and Risk Factors

In 2019, an estimated 5.8 million Americans had AD, 1 in 10 older than 65 years. By 2050, the population of United States over the age of 65 is projected to grow from 55 million to 88 million. With this increase in population, the number of those with AD will also grow. Almost two thirds of Americans with AD are women. Dementia appears to affect all groups, but studies in the United States reveal a higher incidence in African Americans and Hispanics than in whites. Currently, AD is the fifth leading cause of death among older adults in the United States (Alzheimer's Association, 2019a).

General Risk Factors

AD can run in families. Compared with the general population, first-degree biologic relatives of individuals with early-onset AD are more likely to experience the disorder. Studies show that those with fewer years of education or those who have had a prior head injury are at higher risk of developing Alzheimer disease (Alzheimer's Association, 2019a).

Down Syndrome

People with Down syndrome are at higher risk of developing AD than others, most likely because of the additional copy of chromosome 21. The **amyloid precursor protein** (**APP**) is a gene found on this chromosome that is involved in the formation of neurons and their survival. This gene is cut into smaller fragments (peptides) by enzymes. The extra copy of chromosome 21 increases the amount of beta amyloid fragments in the brain, which in turn increases the possibility of formation of beta-amyloid plaques. By age 40, most people with Down syndrome have increased levels of beta-amyloid plaques and tau tangles in their brain (Alzheimer's Association, 2019a).

Metabolic Syndrome

Individuals with metabolic syndrome have a greater risk of developing AD (Alzheimer's Association, 2019a). Metabolic syndrome, a cluster of conditions (hypertension, hyperglycemia, abdominal obesity, and hyperlipidemia) that occur together, increases the risk of heart disease, stroke, and diabetes. Metabolic syndrome is associated with microvascular changes in the brain, which in turn appear to cause mitochondrial dysfunction. Insulin resistance is thought to play a key role in the neuroinflammation and loss of synapses (de la Monte, 2017; Pugazhenthi, 2017; Wang, Norman, Srinivasan, & Rutledge, 2016).

Etiology

Researchers have yet to identify a definitive cause of AD, but a combination of genetic, environmental, and lifestyle factors influences a person's risk for developing the disease. There are multiple factors involved in the development and progression of this disorder (U.S. Department of Health and Human Services [USDHHS], 2015).

Amyloid Precursor Protein

The APP located on the cell membrane appears to have a neuroprotective role in situations of metabolic stress. During an acute stroke, cardiac arrest, or chronic hypoxic-ischemic condition, the APP can promote neuronal survival. When APP is cut or cleaved by the beta-site APP Cleaving Enzyme 1, neurotoxic amyloid-β is released. These peptides can accumulate as amyloid plaques, promoting neurodegeneration (Hefter & Draguhn, 2017).

Beta-Amyloid Plaques

One piece of the puzzle is partially explained by a leading theory that **beta-amyloid plaques**, made up of proteins, clump together in the brain and destroy cholinergic neurons. Research suggests that beta-amyloid deposits impair the normal function of pericytes, which are cells important for controlling the removal of protein from the brain. This leads to further accumulation of the protein. Beta-amyloid is hypothesized to interfere with the process of storing memories through interrupting synaptic connection. Symptoms such as aphasia and visuospatial abnormalities are attributable to plaque formation (USDHHS, 2015).

Neurofibrillary Tangles

Neurofibrillary tangles are made of abnormally twisted protein threads found inside the brain cells. The main component of the tangles is *tau*, a protein that stabilizes the microtubules of transport cells. In AD, tau separates from the microtubules. Loose tau proteins tangle with each other, causing the characteristic neurofibrillary tangles. When microtubules disintegrate, the neuron's transport system collapses, resulting in cell death (USDHHS, 2015) (Fig. 31.2).

Cell Death and Neurotransmitters

In patients with AD, neurotransmission is reduced, neurons are lost, and the hippocampal neurons degenerate. Several major neurotransmitters are affected. Cellular loss leads to reduced **acetylcholine** (ACh) important in cognitive functioning and memory (see Chapter 6). See Figure 31.3. Norepinephrine and serotonin are also affected (USDHHS, 2015).

One of the early hypotheses was that cholinergic dysfunction contributed to cognitive deficits associated with aging and AD. This hypothesis was based on evidence that alterations in the cholinergic systems induced cognitive deficits similar to those in AD and aging. When cholinergic functioning was increased, there were beneficial effects. Today we understand that the pathogenesis of AD is much more complicated than a single cause, even though the primary medications for AD target the cholinergic system (Douchamps & Mathis, 2017).

Genetic Factors

Mutations on three genes are identified as causing AD through altering Aβ processing and are transmitted through genetic inheritance—*APP*, *PSEN1*, *and PSEN2*. These mutations explain 5% to 10% of the occurrence

FIGURE 31.2 Series comparison of elderly control subjects (*top row*) and patients with Alzheimer disease (AD) (*bottom row*). Although some decreases in metabolism are associated with age, in most patients with AD, marked decreases are seen in the temporal lobe, an area important in memory functions. (Courtesy of Monte S. Buchsbaum, MD, The Mount Sinai Medical Center and School of Medicine, New York.)

FIGURE 31.3 Metabolic activity in a subject with Alzheimer disease (*left*) and control subject without AD (*right*). (Courtesy of Monte S. Buchsbaum, MD, The Mount Sinai Medical Center and School of Medicine, New York.)

of early-onset AD. The majority of early-onset AD cases do not have a clear genetic pattern of inheritance. However, genetic predisposition is estimated to be a factor in 60% to 80% of AD cases, including late-onset AD (Van Cauwenberghe, Van Broeckhoven, & Sleegers, 2016).

The APOE gene transports cholesterol in the bloodstream. Three forms of the APOE gene (e2, e3, and e4) are inherited from each parent. The e3 form is the most common and is believed to neither increase or decrease the risk of AD. The e4 is the next most common and is found to increase the risk of developing AD. People with one copy of the e4 form are three times as likely to develop AD compared to those who have the e3 form, and those with two copies of the e4 form have an 8 to 12 times greater risk. The least common APOE gene, e2, is relatively rare and may actually decrease one's risk of AD (Alzheimer's Association, 2019a).

Oxidative Stress, Free Radicals, and Mitochondrial Dysfunction

It is hypothesized that in AD-affected brains, there is a rapid increase in formation of free radicals (i.e., highly reactive molecules) that can lead to **oxidative stress** that damages other cellular molecules such as proteins, lipids, and nucleic acid. Recent studies suggest that oxidative stress may result in changes in chromatin (a complex of DNA and proteins), which may lead to dysfunctional gene expression (Manoharan et al., 2016).

Inflammation

Inflammation is now considered as one of many factors that contribute to the development of AD. The hypothesis is that inflammation may damage small blood vessels and brain cells, initiating a cascade of pathologic events related to oxidative damage and dysregulated amyloid metabolism (Barron, Gartlon, Dawson, Atkinson, & Pardon, 2016).

Family Response to Disorder

Families are the first to be aware of the cognitive problem, often before the patient, who can be unaware of the extent of memory impairment. When finally confirmed, the actual diagnosis can be devastating to the family. Unlike delirium, a diagnosis of AD means long-term care responsibilities while the essence of a family member diminishes day by day. Most families keep their relative at home as long as possible to maintain contact and to avoid costly nursing home placement. The two symptoms that often result in nursing home placement are incontinence that cannot be managed and behavioral problems, such as wandering and aggression.

Recovery-Oriented Care for Persons With AD

Teamwork and Collaboration: Working Toward Recovery

The nature and range of services needed by patients and families throughout the illness can vary dramatically at different stages. As with any other patient, the person with

AD should be the center of the decision-making process. The plan should include educational and supportive programs individualized for the person's self-identified needs. Ideally, plans should be designed to support self-awareness, self-esteem, maintenance of abilities, and management of behavioral symptoms and health promotion (Fortinsky & Downs, 2014).

Treatment efforts currently focus on managing cognitive symptoms, delaying cognitive decline (e.g., memory loss; confusion; and problems with learning, speech, reasoning), treating the noncognitive symptoms (e.g., psychosis, mood symptoms, agitation), and supporting the caregivers to improve the quality of life for both patients and their caregivers.

Safety Issues

The priority of care changes throughout the course of AD. Initially, the priority is delaying cognitive decline and supporting family members. Later, the priority is protecting the patient from injury because of lack of judgment. Near the end, the physical needs of the patient are the focus of care.

Evidence-Based Nursing Care for Persons With Alzheimer Disease

Development and implementation of appropriate, effective, and safe nursing services for the care and support of patients with Alzheimer Disease and their families is a particular challenge because of the complex nature of the illness. See Nursing Care Plan 31.1, available at http://thepoint.lww.com/BoydEssentials.

> **NCLEXNOTE** Needs and problematic behaviors of patients with AD vary throughout the course of the disorder. Early in the disorder, the nurse focuses on support, education, and cognitive interventions for depression. As the Alzheimer disease progresses, priority care becomes safety interventions.

Mental Health Nursing Assessment

Physical Health Assessment

A review of body systems must be conducted on each patient suspected of having AD. Neurologic function of the patient with AD is usually preserved through the early and middle stages of the disease, although seizures, gait disturbances, and tremors may occur at any time. In the later stages of the disease, neurologic signs, such as flexion contractures and primitive reflexes, are prominent features.

Physical Functions. Assessment of physical functions includes ADLs, recent changes in functional abilities, use of sensory aids (e.g., eyeglasses, hearing aids), activity level, and assessment of pain. Eyeglasses and hearing aids may need to be in place before other assessments can be made.

At first, limitations may primarily involve instrumental activities of daily living (IADLs), (e.g., shopping, preparing meals, performing other household chores). Later in the disease process, basic physical dysfunctions occur, such as incontinence, ataxia, dysphagia, and contractures. Incontinence can be a major source of stress and a considerable burden to family caregivers. Evaluation of the patient's functional abilities includes bathing, dressing, toileting, feeding, nutritional status, physical mobility, sleep patterns, and pain.

Self-Care. Alterations in the central nervous system (CNS) associated with AD impair the patient's ability to collect information from the environment, retrieve memories, retain new information, and give meaning to current situations. Therefore, patients with AD often neglect self-care activities. Periodically, biologic assessment parameters need to be reevaluated because patients with AD may neglect activities such as bathing, eating, or skin care.

Sleep–Wake Disturbances. Patients with AD have frequent daytime napping and nighttime periods of wakefulness, with little rapid eye movement (REM) sleep. Lowered levels of REM sleep are associated with restlessness, irritability, and general sleep impairment (Liguori et al., 2016).

Activity and Exercise. One of the earliest symptoms of AD is withdrawal from normal activities. Motor activity is affected in the mild stages of AD and can lead to early problems in functional performance (Alzheimer's Association, 2019a). As the disease progresses, the patient may just sit staring at a blank wall.

Nutrition. Eating can become a problem for a patient with AD and is associated with rapid cognitive decline (Zhao et al., 2016). As the disease progresses, patients may lose the ability to feed themselves or recognize that what is being offered is food. Some patients with Alzheimer Disease are bulimic or hyperoral (eating or chewing almost everything possible and sometimes with an insatiable appetite). Other patients with Alzheimer Disease experience anorexia and have no appetite.

Pain. Although AD is not usually considered a physically painful disorder, patients often have other comorbid physical diseases that may be painful. In the early stages of AD, the patient can usually respond to verbal questions regarding pain. Later, it may be difficult to assess the comfort level objectively, especially if the patient cannot communicate. Some patients in the end stage of AD become hypersensitive to touch.

Subtle behavioral changes, such as lethargy, anxiety, or restlessness, or more obvious physical signs, such as pyrexia, tachypnea, or tachycardia, may be the only indications of actual or impending illness. Observing for changes in patterns of nonverbal communication, such as facial expressions, may help in identifying indicators of pain. Hypervocalizations (disturbed vocalizations), restlessness, and agitation are other possible signs of pain.

Psychosocial Assessment

Personality changes almost always accompany AD. Researchers have identified two contrasting patterns. One is marked by apathy, lack of spontaneity, and passivity. The other involves growing irritability, sarcasm, self-preoccupation, and intolerance of and lack of concern for others.

Cognitive Status. The mental status assessment can be difficult for the patient with AD because cognitive disturbance is the clinical hallmark of AD. However, family members should also be a part of any assessment, especially early in the disease process. There are several screening instruments that can be used in detecting symptoms of dementia. The Mini-Cog is used by clinicians in assessing whether an individual has symptoms of AD (Borson, Scanlan, Chen, & Ganguli, 2003). The AD8 Dementia Screening Interview, which is given to a family member, is a brief, sensitive measure that differentiates between those with and without dementia (Galvin et al., 2005; Galvin, Roe, Xiong, & Morris, 2006). The AD8 contains eight questions asking the family member to rate any change (yes or no) in memory, problem-solving abilities, orientation, and ADLs. The higher the number of changes, the more likely dementia is present (Fig. 31.4). The nurse should

Remember, "Yes, a change" indicates that there has been a change in the last several years caused by cognitive (thinking and memory) problems.	Yes, A change	No, No change	N/A, Don't know
1. Problems with judgment (e.g., problems making decisions, bad financial decisions, problems with thinking)			
2. Less interest in hobbies/activities			
3. Repeats the same things over and over (questions, stories, or statements)			
4. Trouble learning how to use a tool, appliance, or gadget (e.g., VCR, computer, microwave, remote control)			
5. Forgets correct month or year			
6. Trouble handling complicated financial affairs (e.g., balancing checkbook, income taxes, paying bills)			
7. Trouble remembering appointments			
8. Daily problems with thinking and/or memory			

The final score is a sum of the number of items marked "Yes, A change".

Based on clinical research findings from 995 individuals included in the development and validation samples, the following cut points are provided:
- 0–1: Normal cognition
- 2 or greater: Cognitive impairment is likely to be present

Interpretation of the AD8 (Galvin, J. E., Roe, C. M., Powlishta, K. K., Coats, M. A., Muich, S. J., Grant, E., et al. (2005). The AD8: A brief informant interview to detect dementia. *Neurology, 65*(4), 559–564.)

Scores in the impaired range indicate a need for further assessment. Scores in the "normal" range suggest that a dementing disorder is unlikely, but a very early disease process cannot be ruled out. More advanced assessment may be warranted in cases where other objective evidence of impairment exists.

FIGURE 31.4 AD8 tool. (Used with permission from James E. Galvin, MD, MSc, Assistant Professor, Director of the Memory Diagnostic Center, Washington University School of Medicine, St. Louis.)

suspect delirium in instances where cognitive deterioration occurs rapidly.

Memory. The most dramatic and consistent cognitive impairment is in memory. Patients with dementia appear mildly forgetful and repetitive in conversation. They misplace objects, miss appointments, and forget what they were just doing. They may lose track of a conversation or television show. Initially, they may complain of memory problems, but rapidly in the course of the illness, insight is lost, and they become unaware of what is lost. Sometimes they may confabulate, making what appears to be an appropriate explanation of why the information or object is missing. Eventually, all aspects of memory are impaired and even long-term memories are affected. During the interview, short-term memory loss is usually readily evident by the patient's inability to recall three or four words given to him or her at the beginning of the assessment. Often, the earliest symptom of AD is the inability to retain new information.

Language. Language is also progressively impaired. Individuals with AD may initially have agnosia (difficulty finding a word in a sentence or in naming an object). They may be able to talk around it, but the loss is noticeable. Later, fluent aphasia develops; comprehension diminishes; and, finally, they become mute and unresponsive to directions or information.

Visuospatial Impairment. Deficits in visuospatial tasks that require sensory and motor coordination develop early, drawing is abnormal, and the ability to write may change. An inaccurate clock drawing is diagnostic of impairment in this area (Fig. 31.5). Sequencing tasks, such as cooking or other self-care skills, become impaired. The individual becomes unable to complete complex tasks that require calculations, such as balancing a checkbook.

Executive Functioning. Judgment, reasoning, and the ability to problem solve or make decisions are also impaired later in the disorder, closer to the time of nursing home placement. It is hypothesized that as the disease progresses, the degeneration of neurons is spread diffusely throughout the neocortex.

Psychotic Symptoms. Delusional thought content and hallucinations are common in people with AD. These psychotic symptoms differ from those of schizophrenia.

Suspiciousness, Delusions, and Illusions. **Illusions**, or mistaken perceptions, are also common in patients with AD. For example, a woman with AD mistakes her husband for her father. He resembles her father in that he is roughly her father's age when the father was last alive. If an illusion becomes a false fixed belief, it is a delusion.

As the disease progresses, delusions develop in 34% to 50% of the people with AD. These characteristic delusions are different from those discussed in the psychotic disorders. Common delusional beliefs include the following:

- Belief that his or her partner is engaging in marital infidelity
- Belief that other patients or staff are trying to hurt him or her
- Belief that staff or family members are impersonators
- Belief that people are stealing his or her belongings
- Belief that strangers are living in his or her home
- Belief that people on television are real and not actors

Hallucinations. Visual, rather than auditory, hallucinations are the most common in AD. A frequent complaint is that children, adults, or strange creatures are entering the house or the patient's room. These hallucinations may not seem unusual to the patient. If possible, the content and form of hallucination should be ascertained because this information may suggest a treatable disorder. For example, an auditory hallucination commanding the patient to commit suicide may be caused by a treatable depression, not AD. In some cases, hallucinations may be pleasant, such as children being in the room, or the hallucinations may be frightening and uncomfortable.

Mood Changes. A depressed mood is common, but major depression and AD appear to be separate disorders (Zhao et al., 2016). Many people with AD experience one or more depressive episodes with symptoms such as psychomotor retardation, anxiety, feelings of guilt and worthlessness, sadness, frequent crying, insomnia, loss of appetite, weight loss, and suicidal rumination. Depressive symptoms are most prevalent in the early stages of AD, which may be attributed to the patient's awareness of cognitive changes, memory loss, and functional decline.

Anxiety. Moderate anxiety is a natural reaction to the fear engendered by gradual deterioration of intellectual function and the realization of impending loss of control over one's life. Failure to complete a task formerly

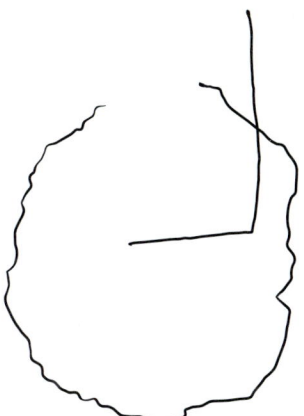

FIGURE 31.5 Clock drawing by a patient with moderate Alzheimer disease. The patient was asked to draw a clock at 3:00 PM.

regarded as simple creates a source of anxiety in patient with AD. As patients with AD become unsure of their surroundings and the expectations of others, they frequently react with fear and distress. It is thought that anxious behavior occurs when the patient is pressed to perform beyond his or her ability.

Catastrophic Reactions. **Catastrophic reactions** are overreactions or extreme anxiety reactions to everyday situations. Catastrophic responses occur when environmental stressors are allowed to continue or increase beyond the patient's threshold of stress tolerance. Behaviors indicative of catastrophic reactions typically include verbal or physical aggression, violence, agitated or anxious behavior, emotional outbursts, noisy behavior, compulsive or repetitive behavior, agitated night awakening, and other behaviors in which the patient is cognitively or socially inaccessible. Factors that contribute to catastrophic responses in patients with progressive cognitive decline include fatigue, a change in routine (e.g., faster pace, caregiver), demands beyond the patient's ability, overwhelming sensory stimuli, and physical stressors (e.g., pain, hunger).

Behavioral Responses

Apathy and Withdrawal. Apathy, the inability or unwillingness to become involved with one's environment, is common in AD, especially in the moderate to late stages. Apathy leads to withdrawal from the environment and a gradual loss of empathy for others. This lack of empathy is very difficult for families and friends to understand.

Restlessness, Agitation, and Aggression. Restlessness, agitation, and aggression are relatively common in the moderate to late stages of AD. Restlessness should be further evaluated to determine its underlying cause. If the restlessness occurs during medication change or adjustment, side effects should be suspected.

Aberrant Motor Behavior. Symptoms such as fidgeting, picking at clothing, wringing hands, loud vocalizations, and wandering may all be signs of such underlying conditions as dehydration, medication reaction, pain, or infection (suggesting delirium). One of the most difficult behaviors for which to determine an underlying cause is **hypervocalization**, a term comprising the screams, curses, moans, groans, and verbal repetitiveness that are common in the later stages of AD in cognitively impaired older adults, often occurring during a hospitalization or nursing home placement. In the assessment of these hypervocalizations, it is important to identify when the behavior is occurring; antecedents of the behavior; and any related events, such as a family member leaving or a change in stimulation.

Disinhibition. One of the most frustrating symptoms of AD is **disinhibition**, acting on thoughts and feelings without exercising appropriate social judgment. In AD, the patient may decide that he or she is more comfortable naked than with clothes. Or the patient may not be able to find his or her clothes and may walk into a room of people without any clothes on. This behavior is extremely disconcerting to family members and can also lead to nursing home placement.

Hypersexuality. A closely related symptom is **hypersexuality**, which is inappropriate and socially unacceptable sexual behavior. The patient begins talking and behaving in ways that are uncharacteristic of premorbid behavior. This behavior is very difficult for family members and nursing home staff.

Stress and Coping Skills. Patients with AD seem extremely sensitive to stressful situations and often do not have the coping abilities to deal with such situations. A careful assessment of the triggers that precede stressful situations will help in understanding a provoking event.

Social Interaction

AD interferes with a person's ability to interact socially as much as it disrupts intellectual functioning. The patient's whole social network is affected by AD and the primary caregiver of a person with AD (usually the partner or offspring in a community setting) is often considered a copatient. It is important to assess the family caregiver's ability to use supportive mechanisms to maintain his or her own integrity throughout the disease process.

If the patient still resides in the community, a home visit will prove useful because it provides information about the patient in the natural environment. From this assessment, the situational and psychosocial stressors that affect the family and patient can be identified, so interventions to strengthen coping strategies, including the ability to seek help from appropriate community resources, can be developed.

Priority of Nursing Care

The unique and changing needs of these patients present a challenge for nurses in all settings. Priorities of care vary according to the stage of the disease. Early on, memory impairment and confusion may be present. An individual may begin to feel less connected and engaged in usual activities. As the disease progresses, the patient may have difficulty with their ADLs. Safety concerns may be present, especially if the patient is agitated, aggressive, or prone to wondering. In late stages of AD, the patient may be completely reliant on others in meeting basic health care needs.

Mental Health Nursing Interventions

Self-Care Interventions

Patients should be encouraged to maintain as much self-care as possible. If eyeglasses and hearing aids are needed but not used, patients are more likely to have false perceptual experiences (hallucinations). Oral hygiene can be a problem and requires excellent basic nursing care. Aging and many medications reduce salivary flow, which can lead to a painfully dry and cracking oral mucosa. For patients with xerostomia (dry mouth) hard candy or chewing gum may stimulate salivary flow or modification of the drug regimen may be necessary. Glycerol mouthwash can provide as much relief from xerostomia as artificial saliva.

During later stages of AD, bathing can be problematic for the patient and nursing staff. Bath time is a high-risk time for agitation and aggression. The person-centered approach focuses on personalizing care to meet residents' needs, accommodating to residents' preferences, attending to the relationship and interaction with the resident, using effective communication and interpersonal skills, and adapting the physical environment and bathing procedures to decrease stress and discomfort.

Physical Health Interventions

Supporting Bowel and Bladder Function. Urinary or bowel incontinence affects many patients with AD. During the middle phases of the disease, incontinence may be caused by the patient's inability to communicate the need to use the toilet or locate a toilet quickly, undress appropriately to use the toilet, recognize the sensation of fullness signaling the need to urinate or defecate, or apathy with lack of motivation to remain continent.

For the patient who is incontinent because of an inability to locate the toilet, orientation may be helpful. Signs and active training should help to modify disorientation. Displaying pictures or signs on bathroom doors provides visual cues; words should use appropriate terminology.

Sleep Interventions. Sedative–hypnotic agents may be prescribed for a short time for restlessness or insomnia, but they may also cause a paradoxic reaction of agitation and insomnia (especially in older adults). Sleep hygiene interventions are appropriate for patients with AD, although morning and afternoon naps (or rest periods for patients who do not nap) may be the most effective intervention for a patient with altered diurnal rhythms.

Activity and Exercise Interventions. Activity and exercise are important nursing interventions for patients with AD. To promote a feeling of success, any activity or exercise plan must be culturally sensitive and adapted to the patient's functional ability and interests. The activity or exercise must be designed to prevent excess stress (both physical and psychological), which means that it must be individualized for each patient with AD based on his or her relative strengths and deficits.

Nutritional Interventions. Maintenance of nutrition and hydration are essential nursing interventions. The patient's weight, oral intake, and hydration status should be monitored carefully. Patients with AD should eat well-balanced meals appropriate to their activity level and eating abilities, with special attention given to electrolyte balance and fluid intake.

Watch for swallowing difficulties that may put the patient at risk for aspiration and asphyxiation. Swallowing difficulties may result from changes in esophageal motility and decreased secretion of saliva.

Pain and Comfort Management. Nursing care of noncommunicative patients who have AD and who also have pain can be challenging. Because of the difficulty in identifying and monitoring the pain, the patients are often undertreated. However, several measures may be used to assess the efficacy of pharmacologic interventions, such as decreased restlessness and agitation. Small doses of oral morphine solution appear to reduce discomfort during routine nursing procedures. The main side effect of morphine is constipation.

Relaxation. Approaching patients in a calm, confident, unhurried manner; maintaining a soothing, quiet environment; avoiding unnecessary noise or chatter around patients and lowering vocal tone and rate when addressing them; maintaining eye contact; and using touch judiciously are likely to promote a sense of security conducive to patient relaxation and comfort. Simple relaxation exercises can be used to reduce stress and should be performed by the patient.

Medications. Medications have two goals: restoration or maintenance of cognitive function and treatment of related psychiatric and behavioral disturbances that cause discomfort for the patient, interfere with treatment, or worsen the individual's cognitive status. Doses must be kept extremely low, and patients should be monitored closely for any side effects or worsening of cognitive status. "Start low and go slow" is the principle guiding the administration of psychopharmacologic agents in older patients.

Cholinesterase Inhibitors. **Acetylcholinesterase inhibitors** (AChEIs) are the mainstay of pharmacologic treatment of AD because they inhibit **acetylcholinesterase** (AChE), an enzyme necessary for the breakdown of acetylcholine. Inhibition of AChE results in an increase in

TABLE 31.3 MEDICATIONS TO TREAT ALZHEIMER DISEASE

Drug	Drug Type and Use	Dose	Common Side Effects	Drug–Drug Interactions
Donepezil (Aricept) Prevents the breakdown of acetylcholine in the brain	Cholinesterase inhibitor treats symptoms of mild, moderate, and severe Alzheimer	5 mg once a day Increase after 4–6 wks to 10 mg/day	Nausea, diarrhea, vomiting	None observed in laboratory studies. NSAIDs should be used with caution in combination with this medication
Galantamine (Razadyne) Prevents breakdown of acetylcholine and modulates nicotinic receptors which release acetylcholine in the brain	Cholinesterase inhibitor treats symptoms of mild and moderate Alzheimer	4 mg bid Titrate to 16–24 mg/day over 8 wks	Nausea, vomiting, diarrhea, weight loss	Some antidepressants, such as paroxetine, amitriptyline, fluoxetine, fluvoxamine, and other drugs with anticholinergic action, may cause retention of excess galantamine in the body. NSAIDs should be used with caution in combination with this medication
Memantine (Namenda) Blocks toxic effects of excess glutamate and regulates glutamate activation	NMDA antagonist to treat moderate to severe symptoms of Alzheimer	Initial dose 5 mg once a day; may increase to 10 mg/day, 15 mg/day, 20 mg/day at weekly intervals	Dizziness, headache, diarrhea, constipation, confusion	A total of 174 drugs (1,401 brand and generic names) are known to interact with memantine. Other prescribed medications and substances should be checked for interactions
Memantine Extended Release and Donepezil (Namzaric) Blocks the toxic effects associated with excess glutamate and prevents the breakdown of acetylcholine in the brain	NMDA antagonist and cholinesterase inhibitor to treat symptoms of moderate to severe Alzheimer	28-mg memantine extended release + 10-mg donepezil once a day	Headache, nausea, vomiting, diarrhea, dizziness	Combined use with NMDA antagonists, anticholinergic medications, succinylcholine, similar neuromuscular blocking agents, or cholinergic agonists
Rivastigmine (Exelon) Prevents the breakdown of acetylcholine and butyrylcholine in the brain	Cholinesterase inhibitor treats symptoms of mild to moderate Alzheimer (patch is also for severe)	1.5 mg bid Titrate to 24 mg/day by increasing 3 mg/day every 2 wks	Nausea, vomiting, weight loss, upset stomach, muscle weakness	None observed in laboratory studies; NSAIDs should be used with caution in combination with this medication

bid, twice a day; NSAIDs, nonsteroidal anti-inflammatory drugs.
Adapted from USDHHS. (2016). *Alzheimer's disease medications fact sheet.* Washington, DC: Alzheimer's Disease Education & Referral (ADEAR) Center, National Institute on Aging, National Institutes of Health, NIH Publication N. 08–3431. Retrieved March 2017, from https://www.nia.nih.gov/alzheimers/publication/alzheimers-disease-medications-fact-sheet#treatment

cholinergic activity. Because these medications have been shown to delay the decline in cognitive functioning but generally do not improve cognitive function after it has declined, it is important that this medication be started as soon as the diagnosis is made. The primary side effect of these medications is gastrointestinal distress, including nausea, vomiting, and diarrhea.

Cholinesterase inhibitors are indicated for the treatment of AD. These drugs may help to delay or prevent symptoms from becoming worse. See Table 31.3. Cholinesterase inhibitors are oral medications usually taken once or twice a day. The earlier in the disease process these medications are initiated, the more likely they will delay cognitive decline. Although there are no special monitors for the cholinesterase inhibitors, the prolonged concurrent use of nonsteroidal anti-inflammatory drugs (NSAIDs) with them can increase the risk of stomach ulcers.

N-Methyl-D-Aspartic Acid Antagonists. In AD, it is hypothesized that the chronic release of glutamate leads to neuronal degeneration. Memantine (Namenda XR) is an *N*-methyl-D-aspartic acid (NMDA) receptor antagonist that has been shown to improve cognition and ADLs in patients with moderate to severe symptoms of AD (Tucci, et al., 2014).

Memantine and Donepezil Combination. Patients stabilized on daily donepezil may be prescribed Namzaric, a combination of memantine and donepezil in one capsule (Box 31.4). This medication is formulated in various strengths of memantine (7, 14, 21, and 28 mg) combined with 10-mg donepezil.

Other Medications. Even though antipsychotics are not approved for the use dementia-related psychosis and have a boxed warning for this population, off-label use of antispsychotics for psychosis is common. The evidence for the use of antidepressants for treating symptoms of depression in individuals with dementia is inconclusive (Leong, 2014), but there is limited research support for their use in reducing agitation (Porsteinsson et al., 2014). Benzodiazepines should be used with caution and only on a short-term basis to treat anxiety in older adults. Anticholinergic medications should be avoided in patients with AD if at all possible. See Box 31.5 for examples of medications that are commonly prescribed in older adults that have anticholinergic properties.

Psychosocial Interventions

The therapeutic relationship is the basis for interventions for the patient and family with dementia. Care of the patient entails a long-term relationship needing much support and expert nursing care. Interventions should be delivered within the relationship context.

Memory Enhancement. The sooner patients begin taking AChEIs, the slower the cognitive decline will be. However, pharmacologic agents are only a small part of the intervention picture. The nursing goal is to maintain memory function as long as possible. When caring for a patient with AD, a concerted effort should be made to reinforce short- and long-term memory. For example, reminding patients what they had for breakfast, which activity was just completed, or who their visitors were a few hours ago will reinforce short-term memory. Encouraging patients to tell the stories of their earlier years will help bring long-term memories into focus. In the earlier stages of AD, there is

---

BOX 31.4
Drug Profile: Memantine and Donepezil (Namzaric)

DRUG CLASS: *N*-methyl-D-aspartate (NMDA) receptor antagonist and cholinesterase inhibitor.

RECEPTOR AFFINITY: Low to moderate affinity uncompetitive (open-channel) NMDA receptor antagonist, which binds preferentially to the NMDA receptor, a reversible inhibitor of the enzyme acetylcholinesterase.

INDICATIONS: For treatment of moderate to severe dementia of the Alzheimer type in patients stabilized on 10 mg of donepezil hydrochloride once daily.

ROUTES AND DOSAGE: 7-, 14-, 21-, and 28-mg tablets.

For patients stabilized on donepezil hydrochloride 10 mg and not currently on memantine hydrochloride, the recommended starting dose of Namzaric is 7/10 mg, taken once a day in the evening. The dose should be increased in 7-mg increments of the memantine hydrochloride component to the recommended maintenance dose of 28/10 mg once daily. The minimum recommended interval between dose increases is 1 week. The dose should only be increased if the previous dose has been well tolerated. The maximum dose is 28/10 mg once daily.

HALF-LIFE (PEAK EFFECT): Terminal half-life, 60–80 hours (peak effect, 3–7 hours). Excreted predominantly in the liver.

SPECIFIC PATIENT AND FAMILY EDUCATION: Caregivers should be instructed in the recommended administration (twice per day for doses above 5 mg) and dose escalation (minimum interval of 1 week between dose increases).
- This drug does not alter the Alzheimer disease process, and the efficacy of the medication may decrease over time.

- Continue using other medications for dementia as prescribed by the health care provider.
- Review the patient information.
- Instruct patients and caregivers to take Namzaric only once daily in the evening, as prescribed.
- If a patient misses a single dose of Namzaric, that patient should not double up on the next dose. The next dose should be taken as scheduled.
- Instruct patients and caregivers that Namzaric capsules should be swallowed whole. Alternatively, Namzaric capsules may be opened and sprinkled on applesauce and the entire contents should be consumed. The capsules should not be divided, chewed, or crushed. Warn patients and caregivers not to use any capsules of Namzaric that are damaged or show signs of tampering.
- Advise patients and caregivers that Namzaric may cause headache, diarrhea, dizziness, anorexia, vomiting, nausea, and ecchymosis.
- Do not discontinue the drug or change the dose unless advised by the health care provider.
- Do not increase the dose of memantine if Alzheimer disease symptoms do not appear to be improving or appear to be getting worse; notify the health care provider.
- Namzaric may cause drowsiness or dizziness. Use caution while driving and performing other activities requiring mental alertness and coordination until tolerance is determined.
- Do not use any prescription or over-the-counter medications, dietary supplements, or herbal preparations unless advised by the health care provider.
- Follow-up visits may be required to monitor therapy and to keep appointments.

> **BOX 31.5**
> **Medications With Anticholinergic Effects**
>
> Amitriptyline
> Captopril (Capoten)
> Codeine
> Cimetidine (Tagamet)
> Citalopram (Celexa)
> Digoxin (Lanoxin)
> Diphenhydramine
> Dipyridamole (Trental)
> Donepezil (Aricept)
> Escitalopram (Lexapro)
> Furosemide (Lasix)
> Fluoxetine (Prozac)
> Isosorbide (Ismotic)
> Mirtazapine (Remeron)
> Nifedipine (Procardia)
> Oxybutynin ER
> Paroxetine (Paxil)
> Phenytoin (Dilantin)
> Prednisolone
> Ranitidine (Zantac)
> Theophylline
> Triamterene and hydrochlorothiazide
> Tolterodine (Detrol LA)
> Warfarin (Coumadin)

considerable frustration when the patient realizes that he or she has short-term memory loss. In a matter-of-fact manner, help "fill in the blanks" and then redirect to another activity. Pictures of familiar people, places, and activities are also important tools in memory retrieval. Using scents (perfume, shaving lotions, spices, different foods) to stimulate memory retrieval and asking patients to relate their memories are also useful. Formalized reminiscence groups also help patients relive their earlier experiences and support maintenance of long-term memories.

Orientation Interventions. To enhance cognitive functioning, attempts should be made to remind patients of the day, time, and location. However, if the patient begins to argue that he or she is really at home or that it is really 1992, the patient need not be confronted by facts. Any confrontation could easily escalate into an argument. Instead, either redirect the patient or focus on the topic at hand (Box 31.6).

Maintaining Language. Losing the ability to name an object (i.e., agnosia) is frustrating. For example, the patient may describe a flower in terms of color, size, and fragrance but never be able to name the flower. When this happens while interacting with a patient, immediately say the name of the item. This reinforces cognitive functioning and prevents disruption in the interaction. Referral to speech therapists may also be useful if the language impairment impedes communication.

Supporting Visuospatial Functioning. The patient with visuospatial impairments loses the ability to sequence automatic behaviors, such as getting dressed or eating with silverware. For example, patients often put their clothes on backward, inside out, or with undergarments over outer garments. After they are dressed, they become confused as to how they arrived at their current state. If this happens, it may help to place clothes for dressing in a sequence for the patient so the patient can move from one article to the next in the correct sequence. This same technique can be used in other situations, such as eating, bathing, and toileting.

Managing Suspicions, Illusions, and Delusions. Delusions often occur when patients are placed in a situation they cannot master cognitively. The principle of nonconfrontation is most important in dealing with formation of suspiciousness and delusion. Efforts should be directed at determining the circumstances that trigger suspicion or delusion formation and creating a means of avoiding these situations.

Frequent causes of suspicion occur when changes in daily routine occur. The common accusations that "Someone has entered my room," or "Someone has changed my room" can be managed by asking, "Do you want to see if anything is missing?" Such accusations usually arise when a patient cannot remember what the room looked like or when the room was rearranged or cleaned.

Patients with AD often have delusions that a spouse, child, or other significant person is an impostor. If this situation occurs, it is important to assert in a matter-of-fact manner, "This is your wife Barbara" or "I am your daughter Jenny." More vigorous assertions, such as offering various types of proof, tend to increase puzzlement as to why a person would go so far to impersonate the spouse or child.

When patients experience illusions, find the source of the illusion and remove it from the environment if possible. For example, if a patient is watching a television program featuring animals and then verbalizes that the animal is in the room, switch the channel and redirect the conversation.

Some patients with AD may no longer recognize the reflections in the mirror as themselves and become agitated, thinking that a stranger is staring at them. Potentially misleading or disturbing stimuli, such as mirrors or art work, can be easily covered or removed from the environment.

Managing Hallucinations. Reassurance and distraction may be helpful for the hallucinating patient. For example, an 89-year-old patient with AD in a residential care facility would get up each night, walk to the nursing station, and whisper to the nurses, "There's a man in my bed who won't let me sleep. You should patrol this place better!" If the hallucination is not too disturbing for the patient, it can often be dismissed calmly with diversion

BOX 31.6 • THERAPEUTIC DIALOGUE • The Patient With Dementia of the Alzheimer Type

Lois's daughter has told the home health agency nurse that on several occasions, Lois has been found cowering and fearful under the kitchen table, saying she was hiding from voices. The nurse also knows that Lois denies having any difficulty with her memory or her ability to care for herself.

INEFFECTIVE APPROACH

Nurse: I'm here to see you about your health problems.
Lois: I have no problems. Why are you here?
Nurse: I'm here to help you.
Lois: I do not need any help. I think there is a mistake.
Nurse: Oh, there is no mistake. Your name is Ms. W, isn't it?
Lois: Yes, but I don't know who you are or why you are here. I'm very tired, please excuse me.
Nurse: OK. I will return another day.

EFFECTIVE APPROACH

Nurse: Hello, my name is Susan Miller. I'm the home health nurse, and I will be spending some time with you.
Lois: Oh, alright. Come in. Sit here.
Nurse: Thank you.
Lois: There is nothing wrong with me, you know.
Nurse: Are you wondering why I am here? (Open-ended statement)
Lois: I know why you are here. My children think that I cannot take care of myself.
Nurse: Is that true? Can you take care of yourself? (Restatement)
Lois: Of course I can care for myself. When people get older, they slow down. I'm just a little slower now, and that upsets my children.
Nurse: You are a little slower? (Reflection)
Lois: I sometimes forget things.
Nurse: Such as…(open-ended statement)
Lois: Sometimes I cannot remember a telephone number or a name of a food.
Nurse: Does that cause problems?
Lois: According to my children, it does!
Nurse: What about you? What causes problems for you?
Lois: Sometimes the radio says terrible things to me.
Nurse: That must be frightening. (Acceptance)
Lois: It's terrifying. Then, my daughter looks at me as if I am crazy. Am I?
Nurse: It sounds like your mind is playing tricks on you. Let's see if we can figure out how to control the radio. (Validation)
Lois: Oh, OK. Will you tell my daughter that I am not crazy?
Nurse: Sure, I would be happy to meet with both you and your daughter if you would like. (Acceptance)

CRITICAL THINKING CHALLENGE

- How did the nurse's underlying assumption that the patient would welcome the nurse in the first scenario lead to the nurse's rejection by the patient?
- What communication techniques did the nurse use in the second scenario to open communication and set the stage for the development of a sense of trust?

or distraction. Because this patient did not seem too concerned by the man in her bed, the nurse may gently respond by saying, "I'm sorry you have to put up with so much. Just wait here (or come with me) and I'll make sure your room is ready for you." The nurse should then take the patient back to her room and help her into bed.

Frightening hallucinations and delusions usually require antipsychotic medications to dampen the patient's emotional reactions, but they can also be dealt with by optimizing perceptual cues (e.g., cover mirrors, turn off the television) and by encouraging patients to stay physically close to their caregivers. For example, one patient complained to her visiting nurse that she was being poisoned by deadly bugs that crawled up and down her arms and legs while she tried to sleep at night. Antipsychotic medication may help this patient sleep at night and she would also likely benefit from reassurance and protection.

Interventions for Mood Changes

Managing Depression. Psychotherapeutic nursing interventions for depression that accompanies AD are similar to interventions for any depression. It is important to spend time alone with patients and to personalize their care as a way of communicating the patient's value. Encouraging expression of negative emotions is helpful because patients can talk honestly to a nonjudgmental person about their feelings. Although depressed patients with AD are likely to be too disorganized to attempt suicide, it is wise to remove potentially harmful objects from the environment.

Managing Stress and Anxiety. Cognitively impaired patients are particularly vulnerable to anxiety. Patients with AD become unsure of their surroundings or of what is expected of them and then tend to react with fear and distress. They may feel lost, insecure, and left out. Failure to complete a task formerly regarded as simple creates anxiety and agitation. Often, they cannot explain the source of their anxiety. In many cases, lowering the demands, simplifying routines, and reducing the number of choices alleviates the anxiety.

Managing Catastrophic Reactions. If a patient reacts catastrophically, remain calm, minimize environmental distractions (quiet the environment), get the patient's attention, and softly assure the patient that he or she is safe. Give information slowly, clearly, and simply, one step at a time. Let the patient know that you understand the fear or other emotional response, such as anger or anxiety.

As nursing skills are developed in identifying antecedents to the patient's catastrophic reactions, it becomes possible to avoid situations that provoke such reactions. Patients with AD respond well to structure but poorly to change. Attempts to argue or reason with them will only escalate their dysfunctional responses.

Managing Apathy and Withdrawal. As the patient withdraws and becomes more apathetic, it becomes more challenging to engage the patient in meaningful activities and interactions. Providing this level of care requires knowing the premorbid functioning level of the patient. Close contact with family helps provide ideas about meaningful activities.

Managing Restlessness and Wandering. Restlessness and wandering are major concerns for caregivers, especially in the community (home) or long-term care setting. The principal means of dealing with restless patients who wander into other patients' rooms or out of the door is to have an adequate number of staff (or caregivers in the home setting) to provide supervision, as well as electronically controlled exits. Wandering behavior may be interrupted in more cognitively intact patients by distracting them verbally or visually. Patients who are beyond verbal distraction can be distracted by physically joining them on their walk and then interrupting their course of action and gently redirecting them back to the house or facility. Many times, wandering is a result of a patient's inability to find his or her own room or may represent other agenda-seeking behaviors such as trying to find a bathroom.

Managing Agitated Behavior. Agitated behavior is likely to occur when patients are pressed to assist in their own care. A calm, unhurried, and undemanding approach is usually most effective. Attempts at reasoning may only aggravate the situation and increase the patient's resistance to care. If unable to determine the source of the patient's anxiety, the patient's restless energy can often be channeled into activities such as walking. Relaxation techniques also can be effective for reducing behavioral problems and anxiety in patients with AD.

Managing Aberrant Behavior. When patients are picking in the air or wringing hands, simple distraction may work. Hypervocalizations are another story. Direct care staff tend to avoid these patients, which only makes the vocalizations worse. In reality, these vocalizations may have meaning to the patient. Instead, develop strategies to try to reduce the frequency of vocalizations (Table 31.4).

Reducing Disinhibition. Anticipation of disinhibiting behavior is the key to nursing interventions for this problem. Disinhibition can take many forms, from undressing in a public setting to touching someone inappropriately to making cruel but factual statements. This behavior can usually be viewed as normal by itself but abnormal within its social context. Keen behavioral assessment of the patient increases the ability to anticipate the likely socially inappropriate behavior and redirect the patient or change the context of the situation. If the patient starts undressing in the dining room, offering a robe and gently escorting him or her to another part of the room might be all that is needed. If a patient is trying to fondle a staff member, having the staff member leave the immediate area or redirecting the patient may alleviate the situation.

Safety Interventions

In the early stages of the illness, safety may not seem to be a prime issue because the individual is cognitively intact.

TABLE 31.4 MESSAGES, MEANINGS, AND MANAGEMENT STRATEGIES

Possible Underlying Meanings	Related Management Strategies
"I hurt!" (e.g., from arthritis, fractures, pressure ulcers, degenerative joint disease, cancer)	• Observe for pain behaviors (e.g., posture, facial expressions, and gait in conjunction with vocalizations). • Treat suspected pain judiciously with analgesics and nonpharmacologic measures (e.g., repositioning, careful manipulation of patient during transfers and personal care, warm or cold packs, massage, relaxation).
"I'm tired." (e.g., sleep disturbances possibly related to altered sleep–wake cycle with day–night reversal, difficulty falling asleep, frequent night awakenings)	• Increase daytime activity and exercise to minimize daytime napping and promote nighttime sleep. • Promote normal sleep patterns and biorhythms by strengthening natural environmental cues (e.g., provide light exposure during the day; avoid bright lights at night), provide large calendars and clocks. • Establish a bedtime routine. • Reduce night awakenings: avoid excess fluids, diuretics, caffeine at bedtime, minimize loud noises, consolidate nighttime care activities (e.g., changing, medications, treatments).
"I'm lonely."	• Encourage social interactions between patients and their family, caregivers, and others. • Increase time the patient spends in group settings to minimize time in isolation. • Provide opportunity to interact with pets.
"I need…" (e.g., food, a drink, a blanket, to use the toilet, to be turned or repositioned)	• Anticipate needs (e.g., assist the patient to toilet soon after breakfast when the gastrocolic reflex is likely). • Keep the patient comfort and safety in mind during care (e.g., minimize body exposure to prevent hypothermia).
"I'm stressed." (e.g., inability to tolerate sensory overload)	• Promote rest and quiet time. • Minimize "white noise" (e.g., vacuum cleaner) and background noise (e.g., televisions and radios). • Avoid harsh lighting and busy, abstract designs. • Limit patient's contacts with other agitated people. • Reduce behavioral expectations of patient, minimize choices, and promote a stable routine.
"I'm bored." (e.g., lack of sensory stimulation)	• Maximize hearing and visual abilities (e.g., keep external auditory canals free from cerumen plugs, ensure that glasses and hearing aids are worn, provide reading material of large print, soften lighting to reduce glare). • Play soft classical music for auditory stimulation. • Offer structured diversions (e.g., outdoor activities).
"What are you doing to me?" (e.g., personal boundaries are invaded)	• Avoid startling patients by approaching them from the front. • Always speak before touching the patient. • Inform patients what you plan to do and why before you do it. • Allow for flexibility in patient care.
"I don't feel well." (e.g., a urinary or upper respiratory tract infection, metabolic abnormality, fecal impaction)	• Identify the etiology through patient history, examination, possible tests (e.g., urinalysis, blood work, chest radiography, neurologic testing). • Treat underlying causes.
"I'm frustrated—I have no control." (e.g., loss of autonomy)	• When possible, allow patient to make their own decisions. • Maximize patient involvement during personal care (e.g., offer the patient a washcloth to assist with bathing). • Treat patients with dignity and respect (e.g., dress or change patients in private).
"I'm lost." (e.g., memory impairment)	• Maintain familiar routines. • Label the patient's room, bathroom, drawers, and possessions with large name signs. • Promote a sense of belonging through displays of familiar personal items, such as old family pictures.
"I feel strange." (e.g., side effects from medications that may include psychotropics, corticosteroids, beta-blockers, NSAIDs)	• Minimize the overall number of medications; consider nondrug interventions when possible. • Begin new medications one at a time; start with low doses and titrate slowly. Suspect a drug reaction if the patient's behavior (e.g., vocal) changes. • Educate caregivers about the patient's medications.
"I need to be loved!"	• Provide human contact and purposeful touch. • Acknowledge or verify the patient's feelings. • Encourage alternative, nonverbal ways to express feelings, such as through music, painting, or drawing. • Stress a sense of purpose in life, acknowledge achievement, and reaffirm that the patient is still needed.

NSAID, nonsteroidal anti-inflammatory drug.
From Clavel, D. S. (1999). Vocalizations among cognitively impaired elders. *Geriatric Nursing*, 20, 90–93. Reprinted with permission from Elsevier.

However, early behaviors suggesting AD are often related to safety, such as the patient getting lost while driving or going the wrong way on the highway. Patients may be prevented from driving even though they can continue to live at home. Safety continues to be an issue in the home when patients engage in unsupervised cooking, cleaning, or household tasks. Day care centers provide a structured yet safe environment for these individuals. Family members should be encouraged to assess continually the abilities of members to live at home safely.

During hospitalizations or nursing home care, the safety issues are different. Most geropsychiatric units are kept locked and a dementia unit often has an electronic alarm system to alert staff about patients attempting to leave the secured floor. Staff and visitors need to be vigilant for perilous situations.

Milieu Management

Overstimulating activities (e.g., social outing, family visit) can result in an outburst of delusional accusations or agitation. The nurse should attempt to determine each patient's optimal level of stimulation at various times of the day. It may be that stimulating environments can be tolerated early in the morning but not in the afternoon when the patient is tired.

Socialization Activities

Overlearned social skills are rarely lost in patients with AD. It is not unusual for patients with dementia to respond appropriately to a handshake or smile well into the disease process. Even patients who are no longer able to communicate coherently will carry on long discussions with people who are willing to listen and respond (to language that does not make sense). The risk for social isolation is strong in patients with AD because of communication difficulties. Reinforcing social remarks and gestures, such as eye contact, smiling, greetings, and farewells, can promote a sense of competency and self-esteem. Pet therapy and "stuffed animal" therapy can also enhance social interaction in cognitively impaired individuals. It is important to remember that patients with AD do not lose their ability to laugh and play and the psychosocial benefits of humor are well known.

Activities that elicit pleasant memories from an earlier time in the patient's life (reminiscence) may produce a soothing effect. Eliciting pleasant memories may be enhanced by gentle stimulation of the patient's senses, for example, viewing and discussing photo albums, looking at personal memorabilia, providing a favorite food item, playing a musical instrument, or listening to music the person preferred in younger years. It may be useful to incorporate movement or dance along with a singing exercise.

If the patient with AD resists structured exercise, it may be because of a fear of falling or injury or of demonstrating to others that his or her health is failing. Patients with AD often forget how to move or how to coordinate their movements in relation to objects. Therefore, exercise should be light and enjoyable. Encourage the patient to take rest periods at intervals throughout the activity in an effort to minimize stress.

Home Visits

The goal of in-home and community-based long-term care services is to maintain patients in a self-determining environment that provides the most home-like atmosphere possible, allows maximum personal choice for care recipients and caregiver and encourages optimal family caregiving involvement without overwhelming the resources of the family network. All services for patients with AD and their families must be provided within a context of continuity of care, a concept that mandates access to various health and supportive services over an unpredictable and changing clinical course.

Community Actions

Nurses working with patients with AD are especially knowledgeable about all aspects of the illness and care. These nurses are often involved in local organizations, such as the Alzheimer's Association. Issues of care and safety and reimbursement for services often require professional expertise and influence.

Family Interventions

Especially in AD, the needs of family members should also be considered. Caring for a family member with dementia takes its toll. Eighty percent of the home care is provided by family caregivers. Two thirds of the caregivers are women, and 34% are over the age of 65 years. Caregivers' health often declines and directly affects their ability to provide care (Alzheimer's Association, 2019a). Caregivers are faced with extreme pressures and often feel isolated, frustrated, and trapped. The potential for patient abuse is significant, especially if agitated and aggressive behaviors are present in the relative.

BOX 31.7

Psychoeducation Checklist: Tips for Caregivers

When caring for the patient with dementia, be sure to include the caregivers, as appropriate, and address the following topic areas in the teaching plan:
- Psychopharmacologic agents, if used, including drug action, dosage, frequency, and possible adverse effects
- Rest and activity
- Consistency in routines
- Nutrition and hydration
- Sleep and comfort measures
- Protective environment
- Communication and social interaction
- Diversional measures
- Community resources

> **BOX 31.8**
>
> **Research for Best Practice: Predictors for Caregiver Burden, Anxiety, and Depression**
>
> Lou, Q., Liu, S., Huo, Y. R., Liu, M., Liu, S., & Ji, Y. (2016). Comprehensive analysis of patient and caregiver predictors for caregiver burden, anxiety and depression in Alzheimer's disease. *Journal of Clinical Nursing, 24*(17–18), 2668–2678.
>
> **THE QUESTION:** Are there characteristics between patient and caregiver characteristics with caregiver burden, anxiety, and depression in Alzheimer disease? What behavioral and psychological symptoms had the greatest impact on caregiver burden, anxiety, and depression in Alzheimer disease?
>
> **METHODS:** A cross-sectional design was used. A total of 310 patients with probable Alzheimer disease and their primary caregivers were assessed. Cognitive impairment and neuropsychiatric symptoms were assessed with several well-validated instruments.
>
> **FINDINGS:** The longer the duration of being the caregiver, the higher the levels of burden. Caregiver burden, anxiety, or depression was not significantly correlated with hours per day of caring for the patient.
>
> **IMPLICATIONS FOR NURSING:** Caregivers are high risk for caregiver burden, anxiety, and depression. Nurses should assess caregivers and provide them support as they care for persons with Alzheimer disease.

Caregivers should be encouraged to attend support groups and carve out personal time. Educational and training programs may help in understanding the complex nature of the disorder (Boxes 31.7 and 31.8). Community resources, such as day care centers, home health agencies, and other community services, can be an important aspect of nursing care for the patient with dementia.

Evaluation and Treatment Outcomes

The objectives of nursing interventions are to help the patient with AD remain as independent as possible and to function at the highest cognitive, physical, emotional, spiritual, and social levels. The maximum level of functional ability can be promoted when nursing care is related to and based on the remaining abilities of the patient.

Continuum of Care

Community Care

It is estimated that more than 60% to 70% of older adults with AD live at home, with 83% of home care provided by family and friends. Unpaid caregivers provide 233.9 billion economic worth (Alzheimer's Association, 2019a). Use of community-based services (e.g., home health aides, home-delivered meals, adult day care centers, respite care, caregiver support groups) often extends the amount of time an individual with AD or a related disorder can safely remain in the home.

Inpatient-Focused Care

Comprehensive admission assessment followed by the development of an individualized (and constantly updated) care plan that involves the patient, significant others, and diverse health care professionals is the foundation of an effective and efficient postdischarge plan. Attention to all aspects of this process is necessary to ensure that the goal of continuity of care is achieved. The hospital-based nurse may initiate family education and counseling as part of discharge planning.

Nursing Home Care

As the AD progresses, many patients are placed in a nursing home for care. Nursing care in a nursing home is usually delivered by nurses' aides, who need support and direction. Interestingly, people with AD require complex nursing care, but the skill level of people caring for these individuals often is minimal. Education and support of the direct caregiver is the focus of most nursing homes.

OTHER DEMENTIAS

Dementia symptoms may occur as a result of a number of disorders and underlying etiologies. The subsequent sections provide a brief description of some of the dementias listed in the *DSM-5*. In each case, the classic symptoms of dementia (e.g., memory impairment with a number of other cognitive deficits) must be present. Nursing interventions for all dementias are similar to those described for individuals with AD.

Vascular Neurocognitive Disorder

Vascular neurocognitive disorder (also known as *vascular dementia*) is a decline in thinking skill caused by conditions that block or reduce blood flow to the brain and the second most common type of dementia. Slightly more men than women are affected. Vascular dementia results when a series of small strokes damage or destroy brain tissue. These are commonly referred to as "ministrokes" or transient ischemic attacks (TIAs) and several TIAs may occur before the affected individual becomes aware of the symptoms of vascular dementia. Most often, a blood clot or plaques (fatty deposits) block the vessels that supply blood to the brain, causing a stroke. However, a stroke can also occur when a blood vessel bursts in the brain (Alzheimer's Association, 2019b).

Symptoms of vascular neurocognitive disorder usually begin more suddenly rather than in AD. Often, the neurologic symptoms associated with a TIA are minimal and may last only a few days, including slight weakness in a limb, dizziness, or slurred speech. Thus, the clinical progression is often described as intermittent and fluctuating or of step-like deterioration, with the patient's cognitive and functional status improving or plateauing for a period of time followed by a rapid decline in function after another series of TIAs. Treatment aims to reduce the primary risk factors for vascular dementia, including hypertension, diabetes mellitus, and additional strokes.

Dementia Caused by Parkinson Disease

In individuals with Parkinson disease, 75% will develop neurocognitive dementia (APA, 2013). Although investigators do not know why, pathologic overlap is considerable between Parkinson disease and AD. The evidence consistently suggests that low cerebrospinal fluid levels of amyloid-β predict future cognitive decline and dementia in Parkinson disease. Cognitive-enhancing medications have some effect, but there is no convincing evidence that the progression of dementia can be delayed (Aarsland et al., 2017).

Dementia Caused by Huntington Disease

Huntington's disease is a progressive, genetically transmitted autosomal dominant disorder characterized by choreiform movements and mental abnormalities. The onset is usually between the ages of 30 and 50 years, but onset occurs before 5 years of age in the juvenile form or as late as 85 years of age in the late-onset form. The disease affects men and women equally. A person with Huntington's disease usually lives for approximately 15 years after diagnosis (APA, 2013). The dementia syndrome of Huntington's disease is characterized by insidious changes in behavior and personality. Typically, the dementia is frontal, which means that the person demonstrates prominent behavioral problems and disruption of attention.

FRONTOTEMPORAL NEUROCOGNITIVE DISORDER

Progressive development of behavioral and personality change and/or language impairment characterizes frontotemporal neurocognitive disorder which has distinct patterns of brain atrophy and distinctive neuropathology. Individuals with this disorder have varying degrees of apathy or disinhibition. They may lose interest in socialization, self-care, and personal responsibilities. Family members report socially inappropriate behaviors, but afflicted individuals show little insight. The cognitive deficits are typically in the areas of planning, organization, and judgments. They are easily distracted (APA, 2013).

NEUROCOGNITIVE DISORDER WITH LEWY BODIES

Progressive cognitive decline with visual hallucination, REM sleep disorder, and spontaneous parkinsonism characterizes dementia with Lewy bodies, a major neurocognitive disorder. Cognitive symptoms occur several months before motor symptoms. These symptoms fluctuate and may resemble delirium. These individuals are at high risk for falls because of periods of syncope and transient episodes of consciousness. Orthostatic hypotension and urinary incontinence may occur. The cause is unknown, but evidence implies a genetic component (Bruni, Conidi, & Bernardi, 2014). The pathology involves Lewy bodies found in the cortical location in the brain which are thought to be responsible for the disorder.

The estimated prevalence of this dementia ranges from 0.1% to 5% of the general elderly population with men slightly more affected (APA, 2013). This onset of disorder is typically in the sixth to ninth decades and is progressive with a 5- to 7-year survival rate. These individuals are more functionally impaired than those with other types of dementia (e.g., AD) and are very sensitive to psychotropic medication, especially antipsychotics.

NEUROCOGNITIVE DISORDER DUE TO PRION DISEASE

Neurocognitive disorder due to prion disease comprises a group of spongiform encephalopathies including Creutzfeldt–Jakob disease, a rare, rapidly fatal, brain disorder, and mad cow disease, which is a bovine disorder. A prion is a small infectious particle composed of abnormally folded protein that causes progressive neurodegeneration. Many of the symptoms seen in Creutzfeldt–Jakob disease are similar to those found in AD and other dementias. However, changes in the brain tissue are different in Creutzfeldt–Jakob disease and are best differentiated with surgical biopsy or during autopsy (APA, 2013). Common symptoms include fluctuating fever, difficulty swallowing, incontinence, tremors, seizures, and sensitivity to touch and environmental noise.

At present, no effective treatment for the disease exists and nothing has been found to slow progression of the illness, although antiviral drug studies are ongoing. Person-to-person transmission of Creutzfeldt–Jakob disease is rare (but possible) and it can be transmitted from people to animals and between animals. Because of the transmissible nature of Creutzfeldt–Jakob disease and because the virus is not easily destroyed, strict criteria for the handling of infected tissues and other contaminated materials have been developed.

NEUROCOGNITIVE DISORDER DUE TO TRAUMATIC BRAIN INJURY

Traumatic brain injury (TBI) affects about 1.4 to 1.7 million people in the United States each year resulting in various symptoms including neurological, cognitive, behavioral, and emotional impairments (APA, 2013). Repeated concussions can lead to brain injury with long-term TBI. Evidence suggests that even mild TBI is a significant risk factor of developing dementia (Mendez, 2017).

SUBSTANCE/MEDICATION-INDUCED NEUROCOGNITIVE DISORDER

If dementia results from the persisting effects of a substance (e.g., drugs of abuse, a medication, exposure to toxins), substance-induced neurocognitive disorder is diagnosed. Other causes of dementia (e.g., dementia caused by a general medical condition) must always be considered even in a person with a dependence on or exposure to a substance. For example, head injuries often result from substance use and may be the underlying cause of the neurocognitive changes (APA, 2013). Prescription drugs are the most common toxins in older adults.

SUMMARY OF KEY POINTS

- Neurocognitive disorders are characterized clinically by significant deficits in cognition or memory that represent a clear-cut change from a previous level of functioning. In some disorders, the loss of cognitive function is progressive, such as in AD. It is important to recognize the differences because the interventions and expected outcomes of the two syndromes are different.
- Delirium is characterized by a disturbance in consciousness and a change in cognition that develops over a short period of time. It requires rapid detection and treatment.
- The primary goal of treatment of individuals with delirium is prevention or resolution of the acute confusion episode with return to previous cognitive status and interventions focusing on (1) elimination or correction of the underlying cause and (2) symptomatic and safety and supportive measures.
- Dementia is characterized by the gradual onset of decline in cognitive function, especially memory, usually accompanied by changes in behavior and personality.
- AD is an example of a progressively degenerative dementia. Treatment efforts currently focus on reduction of cognitive symptoms (e.g., memory loss; confusion; and problems with learning, speech, and reasoning) in attempts to improve the quality of life for both patients and their caregivers.
- Research efforts continue to focus on understanding the relationship among the development of the beta-amyloid plaques, neurofibrillary tangles, and cell death.
- Nursing care of a person with dementia depends on the stage of the disease and the availability of family caregivers.
- Educating and supporting families and caregivers through the progressive cognitive decline and behavior changes is essential to ensuring proper care.
- Several mental health strategies (exercise, education, cognitive stimulation) support and protect a person's cognitive reserve. A healthy cognitive reserve is thought to be protective against neuropathologic insults.
- Other neurocognitive disorders may be related to specific brain changes (Lewy bodies), infections (prion disease), genetic diseases (Huntington), and substances/medications.

CRITICAL THINKING CHALLENGES

1. What factors should be considered in differentiating AD from vascular dementia?
2. Suggest reasons that older adults are particularly vulnerable to the development of neurocognitive disorders.
3. Compare the nursing care of a person with delirium versus one with dementia. What are the similarities and differences in the care?
4. The physical environment is particularly important to the patient with dementia. Visualize your last experience in a health care setting (e.g., hospital, nursing home, day care program, home care setting). Identify environmental factors that could be misleading or stress producing to a person with impaired cognition (dementia), and identify ways to modify this environment to alleviate some of the stressors or misleading stimuli.
5. Mr. J. has been recently diagnosed with mild AD and is asking for advice about deciding on his care in the future. His wife and daughter believe that he does not have the ability to make these decisions and asks for the nurse's advice. How should the nurse respond? Explain the rationale.

2001: *Iris*

This film tells the story of British novelist Iris Murdoch (played by Kate Winslet and then by Judi Dench when Iris is much older) and her relationship with her husband John Bayley (played by Hugh Bonneville and Jim Broadbent) during the last 5 years of her life. Based on Bayley's memoir, *Elegy for Iris*, the film depicts Ms. Murdoch's decline into dementia and the stress associated with caregiving. This wonderful movie shows the suffering of AD but also shows the strength of relationships. The film contrasts the start of their relationship when Iris was an outgoing but dominant individual and John was a timid, shy, scholarly partner with the two older adults who created a loving bond that provided the fabric of the last days of Iris' life.

Viewing Points: Identify the symptoms of the progressive illness throughout the film. Were there any "breaking points" for the caregiver? Were there aspects of Iris' personality that were sustained throughout the course of her life that were evident at the end? What nursing interventions would have been helpful to support her cognitive functioning?

REFERENCES

Aarsland, D., Creese, B., Politis, M., Chaudhuri, K. R., Ffytche, D. H., Weintraub, D., et al. (2017). Cognitive decline in Parkinson disease. *Nature Reviews Neurology*, 13(4), 217–231.

Agar, M. R., Lawlor, P. G., Quinn, S., Draper, B., Caplan, G. Z., Rowett, D., et al. (2017). Efficacy of oral risperidone, haloperidol, or placebo for symptoms of delirium among patients in palliative care: A randomized clinical trial. *JAMA Internal Medicine*, 177(1), 34–42.

Alzheimer's Association. (2019a). *2019 Alzheimer's disease facts and figures*. Chicago: Alzheimer's Association. Retrieved March 25, 2019, from https://www.alz.org/media/Documents/alzheimers-facts-and-figures-2019-r.pdf

Alzheimer's Association. (2019b). *Vascular dementia*. Retrieved May 9, 2019, from https://alz.org/alzheimers-dementia/what-is-dementia/types-of-dementia/vascular-dementia

American Psychiatric Association. (2013). *Diagnostic and Statistical Manual of Mental Disorders* (5th ed.). Arlington, VA: Author.

Barron, M., Gartlon, J., Dawson, L. A., Atkinson, P. J., & Pardon, M. C. (2016). A state of delirium: Deciphering the effect of inflammation on tau pathology in Alzheimer's disease. *Experimental Gerontology*, 94, 103–107.

Bateman, R. J., Xiong, C., Benzinger, T. L., Fagan, A. M., Goate, A., Fox, N. C., et al. (2012). Clinical and biomarker changes in dominantly inherited Alzheimer' Disease. *The New England Journal of Medicine*, 367(9), 795–804.

Borson, S., Scanlan, J. M., Chen, P., & Ganguli, M. (2003). The Mini-Cog as a screen for dementia: Validation in a population-based sample. *Journal of the American Geriatrics Society*, 51, 1451–1454.

Bruni, A. C., Conidi, M. E., & Bernardi, L. (2014). Genetics in degenerative dementia: Current status and applicability. *Journal of Alzheimer Disease and Associated Disorders*, 28(3), 199–205.

Clavel, D. S. (1999). Vocalizations among cognitively impaired elders: What is your patient trying to tell you? *Geriatric Nursing*, 20, 90–93.

Csulky, G., Sirály, E., Fodor, Z., Horváth, A., Salacz, P., Hidasi, Z., et al. (2016). The differentiation of amnestic type MCI from the non-amnestic types by structural MRI. *Frontiers in Aging Neuroscience*, 8, 52.

Davis, D. H., Muniz-Terrera, G., Keage, H. A., Stephan, B. C., Fleming, J., Ince, P. G. et al. (2017). Association of delirium with cognitive decline in late life: A neuropathologic study of 3 population-based cohort studies. *JAMA Psychiatry*, 74(3), 244–251.

de la Monte, S. M. (2017). Insulin resistance and neurodegeneration: Progress towards the development of new therapeutics for Alzheimer's disease. *Drugs*, 77(1), 47–65.

Douchamps, V., & Mathis, C. (2017). A second wind for the cholinergic system in Alzheimer's therapy. *Behavioural Pharmacology*, 28,(2 and 3-Spec Issue), 112–123.

Fortinsky, R. H., & Downs, M. (2014). Optimizing person-centered transitions in the dementia journey: A comparison of national dementia strategies. *Health Affairs*, 33(4), 566–573.

Galvin, J. E., Roe, C. M., Powlishta, K. K., Coats, M. A., Muich, S. J., Grant, E., et al. (2005). The AD8: A brief informant interview to detect dementia. *Neurology*, 65(4), 559–564.

Galvin, J. E., Roe, C. M., Xiong, C., & Morris, J. C. (2006). Validity and reliability of the AD8 informant interview in dementia. *Neurology*, 67(11), 1942–1948.

Gorski, S., Piotrowicz, K., Rewiuk, K., Halicka, M., Kalwak, W., Rybak, P., et al. (2017). Nonpharmacological interventions targeted at delirium risk factors, delivered by trained volunteers (medical and psychology students), reduced need for antipsychotic medications and the length of hospital stay in aged patients admitted to an acute internal medicine ward: Pilot study. *BioMed Research International*, 2017, 1297164.

Gray, S. L., & Hanlon, J. T. (2016). Anticholinergic medication use and dementia: Latest evidence and clinical implications. *Therapeutic Advances in Drug Safety*, 7(5), 217–224.

Gray, S. L., & Hanlon, J. T. (2017). Anticholinergic medication use and dementia: Latest evidence and clinical implications. *Therapeutic Advances in Drug Safety*, 7(5), 217–224.

Hefter, D., & Draguhn, A. (2017). APP as a protective factor in acute neuronal insults. *Frontiers in Molecular Science*, 10(22), 1–15.

Leong, C. (2014). Antidepressants for depression in patients with dementia: A review of the literature. *The Consultant Pharmacist*, 29(4), 254–263.

Levy, I., Attias, S., Ben-Arye, E., Bloch, B., & Schiff, E. (2017). Complementary medicine for treatment of agitation and delirium in older persons: A systematic review and narrative synthesis. *International Journal of Geriatric Psychiatry*, 32(5), 492–508.

Lewis, M. L., Hobday, J. V., & Hepburn, K. W. (2010). Internet-based program for dementia caregivers. *American Journal of Alzheimer's Disease and Other Dementias*, 25(8), 674–679.

Liguori, C., Nuccetelli, M., Izzi, F., Sancesario, G., Romigi, Al, Martorana, A., et al. (2016). Rapid eye movement sleep disruption and sleep fragmentation are associated with increased orexin-A cerebrospinal-fluid levels in mild cognitive impairment due to Alzheimer's disease. *Neurobiology of Aging*, 40, 120–126.

Manoharan, S., Guillemin, G. J., Abiramasundari, R. S., Essa, M. M., Akbar, M., & Akbar, M. D. (2016). The role of reactive oxygen species in the pathogenesis of Alzheimer's disease, Parkinson's disease, and Huntington's disease: A mini review. *Oxidative Medicine and Cellular Longevity*, 2016, 8590578.

Mendez, M. F. (2017). What is the relationship of traumatic brain injury to dementia. *Journal of Alzheimer's Disease*, 57(3), 667–681.

Porsteinsson, A. P., Drye, L. T., Pollock, B. F., Devannand, D. P., Frangakis, C., Ismail, Z., et al. (2014). Effect of citalopram on agitation in Alzheimer disease: The CitAD randomized clinical trial. *The Journal of the American Medical Association*, 311(7), 682–691.

Pugazhenthi, S. (2017). Metabolic syndrome and the cellular phase of Alzheimer's disease. *Progress in Molecular and Biology Translational Science*, 146, 243–258.

Slooter, A. J., Van De Leur, R. R., & Zaal, I. J. (2017). Delirium in critically ill patients. *Handbook of Clinical Neurology*, 141, 449–466.

Stelmokas, J., Gabel, N., Flaherty, J. M., Rayson, K., Tran, K., Anderson, J. R., et al. (2016). Delirium detection and impact of comorbid health conditions in a post-acute rehabilitation hospital setting. *PLoS One*, 11(11), e0166754.

Todd, O. M., & Teale, E. A. (2017). Delirium: A guide for the general physician. *Clinical Medicine (Lond)*, 17(1), 48–53.

Tucci, P., Mhillaj, E., Morgese, M.G., Colaianna, M., Zotti, M., Schiavone, S., et al. (2014). Memantine prevents memory consolidation failure induced by soluble beta amyloid in rats. *Frontiers in Behavioral Neuroscience*, 8, 332.

U.S. Department of Health and Human Services. (2015). *2014–2015 Alzheimer's disease progress report: Advancing research toward a cure*. Washington DC: Alzheimer Disease Education and Referral (ADEAR) Center, National Institute on Aging, National Institutes of Health.

Van Cauwenberghe, C., Van Broeckhoven, C., & Sleegers, K. (2016). The genetic landscape of Alzheimer disease: Clinical implications and perspectives. *Genetics in Medicine*, 18(5), 421–430.

Wang, M., Norman, J. E., Srinivasan, V. J., & Rutledge, J. C. (2016). Metabolic, inflammatory, and microvascular determinants of white matter disease and cognitive decline. *American Journal of Neurodegenerative Disease*, 5(5), 171–177.

Zhao, Q. F., Tan, L., Wang, H. F., Jiang, T., Tan, M. S., Tan, L., et al. (2016). The prevalence of neuropsychiatric symptoms in Alzheimer's disease: Systematic review and meta-analysis. *Journal of Affective Disorders*, 190, 264–271.

Appendices A, B, and the Glossary

Appendix A, Brief Psychiatric Rating Scale; Appendix B, Abnormal Involuntary Movement Scale (AIMS); and the **Glossary** are available at http://thepoint.lww.com/BoydEssentials2e and in the CoursePoint ebook.

Index

NOTE: Locators followed by 'b', 'f' and 't' refer to boxes, figures and tables respectively. Page numbers preceded by "e-" indicate pages from Chapters 7 and 28, which can be found at http://thepoint.lww.com/BoydEssentials2e and in the CoursePoint ebook.

A

Abandonment fears, 405
ABCs of psychological first aid, 220
Abnormal Involuntary Movement Scale (AIMS), 144
Absorption, 134
Abuse. *See also* Violence and abuse, types of
  alcohol, long-term, effects, 429–430, 430b
  assessment, 246b
  child, and neglect, 242
  history/physical findings suggestive of, 249b–250b
  of older adults, 242–243
  physical, 240, 241f
  psychoeducation for, 253, 253b
  violence and, screening for, 245–246, 246b, 247b
Abuser, treatment for, 254
Acamprosate calcium, for alcoholism, 432
Accountability issues
  lawsuits in psychiatric mental health care, 25
  legal liability in psychiatric nursing practice, 25
  nursing documentation, 26
Acculturation, 8
Acetylcholine (ACh), 67, 541
Acetylcholine receptor blockade (muscarinic), 133t
Acetylcholinesterase inhibitors (AChEIs), 547–548
Acquired capability for suicide, 228
Acrophobia, 278b
Activities of daily living (ADLs), 248
Activity and exercise, 109
Acupressure, 436
Acute dystonia, 142
Acute extrapyramidal symptoms, 142
Acute stress, 178
Adaptation, 186
Adaptive behavior, 512
Addiction, defined, 426
Addiction and substance-related disorders
  age of onset, 426
  chemical dependency and professional nurses, 451
  comorbidity, 427
  diagnostic criteria, 426
  emerging drugs and trends, 442
  ethnicity and culture, 426–427
  etiology, 427
  family responses to substance use/abuse, 427
  gambling (non-substance-related disorder), 442–443
  overview of substance use/abuse, 425
  substances and related disorders
    alcohol, 427–434, 428t–429t, 430b, 430t, 431b, 433t
    cannabis, 437
    evidence-based nursing care for, 443–451
    hallucinogens and dissociative drugs, 437–438
    inhalants, 441
    opioids and morphine derivatives, 438–441, 439t, 440t
    prescription and over-the-counter drugs, 438
    steroids, 441–442
    stimulants, 434–437
  treatment and recovery, 427
Adherence, 159–160
Adler's foundation, for individual psychology, 42
Adolescents
  anxiety disorders among, 261
  OCD among, 298
  suicide/suicide attempt among, 224–225
Adults, suicide/suicide attempt among, 225
Advanced Practice Psychiatric–Mental Health Registered Nurses (PMH-APRN), 31
Adverse reactions, psychiatric medications, 129
Advocacy, e-5
Aerosols, 441
Affective instability, 396
Affinity, 131
African Americans with mental illness
  racial discrimination against, 10–11
  stigma, 10
  views about mental illnesses, 10–11
Age
  albumin production, 137
  drug effects and, 137
  gastric absorption changes, 137
  related groups, 173
  renal function, 137
Aggression and violence
  assessment for, 199–200
  characteristics predictive of, 199
  evaluation and treatment outcomes, 204
  gender differences in aggressive behavior, 198
  impaired communication, 199–200
  influencing factors, 197
  interventions for promoting safety
    administering and monitoring PRN medications, 203
    aggression-prevention strategies, 202
    communication and development of nurse–patient relationship, 200–202
    de-escalation, 203
    empathic responding, 201
    listening to patients, 200–201
    milieu and environmental interventions, 202b
    providing choices, 201–202
    providing patient education, 202
    reducing stimulation strategy, 203
    seclusion and restraint, avoiding use of, 203–204
  milieu and environmental factors and, 200
  physical condition and, 200
  priority of nursing care for, 200
  research and policy initiatives, 205
  responding to assault on nurses, 204–205, 204t
  social factors and, 200
  theories
    behavioral, 198
    biologic, 197–198
    general aggression model (GAM), 198–199, 199f
    psychoanalytic, 198
    psychological, 198–199
    social learning theory, 198

Agonists, 131, 131f
Agoraphobia, 265, 277, 278b
Agranulocytosis, 141
Ailurophobia, 278b
Akathisia, 142, 143
Akinesia, 142
Alcohol
  alcohol-induced amnestic disorders, 432
  blood alcohol levels and behavior, 429t
  effects/withdrawal syndrome/prolonged use, 428, 429t–430t
  long-term abuse, effects of, 429–430, 430b
  multivitamins and adequate nutrition, 432, 434
  relapse prevention, 432, 433b
  withdrawal and detoxification, 430–432, 430t, 431b
Alcoholics anonymous (AA), 450, 450b
Alcohol-induced amnestic disorders, 432
Alcohol withdrawal syndrome, 430, 430t
Algophobia, 278b
Allostasis, 178
Allostatic load, 179, 179f, 180b
Alprazolam (Xanax), 152, 152t
Altruism, 173t
Alzheimer disease, 541f–542f
  behavioral responses, 546
  bursing home care, 555
  cell death in, 541
  clinical course, 539, 539f
  continuum of care, 555
  diagnosis of, 540
  epidemiology, 540
  etiology, 540
  evaluation and treatment outcomes, 555
  evidence-based nursing care for, 543–555
    activity and exercise interventions, 547
    by caregivers, 554b–555b
    community actions, 554
    family interventions, 554
    home visits, 554
    medications, 547, 548t, 550b
    messages, meanings, and management strategies, 553t
    milieu management, 554
    for mood changes, 552
    nutritional interventions, 547
    pain and comfort management, 547
    physical health interventions, 547–549
    priority of nursing care, 546
    psychosocial interventions, 549–552
    relaxation, 547
    self-care interventions, 547
    sleep interventions, 547
    social interaction, 546
    socialization activities, 554
    therapeutic dialogue, 551b
  family response to, 542
  genetic factors of, 541–542
  inflammation and, 542
  inpatient-focused care, 555
  mental status assessment, 544–545
  metabolic syndrome and, 540
  neurofibrillary tangles in, 541
  neurotransmission in, 541
  oxidative stress and, 542
  physical health assessment, 543–544
  psychosocial assessment, 544–546
  risk factors, 540
  safety interventions, 552–554
  safety issues, 543
  working toward recovery, 542–543
Amantadine (Symmetrel), 143t
American Association of Suicidology, 230
American Health Care Association, 18
American Hospital Association, 18
American Indians/Alaska Natives
  suicide rates among, 227
American Nurses Association (ANA), 30
American Nurses Credentialing Center (ANCC), 32
American Psychiatric Nurses Association (APNA), 33
American Public Health Association, 18
American Recovery and Reinvestment Act of 2009, 22
Americans With Disabilities Act of 1990 (ADA), 18
Amino acids, 70–71
Amitriptyline (Elavil), 148t, 550b
Amnestic disorders, alcohol-induced, 432
Amnestic MCI, 540
Amoxapine, 148t
Amphetamine–dextroamphetamine (Adderall, Adderall XR), 154, 155t, 521
Amphetamines, 154, 435
Amygdala, 62
Amyloid precursor protein (APP), 540
Anabolic steroid, 441, 442
Analytical psychology, 42
Anatomic barriers, in distribution of drug, 134, 136t
Androstenedione, 442
Anger
  assessment of, 195–196
    culture and gender considerations, 196
  cultural myths about, 193t
  experience of, 193–194
  expression of, 194–195
  intensity of, 198b
  inwardly directed, 195
  maladaptive, 192–193
  management, 196–197
    calming strategies, 193
    cognitive-behavioral therapy (CBT), 197
    nurse–patient relationship, role of, 195
  negative outcomes of, 196
  outwardly directed, 195
  suppressed, 193
Anger management, 252, 413
  groups, 175
Anger-related disorder, 195
Anorexia nervosa. *See also* Eating disorders
  biologic theories, 458–459
  body distortion, 456–457
  clinical course, 455–456
  comorbidity, 458
  diagnostic criteria, 457
  epidemiology, 457–458
  ethnicity and culture, 458
  family response to disorder, 460–461, 461b
  gender, 458
  psychological theories, 459
  recovery-oriented care for
    integration with primary care, 462
    safety issues, 462
    teamwork and collaboration, 461–462, 461b
  risk factors, 460
  social theories, 459, 460b
Anorgasmia, 149, 499
Antagonists, 131, 131f
Antianxiety medications, 152t
Anticholinergics, 143t
  delirium and, 537t
Anticonvulsants, 146–147
  delirium and, 537t
  indications, 146
  mechanisms of action, 146
  pharmacokinetics, 146–147
  side effects, 147
  teaching points, 147
  toxicity in, 147
Antidepressants
  FDA-approved, 149
  monoamine oxidase inhibitors, 150–151
  norepinephrine–dopamine reuptake inhibitors, 149
  for OCD, 303, 304t
  selective serotonin reuptake inhibitors, 147–149
  serotonin norepinephrine reuptake inhibitors, 149
  tricyclic, 149–150
Antihistamines, 143t, 154
Antipsychotic medications, 138–144
  absorption, 140
  anticholinergic side effects, 141
  atypical, 138, 139t
  blood disorders, 141
  cardiovascular side effects, 140
  clinical effects, 140
  conventional, 138, 139t
  excretion of drugs, 140
  indications and mechanism of action, 139–140
  long-acting preparations, 140
  medication-related movement disorders, 142–144, 143t
  metabolism of drugs, 140
  neuroleptic malignant syndrome (NMS), 141–142
  pharmacokinetics, 140
  photosensitivity reactions, 142
  recommended assessments before and during, 141b

risk for type II diabetes, 141
sexual side effects, 141
for tics, 523
weight gain, 141
Antisocial personality disorder (ASPD)
age of onset, 408–409
biologic theories, 409
clinical course/diagnostic criteria, 408, 409
comorbidity, 409
continuum of care, 413
defined, 408
epidemiology/risk factors, 408–409
evaluation/treatment outcomes, 413
evidence-based nursing care of, 410–413, 412b
family response to, 410
psychosocial theories, 409–410
safety issues, 410
Anxiety, 41, 51
defined, 258
degrees of, 258t
levels of, 52b
management, 252
symptoms of, 259b
Anxiety disorders
across life span
children and adolescents, 261
older adults, 261
case study, 257
defined, 258
generalized anxiety disorder (GAD)
agoraphobia, 277
clinical course, 276–277
diagnostic criteria, 277
nursing care, 277, 277b
social anxiety disorder (social phobia), 278–279
specific phobia, 277–278, 278b
normal vs. abnormal anxiety response, 258, 258t, 259b
overview of, 260–261
panic disorder
clinical course, 261–262, 262b
comorbidity, 262–263
continuum of patient care, 274
diagnostic criteria, 262, 263
epidemiology/risk factors, 40
etiology, 263–264
evaluation/treatment outcomes, 274
evidence-based nursing care for, 265–268, 267b, 268t, 269t
family response to disorder, 264
mental health nursing interventions, 269–273, 270b, 271b, 271t, 272b
primary care, integration with, 274, 276
psychosocial interventions, 273–274, 273t, 275b, 276b
recovery-oriented care for persons, 264–265
therapeutic relationship, 268–269
phobias
defense mechanisms and anxiety, 260, 260t
Anxiolytics, 151–154, 421

Appetite and nutrition, 110
Appraisal, 180–181
personality influences, 182
primary, 181
secondary, 181
Arab Americans, 11
Arachnophobia, 278b
Aripiprazole (Abilify), 139t, 141
Aripiprazole lauroxil (Aristada), 139t
Armodafinil (Nuvigil), 154, 155
Asenapine (Saphris), 139t
Asian Americans
culture-bound syndrome, 11
living in United States, 11
views about mental illnesses, 11
Asian/Pacific Islanders
suicide rates among, 227
ASPD. See Antisocial personality disorder (ASPD)
Assessment, 105
Association cortex, 60
Association of Child and Adolescent Psychiatric Nurses, 33
Ataque de nervios, 3b
Atomoxetine (Strattera), 521
Attachment, 410
Attention, 517
Attention-deficit hyperactivity disorder (ADHD), 299, 517–522
across life-span, 517
biologic theories, 518
clinical course and diagnostic criteria, 517
continuum of care, 522
epidemiology and risk factors, 517–518
etiology, 518
evaluation and treatment outcomes, 522
family response to, 518
long-term outcomes of optimal treatment for, 522f
nursing interventions
pharmacologic interventions, 520–521
physical health interventions, 520–521
priorities of nursing care, 520
psychosocial interventions, 522
patient education, 521
pharmacologic interventions, 520–521
Atomoxetine (Strattera), 521
psychostimulants, 521
phychosocial assessment, 519–520
physical health assessment, 519
physical health interventions
few foods diet, 520
modification of nutrition, 520
restricted elimination diet, 520
sleep hygiene and behavior therapy, 520
psychosocial interventions, 522
psychosocial theories, 518
psychostimulants for, 155
safety issues, 518–519
tools for diagnosis, 519b
working toward recovery, 518

Attitude
influence on African American and Latino population, 10b
Atypical antipsychotics, 138, 139t
Auditory hallucinations, 225
Augmentation, 138
Auricular therapy, 136
Autism spectrum disorder (ASD), 513–517, 514f
behavioral interventions, 516
epidemiology, 514–515
etiology, 514–515
evaluation and treatment outcomes, 517
evidence-based nursing care for, 515–517
family interventions, 516–517
nursing interventions
physical health assessment, 515
physical health interventions, 516
priority of nursing care, 515
psychosocial assessment, 515
psychosocial interventions, 516
pattern of intellectual strengths and weaknesses, 513
physical health interventions, 516
psychosocial interventions
ensuring predictability and safety, 516
structuring interventions for social isolation, 516
working toward recovery, 514
Autonomic nervous system, 63, 64f
peripheral organ response in, 63t
Autonomy, 30
Avanafil (Stendra), 504
Avoidance and numbing (dissociative symptoms), 284
Avoidant personality disorder
clinical course/diagnostic criteria, 416
continuum of care, 416
epidemiology/risk factors, 416
etiology, 416
nursing care, 416
Ayahuasca, 438

B

Bandura's social cognitive theory, 45
Barbiturates, 438
Bath salts, 442
Beck's theory, 45
Beginning stage of group, 166–167
Behavioral theories, 43–45
early stimulus–response theories, 44
reinforcement theories, 44–45
Behaviorism, 44
Behavior modification, 121–122
Behavior therapy, 121
Belief forms and religions, 12t, 13t
Beneficence, 30
Benzodiazepines, 143t, 154, 549
individual reactions to, 153
pharmacokinetics, 152
side effects, 152
toxicity, 152

Benzodiazepine therapy
  administering/monitoring benzodiazepines, 272–273
  for panic disorder
    drug interactions, monitoring for, 273
    side effect management, 273
Benztropine (Cogentin), 143t
Bereavement
  complicated, 212
  dual process model of coping with, 211, 212f
  uncomplicated, 211–212
Beta-amyloid plaques, 540–541
Bibliotherapy, 121
Binge-eating disorder (BED), 454, 474
Bioavailability, 134
Biogenic amines (bioamines), 69–71
Biologic domain, 33–34. *See also* Psychiatric-mental health nursing
  interventions for
    electroconvulsive therapy, 233
    medication management, 233
Biologic foundations, of psychiatric nursing
  central nervous system
    neuroanatomy of, 58–63
    neurophysiology of, 63–73
  diagnostic approaches, 76–78
  studies of biologic basis of mental disorders, 73–76
Biologic perspectives of stress
  acute stress, 178
  allostasis, 178
  allostatic load, 179, 179f, 180b
  chronic stress, 178–180
  homeostasis, 178
Biologic theories
  for anorexia nervosa
    genetic theories, 458
    neuroendocrine/neurotransmitter changes, 458–459
  antisocial personality disorder, 409
  for BPD, 397
  for bulimia nervosa, 469–470
  OCD
    biochemical theories, 300
    genetic factors, 300
    neuropathologic theories, 300
  panic disorders, 263
    gamma-aminobutyric acid (GABA), 264
    hypothalamic–pituitary–adrenal (HPA) axis, 264
    norepinephrine, 264
    serotonin, 264
Biopsychosocial framework, 33–34, 33f
  biologic domain, 33–34
  psychological domain, 34
  social domain, 34
Bipolar disorder
  across life span, 336
  bipolar I disorder, 336–351
  bipolar II disorder, 351
  in children and adolescents, 336
  clinical course, 336

comorbidity, 337
continuum of care, 350–351
  inpatient-focused care, 350
  intensive outpatient programs, 350
  spectrum of care, 351
cyclothymic disorder, 351
diagnostic criteria, 336, 337b
epidemiology, 336
  age of onset, 337
  ethnicity and culture, 337
  gender, 337
etiology, 337–338
  chronic stress, 338
  chronobiologic theories, 338
  genetic factors, 338
  inflammation, 338
  kindling, 338
  psychosocial theories, 338
  social theories, 338
family response to, 338
hypomania, 351
interventions
  antipsychotics, 347
  carbamazepine, 346
  divalproex sodium (Depakote), 344–346
  electroconvulsive therapy (ECT), 348
  for family members, 350
  lamotrigine (Lamictal), 346–347, 347b
  lithium in, 344
  medications, 342–344
  mood-stabilizing drugs, 342–347
  psychosocial, 349
  self-care, 342–344
  support groups, 350
  teaching patients and family, 349–350, 349b
mental health nursing assessment
  nursing care, 341
  nursing interventions, 341
  physical health assessment, 340
  psychosocial assessment, 340–341
  social and occupational functioning, 341
  strength assessment, 341
mental health promotion, 351
and mood, 340
nursing care of, 339–340
in older adults, 336
recovery goal, 339
risk assessment, 341
risk factors, 336
stress and coping, 340–341
thought distortions in, 340
Bipolar I disorder, 336–351
Bipolar II disorder, 351
Bleuler, Eugen, 355
Biosexual identity, 496
Biosocial theories, 398
Biotransformation, 136
Biperiden (Akineton), 143t
Blood alcohol level (BAL) and behavior, 429, 429t
Blood disorders, antipsychotic medications and, 141

Body dissatisfaction, 459
Body dysmorphic disorder (BDD), 297t, 307–308, 308b
Body image, 113
Body image distortion
  drive for thinness, 456
  guilt and anger, 456, 457
  outcomes, 457
  perfectionism, 456–457
Body systems review, 107
Borderline emotions, 184
Borderline personality disorder (BPD). *See also* Personality/impulse-control disorders
  across life span, 397
  behavioral patterns in, 398b
  biologic theories, 397
  clinical course, 395
  cognitive dysfunctions, 396
  comorbidity, 397
  continuum of care, 407, 408b
  defined, 395
  diagnostic criteria, 395–397
  epidemiology/risk factors, 397
  evaluation/treatment outcomes, 407
  evidence-based nursing care for, 399–407, 400b, 403b, 406t, 407t
  family response to, 399
  psychosocial theories, 397–399, 398b
  safety issues, 399
  teamwork and collaboration, 399
  unstable affect, 396
  unstable interpersonal relationships, 396
  unstable self-image, 396
Boxed warning in PI, 129
BPD. *See* Borderline personality disorder (BPD)
Brady Handgun Violence Prevention Act of 1993, 25
Breathing control, teaching, 269–270
Brexpiprazole (Rexulti), 139t
Brief intervention, 447, 449
Brontophobia, 278b
Bulimia nervosa. *See also* Eating disorders
  across lifespan, 469
  age of onset, 469
  biologic theories, 469–470
  clinical course, 468
  comorbidity, 469
  diagnostic criteria, 468–469, 468b
  epidemiology, 469
  ethnicity and culture, 469
  evidence-based nursing care for, 471–474
  gender, 469
  psychosocial theories, 470
  risk factors, 470
  safety issues, 471
  teamwork and collaboration, 470
Buprenorphine, 440, 441
Bupropion
  nicotine prevention, 436
Bupropion (Wellbutrin, Zyban), 148t, 149, 150t
Burgess-Partner abuse scale for teens, 247b

Buspirone (BuSpar), 152t
　indications for, 153
　mechanisms of actions, 153
　pharmacokinetics, 153
　side effects, 153
　toxicity, 153

C

Caffeine, 436–437
Cannabidiol (CBD), 437
Cannabis sativa, 437
Captopril (Capoten), 550b
Carbamazepine (Equetro), 146–147
Cariprazine (Vraylar), 139t
Carrier proteins, 132, 132f
Catharsis, 173t
CDC. *See* Centers for Disease Control and Prevention (CDC)
Centers for Disease Control and Prevention (CDC), 2
Centers for Medicare & Medicaid Services (CMS), 19
Central nervous system (CNS), 57
　neuroanatomy of, 58–63
　neurophysiology of, 63–73
Cerebrum, 58–60, 58f
　association cortex, 60
　frontal lobes, 59
　left and right hemispheres, 58–59
　lobes of brain, 58f, 59–60
　occipital lobes, 60
　parietal lobes, 59–60
　temporal lobes, 60
Challenge test, 77
Chemical dependency and professional nurses, 451
Chemical restraint, 21
Child abuse, 242
Child Behavior Checklist (CBCL), 519b
Childhood schizophrenia, 529
Childhood trauma, 227
Child management skills, 253
Child neglect, 242
Children
　anxiety disorders among, 261
　OCD among, 298
　suicide/suicide attempt among, 224–225
Chlordiazepoxide (Librium), 152, 152t, 432
Chlorpromazine, 139t
Cholinergic pathways, 67f
Chronic stress, 178–180
　consequences, 179
　mental illness and, 180
Chronic syndromes, 144
Chronobiology, 76
Cigarette smoking
　cause of premature death, 436
Cimetidine (Tagamet), 550b
Citalopram (Celexa), 148t, 150t, 550b
Classical conditioning. *See* Pavlovian Theory
Claustrophobia, 278b
Clearance, 136

Clinical Institute Withdrawal Assessment for Alcohol Scale (CIWA-Ar), 430, 431b
Clinical reasoning, 34, 34b
Clomipramine (Anafranil), 148t
Clonazepam (Klonopin), 143t, 152t
Clorazepate (Tranxene), 152t
Closed groups, 165
Clozapine (Clozaril, FazaClo, Versacloz), 139t, 141
Club drugs, 435
Cluster A personality disorders, 392
Cluster B personality disorders, 392
Cluster C personality disorders, 392
CNS. *See* Central nervous system (CNS)
Cocaine. *See also* Stimulants
　biologic responses to, 434
　intoxication, 434
　types of, 434
　withdrawal, 434
Codeine, 550b
Codependence, 445
Cognition, 45, 120, 199, 285, 534
　and intellectual performance, 112
Cognitive-behavioral theories, 45t
　applicability to psychiatric-mental health nursing, 45–46
　behavioral theories, 43–45, 44t
　　early stimulus–response theories, 44
　　reinforcement theories, 44–45
　cognitive theories, 45
　　Bandura's social cognitive theory, 45
　　Beck's theory, 45
Cognitive behavioral therapy (CBT), 264, 265, 287, 287b
Cognitive-behavioral therapy (CBT), 197, 506
Cognitive disturbances, 401
Cognitive dysfunctions. *See also* Borderline personality disorder (BPD)
　impaired problem solving, 396
　impulsivity, 396
　self-harm behaviors, 396–397
Cognitive interventions, 120
Cognitive restructuring, 305
Cognitive schemata, 398
Cognitive theories
　for suicide prevention, 228
Cognitive thought patterns, 266–267
Cohesion, 170
Coleadership, 166
Combat exposure, 225
Commitment to treatment statement (CTS), 234
Communication
　blocks, 93–94
　skills, 407
Communication disorders, 527–528
Communication pathways, 169
Community
　care
　　for OCD patients, 306–307
　　for panic disorder, 276
　　for person with PTSD, 293
　　for survivors of violence/abuse, 253

disorganization, 243
　interventions
　　for bulimia nervosa, 474
Comorbidity, 240, 299
　addiction and substance related disorders, 427
　anorexia nervosa, 458
　for antisocial personality disorder, 409
　for BPD, 397
　bulimia nervosa, 469
　panic disorder, 262–263
Competency, 19. *See also* Patient rights and legal issues
　determination of, 19t
Compliance, 159–160
Complicated bereavement, 212
Compromiser, 170
Compulsions
　defined, 297
　diagnostic criteria, 298
　obsessions and, 296–297
Compulsive gamblers, 443
Compulsive hoarding disorder, 308, 308b
Concordance rate, 73
Conditioned stimuli, 300
Confabulation, 432
Confidentiality, 22
Conflict resolution, 120–121
Confrontation, 447
Connections, 48
Conners Parent Questionnaire, 519b
Containment, 124
Content themes, 93, 93b
Continuum of care, 421
　for anorexia nervosa
　　emergency care, 467
　　family interventions, 467, 467b
　　inpatient, 467
　　outpatient treatment, 467
　　school interventions, 467–468
　bipolar disorder
　　inpatient-focused care, 350
　　intensive outpatient programs, 350
　　spectrum of care, 351
　for antisocial personality disorder, 413
　for BPD, 407, 408b
　for bulimia nervosa, 474
　for disruptive, impulse-control disorders, 422
　for histrionic personality disorder, 415
　for narcissistic personality disorder, 415
　for OCD
　　community treatment, 306–307
　　emergency care, 306
　　family interventions, 306
　　inpatient-focused care, 306
　for panic disorder, 274
　for paranoid personality disorder, 393
　for PTSD
　　community treatment, 293
　　emergency care, 292–293
　　family interventions, 292
　　inpatient-focused care, 293
　for schizoid personality disorder, 394
　for schizotypal personality disorder, 394–395

Conventional antipsychotics, 138, 139t
Coordinator, 170
Coping skills, 402, 449, 450b
Cortical blindness, 60
Cortical dementia, 535
Cough medicine, OTC, 438
Counseling interventions, 120
Countertransference, 41, 99, 445, 445t
Crack cocaine, 434
Craving, 432
Creutzfeldt–Jakob disease, 556
Criminal judicial processes
  fitness to stand trial, 23–24
  guilty but mentally ill, 24
  gun laws and mental illness, 25
  misconceptions regarding insanity pleas, 24, 25b
  not guilty by reason of insanity, 24
  probation, 24
  stigma of criminality, 23
Crisis, 208–209
  evidence-based nursing care
    emotional and behavioral responses, 213
    evaluation and treatment outcomes, 216
    maintaining health, 213
    priority nursing care, 213–214
    social functioning and support, 213
    therapeutic relationship, 214
  guidelines for intervention, 214t
  historical perspectives of, 209
  loss and bereavement, 210–213
  mental health nursing interventions, 214–216
    counseling, 216
    medications, 215
    residential crisis services, 216
    self-care, 215
    social support strategies, 216
    telephone hotlines, 216
  types of
    developmental crisis, 209–210
    situational crisis, 210
    traumatic crisis, 210
  working towards recovery, 212–213
CTS. See Commitment to treatment statement (CTS)
Cultural brokering, 120–121
Cultural competence, 8
  and mental health, 10b
Cultural expectations and role strain, 183
Cultural explanation, 3
Cultural groups
  linguistic variations within, 9
  values and beliefs on mental illness, 8
Cultural identity, 9
Cultural idiom of distress, 3, 9
Culture, 8–9
Culture-bound syndrome, 11
Cycle of violence, 244, 244f
Cyclothymic disorder, 335
Cynophobia, 278b
Cytochrome P450 (CYP450) system, 136
  metabolism of common antidepressants, 150t

D

d-amphetamine (Dexedrine), 154
Danger assessment, 246b
Debriefing, 220
Decision-making groups, 172–173
De-escalation, 125
Defense mechanisms, 41
Defensive, 51
Dehydroepiandrosterone (DHEA), 442
Delay or absence of ejaculation (DE), 503
Delirium, 535
  clinical course, 535
  continuum of care, 539
  diagnosis, 535
  differentiating from dementia, 536t
  drug-induced, 537t
  epidemiology, 535
  etiology, 535–536
  evaluation and treatment outcomes, 539
  evidence-based nursing care, 537–539
    complementary and alternative medicine, 538
    medications, 538
    psychosocial interventions, 538–539
    safety interventions, 538
  nursing interventions, 538–539
    family environment assessment, 538
    mental health nursing assessment, 537
    mental status evaluation, 537–538
    physical health assessment, 537
    psychosocial assessment, 537–538
  risk factors, 535, 536t
  safety issues, 536–537
  working toward recovery, 536
Delirium tremens, 430
Dementia, 535
  caused by Huntington's disease, 556
  caused by Parkinson disease, 556
Denial, defined, 443
Denial of problem, 443–444
Dependent personality disorder. *See also* Personality/impulse-control disorders
  clinical course/diagnostic criteria, 416
  continuum of care, 417
  epidemiology/risk factors, 417
  etiology, 417
  nursing care, 417
Depersonalization, 261, 284, 293
Depression
  defined, 312
  mood and, 311–312
  overview, 312–313
  in schizophrenia, 343
Depression and Bipolar Support Network (DBSA), 329
Depressive disorders
  across life span, 312–313
  in children and adolescents, 312
  clinical course, 313
  cognition and memory, 319
  comorbidity, 314
  continuum of care, 329–330
  deep-breathing exercises, 321, 322b
  diagnostic criteria, 313
  disruptive mood dysregulation disorder, 330
  epidemiology, 313
    age of onset, 337
    culture, 313
    ethnicity, 313
    gender, 337
  etiology
    behavioral factors, 315
    biologic theories, 314
    cognitive factors, 315
    developmental factors, 315
    environmental factors, 316
    family factors, 315–316
    genetic, 314
    neurobiologic theories of, 315
    neuroendocrine hypothesis, 315
    neuropeptide hypothesis, 315
    psychodynamic factors, 315
    psychological theories, 315
    psychoneuroimmunology, 315
    social theories, 315
  evaluation and treatment outcomes, 350–351
  evidence-based nursing care of behavior, 319
    mental health nursing assessment, 340
    psychosocial assessment, 318–319
    therapeutic relationship320
  family response to, 316
  genetic factor, 298
  interventions
    antidepressants, 321–322
    behavioral, 328
    cognitive, 328
    electroconvulsive therapy, 327
    family, 329
    group, 328
    light therapy (phototherapy), 327
    milieu therapy, 329
    monoamine oxidase inhibitors, 322
    pharmacological, 321–326
    physical care, 320–321
    psychoeducation, 328–329, 328b
    psychosocial, 328–313
    repetitive transcranial magnetic stimulation (rTMS), 327–328
    safety, 329
    selective serotonin reuptake inhibitors, 322
    serotonin norepinephrine reuptake inhibitors, 322, 324
    support groups, 329
    tricyclic antidepressants, 322
  medication assessment for, 318
  mood and affect, 318–319
  neurobiologic hypotheses, 319
  overview of, 312–313
  persistent depressive disorder (dysthymia), 330
  physical health assessment for, 340
  premenstrual dysphoric disorder, 330

recovery, 316–317
    alternative/complementary
        therapies, 317
    cognitive behavioral therapy (CBT),
        316
    combination therapies, 317
    interpersonal therapy, 316
risk factors, 336–337
safety issues, 317
self-report scales for, 319
strength assessment for, 320
suicidal behavior in, 319
therapeutic relationship, 320, 321b
thought content, 319
Depressive episodes, 336
Derealization disorder, 284, 293
Desensitization, 72, 133
Desipramine (Norpramin), 148t, 149
Desmopressin (DDAVP), 529
Desvenlafaxine (Pristiq), 149, 150t
Desvenlafaxine (Pristiq Extended
    Release), 148t
Detoxification, 426, 430, 440
    alcohol, 430–432, 430t, 431b
Deutetrabenazine (AUSTEDO), 144
Developmental crisis, 209–210
Developmental theories
    Erikson's psychosocial development,
        46–47, 46t
    Gilligan's gender differentiation, 48
    Miller's theory, 48
    Piaget's theory, 47–48
    and psychiatric–mental health nursing,
        48
Dexmethylphenidate (Focalin), 154
Dexmethylphenidate Extended Release
    (Focalin XR), 155t
Dextroamphetamine (Dexedrine), 155t
*Diagnostic and Statistical Manual of Mental
    Disorders–5 (DSM-5)*, 3, 9
Dialectical behavior therapy (DBT), 399
Diathesis, 180
Diazepam, 432
Diazepam (Valium), 132, 143t, 152, 152t
Dichotomous thinking, 396
Dietary restraint, 469
Dietary supplements, 157
Digoxin (Lanoxin), 550b
Diphenhydramine (Benadryl), 143t, 550b
Dipyridamole (Trental), 550b
Direct leadership, 166
Disaster
    definition, 216
    evidence-based nursing care
        community care, 220–221
        counseling, 220
        evaluation and treatment outcomes,
            221
        family support systems, 220
        medications, 220
        mental health nursing assessment,
            218–219
        mental health nursing interventions,
            219–221
        psychoeducation, 220
        self-care, 219–220

historical perspectives of, 216–217
long-term mental health
    consequences, 217
phases of, 217
priority care issues, 218
responses to, 217–218
working toward recovery, 218
Disconnections, 48
Discontinuation phase, drug therapy, 138
Disinhibited social engagement disorder,
    293
Disliked member, 171
Disruptive, impulse-control, and conduct
    disorders
    continuum of care, 421
    continuum of care for, 422
    epidemiology, 418–419
    etiology, 419–420, 420b
    evaluation/treatment outcomes, 421
    intermittent explosive disorder, 421
    kleptomania, 421
    mental health nursing assessment, 419
    mental health nursing interventions
        for biologic domain, 420
    oppositional defiant disorder, 418,
        419b
    priority of care, 419–420
    psychosocial interventions, 420
    pyromania, 421–422
Disruptive mood dysregulation disorder,
    330
Dissociation, 284, 396, 401
Dissociative amnesia, 293
Dissociative disorders, 293. *See also*
    Trauma-/stressor- related
    disorders
Dissociative drugs, 438
    hallucinogens and, 437–438
Dissociative identity disorder (DID), 293
Distraction, 273
Distribution of drug, 134–136
    factors affecting, 136t
        anatomic barriers, 134, 136t
        blood–brain barrier, 134, 136t
        blood flow of organ, 134, 136t
        plasma protein binding, 134, 136,
            136t
        size of organ, 134, 136t
        solubility of drug, 134, 136, 136t
Disulfiram (Antabuse), for alcoholism,
    432, 433b
Divalproex sodium (Depakote), 344–346
DMT (dimethyltryptamine), 438
Doctorate in nursing practice (DNP), 33
Documentation, for suicidal patients, 235
Donepezil (Aricept), 550b
Donepezil (Namzaric), 549b
Dopamine, in mental disorder, 69, 69f
Dopamine agonists, 143t
Dopamine receptor blockade (D_2), 133t
Dopamine reuptake inhibition, 133t
Dosing, 136–137
Downregulation, 72
Down syndrome, 540
Doxepin, 148t
Doxylamine (Unisom), 154t

Drive for thinness, 456
Dronabinol (Marinol), 437
Drug–drug interaction, 136, 138
Drug effects, individual variations in
    age, 137
    ethnopsychopharmacology, 137
    pharmacogenomics, 137
Drug-induced parkinsonism, 142
Drug regulation and use
    psychiatric medications, 129
D-9-tetrahydrocannabinol (THC), 437
Duloxetine (Cymbalta), 148t, 149, 150t
Dyad, 165
Dysfunctional thinking, 405–406, 406b,
    406t
Dyslexia, 527
Dyspareunia, 506
Dystonia, 142

E

Eating disorders
    anorexia nervosa
        biologic theories, 458–459
        body distortion, 456–457
        clinical course, 455–456
        comorbidity, 458
        diagnostic criteria, 457
        epidemiology, 457–458
        ethnicity and culture, 458
        evidence-based nursing care for,
            463–468
        family response to disorder,
            460–461, 461b
        gender, 458
        psychological theories, 459
        recovery-oriented care for, 461–462
        risk factors, 460
        social theories, 459, 460b
    binge-eating disorder (BED), 474
    bulimia nervosa
        across lifespan, 469
        age of onset, 469
        biologic theories, 469–470
        clinical course, 468
        comorbidity, 469
        diagnostic criteria, 468–469, 468b
        epidemiology, 469
        ethnicity and culture, 469
        evidence-based nursing care for,
            471–474
        gender, 469
        psychosocial theories, 470
        risk factors, 470
        safety issues, 471
        teamwork and collaboration, 470
    complications of, 462t
    night eating syndrome, 474
    overview, 454–455
    purging disorder, 474
    symptoms, 455f
Ecstasy, 435
ECT. *See* Electroconvulsive therapy
    (ECT)
The Education for the Handicapped Act
    (Public Law 94–142), 524
Efficacy, 132

Ejaculatory dysfunction, 502–503
  delay or absence of ejaculation (DE), 503
  epidemiology, 503
  etiology, 503
  evidence-based nursing care, 503
  integration with primary care, 503
  premature ejaculation (PE), 502–503
  working toward recovery, 503
Elation, 336
Electroconvulsive therapy (ECT), 129, 157–158, 233, 301
Electroencephalography (EEG), 77
Electrolytes, 464
Electronic cigarettes (e-cigarettes), 436
Elevated mood, 336
Elimination, 109
Elimination disorders, 529–530
Emergency care
  alert, 230
  for anorexia nervosa, 467
  for OCD patients, 306
  for panic disorder, 276
  for person with PTSD, 292–293
Emotional dysregulation, 456
  defined, 398
Emotional factors
  and suicide prevention, 228
Emotional regulation, 406
Emotion-focused coping, 185
Emotions, 184, 185t
Empathic linkage, 51
Empathic linkages, 97
Empathy, 43, 96
Employment, 183
Encopresis, 529–530
Endorphin, 71
Enmeshment, 460
Entomophobia, 278b
Enuresis, 529
Enzymes, 132
Epidemiology, 2–3, 3b
Epinephrine, in mental disorder, 69
Erectile dysfunction (ED)
  biologic theories, 503–504
  diagnostic criteria, 503
  epidemiology, 503
  etiology, 503–504
  medical problems and, 504
  mental health nursing assessment, 504
  priority of nursing care, 504
  psychological theories, 504
  working toward recovery, 504
Erikson's psychosocial development, 46–47, 46t
Erythroxylon coca plant, 434
Escitalopram (Lexapro), 148t, 150t, 550b
Escitalopram oxalate (Lexapro), 148
Estazolam (ProSom), 154t
Eszopiclone (Lunesta), 154t
Ethnicity and culture
  on addiction/substance-related disorders, 426–427
  on anorexia nervosa, 458
  on bulimia nervosa, 469
Evidence-based nursing care
  for OCD
    continuum of care, 306–307
    evaluation/treatment outcomes, 306
    interventions for hospitalized patients, 305–306, 306b
    mental health nursing assessment, 302–303, 303t
    nursing interventions, 303–305, 304b
  for PTSD
    continuum of care, 292–293
    evaluation/treatment outcomes, 292
    mental health nursing assessment, 288–289, 289b
    mental health nursing interventions, 289–291
    priority of nursing care, 289
    psychosocial nursing interventions, 292, 292b
    therapeutic relationship, 289, 290b
  for survivors of violence/abuse
    evaluation/treatment outcomes, 253–254
    mental health nursing assessment, 245–251, 246b, 247b, 248b, 249b–250b
    nursing interventions, 251–253, 253b
    priority of nursing care, 251
  for trichotillomania, 307
Evidence-based nursing care, for anorexia nervosa
  continuum of care, 467
  evaluation/treatment outcomes, 466
  mental health nursing assessment
    behavioral responses, 463
    physical health assessment, 463
    self-concept, 463
    social assessment, 463
    stress and coping patterns, 463
  mental health nursing interventions
    mental health and wellness goals, 464
    physical health interventions, 464–465
    psychosocial interventions, 465–466, 465b, 466t
  priority of nursing care, 464
  strengths assessment, 463–464
  therapeutic relationships, 464
Evidence-based nursing care, for ASPD
  mental health nursing assessment, 410–411
  mental health nursing interventions
    anger management, 413
    group interventions, 412–413
    interventions for family members, 413
    milieu interventions, 413
    patient education efforts, 411–412, 412b
    self-awareness, enhancing, 411
    self-responsibility, facilitating, 411
    social support, 413
  priority of care, 411
  therapeutic relationships, 411
Evidence-based nursing care, for BPD
  mental health nursing assessment
    medication assessment, 400
    physical health assessment, 399–400
    psychosocial assessment, 401–402
    risk assessment (suicide or self-injury), 402
    self-injurious behaviors, physical indicators of, 400
    strength assessment, 402
  mental nursing interventions
    pharmacologic interventions, 404–405
    physical care, 403–404
  priority in care, 402
  psychosocial interventions
    abandonment and intimacy fears, 405
    behavioral interventions, 405
    dysfunctional thinking, 405–406, 406b, 406t
    personal boundaries/limitations, 405
    psychoeducation, 406–407, 407b
  response patterns, 400b
  therapeutic relationship, 402–403, 403b
Evidence-based nursing care, for bulimia nervosa
  community interventions, 474
  continuum of care, 474
  evaluation/treatment outcomes, 473–474
  mental health nursing assessment
    physical health assessment, 471
    priority of nursing care, 471
    psychosocial assessment, 471
    strengths assessment, 471
    therapeutic relationship, 471, 472b
  mental health nursing interventions
    medication interventions, 472
    physical health interventions, 472
  psychosocial interventions
    behavioral strategies, 472–473
    group interventions, 473
    psychoeducation, 473, 473b
Evidence-based nursing care, for panic disorder
  mental health nursing assessment, 265
  panic attack assessment, 265–266
  physical health assessment
    medications, 266
    physical activity, 266
    sleep patterns, 266
    substance use, 266
  priority of nursing care, 267–268
  psychosocial assessment
    cognitive thought patterns, 266–267
    cultural factors, 267
    family factors, 267
    mental status examination, 266
    self-report scales, 266, 267b, 268t
    strength identification, of patient, 267
Evidence-based nursing care, for substances-related disorders

mental health nursing interventions, 447, 447b, 448t
brief intervention, 447, 449
cognitive and cognitive behavioral interventions, 449, 449b
coping skills, enhancing, 449, 450b
family interventions, 450
group interventions and early recovery, 449–450
harm-reduction, 450
individual therapy, 450
peer support self-help group, 450–451, 450b
psychoeducation, 449, 449b
nursing assessment, 443b, 444b
codependence, 445
countertransference, 445, 445t
denial of problem, 443–444
motivation for change, 444–445, 445b
priority of care, 446
therapeutic relationship, 446–447, 446t
Evoked potentials (EP), 78
Excitatory neurotransmitters, 66
Excitotoxicity, 71
Excoriation disorder. *See also* Trichotillomania and excoriation disorder
body dysmorphic disorder (BDD), 307–308, 308b
hoarding disorder, 308, 308b
Exercise and yoga, 291
Exhibitionism, 507t
Existential and humanistic theoretical perspectives
Parse's theory, 52
Watson's theory, 52–53
Expansive mood, 336
Exposure and response prevention (ERP), 305
Exposure therapy, 265
External advocacy systems, 18–19
Extrapyramidal symptoms (EPS), 142–143
Eye movement, desensitization, and reprocessing (EMDR), 287

F

False imprisonment, 25
Family dynamics, 48–49
Family interventions
for survivors of violence/abuse, 253
Family response
to anorexia nervosa, 460–461, 461b
to antisocial personality disorder, 410
to BPD patients, 399
to OCD, 300–301
to panic disorder, 264
to substance use and abuse, 427
Family therapy, 287
Fear, 248
Federal Emergency Management Agency (FEMA), 220
Female orgasmic disorder
diagnostic criteria, 499

epidemiology and risk factors, 499
etiology, 499–500
evaluation and treatment outcomes, 502
evidence-based nursing care for, 500–502
integration with primary care, 500
mental health nursing assessment, 500, 501t
nursing interventions for, 502
priority of nursing care, 502
self-care and wellness activities for, 502, 502b
working toward recovery, 500
Female sexual interest/arousal disorder, 505–506
Fetal alcohol syndrome (FAS), 427
Fetishism, 507t
Fever phobia, 278b
Fidelity, 30
"Fight-or-flight" response, 178, 178t
Firearm ownership
suicide rates among, 227
First-pass effect, 134
Fissures, 58
Fitness to stand trial, 23–24
Flooding, 265
Fluoxetine, 303
for bulimia nervosa, 472
Fluoxetine (Prozac), 148, 148t, 150t, 550b
Fluoxetine hydrochloride (Prozac)
for anorexia nervosa, 465, 465b
Fluphenazine, 139t, 140
Fluphenazine decanoate, 139t
Flurazepam (Dalmane), 152, 154t
Fluvoxamine, 303, 304t
Fluvoxamine (Luvox), 148, 148t, 150t
Folic acid deficiency
withdrawing from alcohol, 432
Forensic, 23
Formal group roles, 170
Formal support system, 49, 49b
Free-base cocaine, 434
Fromm's societal needs, 42
Frontal lobe, 59
syndrome, 59b
Frontotemporal neurocognitive disorder, 556
Frotteurism, 507t
Furosemide (Lasix), 550b

G

GABA enhancers, 154
GAD. *See* Generalized anxiety disorder (GAD)
Gambling. *See also* Addiction and substance-related disorders
non-substance-related disorder, 442–443
Gamma-aminobutyric acid (GABA), 71, 264
Gastric motility, 137
Gender
and anorexia nervosa, 458
and bulimia nervosa, 469
and suicide risk, 226

Gender dysphoria, 506
Gender identity, 496
General aggression model (GAM), 198–199, 199f
Generalized anxiety disorder (GAD). *See also* Anxiety disorders
agoraphobia, 277
clinical course, 276–277
diagnostic criteria, 277
nursing care, 277, 277b
social anxiety disorder (social phobia), 278–279
specific phobia, 277–278, 278b
Generativity, 47
Genetic, 73–74
molecular, 73–74
population, 73
susceptibility, 74
Genetic factors on suicidal behavior, 228
Genitopelvic pain/penetration disorder, 506
Geropsychiatric–Mental Health Nurses, 33
Gestalt therapy, 43
Gilligan's gender differentiation, 48
Global Burden of Disease 2010, 2
Glutamate, 71
Goals, 181
Gray matter, 58
Group, 164
communication
encouraging interaction, 167–168
group themes, 169
nonverbal, 169–170
pathways, 169
tracking, 170
verbal, 169
Group cohesiveness, 173t
Group conflict, 171
Group dynamics, 166
Group interventions, 412–413
for bulimia nervosa, 473
comparison of models, 167t
and early recovery, 449–450
guidelines for, 166b
leading a group, 168t
beginning stage, 166–167
dealing with challenging group behaviors, 170–172
determining roles of group members, 170
termination stage, 172
working stage, 167–170
nursing intervention groups
anger management groups, 175
medication groups, 174–175, 174b
reminiscence groups, 175
self-care groups, 175
symptom management groups, 175
preparing to lead a group
determining group composition, 165
forming open or closed group, 165
planning first meeting, 166
seating arrangement, 166
selecting leadership style, 165–166
selecting members, 165

Group interventions (Continued)
　roles and functions of group members, 171b
　types of groups
　　age-related groups, 173
　　decision-making groups, 172–173
　　psychoeducation groups, 172
　　psychotherapy groups, 173
　　self-help groups, 173
　　support groups, 173
　working with older people, 174b
Group process, 166
Group psychoeducation, 172
Group themes, 169
Group therapy, 287
Groupthink, 172
Guilt
　and anger, 456, 457
　and shame, 250
Guilty but mentally ill (GBMI), 24
Gun laws and mental illness, 25
Gyri, 58

H

Halazepam (Paxipam), 152t
Half-life of drug, 136
Hallucinogens and dissociative drugs, 437–438
Haloperidol (Haldol), 139t, 140
Haloperidol decanoate (Haldol D), 139t
Hamilton rating scale for anxiety, 268t
Harmonizer, 170
Harm-reduction, 450
Hashish, 437
Health Insurance Portability and Accountability Act of 1996 (HIPAA), 105
Health Insurance Portability and Accountability Act (HIPAA) of 1996, 22
Health teaching, 122–123, 123f
Healthy coping, 186
Hearing, 404
Hearing impairment, 157
Hematophobia, 278b
Hemp. See Cannabis
Heroin, 438
Hippocampus, 61
Hispanic Americans
　beliefs about mental illness, 10
　living in United States, 10
Histamine, 71
Histamine receptor blockade (H_1), 133t
Histrionic personality disorder
　clinical course/diagnostic criteria, 413–414
　continuum of care, 415
　epidemiology/ risk factors, 414
　etiology, 414
　nursing care, 414–415
Hoarding disorder, 297t, 308, 308b. See also Trichotillomania and excoriation disorder
Homeostasis, 178
Homicidal ideation, 114–115
Hopelessness, 228

Horney's feminine psychology, 42
Hospitalized patients with OCD, interventions for
　Psychoeducation, 305–306, 306b
Household organization training, 253
Humanbecoming Theory, 52
Humanistic theories
　Gestalt therapy, 43
　Maslow's hierarchy of needs, 43, 43f
　Rogers' client-centered therapy, 43
Human sexual response cycle, 498
Hwa-byung, 11
Hydration, 110
　interventions, 119
Hydroxyzine (Vistaril), 154t
Hyperarousal, 285
Hyperarousal symptoms, 286
Hypersalivation, 142
Hyperventilation, 269
Hypnotics, 154
　for insomnia, 154t
Hypothalamic-pituitary-adrenal (HPA) axis
　in panic disorders, 264
Hypothalamus, 61–62
Hypothyroidism, 75

I

Ideation-to-action theories. *See also* Suicide prevention
　IMV model, 228–229
　IPTS, 228
Identity diffusion, 401
Idioms and cultural syndromes, 3b
Illusions, 545
Iloperidone (Fanapt), 139t
Illness anxiety disorder, 488–489
Insomnia disorder, e-13–e-14
Imipramine (Tofranil), 148t
Imitative behavior, 173t
Imminent risk for suicide, interventions for
　inpatient safety considerations, 233
　patient safety, ensuring, 232–233
Impaired consciousness, 535
Impaired problem solving, 396
Implosive therapy, 265
Impulse-control disorders, defined, 418
Impulsive aggression, 197
Impulsiveness, 517
Impulsivity, 396, 401
　defined, 418
IMV model. *See* Integrated motivational volitional (IMV) model
Incidence, epidemiology, 3b
Indirect leadership, 166
Individual roles, 170
Individual therapy, 450
Informal group roles, 170
Informal support system, 49 , 49b
Information seeker, 170
Informed consent, 20
Inhalants. *See also* Substances and related disorders
　aerosols, 441
　gases, 441

　intoxication, 441
　long-term complications, 441
　nitrites, 441
　volatile solvents, 441
Inhibited grieving, 401
Inhibitory neurotransmitters, 66–67
Initial opioid detoxification, 439
Initiation phase, drug therapy, 137–138
Inpatient-focused care, 276
　for OCD patients, 306
　for person with PTSD, 293
Inpatient safety, 233
Instrumental aggression, 197
Integrated motivational volitional (IMV) model, 228–229
Integrative health care, 156–157
Intellectual disability, 512–513
　clinical course, 512
　continuum of care, 513
　diagnosis of, 512
　epidemiology, 512–513
　etiology, 512–513
　nursing care, 513
Intermediate suicide risk, interventions for, 233
Intermittent explosive disorder, 421
Intermittent explosive disorder (IED), 195–196
Internalization of peer pressure, 459
Internal rights protection systems, 18
International Nurses Society on Addictions (IntNSA), 33
International Society of Psychiatric Consultation Liaison Nurses, 33
International Society of Psychiatric Nursing (ISPN), 33
Interoceptive conditioning, 264
Interpersonal learning, 173t
Interpersonal psychological theory of suicidal behavior (IPTS), 228
Interpersonal relations, 42
Interpersonal Relations in Nursing, 51
Interpersonal relations models
　Orlando's theories, 52
　Peplau's theories, 51–52
Interpersonal skills, 401–402
Interventions
　behavioral, 405
　for biologic domain
　　electroconvulsive therapy, 233
　　medication management, 233
　for bipolar disorder
　　antipsychotics, 347
　　carbamazepine, 346, 347t
　　divalproex sodium (Depakote), 344–346
　　electroconvulsive therapy (ECT), 348
　　lamotrigine (Lamictal), 346–347mood-stabilizing drugs, 342–347
　　support groups, 350
　　teaching patients and family, 349
　for family members, 413
　for hospitalized patients, OCD, 305–306, 306b
　for imminent suicide risk, 232–233

for intermediate suicide risk, 233
for long-term suicide risk, 233
pharmacologic, for BPD, 404–405
pharmacologic, in panic disorder, 271–273, 271t
physical health
  healthy daily activity promotion, 251
  for mental health/substance abuse issues, 252
physical health, for PTSD, 290–291
for psychological domain
  CTS, 234
  new coping strategy development, 234
  suicidal mindset, challenging, 234, 234b
psychosocial (See Psychosocial interventions)
psychosocial, for BPD, 405–406
Psychosocial, in panic disorder, 273–274, 275b, 276b
psychosocial nursing, 292, 292b
for social domain, 234–235
Intimacy
  fears, 405
  problems with, 250
Intimate partner violence (IPV)
  comorbidities, 240
  defined, 240
  overview, 239–240
  physical abuse, 240, 241f
  risk factors for, 240
Intoxication
  cocaine, 434
  inhalants, 441
Intrusion, defined, 284
Inwardly directed anger, 195
Ion channels, 131–132
IPTS. See Interpersonal psychological theory of suicidal behavior (IPTS)
Isocarboxazid (Marplan), 148t, 150
Isosorbide (Ismotic), 550b

J
Jung's analytical psychology, 42
Justice, 30

K
Kava, 156, 157
Ketamine, 435
Khat plant (Catha edulis), 442
King model, 53–54, 53f
Klein's play therapy, 42
Kleptomania, 421
Korsakoff's amnestic syndrome, 432
Kraepelin, Emil, 355

L
Label avoidance, 4
Lamotrigine (Lamictal), 146–147
Lability, mood, 335
Lamotrigine (Lamictal), 346–347
Leader-to-member conflict, 171
Learning disorders, 527
  continuum of care in, 528
  evidence-based nursing care, 527–528

Lecithin, 157
Leininger's theory, 50–51, 50f
Leisure skills, 253
Lesbian, gay, bisexual, and transgender (LGBT)
  and risk for suicide, 226
Lethality, 224
Leukopenia, 157
Levomilnacipran (Fetzima), 148t
Libido, 41
Life changes questionnaire, 184t
Life events, 183
Light therapy, 129, 158–159
  morning phototherapy, effects of, 159
  side effects of, 159
Limbic midbrain nuclei, 62
Limbic system, 61–62, 61f
  amygdala, 62
  hippocampus, 61
  hypothalamus, 61–62
  limbic midbrain nuclei, 62
  thalamus, 61
Linguistic competence, 8
Lisdexamfetamine (Vyvanse), 154, 155t
Lithium
  indications for, 144–145
  mechanisms of action, 144–145
  pharmacokinetics, 145
  side effects, 145–146
  toxicity, 145–146
Lithium carbonate, 344
Long-term suicide risk, interventions for, 233
Lorazepam (Ativan), 143t, 152, 152t, 215b, 272
  for panic disorder, 272
Loxapine (Adasuve), 139t
Lurasidone HCl (Latuda), 139t, 140, 141

M
Magnesium sulfate, 434
Magnetic resonance imaging (MRI)
  of schizotypal personality disorder, 394
Maintenance phase, drug therapy, 138
Maintenance roles, 170
Maladaptive anger, 192–193
Maladaptive cognitive processes, 398
Male hypoactive sexual desire disorder, 506
Mandatory reporting, in violence, 245
Mania, 334–335
  defined, 335, 335b
Manic episode, 335
MAOIs. See monoamine oxidase inhibitors
Maprotiline (Ludiomil), 148t
Marijuana, 437
Maslow's hierarchy of needs, 43, 43f
Master gland, 62
MDMA. See 3,4-methylenedioxymethamphetamine (MDMA)
Mead's theory, 50
Medication groups, 174–175, 174b
Medications
  for anorexia nervosa, 465
  for OCD, 303–305
  for suicidal behavior, 233

Melatonergic hypnotics, 154
Melatonin, 154t, 157
Melatonin, in mental disorder, 69
Memantine, 549b
Mental disorders
  barriers to treatment of, 3–4
  case studies, 7
  definition, 2
  diagnosis, 3
  epidemiologic studies, 2–3, 3b
  impact on health and productivity, 2
  negative views of, 4
  prevalence of, 2
  recovery, 6
    benefits, 4
    definition, 4
    dimensions supporting, 4
    guiding principles of, 4, 5b
    oriented care, 4, 5b
    process, 3
  stigma, 3
    label avoidance, 4
    public, 4
    self, 4
  symptoms, 3
Mental disorders, studies of biologic basis of, 73–76
  chronobiology, 76
  genetics, 73–74
  psychoneuroimmunology, 74–76
Mental disorders and suicide attempt, 224, 225
Mental health
  definition, 1–2
  importance, 2
  problems, 2
Mental health care delivery systems, 19
Mental health care for violence survivors
  abuser, treatment for, 254
  evidence-based nursing care
    evaluation and treatment outcomes, 253–254
    mental health nursing assessment, 245–251, 246b, 247b, 248b, 249b–250b
    nursing interventions, 251–253, 253b
    priority of nursing care, 251
  therapeutic relationship, 245
  violence, theories of
    community disorganization, 243
    cycle of violence, 244, 244f
    economic disadvantage, 243
    imbalances in relationship power, 243–244
    leaving vs. staying in violent relationship, 244–245
    safety issues and mandatory reporting, 245
    social learning theory, 243
  violence and abuse, types of
    abuse of older adults, 242–243
    child abuse and neglect, 242
    intimate partner violence (IPV), 239–240, 241f
    rape and sexual assault, 241–242
    stalking, 242

Mental health nursing assessment, 419
  for anorexia nervosa
    behavioral responses, 463
    physical health assessment, 463
    self-concept, 463
    social assessment, 463
    stress and coping patterns, 463
  for bulimia nervosa
    physical health assessment, 471
    priority of nursing care, 471
    psychosocial assessment, 471
    strengths assessment, 471
    therapeutic relationship, 471, 472b
  for OCD
    physical health assessment, 302
    psychosocial assessment, 302–303, 303t
    strength assessment, 303
  in panic disorder, 265
  pharmacologic assessment, 187
  physical assessment, 187
  physical functioning, 187
  physical health assessment, 247–248, 248b, 249b–250b
  psychosocial assessment, 187–188
    economic/emotional dependency, 251
    fear, 248
    guilt and shame, 250
    low self-esteem, 248
    problems with intimacy, 250
    revictimization, 250
    social isolation, 250–251
    social networks, 250
  for PTSD
    physical health assessment, 288
    psychosocial assessment, 289
    strength assessment, 289
    trauma, 288
  safety assessment, conducting, 245, 246b
  screening for violence and abuse, 245–246, 246b, 247b
  systems review, 187
Mental health nursing interventions
  for anorexia nervosa
    mental health and wellness goals, 464
    physical health interventions, 464–465
    psychosocial interventions, 465–466, 465b, 466t
  for ASPD
    anger management, 413
    group interventions, 412–413
    interventions for family members, 413
    milieu interventions, 413
    patient education efforts, 411–412, 412b
    self-awareness, enhancing, 411
    self-responsibility, facilitating, 411
    social support, 413
  for biologic domain, 420
  for bulimia nervosa
    medication interventions, 472
    physical health interventions, 472
    pharmacologic interventions, 404–405
    physical care, 403–404
    physical health interventions
      exercise and yoga, 291
      nutrition interventions, 291
      sleep enhancement, 290–291
      smoking cessation, 291
    for substances-related disorders, 447, 447b, 448t
      cognitive and cognitive behavioral interventions, 449, 449b
      coping skills, enhancing, 449, 450b
      family interventions, 450
      group interventions and early recovery, 449–450
      harm-reduction, 450
      individual therapy, 450
      peer support self-help group, 450–451, 450b
      psychoeducation, 449, 449b
    and wellness goals, 289
    wellness strategies, 289–290
Mental health nursing interventions, in panic disorder
  breathing control, teaching, 269–270
  nutritional planning, teaching, 270
  pharmacologic interventions
    benzodiazepine therapy, 272–273
    medication for, 271, 271t
    selective serotonin reuptake inhibitors, 271–272
    serotonin–norepinephrine reuptake inhibitors, 272
  physical activity promotion, 270–271
  relaxation techniques, teaching, 270, 271b
  wellness challenges, 269, 270b
Mental Health Parity and Addiction Equity Act (MHPAEA), 18
Mental health patients, bill of rights for, 17–18
Mental health problems, 110
Mental health services, access to, 18
Mental Health Systems Act, 17–18
Mental illness
  cultural and social factors and beliefs about, 9–12
    African Americans, 10–11
    Arab Americans, 11
    Asian Americans, 11
    cultural idiom of distress, 9
    Hispanic Americans, 10
    Native Americans, 11
    Pacific Islanders, 11
    Polynesians, 11
    poverty, 9–10
    rural cultures, 11–12
    women within minority groups, 11
  spirituality and religion, 12, 12t, 13t, 14, 14b
Mentalization-based therapy (MBT), 399
Mental status examination, 111
Mesocortical pathway, 69
Mesolimbic pathway, 69
Metabolites, 136

Methadone (Dolophine) maintenance, 439–441, 440b
Methamphetamine, 435
Methylphenidate, 154–155
Methylphenidate (Ritalin, Methylin, Metadate), 154, 155t, 521, 521b
Microphobia, 278b
Mild neurocognitive impairment (MCI), 540
Milieu interventions, 413
Milieu therapy, 124
Miller's theory, 48
Mirtazapine (Remeron), 148t, 149, 150t, 550b
Modafinil (Provigil), 154, 155
Modeling, 45
Molecular genetics, 73–74
Molindone, 139t
Molly, 435
Monoamine, in mental disorder, 69
Monoamine oxidase (MAO), 132
Monoamine oxidase A (MAO A), 198
Monopolizer, 170
Mood, 285
Mood and affect, 111
Mood disorders, 528–529
Mood lability, 335
Mood stabilizers
  anticonvulsants, 146–147
  lithium, 144–146
Morphine derivatives. See Opioids and morphine derivatives
Motivation, defined, 444
Motivational interviewing (MI), 101, 445
Motivation for change, 444–445, 445b
Motor tics, 522
Multiple personality disorder, 293
Multivitamins and adequate nutrition, 432, 434

N

Nabilone (Cesamet), 437
Naltrexone, 440
  for alcoholism, 432, 433b
Namzaric, 549
Narcissistic personality disorder. See also Personality/impulse-control disorders
  clinical course/diagnostic criteria, 415
  continuum of care, 415
  epidemiology, 415
  etiology, 415
  nursing care, 415
Narcolepsy, e-20–e-21
Narcotics Anonymous, 440
National Alliance on Mental Illness (NAMI), 329
Native Americans
  views about mental illnesses, 11
Natural killer (NK) cells, 74
Nefazodone (Serzone), 148t, 149, 150t
Negative emotions, 184
Neo-Freudian models
  Adler's foundation for individual psychology, 42
  Fromm's societal needs, 42

Horney's feminine psychology, 42
Jung's analytical psychology, 42
Klein's play therapy, 42
Rank's birth trauma, 42
Sullivan's interpersonal relations, 42
Nervios, 9
Neuman model, 54
Neurasthenia, 11
Neuroanatomy, of CNS, 58–63
 autonomic nervous system, 63
 cerebrum, 58–60
 limbic system, 61–62
 subcortical structures, 60–61, 60f
Neurocognitive disorders, 535
 due to prion disease, 556
 due to traumatic brain injury (TBI), 557
 with Lewy bodies, 556
Neurodevelopmental delay, 512
Neurodevelopmental disorders of childhood
 attention-deficit hyperactivity disorder (ADHD), 517–522
 autism spectrum disorder (ASD), 513–517
 communication disorders, 527–528
 history of childhood and adolescent disorders, 513b
 intellectual disability, 512–513
 learning disorders, 527
 neurodevelopmental delay, 512
 obsessive-compulsive disorder (OCD), 526–527
 separation anxiety disorder, 524–525
 tics disorder, 522–524
 Tourette disorder, 522–524
Neurofibrillary tangles, 541
Neurologic status, 107
Neurons and nerve impulses, 65–66, 65f, 66f
Neuropeptides, 71
 nonopioid, 71
 opioid, 71
Neurophysiology, of CNS, 63–73
 neurons and nerve impulses, 65–66
 neurotransmitters, 66–71
 receptors, 71–73
 synaptic transmission, 66
Neuroplasticity, 63
Neurotransmitters, 66–71, 157
 classic and putative, 68t
 physiologic effects from drug actions on, 133t
Nicotine. *See also* Stimulants
 about, 435–436
 biologic response to, 436
 withdrawal and smoking cessation, 436
Nifedipine (Procardia), 550b
Night eating syndrome, 474
Nightmare disorder, e-24–e-25
Nigrostriatal pathway, 69
Nitrites, 441
N-methyl-d-aspartic acid antagonists, 549
Nonadherence, reasons for, 160t
Nonamnestic MCI, 540

Nonemotions, 184
Nonmaleficence, 30
Nontherapeutic relationships, 99
Nonverbal communication, 83–84, 85f
Noradrenergic, 69, 70f
Norepinephrine
 depletion, 434
 in mental disorder, 69–70
 in panic disorder, 264
Norepinephrine–dopamine reuptake inhibitor, 148t
Norepinephrine receptor blockade (a_1 and a_2 receptor), 133t
Norepinephrine receptor blockade (b_1 receptor), 133t
Norepinephrine reuptake inhibition, 133t
Nortriptyline (Aventyl, Pamelor), 148t
No-suicide contracts, 233
Not guilty by reason of insanity (NGRI), 24
Numbing, 284
Nurse-patient relationship
 empathic linkages, 97
 empathy, 96
 motivational interviewing (MI), 101
 nontherapeutic relationships, 99
 orientation phase, 97–98
 rapport, 96
 resolution phase, 99
 therapeutic relationships, examples of working phase, 98
Nursing documentation, 26
Nursing intervention groups
 anger management groups, 175
 medication groups, 174–175, 174b
 reminiscence groups, 175
 self-care groups, 175
 symptom management groups, 175
Nursing interventions, for OCD
 cognitive restructuring, 305
 exposure and response prevention, 305
 medications, 303, 304t, 305
 relaxation techniques, 305
 skin integrity, maintaining, 303
 thought stopping, 305
Nursing interventions, for survivors of violence/abuse
 physical health interventions
  healthy daily activity promotion, 251
  mental health/substance abuse issues, 252
 psychosocial interventions
  anger management, 252
  anxiety, coping with, 252
  community involvement, 253
  family interventions, 253
  psychoeducation, 253, 253b
  strength and hope, finding, 252
  working with children, 252
 safety planning, 251
Nursing Interventions Classification (NIC), 33, 118
Nursing Outcomes Classification (NOC), 33

Nursing theories
 Calista Roy's adaptation model, 54
 existential and humanistic theoretical perspectives
  Parse's theory, 52
  Watson's theory, 52–53
 interpersonal relations models
  Orlando's theories, 52
  Peplau's theories, 51–52
 systems models
  King model, 53–54, 53f
  Neuman model, 54
  Orem's model, 54
Nutritional balance, 404
Nutritional planning, 270
Nutrition interventions, 291
Nyctophobia, 278b

O

Object relations, 41
Obsessions
 and compulsions, 296–297
 defined, 296
 diagnostic criteria, 298
Obsessive-compulsive and related disorders
 obsessions and compulsions, 296–297
 overview of, 297, 297t
Obsessive-compulsive disorder (OCD), 526–527. *See also* Trichotillomania and excoriation disorder
 across life span
  children and adolescents, 298
  older adults, 299
 clinical course, 297–298
 comorbidity, 299
 diagnostic criteria
  compulsions, 298
  obsessions, 298
 epidemiology, 526
 epidemiology/risk factors, 299, 299b
 etiology, 526
  biologic theories, 300
  psychological theories, 300
 evidence-based nursing care, 526–527
 evidence-based nursing care, for OCD
  continuum of care, 306–307
  evaluation/treatment outcomes, 306
  interventions for hospitalized patients, 305–306, 306b
  mental health nursing assessment, 302–303, 303t
  nursing interventions, 303–305, 304b
 family response to, 300–301
 family's response to, 526–527
 safety issues, 302
 teamwork and collaboration, 301, 301b
  electroconvulsive therapy (ECT), 301
  psychosurgery, 302
  transcranial magnetic stimulation (TMS), 301–302
 working toward recovery, 526

Obsessive-compulsive personality disorder (OCPD)
  clinical course/diagnostic criteria, 417
  continuum of care, 418
  epidemiology/risk factors, 417–418
  etiology, 418
  nursing care, 418
Obstructive sleep apnea syndrome
  clinical course, e-21–22
  diagnosis, e-22
  epidemiology, e-22
  etiology, e-22
  risk factors, e-22
Occipital lobes, 60
OCD. See Obsessive-compulsive disorder (OCD)
OCPD. See Obsessive-compulsive personality disorder (OCPD)
Olanzapine (Zyprexa, Relprevv), 139t, 141
Older adults
  abuse of, 242–243
  anxiety disorders among, 261
  OCD among, 299
  suicide/suicide attempt among, 225
Omaha System, 33
Omnibus Budget Reconciliation Act of 1990, 17
Open communication, 124
Open groups, 165
Operant behavior, 44
Ophidiophobia, 278b
Opioids and morphine derivatives. See also Substances and related disorders
  effects of, 438
  initial opioid detoxification, 439
  methadone maintenance, 439–441, 440b
  opioid intoxication or overdose, 439
  withdrawal symptoms, 438, 439t
Oppositional defiant disorder, 418, 419b
Orem's model, 54
Orexin receptor antagonists, 154
Orientation, 111
Orlando's theories, 52
Other Specified Feeding and Eating Disorders (OSFED), 455
Outwardly directed anger, 195
Overprotectiveness, defined, 460
Over-the-counter (OTC) drugs, 438
  herbal remedies, 267
  for pain, 291
Oxazepam (Serax), 152t
Oxidative stress, 542
Oxybutynin ER, 550b

P

Pacific Islanders, 11
Pain management, 120
Paliperidone (Invega Extended Release), 139t
Paliperidone palmitate (Invega Sustenna), 139t, 140
Panic, defined, 261
Panic attack
  assessment, 265–266
  defined, 261
  physical symptoms of, 262
Panic control treatment, 264
Panic disorder. See also Anxiety disorders
  clinical course, 261–262, 262b
  comorbidity, 262–263
  continuum of patient care, 274
  diagnostic criteria, 262, 263
  epidemiology/risk factors, 40
  etiology, 263–264
  evaluation/treatment outcomes, 274
  evidence-based nursing care for, 265–268, 267b, 268t, 269t
  family response to disorder, 264
  mental health nursing interventions, 269–273, 270b, 271b, 271t, 272b
  primary care, integration with, 274, 276
  psychosocial interventions, 273–274, 273t, 275b, 276b
  recovery-oriented care for persons, 264–265
  therapeutic relationship, 268–269
Paranoid personality disorder. See also Personality/impulse-control disorders
  clinical course/diagnostic criteria, 392
  continuum of care, 393
  epidemiology/risk factors, 392–393
  etiology, 393
  nursing care, 393
Paraphilias, 506, 507t
Parasuicidal behavior, 396
Parasuicide, 224
Parenting skills, 253
Parent management training/education, 420, 420b
Parietal lobes, 59–60
Parkinson disease, 142
Paroxetine (Paxil), 148, 148t, 150t, 291, 303, 304t, 550b
Parse's theory, 52
Partial adherence, 160
Partial agonists, 131
Paternalism, 30
Patient Protection and Affordable Care Act, 18
Patient rights and legal issues
  criminal judicial processes
    fitness to stand trial, 23–24
    guilty but mentally ill, 24
    gun laws and mental illness, 25
    misconceptions regarding insanity pleas, 24
    not guilty by reason of insanity, 24
    probation, 24
    stigma of criminality, 23
  nurses and other health care professionals, accountability for
    lawsuits in psychiatric mental health care, 25
    legal liability in psychiatric nursing practice, 25
    nursing documentation, 26
  privacy and confidentiality
    HIPAA and protection of health information, 22
    mandates to inform, 22–23
  protection of, 17
    accreditation of mental health care delivery systems, 19
    advance care directives in mental health, 17
    Americans With Disabilities Act of 1990, 18
    bill of rights for mental health patients, 17–18, 18b
    external advocacy systems, 18–19
    internal rights protection systems, 18
    mental health services, 18
    Self-Determination Act, 17
  self-determinism in, 16–17
  treatment and patient rights
    competency, 19, 19t
    informed consent, 20
    least restrictive environment, 20
    seclusion and restraint, 20–21
    voluntary and involuntary treatment, 21–22
Patient safety, 232
Patient Self-Determination Act (PSDA), 17
Patients' Rights Condition of Participation, 21
Pavlovian Theory, 44
PDE5 inhibitors, 504–505
Pedophilia, 507t
Peer pressure, internalization of, 459
Peer support self-help group, 450–451, 450b
Peplau's theories, 51–52
Perceived burdensomeness, 228
Perfectionism, 456–457
  defined, 457
Perioperative Nursing Data Set (PNDS), 36
Peripheral nervous system (PNS), 57
Perphenazine, 139t
Personal identity, 114
Personality disorder, defined, 392
Personality factors
  and suicide prevention, 228
Personality/impulse-control disorders
  antisocial personality disorder (ASPD)
    biologic theories, 409
    clinical course/diagnostic criteria, 408, 409
    comorbidity, 409
    continuum of care, 413
    defined, 408
    epidemiology/risk factors, 408–409
    evaluation/treatment outcomes, 413
    evidence-based nursing care of, 410–413, 412b
    family response to, 410
    psychosocial theories, 409–410
    safety issues, 410
    teamwork and collaboration, 410
  avoidant personality disorder
    clinical course/diagnostic criteria, 416
    continuum of care, 416
    epidemiology/risk factors, 416

etiology, 416
nursing care, 416
borderline personality disorder (BPD)
across life span, 397
behavioral patterns in, 398b
biologic theories, 397
clinical course, 395
cognitive dysfunctions, 396
comorbidity, 397
continuum of care, 407, 408b
defined, 395
diagnostic criteria, 395–397
epidemiology/risk factors, 397
evaluation/treatment outcomes, 407
evidence-based nursing care for, 399–407, 400b, 403b, 406t, 407t
family response to, 399
psychosocial theories, 397–399, 398b
safety issues, 399
teamwork and collaboration, 399
unstable affect, 396
unstable interpersonal relationships, 396
unstable self-image, 396
dependent personality disorder
clinical course/diagnostic criteria, 416
continuum of care, 417
epidemiology/risk factors, 417
etiology, 417
nursing care, 417
disruptive, impulse-control, and conduct disorders
continuum of care, 421
continuum of care for, 422
epidemiology, 418–419
etiology, 419–420, 420b
evaluation/treatment outcomes, 421
intermittent explosive disorder, 421
kleptomania, 421
mental health nursing assessment, 419
mental health nursing interventions for biologic domain, 420
oppositional defiant disorder, 418, 419b
priority of care, 419–420
psychosocial interventions, 420
pyromania, 421–422
histrionic personality disorder
clinical course/diagnostic criteria, 413–414
continuum of care, 415
epidemiology/ risk factors, 414
etiology, 414
nursing care, 414–415
narcissistic personality disorder
clinical course/diagnostic criteria, 415
continuum of care, 415
epidemiology, 415
etiology, 415
nursing care, 415

obsessive-compulsive personality disorder (OCPD)
clinical course/diagnostic criteria, 417
continuum of care, 418
epidemiology/risk factors, 417–418
etiology, 418
nursing care, 418
paranoid personality disorder
clinical course/diagnostic criteria, 392
continuum of care, 393
epidemiology/risk factors, 392–393
etiology, 393
nursing care, 393
personality disorder, defined, 392
schizoid personality disorder
clinical course/diagnostic criteria, 393
continuum of care, 394
epidemiology, 393
etiology, 393
nursing care, 393–394
schizotypal personality disorder
clinical course/diagnostic criteria, 394
continuum of care, 394–395
epidemiology/risk factors, 394
etiology, 394
nursing care, 394
Personality traits, 392
Peyote (Mescaline), 438
Pharmacodynamics, 129–132
affinity, 131
carrier proteins, 132, 132f
enzymes, 132
intrinsic activity, 131
ion channels, 131–132
receptors, 131
selectivity, 131
Pharmacogenomics, 137
Pharmacokinetics
distribution, 134–136
drug effects, individual variations in, 137
excretion, 136–137
metabolism, 136
Pharmacologic assessment, 110
Phenelzine (Nardil), 148t, 150
Phenytoin (Dilantin), 550b
Phobia. See also Anxiety disorders
defense mechanisms and anxiety, 260, 260t
fever, 278b
social, 278–279
specific, 277–278, 278b
Phonic tics, 522
Phonologic processing, 527
Phonophobia, 278b
Photophobia, 278b
Phototherapy, 158–159
Physical abuse, 240, 241f
Physical activity promotion, 270–271
Physical care, for BPD, 403–404
Physical health assessment
for OCD patients, 302

in panic disorder
medications, 266
physical activity, 266
sleep patterns, 266
substance use, 266
for survivors of violence and abuse, 247–248, 248b, 249b, 250b
Physical health interventions
healthy daily activity promotion, 251
for mental health/substance abuse issues, 252
Physiologic stability, 178
Piaget's periods, of intellectual development, 47t
Piaget's theory, 47–48, 47t
Pia mater, 70
Pimavanserin (Nuplazid), 139t
Pimozide (ORAP), 139t
Plasma protein binding, 134, 136, 136t
Point prevalence, 3b
Polynesians, 11
Polypharmacy, 138
Polysomnography, 77–78
Population genetics, 73
adoption studies, 73
family studies, 73
twin studies, 73
Positive emotions, 184
Positive self-talk, 274, 275b
Posttraumatic stress disorder (PTSD), 179, 180, 195, 204, 212, 216–220. See also Trauma-/stressor- related disorders
defined, 284
following disaster, 218b
and risky sexual behavior, 286b
symptoms in children/adolescents, 284t
Potassium depletion, 464
Potency, 132
Potentially aggressive patient, 201b
Poverty and psychiatric impairments, link between, 9–10
Power of attorney, 17
Prazepam (Centrax), 152t
Preadolescent children, 459
Preconscious, 39
Prednisolone, 550b
Premature ejaculation (PE), 502–503
Preoccupation with body image, 459
Prescribing information (PI), 129
Prescription medications
opioids as, 438
Prevalence, epidemiology, 3b
Primary appraisal, 181
Primary care, integration with
anorexia nervosa, 462
in anxiety disorders management, 265
in panic disorder
community care, 276
emergency care, 276
family interventions, 274, 276
inpatient-focused care, 276
for PTSD, 287
Principle of frequency, 44
Principle of recency, 44

Priority care issues, suicide prevention assessment
    case finding, 230–232, 230b, 231b
    of suicide risk, 232, 232b
  biologic domain, interventions for
    electroconvulsive therapy (ECT), 233
    medication management, 233
  imminent risk for suicide, interventions for, 232–233
  intermediate suicide risk, interventions for, 233
  long-term suicide risk, interventions for, 233
  psychological domain, interventions for
    commitment to treatment statement (CTS), 234
    new coping strategy development, 234
    suicidal mindset, challenging, 234, 234b
  social domain, interventions for, 234–235
Privacy, 22
Probation, 24
Problem-focused coping, 185
Problem-solving therapy, 420
Professional rescuers, 217
Projective identification, 397
Propranolol (Inderal), 143t
Protection and Advocacy for Mentally Ill Individuals Act of 1986, 18
Protriptyline (Vivactil), 148t
Prozac, 70
Pseudoparkinsonism, 142
Psilocybin (4-phosphoryloxy-*N*,*N*-dimethyltryptamine), 438
Psychiatric advance directives (PAD), 17
Psychiatric hospitals, 4
Psychiatric medications
  drug regulation and use, 129
  managing common side effects of, 130t
  phases of drug treatment and nurse's role
    discontinuation phase, 138
    initiation phase, 137–138
    maintenance phase, 138
    stabilization phase, 138
  phases of new drug testing, 129b
    implications for mental health nurses, 129b
  side effects, 129
  target symptoms, 129
Psychiatric-mental health nursing
  biopsychosocial framework, 33–34, 33f
    biologic domain, 33–34
    psychological domain, 34
    social domain, 34
  challenges of, 35–36
    health care delivery system challenges, 35–36
    holistic nursing care, 35
    impact of technology and electronic health records, 36, 36t
    knowledge development, dissemination, and application, 35
    overcoming stigma, 35
  ethics of, 29–30
    autonomy, 30
    beneficence, 30
    code, 29, 30b
    fidelity, 30
    justice, 30
    nonmaleficence, 30
    paternalism, 30
    questions for ethical decision making, 30b
    veracity, 30
  psychosocial theoretic basis of
    cognitive-behavioral theories, 43–46
    developmental theories, 46–48
    nursing theories, 51–54
    psychodynamic theories, 39–43
    social theories, 48–51
  scope and standards of practice, 30–33
    areas of concern for psychiatric-mental health nurse, 31
    levels of practice, 32–33, 32b
    psychiatric-mental health nursing organizations, 33
    standards of practice, 31, 31b
    standards of professional performance, 31–32, 32t
  tools of, 34–35
    clinical reasoning, 34
    interdisciplinary care, 34–35
    plan of care, 35
    reflection, 34
    self, 34
Psychiatric-mental health nursing process, 104–105
  assessment interview behaviors, 107b
  of biologic domain
    activity and exercise, 109
    appetite and nutrition, 110
    body systems review, 107
    elimination, 109
    hydration, 110
    laboratory results, 107
    neurologic status, 107
    pharmacologic assessment, 110
    self-care, 110
    sexuality, 110
  biopsychosocial psychiatric nursing assessment, 106b
  developing recovery outcomes, 117, 117t
  hematologic measures, 108t–109t
  narrative mental status examination note, 111b
  nursing care, priorities of, 117
  patient interviews, 105
  physical domain, 105–110
  psychological assessment, 110–115
  of psychological domain
    behavior, 112–113
    mental health problems, 110
    mental status examination, 111–112
    risk assessment, 114–115
    self-concept, 113–114
    stress and coping patterns, 114
  recovery-oriented nursing interventions, 117–118, 117b
    physical interventions, 118–120
    psychological interventions, 120–123
    social domain, 123–126
  self-concept awareness, 107b
  social domain, 115–116
  of social domain
    economic status, 116
    functional status, 115
    legal status, 116
    occupational status, 115–116
    quality of life, 116
    social systems, 115
    spiritual assessment, 116
  spiritual assessment, 116
Psychiatric–Mental Health Registered Nurse (PMH-RN), 31
Psychoanalysis, 41
Psychoanalytic theories, 264
Psychodynamic theories, 40t, 264
  humanistic theories
    Gestalt therapy, 43
    Maslow's hierarchy of needs, 43, 43f
    Rogers' client-centered therapy, 43
  neo-Freudian models
    Adler's foundation for individual psychology, 42
    Fromm's societal needs, 42
    Horney's feminine psychology, 42
    Jung's analytical psychology, 42
    Klein's play therapy, 42
    Rank's birth trauma, 42
    Sullivan's interpersonal relations, 42
  and psychiatric–mental health nursing, 43
  psychoanalytic theory
    of anxiety mechanism, 41
    countertransference, 41
    of defense mechanisms, 41
    object relations and identification, 41
    personality development, 41
    psychoanalysis, 41
    sexuality, 41
    transference, 41
    unconscious, study of, 39
Psychoeducation, 122, 253, 253b
  for anorexia nervosa, 465–466, 466b
  for antisocial personality disorder, 412
  for BPD, 406–407, 407b
  for bulimia nervosa, 473, 473b
  for GAD, 277b
  for OCD patients, 305–306, 306b
  for panic disorder, 274, 276b
  Program, 122b
  for PTSD, 292, 292b
  for substances-related disorders, 449, 449b
Psychoeducation groups, 172
Psychological abuse, 240
Psychological domain, 34. *See also* Psychiatric-mental health nursing interventions for
  commitment to treatment statement, 234

new coping strategy development, 234
suicidal mindset, challenging, 234, 234b
Psychological theories
　for anorexia nervosa
　　body dissatisfaction, 459
　　internalization of peer pressure, 459
　in OCD
　　behavioral factors, 300
　　psychodynamic factors, 300
　for suicide prevention
　　cognitive theories, 228
　　emotional factors, 228
　　Ideation-to-action theories, 228–229
　　personality factors, 228
Psychological well-being, 186
Psychoneuroimmunology (PNI), 73–76, 74–76, 74f–76f
Psychopharmacologic drug classes
　antianxiety and sedative–hypnotic medications, 151–154
　antianxiety medications
　　benzodiazepines, 152–153
　　buspirone, 153
　antidepressants
　　a_2-antagonist, 149
　　FDA-approved, 149
　　monoamine oxidase inhibitors, 150–151
　　norepinephrine–dopamine reuptake inhibitors, 149
　　selective serotonin reuptake inhibitors, 147–149
　　serotonin norepinephrine reuptake inhibitors, 149
　　tricyclic, 149–150
　antipsychotic medications, 138–144
　　absorption, 140
　　anticholinergic side effects, 141
　　atypical, 138, 139t
　　blood disorders, 141
　　cardiovascular side effects, 140
　　clinical effects, 140
　　conventional, 138, 139t
　　excretion of drugs, 140
　　indications and mechanism of action, 139–140
　　long-acting preparations, 140
　　medication-related movement disorders, 142–144, 143t
　　metabolism of drugs, 140
　　neuroleptic malignant syndrome (NMS), 141–142
　　pharmacokinetics, 140
　　photosensitivity reactions, 142
　　recommended assessments before and during, 141b
　　risk for type II diabetes, 141
　　sexual side effects, 141
　　weight gain, 141
　mood stabilizers
　　anticonvulsants, 146–147
　　lithium, 144–146
　sedative–hypnotic medications, 154

stimulants and wakefulness-promoting agents, 154–156
Psychopharmacology
　clinical concepts, 132–134
　　mechanisms effecting medication, 133b
　　physiologic effects from drug actions on neurotransmitters, 133t
　pharmacodynamics, 129–132
　　affinity, 131
　　carrier proteins, 132, 132f
　　enzymes, 132
　　intrinsic activity, 131
　　ion channels, 131–132
　　physiologic effects from drug actions on neurotransmitters, 133t
　　receptors, 131
　　selectivity, 131
　pharmacokinetics, 134–137
　　absorption, 134
　　administration routes of, 134, 135t
　　distribution, 134–136
　　drug effects, individual variations in, 137
　　excretion, 136–137
　　metabolism, 136
Psychosis, 355
Psychosocial assessment
　for BPD
　　cognitive disturbances, 401
　　dissociation and transient psychotic episodes, 401
　　functional assessment, 402
　　identity diffusion, 401
　　Impulsivity, 401
　　interpersonal skills, 401–402
　　self-esteem and coping skills, 402
　　social support systems, 402
　cognitive thought patterns, 266–267
　cultural factors, 267
　economic/emotional dependency, 251
　family factors, 267
　fear, 248
　guilt and shame, 250
　low self-esteem, 248
　mental status examination, 266
　for OCD, 302–303, 303t
　problems with intimacy, 250
　revictimization, 250
　self-report scales, 266, 267b, 268t
　social isolation, 250–251
　social networks, 250
　strength identification, of patient, 267
Psychosocial interventions
　abandonment and intimacy fears, 405
　anger management, 252
　for anorexia nervosa
　　cognitive interventions, 465
　　feelings, identifying, 465
　　Psychoeducation, 465–466, 466b
　　wellness strategies, 466
　anxiety, coping with, 252
　behavioral interventions, 405
　community involvement, 253

disruptive, impulse-control, and conduct disorders
　parent management training/education, 420, 420b
　problem-solving therapy, 420
　referral to family therapy, 420
　social skills training, 420
dysfunctional thinking, 405–406, 406b, 406t
family interventions, 253
in panic disorder
　distraction, 273
　positive self-talk, 274, 275b
　psychoeducation, 274, 276b
　reframing, 273–274
　therapeutic interactions, 273, 273t
　wellness strategies, 274
personal boundaries/limitations, 405
psychoeducation, 253, 253b, 406–407, 407b
strength and hope, finding, 252
working with children, 252
Psychosocial nursing interventions
　psychoeducation, 292, 292b
　trauma-informed care, 292
Psychosocial perspectives of stress, 180–183
　appraisal, 180–181
　life events, 183
　social network, 182–183
　transactional stress model, 180
　values and goals, 181–182
Psychosocial theories
　ASPD
　　attachment, 410
　　family issues, 410
　　temperament, 409–410
　for BPD
　　maladaptive cognitive processes, 398
　　psychoanalytic theories, 397
　　social theories, 398–399, 398b
　for bulimia nervosa
　　cognitive theory, 470
　　family factors, 470
　in panic disorders
　　cognitive behavioral theories, 264
　　psychoanalytic and psychodynamic theories, 264
Psychostimulants
　indications and mechanisms of action, 154–155
　pharmacokinetics, 155–156
　side effects, 156
　toxicity, 156
Psychosurgery, 302
Psychotherapy, for BPD, 399
Psychotherapy groups, 173
PTSD. See Posttraumatic stress disorder (PTSD)
Public stigma, 4
Purging disorder, 474
Pyridoxine (vitamin B_6), 157
Pyromania, 421–422
Pyrophobia, 278b

Q

Quazepam (Doral), 154t
Quetiapine fumarate (Seroquel), 139t

R

Race and ethnicity
   and suicide rates, 226–227
Racial differences
   disease susceptibility, 137
Racial discrimination, 10–11
Rameltoon (Rozerem), 154t
Ranitidine (Zantac), 550b
Rank's birth trauma, 42
Rape and sexual assault, 241–242
Rapid eye movement (REM), 70
   sleep, 434
Rate, epidemiology, 3b
Reactive attachment disorder, 293
Reappraisal, 186
Recent Life Changes Questionnaire, 183, 184t
Receptors, 71–73, 131
   blockade, 133t
   lock and key, 71–72
   sensitivity, 72
   subtypes, 72–73, 72f, 72t
Recorder, 170
Recovery, 427
Recovery from mental disorders, 6
   benefits, 4
   definition, 4
   dimensions supporting, 4
   guiding principles of, 4, 5b
   movie on, 6
   oriented care, 4, 5b
   process, 3
Recovery-oriented care, 4, 5b
Recovery-oriented care, for PTSD
   primary care, integration of, 287
   safety issues, 287–288
   teamwork and collaboration, 286–287, 287b
Refeeding, 464
Referral, decision tree for determining, 210–213
Referral to family therapy, 420
Reflection, 34
Refractoriness, 72
Reframing, 273–274
Reinforcement theories, 44–45
   Skinner, 44–45
   Thorndike, 44
Relapse, 138
Relapse prevention, 432, 433b
Relaxation
   interventions, 119
   techniques, 119b
Relaxation techniques, 270, 271b, 305
Religion
   and belief forms, 12t, 13t
   and mental illness, 12, 12t, 13t, 14, 14b
Religiousness, 12
Reminiscence, 121
Reminiscence groups, 175
Reminiscence therapy, 175
Repetitive transcranial magnetic stimulation (rTMS), 129, 159
Resilience
   defined, 283
   trauma and, 282–283, 283b
Restraint, 20–21, 20b
Retraumatization, 5
Revictimization, 250
Rigidity, 461
Risk assessment of suicide, 232, 232b
Risperidone (Risperdal, Risperdal Consta, Perseris), 139t
Rogers' client-centered therapy, 43
Rohypnol gamma-hydroxybutyrate (GHB), 435
Role theories, 49–50
Rural cultures, 11–12

S

Safety issues
   for anorexia nervosa, 462
   antisocial personality disorder, 410
   for BPD, 399
   for bulimia nervosa, 471
   for OCD patients, 302
   for PTSD, 287–288
   for violence survivors, 245, 246b
Safety planning, 251
SANE (sexual assault nurse examiner), 248
Schizoid personality disorder. *See also* Personality/impulse-control disorders
   clinical course/diagnostic criteria, 393
   continuum of care, 394
   epidemiology, 393
   etiology, 393
   nursing care, 393–394
Schizophrenia, 233, 355
   across life-span, 359
   in children, 359
   clinical course
     acute illness, 356
     prodromal period, 355
     recovery, 356
     relapses, 356
     stabilization, 356
   comorbidity
     depression, 361
     diabetes mellitus, 361
     obesity, 361
     substance abuse, 361
   diagnostic criteria, 356
     disorganized behavior, 359
     negative symptoms, 358
     neurocognitive impairment, 358–359
     positive symptoms, 357
   disorganized symptoms, 358
   epidemiology
     age of onset, 360
     ethnic and cultural differences, 360
     familial differences, 360
     gender differences, 360
     risk factors, 360
   etiology, 360
     biologic theories, 361
     genetic associations, 361
     neuroanatomic findings, 361
     neurodevelopmental hypothesis, 361–362
     neurotransmitters, pathways, and receptors, 362–364
     psychosocial theories, 364
   in older adults, 359–360
   recovery, 356
   safety issues, 365
Schizophrenia spectrum disorders, 355
Schizotypal personality disorder
   clinical course/diagnostic criteria, 394
   continuum of care, 394–395
   epidemiology/risk factors, 394
   etiology, 394
   nursing care, 394
Schizotypy, 394
School phobia, 525
Screening, brief intervention, and referral to treatment (SBIRT), 447
Seclusion, 20–21, 20b
Secondary appraisal, 181
sedative–hypnotics, 152t, 154
Sedatives, 154
Selective serotonin reuptake inhibitors (SSRI)
   for anorexia nervosa, 465
   for BPD, 400
   for OCD patients, 303
   for panic disorder, 271–272
   for PTSD, 287
Selective serotonin reuptake inhibitors (SSRIs), 148t, 196, 529
Selectivity, 131
Selegiline (Emsam), 148t, 150t
Self-awareness, 81–82, 82b
Self-care, 110
Self-Care Deficit Nursing Theory, 54
Self-care groups, 175
Self-concept, 113–114
Self-determinism, 16–17
Self-efficacy, 45
Self-esteem, 114, 402, 407
Self-harm, 232, 235
   behaviors, 396–397
   defined, 396
   prevention, 404
Self-help groups, 173
Self-help groups/services, 234
Self-monitoring, in bulimia nervosa, 472
Self-report scales, for panic disorder assessment, 266, 267b, 268t
Self-responsibility, facilitating, 411
Self-stigma, 4
Sensate focus, 500
Separation anxiety disorder, 524–525
   epidemiology, 525
   etiology, 525
   evidence-based nursing care for, 525
   family response to, 525
   working toward recovery, 525
Separation-individuation, 397

Serotonergic antidepressants, 421
Serotonin, 70, 264
   in mental disorder, 69
   in OCD, 300
Serotonin syndrome, 309, 326, 326b
Serotonin-norepinephrine reuptake inhibitors (SNRI), 272, 287
Serotonin syndrome, 147
Sertraline, 303
Sertraline (Zoloft), 148, 148t, 150t
Sex role identity, 496
Sex therapist, 500
Sexual assault, rape and, 241–242
Sexual continuity, 497
Sexual development
   gender identity, 496
   genes and sex determination, 496
   sex role identity, 496
   sexual behaviors
      in adults, 497
      age-appropriate solitary, 496
      in children and adolescents, 496–497
      estrogen deficiency during menopause and, 497
      testosterone production and, 497
   sexual desire and arousal, 497–498
   sexual maturation, 496
   sexual orientation, 496
   theoretical models of sexual response, 498
      circular model, 498
      dual-control model, 498
      excitement phase, 498
      linear model, 498
      orgasmic phase, 498
      plateau phase, 498
      resolution, 498
Sexual dysfunctions and problematic behaviors
   antipsychotic medications and, 141
   DSM-5 classification, 499
   ejaculatory dysfunction, 502–503
      delay or absence of ejaculation (DE), 503
      epidemiology, 503
      etiology, 503
      evidence-based nursing care, 503
      integration with primary care, 503
      premature ejaculation (PE), 502–503
      working toward recovery, 503
   erectile dysfunction (ED), 503–505
      biologic theories, 503–504
      diagnostic criteria, 503
      epidemiology, 503
      etiology, 503–504
      evaluation and treatment outcomes, 505
      medical problems and, 504
      mental health nursing assessment, 504
      nursing interventions, 504–505
      pharmacologic interventions, 504–505
      priority of nursing care, 504
      psychoeducation for, 505, 505b
      psychological theories, 504
      wellness strategies for, 504
      working toward recovery, 504
   female orgasmic disorder
      diagnostic criteria, 499
      epidemiology and risk factors, 499
      etiology, 499–500
      evaluation and treatment outcomes, 502
      evidence-based nursing care for, 500–502
      integration with primary care, 500
      mental health nursing assessment, 500, 501t
      nursing interventions for, 502
      priority of nursing care, 502
      self-care and wellness activities for, 502, 502b
      working toward recovery, 500
   female sexual interest/arousal disorder, 505–506
   gender dysphoria, 506
   genitopelvic pain/penetration disorder, 506
   male hypoactive sexual desire disorder, 506
   medical conditions and substances affecting sexual function, 501b
   paraphilias, 506, 507t
   SSRIs and, 149
Sexual health and wellness, 498–499
   of LGBTQ, 499
   woman's sexual knowledge, assessment of, 500
Sexuality, 110, 495–496
Sexual masochism, 507t
Sexual maturation, 496
Sexual orientation, 496
Sexual sadism, 507t
Short-acting benzodiazepines for panic disorder, 272
Side effects, psychiatric medications, 129
Sildenafil citrate (Viagra), 504
Silent member, 171
Simple relaxation techniques, 119
Situational crisis, 210
Skin integrity maintenance, 303
Skin-picking disorder. See Excoriation disorder
Sleep, 109–110, e-9
   architecture, e-10
   assessment, e-15
   enhancement, 290–291
   homeostasis, e-11
   hygiene, 251, 404
   latency, e-10
   patterns, panic disorder and, 266
   promotion, 465
   sleepwalking, e-24
   stages of, e-11
   terrors, e-24
   wake cycle, e-10
Sleep-deprived individuals, 472
Sleep pattern, e-12
   age, e-12
   environment, e-12–e-13
   gender, e-12
   lifestyles, e-13
Smell, 404
Smoking cessation, 291
   nicotine withdrawal and, 436
SNRI. See Serotonin-norepinephrine reuptake inhibitors (SNRI)
Social anxiety disorder (social phobia), 278–279
Social distance, 49
Social distress, 226
   and suicidal behavior, 229
Social domain, 34. See also Psychiatric–mental health nursing
   assessment of, 115
      economic status, 116
      functional status, 115
      legal status, 116
      occupational status, 115–116
      psychosocial strengths, 116
      quality of life, 116
      social systems, 115
   interventions for, 123–126
Social factors, 9
Social functioning, 186
Social gambling, 442
Social identity, 182
Social isolation, 226, 250–251
Socialization process, 8
Social learning theory, 198, 243
Social media, 121
Social network, 182–183
Social networks, 250
Social risk factors for suicide, 226
Social skills, 407
   training, 420
Social support, 182–183, 183t, 402, 413
Social theories
   for anorexia nervosa, 459, 460b
   applicability of social theories to psychiatric–mental health nursing, 51
   for BPD, 398–399, 398b
   family dynamics, 48–49
   formal and informal social support, 49, 49b
   role theories, 49–50
   sociocultural perspectives
      Leininger's theory, 50–51
      Mead's theory, 50
   for suicide prevention
      economic disadvantage, 229
      social distress, 229
      suicide contagion, 229
Society for Education and Research in Psychiatric–Mental Health Nursing, 33
Solubility of drug, 134, 136, 136t
Somatic symptom disorder (SSD), 478
Somatic Symptom Disorder and Stress, 482b
Somatic Symptom Disorder, 488b
Speech, 111–112
Spielberger State-Trait Anger Expression Inventory (STAXI), 195

Spiritual assessment, 116
Spiritual care assessment, 116
Spiritual interventions, 123
Spirituality and mental illness, 12, 12t, 13t, 14, 14b
Splitting, 399
SSRI. *See* Selective serotonin reuptake inhibitors (SSRI)
St. John's Wort, 150t, 156
Stabilization phase, drug therapy, 138
Stalking, 242
Standardized nursing language, 36
Standard setter, 170
Steady-state plasma concentration, 137
Stereotypes
  public stigma, 4
  self-stigma, 4
Steroids, 441–442
Stigma, e-5
  influence on African American and Latino population, 10b
  label avoidance, 4
  public, 4
  self, 4
Stimulants. *See also* Substances and related disorders
  amphetamines, 435
  caffeine, 436–437
  cocaine
    biologic responses to, 434
    intoxication, 434
    types of, 434
    withdrawal, 434
  MDMA and club drugs, 435
  methamphetamine, 435
  nicotine
    about, 435–436
    biologic response to, 436
    withdrawal and smoking cessation, 436
Strength
  assessment
    for BPD, 402
    for OCD, 303
  and hope, 252
  identification, of patient, 267
Strengths and wellness assessment, 110
Stress, 177–178
  acute, 178
  adaptation
    healthy coping, 186
    psychological well-being, 186
    social functioning, 186
  biologic perspectives of, 178–180
  chronic, 178–180
  coping, 184–186
    emotion-focused, 185
    ways of, 185
  nursing care of person experiencing
    evaluation and treatment outcomes, 189
    family interventions, 189
    mental health nursing assessment, 187–189
    nursing interventions, 188
    priorities, 188
    problem-solving strategies, 188–189
    psychosocial nursing interventions, 188–189
  psychosocial perspectives of, 180–183
  responses to, 183–184
Stress and coping patterns, 114
Stress-reduction technique, 253
Striatum, 69
Structured interaction, 124
Subcortical dementia, 535
Subcortical structures, 60–61, 60f
Substance Abuse and Mental Health Services Administration (SAMHSA), 18, 220, 297
Substance abuse interventions, 291–292
Substance-induced disorders, 426
Substance/medication-induced neurocognitive disorder, 557
Substances and related disorders
  alcohol, 427–434, 428t–429t, 430b, 430t, 431b, 433t
  cannabis, 437
  hallucinogens and dissociative drugs, 437–438
  inhalants, 441
  opioids and morphine derivatives, 438–441, 439t, 440t
  prescription and over-the-counter drugs, 438
  steroids, 441–442
  stimulants, 434–437
Substance Abuse and Mental Health Services Administration (SAMHSA), e-5
Substance use disorder (SUD), 299, 426
Sudden sniffing death, 441
Suicidal ideation, 114, 224
Suicidality, 224, 326
Suicidal mindset, challenging, 234, 234b
Suicide
  across life span
    adults and older adults, 225
    children, adolescents, and young adults, 224–225
  assessment, 232
  attempt, defined, 224
  contagion, 229
  definition of, 224
  therapeutic dialogue, 231b
  warning signs for, 230
Suicide prevention
  definition of suicide, 224
  epidemiology/risk factors, 225, 225b
    gender, 226
    psychological risk factors, 226
    race and ethnicity, 226–227
    sexuality, 226
    social risk factors, 226
  etiology
    biologic theories, 227–228
    psychological theories, 228–229
    social theories, 229
  family response to suicide, 229
  myths/facts about suicide, 224b
  nurses' reflection, 235
  overview, 223
  parasuicide, 224
  protective factors, 230
  psychoeducation checklist for, 234b
  rate of suicide, in US, 224, 225f
  suicidality, 224
  suicide across life span
    adults and older adults, 225
    children, adolescents, and young adults, 224–225
  suicide attempt, 224
  treatment/nursing care for
    continuum of care, 235
    documentation and reporting, 235
    evaluation and treatment outcomes, 235
    interdisciplinary treatment and recovery, 230
    priority care issues, 230
    and promoting mental health, 230–235, 232b
Sullivan's interpersonal relations, 42
Support groups, 173
Suppressed anger, 193
Suppressed anger syndrome, 11
Suprachiasmatic nucleus, e-10
Susto, 3b, 9
Suvorexant (Belsomra), 154t
Symbolism, 92–93, 93t
Symptom management groups, 175
Synaptic transmission, 66, 67f
Synthetic hallucinogens, 442
Systematic desensitization, 265
Systemic lupus erythematosus (SLE), 74
Systems models
  King model, 53–54, 53f
  Neuman model, 54
  Orem's model, 54

T

Tadalafil (Cialis), 504
Tardive dyskinesia, 144
  risk factors for, 144t
Target symptoms, psychiatric medications, 129
Taste, 404
Teamwork and collaboration, 301, 301b
  anorexia nervosa, 461–462, 461b
  antisocial personality disorder, 410
  for BPD, 399
  for bulimia nervosa, 470
  electroconvulsive therapy (ECT), 301
  in panic disorder, 264–265
  psychosurgery, 302
  for PTSD, 286–287, 287b
  transcranial magnetic stimulation (TMS), 301–302
Teen partner abuse, 240
Temazepam (Restoril), 154t
Temperament, 409–410
  defined, 410
  difficult, 410
Temporal lobes, 60
Termination stage of group, 172
Terrorism
  psychological effects of, 218

responses to, 217–218
September 11, 2001 attack, 217
Thalamus, 61
The Mental Health Parity and Addiction
    Equity Act (MHPAEA), 18
Theophylline, 550b
Therapeutic communication, 9, 84–87
    boundaries and body space zones
        personal boundaries, 88–89, 89f
        professional boundaries and ethics,
            89
    defense mechanisms, 89, 90t–91t
    effective communication, 82–84, 83b
    for patients with mental health
        challenges, 89–94, 92t
    relationships examples
        motivational interviewing, 101
        Transitional Discharge Model, 101
        Transitional Relationship Model,
            101
    self-awareness, 81–82, 82b
    therapeutic communication strategies
        and techniques, 84–87
        active listening, 84–85, 85f
        avoiding blocks to communication,
            87, 87t
        limiting self-disclosure, 84, 84t
        selection of, 85–87
        silence, 86
        strength-based communication, 87
        validation, 86–87
Therapeutic drug monitoring, 138
Therapeutic index, 134
Thermoregulation interventions,
    119–120
Thiamine
    withdrawing from alcohol, 432
Thiothixene (Navane), 139t
Thought processes, 112
Thought stopping, 305
Three-step theory (3ST), 229. *See also*
    Ideation-to-action theories
Thrombocytopenia, 157
Thwarted belongingness, 228
Thyrotropin-releasing hormone (TRH),
    71
Tics disorder, 522–524
    age of onset for, 522
    epidemiology, 523
    etiology, 523
    evaluation and treatment outcomes,
        524
    family disorder to, 523
    mental health nursing assessment, 523
    nursing interventions
        pharmacologic, 523–524
        priority of nursing care, 523
        psychoeducation, 524
        therapeutic dialogue, 524b
Token economy, 122
Tolerance, 134, 154
Tolterodine (Detrol LA), 550b
Topophobia, 278b
Touch, 404
Tourette disorder, 522–524
    course of, 522

epidemiology, 523
etiology, 523
evaluation and treatment outcomes,
    524
evidence-based nursing care for,
    523–524
family disorder to, 523
mental health nursing assessment, 523
nursing interventions
    pharmacologic, 523–524
    priority of nursing care, 523
    psychoeducation, 524
    therapeutic dialogue, 524b
underlying pathophysiology, 523
Toxicity, 134
Transaction, 54
Transcranial magnetic stimulation, 159
Transcranial magnetic stimulation
    (TMS), 301–302
Transference, 41
Transient psychotic episodes, 401
Transvestic fetishism, 507t
Tranylcypromine (Parnate), 148t, 150
Trauma, 5
    associated with PTSD, 288
    childhood, 227
    and resilience, 282–283, 283b
Trauma-informed care, 5, 21
    PTSD and, 286, 292
Trauma-/stressor- related disorders
    across lifespan, 283
    clinical course, 284, 284b
    diagnostic criteria
        avoidance/numbing, 284
        for children 6 years and younger,
            285
        hyperarousal, 285
        intrusion, 284
        mood and cognition, 285
    dissociative disorders, 293
    epidemiology/risk factors, 285–286,
        286b
    etiology, 286
    evidence-based nursing care, for
        PTSD
        continuum of care, 292–293
        evaluation/treatment outcomes, 292
        medication interventions, 291–292,
            291b
        mental health nursing assessment,
            288–289, 289b
        mental health nursing interventions,
            289–291
        priority of nursing care, 289
        psychosocial nursing interventions,
            292, 292b
        therapeutic relationship, 289, 290b
    posttraumatic stress disorder (PTSD),
        284
    recovery-oriented care for persons
        with PTSD
        primary care, integration of, 287
        safety issues, 287–288
        teamwork and collaboration,
            286–287, 287b
    trauma and resilience, 282–283, 283b

Traumatic brain injury (TBI), 557
Traumatic crisis, 210
Traumatic events, 284
Traumatic grief, 212
Trazodone (Desyrel), 148t, 149, 150t
Triad, 165
Triamterene and hydrochlorothiazide,
    550b
Triazolam (Halcion), 152, 154t
Trichotillomania and excoriation
    disorder. *See also* Obsessive-
    compulsive disorder (OCD)
    clinical course, 307
    diagnostic criteria, 307
    etiology and treatment, 307
    evidenced-based nursing care for, 307
    excoriation (skin-picking) disorder
        body dysmorphic disorder (BDD),
            307–308, 308b
        hoarding disorder, 308, 308b
Tricyclic antidepressants, 149–150, 150t
Trifluoperazine, 139t
Trihexyphenidyl (Artane), 143t
Tryptophan, 157
Tryptophan, in mental disorder, 69
Tuberoinfundibular pathway, 69
Type A personalities, 182
Type B personalities, 182
Type C personalities, 182
Type D (distressed) personalities, 182
Tyramine-restricted diet, 151t

U

Uncomplicated bereavement, 211–212
Unconditional positive regard, 43
Unfit to stand trial (UST), 24
United States, cultural and social factors
    and beliefs (mental illness), 9–12
    African Americans, 10–11
    Arab Americans, 11
    Asian Americans, 11
    cultural idiom of distress, 9
    Hispanic Americans, 10
    Native Americans, 11
    Pacific Islanders, 11
    Polynesians, 11
    poverty, 9–10
    rural cultures, 11–12
    women within minority groups, 11
Universal Bill of Rights for Mental
    Health Patients, 26
Universality, 173t
Unspecified Feeding and Eating
    Disorders (UFED), 455
Unstable interpersonal relationships, 396
Unstable self-image, 396
Uptake receptors, 132, 132f
U.S. Food and Drug Administration
    (FDA)
    drug regulation and use, 129

V

Vaginismus, 506
Vagus nerve stimulation (VNS), 129, 159
Valbenazine (INGREZZA), 144
Valerian (*Valeriana officinalis*), 157

Validation, 124
Valproate (valproic acid), 146–147
Values, 181
Vardenafil HCl (Levitra), 504
Varenicline tartrate (Chantix)
    nicotine prevention, 436
Vascular neurocognitive disorder, 555–556
Venlafaxine (Effexor), 148t, 149, 150t
Veracity, 30
Verbal communication, 83, 83f, 86t
Vilazodone (Viibryd), 148t, 149, 150t
Violence
    and abuse
        child abuse and neglect, 242
        intimate partner violence (IPV), 239–240, 241f
        of older adults, 242–243
        rape and sexual assault, 241–242
        screening for, 245–246, 246b, 247b
        stalking, 242
    attitudes supportive of, 243
    theories of
        community disorganization, 243
        cycle of violence, 244, 244f
        economic disadvantage, 243
        imbalances in relationship power, 243–244
        leaving *vs.* staying in, 244–245
        safety issues and mandatory reporting, 245
        social learning theory, 243
    vocabulary, 252
Virtual Reality Exposure Therapy (VRET), 287
Vision, 404
Vivitrol
    for alcoholism, 432
Volatile substances. *See* Inhalants
Volitional factors for suicide attempt, 228
Vortioxetine (Brintellix), 148t, 149, 150t
Voyeurism, 507t

W

Warfarin (Coumadin), 550b
Watson's theory, 52–53
Wellness
    concept, 2
    definition, 2
    dimensions of, 2, 2f
Wellness strategies
    for anorexia nervosa, 466
    in panic disorder, 269, 270b, 274
    for person with PTSD, 289–290
Wernicke encephalopathy, 432
Wernicke–Korsakoff syndrome, 432
Whites, in US
    suicide rates among, 227
WHO Disability Assessment Schedule 2.0, 3
Withdrawal and detoxification
    of alcohol, 430–432, 430t, 431b
Women of minority groups, 11
Working stage of group, 167–170

X

Xenophobia, 278b

Y

Yalom's therapeutic factors, 173t
"Yes, but ..." reponse, 170–171
Yoga, exercise and, 291
Young adults
    suicide/suicide attempt among, 224–225

Z

Zaleplon (Sonata), 154t
Ziprasidone (Geodon), 141
Ziprasidone HCl (Geodon), 139t
Zoloft, 70
Zolpidem (Ambien), 154t
Zolpidem CR (Ambien CR), 154t
Zoophobia, 278b
Zyban, nicotine prevention, 436